PSYCHIATRIC MENTAL HEALTH NURSING

PSYCHIATRIC MENTAL HEALTH NURSING

ELLEN H. JANOSIK, R.N., M.S.

Associate Professor Emeritus
Alfred University
Alfred, New York

Adjunct Professor
Roberts Wesleyan College
Rochester, New York

JANET L. DAVIES, R.N., PH.D.

Assistant Chief, Nursing Service
Veteran's Administration Medical Center
Batavia, New York

Adjunct Assistant Professor
University of Rochester
Rochester, New York

Jones and Bartlett Publishers, Inc.
Boston/Monterey

Editorial offices: Jones and Bartlett Publishers, Inc., 23720 Spectacular Bid, Monterey, CA 93940
Sales and customer service offices: Jones and Bartlett Publishers, Inc., 20 Park Plaza, Boston, MA 02116

Printed in the United States of America

10 9 8 7 6 5 4 3 2 1

Library of Congress Cataloging-in-Publication Data

Janosik, Ellen Hastings.
    Psychiatric mental health nursing.

    Includes bibliographies and index.
    1. Psychiatric nursing.   I. Davies, Janet L.
II. Title. [DNLM: 1. Psychiatric Nursing.
WT 160 J34p]
RC440.J29   1986   616.89′0024613   85-22524

ISBN 0-86720-352-8

Sponsoring Editor: James Keating
Project Coordinator: David Hoyt
Project Development Editor: Mary Beth McDavid
Editorial Assistant: Corinne Kibbe
Production: Del Mar Associates
Manuscript Editors: Jackie Estrada, Katalin Wolff
Design: John Odam
Cover Design: Jamie Sue Brooks
Illustrations: John Odam, David Diaz
Permissions: Mary Kay Hancharick
Typesetting: Boyer and Brass, Inc., San Diego, California
Printing: Malloy Lithographing, Inc., Ann Arbor, Michigan

The selection and dosage of drugs presented in this book are in accord with standards accepted at the time of publication. The authors and publisher have made every effort to provide accurate information. However, research, clinical practice, and government regulations often change the accepted standard in this field. Before administering any drug, the reader is advised to check the manufacturer's product information sheet for the most up-to-date recommendations on dosage, precautions, and contraindications. This is especially important in the case of drugs that are new or seldom used.

Cover photo: Cross-section of a nerve; courtesy of Dr. J. Robert Troyer, School of Medicine, Temple University
Photos on pages 9, 10, 11, 26, and 33: The Bettmann Archive, Inc.
Poems on pages 205 and 209: From *Salt and Bitter and Good* by Dorothy Parker, pages 269 and 270. Copyright © 1936 by Viking Press. Reprinted by permission.
Poem on page 285: Copyright © 1977 by Elise Maclay. Reprinted by permission of the publisher, Reader's Digest Press.

For Charles Edward and Elizabeth Ann
For Kimberly and Klaus

CONTRIBUTORS

MARY L. BELENCHIA, R.N., M.S.N.
HSRO Coordinator
Veteran's Administration Medical Center
Memphis, Tennesee

SANDRA ANN CHENELLY, R.N., M.S.
Clinical Nurse Specialist in Gerontology
Veteran's Administration Medical Center
Batavia, New York

CHERYL L. COX, R.N., PH.D.
Assistant Professor of Nursing
University of Illinois College of Nursing
Chicago, Illinois

SUE C. DeLAUNE, R.N., M.S.
Assistant Professor of Nursing
Nicholls State University
Thibodaux, Louisiana

KAREN LEE FONTAINE, R.N., M.S.N.
Assistant Professor of Nursing
Purdue University Calumet
Hammond, Indiana

LOY W. HAMANN, R.N., M.S.
Professor of Nursing
Denver Auraria Community College
Denver, Colorado

MICHELLE HARDMAN, R.N., M.S.
Psychiatric Nurse Clinician
United States Army Nurse Corps

LINDA VASANT LEON, PH.D.
Assistant Professor
St. John Fisher College
Rochester, New York

BARBARA S. MASIULIS, R.N., M.S.
Instructor and Pediatric Clinician
Birth Defects Center
University of Rochester Medical Center
Rochester, New York

KATHLEEN A. POWERS, R.N., ED.D.
Associate Professor and Chairperson
College of Nursing, Rochester Division
Alfred University
Alfred, New York

BARBARA SMULLEN, R.N., ED.D.
Associate Professor and Chairman
Department of Nursing
Nazareth College
Rochester, New York

MARY S. TURNER, R.N., M.S., C.S.
Assistant Professor of Nursing
University of Rochester School of Nursing
Rochester, New York

A. PETER ZIARNOWSKI, PH.D.
Chief, Day Treatment Center
Veteran's Administration Outpatient Clinic
Rochester, New York

This comprehensive textbook in psychiatric mental health nursing is intended for undergraduate nursing students in baccalaureate, associate-degree, and diploma programs. The book may be used in its entirety or selectively, depending on time constraints imposed by the curriculum. It was the purpose of the authors to write a text that is clear, well organized, and definitive but not redundant.

Although nursing includes such speciality areas as adult health, psychiatric mental health, and maternal and child health, there is a current trend toward integration across speciality areas. This trend received impetus from the adoption of a single comprehensive examination for professional licensure. Therefore, there is a genuine need for nursing texts that may be specialized but that use a broad rather than a limited perspective. At the same time, adequate attention must be paid to concepts necessary to understand intrapsychic, interpersonal, behavioral, and cultural influences on mental health. In this text, the framework of holistic interaction across the life cycle span is used to explain adaptive and maladaptive alterations manifested by individuals, families, and communities as they function throughout the life cycle.

The authors of this text acknowledge a responsibility to undergraduate nursing students, to instructors trying to make a vast body of knowledge comprehensible and relevant for students, and to the individuals, families, and communities who are consumers of health care.

In discharging their responsibility to students, the authors have included those theories and concepts that seem most useful to beginners in the field of psychiatric mental health nursing and have tried to present them in a meaningful way. Consistent with prevailing philosophy in nursing, the medical model is neither emphasized nor ignored but is recognized. Exclusion of any treatment modality from the repertoire of nursing would be unrealistic. Nursing actions may be independent or interdependent. Those actions that consist solely of nursing measures are independent; those actions that require collaboration with other disciplines are interdependent. Attention to the three levels of prevention requires that contributions from many interdependent disciplines be acknowledged.

As educators and clinicians, the authors have found students to be more receptive to information that is placed near related content rather than fragmented or isolated. Somatic interventions, for example, are more easily understood when taught in the context of the particular alteration for which they are appropriate. Thus, in this text nursing approaches and interventions appropriate for various alterations are placed in the appropriate chapter.

The authors interpret decision making as a collaborative process between the nurse and the client, and they have tried not to patronize students by presenting simplistic or mechanical explanations of complex processes. The authors believe that the practice of psychiatric mental health nursing must build on a strong theoretical foundation. Wherever possible, the authors have attempted to show students the "why" of psychiatric nursing before moving on to the "how."

In discharging their responsibility to clinical and classroom instructors, the authors have gathered a body of knowledge from a variety of theories and a range of disciplines, including nursing. In this text the contributions of nurse theorists mingle with those of theorists representing the physical sciences, the social sciences, the arts, and the humanities. The ideas of a number of nurse theorists are presented, their strengths and weaknesses are noted, and their applicability is compared. Because the nursing process is essential to professional nursing practice, the evolution of the nursing process is traced and its current directions are described so that instructors can indicate to students the growing scientific base of nursing theory. The authors interpret the nursing process as a scientific tool and a humanistic art.

In discharging their responsibility to consumers of health care, the authors call attention to the needs of individuals as clients, families as clients, and communities as clients. The text adopts a holistic viewpoint that is illuminated by the life cycle focus. This expanded vision of holism reveals dimensions that most other texts have neglected or have presented in cursory fashion.

Human functioning takes place at multiple levels that are interdependent and reciprocal as people struggle to meet universal needs for biological integrity, security, individuation, self-esteem, and fulfillment. Adaptive and maladaptive patterns of functioning exist on a continuum; altered patterns of functioning do not necessarily represent extremes of a continuum but movements toward or departures from optimum health. Martha Rogers described the goal of the nursing process as the "repatterning" of human functioning in order to promote optimum health. Consistent with this viewpoint, the authors present patterns of holistic interaction, alterations in patterns, and responsive nursing activities.

In organizing the text, the authors have used a unified and internally consistent format. The book is divided into five parts. Part I presents an overview of psychiatric mental health nursing that covers historical and contemporary issues and that emphasizes the role expansion and current ramifications of psychiatric mental health nursing. Chapters in Part I also encourage student awareness of collaborative data collection, nursing diagnoses, assessment, problem identification, and resolution. Although approved nursing diagnoses continue to be subject to refinement, they are extensive enough to facilitate documentation and communication. Moreover, nursing diagnoses are compatible with the multiaxial classification of DSM-III. Students using this text can learn how each diagnostic method augments and enriches the other. Out of the discussion of assessment and nursing diagnoses, guidelines for nursing care plans emerge. In addition to general explanations of how to compile a nursing care plan, the authors have provided a number of generic or standardized care plans that

employ nursing diagnoses and are oriented toward the nursing process. The generic care plans are not blueprints but rather offer guidance in the formulation of plans for specific clients.

Part II, titled "Holistic Interactional Patterns," deals with adaptive and maladaptive alterations that human beings engage in as they respond to internal and external demands. The chapters in Part II examine altered patterns of functioning in a way that permits such alterations to be regarded in terms of nursing diagnoses as well as psychiatric diagnoses. Nursing diagnoses evolve from systematic, thorough data collection, followed by recognition and identification of problematic patterns of functioning. The nursing diagnoses then direct the planning and implementation of nursing interventions, along with ongoing evaluation.

Each of the chapters in Part II contains dynamic and clinical explanations of the alterations being discussed. Biological, psychological, and social treatment approaches are included in each chapter. For example, the chapter on altered patterns of mood and affect includes discussions of antidepressants, electroconvulsive therapy, cognitive therapy, and lithium therapy, while the chapter dealing with altered patterns of thought and perception contains material on antipsychotic medications—their therapeutic effects, side effects, and related nursing responsibilities.

Part III comprises two chapters concerned with maturational and situational alterations in functioning. The chapter on maturational tasks and challenges presents the theories of Piaget and Kohlberg, among others. The chapter on situational alterations looks at crises that are not maturational and therefore cannot be anticipated. Organizationally, this section follows the life cycle span of individuals and families.

Part IV examines various therapeutic approaches. Each chapter begins with a theoretical rationale for a specific approach, contrasts the strengths and weaknesses of the approach, and views the approach in the context of the nursing process and nursing role.

Part V addresses current issues in psychiatric mental health nursing. Here the authors present content related to the nurse's responsibility, not only to the client but also to the profession, to the health care system, and to the community. The need for nurses to be enlightened consumers of research, to refute or validate findings, and to participate in clinical and laboratory investigation is emphasized.

The organizational features of the book that enhance its usefulness include its:

Emphasis on holistic interaction across the life cycle span.

Unified, internally consistent structure.

Clinical content placed in the relevant chapters.

Integration of nursing diagnoses with DSM-III.

Comprehensive clinical examples based on nursing process in every chapter.

Content outline for every chapter.

Summary for every chapter.

Review questions for every chapter.

Supplementary reading list for every chapter.

Comprehensive glossary.

Appendixes.

An instructor's manual is provided. Its organization is based on the premise that learning should take place in the cognitive, affective, and psychomotor domains. For cognitive learning, each chapter of the manual contains a brief outline of the textbook content for the corresponding chapter. The affective/psychomotor section of each manual chapter includes suggestions for introducing related topics that may lead to affective or attitudinal change. It also presents ideas for role playing and checklists to encourage self-evaluation as well as to assess such activities as films and simulated interviews. If time pressures are too great, some of the affective/psychomotor activities can be assigned as homework or can be adapted to the clinical conference that is an important part of courses in psychiatric mental health nursing.

The manual contains a bank of test questions that instructors may wish to adapt for the evaluation of their students. The test bank is also available on MICRO-PAC®, a test-authoring software package compatible with IBM-PC® and Apple II® series computers.

The authors wish to acknowledge their indebtedness to a number of people without whom their task might not have been accomplished. Foremost among them is James Keating, our executive editor, whose unfailing good humor and faith in the project encouraged us when confidence lagged. We are also indebted to all the individuals and families we encountered over the years in the course of our clinical practice who shared their joys and tribulations with us and paid us the high compliment of allowing us to help. Our students have assisted us by expressing with clarity and frankness their reactions to various educational material included in the book.

The authors also recognize their indebtedness to Jackie Estrada for her careful and gifted editing that so greatly improved the quality and coherence of this manuscript. Mary Beth McDavid of Wadsworth Health Sciences deserves special mention for the sensitivity and helpfulness she consistently extended to the authors. Completion of the manuscript was facilitated by the skills and interest of our secretaries, Lilliam Harris and Barbara Weigand. The chapter on altered patterns of mood and affect benefited from a literature search by Kristin Huckabone, and the chapter on crisis theory and practice was enhanced by material compiled by Lisa deBergh, both of whom are graduates of Alfred University. The chapter on trends and research was enriched by the research projects of Susan Soanes on remotivation and Elizabeth Malone on obesity control among psychiatric patients. Professor Mary Koval reviewed medical content of the text.

The authors also wish to pay tribute to the following external reviewers who provided constructive examinations of the manuscript:

Lorna Barrell, School of Nursing, Medical College of Virginia

Dorothy Brockopp, School of Nursing, McMaster University

Verna Carson, School of Nursing, University of Maryland

Lynne Faulk, Community Mental Health Department, University of Alabama

Laina Gerace, College of Nursing, University of Illinois

Karolyn Godbey, College of Nursing, University of Florida

Thelma Hostetter, College of Nursing, University of Arizona

Florence Munoz, School of Nursing, Pasadena City College

Carol Wurzell, College of Nursing, Arizona State University

The statements made in this work represent the opinions of the respective authors and contributors and do not necessarily reflect the views of the institutions or agencies with which they are affiliated.

Finally, the authors are sensitive to the use of sexist pronouns. Where possible, plural nouns and pronouns have been used. In those instances where the use of plural wording would cause ambiguity or awkwardness, the authors have used gender pronouns alternately.

Ellen H. Janosik
Janet L. Davies

xi

BRIEF CONTENTS

PART ONE
INTRODUCTION TO PSYCHIATRIC MENTAL HEALTH NURSING 1
CHAPTER 1
OVERVIEW AND INTRODUCTION TO PSYCHIATRIC NURSING 3
Ellen H. Janosik, R.N., M.S.

CHAPTER 2
THEORETICAL FRAMEWORKS IN PSYCHIATRIC MENTAL HEALTH NURSING 23
Ellen H. Janosik

CHAPTER 3
HOLISTIC INTERACTION AS A UNIFYING FRAMEWORK 51
Ellen H. Janosik

CHAPTER 4
THE PRINCIPLES AND PRACTICE OF PSYCHIATRIC MENTAL HEALTH NURSING 73
Janet L. Davies, R.N., Ph.D.

CHAPTER 5
COMMUNICATION AND INTERACTIONS IN PSYCHIATRIC MENTAL HEALTH NURSING 103
Barbara Smullen, R.N., Ed.D.

PART TWO
HOLISTIC INTERACTIONAL PATTERNS 127
CHAPTER 6
ALTERED PATTERNS OF THOUGHT AND PERCEPTION 129
Michelle Hardman, R.N., M.S.

CHAPTER 7
ALTERED PATTERNS OF MOOD AND AFFECT 161
Ellen H. Janosik

CHAPTER 8
ALTERED PATTERNS OF SOCIAL RELATEDNESS 193
Janet L. Davies

CHAPTER 9
ALTERED PATTERNS OF SOCIETAL ADJUSTMENT 217
Janet L. Davies

CHAPTER 10
ALTERED PATTERNS OF CONGENITAL ORIGIN 249
Barbara Masiulis, R.N., M.S.

CHAPTER 11
ALTERED PATTERNS OF DEGENERATIVE ORIGIN 277
Sue C. DeLaune, R.N., M.S.
Sandra Ann Chenelly, R.N., M.S.

CHAPTER 12
ALTERED PATTERNS OF ADAPTATIONAL ORIGIN 301
Ellen H. Janosik

CHAPTER 13
ALTERED PATTERNS OF SEXUALITY 335
Karen Lee Fontaine, R.N., M.S.N.

PART THREE
CRITICAL TASKS AND CHALLENGES 367
CHAPTER 14
ALTERED MATURATIONAL PATTERNS 369
Linda Vasant Leon, Ph.D.

CHAPTER 15
SITUATIONAL ALTERATIONS: THE CRISES OF SUICIDE AND VIOLENCE 403
Janet L. Davies

PART FOUR
THEORY AND PRACTICE OF PSYCHIATRIC MENTAL HEALTH NURSING 435
CHAPTER 16
CRISIS THEORY AND PRACTICE 437
Ellen H. Janosik

CHAPTER 17
BEHAVIORAL THEORY AND PRACTICE 459
A. Peter Ziarnowski, Ph.D.

CHAPTER 18
FAMILY THEORY AND PRACTICE 477
Ellen H. Janosik

CHAPTER 19
GROUP THEORY AND PRACTICE 511
Ellen H. Janosik

CHAPTER 20
COMMUNITY THEORY AND PRACTICE 543
Kathleen A. Powers, R.N., Ed.D.

CHAPTER 21
ECLECTIC THEORY AND PRACTICE 567
Loy W. Hamann, R.N., M.S.

PART FIVE
ISSUES IN PSYCHIATRIC MENTAL HEALTH NURSING 593
CHAPTER 22
CASE MANAGEMENT AND COLLABORATION 595
Mary S. Turner, R.N., M.S., C.S.

CHAPTER 23
ADVOCACY, LEGALITY, AND ETHICAL VALUES 615
Cheryl L. Cox, R.N., Ph.D.
Mary L. Belenchia, R.N., M.S.N.

CHAPTER 24
TRENDS AND RESEARCH IN NURSING 633
Janet L. Davies

CONTENTS

PART ONE
INTRODUCTION TO PSYCHIATRIC MENTAL
HEALTH NURSING 1

CHAPTER 1
OVERVIEW AND INTRODUCTION TO
PSYCHIATRIC NURSING 3

Defining Health and Mental Health 5
Holistic Definitions 5
Health as Adaptation 6
Definitions of Mental Health 7

Historical Perspectives on Psychiatric Care 8
Mental Disturbance as Supernatural 8
Mental Disturbance as Affliction 10
Mental Disturbance as Psychodynamic 11

Emergent Trends in Psychiatric Care 11
Somatic Therapies 11
Government Involvement in Health Care 11
Deinstitutionalization 12
The Community Mental Health Movement 12

Expanded Nursing Functions and Roles 13
Client-Nurse Relationships 14
The Psychiatric Mental Health Nurse 15

Convergent Trends in Psychiatric Care 15
Psychiatric Diagnoses 15
Nursing Diagnoses 17

CHAPTER 2
THEORETICAL FRAMEWORKS IN PSYCHIATRIC
MENTAL HEALTH NURSING 23

Psychogenic Framework 25
Psychosexual Theory 25
Psychosocial Theory 31

Interpersonal Framework 34
Self System 34
Modes of Experience 35
Nursing Implications of Sullivan's Theory 36

Sociological Framework 37
Social Institutions 37
Symbolic Interactionism 37
Social Roles 38
Social Stratification 38
Nursing Implications of Sociological
 Approaches 38

Biogenic Framework 39
Constitutional Factors 39
Genetic Factors 39
Chemical Imbalance 40
Biological Rhythms 40
Nursing Implications of Biogenic Approaches 43

Other Frameworks 44
Existential Framework 44
Cognitive Framework 47

CHAPTER 3
HOLISTIC INTERACTION AS A UNIFYING FRAMEWORK 51

Holistic Interaction 53
Reciprocal Interaction 54
Reciprocal Interaction 54
Assignment of Meanings 54

Adaptation 55
Coping and Defensive Behaviors 56
Adaptation to Life Changes 57

Systems Theory Approaches 58
Basic Concepts of Systems Theory 58
Nursing Models 59
The Roy Model 59

Clinical Testing and Assessment 61
Intelligence Testing 61
Mental Status Assessment 62
Personality Assessment 64

CHAPTER 4
THE PRINCIPLES AND PRACTICE OF PSYCHIATRIC
MENTAL HEALTH NURSING 73

Theoretical Bases of Psychiatric Nursing 75
Peplau's Theory 75
Leininger's Theory 76
Orem's Theory 76
Kinlein's Theory 76
Newman's Theory 76
Johnson's Theory 77
Aguilera's Theory 77
King's Theory 77

The Nursing Process 77
The Components of the Nursing Process 78
The Nursing Care Plan 81
Generic Nursing Care Plans 82

The Practice of Psychiatric Nursing 84
The Anxious Client 84
The Delusional Client 86
The Demanding Client 87
The Hallucinating Client 89
The Angry Client 89
The Hypochondriacal Client 91
The Manipulative Client 92
The Regressed Client 93
The Ritualistic Client 95
The Suspicious Client 96
The Withdrawn Client 97

CHAPTER 5
COMMUNICATION AND INTERACTIONS IN
PSYCHIATRIC MENTAL HEALTH NURSING 103

Establishing a Therapeutic Relationship 105

Elements in the Therapeutic Communication Process 106

Characteristics of Therapeutic Communication 108

xv

Client-Centeredness 108
Goal-Directedness 108
Authenticity 109
Self-disclosure 109
Confidentiality 109
Acceptance 109
Collaboration 109
The Collaborative Continuum 110
The Therapeutic Contract 110
Facilitating Therapeutic Communication 111
Affective Characteristics of Therapeutic
　Communication 112
Cognitive Processes in Therapeutic
　Communication 113
Therapeutic Communication and the Nursing
　Process 117
Documentation of Care 118
The Health Status Profile 118
The Problem List 119
Progress Notes 119
Discharge Plans and Summary 120
Process Recording 120

PART TWO
HOLISTIC INTERACTIONAL PATTERNS 127

CHAPTER 6
ALTERED PATTERNS OF THOUGHT AND
PERCEPTION 129

Etiologic Theories of Thought Disturbance 132
Genetic Theories 132
Biochemical Theories 133
Developmental Theories 133
Psychodynamic Theories 137
The Process of Thought Disturbance 138
Types of Thought Disturbances 139
Primary Manifestations of Thought
　Disturbance 140
Secondary Manifestations of Thought
　Disturbance 141
**Therapeutic Approaches for Clients with Thought
　Disturbance** 144
Psychotropic Drug Therapy 145
Relationship Therapy 148
Milieu Therapy 151
Family Therapy 153
Predictive Factors 153

CHAPTER 7
ALTERED PATTERNS OF MOOD AND AFFECT 161

Depression as a Maladaptive Response 163

**Classification of Altered Patterns of Mood and
　Affect** 164

Etiology of Affective Disturbance 165
Psychodynamic Factors 165
Biochemical Factors 166
Genetic Factors 167
Existential Factors 167

Working with Depressed Clients 168
Assessment 168

Planning 170
Implementation 171
Evaluation 172
Working with Elated Clients 172
Assessment 172
Planning 174
Implementation 174
Evaluation 175
Somatic Treatment Measures 175
Electroconvulsive Therapy 175
Antidepressant Medication 176
Lithium Therapy 179
Grief and Mourning 181
Adaptive and Maladaptive Grief 182
Phases of Grief 183
Anticipatory Grief 184
Helping the Grief Stricken 184

CHAPTER 8
ALTERED PATTERNS OF SOCIAL RELATEDNESS 193
**Comparison of Healthy and Altered Sense of
　Self** 196
The Healthy Self 196
The Altered Self 196
The Role of Anxiety and Fear 197
Theoretical Frameworks 197
Psychosexual or Psychodynamic Model 197
Psychosocial Model 198
Interpersonal Model 198
**Comparison of Altered Patterns of
　Functioning** 199
**Altered Patterns of Relatedness: Neurotic
　Patterns** 200
Anxiety Reactions 202
Obsessive-Compulsive Reactions 203
Posttraumatic Stress Syndrome 203
Phobic Reactions 204
Conversion Reactions 206
Dissociative Reactions 207
Hypochondriacal Reactions 207
**Altered Patterns of Relatedness: Personality
　Patterns** 208
Schizoid Type 208
Compulsive Type 209
Histrionic Type 209
Antisocial Type 209
Passive-Aggressive/Passive-Dependent Type 210
Paranoid Type 210
General Nursing Approaches 213
Borderline Conditions 213
Pharmacological Approaches 213

CHAPTER 9
ALTERED PATTERNS OF SOCIETAL ADJUSTMENT 217
Drug Terminology 219
Nursing Attitudes 220
Use and Abuse of Alcohol 220
Classification and Diagnosis of Alcoholism 220
Causes of Alcoholism 223

Psychological Theories 224
Sociocultural Theories 225
Learning Theory 225

Physiological Consequences of Alcohol Abuse 225
Alcohol and the Brain 226
Alcohol and the Liver 226
Alcohol and the Gastrointestinal Tract 227
Alcohol and the Heart 227
Alcohol and the Muscles 227
Alcohol and the Endocrine System 227
Alcohol and the Reproductive System 227

The Progression of Alcoholism 227

Alcoholism and the Nursing Process 228
Acute Stage 228
Rehabilitation Stage 229

Use and Abuse of Drugs 231

Commonly Abused Drugs 233
Stimulants 233
Opiates and Related Analgesics 234
Depressants 234
Cannabinols (Marijuana) 235
Hallucinogens 235
Inhalants 236

Causes of Drug Abuse 236
The Role of the Host 237
The Role of the Environment 238
The Role of the Agent 238

Physiological Consequences of Drug Abuse 238
Circulatory and Respiratory Complications 239
Hepatic Dysfunction 239
Gastrointestinal Disturbances 239
Skin Complications 239
Muscular Disorders 239
Miscellaneous Complications 239

Drug Abuse and the Nursing Process 239
Acute Stage 239
Rehabilitation Stage 239

CHAPTER 10
ALTERED PATTERNS OF CONGENITAL ORIGIN 249

**Etiology of Altered Patterns of Congenital
   Origin** 251
Prenatal Factors 252
Perinatal Factors 252
Postnatal Factors 252

**Types of Altered Patterns of Congenital
   Origin** 253
Mental Retardation 253
Down's Syndrome 255
*Learning Disabilities: Attention Deficit
   Disorders* 257
Phenylketonuria 258
Tay-Sachs Disease 259
Cystic Fibrosis 259
Hemophilia A 260
Sickle Cell Anemia 261
Cerebral Palsy 261
Spina Bifida 262
Klinefelter's Syndrome 264
Turner's Syndrome 264

**The Impact of Altered Patterns of Congenital
   Origin** 264
Changes in Family Roles 264
Stress and Coping 266
Adapting to Specific Disabilities 267
Genetic Counseling 268

**The Nursing Process in Altered Patterns of
   Congenital Origin** 269
Assessment 269
Planning 270
Implementation 270
Evaluation 274

CHAPTER 11
ALTERED PATTERNS OF DEGENERATIVE ORIGIN 277

Definitions of Key Terms 279

**The Relationship Between Aging and Altered
   Patterns of Degenerative Origin** 281

Major Degenerative Alterations 282
Alzheimer's Disease 282
Parkinson's Disease 285
Huntington's Chorea 286

**Impact of Degenerative Alterations on the
   Client** 287
Memory Impairment 287
Cognitive and Behavioral Alterations 288
Impaired Reality Testing 288
Impaired Judgment 289
Impaired Communication 289
Self-care Deficits 289
Social Alterations 290

**Impact of Degenerative Alterations on the
   Nurse** 292

**The Nursing Process in the Care of Clients with
   Altered Patterns of Degenerative Origin** 292
Assessment 292
Planning 293
Implementation 293
Evaluation 293

CHAPTER 12
ALTERED PATTERNS OF ADAPTATIONAL ORIGIN 301

Holistic Perspectives 303

Theories of Stress and Adaptation 304

Disorders of Adaptation 309
Gastrointestinal Responses to Stress 309
Respiratory Responses to Stress 313
Cardiovascular Responses to Stress 316
Skeletomuscular Responses to Stress 320
Behavioral Responses to Stress 322
Psychogenic Pain Responses to Stress 325
Neoplastic Responses to Stress 326

CHAPTER 13
ALTERED PATTERNS OF SEXUALITY 335

Physiological Aspects of Human Sexuality 337
Anatomical Structures 337
Physiological Responses 339

xvii

Intrapersonal and Interpersonal Dimensions 341
Socially Conditioned Sexual Expectations 341
Sexual Activity as a Coping Mechanism 342
Alternative Sex Role Enactment 343
Homosexuality 343
Bisexuality 347
Celibacy 347
Transvestism 348
Transsexualism 348
Sexual Dysfunctions 349
Decreased Sexual Interest 349
Increased Sexual Interest 350
Inhibitions 350
Orgasm Difficulties 350
Problems with Satisfaction 351
Sexual Deviance 351
Fetishism 351
Zoophilia 351
Pedophilia 352
Exhibitionism 352
Voyeurism 353
Necrophilia 353
Sexual Abuse 353
Sadomasochism 353
Incest 354
Sexual Harassment 355
Counseling 355
Premarital Counseling 355
Marital Counseling 357
Sexual Counseling 358
The Nursing Process in Sexual Health Care 360

PART THREE
CRITICAL TASKS AND CHALLENGES 367

CHAPTER 14
ALTERED MATURATIONAL PATTERNS 369
Developmental Theories 371
Erikson's Psychosocial Theory 371
Kohlberg's Theory of Moral Development 372
Piaget's Cognitive Development Theory 375
Duvall's Theory of Family Development 376
*Nursing Implications of Developmental
   Theories* 378
Altered Maturational Patterns of Childhood 379
Sleep Disturbances 379
Eating Disturbances 381
Urinary and Excretory Disturbances 382
Fears and Phobias 383
Working with Children 385
Altered Maturational Patterns of Adolescence 385
Identity Confusion 386
Antisocial Behavior 386
Body Image Distortion 387
Working with Adolescents 388
Altered Maturational Patterns of Adulthood 390
Career Crises 390
Marital Crises 391
Parental Crises 394
Working with Adults 394

Altered Maturational Patterns of Old Age 395
The Empty Nest Syndrome 395
Retirement Crises 395
Health-Related Crises 396
Terminal Crises 397
Working with the Elderly 398

CHAPTER 15
SITUATIONAL ALTERATIONS: THE CRISES OF
SUICIDE AND VIOLENCE 403
The Crisis of Suicide 405
Theoretical Approaches 406
Nursing Attitudes 409
The Nursing Process and the Suicidal Client 409
The Crisis of the Violent Individual 412
Aggression, Alcohol, and Violence 412
The Violent Individual 413
*The Nursing Process and the Violent
   Individual* 413
The Crisis of Rape 415
Motivation to Rape 415
Reaction of Rape Victims 415
Attitudes Toward Rape 416
The Nursing Process and the Rape Victim 416
The Crisis of the Violent Family 417
Spouse Abuse 417
Child Abuse 422
Alcohol and Family Violence 424
Implications for Nursing 425
The Nursing Process and the Violent Family 426

PART FOUR
**THEORY AND PRACTICE OF PSYCHIATRIC MENTAL
HEALTH NURSING** 435

CHAPTER 16
CRISIS THEORY AND PRACTICE 437
Characteristics of Crisis 439
Opportunities in Crisis 440
Crisis and Emergency 441
Duration of Crisis 442
Patterns of Crisis Behavior 443
Crisis Assessment and Intervention 444
Crisis Counseling 445
Types of Crisis Work 448
Typology of Crises 449
Dispositional Crisis 450
Transitional Crisis 450
Traumatic Crisis 450
Developmental Crisis 451
Psychopathological Crisis 451
Psychiatric Emergency 452
Staff Burnout as Crisis 452

CHAPTER 17
BEHAVIORAL THEORY AND PRACTICE 459
Behavior Modification 462
The Scientific Method in Psychology 462
Classical Conditioning 463
Operant Conditioning 465

xviii

Learning Theorists 467

Behavior Modification Techniques 467
Systematic Desensitization 467
Aversion Techniques 468
Operant Techniques 470

Basic Guidelines for the Use of Behavior Modification 471

Limitations of Behavior Therapy 472

CHAPTER 18
FAMILY THEORY AND PRACTICE 477

Origins of Family Theory and Therapy 479

Conceptual Approaches 481
Developmental Concepts 482
Systems Theory Concepts 483
Psychodynamic Concepts 486
Structural Concepts 488
Functional Concepts 489
Communication Concepts 495
Learning Theory Concepts 499

Some Practicalities in Family Intervention 502

CHAPTER 19
GROUP THEORY AND PRACTICE 511

Categories of Groups 513

Historical Influences on Group Treatment 514

Psychodynamic Issues 517

Organizing the Group 518
Assessing Needs and Resources 519
Planning the Group 519
Implementing the Plan 521
Evaluating Group Progress 521

Stages of Group Development 522
Initial Stage 522
Middle Stage 523
Final Stage 524

Leadership in Groups 525
Leadership Styles 526
Coleadership 529

Membership Roles in Groups 530

Curative Factors in Groups 533

Group Research Issues 534

CHAPTER 20
COMMUNITY THEORY AND PRACTICE 543

The Dimensions of Community 545
Community as Group 545
Community as Place 547
Community as Culture 548

Epidemiological Concepts 550
Host, Agent, and Environment 551
Epidemiological Terminology 552
Risk Factors 552

Community Health Care Delivery 554

The Impact of Deinstitutionalization 555

The Role of the Community Mental Health Nurse 557

Community Program Evaluation 558

CHAPTER 21
ECLECTIC THEORY AND PRACTICE 567

Reality Therapy 569

Rational Emotive Therapy 571

Implosive Therapy 575

Primal Therapy 576

Milieu Therapy and the Therapeutic Community 578

Client-Centered Therapy 581

Relationship Therapy as Nursing Process 582
Assessment in Relationship Therapy (The Introductory Phase) 583
Planning in Relationship Therapy (The Testing Phase) 584
Intervention in Relationship Therapy (The Working Phase) 585
Evaluation in Relationship Therapy (The Termination Phase) 586

PART FIVE
ISSUES IN PSYCHIATRIC MENTAL HEALTH NURSING 593

CHAPTER 22
CASE MANAGEMENT AND COLLABORATION 595

Health Care Team Structure 597

Models of Nursing Care Delivery 598
Team Nursing in Mental Health Settings 598
Primary Nursing in Mental Health Settings 599

Consultation and Liaison Work 601
Types of Mental Health Consultation 602
Implementation of Consultation and Liaison Work 603
Implications of Consultation and Liaison Work 605

The Referral Process in Psychiatric Nursing 607
Sequence of Referrals 608
Themes of Referrals 609

Collaboration and Coordination in Health Care Delivery 610

CHAPTER 23
ADVOCACY, LEGALITY, AND ETHICAL VALUES 615

Nursing and Ethics 617
The Rights of Mental Health Clients 618
Institutional Responsibilities Regarding Client Rights 620
The Right to Refuse Treatment 620
Restrictive Treatment 621
Involuntary Commitment 621
Nursing Implications of Clients' Rights 622

Professional Accountability and Liability 623
Standards of Practice 623
Peer Review 624
Professional Liability 625

Advocacy 626
The Nurse as Client Advocate 627
Cautions Relative to the Advocacy Role 630

The Mental Health Nurse as Change Agent 630

CHAPTER 24
TRENDS AND RESEARCH IN NURSING 633

Nursing and the DRGs 635
Historical Perspectives 635
The Yale Study 635
Implications for Nursing 636
Nursing and Quality Assurance 637
Components of Quality Assurance 638
Establishing a Quality Assurance Program 638
Nursing Research 641
Historical Perspectives 642
The Research Process 643
The Importance of Writing 647

APPENDIX A
NURSING DIAGNOSES ACCORDING TO PATTERNS OF
ALTERATION 653

APPENDIX B
DSM-III CLASSIFICATION: AXES I AND II
CATEGORIES AND CODES 656

APPENDIX C
STANDARDS OF PSYCHIATRIC AND MENTAL
HEALTH NURSING PRACTICE 660

APPENDIX D
ETHICAL CODE FOR NURSES 662

APPENDIX E
MENTAL HEALTH PATIENTS' LIBERATION PROJECT 663

APPENDIX F
LEGISLATION PROTECTING MENTAL
PATIENTS 664

APPENDIX G
STATEMENT OF THE RIGHTS OF MENTAL
PATIENTS 665

APPENDIX H
PSYCHOLOGICAL TESTS: PURPOSES AND AGE
RANGE OF SUBJECTS 666

APPENDIX I
HEALTH-RELATED ORGANIZATIONS 667

APPENDIX J
CONTROLLED DRUGS 668

APPENDIX K
COMPENDIUM OF COMMON DRUGS IN
PSYCHIATRIC NURSING 669

GLOSSARY 733

INDEX 749

xx

PSYCHIATRIC MENTAL HEALTH NURSING

P   A   R   T

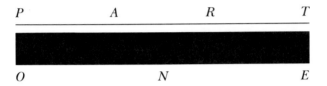

O   N   E

INTRODUCTION TO PSYCHIATRIC MENTAL HEALTH NURSING

DEFINING HEALTH AND MENTAL HEALTH
Holistic Definitions
Health as Adaptation
Definitions of Mental Health

HISTORICAL PERSPECTIVES ON
PSYCHIATRIC CARE
Mental Disturbance as Supernatural
Mental Disturbance as Affliction
Mental Disturbance as Psychodynamic

EMERGENT TRENDS IN PSYCHIATRIC CARE
Somatic Therapies
Government Involvement in Health Care
Deinstitutionalization
The Community Mental Health Movement

EXPANDED NURSING FUNCTION AND ROLES
Client-Nurse Relationships
The Psychiatric Mental Health Nurse

CONVERGENT TRENDS IN PSYCHIATRIC CARE
Psychiatric Diagnoses
Nursing Diagnoses

C H A P T E R

1

Overview and Introduction to Psychiatric Nursing

Learning Objectives

After reading this chapter, the student should be able to:

1. Identify major historical developments in psychiatric care and psychiatric mental health nursing.

2. Evaluate the impact of the community mental health movement on psychiatric mental health nursing.

3. Describe the concepts of primary, secondary, and tertiary levels of prevention as they relate to psychiatric mental health nursing.

4. Trace the various developments that influenced the roles and functions of psychiatric mental health nurses.

5. Compare the educational preparation and clinical responsibilities of generalists and clinical specialists in psychiatric mental health nursing.

6. Recognize the convergent trends in psychiatric care and psychiatric mental health nursing by contrasting nursing diagnoses with the diagnoses of DSM-III.

Overview

Nursing is a health-oriented profession. This chapter therefore begins by presenting a number of definitions of health that are used by nurses to focus and direct their professional activities. Definitions of health range from narrow, reductionistic formulations to broad, holistic ones. Comprehensive definitions of health that consider the individual and family in the context of the environment have been developed by nurse theorists endeavoring to expand the functions and scope of professional nursing. The chapter is also concerned with definitions of mental health and with the influence of social and cultural attitudes on the identification and care of persons with mental disorders.

In order to understand the evolution of psychiatric mental health nursing, it is necessary to examine historical attitudes toward persons thought to be mentally disturbed. This chapter traces historical developments chronologically, beginning with early beliefs that mental disorders were supernatural in origin and proceeding to beliefs that they were medical afflictions. The dramatic changes introduced by the community mental health movement are described, as are contributions made by nurses to the deinstitutionalization of long-term psychiatric clients.

The chapter also examines trends toward a multidimensional diagnostic approach in psychiatry, as demonstrated in the third edition of the American Psychiatric Association's *Diagnostic and Statistical Manual of Mental Disorders* (DSM-III), and trends toward systematic problem solving in nursing, as demonstrated in the accepted nursing diagnoses used to identify problems and to plan and implement nursing care. The DSM-III diagnostic categories and the growing list of nursing diagnoses represent converging trends that promote collaboration between nurses and other health care professionals.

What a piece of work is man! How noble in reason!
How infinite in faculty! In form, in moving,
how express and admirable! In action how like an angel!
In apprehension how like a god!

WILLIAM SHAKESPEARE

DEFINING HEALTH AND MENTAL HEALTH

The future of nursing as a profession depends to a great extent on building a knowledge base for nursing practice. Such a knowledge base requires developing operational definitions of relevant terms used by nurses who are engaged in teaching, research, and clinical practice (Evans, 1979). Of particular importance is arriving at suitable definitions for *health* and *illness*. One interesting but limited definition was offered by Susan Sontag (1978), who wrote that illness is the "dark side of existence" and that every human being holds "dual citizenship" in the realm of the well and the realm of the sick. Even though most people prefer to live in the kingdom of the well, all of us, according to Sontag, must sometimes emigrate to the darker side of life. This definition is problematic in that it totally externalizes health and illness, describing neither as an inner experience.

Holistic Definitions

A less narrow definition was proposed by the World Health Organization (WHO), which described health not merely as the absence of disease or infirmity but as a state of optimal physical, mental, and social well-being (Dubos, 1965). The WHO definition of health, which refers to biopsychosocial experience, has the advantage of being holistic. A *holistic* view of human existence includes all physiological, psychological, and interpersonal transactions that occur throughout the life cycle of individuals, families, and communities. Holism not only includes all aspects of existence but is also concerned with the unity or wholeness of experience rather than its separate components.

The most positive implication of the WHO definition is that it emphasizes health as being something more than the absence of disease or infirmity. Its chief deficiency lies in the fact that it perceives health and illness as opposite extremes and as conditions distinct in themselves rather than as integral aspects of the human experience. An integrated definition was offered by Engel (1960), who noted that disease is "failure or disturbance in the growth, development, functions, or adjustments of the organism as a whole or any of its systems" (p. 459). This statement encompasses failures at any level—biochemical, cellular, organic, psychological, interpersonal, social—as well as failures in relationships between levels. It describes disease not as an isolated entity but as an interaction within the organism or between the organism and the external environment. This view is compatible with Martha Rogers's (1970) idea that the individual and the environment inhabited by the individual are one and the same.

Also moving away from a polarized view of health and illness as two extremes, Dunn (1961) described health in terms of levels of wellness, explaining that *high-level wellness* is a mode of functioning that requires internal balance and integration. At different periods during their lives people may operate at different levels of wellness. Optimal wellness consists not merely of coping but of handling life's demands with energy and a sense of purpose. Thus, high-level wellness can be seen as both a process and a goal.

Another theorist who did not see health and illness as an absolute dichotomy was Abraham Maslow (1970), who identified a hierarchy of human needs that must be satisfied if health is to be achieved or

SUCCESSFUL ADAPTATION

Every organism, human or otherwise, must deal repeatedly with changing internal and external conditions. Response to change may be functional or dysfunctional, depending on a variety of factors. Successful adaptation depends on the resources available to the individual and on the ability to make use of those resources. Available resources include the physiological and psychological characteristics of individuals, as well as their coping skills, social supports, and life experiences. Coping skills and problem-solving ability may be weakened or strengthened by responses to life experiences. Successful adaptation in one situation is likely to promote successful adaptation in subsequent situations, when customary methods of adaptation are improved or new methods acquired.

6

maintained (see Figure 1-1). This hierarchy of needs may be explained simply. Satisfaction of basic needs (at the bottom of the hierarchy) leads to desire for gratification of higher needs. As lower needs are met, the next level of needs becomes dominant. According to Maslow, the desire for higher levels of need fulfillment is a powerful motivating force.

Maslow's hierarchy is not rigid or even sequential, for needs become more or less urgent depending on the individual and the circumstances. For example, a person who has been concerned with meeting high-level needs such as self-actualization (at the top of the hierarchy) may drop down to a lower level because of failing physiological functioning. Preoccupation with relieving current physical distress replaces efforts to achieve self-actualization, at least momentarily. Thus, any consideration of levels of needs must take into account motivation and current situation as important factors. When the entire list of needs is considered, Maslow's hierarchy suggests a holistic view of health, although the idea of holism is implied, rather than clearly stated.

Among nurse theorists, King (1971) proposed a holistic definition that envisions health as a dynamic process characterized by continuous adaptation to conditions in the internal and external environment. This definition implies that organisms undergo growth and change during their life cycle as they respond to diverse psychological, biological, and social influences in their daily lives. Existence is never static but rather an ongoing cyclical process in which freedom from struggle and adaptation is rarely complete, even when conditions of optimal well-being are present.

Health as Adaptation

Whenever health and illness are described as absolute opposites, the result is adherence to a restrictive medical model that is chiefly concerned with differentiating the normal from the abnormal. In the medical model, diseases and infirmities are classified and labeled according to certain signs and symptoms. Because the medical model is not central to nursing theory and practice, nurses avoid approaches that emphasize illness as opposed to health. Instead of basing their practice on simplistic distinctions between normality and abnormality, nurses have become increasingly concerned with the adjustments or *adaptations* that individuals, families, and communities must make to meet the demands of everyday life. From this viewpoint, health is seen as a *functional* form of adaptation to internal and external conditions.

Based on this functional model of health, a basic concept of this book is *adaptation*, which may be described as the ability of living organisms to respond to change. Every organism, human or otherwise, must deal repeatedly with changing internal and external conditions. Response to change may be functional or dysfunctional, depending on a variety of factors. Dysfunctional adaptation can be explained as the physiological, psychological, and social alterations that may appear detrimental to the well-being of individuals, families, and communities but that nevertheless represent their efforts to respond to the circumstances in which they find themselves.

Figure 1-1. Maslow's hierarchy of needs.
SOURCE: Based on Maslow (1970).

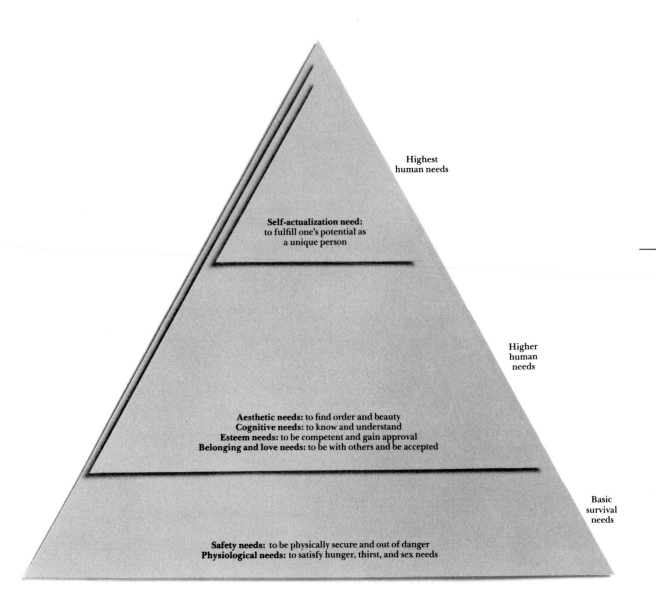

Highest
human needs

Self-actualization need:
to fulfill one's potential as
a unique person

Higher
human
needs

Aesthetic needs: to find order and beauty
Cognitive needs: to know and understand
Esteem needs: to be competent and gain approval
Belonging and love needs: to be with others and be accepted

Basic
survival
needs

Safety needs: to be physically secure and out of danger
Physiological needs: to satisfy hunger, thirst, and sex needs

7

Successful adaptation depends on the resources available to the individual and on the ability to make use of those resources. Available resources include not only the physiological and psychological characteristics of individuals but also their coping skills, social supports, and life experiences. Coping skills and problem-solving ability may be weakened or strengthened by responses to life experiences. Successful adaptation in one situation is likely to promote successful adaptation in subsequent situations, especially when customary methods of adaptation are improved or better methods are acquired. When resources are adequate and indi-

viduals use them effectively, adaptational patterns are wholesome and gratifying to the individual and society. But in circumstances where resources are inadequate or individuals are unable or unwilling to use available resources, the result is *altered patterns* of adaptation that may be questionable.

Definitions of Mental Health
If definitions of health and illness are complex, definitions of mental health and mental illness are even more so. Definitions of mental disorders as disease entities have proved inadequate, but definitions of mental disorders as behavioral or

8

THE FIRST AMERICAN
PSYCHIATRIC TEXTBOOK

A year before his death in 1813, Dr. Benjamin Rush published a compilation of his observations and conclusions regarding mental illness based on his work at Pennsylvania Hospital and as medical professor at the University of Pennsylvania. Rush regarded insanity as a disease of the brain, noting that the cause of madness was seated primarily in the blood vessels of the brain and was a chronic illness attacking that part of the brain containing the mind. This volume was published in Philadelphia, was well regarded in most quarters, and for seventy years was the only available American textbook on the subject of mental illness.

psychological deficiencies have been equally unsatisfactory. As with health in general, holistic definitions have proved to be the most useful and meaningful for nurses.

Holistic approaches to mental health have their roots in the nineteenth century, in the theories of people such as Amariah Brigham (1798–1849), the founder and editor of the *American Journal of Insanity*, which eventually became the *American Journal of Psychiatry*. He wrote that the mind depends on the healthy state of the body, which is in turn influenced in health and illness by the state of the mind. Brigham (1832) went on to describe insanity as a disease of the brain caused by mental or moral factors. During the interval between World Wars I and II, William A. White (1921), an eminent American psychiatrist, emphasized the relationships between physiological and psychological factors in health and illness. His writings and those of Dunbar (1935) in the area of psychosomatic investigation supported multifactorial explanations for illness and led to the recognition that mental disorders involve total rather than partial responses of the individual. Awareness grew that people are social beings who can be understood only if their social relationships are taken into account. Most recently, mental illness has been conceptualized as a complex disruption of mind-body integrity that alters the interface between the individual and the social group (Lipowski, 1981).

Definitions of mental health and mental illness can have far-reaching cultural and political implications. Labeling people as mentally ill has been criticized by Thomas Szasz (1961, 1970, 1974), who alleges that "mental illness" is in fact a myth perpetuated by society and that individuals presumed to be mentally ill merely have "problems in living" that are not acceptable to society. Although some of Szasz's allegations are questionable, there is historical evidence that prevailing cultural beliefs do indeed determine what constitutes mental health and illness. Historically, such beliefs have affected popular attitudes toward those considered mentally ill, and popular attitudes in turn have affected the treatment received by those labeled mentally ill, as we shall see in the next section.

HISTORICAL PERSPECTIVES ON PSYCHIATRIC CARE

Mental Disturbance as Supernatural

In early times mental disturbance was thought to be sent from the gods and was considered beyond the control of mortals. Feelings of powerlessness led to the belief that disturbed people could be cured only when and if the gods were willing. Accordingly, little was provided in the way of treatment except in the form of physical restraint for those whose behavior was considered violent or dangerous. Acceptance of the idea that mental disturbance is a supernatural phenomenon caused the ancient Greeks to consider disorganized individuals as not being legally responsible for their actions. This belief led most societies to delegate responsibility for the mentally disturbed to priests and legal authorities.

The Greek physician Hippocrates attempted to contradict the popular idea that mental illness came from the gods. He wrote that epilepsy, which was

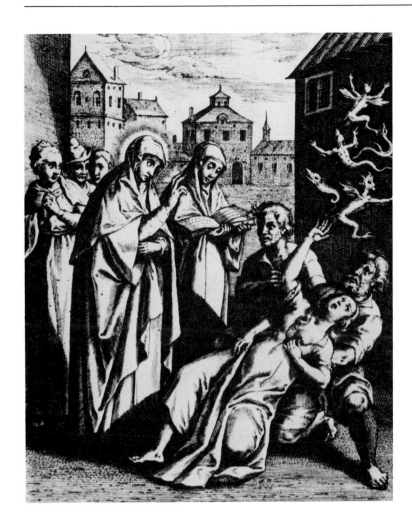

*Exorcism of devils from the
mentally ill, as envisioned in
medieval times.*

generally thought to be divinely caused, was much like any other illness, with its own identifiable symptoms. In addition, Hippocrates described the interaction of four body fluids, or *humors*—blood, black bile, yellow bile, and phlegm—and suggested that each humor was associated with a particular temperament or disposition: sanguine, choleric, melancholic, or phlegmatic. In current terminology, the sanguine temperament might be characterized by hopefulness, the choleric by anger, the melancholic by sadness, and the phlegmatic by passivity. Conflict between the body humors was thought to create a state of imbalance called *dyscrasia*, the treatment for which was purging with strong cathartic drugs.

Like members of most other early societies, the Romans allowed fear and superstition to dominate their attitudes toward persons thought to be mentally disturbed. It was in the area of legal or forensic psychiatry that the Romans made an original contribution. Not only were the mentally disturbed neglected or mistreated, but they were also deprived of freedom and often deemed incompetent to manage their own affairs. Relatives or court-appointed guardians were made custodians of persons judged incompetent or irresponsible. At the

same time, however, the Romans were tolerant of excess alcohol consumption, and drunkenness was considered an acceptable reason for overlooking otherwise reprehensible behavior.

During the Middle Ages, belief persisted that mental illness had a supernatural cause, although by this time devotion to many gods had been replaced by devotion to one god.

From 500 to 1500, there was widespread interest in demonology and witchcraft. The medieval church recognized human beings as having a body (soma) and a soul (psyche). Individuals were often seen as arenas in which evil forces contended for control of the soul. When evil forces seemed to possess a human being, various tactics were used to exorcise or drive them out. Sometimes the methods of exorcism were benign, but more often they were brutal. It was considered advisable to deal forcefully with any person inhabited by a demon in order to punish the malignant spirit dwelling within. Beatings, starvation, exposure, and similar procedures were used.

Exorcism was based on the assumption that the person possessed was an unwilling victim. No such assumption was made for persons accused of witchcraft. These unfortunates were generally

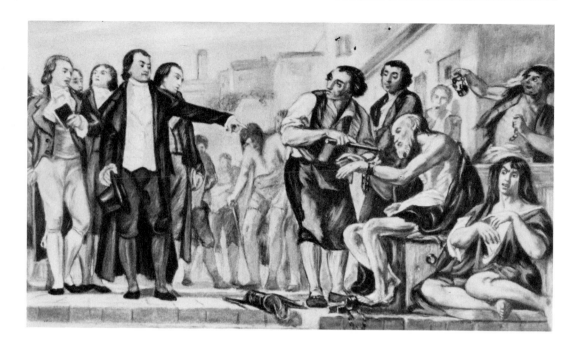

10

accused of willingly making a pact with the devil and were treated accordingly. Preoccupation with witchcraft continued through the eighteenth century and traveled from Europe to colonies in the New World. Witch hunting ultimately abated, but belief that mental illness represented an association with demons aggravated the inhuman treatment endured by those afflicted (Coleman, Butcher and Carson, 1984).

During this period, ostracism or segregation of the mentally disturbed also became frequent. Occasionally, mentally disturbed persons were placed on sailing ships and sent forth in search of their lost reason, thus giving rise to the expression "ship of fools." Confinement became the customary treatment, effectively isolating the mentally disturbed from the rest of the community. Also included within the ranks of the mentally disturbed at this time were the poor, the physically handicapped, the developmentally impaired, and often the unproductive elderly (Mora, 1980).

Mental Disturbance as Affliction

During the seventeenth and eighteenth centuries, society gradually relinquished exclusive belief in supernatural and religious forces for an interest in scientific investigation. In England, Thomas Sydenham (1624–1689) introduced to medicine the systematic clinical observation of patients, and Robert Burton (1577–1640), in *The Anatomy of Melancholy*, identified the causative factors of such mental disturbances as jealousy, solitude, unrewarded affection, and religiosity. Some years later the Society of Friends opened a facility in York, England for about thirty mentally disturbed persons, who were treated kindly and were not subjected to physical restraint or purely medical procedures. Across the English Channel, Philippe Pinel (1745–1826), a superintendent of French institutions that housed criminals, the mentally retarded, and the mentally disturbed, introduced humane treatment, classified the symptoms of his charges, and arranged for the participation of inmates in structured activities (Freedman, Kaplan, and Sadock, 1972).

About the same time, Benjamin Franklin encouraged the Pennsylvania Hospital in Philadelphia to become the first public institution in the United States to admit mentally disturbed persons. Benjamin Rush (1745–1813), a physician at the hospital (and a signer of the Declaration of Independence), is considered the father of American psychiatry. Although he adopted some moderate practices in his work at Pennsylvania Hospital, he also used harsh methods, such as the use of a specially designed chair in which agitated patients were tied and suspended.

The nineteenth century saw the establishment of a number of small mental hospitals and larger state institutions. Among them was McLean Asylum in Massachusetts, which was founded in 1818 and which opened the first school for psychiatric nurses in 1882. The school offered a two-year program that stressed training rather than education, and it established the precedent of preparing psychiatric nurses in psychiatric institutions. The woman acknowledged to be the first American psychiatric nurse was Linda Richards, an 1873 graduate of the nursing program of the New England Hospital for Women and Children in Boston. She was noted for her work in improving nursing care in state mental hospitals in the United States.

Philippe Pinel (opposite) demanding the removal of chains from those institutionalized at Bicetre Hospital in Paris (eighteenth century).

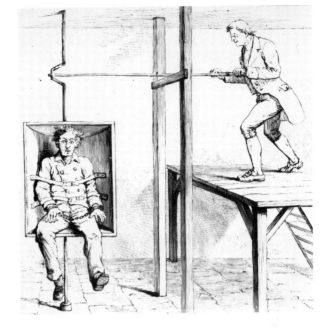

A circulatory chair, one of many devices used to treat the mentally disordered in the early nineteenth century.

11

Much of the impetus for placing the mentally disturbed in large state institutions came from Dorothea Lynde Dix (1802–1887), a teacher and social reformer. Her efforts were well intended but ultimately fostered a system of impersonal, segregated care in specialized facilities. A redeeming event at this time was the publication in 1908 of Clifford Beers's account of his own mental breakdown, *A Mind That Found Itself,* in which he emphasized the importance of social factors in his recovery. A year later, Beers founded the Mental Hygiene Movement, which was concerned with improving conditions and eradicating abuses in asylums and state mental hospitals.

Mental Disturbance as Psychodynamic

Around the turn of the century, Sigmund Freud (1856–1939) introduced the school of psychodynamic psychiatry, which greatly altered treatment of the mentally disturbed and brought new optimism to clinical practice. In contrast to the belief that mental disorders are afflictions, Freud believed that individuals possess drives and instincts that are gradually modified by childhood experiences. Unresolved conflict between instinctual forces and the expectations of family and society can lead to maladaptive behavior in adulthood: the person behaves in ways that perpetuate childhood patterns even when these behaviors do not produce the desired results. Freud devised the therapeutic technique of *psychoanalysis* to explore, analyze, and eventually correct such maladaptive patterns.

Freud's insistence on the absolute importance of the relationship between psychoanalyst and client had the effect of reducing the importance of other therapeutic relationships. In addition, psy-

choanalysis could only be afforded by persons of means. Moreover, many individuals undergoing psychoanalysis remained unhospitalized or received care in private facilities. Thus, the number of nurses using a psychodynamic approach with clients was limited. The influence of psychoanalysis as therapy has diminished in recent years, although it continues to be important theoretically (Adams, 1979; Blumenthal, 1981). The details of Freud's theory are discussed in Chapter 2.

EMERGENT TRENDS IN PSYCHIATRIC CARE

Somatic Therapies

From 1917 through the 1930s, the introduction of various somatic therapies expanded the responsibilities of nurses, even though the medical model was reinforced by these innovations. Malarial therapy, insulin shock treatment, electroconvulsive therapy, and psychosurgery were procedures that required the assistance of nurses who were technically proficient and capable of more than custodial care. However, the tasks of nurses at this time were primarily administrative and managerial. Medical regimens were prescribed by physicians and were carried out by nurses who performed numerous dependent but few independent functions.

Government Involvement in Health Care

One of the lasting effects of the Depression was to bring the federal government into greater involvement with the American health care system. The first milestone of this involvement was the passage of the Social Security Act in 1935, which increased the revenues of the federal government as it assumed new responsibilities for aid to the blind and to dependent children as well as for old age and survivors insurance. World War II was another milestone, when 1,767,000 Americans were excused from military service for mental disorders or related reasons. Furthermore, the war itself produced many psychiatric casualties who needed treatment on returning to civilian life (Lancaster, 1980).

In 1946 President Truman signed the National Mental Health Act, which enabled the National Institute for Mental Health (NIMH) to be established three years later. The first purpose for establishing NIMH was to explore the causes and treatment of mental disorders. The second purpose was to provide federal funds for training grants for nurses and other professionals committed to working in the field of mental health.

The need for additional mental health services was confirmed in a classic study conducted by Hollingshead and Redlich (1958). They found wide discrepancies in the care received by members of various social classes. Persons with fewer socioeconomic resources tended to be labeled readily, to be stigmatized, and to receive mental health services as a result of referral from social agencies or the legal system. Such referral methods tended to reduce these clients' autonomy in the choice of treatment methods. This is significant, since the mode of treatment drastically influences the extent to which the need for mental health care is accepted by clients, families, and community. For example, outpatient care and group treatment are usually less embarrassing for clients and their families than is inpatient hospitalization.

Deinstitutionalization

Until the 1950s, persons suffering psychiatric disorders were hospitalized for many years. Hospitalization often carried the added burden of separation from friends and family, since most mental hospitals were located at some distance from urban centers. Public awareness of poor conditions in mental hospitals was heightened by writers such as Erving Goffman (1961), who movingly described the detrimental effects of institutionalization, especially when the convenience of staff members was given priority over the needs of clients.

A new trend toward deinstitutionalization began with the development of effective psychotropic drugs, particularly the major tranquilizers, which alleviated long-standing maladaptive alterations of thought, mood, and behavior. Clients who had previously been inaccessible to communication became responsive to therapeutic interaction with staff members, and functioned well enough to be released.

The success of deinstitutionalization varied greatly from one locality to another. When clients were carefully prepared for returning to the community and when adequate follow-up care was available, outcomes were relatively successful. In other instances, large numbers of clients were denied much-needed support and became victims of a "revolving door" policy in which discharge to community care was followed by repeated hospitalization, release, and rehospitalization.

During World War II, American and English psychiatrists working together in military installations in England discarded army regulations and established community support systems in which friends, relatives, and care providers interacted with mentally disabled soldiers in a nonthreatening environment. This *milieu therapy* encouraged equalitarian interaction between clients and staff members and expanded the functions and responsibilities of nurses working in psychiatric settings. Milieu therapy as a formal treatment modality continues to be used; it is discussed extensively in Chapter 19.

The Community Mental Health Movement

The Joint Commission on Mental Health and Mental Illness, appointed by President John F. Kennedy, in 1961 published *Action for Mental Health*. Prompted by the commission's disclosures of great inadequacy in mental health services available to the general population, President Kennedy asked Congress for a new approach in caring for the mentally disturbed. The response was enactment of the Community Mental Health Act of 1963, which provided financial support for the construction and staffing of mental health centers in communities throughout the United States. It was this legislation that ultimately opened the doors of state mental institutions and returned many clients to the community.

The purpose of the Community Mental Health Act was to provide full service to all persons living within a geographic region known as a *catchment area*. Depending on population density, catchment areas contain from 75,000 to 200,000 people. In many cases the boundaries of the catchment area do not coincide with other geographic divisions because of efforts to ensure socioeconomic diversity in the population served. Such attempts at diversity have been made to increase community acceptance and to present an image of the community mental health center as care provider for all segments of the population. The communities themselves have some discretion in setting up mental health programs that suit the particular needs of the catchment area.

Federal legislation stipulated that five essential

services be included in community mental health programs:

1. Emergency care offered on a twenty-four-hour basis.
2. Inpatient care for clients needing short-term hospitalization.
3. Partial hospitalization in the form of day treatment centers for clients who returned home at night; partial hospitalization in the form of night treatment centers for clients who worked during the day but needed some care at night.
4. Outpatient care for clients who could live at home but required follow-up care at designated intervals.
5. Consultation and education for the community served by the center.

Inherent in the community mental health movement is commitment to comprehensive care, the use of indigenous residents as paraprofessionals, and reliance on team efforts. Schmitt (1982) has described three types of team approaches: unidisciplinary, multidisciplinary, and interdisciplinary. A *unidisciplinary team* is composed of members of the same discipline. A *multidisciplinary team* is composed of representatives of more than one discipline who work in parallel or sequential ways, with each team member contributing specialized disciplinary skills. For example, a physician might be concerned strictly with medical problems, a social worker with economic and social problems, and a nurse with nursing interventions and procedures. In addition, the nurse or the social worker might be charged with coordinating the various facets of care. An *interdisciplinary team* works together toward a common goal, with representatives of various disciplines sharing responsibilities in a way that bridges intradisciplinary functions. In this approach, team members are less specialized and less restricted in the contributions they can make.

LEVELS OF PREVENTION The prevention concepts formulated by Gerald Caplan (1964) have been important in the community mental health movement. According to Caplan, a major goal in community mental health work is *primary prevention*, which is designed to reduce the incidence of new cases of mental disturbance. Another goal is *secondary prevention*, which is accomplished through case finding, diagnosis, and treatment. *Tertiary prevention* is concerned with reducing residual disabling effects of mental disturbance by promoting physical, psychological, vocational, and social rehabilitation. These three levels of prevention are no longer

limited to community mental health work and have become fundamental principles used extensively by nurses in clinical and community settings.

NURSES' CONTRIBUTIONS TO COMMUNITY MENTAL HEALTH The community mental health movement led to the release of many clients from institutional care and at the same time enlarged the spheres in which nurses worked. As nurses moved out of the relatively protected environment of inpatient facilities and assumed more independent roles, nursing leaders and clinical nurses expressed concerns about nurses' qualifications and preparation for meeting the new demands created by the community mental health movement.

Nurses were in the vanguard of the community mental health movement, and they often made the difference between happy and unhappy outcomes of deinstitutionalization. Working as unidisciplinary, multidisciplinary, and interdisciplinary team members, they organized and coordinated the activities related to discharge into community care. They led predischarge groups in psychiatric hospitals and postdischarge groups in halfway houses and other community settings. Such groups were a means of resocializing clients and reactivating long-forgotten skills. Clients were taught to practice such ordinary activities as shopping and handling money, using a laundromat, and riding a bus, and nurses reassured clients made anxious by impending change. The community mental health movement has not been equally successful everywhere, but for many nurses and clients it has brought new challenges and new opportunities for growth.

EXPANDED NURSING FUNCTIONS AND ROLES

Many principles advocated by Florence Nightingale (1820–1910) remain part of current nursing practice. Among these principles are informed observation, concern for the client as a person, maintenance of a therapeutic environment, and implementation of preventive health measures. The founder of modern nursing considered the duties of an administrator, nutritionist, spiritual counselor, and social worker to be appropriate to nursing. She was sharply critical of the handmaiden role for nurses, stating that nursing "is the skilled servant of medicine, surgery, and hygiene, not the skilled servant of physicians, surgeons, or health officers" (Woodham-Smith, 1951, p. 61).

This gifted woman spent a great deal of time and energy delineating the purpose of nursing, and the process she began has not yet been completed. The uniqueness of nursing is valued by most members of the profession, some of whom have opposed

13

role expansion in order to protect this uniqueness. In the last decade there has been greater agreement within the profession on what constitutes nursing and less fear that the essence of nursing will be jeopardized by expansion and change.

Three recurrent themes have been used by nursing leaders to describe the essence or core of professional nursing (Donaldson and Crowley, 1978):

1. Concern with principles and laws governing life processes and the optimal functioning of all persons, sick or well. This concern is expressed through primary and secondary prevention measures and through tertiary prevention programs used to reduce residual disability.

2. Concern with patterned interactions between individuals and their external environment in critical life situations. This concern is demonstrated in the maintenance of a therapeutic environment and the reinforcement of clients' adaptive coping skills and behaviors.

3. Concern with support systems and interpersonal processes that promote functional adaptation in individuals, families, and communities. This concern is reflected in the interpersonal transactions between nurses and clients, in the self-monitoring and self-awareness of nurses, and in the utilization of family and community resources.

This description of the essence of professional nursing can accurately be applied to psychiatric mental health nursing as it is practiced today. Not too many years ago, the same statement would have been criticized by influential nurses who were afraid that the uniqueness of nursing would be lost if nurses did not leave psychotherapeutic work to members of other disciplines.

Client-Nurse Relationships

One of the most significant figures in the expansion of roles in psychiatric mental health nursing was Hildegarde Peplau (1962), who outlined the scope of psychiatric nursing and asserted that nurses should be counselors of clients, not mothers or managers. In her book *Interpersonal Relations in Nursing* (1952), Peplau wrote that "counseling in nursing has to do with helping the client to remember and to understand fully what is happening to him in the present situation so that the experience can be integrated with, rather than dissociated from, other experiences in life" (p. 64). In

other words, Peplau envisioned mental health nurses actively performing psychotherapeutic tasks with clients. She went on to differentiate surface from in-depth psychotherapeutic work, insisting that both types of intervention are within the capacity of well-prepared nurses. According to Peplau (1962), nursing interventions should consist of aiding clients in recognizing their maladaptive behavior, in describing the behavior verbally, in connecting the causes and consequences of the behavior, in searching for alternative behaviors, and in generalizing the improved behavior to other situations. In her opinion, nursing is an educative instrument and a force designed to promote progress toward constructive and productive personal and social living.

By the middle of the 1960s, the controversy over nurses functioning as counselors and psychotherapists had abated. Psychotherapeutic intervention as performed by nurses was now presented as a one-to-one relationship, and relationship therapy was accepted in most quarters as the basis of psychiatric mental health nursing.

A second nurse theorist concerned with psychotherapeutic relationships was June Mellow (1968), who worked with schizophrenic clients and advocated an intense, close experience between nurse and client. Although Mellow based her work on psychoanalytic principles, she did not believe in maintaining the detachment and aloofness of a psychoanalyst. Rather, she felt that a warm emotional relationship should be established by the nurse through routines of helping the client bathe, dress, and engage in planned activities. Mellow thought that by building trust and exhibiting nurturing behaviors toward the client, the nurse would become a positive identification figure and help provide a corrective emotional experience.

Ida Orlando's (1961) conceptualization of the dynamic nurse-client relationship is applicable to all nurse-client interactions, not just those in psychiatric settings. The nurse, whatever the clinical setting, helps clients explore their behavioral patterns to identify underlying causes and motives. Within the dimensions of the dynamic relationship, the nurse assesses the meaning of the client's behavior and shares the nature of the assessment with the client. The nurse's reactions to the client's behaviors may be disclosed to facilitate change. In the dynamic nurse-client relationship, interactions require adaptation from both participants.

Nursing intervention follows observation of behavior and assessment of needs expressed by that behavior. For example, a client suffering from ulcerative colitis and being cared for on a medical unit might be observed making excessive demands on the nursing staff while bitterly criticizing the care received. On observing this, the nurse might conclude that the underlying need of the client is to be reassured that the nursing staff is concerned and that he will be allowed to control most aspects of the care being given. Thereafter, nursing interventions would be designed to meet the client's needs for reassurance and control rather than to confront the seemingly unreasonable behavior. When the nurse sees improvement after an intervention, this change denotes that the client's needs have been understood and gratified. If improvement does not follow an intervention, the nurse must again observe behaviors, validate observations with the client, try to assess the needs being met by the behavior, and, if possible, respond effectively to the client's underlying needs.

The Psychiatric Mental Health Nurse

Psychiatric mental health nurses may be either generalists or clinical specialists.

THE GENERALIST NURSE The generalist nurse is most often a staff member of a hospital or facility in which the clients are treated for acute or chronic psychiatric disabilities. Most nurses who work with psychiatric clients are generalists, even though they may be called psychiatric nurses or mental health nurses. As generalists, they have received undergraduate education in nursing in a two-year associate degree program, a three-year diploma program, or a four-year baccalaureate program. They have passed a state board examination and are licensed in the state in which they practice as professional nurses. Whether graduates of a two-, three-, or four-year program, they have completed an introductory course in mental health nursing that combines classroom instruction with supervised clinical practice. In addition to this basic course in mental health nursing, most programs integrate mental health concepts throughout the curriculum, particularly in schools that emphasize biopsychosocial nursing.

At the generalist level, registered nurses participate in the activities of a therapeutic community that may be a day treatment program or in an inpatient unit. Community mental health nurses and community health nurses are generalist nurses who make frequent home visits to monitor the progress of clients. Most regions require community health nurses to have a minimum of a baccalaureate degree. Generalist nurses may function as formal or informal leaders of short-term groups, may engage in some forms of family guidance or teaching, and may evaluate the effects of prescribed medication. Often, the generalist is concerned with communication issues, problems of daily living, and health teaching in the form of primary, secondary,

and tertiary prevention. The generalist nurse in a mental health setting is usually a member of a health care team. Although a member from another discipline, such as medicine or psychology, may head the team, the generalist nurse is usually also accountable to a supervisory nurse with graduate education in psychiatric mental health nursing.

THE CLINICAL SPECIALIST The clinical specialist in mental health nursing usually has a master's degree that represents two years of education beyond the baccalaureate level. Nurses with such advanced training provide direct care to clients and families in addition to overseeing the clinical performance of generalist nurses. The American Nurses' Association, recognizing the differing levels of expertise among nurses working in mental health settings, has offered certificates to both generalists and clinical specialists who meet certain standards. Certification at the generalist level means that the nurse has a minimum of two years' experience as a registered nurse working in a mental health facility, is currently engaged in practice, and has given evidence of theoretical knowledge and clinical skills. Certification as a clinical specialist means that the nurse has at least a master's degree in psychiatric mental health nursing, has a minimum of two years of postgraduate clinical experience, and has demonstrated by examination and peer review a superior level of theoretical knowledge and clinical skills (O'Toole, 1980).

CONVERGENT TRENDS IN PSYCHIATRIC CARE

Revisions in psychiatric diagnostic classification systems and a growing list of nursing diagnoses represent converging trends that enhance the effectiveness of health care teams.

Psychiatric Diagnoses

The first official *Diagnostic and Statistical Manual of Mental Disorders* prepared by the American Psychiatric Association (APA) appeared in 1952. In 1968 a second edition, known as the DSM-II, was published and served as the standard diagnostic guide until 1979, when the third edition was approved by the APA. Although faithful to the medical model in some respects, this most recent revision (DSM-III) has moved toward a functional, behavioral, and social understanding of the manifestations of mental disorders. Without presenting any particular theoretical approach, DSM-III assists in the collection of extensive data that may be used by care providers from several disciplines, including nursing.

> ### *DSM-III AXES*
>
> Axis I   Clinical Syndromes or Disorders
> Conditions Not Attributable to a
> Mental Disorder That Are a
> Focus of Attention or Treatment
> Additional Codes
>
> Axis II   Personality Disorders
> Specific Developmental Disorders
>
> Axis III   Physical Disorders or Conditions
>
> Axis IV   Severity of Psychosocial Stressors
>
> Axis V   Highest Level of Adaptive
> Functioning in the Past Year

The preparation of DSM-III, which took five years, was an effort to resolve a number of problematic issues that had plagued the first two versions:

1. Tendencies among psychiatric clinicians, researchers, and educators to classify *people* rather than disorders. Instead of discussing clients as having various symptoms, they used labels such as "schizophrenic" or "alcoholic."

2. The inaccurate but widespread belief that all persons with the same disorder are similar, tend to behave alike, and tend to respond in the same way to similar interventions.

3. Lack of concordance or agreement regarding diagnosis even among experienced professionals.

4. Inadequate criteria in DSM-I and DSM-II on which to base a reliable diagnosis.

5. Discrepancies in treatments offered persons with the same psychiatric diagnosis, and inconsistent outcomes even when similar treatment was offered to clients with the same diagnosis.

6. Attempts of DSM-I and DSM-II to explain the *causes* of symptoms. In other words, theoretical explanations were offered even though they were untested and unproven.

In response to these problems, the task force appointed to revise the DSM took upon itself the following objectives:

1. Formulation of reliable diagnostic categories acceptable to professionals with different orientations.

2. Clinical testing of new diagnostic categories before final approval.

3. Development of mechanisms for data collection and for describing degrees of psychiatric disturbance, biopsychosocial influences, and complicating factors.

The result of this effort was a descriptive multiaxial framework. DSM-III requires each client to be assessed on five *axes*, each of which provides specific information. The first three axes constitute the official psychiatric diagnosis; the last two permit rating of psychosocial stressors and levels of adaptive function. Every client is assessed on each axis.

Axes I and II include all the clinical entities known as mental disorders. Sometimes multiple diagnoses are necessary, as when substance abuse is superimposed on another psychiatric disorder. Personality disorders are recorded on Axis II; notation of a code number on Axis II indicates that a specific personality *disorder* is present, not merely a trait. Any current physical disability that has a bearing on treatment management is recorded on Axis III.

Axis IV enables the clinician to report the severity of psychosocial stressors on a scale from 1 (no apparent psychosocial stressor) to 7 (catastrophic psychosocial stressor). A rating of 0 is given if severity of psychosocial stressors is unspecified, unknown, or not applicable. Axis V indicates the clinician's opinion of the highest level of adaptive function in the past year, using a scale ranging from 1 (superior) to 7 (grossly impaired). A rating of 0 is given if the highest level of adaptive function is unspecified, unknown, or not applicable. A complete listing of DSM-III diagnoses is provided in the appendix.

DSM-III helps clinicians to assess the biopsychosocial status of the client and to report data in an organized fashion. Data collection along the five axes provides an informed basis for making clinical decisions about target symptoms and treatment goals. The collected data are descriptive rather than theoretical and are not unduly influenced by the preferences and orientation of the clinician. Like its predecessors, DSM-III is not entirely satisfactory, but it represents a broader, more objective approach to mental disorder than was previously available.

The DSM-III axes most relevant for nurses are Axes IV and V, psychosocial stressors and adaptive functioning levels. It has been proposed that psychiatric nurses extend the DSM-III to include a sixth axis that could be used by members of the mental health disciplines to design a treatment plan based on multiaxial assessment. This is already being done informally, and there is some justification for suggesting that nurses become involved in refining DSM-III so that working relationships among members of the health care disciplines may become less territorial and more collegial (Williams and Wilson, 1982).

Nursing Diagnoses

Johnson (1974) described *nursing diagnosis* as identifying and defining real or potential nursing problems. She went on to define *nursing problems* as any behavioral imbalances or instabilities considered to be within the scope of nursing, and further classified them as problems of insufficiency, discrepancy, dominance, and incompatibility. The

---

NURSING DIAGNOSES ACCEPTED BY THE NORTH AMERICAN NURSING DIAGNOSIS ASSOCIATION

Activity intolerance
Anxiety
Bowel elimination, alteration in:
    Constipation
    Diarrhea
Cardiac output, alteration in: Decreased
Comfort, alteration in: Pain
Communication, impaired verbal
Coping, ineffectual individual
Coping, ineffective family
Diversional activity deficit
Family processes, alteration in
Fear
Fluid volume deficit
Fluid volume excess
Grieving
Health maintenance, alterations in
Home maintenance management, impaired
Injury, potential for
Knowledge deficit (specify)
Mobility, impaired physical
Noncompliance (specify)
Nutrition, alterations in: Less than body requirements
Nutrition, alterations in: More than body requirements
Oral mucous membrane, alterations in
Parenting, alteration in
Powerlessness
Rape trauma syndrome
Self-care deficit (specify)
Self-concept, disturbance in
Sensory perceptual alteration
Sexual dysfunction
Skin integrity, impairment of
Sleep pattern disturbance
Social isolation
Spiritual distress
Thought processes, alterations in
Tissue perfusion, alterations in
Urinary elimination, alterations in patterns of
Violence, potential for

SOURCE: Reprinted with permission of the North American Nursing Diagnosis Association and the American Nurses' Association.

17

Table 1-1. Nursing Problems and Nursing Responses

Problems	Responses
Problems of insufficiency	Increase the functioning ability of the client and of associated subsystems and suprasystems
Problems of discrepancy	Offer choices and actions so the client, subsystems, and suprasystems can function harmoniously and evenly
Problems of dominance	Strengthen weaker clients and associated systems, and modify dominant clients and associated systems
Problems of incompatibility	Moderate conflicting behaviors to promote stability

Adapted from Johnson (1974).

four classifications, shown in Table 1-1, form a tentative blueprint for nurses engaged in assessment, planning, and implementation.

Nursing diagnoses are systematic efforts to establish a better knowledge base for informed practice. Although less extensive than the DSM-III categories, official nursing diagnoses (see box on page 17) are part of the scientific direction that nursing is pursuing. Any diagnoses tentatively approved by the North American Nursing Diagnosis Association are subjected to clinical testing and validation. Nursing diagnoses identify some etiologic factors, list certain characteristics, and suggest general nursing responses. Additional work is needed to refine terminology, delineate criteria, and test the diagnoses in clinical and laboratory situations. The formulation of nursing diagnoses is an indication of progress in developing and applying nursing theory.

There are many similarities and few real discrepancies between the DSM-III diagnostic categories and the list of approved nursing diagnoses. Like the DSM-III categories, the nursing diagnoses make client assessment more specific and consistent. Additionally, the use of nursing diagnoses enables nurses to function autonomously within the dimensions of the nursing process.

SUMMARY

A review of the history of psychiatric care and psychiatric nursing reveals certain trends. Over the ages, mental disturbance has been seen in turn as supernatural in origin, as a mental and moral affliction, as a product of psychodynamic factors, and finally as a social and community responsibility. For many years psychiatry and psychiatric nursing remained separate and divisible, with the scope of psychiatric nursing limited by the nature of whatever treatment approaches were adopted. Out of the community mental health movement came influences that expanded the roles and responsibilities of psychiatric nurses. When long-term psychiatric clients left institutions and reentered the community, this radical change was facilitated by the discovery of somatic treatments, by the use of milieu therapy, and by the contributions of a number of nurse theorists, most notably Peplau, Mellow, and Orlando, who advocated psychotherapeutic work by nurses.

Many health care professionals are afraid of be-

CLINICAL EXAMPLE

CONVERGENCE OF PSYCHIATRIC ND NURSING DIAGNOSES

Mrs. Stevens is a sixty-year-old woman who suffered a cardiovascular accident. She has residual paralysis of the left side severe enough to require the use of a walker. Prior to the cardiovascular accident, Mrs. Stevens had lived alone in a small apartment, but afterward she had to be admitted to a skilled nursing facility subsequent to spending several weeks' stay in a general hospital.

While in the nursing facility, Mrs. Stevens became seriously depressed and was then transferred to an inpatient psychiatric unit where she could be observed more closely. Because she was so depressed, suicide precautions were instituted. Mrs. Stevens was distrustful and suspicious of everyone with whom she came in contact. She was afraid that staff members and other clients would disturb her possessions and steal her belongings if she left her room even to attend physical therapy. At the same time, she refused to allow staff members to lock the door of her room.

Mrs. Stevens had few friends and no visitors except for her landlady. Her husband was dead and her only son lived many miles away. In general, her behavior was withdrawn and seclusive. Most of her time was spent in her room, where she would lie in her bed or sit staring into space. Her daytime inactivity contributed to nighttime insomnia. She was indifferent to her appearance, often objecting to taking a bath or combing her hair even with assistance. Mrs. Stevens never initiated conversations and responded with monosyllables when others spoke to her. At times she was abrupt and rude toward the staff and fellow clients. She never attended activities or programs organized for clients in the facility. Because of her extreme resistance to involvement of any kind, her physical and social rehabilitation was impeded.

Psychiatric and nursing assessments of the client led to the formulation of the following nursing and psychiatric diagnoses:

Nursing Diagnoses
Comfort, alterations in
(related to immobility and impaired motor function)

Coping, ineffectual individual
(related to loss of independence and to social isolation)

Coping, ineffective family
(related to geographic distance separating client from son)

Diversional activity deficit
(related to client's resentment of psychiatric hospitalization and her depressed mood)

Fear
(related to physical disability and loneliness)

Knowledge deficit
(related to ignorance regarding prognosis and expectations of recovery)

Mobility, impaired physical
(related to residual paralysis following the cardiovascular attack)

Self-care deficit
(caused by combination of factors related to physical impairment, social isolation, and psychological distress)

Multiaxial Psychiatric Diagnoses

Axis I   Clinical Syndromes
296.23 Major depression, single episode, with melancholia
V15.81 Noncompliance with medical regimen
V62.89 Life circumstance problem

Axis II   Personality and Developmental Disorders
Atypical paranoid disorder
(Code number is not used in Axis II except to indicate personality disorder rather than a trait)

Axis III   Physical Disorders or Conditions
Cardiovascular accident

Axis IV   Code 5—Severe psychosocial stressors
Psychological factors affecting physical condition
Psychiatric hospitalization
Lack of support networks
Loss of autonomy

Axis V   Level 5—Poor
Social relationships impaired
Use of leisure time impaired

It is evident from these classifications of Mrs. Stevens's problems that there is wide agreement between her psychiatric diagnoses and her nursing diagnoses, which supplement and reinforce one another. Both diagnostic approaches are comprehensive and objective. Each approach in its own way assists in planning, implementing, and evaluating interventions designed to meet the specific needs of the client.

19

coming involved with clients identified as having mental disorders. This attitude is generated by belief that mental disorders are intractable diseases that are difficult to diagnose and treat. What is often overlooked is that diagnostic categories or labels have little relevance in psychiatric nursing. It is much more useful for nurses to think of mental disorders as reactions to overwhelming conditions of daily life. The person with a psychiatric problem is less mysterious and easier to understand if nurses rely on their powers of observation and on systematic assessment. Such observation and assessment are activities that are facilitated by the use of nursing diagnoses.

Review Questions

1. What are the major characteristics of nursing definitions of health and illness?

2. What influence does motivation play in Maslow's hierarchy of needs?

3. What divergent historical trends have been evident in psychiatric care?

4. What effects did the following developments have on the roles and functions of psychiatric mental health nurses?
   a. Psychoanalytic theory.
   b. Somatic therapies.
   c. State mental hospitals.
   d. Community Mental Health Act.
   e. Milieu therapy.

5. What were the mandated services of community mental health centers? Which of the mandated services represent primary prevention? secondary prevention? tertiary prevention?

6. Differentiate the educational levels and clinical responsibilities of generalists and clinical specialists in psychiatric mental health nursing.

7. What were the innovative contributions of Hildegarde Peplau to role expansion in psychiatric mental health nursing? of June Mellow? of Ida Orlando?

8. Describe the converging trends evident in DSM-III and in approved nursing diagnoses.

9. How might the converging trends of the DSM-III and the approved nursing diagnoses affect the practice of psychiatric mental health nursing?

References

Adams, V. A. 1979. Freud's Work Thrives as Theory Not Therapy. *The New York Times*, August 14.

American Psychiatric Association. 1981. *Diagnostic and Statistical Manual of Mental Disorders*, 3rd ed. Washington, D.C.: Amerian Psychiatric Association.

Blumenthal, R. 1981. Did Freud's Isolation (and) Peer Rejection Prompt Key Theory Reversal? *The New York Times*, August 25.

Brigham, A. 1832. *Remarks on the Influence of Mental Cultivation Upon Health*. Hartford, Conn.: Huntington Press.

Caplan, G. 1964. *Principles of Preventive Psychiatry*. New York: Basic Books.

Coleman, J. C.; Butcher, J. N.; and Carson, R. C. 1984. *Abnormal Psychology and Modern Life*. Glenview, Ill.: Scott Foresman.

Donaldson, S. K., and Crowley, D. M. 1978. The Discipline of Nursing. *Nursing Outlook*, 26 (Feb.): 113–120.

Dubos, R. 1965. *Man Adapting*. New Haven, Conn.: Yale University Press.

Dunbar, H. 1935. *Emotions and Bodily Changes: A Survey of Literature on Psychosomatic Interrelationships: 1910–1933*. New York: Columbia University Press.

Dunn, H. 1961. *High Level Wellness*. Arlington, Va.: R. W. Beatty.

Engel, G. L. 1960. A Unified Concept of Health and Disease. *Perspectives in Biology and Medicine*. Chicago: University of Chicago Press, Summer: 459.

Evans, S. K. 1979. Descriptive Criteria for the Concept of Depleted Health Potential. *Advances in Nursing Science*, 1(4):67–74.

Freedman, A. M.; Kaplan, H. I.; and Sadock, B. J. 1972. *Modern Synopsis of Psychiatry*. Baltimore: Williams & Wilkins.

Goffman, E. 1961. *Asylums*. New York: Doubleday.

Gordon, M. 1982. *Nursing Diagnosis: Process and Application*. New York: McGraw-Hill.

Hollingshead, A., and Redlich, F. C. 1958. *Social Class and Mental Illness*. New York: John Wiley & Sons.

Johnson, D. E. 1974. Development of Theory: A Prerequisite for Nursing As a Primary Health Profession. *Nursing Research*, 23(5):372–377.

King, I. M. 1971. *Toward a Theory of Nursing*. New York: John Wiley & Sons.

Lancaster, J. 1980. *Adult Psychiatric Nursing*. New York: Medical Examination Publishing.

Lipowski, Z. J. 1981. Holistic Medical Foundations of American Psychiatry. *American Journal of Psychiatry*, 138(7):888–897.

Maslow, A. H. 1968. *Toward a Psychology of Being*, 2nd ed. New York: Van Nostrand Reinhold.

Maslow, A. H. 1970. *Motivation and Personality*, 2nd ed. New York: Harper & Row.

Mellow, J. 1968. Nursing Therapy. *American Journal of Nursing*, 11:2365–2369.

Mora, G. 1980. Historical and Theoretical Trends in Psychiatry. In *Comprehensive Textbook of Psychiatry*, 3rd ed., eds. H. I. Kaplan, A. M. Freedman, and B. J. Sadock. Baltimore: Williams & Wilkins.

Orlando, I. 1961. *The Dynamic Nurse-Patient Relationship*. New York: Putnam's.

O'Toole, A. W. 1980. Psychiatric Nursing. In *Comprehensive Textbook of Psychiatry*, 3rd ed., eds. H. I. Kaplan, A. M. Freedman, and B. J. Sadock. Baltimore: Williams & Wilkins.

Peplau, H. E. 1952. *Interpersonal Relations in Nursing*. New York: Putnam's.

20

Peplau, H. E. 1962. Interpersonal Techniques: The Crux of Psychiatric Nursing. *American Journal of Nursing*, 6:53–54.

Rogers, M. 1970. *An Introduction to the Theoretical Basis of Nursing*. Philadelphia: F. A. Davis.

Schmitt, M. 1982. Working Together in Health Teams. In *Life Cycle Group Work in Nursing*, eds. E. H. Janosik and L. B. Phipps. Monterey, Calif.: Wadsworth Health Sciences.

Sontag, S. 1978. *Illness as Metaphor*. New York: Farrar, Straus & Giroux.

Spingarn, N. D. 1982. Primary Nurses Bring Back One-on-One Care. *The New York Times Magazine*. December 26:26.

Szasz, T. S. 1961. *The Myth of Mental Illness*. New York: Dell.

Szasz, T. S. 1970. *Ideology and Insanity*. New York: Doubleday.

Szasz, T. S. 1974. *The Second Sin*. New York: Doubleday.

White, W. A. 1921. *Foundations of Psychiatry*. New York: Nervous and Mental Disease Publishing.

Williams, J. B. W., and Wilson, H. S. 1982. A Psychiatric Nursing Perspective on DSM-III. *Journal of Psychosocial Nursing and Mental Health Services*, 20(4):14–20.

Woodham-Smith, C. 1951. *Florence Nightingale, 1820–1910*. New York: McGraw-Hill.

Supplementary Readings

Alexander, F. G., and Silesnick, S. T. *The History of Psychiatry: An Evaluation of Psychiatric Thought and Practice from Prehistoric Times to the Present*. New York: Harper & Row, 1966.

Angrest, S. The Mental Hospital: Its History and Destiny. *Perspectives in Psychiatric Care*, 11(1963):20.

Birnbach, N. Political Activism in Nursing: A Historical Overview. *Society for Nursing History Gazette*, 3(1983):2.

Bruce, N. G. Searching the History of the Health Sciences. *Medical Reference Services Quarterly*, 1(1982):13–35.

Curtis, D. E. Nurses and War: The Way It Was, December 1944. *American Journal of Nursing*, 84(1984):1253–1254.

Chamberlain, J. G. The Role of the Federal Government in the Development of Psychiatric Nursing. *Journal of Psychiatric Nursing and Mental Health Services*, 21(1983):11–18.

Donahue, P. M. *Nursing: The Oldest Art*. St. Louis: C. V. Mosby, 1985.

Doona, M. E. At Least as Well Cared For: Linda Richards and the Mentally Ill. *Image*, 16(1984):51–56.

Dopson, L. The Cut-Throat World of Nursing Politics, 19th Century Style. *Nursing Times*, 80(1984):19–20.

Dumas, R. G. Social, Economic, and Political Factors and Mental Illness. *Journal of Psychiatric Nursing and Mental Health Services*, 21(1983):31–35.

Hall, C. A. Time for Reflection. *Journal of Advanced Nursing*, 8(1983):457–472.

Ham, L. M. Nursing History: Our Wasted Asset. *Nursing and Health Care*, 3(1982):434–437.

Hanric, A. B., and Spros, J. *The Clinical Nurse Specialist in Theory and Practice*. Orlando, Fla.: Grune & Stratton, 1983.

Henderson, V. Is the Study of History Rewarding for Nurses? *Society for Nursing History Gazette*, 2(1982):1–2.

Hepplethwaite, A. Nursing in the Thirties. *Nursing Times*, 80(1984):40–42.

Jackson, B. S. Nurses at Work in America: A History of Nursing's Economic and General Welfare Posture. *Nursing Leadership*, 6(1983):93–99.

Kalisch, B. J. Image Making in Nursing. Anatomy of the Image of the Nurse: Dissonant and Ideal Models. *ANA Publication American Academy of Nursing*, #G161 (1983):3–23.

Menninger, W. *Psychiatry: Its Evolution and Present Status*. New York: Cornell University Press, 1948.

Mitsunaga, B. K. Designing Psychiatric/Mental Health Nursing for the Future: Problems and Prospects. *Journal of Psychiatric Nursing and Mental Health Services*, 20(1982):15–21.

Norman, E. M. Who and Where are Nursing Historians? *Nursing Forum*, 20(1981):138–152.

Palmer, I. S. Nightingale Revisited. *Nursing Outlook*, 31(1983):229–233.

Parsons, M. E. Mothers and Matrons: The Origins of Modern American Nursing. *Nursing Outlook*, 31(1983):274–278.

Perry, D. S. The Early Midwives of Missouri. *Journal of Nurse Midwifery*, 28(1983):15–22.

Rosen, G. *Madness in Society*. New York: Harper & Row, 1968.

Sabin, L. E. The French Revolution: The Forgotten Era in Nursing History. *Nursing Forum*, 20(1981):225–243.

Stainton, M. C. The Birth of Nursing Science. *Canadian Nurse*, 78(1982):24–28.

Talbott, J. A. The Chronically Mentally Ill: A Look at the Past Five Years with an Eye to the Future. *Psychosocial Rehabilitation Journal*, 6(1983):12–21.

PSYCHOGENIC FRAMEWORK
Psychosexual Theory
Psychosocial Theory

INTERPERSONAL FRAMEWORK
Self System
Modes of Experience
Nursing Implications of Sullivan's Theory

SOCIOLOGICAL FRAMEWORK
Social Institutions
Symbolic Interactionism
Social Roles
Social Stratification
Nursing Implications of Sociological Approaches

BIOGENIC FRAMEWORK
Constitutional Factors
Genetic Factors
Chemical Imbalance
Biological Rhythms
Nursing Implications of Biogenic Approaches

OTHER FRAMEWORKS
Existential Framework
Cognitive Framework

C H A P T E R

2

Theoretical Frameworks in Psychiatric Mental Health Nursing

Learning Objectives

After reading this chapter, the student should be able to:

1. Contrast the strengths and limitations of theoretical frameworks used in psychiatric mental health nursing.

2. Trace the major contributions of Freud to our understanding of personality development.

3. Trace the major contributions of Erikson to our understanding of personality development and compare his framework with that of Freud.

4. Discuss the differences between the experiential states of shame and guilt.

5. Describe the development of the self system and explain its importance in social interactions.

6. Discuss the applications of sociological theory to psychiatric nursing practice.

7. Describe the influence of biogenic approaches on psychiatric nursing practice.

Overview

In psychiatric mental health nursing, the contributions of a number of major theoretical frameworks enhance the understanding of biopsychosocial development and adaptation. The major approaches discussed in this chapter include the psychogenic framework, the interpersonal framework, the sociological framework, the existential framework, the cognitive framework, and the biogenic framework. Systems theory is discussed in Chapter 3.

Much madness is divinest sense
To a discerning eye
Tis the majority
In this, as all, prevails.
Assent and you are sane
Demur—you're straightway dangerous
And handled with a chain.

EMILY DICKINSON

25

Factual knowledge is the basis of psychiatric nursing, but isolated facts tend to seem irrelevant and to be easily forgotten. Knowledge must therefore be organized systematically into a coherent pattern, using theoretical frameworks. A *theory* may be defined as a set of related principles that can be used to explain, predict, or analyze certain phenomena. Theories permit inferences or generalizations to be made on the basis of principles that are applicable to more than one situation. *Theoretical frameworks* are organizing structures that reveal relationships and connections and that therefore increase our understanding of phenomena. No theoretical framework is all inclusive. Rather, each offers a particular perspective that helps illuminate a part of the whole.

Theoretical frameworks are composed of selected concepts and constructs. *Concepts* are general abstract ideas. They are not "objects" that can be perceived or witnessed, because they exist only in the mind. Most concepts have a collective meaning that is shared by the people who use them. *Constructs* are collections or syntheses of concepts, but the terms are sometimes used interchangeably.

Theoretical frameworks promote the analysis and synthesis of knowledge in a way that mere facts do not. For these reasons, many nurse educators rely on theoretical frameworks to transmit the knowledge on which professional expertise depends.

Theoretical frameworks are also important in the research conducted by nurses working in clinical and laboratory settings. Although there is a growing body of nursing theory based on research, many theoretical formulations in nursing remain "a synthesis of principles, concepts, laws, and theories drawn from the natural and social sciences" (King,

1971, p. 3). However, nurse researchers continue to be involved in building a theory base that is unique to nursing.

Every theoretical framework has a particular viewpoint that reveals some phenomena but excludes others. The same concepts may appear in more than one framework, but they are interpreted differently in each. Because psychiatric nursing is a complex field in which there are few definitive answers, no single framework is fully satisfactory. It is important, therefore, for nurses to be familiar with those theories of biopsychosocial functioning that are the most influential.

PSYCHOGENIC FRAMEWORK

The psychogenic framework is represented by Freud's psychosexual theory and Erikson's psychosocial theory.

Psychosexual Theory

Psychosexual theory is a term applied to the developmental aspects of the psychoanalytic approach developed by Sigmund Freud (1856–1939). Freud believed that civilization depends on the control of sexual impulses. Energy that is diverted from sexual gratification becomes available for cultural and social improvement. He thought that society is repressive because it frustrates human sexual desires and that there is always danger that primitive sexual impulses will be released and threaten social stability. His idea of sexuality beginning in infancy created a great deal of hostility, which he attributed to fear on the part of society (Freud, 1961).

FREUD ON DREAMS

Freud suggested that dreams protect the sleeper by disguising aggressive or sexual images that might otherwise prove disturbing. He was interested in both the apparent (manifest) content of dreams and in the hidden (latent) content. A partial list of Freudian dream symbolism follows.

Dream Symbols	Signify	Dream Symbols	Signify
Steps, ladders, stairways, riding horseback	Sexual intercourse	Balloons, airplanes, flying	Erection
Candles, snakes, tree trunks, reptiles, fish, hands or feet	Penis and other aspects of male genitals	Water	Birth
		Journeys, travel	Death
Boxes, doors, balconies, caves, jars, ships, chests, bottles, tunnels	Female genitals	Small animals	Children (siblings, self, or offspring)
Apples, peaches, pears	Female breasts	Kings and queens	Parents

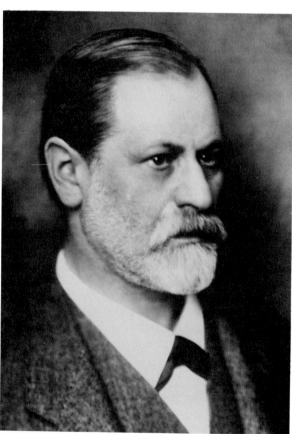

Sigmund Freud.

Freud asserted that human beings, like lower animals, possess instinctual drives that influence behavior patterns. Drives are the source of psychic energy; they operate from birth and promote personality development. Two opposing drives, erotic and aggressive, are part of the *id*, which is the primitive or instinctual part of the personality. Every individual possesses erotic (libidinous) and aggressive drives that operate simultaneously, so that many human acts have both loving and destructive components. Freud's description of the duality of drives helps explain the ambivalence that individuals feel in many situations. A good example is the mother who is devoted to the welfare of her family but sometimes wishes to be free of responsibility.

Freud explained that psychic energy, like physical energy, is limited in quantity. When one individual bestows affection on someone else, this results in a loss of psychic energy unless the affection is returned. Love that is returned restores psychic energy, but unreturned love depletes the lover. The fact that psychic energy can be exhausted helps explain the fatigue that follows excessive psychologic demands on an individual.

In his theory, Freud distinguished between two different ways of thinking and relating: primary and secondary. *Primary process thinking* is not rooted in reality but is controlled by impulsive id forces that seek instant gratification. This way of thinking sometimes enhances the creative processes that produce art, literature, and music. Primary process may also include psychotic thinking and can be discerned in the thought patterns of persons who are in acute states of mental disturbance. *Secondary process thinking* originates in the ego and is rooted in reality. It utilizes conscious reasoning, comprehension, logic, and judgment.

PERSONALITY STRUCTURES According to Freud, in the first months of life the infant is motivated entirely by id or instinctual forces. Contact with the environment modifies the id; maturation is achieved through both frustration and gratification

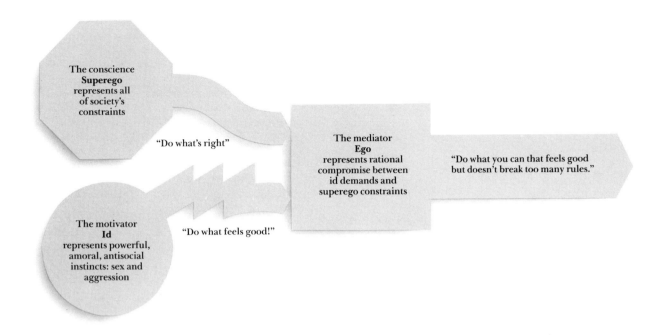

The conscience
Superego
represents all
of society's
constraints

"Do what's right"

The mediator
Ego
represents rational
compromise between
id demands and
superego constraints

"Do what you can that feels good
but doesn't break too many rules."

The motivator
Id
represents powerful,
amoral, antisocial
instincts: sex and
aggression

"Do what feels good!"

27

of the id, provided always that frustration is not excessive. The *ego* begins to develop when the infant is about six months old. The primary purpose of the ego is to maintain a sense of reality, to negotiate with reality, and to adapt to reality. Development of the ego is assisted by the increasing perceptual, cognitive, and language ability of the child (Brenner, 1955).

Besides dealing with reality, additional ego functions include (Bellak, Hurvick, and Gediman, 1973):

1. Reality testing, or the ability to differentiate internal stimuli from external stimuli. Hallucinations and delusions indicate failure of reality testing.

2. Judgment, or the ability to control impulses and predict the consequences of one's behavior. Inability to tolerate delayed gratification is a sign of poor judgment.

3. Subjective awareness of what reality is and where selfhood begins and ends. When this awareness is impaired, individuals feel isolated from reality or merged with reality.

4. Regulation of moods and drives without acting them out behaviorally.

5. Establishment of object relatedness, or the ability to form and maintain relationships.

6. Maintenance of thought processes such as memory, concept formation, and language skills.

7. Regression in the service of the ego, or the ability to reduce functioning temporarily in order

to rest, feel pleasure, or engage in creative work. Sleep, vacations, and orgasm are examples of regression in the service of the ego.

8. Maintenance of a stimulus barrier to permit concentration or prevent being overwhelmed by stimuli. Inadequacies in the stimulus barrier lead to confusion and feelings of disorientation.

9. Performance of complex mental functions related to learning, perception, logical thinking, and complex skills.

10. Integration and synthesis of contradictory values and attitudes in order to establish meaningful relationships and attain appropriate goals.

11. Maintenance of mastery and competence related to self-control and control of one's environment.

The third personality structure to develop is the *superego* (see Figure 2-1). The superego represents the internalized attitudes of the parents and of society. It includes the *ego ideal*, which is the self as one would like to be. Because much of the superego is controlled by unconscious attitudes, it is not a reliable means of dealing with reality. It is the emergence of the superego at about age six that leads to the feeling of guilt. *Shame* is an earlier experience that results from one's failure to live up to the ego ideal. Shame is rarely felt unless one's unacceptable behavior is discovered by others. *Guilt* is an internal experience caused by failure to conform to the standards of the superego, and it is felt even when one's inner thoughts and desires are unknown to others.

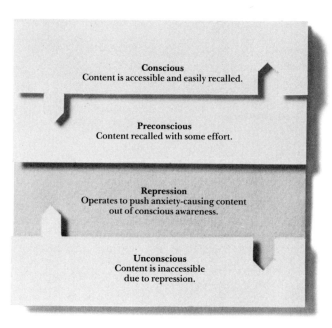

Figure 2-2. Levels of mental awareness.

Table 2-1. Personality Structures and Level of Consciousness

Structure	Basis	Level of Consciousness	Principle Followed	Process Used
Id	Instincts for sex and aggression	Unconscious	Pleasure principle	Primary process thinking
Ego	Learned behaviors in response to reality	Mostly conscious	Reality principle	Secondary process thinking
Superego	Learned social inhibitions	Partly conscious	—	—

Freud also described three levels of mental activity: the *unconscious*, the *preconscious*, and the *conscious* (see Figure 2-2). Of the three, the unconscious is by far the largest. Memories and feelings that are unacceptable to the individual are pushed out of awareness into the unconscious by means of a mental process called *repression*. Unacceptable memories and feelings are *ego alien* or *ego dystonic* and produce anxiety unless they are repressed. Acceptable memories and feelings are *ego syntonic* and do not produce anxiety. The preconscious level contains material not immediately available but subject to recall if one tries. The conscious level is the smallest and contains material that is accessible and easily remembered. Table 2-1 outlines the relationship between personality structures and levels of consciousness.

PSYCHOSEXUAL STAGES Freud suggested that each person, beginning at birth, undergoes a uniform, predetermined sequence of *psychosexual stages* and that each developmental stage is related to a particular psychosexual conflict. In psychoanalytic theory, a conflict is explained as a wish for something and a simultaneous fear of the consequences

if that wish is fulfilled. For example, a person who is in conflict about dependency might want to depend on others but fears the loss of freedom that dependency often brings. Individuals can progress from one psychosexual phase to another, can be *fixated* in one phase without advancing further, or can progress and later *regress* to an earlier developmental phase. Within each phase, specific body orifices (mouth, anus, or genitals) are the objects of erotic interest and instinctual energy. Table 2-2 outlines the psychosexual stages, chronologic ages, and related conflicts formulated by Freud.

In Greek mythology, Oedipus was a ruler who unknowingly killed his father, wed his mother, and suffered for his misdeeds. According to Freud, the

Table 2-2. Psychosexual Stages

Psychosexual Stage	Age	Related Conflict
Oral	Birth to 1 year	Dependency
Anal	1 to 3 years	Control
Phallic (Oedipal)	3 to 5 or 6 years	Competition
Latency	5 or 6 years to puberty	Mastery
Genital	Puberty and onward	Intimacy

HIERARCHY OF
DEFENSE MECHANISMS

The following hierarchy of defense mechanisms is ordered from least primitive to most primitive based on extent of reality distortion:

1. Rationalization.
2. Repression.
3. Displacement.
4. Identification.
5. Conversion.
6. Isolation/Intellectualization.
7. Reaction Formation/Compensation.
8. Undoing.
9. Introjection.
10. Projection.
11. Denial.

Oedipal romance is enacted in every family during the phallic phase of childhood. For all infants the mother is the first love object. As the child matures, the parent of the opposite sex becomes a love object and the parent of the same sex becomes a rival in the mind of the child. The task of the boy is considered to be less complicated because for him the mother can remain the primary love object, but girls must cope with the transformation of mother from love object into rival.

Sexual feelings for one parent and resentment for the other create a fear of punishment in the child. Freud called this fear of impending punishment *castration anxiety*, and out of this fear emerges the *superego*, the conscience or censor of the personality. Freud believed that because girls have no penis, they suffer less castration anxiety. The effect is to prolong the Oedipal conflict in girls and to make the female's superego less strict and punitive than the male's.

Freud saw the Oedipal conflict as an explanation for the adult fantasies of childhood seduction that he encountered in his practice. He hypothesized that such fantasies of parental rape and seduction arose out of sexual interest in the parent of the opposite sex. Many clinicians working in the field of child abuse today feel that the Freudian viewpoint has seriously damaged the credibility of children who have been victims of actual sexual abuse.

ANXIETY Freud described several causes and manifestations of anxiety. He attributed castration anxiety, which surfaces during the Oedipal conflict, to unacceptable erotic wishes and saw superego anxiety as arising from internalized guilt. *Separation anxiety* is triggered first by the trauma of birth and

later by separation from beloved persons, places, and possessions. The concept of separation anxiety helps explain the difficulties many people experience when they must relinquish familiar surroundings and friendships. Extreme forms of separation anxiety are felt by persons dealing with death, either their own or that of loved ones. *Anaclitic* separation anxiety is caused by early loss of the mothering figure. When this happens in the first year of life, the child may react by withdrawing and by failing to thrive, behaviors considered by some theorists to be a form of depression (Engel, 1964). *Signal* or *anticipatory anxiety* is based on the memory of early experiences that had produced anxiety. Repetitions or recollection of the early experiences reactivate feelings of anxiety. Freud believed that anxiety is generally useful because it calls into play defenses that help control irrational impulses and reactions (Brenner, 1955).

DEFENSE MECHANISMS Freud considered the ego to be a defensive structure that mediates between the excessive demands of the id and the excessive restrictions of the superego. It was Freud's daughter, Anna (1953), who formulated a comprehensive list of *defense mechanisms* employed by the ego. Anna Freud contended that everyone uses a variety of defenses, some of which are more functional than others. The major defense mechanisms she identified are as follows:

1. *Repression*, the central defense mechanism, is the inability to remember material that is unacceptable to the individual. By means of repression, ideas, impulses, and affects pass out of conscious awareness. For example, the individual who

cannot acknowledge hostile feelings toward an old friend may "forget" the friend's name.

2. *Displacement* is the transferral of emotion from one target to another. The man who is angry with his employer but does not want to lose his job may displace his anger by yelling at family members.

3. *Reaction formation* is the transformation of unacceptable impulse into opposite behavior. For example, hostile feelings toward someone may be expressed by behaviors that are excessively kind and loving.

4. *Isolation* is the separation of an idea from the emotion surrounding it. The idea itself may or may not be forgotten, but the accompanying emotion always is. Thus, a college freshman may ignore feelings of homesickness even though she often has thoughts of returning home.

5. *Undoing* is an effort to cancel out certain actions, real or imaginary. Undoing may be accomplished through apologies, atonement, or ceremonies and rituals. An adolescent who engages in masturbation may try to undo the behavior by repeated, ritualistic handwashing, for example.

6. *Rationalization* is the formation of reasonable explanations, which may or may not be valid, for certain events or behaviors. Rationalization is used to conceal one's real motives or shortcomings from oneself or from others. An example is the alcoholic who says that he needs to drink in order to "wind down" from daily pressures.

7. *Intellectualization* is similar to rationalization and involves the use of intellectual processes to avoid emotional expression. An incompatible couple may use intellectualization to avoid discussing their actual feelings about each other.

8. *Denial* is a partial or complete rejection of something. That is, one may deny a total experience or only the emotion that accompanies the experience. Denial is quite common and may be adaptive or maladaptive, depending on the circumstances. Dealing with loss often begins by denying the reality of the loss.

9. *Projection* is a mechanism by which individuals attribute their own feelings and desires to others. Thus, a student with hostile feelings toward a certain instructor may assume that the instructor is in fact hostile toward her.

10. *Regression* enables people to return to an earlier stage of functioning in order to avoid the tension and demands of a later stage. The five-year-old whose world is invaded by a new sibling may, for example, return to the oral or anal stage, where gratification was assured.

11. *Introjection* is the eradication of distinctions between the individual and an early love object.

When all the characteristics of a love object are internalized, the sense of being a separate entity is lost. Thus, a child who adopts all the characteristics of a parent may lose his sense of being separate or different from the parent.

12. *Identification* is the imitation or acquisition of certain attributes of a significant person. The son of a famous baseball player who tries to emulate his father is using the mechanism of identification.

13. *Sublimation* is the expression of psychic energy in socially acceptable ways by controlling or delaying instinctual drives. Sublimation of the erotic drive may be seen in the behavior of a childless woman who expresses her mothering capacities by teaching preschool children. Sublimation of the aggressive drive may be seen in the behavior of an adolescent who becomes a competitive and successful athlete.

PSYCHOANALYSIS Freud's theory is the basis of *psychoanalysis*, a treatment whose ambitious goal is the restructuring of personality. Classical psychoanalysis assumes that a great deal of mental activity is outside our conscious awareness, that human beings experience psychological conflicts, and that people tend to continue behaving in familiar ways even if the results produce unhappiness. In psychoanalytic treatment, conflicts of early life are explored so that the client can understand and resolve them. Because of the time and expense required, relatively few people undergo complete psychoanalysis. However, psychoanalytic concepts continue to be important not only within the health professions but in literature, history, social sciences, and the arts (Adams, 1979).

During this early part of his career Freud introduced the concept of *psychic determinism*, which states that all behavior is meaningful even when it seems accidental. At this time, Freud was using hypnosis to eradicate the symptoms of his clients. Inconsistent results obtained with hypnosis caused him to substitute the technique of *free association*, in which clients reconstruct disturbing events they have "forgotten." In free association the psychoanalyst remains silent so as not to interfere with the clients' flow of associated thoughts.

The detachment of the psychoanalyst promotes powerful transferences on the part of the client. *Transference* is a distortion in which the client acts as if the therapist were a significant person from the client's own life. For example, a client might react as if the therapist were a parent or other authority figure from the past. Exploring the transference helps clients bring irrational feelings and conflicts into conscious awareness so that a corrective emotional experience can occur. *Countertransference* occurs when transference is felt by the psychoanalyst toward the client. Countertransference can be dealt with by introspection on the part of the psychoanalyst and by a personal training analysis.

Freud described psychoanalysis as a treatment carried out through an exchange of words:

Words and magic were in the beginning one and the same thing, and even today words retain much of their magic power. By words one of us can give to another the greatest happiness or bring about utter despair; by words the teacher imparts his knowledge to the student; by words the orator sweeps his audience with him and determines its judgments and decisions. Words call forth emotions and are universally the means by which we influence our fellow creatures. Therefore, let us not despise words in psychotherapy . . . (Freud, 1953, p. 22)

Freud admitted the absence of objective data in his work. He was an astute observer, but his clinical experience was limited to persons exhibiting hysterical, obsessive-compulsive, and phobic behavior. Much of his data are intuitive in the sense of not being tested or validated systematically. Freud defended his methods by saying that at least he was present in the clinical sessions he described, which is not true of historians, who recount events that happened outside their own lifetimes. He expected psychoanalysts to undergo personal analysis in order to increase their reliability, and advised them to examine their own reactions and personality traits. This advice is similar to the introspection and self-awareness recommended for all nurses working with clients.

Modern feminists find many of Freud's statements objectionable, particularly his insistence that females should adopt passive behaviors that enable them to replace immature clitoral sexuality with mature vaginal sexuality. Freud stated that active, assertive women were motivated by penis envy, the result of which was to make them resentful of their own womanhood. He believed that women felt inferior to men and were treated accordingly, and he attributed these feelings of inferiority to biology rather than to cultural influences. Although criticism of these views is valid, it should be remembered that Freud was a Victorian, conventional in his own life, who was convinced that the formal city of Vienna was typical of the whole world (Thompson, 1950). A prominent feminist writer wrote that women need to remember that their status has improved only in recent years and remains insecure. In her opinion, the masculine vision of the world still prevails (Janeway, 1983). It would be foolish to reject all Freud's insights and equally foolish to accept them without question. There is no doubt that he was a man of his times and that his view of behavior and of personality development was colored by this.

NURSING IMPLICATIONS OF PSYCHOSEXUAL THEORY Although nurses do not engage in classical psychoanalytic work, many of Freud's concepts are useful to nurses working with clients. The idea that human behavior has purpose and meaning is extremely important in psychiatric nursing. The theories of the conscious, preconscious, and unconscious levels of awareness help explain the underlying dynamics of some behaviors. Freud's descriptions of various forms of anxiety have proved durable, particularly the concepts of separation anxiety and of anaclitic depression generated when the infant is separated from his or her mother in the first year of life. The idea that psychological energy is limited can be validated by clinical observation and personal experience. Depletion of psychological energy as a factor in the onset and course of physical illness has been documented in many clinical and experimental situations. In some respects psychoanalytic theory is narrow and restrictive, but its emphasis on the importance of early childhood experiences cannot be entirely discounted.

Psychosocial Theory

Erik Erikson (1963) developed a *psychosocial* theory of personality development in which he stressed external as well as internal influences. He suggested that a triad of forces shapes personality development: constitutional factors, psychological factors, and social factors. As these three types of factors converge on an individual, a period of ascendance or urgency occurs during which essential life tasks must be accomplished.

Erikson divided the life cycle into eight successive stages, all of which have their own critical task. Each of the eight stages contains two opposing poles representing success or failure in accomplishing the critical task (see Table 2-3). If tasks are not completed at the appointed time, they may never be fully resolved. Furthermore, faulty resolution of

31

Table 2-3. Stages and Critical Tasks of Erikson's Psychosocial Framework

Stage	Task
Oral-sensory (Birth to 1 year)	Trust versus mistrust
Muscular-anal (1 to 3 years)	Autonomy versus shame and doubt
Locomotor-genital (3 to 6 years)	Initiative versus guilt
Latency (6 to 11 years)	Industry versus inferiority
Puberty and adolescence (11 to 19 years)	Ego identity versus role confusion
Young adulthood	Intimacy versus isolation
Adulthood	Generativity versus stagnation
Old age	Ego integrity versus despair

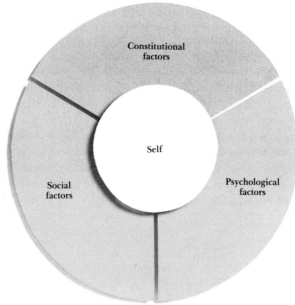

Defensive Ego Functioning (Freud)

Id

Ego

Unacceptable
(ego-dystonic)
thoughts and
feelings

Acceptable
(ego-syntonic)
thoughts and
feelings

Ego ideal

Superego

The ego mediates instinctual drives of the id and
the imposed restrictions of the superego

Integrative Ego Functioning (Erikson)

Constitutional
factors

Self

Social
factors

Psychological
factors

The ego is the integrating aspect of the self and
maintains balance between social, psychological, and constitutional
influences on the self

Figure 2-3. Comparison of ego functioning in Freud's and Erikson's theories.

early tasks endangers the resolution of later ones. The bipolar aspect of Erikson's framework helps explain the progressive (positive) and regressive (negative) trends in the recurrent behaviors of many individuals.

In Erikson's view, society alternately grants and witholds, thus giving children messages out of which they must build *ego strength*. The ego is seen as an integrator of multiple factors operating throughout the life cycle. Figure 2-3 compares the ego functions presented by Freud with those described by Erikson.

ERIKSON'S DEVELOPMENTAL STAGES Erikson's stages extend through the complete life cycle, from birth to old age.

Trust versus Mistrust. In the first months of life, the interaction between infant and mother is crucial. From this interaction the infant develops a sense of trust that basic needs will be gratified. If needs are frustrated more often than gratified, the infant will be disappointed and basic trust will not be established. During the second six months of life, the infant adds biting to its initial sucking activities. In psychoanalytic terms, dual drives are operating: erotic (sucking) and aggressive (biting) (Abraham, 1953). Gradually, the infant realizes the separateness of himself from his mother, and if early experiences have been positive, he has developed a reservoir of trust and hopefulness from which to draw.

Autonomy versus Shame and Doubt. As children learn to walk, talk, and control excretory processes, they are given a choice between holding on and letting

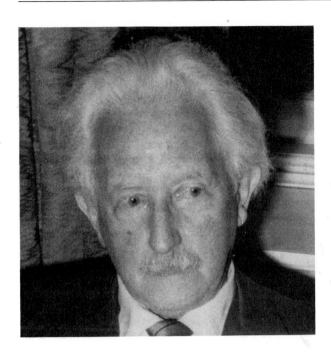

Erik Erikson.

33

go. According to Erikson, the period of toilet training is one of madness and mystery for the child and he warns against excessive parental expectations. If toilet training is not accompanied by shaming tactics, and if parenting is consistent and moderate, the child gains confidence and takes pleasure in autonomous actions. Children subjected to excessive control, on the other hand, become prone to self-doubt.

Initiative versus Guilt. The child's growing initiative may produce conflict between her desires and her parents' restrictions. Gradually, she accepts parental values, identifies with them, and eventually internalizes them. However, a compromise is necessary so that the child is protected from risk but is permitted experimentation and innovation. Otherwise, her capacity for initiative is impaired and she may experience guilt. The accompanying box contrasts the shame of the previous period with the guilt that can occur at this stage.

Industry versus Inferiority. At this point the child can become confident of the ability to work productively, or, losing confidence, can sacrifice industriousness. The child who feels inferior becomes afraid of tasks and enterprises and is reluctant to try. In addition, as the child's world expands, it becomes necessary to reconcile parental values with those of the outside world.

Ego Identity versus Role Confusion. During the teen years, the child is less inclined to accept the guidance of parents and is greatly influenced by peers. Confusion and indecision may be concealed by a facade of rebelliousness. Erikson was sym-

---

EXPERIENTIAL STATES OF SHAME AND GUILT

Shame

Early experiential state, occurring first at about two years of age during the toilet-training period and before the superego begins to emerge.

Transitory state resulting from being discovered as incompetent and perceived by others as unworthy.

Based on external reality.

Ashamed individuals try to overcome their feelings through acts of aggression.

Often results in angry, hostile behaviors.

Represents conflict between the ego and the ego ideal.

Guilt

Later experiential state occurring first between five and six years of age, when the Oedipal conflict is enacted and the superego begins to develop.

Durable or persistent state resulting from failure to live up to internalized values; failures and transgressions may be known only to the self.

Based on internal principles.

Guilty individuals try to atone for their behavior or thoughts through suffering or punishment.

Often results in passive, repentent behaviors.

Represents conflict between the ego and the superego.

pathetic toward the dilemma of adolescence and called these years a "moratorium" between parental values that were once accepted by the child and a new adult code of ethics not yet determined.

Intimacy versus Isolation. A meaningful relationship with another person is needed in order to avoid the egocentricity or self-centeredness that is fostered by social isolation. In genuine intimacy there is giving as well as taking. Ideally, love and sexuality are not isolated from each other but rather are fundamental to establishing reciprocal adult relationships.

Generativity versus Stagnation. Generativity refers not to procreation but to constructive activities performed for the betterment of society. Stagnation results when middle-aged adults become self-engrossed, living only for their own pleasure and comfort. In Erikson's view, preoccupation with self is detrimental to society and to the individual.

Ego Integrity versus Despair. As people grow old, they must come to terms with their own mortality. The idea of death—their own and that of loved ones—brings despair unless they can achieve a sense of purpose and acceptance of their own place in the progression of generations. A backward look at one's own life and accomplishments can promote ego integrity if the retrospective view is positive. However, if retrospection focuses on failures and disappointments in life, the result is despair.

NURSING IMPLICATIONS OF PSYCHOSOCIAL THEORY Erikson's work has been extremely influential in nursing education, practice, and research. The comprehensive life cycle approach, the focus on converging constitutional, social, and psychological forces in development, and the idea of a period of ascendance or urgency for accomplishing critical tasks all provide a holistic view of humankind. Application of psychosocial formulations is appropriate in primary, secondary, and tertiary prevention and helps promote a biopsychosocial approach to health care.

INTERPERSONAL FRAMEWORK

Harry Stack Sullivan (1892–1949) disagreed with the psychoanalytic view that mental disturbance lies within the individual. He believed instead that interpersonal and environmental conditions are the source of emotional difficulties. Sullivan called his work a theory of *interpersonal relationships* because of the vast influence of such relationships on personality development. He admitted that individual differences exist among people but insisted that

everyone shares attributes and experiences that are uniquely human. According to Sullivan, all human beings are guided by two goals: the pursuit of satisfaction and the pursuit of security. The goal of satisfaction is biological, whereas the goal of security is social and cultural.

The notion that we are all uniquely human, called the *one genus postulate,* is central to interpersonal theory. Because of this common humanity, Sullivan objected to professionals who consider themselves superior to or even different from clients. He claimed that many professionals do things *to* clients and do not try to be in touch *with* clients. In his opinion, the restoration of self-respect and self-esteem should be the objective of all health care (Sullivan, 1953).

Self System

According to Sullivan, the sense of self, or *self system,* begins to evolve during the first year of life as a consequence of interpersonal experiences between child and mother. Everyone is born with the need for self-esteem, and self-esteem is an outgrowth of the emerging self system. Personality evolves from the interaction between interpersonal relationships and defensive operations that the individual uses to reduce anxiety and maintain self-esteem.

As a result of early interaction, the self system acquires three main components: the "good me," the "bad me," and the "non-me" (see Table 2-4). Sullivan used the word "mother" in describing the early interactions of infants, but the mothering person might not be the biological parent or even female. It is the primary nurturer of the child. A mother who is warm and nurturing gives her child a feeling of acceptance so that he experiences the self as the "good me." A tense, rejecting mother gives her child a feeling of being a "bad me." When there are few affectionate gestures from the mother, the child perceives the self as more bad than good; good self-appraisals are lost and bad self-appraisals dominate. When the mother uses forbidding or disapproving gestures against certain activities of the child, such as thumbsucking or genital exploration, the effect is

Table 2-4. Components of Sullivan's Self System

Component	Description
Good me	Self-personification of experiences in which the child received nurture and tenderness.
Bad me	Self-personification of experiences in which the child failed to receive nurture and tenderness.
Non-me	Self-personification of experiences in which the child experienced excessive anxiety due to disapproving emotions transmitted by the mother.

to separate or dissociate the genital and oral regions from the child's sense of what is good and acceptable. Sometimes a child will isolate or separate these forbidden regions and behaviors, disown them, and make them part of the "non-me" aspect of the self system.

Sullivan described an undesirable process called *malevolent transformation* in which a child who feels "bad" sees badness in everyone else. Because the child is so aware of being bad, the only way for him to feel human like everyone else is to search for the worst in others. In this, the child is rarely disappointed; the result is that he believes the world is full of enemies. This line of reasoning helps explain suspiciousness and paranoid thinking as outcomes of low self-esteem. Another implication of this theory is that self-love and self-respect are necessary if one is to be able to love and respect others.

Communication between mother and child occurs through a process called *empathy*, which allows one person to understand and identify with the feelings of another. When the mother feels anxiety, it is transmitted by empathy to the child. Thus, for Sullivan, feelings of anxiety arise out of dependency on others for security. Generated first in the interaction between mother and child, anxiety becomes part of every subsequent interpersonal transaction and is the primary cause of problematic relationships and difficulties in living.

Modes of Experience

Sullivan's conceptualization of *experience* included the inner meaning of everything people live through or undergo. He described three distinct modes of experience: prototaxic, parataxic, and syntaxic.

The *prototaxic* mode of experience is that known to the very young infant. It is a continuous flow with no differentiation; there are no connections, no causes or effects, and there is no awareness of self as distinct from others. The separate world does not exist; the infant is the entire world.

The *parataxic* mode of experience is broken, but the fragments are unconnected and unrelated. Parataxic experience belongs only to the person involved in it, and its uniqueness cannot be shared with others. Older infants, many children, and some creative people engage in parataxic experience. At times of acute mental disturbance the subjective experience of a client may become a parataxic distortion. The transference that can develop in psychoanalysis and in everyday life is one example of parataxic distortion.

Syntaxic experience can be validated consensually by means of language and symbols. In syntaxic experience, meanings and principles can be shared with others and can be accepted by others as true or untrue based on common understanding. In general, syntaxic experience is accepted as valid by a group (Sullivan, 1953).

Elaboration of the three modes of experience led Sullivan to describe several strategies people use to handle interpersonal transactions. *Consensual validation* is an efficient strategy that involves measuring one's perceptions against the perceptions of others in order to reduce any distortions. *Selective inattention* is the screening out of anxiety-provoking content so that it can be overlooked or forgotten. Thus, selective inattention actually operates to *prevent* consensual validation of perceptions and interpretations. Persons denying the significance of a serious illness often resort to the anxiety-reducing technique of selective inattention. *Focal awareness* is a means by which people see and hear what they want to and emphasize content that is reassuring. The parents of developmentally impaired children will often use focal awareness and direct all their attention to small signs of progress, thereby fostering unrealistic hopes (Griffin, 1980).

Like Freud and Erikson, Sullivan described a developmental progression of stages (see Table 2-5). The first period, *infancy*, lasts from birth to one and a half years and is characterized by the dominant influence of the mother. During this period experience is prototaxic. The infant can rarely be "spoiled," as mothers sometimes fear, since the idea of cause and effect has not yet evolved. *Childhood* lasts from the end of infancy until the time

35

Table 2-5. Stages and Tasks of Sullivan's Interpersonal Framework

Period	Age	Characteristics
Infancy	Birth to 1½ years	Dominant maternal influence
Childhood	1½ to 6 years	Increasing peer influence
Juvenile	6 to 9 years	Gradual movement into the world
Preadolescent	9 years to puberty	Decreasing egocentricity; increasing socialization
Early adolescence	12 to 14 years	Increasing independence, interest in opposite sex
Late adolescence	15 to 21 years	Increasing sexuality; increasing intimacy

SOURCE: Adapted from Sullivan (1953).

*I want to stress from the very beginning the paralyzing power of anxiety.
I believe that it is fairly safe to say that anybody and everybody devotes
much of his lifetime, a great deal of his energy . . . and a good part of his
effort in dealing with others, to avoiding more anxiety than he already
has and, if possible, to getting rid of this anxiety. Many things which seem
to be independent entities, processes, or whatnot, are . . . various
techniques for minimizing or avoiding anxiety in living.*

HARRY STACK SULLIVAN (1953)

36

when the child begins to cooperate with peers. This period, from age one and a half to six, is marked by clashes between the wishes of the child and those of the parents. Consistent limit setting is necessary if the child is to have a realistic perception of the world. The *juvenile* period, which lasts from age six to nine, sees the child move further from the home into the world. *Preadolescence*, which lasts from age nine to puberty, introduces movement from what is termed egocentricity toward a more socialized orientation. In the preadolescent period, peer influence is important, and having a best friend reinforces the effect of interpersonal experiences on personality development.

Adolescence is divided into early and later stages. *Early adolescence* lasts from age twelve to fourteen and is usually characterized by growing independence and interest in the opposite sex. *Late adolescence* lasts from fifteen to twenty-one years of age and is a time in which sexuality is enriched by establishing a lasting, satisfying intimacy. In discussing sexuality Sullivan expressed concern that the biological sexuality of young people was inhibited by social factors that discouraged sexual expression—a concern that may be less true now than it was in his day.

Nursing Implications of Sullivan's Theory

Sullivan devoted a great deal of attention to specific therapeutic techniques, for he considered himself primarily a clinician. He objected to remote, authoritarian attitudes on the part of professionals and preferred the role of participant-observer. Moreover, he thought that clients should be helped to understand just how their problems developed. He

extended kindness and acceptance to clients, allowing them to sit, stand, or walk as they chose during therapeutic sessions. When anxious clients were distracted from the topic at hand, Sullivan was not reluctant to reintroduce pertinent issues. He termed these digressions by anxious clients "substitute systems of thought" and considered them to be security operations (Thompson, 1950). The purpose of security operations such as digressions is to reduce anxiety.

Unlike Freud, who believed that only neurotic clients could be helped by techniques of psychoanalysis, Sullivan was willing to work with clients who were psychotic or out of touch with reality. He defined "cure" as the gradual realization by clients of the nature of their problems in interpersonal relationships.

Sullivan's interpersonal framework has been used as a basis for building nursing theory. Peplau (1952) described nursing as an interpersonal process that has as its chief purpose promoting the health of individuals and communities. In her view, conflict and anxiety cause tension that results in either actions to confront and solve the problem or actions to avoid the problem. Along with Sullivan, Peplau believed that anxiety is nonspecific and that security represents freedom from anxiety. Because one of the most compelling human desires is to be anxiety free, a great deal of human behavior is directed toward reaching this goal. In addition to defining anxiety operationally, Peplau expanded and refined this concept. She developed a paradigm showing the effects and manifestations of anxiety and suggested appropriate nursing responses (see Table 2-6). Her work in this area constitutes a major contribution to nursing theory.

Table 2-6. Effect of Anxiety on Perception and Behavior

Levels of Anxiety	Perception	Behaviors	Nursing Interventions
Mild anxiety	Sounds seem louder; irritability increases; restlessness increases; energy increases	Alertness increases; vigilance increases	1. Observe what is occurring. 2. Describe what is occurring. 3. Compare what was expected with what actually occurred. 4. Validate impressions with others. 5. Determine whether the situation or expectations can be changed.
Moderate anxiety	Concentration decreases; communication decreases; perception decreases; tension increases; somatic discomforts (sweating, rapid pulse, etc.) occur	Visual and auditory attention to details decreases; selective inattention occurs	1. Recognize that attention is decreased. 2. Recognize that meanings and connections may be lost. 3. Try to identify precipitators or causes. 4. Try to reduce anxiety to mild levels.
Severe anxiety	Feelings of dread, awe, loathing arise; emotional discomfort increases; physical discomfort increases	Details and occurrences are incomprehensible; focal awareness increases distortion	1. Encourage severely anxious people to talk to a willing listener. 2. Encourage severely anxious people to work at a simple task. 3. Provide opportunity for motor activities such as walking, games, etc. 4. Permit emotional outlet of tears.
Panic	Details and occurrences are distorted by being exaggerated or overlooked	Rational communication and behavior is lost; fight/flight actions occur; herd instincts prevail	1. Provide structure and firm direction—people in panic obey a strong leader. 2. Increase safety and comfort by taking charge of the situation.

SOURCE: Adapted from Sullivan (1953) and Peplau (1952).

SOCIOLOGICAL FRAMEWORK

The sociological framework deals with the relationships of individuals and families to social institutions and to society at large. A number of theorists from the health professions and the social sciences agree that the self emerges through social interaction taking place within the individual's social milieu. Sociological theory acknowledges the contradictory norms and values that exist in society and the confusion that these contradictions sometimes create.

Social Institutions

A major focus of sociological theories is social institutions. Such institutions exhibit both manifest and latent functions that often exist side by side. *Manifest functions* include all the acknowledged and obvious reasons for the existence of an institution; *latent functions* include the unacknowledged and hidden reasons for its existence. For example, state mental hospitals have the manifest function of pro-

viding care for persons suffering a mental disorder. However, their latent function may be to isolate clients and permit society at large to ignore their existence as much as possible (Clausen, 1980). The express purpose of psychiatric facilities—to care for clients—is often incompatible with its unacknowledged purpose, which is to label and segregate clients. This chasm between express purpose and unacknowledged purpose has been widened by the subordinate positions in which psychiatric clients are placed. Sociologists have been highly critical of this situation, with many citing the degrading practices sometimes imposed on psychiatric clients by care providers (Goffman, 1961).

Symbolic Interactionism

An important sociological perspective from which to explain the behavior of individuals in a society is *symbolic interactionism* (Mead, 1933; Blumer, 1969). The focus of this perspective is *socialization*, which is considered a process of interpreting and responding to social meanings (the intentions underlying the acts of others). Social organization and social meanings are culturally determined. Every individual analyzes others' intentions and responds on the basis of these analyses. It is therefore important to understand the behavior of others in order to guide one's own responses. Social stability depends on accurate analysis of the behavior of other people and on the capacity to regulate one's own behavior.

The enactment of social roles always requires the participation of more than one person. One can only be a mother if one has children; one can only be a teacher if one has students. Small children see themselves as different people depending on what role they are enacting. The same child may well be the oldest child at home but the smallest child in the classroom, and behave accordingly. Group attitudes greatly determine what role the child enacts, and role enactment helps children integrate all the diverse aspects of selfhood.

Integration of self results from the way others appraise and evaluate us. The term *reference group* is applied to groups whose standards are used to evaluate some aspects of ourselves (Mead, 1933). Our college or university, profession, or religious denomination may function as a reference group. The term *generalized other* has been used to describe group attitudes; our internalized social attitudes are derived from generalized others. It is our internalized attitudes regarding the meaning of events that establish our social environment and influence how we behave.

Social Roles

Role theory is indebted to Talcott Parsons (1951) for describing attributes and expectations attached to the *sick role*. Enactment of the sick role entails privileges and obligations. When persons assume the sick role, they are exempted from certain duties and allowed certain rights. They have the right to receive care, but they also have an obligation to accept help, to cooperate, and to try to recover. Clients with some types of disorders, such as substance abuse, may be rejected by care providers because they do not fully accept sick role obligations. Many persons with mental disorders seem to defy customary enactment of the sick role. As a result, their motivation to seek help, to follow a treatment regimen, and to try to recover is questioned by relatives, friends, and health professionals.

Social Stratification

Social class differences can have a significant impact on childrearing practices and therefore on individual personality development. For example,

many working-class parents emphasize external standards and encourage conformity, whereas middle-class parents are more likely to stress internal standards and to encourage individuality (Scheinfeld, 1983). In middle-class families, praise and encouragement are more generously bestowed, fathers are more involved in childrearing, and less authoritarian measures are used (Miller and Janosik, 1980). Lower-class children may suffer reality shock early in life as they move from disadvantaged homes into schools and communities, whereas middle-class children are less likely to find a great discrepancy between standards inside and outside the home, so for them adjustment is usually less difficult.

Deviant behavior and society's reaction to it are also influenced by social class. Lower-class status increases the likelihood of being sent to prison for legal infractions, of being hospitalized for mental disorders, and of being hospitalized for longer periods. Furthermore, the possibility of being diagnosed with a serious psychiatric disorder greatly depends on the person's social status and on his or her support network (Hollingshead and Redlich, 1958).

The well-known Midtown Manhattan investigation found symptoms of mental disorder to be more prevalent in the lower social classes (Srole et al., 1962). Upward and downward social mobility were also found to be related to the prevalence of psychiatric symptoms. That is, individuals whose education and achievements exceeded those of their parents and individuals whose education and achievements did not reach those of their parents were more likely to suffer mental disorders than persons who had attained but not surpassed the status of their parents.

Nursing Implications of Sociological Approaches

The viewpoint of sociologists is that mental disorders result from the interplay of many factors on individuals and families. Therefore, they tend to be distrustful of purely medical approaches. As members of a discipline that concentrates on social issues, they often become involved in examining public policies and public programs related to mental health.

A number of nurse scientists trained at the doctoral level are currently engaged in health-related research that uses sociological and anthropological approaches. Even though social and cultural factors do not fully explain the occurrence and course of mental disturbance, they are essential to a holistic perspective. Nurses who are sensitive to cultural variations, who are interested in community organization, and who hope to influence public

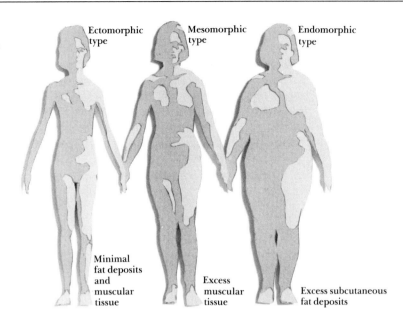

Figure 2-4. Constitutional typology according to Sheldon.

Ectomorphic type

Mesomorphic type

Endomorphic type

Minimal fat deposits and muscular tissue

Excess muscular tissue

Excess subcutaneous fat deposits

39

health policy will incorporate sociological concepts into their enactment of their professional role.

BIOGENIC FRAMEWORK

Biogenic approaches are those that emphasize the role of biological factors in mental disorders. They look to constitutional, genetic, and chemical factors in an effort to explain the causes of psychological difficulties.

Constitutional Factors

In the late nineteenth century, the prevailing view was that mental disorders could be explained on the basis of physiological imbalance. As a result, physicians and others with a medical orientation dominated psychiatric treatment and research. The work of Emil Kraepelin (1856–1926) in describing and classifying mental disorders did much to reinforce biological explanations of mental disturbance. In a classic textbook published in 1883 and revised many times thereafter, Kraepelin classified mental disorders according to symptomatology. For example, he observed the return to normalcy of persons suffering episodes of manic-depressive illness (bipolar affective disorder in DSM-III), contrasted this with the chronic deterioration of persons suffering from dementia praecox (schizophrenic disorders in DSM-III) and considered the latter group to have a less hopeful prognosis.

About this time attempts were made to correlate physical endowment with personality traits and with predisposition to mental disorders. William Sheldon developed a constitutional typol-ogy that classified people according to three main body types: ectomorphs, endomorphs, and meso-morphs (see Figure 2-4). Not only was each body type associated with particular personality traits, but ectomorphs were assumed to be more susceptible to schizophrenic disorders, and endomorphs were assumed to be more susceptible to manic-depressive episodes (Freedman, Kaplan, and Sadock, 1973). Mesomorphs were seen as the least susceptible to mental disorders of all types.

Genetic Factors

Another biogenic approach has been to focus on the role of genetic factors in mental disorders. Kallmann (1953, 1962) found the concordance rate (a measure of correlation) for schizophrenia to be 14.7 percent for nonidentical twins, 14.3 percent for full siblings, 7.1 percent for half-siblings, and a whopping 85.8 percent for identical twins. Even when identical twins were reared apart, the schizophrenia concordance rates remained significantly high. Other studies of schizophrenia have produced similar results (Cohen et al., 1972; Gottesman and Shields, 1972).

These findings indicate that some mental disorders are familial, even though data pointing specifically to heredity are inconclusive. Heredity and environment are influences that moderate or intensify each other. Genetic predisposition can be altered by life experiences, and inherited tendencies can modify environmental factors. The nature versus nurture controversy has yet to be resolved to everyone's satisfaction. At best one can state that heredity and environment are interactive influences on physical and mental well-being.

Implicit in much of the current research . . . is the hypothesis that disturbances in periodic processes . . . may not be apparent at the surface level of clinical description and observation, and that measurement and elucidation of such latent periodic processes may be crucial. The rationale for the hypothesis is the observation that virtually every physiological process, when studied with repeated measurements of sufficient accuracy over time, has demonstrated a 24 hour periodicity. It is inconceivable that human behavior could be totally independent of these pervasive rhythmic fluctuations.

CHARLES F. STROEBEL (1980)

Chemical Imbalance

Neurochemical imbalance is suspected as a factor in some mental disorders. Kety (1959), for example, showed that schizophrenia may result from defective transmethylation, the molecular transformation of one catecholamine to another. There are three major catecholamines that serve as neurotransmitters in the body: dopamine, serotonin, and norepinephrine. In persons with schizophrenia, transmethylation of catecholamines produces a hallucinogenic, mescalinelike substance that is detectible in the urine. Furthermore, the antipsychotic (neuroleptic) drugs used to treat schizophrenia block central nervous system dopamine receptors—an action that helps explain the Parkinsonian symptoms that are frequent side effects of these drugs. Research on neurochemical imbalance as a factor in schizophrenia is promising, but the results are not yet definitive (Morgan and Morgan, 1980).

Research on neurochemical imbalance as a causative factor in affective or mood disorders has been more conclusive. Depressive states have been correlated with deficits of neurotransmitters, especially norepinephrine, while manic or elated states have been correlated with excesses of norepinephrine. It is possible that alterations in catecholamine metabolism may be partly responsible for some of the drastic mood swings of adolescents, of women experiencing menopause, and of elderly people, but this has not been substantiated as yet. In these stressful periods of the life cycle, many individuals experience strong feelings of depression or elation that could be related to natural chemical changes occurring in the body. It must be acknowledged that

this is a rather simplistic explanation considering the complex processes involved, and much additional research on neurochemical imbalances remains to be done.

Biological Rhythms

"Biorhythms," which supposedly predict an individual's good and bad days on the basis of cycles computed from date of birth, are of dubious value, in spite of the popular attention they have received. The cyclical changes of *chronobiology* are another matter. Every process and system in the body, including blood cell levels, blood pressure, hormone levels, body temperature, heartbeat, renal function, and sleep, has its own rhythm that fluctuates regularly within intervals of a second, minute, day, week, month, or year. An excellent example is the monthly menstrual cycle of women that begins at menarche and ends at menopause. Cycles that occur more often, on a daily, or *circadian*, rhythm are shown in Figure 2-5.

Reputabl studies indicate that biological rhythms can profoundly affect physical and psychological well-being. Studies performed at the University of Minnesota, for example, raise questions about the optimal timing of diagnostic and treatment procedures, traditional methods for arranging shift rotations, and the usual sleeping and eating patterns of the general population. Usually practical considerations such as convenience outweigh attention to biological cycles in such matters. According to investigators of chronobiology, ignorance of biological rhythms is detrimental because "working with the body's rhythms

Figure 2-5. Biological rhythms. Many aspects of human physiology show clear-cut circadian cycles, changing regularly over each 24-hour period. Some of the more important ones are shown here.

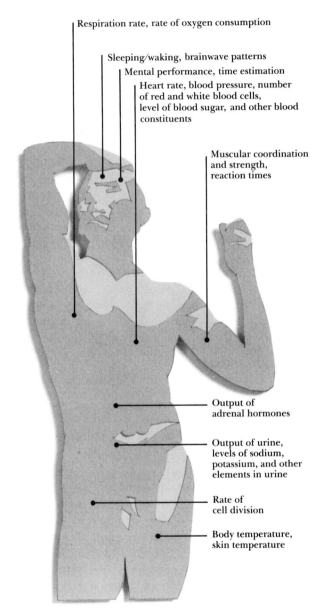

Respiration rate, rate of oxygen consumption

Sleeping/waking, brainwave patterns

Mental performance, time estimation

Heart rate, blood pressure, number of red and white blood cells, level of blood sugar, and other blood constituents

Muscular coordination and strength, reaction times

Output of adrenal hormones

Output of urine, levels of sodium, potassium, and other elements in urine

Rate of cell division

Body temperature, skin temperature

can tip the scale between health and disease, even between survival and death" (Brody, 1981).

Studies of biological rhythms challenge the concept of homeostasis, which assumes that internal physiological conditions remain constant and that any fluctuations are insignificant and self-correcting. Chronobiological studies show that white blood cell counts may vary by as much as 50 percent in a day, blood hormones by 80 percent, and blood pressure by 20 percent. Figure 2-6 shows the peak times of various daily biological rhythms. Changes are determined by a part of the brain called the

suprachiasmatic nucleus, which responds to eating and sleeping changes, travel across time zones, exposure to light and darkness, and incipient illness. Once disturbed, biological rhythms require significant amounts of time to readjust (Stroebel, 1980).

Documented fluctuations in the efficiency of mind and body may be an avenue of research that increases understanding of the etiology of some mental disorders, especially those that are episodic or cyclical. In addition, psychotherapeutic measures and physiological interventions might be employed at times and in ways that increase their range and effectiveness. For example, chronobiology is being used to improve the results of drug and radiation therapy. It has been found that, depending on when an anticancer drug is administered, animals may be relieved of symptoms or may succumb to the side effects of the drug. Similarly, the same amount of alcohol administered to animals may have minimal or drastic effects, depending on the time of day. In a study of radiation therapy used to alleviate malignant tumors of the head and neck, the radiation was found to be more effective when given at times when the internal temperature of the tumors peaked (Brody, 1981).

Chronobiology is also being used to monitor a range of human functions, including blood pressure, pulse, muscle strength, motor coordination, mental skills, energy, and mood, in order to plot characteristic patterns for each individual. Because every individual pattern is unique, deviations may provide guidance in preventing, detecting, or alleviating maladaptive internal conditions. A number of economical procedures have been devised for recording an individual's many biological rhythms.

Figure 2-6. Chronobiological rhythms: peak circadian times. (Curves are idealized).

42

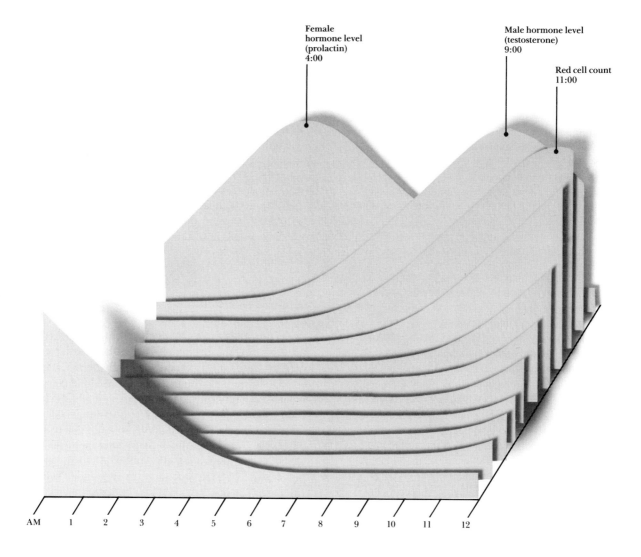

Female hormone level (prolactin) 4:00

Male hormone level (testosterone) 9:00

Red cell count 11:00

AM   1   2   3   4   5   6   7   8   9   10   11   12

One is autorhythmometry, a technique in which individuals are taught to record their own blood pressure, temperature, pulse, grip strength, and mood by means of ratings that can then be computerized. Another technique is the psychophysiological diary, which enables individuals to record quantitative information about physiological processes and about subjective experiences such as mood, hunger, and satiation. When such information is computerized, it becomes possible to detect individual changes in patterns of living and functioning and to make comparisons within and between groups.

Chronobiologic techniques have a number of nursing applications. At the Institute for Living in Hartford, Connecticut, computerized recording of psychiatric nursing observations has been instituted (Stroebel, 1980; Stroebel and Glueck, 1978). Eleven

areas of client behavior are rated by means of a factor analysis, which avoids having the recorders make interpretations. Self-reports of physiological and psychological conditions are also obtained from the clients themselves. Of special interest are the relationships that have been noted between mood, behavior, and biological rhythms. In an analysis of data for 2,400 psychiatric clients, each of whom was observed for a period of three to four weeks, abnormal biological rhythms were found in 30 percent of the subjects. Clinical improvement in the subjects was accompanied by biological rhythms that more closely approached normal.

Chronobiology is a relatively new field of investigation that may provide useful insights in health care. It can serve as a predictive tool as well as a method for collecting current data. Thus, chronobiology has potential as a form of primary preven-

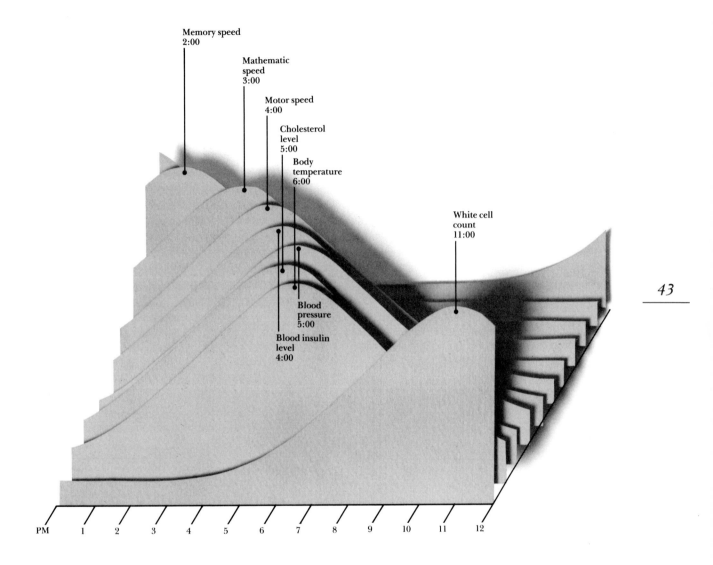

Memory speed
2:00

Mathematic
speed
3:00

Motor speed
4:00

Cholesterol
level
5:00

Body
temperature
6:00

White cell
count
11:00

Blood
pressure
5:00

Blood insulin
level
4:00

PM   1   2   3   4   5   6   7   8   9   10   11   12

tion, in that it can be used to avoid maladaptive alterations in persons whose biological rhythms show unusual fluctuations.

Nursing Implications of Biogenic Approaches

As might be expected, proponents of the biogenic framework favor somatic forms of treatment, which include chemotherapy, psychosurgery, and shock therapy induced by insulin or electrical current. Some clients have been helped by such treatments, while others have been hurt by somatic treatments that are popular for a time and later discarded. Treatments that alter moods, thoughts, and behaviors continue to be used despite the fact that the underlying reasons for their effects are largely unknown. The biological causes of mental disorders remain a matter for conjecture and study, and understanding of how and why somatic treatments

work awaits further investigation. Because somatic intervention demands the skills of knowledgeable, competent nurses, this approach in some respects enhances the role of the psychiatric nurse. In other respects, however, a reliance on somatic measures restricts the scope of nursing intervention.

A significant effect of the biogenic framework is its tendency to reduce the stigmatization that many psychiatric clients endure. If mental disorders are considered the result of physiological dysfunction, the client is less likely to be blamed for her symptoms. The other side of the coin, however, is that biogenic explanations also tend to reduce the client's responsibility for changing maladaptive behavior. Furthermore, adherence to such a medical model changes the focus of care, making clients passive recipients of treatment rather than active participants in their own recovery. Another

44

drawback to the biogenic approach is that it increases distances between clients and care providers. Interventions take the form of procedures done *to* the client rather than *with* the client and reinforce the medical model.

The medical model also helps perpetuate the position of the physician as director of the therapeutic program, making health care teams hierarchical rather than egalitarian and multidisciplinary rather than interdisciplinary. A physician is usually in charge of the health team, with members working according to the traditional scope of their respective disciplines. As a consequence, the dependent functions of psychiatric nurses are likely to be emphasized, while their independent nursing functions are given less opportunity for expression. Psychotherapeutic interactions between clients and nurses may then become secondary to administrative and managerial responsibilities. In a study of four health care teams, each composed of a physician, two nurses, and a dietitian, investigators found that although the physicians enjoyed dominant status in all cases, the team that produced the most successful outcomes for clients scored highest on "collegiality" between members. Interactions on the most successful team were characterized by mutual sharing of information and opinions (Schmitt, 1982).

In general, the medical model tends to use a specific problem-solving rather than a holistic approach to care. However, the model has provided some benefits to nursing in that many somatic measures that are part of the medical model require careful monitoring by professional nurses who must observe, explain, teach, and reassure clients undergoing such treatment.

OTHER FRAMEWORKS

A number of other frameworks are also used in explaining human behavior. Among them are the existential and cognitive approaches.

Existential Framework

Existential theory is relatively unstructured. Its basic premise is that individuals do not exist separately in the world; rather, the world exists only because there are people to experience it. Behavior is not merely the result of external forces acting on the individual but is a complicated response to the individual's interpretation of external events (Gendlin, 1968). Individual existence is not predetermined, nor is it instinctual or biologic; instead, it depends entirely on the daily choices the person makes. Self-determination lies within the grasp of everyone.

Marram (1978) outlined the following existential beliefs:

1. Every individual has the freedom to reach maximum potential.

2. Recognition of immediate reality increases and enhances the potential for change.

3. For an individual to resolve problems it is necessary only to know what they are and not why they exist.

The fundamental problem facing individuals is to determine whether their existence is authentic (based on truth) or inauthentic (based on deception). According to existential theory, few people

C L I N I C A L   E X A M P L E

THEORETICAL FRAMEWORKS IN NURSING ASSESSMENT

Edith Bailey was brought to a mental health facility by her husband at the suggestion of a community health nurse who had visited their home. Three months earlier Mrs. Bailey had given birth to a baby boy after a long and difficult labor. She was thirty-two years old and was the mother of another son, Jimmy, age four. Because Mrs. Bailey was uncommunicative, most of the information given to the intake nurse was obtained from her husband, Bob. He reported that after the birth of their first child, Edith had seemed tired and upset but gradually recovered without hospitalization or specific treatment. She seemed to improve steadily as her first child progressed through the toddler years.

The second child had been planned, but Mrs. Bailey had hoped for a daughter and was disappointed when it turned out to be a boy. Upon returning home after the birth, she had seemed silent and withdrawn. She was indifferent about her appearance and seldom bothered to dress or comb her hair. She ate little but slept for long periods of time. When awake, she smoked constantly and ignored the crying of the baby. The older boy was being cared for by his maternal grandmother. Mr. Bailey took time off from work to help his wife and arranged for a community health nurse to visit daily and a housekeeper to come in a few hours a day. Mr. Bailey cared for the baby and did the cooking when he was not at work. In his free moments he visited Jimmy.

During the initial assessment interview, the nurse observed that Mrs. Bailey was oriented as to time, place, and person. However, she appeared apathetic and indifferent to her surroundings. She did not look at her husband or at the nurse but fixed her eyes on the floor. Often she did not seem to hear what was being said to her. When she did respond, her words were hard to understand. Several times she mumbled that she felt bad because she deserved to feel bad.

Mr. Bailey explained that his wife had experienced an unhappy childhood because her father drank too much. The family was poor and Edith had to take care of her younger brothers while her mother worked. Mr. Bailey added that his own childhood had not been a bed of roses. He had married in the hope of enjoying a happy family life, and he felt that he had always been a good provider. Prior to Jimmy's birth, he believed that he and his wife had had a good relationship. Although Edith was distant and aloof after Jimmy's birth, he tried to be understanding. He said that after his wife had "pulled herself together" their relationship was again harmonious. Although concerned about his wife and children, Mr. Bailey was beginning to feel angry about the heavy burden he was assuming. He was particularly worried about the new baby, in whom no one but himself seemed interested.

Based on Mrs. Bailey's behavior and level of functioning, a decision was made to admit her for observation. Since Edith's mother was willing, plans were made for her to care for the new baby as well as for Jimmy, who seemed delighted to welcome his new brother. It was considered important by the health care team for Mr. Bailey to stay in close touch with the children and for Mrs. Bailey to see them as soon as her condition permitted.

Members of the health team used a number of theoretical frameworks in assessing Mrs. Bailey and in trying to understand her behavior. Although the frameworks differed in focus, they yielded few genuine contradictions. In many respects the various frameworks supported and supplemented one another, as can be seen in the following applications.

PSYCHOGENIC FRAMEWORK

Assessment of Mrs. Bailey: (1) regression to early developmental levels, (2) conflict related to dependency needs, (3) repressed aggression, (4) failure to achieve basic trust, and (5) failure to achieve autonomy.

As a child Edith Bailey had taken on many adult responsibilities. Her mother was not unkind, but she had to work hard to support her daughter and three sons. Edith's irresponsible father had left a residue of distrust in her that a successful marriage had failed to overcome. She had enjoyed the childless years of her marriage, and after a period of adjustment she was able to respond warmly to her first little boy. However, the arrival of a second son reactivated her sense of resentment for her lost childhood.

Edith was a woman with strong dependency needs that had never been fully met. As a result she was torn between her wish to be cared for and the current demands being made on her. Consequently, she regressed to an immature level of functioning where her helplessness was apparent to all.

INTERPERSONAL FRAMEWORK

Assessment of Mrs. Bailey: (1) feelings of low self-esteem, (2) excessive interpersonal insecurity, and (3) poorly integrated self system.

Mrs. Bailey's self-esteem depended on being considered loving and good. In childhood she had performed the tasks her mother expected of her and

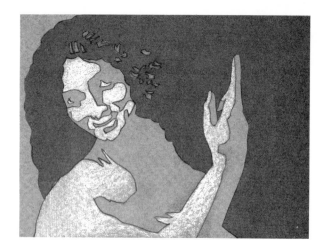

was rewarded by her mother's approval. As a married woman, she had continued to seek approval by doing whatever was asked of her, even if it meant sacrificing her own wishes. At the age of ten she had been expected to cook, clean, and care for her little brothers. After marrying and becoming a parent, she had doubts about having a second child but was reluctant to oppose her husband. When her pregnancy advanced, she began to hope for a baby girl. The birth of a second son disappointed her—looking at the new baby and thinking of her other boy, she was reminded of the constant care that her little brothers had required. Her mood did not improve after she returned home from the hospital. She was irritated by her husband's attentions, and his pride in the new baby annoyed her even more. Unable to break the habits of a lifetime, she did not disclose her feelings to anyone but retreated into a world where no one could intrude.

For years Mrs. Bailey had concealed inner anxiety and insecurity. The self system she had constructed was neither integrated nor realistic. When she asked for something she wanted, she felt like the "bad me." She disclaimed negative emotions and considered herself "good" only when she sacrificed herself for others.

BIOGENIC FRAMEWORK

Assessment of Mrs. Bailey: (1) physical exhaustion, (2) hormonal changes, and (3) possible biochemical imbalance.

Mrs. Bailey suffered from depression following the birth of her second child. A difficult labor and delivery drained her physically and made her dread the demands of running a household and caring for two small children. After the birth of her first child she had experienced similar feelings but had rallied and managed to function fairly well. Because of the two recurrent episodes, it was apparent that the stress of parturition made Mrs. Bailey susceptible to depression. The biological explanation for her depression was physical exhaustion aggravated by postpartal hormonal and biochemical changes and by the stresses of her life situation.

EXISTENTIAL FRAMEWORK

Edith Bailey had spent her life trying to please everyone else and ignoring her own feelings. Trying first to be the perfect daughter and later the perfect wife, she had lost the ability to speak up for herself and state what she truly wanted. She had no confidence in herself and no confidence in anyone else. Her disappointment in her father had caused her to turn inward and to expect little for herself. Although outwardly well adjusted, she based her life on self-sacrifice and self-deception, always concealing her inner resentment. Her relationships with her husband and her mother were essentially dishonest. She pretended to herself and others that she was happy until she eventually became incapable of continuing the pretense. When that point was reached, Edith engaged in extreme withdrawal, abandoning her family just as surely as her father had abandoned her so many years before.

PSYCHIATRIC AND NURSING DIAGNOSES

The following nursing and psychiatric diagnoses were made for Mrs. Bailey:

Nursing Diagnoses
Coping, ineffectual individual
(related to client's indifference to assuming daily tasks and responsibilities)

Home maintenance management, impaired
(related to client's abdication of home management to her husband and her mother)

Parenting, alteration in
(related to neglect of baby and disinterest in the return home of older son)

Self-care deficit
(related to client's neglect of own physical care and an indication of her regression)

Self-concept, disturbance in
(related to impaired role performance as wife and mother that reduced client's self-esteem and jeopardized her sense of identity)

Multiaxial Psychiatric Diagnoses
Axis I   Clinical Syndrome
         296.33 Major depression,
         recurrent, with melancholia

Axis II   Personality Disorders
          301.60 Dependent personality

Axis III Physical Disorders and Conditions
          Postpartum maladjustment

Axis IV Code 5—Severe

Axis V   Level 4—Fair: Moderate impairment of
         function and social relationships before
         birth of second child; Level 5: marked
         impairment in function and social
         relationships after birth of second child

reach their full potential, but anyone who chooses to try can achieve a more authentic existence (Hall and Lindzey, 1970). The search for an authentic existence requires courage, and few people are courageous all the time. Most individuals vacillate between progressing and regressing. For an existentialist, however, regression may not always be detrimental; in fact, it may become a new beginning. For example, an alcoholic who loses his job, his family, and his self-respect may be inspired by desperation to begin again.

Children in particular have great potential unless they are damaged by adverse conditions early in life. Whenever a child is greatly burdened with guilt or anxiety, he or she is likely to become an adult who avoids responsibility and whose life lacks truth or authenticity. But even persons damaged in childhood can be aided by receiving love and acceptance from other people—provided always that they accept responsibility and self-determination.

Existentialism is a humanistic philosophy that respects the potential of people to solve their problems in a manner that enhances their own lives and contributes to society. In reinforcing responsibility and self-determination, humanists oppose rigid beliefs about psychic determinism, asserting that most people have the capacity to grow, to progress, and to break away from the chains of the past, if they so choose.

Existential theory has had an impact on a number of therapeutic modalities, including rational-emotive therapy (Ellis and Harper, 1961), logo therapy (Frankl, 1959), and reality therapy (Glasser, 1965). These treatment approaches differ in detail, but all emphasize personal responsibility and self-determination.

Cognitive Framework

The cognitive framework is based primarily on principles formulated by the Swiss psychologist Jean Piaget (1974). Piaget identified four variables that influence the development of cognitive processes: (1) biological development, (2) interaction with the physical world, (3) interaction with the social world, and (4) integration of new and past experiences as the child proceeds toward maturation.

Piaget traced the cognitive progress of children from the primitive concrete thought of infancy to the mature abstract thinking of adolescence. He saw biological, social, and environmental influences as all playing roles in the emergence of selfhood in children. A more extensive treatment of Piaget's theory is provided in Chapter 14, which deals with the critical tasks and challenges of maturation and development.

SUMMARY

Theoretical frameworks organize knowledge systematically by means of related concepts and constructs. No one framework is all inclusive; each offers a distinct but limited perspective. A number of major frameworks provide insights into biopsychosocial development, adaptation, and maladaptation.

The theories of Freud and Erikson are representative of the psychogenic framework. Freud emphasized psychic determinism, the belief that all behavior is meaningful and purposeful. He described personality as composed of id, ego, and superego and identified three levels of mental awareness: conscious, unconscious, and pre-conscious. A major ego function is reality testing, or the ability to differentiate internal stimuli from external stimuli. Hallucinations and delusions are internal stimuli that are mistakenly thought to be external; they are indicative of failure in reality testing. Freud considered the ego to be a defensive structure that mediates between the demands of the id and the restrictions of the superego. Freud outlined five psychosexual stages of development, each characterized by a conflict to be resolved if development is to progress. His initial work on defense mechanisms was elaborated by his daughter, Anna, who developed a comprehensive list of adaptive and maladaptive defense mechanisms utilized by the ego.

Erikson accepted some of Freud's ideas but modified others. He believed that the ego has an integrative rather than a defensive purpose. He explained that constitutional, psychological, and social factors create a compelling period of urgency during which critical life tasks should be accomplished. Erikson's framework encompasses the entire life cycle, which he divided into eight stages, each of which has its own maturational task.

Sullivan developed the interpersonal framework for explaining personality. He described a self system that evolves as a consequence of interpersonal experiences between mother and child. Everyone engages in interpersonal security operations designed to reduce anxiety. These security operations include selective inattention and focal awareness, both of which allow individuals to overlook information that threatens security. Peplau refined and expanded interpersonal definitions of anxiety and applied them to the nursing process.

Sociologists are interested in the relationships of individuals and families to society. They focus on the effects of such social factors as institutions, socialization, social roles, and stratification. Social institutions may have both manifest and latent functions that justify their existence. Symbolic interactionism explains how our interpretation of underlying social meanings enables us to regulate our behaviors. Roles and attitudes are acquired from interaction with others. Social class influences have a deep effect on childrearing practices and on how mental disorders are diagnosed and treated. It is the opinion of many sociologists that mental disorders result from the interplay of diverse variables. Although social and cultural factors do not fully explain the occurrence or course of mental disorders, they cannot be discounted.

Proponents of the biogenic framework favor somatic treatments, such as psychosurgery, insulin shock therapy, electroconvulsive therapy, and chemotherapy. Many of the currently used somatic treatments are effective, even though the rationale for their use is not clearly understood. Among biogenic sources of mental disorders currently being explored are genetic factors and chemical imbalance. Chronobiology (the study of biological rhythms) is used to monitor a range of human functions and to record characteristic patterns. Because every individual pattern of biological rhythms is unique, deviations may provide guidelines in preventing, detecting, or alleviating internal maladaptations.

Additional frameworks for explaining bio-psychosocial development include the existential approach, which emphasizes self-determination and striving for authentic existence, and the cognitive approach, which emphasizes cognitive factors in emergence of the self.

Review Questions

1. Define the following terms and explain their relevance to psychiatric mental health nursing: theories; theoretical frameworks; concepts.

2. What do the terms ego alien (dystonic) and ego syntonic mean? What is their relationship to repression?

3. Describe the ego function known as reality testing. What manifestations frequently indicate failure of reality testing?

4. What role does the unconscious play in mental life, according to Freud?

5. What Freudian explanations of rape fantasies and female sexuality are rejected by feminist groups?

6. What are the major differences between the formulations of Freud, Erikson, and Sullivan?

7. How did Peplau adapt Sullivan's interpersonal framework to nursing theory and practice?

8. What is meant by symbolic interactionism? How does symbolic interactionism affect human behavior?

9. What does the term concordance mean? Explain the significance of concordance as a factor in the genetic etiology of mental disorders.

10. What advantages are derived from viewing mental disorders as physiological in origin? What are the disadvantages of this viewpoint?

References

Abraham, K. 1953. *Selected Papers on Psychoanalysis.* New York: Basic Books.

Adams, V. A. 1979. Freud's Work Thrives as Theory, Not Therapy. *The New York Times*, August 14.

Bellak, L.; Hurvick, M.; and Gediman, H. K. 1973. *Ego Functions in Schizophrenics, Neurotics, and Normals.* New York: John Wiley & Sons.

Blumer, H. 1969. *Symbolic Interaction: Perspective and Method.* Englewood Cliffs, N.J.: Prentice-Hall.

Brenner, C. 1955. *An Elementary Textbook of Psychoanalysis.* New York: International Universities Press.

Brody, J. E. 1981. Body's Many Rhythms Send Messages on When to Work and Play. *The New York Times*, August 11.

Burgess, A. W., and Lazare, A. 1976. *Psychiatric Nursing in the Hospital and Community*, 2nd ed. Englewood Cliffs, N.J.: Prentice-Hall.

Clausen, J. A. 1980. Sociology and Psychiatry. In *Comprehensive Textbook of Psychiatry*, 3rd ed., eds. H. I. Kaplan, A. M. Freedman, and B. J. Sadock. Baltimore: Williams & Wilkins.

Cohen, S. M.; Allen, M. G.; Pollin, W.; and Hrubec, Z. 1972. Relationship of Schizo-affective Psychosis to Manic-Depressive Psychosis and Schizophrenia. *Teaching of General Psychiatry*, 26:539–546.

Ellis, A., and Harper, R. A. 1961. *A Guide to Rational Living.* Englewood Cliffs, N.J.: Prentice-Hall.

Engel, G. L. 1964. Grief and Grieving. *American Journal of Nursing*, 64:93–98.

Erikson, E. H. 1963. *Childhood and Society*, 2nd ed. New York: W. W. Norton.

Frankl, V. 1959. *Man's Search for Meaning.* New York: Beacon Press.

Freedman, A. M.; Kaplan, H. I.; and Sadock, B. J. 1973. *Modern Synopsis of Psychiatry.* Baltimore: Williams & Wilkins.

Freud, A. 1953. *The Ego and Mechanisms of Defense.* New York: International Universities Press.

Freud, S. 1953. *A General Introduction to Psychoanalysis.* New York: Simon & Schuster.

Freud, S. 1961. Civilization and Its Discontents. In *Standard Edition of Psychological Works of Sigmund Freud*, Vol. 21. London: Hogarth Press.

Gendlin, E. T. 1968. The Experiential Response. In *Use of Interpretation in Treatment*, ed. E. J. Hammer. New York: Grune & Stratton.

Glasser, W. 1965. *Reality Therapy: A New Approach to Psychiatry.* New York: Harper & Row.

Goffman, E. 1961. *Asylums.* New York: Doubleday.

Gottesman, I. I., and Shields, J. 1972. *Schizophrenia and Genetics.* New York: Academic Press.

Griffin, J. Q. 1980. Physical Illness in the Family. In *Family-Focused Care*, eds. J. R. Miller and E. H. Janosik. New York: McGraw-Hill.

Hall, C. S., and Lindzey, G. 1970. *Theories of Personality.* New York: John Wiley & Sons.

Hartman, H. 1964. *Essays on Ego Psychology.* New York: International Universities Press.

Hollingshead, A., and Redlich, F. C. 1958. *Social Class and Mental Illness.* New York: John Wiley & Sons.

Janeway, E. 1983. *Cross Sections: From a Decade of Change.* New York: William Morrow.

Kallmann, F. J. 1953. *Heredity in Health and Mental Disorder.* New York: W. W. Norton.

Kallman, F. J. 1962. *Expanding Goals of Genetics in Psychiatry.* New York: Grune & Stratton.

Kety, S. S. 1959. Biochemical Theories of Schizophrenia. *Science*, 129:1528, 1590.

King, I. M. 1971. *Toward a Theory of Nursing.* New York: John Wiley & Sons.

Marram, G. 1978. *The Group Approach in Nursing Practice*, 2nd ed. St. Louis: C. V. Mosby.

Mead, G. H. 1933. *Mind, Self, and Society.* Chicago: University of Chicago Press.

Meissner, W. W. 1980. Theories of Personality and Psychopathology: Classical Psychoanalysis. In *Comprehensive Textbook of Psychiatry*, 3rd ed., eds. H. I. Kaplan, B. J. Sadock, and A. M. Freedman. Baltimore: Williams & Wilkins.

Miller, J. R., and Janosik, E. H., eds. 1980. *Family-Focused Care.* New York: McGraw-Hill.

Morgan, A. J., and Morgan, M. D. 1980. *Manual of Primary Mental Health Care.* Philadelphia: J. B. Lippincott.

Parsons, T. 1951. *The Social System.* New York: Free Press.

Peplau, H. E. 1952. *Interpersonal Relations in Nursing.* New York: Putnam.

Piaget, J. 1974. *The Origins of Intelligence in Children.* New York: International Universities Press.

Scheinfeld, D. R. 1983. Family Relationships and School Achievement Among Boys of Lower Income Urban Black Families. *American Journal of Orthopsychiatry*, 53(1):127–143.

Schmitt, M. 1982. Working Together in Health Teams. In *Life Cycle Group Work in Nursing*, eds. E. H. Janosik and L. B. Phipps. Monterey, Calif.: Wadsworth Health Sciences.

Srole, L.; Langer, T. S.; Apler, M. L.; and Rennie, T. A. C. 1962. *Mental Health in the Metropolis.* New York: McGraw-Hill.

Stroebel, C. F. 1980. Biological Rhythms in Psychiatry. In *Comprehensive Textbook of Psychiatry*, 3rd. ed., eds. H. I. Kaplan, B. J. Sadock, and A. M. Freedman. Baltimore: Williams & Wilkins.

Stroebel, C. F., and Glueck, B. C. 1978. *The Psychophysiological Diary: A Computer Scored Method of Moods, Body Changes, and Life Events.* Hartford, Conn.: Institute of Living.

Sullivan, H. S. 1953. *The Interpersonal Theory of Psychiatry.* New York: W. W. Norton.

Thompson, C. 1950. *Psychoanalyses: Evolution and Development.* New York: Grune & Stratton.

49

Supplementary Readings

Brady, J. P.; Mendels, J.; Orne, M. T.; and Rieger, W., eds. *Psychiatry: Areas of Promise and Advancement.* New York: Spectrum, 1977.

Chesler, P. *Women and Madness.* Garden City, N.Y.: Doubleday, 1972.

Coan, R. W. *Psychology of Adjustment: Personal Experience and Development.* New York: John Wiley & Sons, 1983.

Coelho, H. *Coping and Adaptation.* New York: Basic Books, 1974.

Deutsch, H. *The Psychology of Women.* 2 vols. New York: Grune & Stratton, 1944, 1945.

Frisanch, A. R. *Human Adaptation: A Functional Interpretation*. Ann Arbor: University of Michigan Press, 1981.

Fromm, E. *Escape from Freedom*. New York: Irvington, 1941.

Horney, K. *Neurosis and Human Growth*. New York: W. W. Norton, 1950.

Jones, M. *The Life and Work of Sigmund Freud*. New York: Basic Books, 1957.

Kaufman, W. *Discovering the Mind. Vol. 3: Freud Versus Adler and Jung*. New York: McGraw-Hill, 1981.

Laing, R. D. *The Politics of Experience*. New York: Ballantine Books, 1967.

Lazarus, R. *Patterns of Adjustment*. New York: McGraw-Hill, 1976.

Menninger, K. *The Vital Balance*. New York: Viking Press, 1963.

Mitchell, J. *Psychoanalysis and Feminism*. New York: Vintage Books, 1974.

Ordall, P. *High Level Wellness*. Emmaus, Penn.: Rodale Press, 1977.

Strachey, J., ed. *The Standard Edition of the Complete Psychological Works of Sigmund Freud*. 24 vols. London: Hogarth Press, 1962.

Szasz, T. S. *The Myth of Mental Illness*. New York: Harper & Row, 1974.

HOLISTIC INTERACTION
Reciprocal Interaction
Assignment of Meanings

ADAPTATION
Coping and Defensive Behaviors
Adaptation to Life Changes

SYSTEMS THEORY APPROACHES
Basic Concepts of Systems Theory
Nursing Models
The Roy Model

CLINICAL TESTING AND ASSESSMENT
Intelligence Testing
Mental Status Assessment
Personality Assessment

C H A P T E R

3

Holistic Interaction as a Unifying Framework

Learning Objectives

After reading this chapter, the student should be able to:

1. Describe the nature of holistic interaction and recognize its relevance to psychiatric mental health nursing.

2. Explain symbolism and describe its influence on human behavior.

3. Define and differentiate defense mechanisms and evaluate the effectiveness of various defense mechanisms as adaptive or maladaptive behavioral responses.

4. Discuss adaptation as a general behavioral concept and the implications of adaptation as a nursing theory.

5. Trace the development of nursing models used to define and conceptualize nursing practice and identify the holistic aspects of nursing practice models.

6. Recognize the usefulness of assessment guidelines that adopt a holistic perspective.

7. Identify major tests and measures developed to facilitate data collection and comprehensive assessment of clients' needs.

52

Overview

In this chapter holistic interaction is presented as a unifying framework for psychiatric mental health nursing. Attention to holism requires nurses to reach beyond the mind-body paradigm and consider all the ramifications of human interaction: physical, psychological, social, political, cognitive, and spiritual. The chapter differentiates the characteristics of functional and dysfunctional interactional patterns and explores the reciprocal and holistic nature of human interaction. Holistic interaction encompasses a variety of adaptational behaviors that have been described in different ways by different nurse theorists. One nurse theorist, Callista Roy, has developed an adaptational model

that is highly regarded and widely used by many nurses. This comprehensive model includes assessment guidelines that examine behavior in several dimensions in order to help nurses assess client needs in a holistic manner. In addition to assessment guidelines proposed by nurse theorists such as Roy, a number of well-known tests and measures have been developed by members of other disciplines to facilitate clinical data collection for purposes of assessment. Since many of these procedures are widely used and provide useful information, they are described briefly in this chapter.

Human felicity is produced not so much by great pieces of
good fortune that seldom happen, as by little
advantages that occur every day.
BENJAMIN FRANKLIN

53

HOLISTIC INTERACTION

People do not exist as separate beings in the world but as acting, reacting, and interacting organisms that must respond to changing conditions at all levels of existence: physical, psychological, and social. From this *holistic* viewpoint, the individual and the environment are a single but changing configuration shaped by the individual's ability to bring order and meaning into life experiences. According to Maslow (1968), individual response to internal and external events requires not merely the acquisition of new habits but a shifting of the whole organism as it continues to interact with its inner and outer worlds. Thus, a holistic approach to biopsychosocial development focuses on the individual's ability to *adapt* in his or her ongoing interactions.

Interactions may be functional or dysfunctional. *Functional interaction* has been defined as the "constant, positive alterations which individuals make in their pattern of interaction to stimuli within the environment. These alterations perpetuate the survival of the individual and increase the individual's utility, performance, and pleasure within the chosen environment" (Goosen and Bush, 1979, p. 66). In contrast, *dysfunctional interaction* consists of responses to environmental stimuli that result in conditions of disruption, disorganization, and displeasure. Functional interaction is achieved when responses to internal and external conditions preserve the integrity and well-being of the individual, family, or community. Dysfunctional interaction results from responses that threaten or destroy this integrity and well-being.

Functional and dysfunctional interaction patterns can be found at every level of human existence. A physiological example is the fight-or-flight response. When people face conditions that require high expenditures of energy, adrenocorticotropic hormone (ACTH) is released from the hypothalamus. The sympathetic nervous system is then activated, causing large amounts of epinephrine and norepinephrine to be produced. Increased amounts of these hormones help prepare the individual for fight-or-flight. Mobilization for fight-or-flight behavior was functional for primitive humans, but this form of physiological response is less adaptive and less functional in the modern world, where more selective responses are needed. For example, the employee who reacts by venting anger or by leaving whenever things go wrong on the job is not likely to be highly regarded by her employer or her coworkers (Cooper, 1981).

In the realm of interpersonal relationships, Horney (1937, 1950) has described three dysfunctional patterns of psychosocial interaction: (1) moving toward other people, (2) moving away from other people, and (3) moving against other people. In moving *toward* other people, the individual reveals dependency by becoming clinging and placating and by constantly searching for approval and acceptance. Moving *away* from others is the response of the individual who dreads closeness, disengages from social interaction, and appears withdrawn. Moving *against* others can be seen in the aggressive, angry individual who expresses hostility toward others.

Moving away from others is a form of flight behavior; moving against others is a form of fight behavior. The pattern of moving toward others is not an intrinsic part of fight-flight behavior, but it does

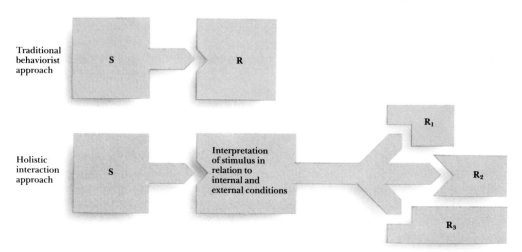

Figure 3-1. *A holistic interaction approach to behavior. Whereas the behavioral approach allows for a single response to a stimulus, the holistic approach allows for a range of alternative responses.*

provide a third psychosocial option. All three response patterns are dysfunctional when used exclusively or in exaggerated forms, because a fragile sense of interpersonal safety is won at the expense of healthy personality development. Well-adjusted individuals are not restricted to any single pattern but alter their responses as situations unfold.

Reciprocal Interaction

Reciprocal interaction is the capacity of organisms to adjust to external change by altering internal conditions and, conversely, to cause external change by means of internal modifications. Changes within a system may also be reciprocal in that such changes inevitably have an effect on other systems coexisting in the environment. In the natural world examples of reciprocal interaction are endless. Plants adjust to external conditions by turning their leaves toward the sun and sending their roots in search of moisture. Reciprocally, the leafy foliage shields the soil from water evaporation and healthy roots prevent soil erosion. Another example of reciprocal interaction is the ability of some animals to camouflage themselves by changing color so that they seem to merge with their seasonal environment.

Human beings engage in holistic interactions that are reciprocal and extremely complex. On a physiological level, the human fetus is accustomed to the uterine environment, but with its first breath it interacts in response to extrauterine conditions. Psychologically, reciprocal interaction can be seen in adjustment to separation or loss, in which grieving is followed by a willingness to establish new relationships. An example of reciprocal sociocultural interaction is the immigrant who begins to master English as a second language. The immigrant's response to conditions within the dominant culture is to master a new language; her way of experiencing and acting upon the culture will alter as her mastery of the English language grows.

For most individuals, internal conditions may be altered in response to existing, remembered, or anticipated environmental changes. A ballplayer warming up before a big game is displaying reciprocal interaction designed to meet the demands being made upon him or about to be made upon him. If the athlete proves unequal to the demands of the situation, this failure will affect the conditions surrounding his next game. And the memory of a satisfactory or unsatisfactory experience will affect future interactions in positive or negative ways.

Assignment of Meanings

The holistic interactional approach goes well beyond the purely behavioristic approach of analyzing relationships between stimuli and responses. For behaviorists, S is used to represent the sum of sensory stimuli affecting an organism at a specific point in time and R refers to the organism's response. Holistic interaction suggests that there is more than a simple, direct connection between S and R. There is, instead, an intervening process in which the person involved attaches meaning to S and responds on the basis of the perceived meaning (see Figure 3-1). In short, the interactions of human beings have a complexity beyond stimuli and overt, observable responses. The link between S and R exists, but the individualistic meanings assigned to S greatly alter responsive behaviors.

A holistic view of human interaction assumes

CHARACTERISTICS OF ADAPTATION

Adaptation is an essential process in the life cycle, involving conscious and unconscious responses.

The same conditions will elicit different adaptive responses from different individuals.

The same conditions will elicit different adaptive responses from the same individual at different times.

The same conditions will be perceived and interpreted differently by different individuals.

Table 3-1. Nature of Holistic Interaction

Dimensions	Chronology	Structure	Characteristics
Physical	Past	Individual	Reciprocal
Psychological	Present	Family	Differentiated
Social	Future	Community	Selective
Symbolic			Circumstantial

that people live in a symbolic as well as a physical, psychological, and social environment. Our behaviors therefore reflect the meanings we assign to our own actions and to the actions of others (Mead, 1933). Table 3-1 summarizes the various aspects of holistic interaction. Table 3-2 elaborates on the four main characteristics of holistic interaction by defining their S–R relationships and providing examples for each.

ADAPTATION

Because human existence is dynamic, not static, people must accept the inevitability of recurrent change in themselves, in their environment, and between themselves and their environment. This means that *adaptation* takes place continuously, despite great variability in the adaptive capacities of individuals. Adaptive ability depends on a number of factors, including personality traits, life experiences, and learned behaviors. Some basic characteristics of adaptation are listed in the accompanying box.

As a rule, successful adaptation depends on congruence between the adaptive capacities of individuals and the nature of the demands made on them (Mechanic, 1976). For example, an elderly

Table 3-2. Characteristics of Holistic Interaction

Characteristic	S–R Relationships	Example
Reciprocal	Stimuli influence responses; responses in turn influence stimuli	A neighborhood suffers a series of robberies: additional police are assigned; householders become more vigilant, and the robberies cease
Differentiated	Responses to stimuli are idiosyncratic and different for each individual, family, and community	One pregnant teenager runs away from home; a second turns to her family for help and is able to finish high school
Selective	Similar stimuli evoke different responses in the same individual, family, and community	A mother welcomes the marriage of a daughter but opposes an equally suitable marriage for a son
Circumstantial	Responses to similar stimuli are influenced by context, perception, attitudes, and other variables	A devoted father forgets a child's birthday after suffering a business disappointment

56

person who must give up an independent lifestyle for supervised residential placement may react adaptively or maladaptively. An angry or bitter reaction is likely to evoke resentment in others and prevent an easy adjustment to the new situation, whereas a reaction of acceptance will probably elicit positive gestures from staff and fellow residents, thereby promoting adjustment.

Some individuals are capable of displaying adaptive behaviors as long as the demand is not prolonged. For example, a divorced father or mother may be willing to take care of the children on occasional weekends but may be unwilling to accept sustained parental responsibility. The presence or absence of rewards for certain behaviors may determine whether adaptive or maladaptive behaviors occur. A child whose efforts to succeed are acknowledged only by greater parental demands may become discouraged and fearful of ultimate failure and may stop trying. When demands exceed the capacities of the individual, or when adaptive behaviors are unrewarded, maladaptive responses usually follow. In other words, every individual, family, and group has a certain point at which they become overwhelmed by the conditions in which they must try to function. Whenever this breaking point is reached, responsive behavior is likely to be maladaptive.

Coping and Defensive Behaviors

Adaptation to change can occur at various levels, from functional coping behaviors to dysfunctional defense mechanisms. *Coping behaviors* are reality-based, task-oriented, problem-solving activities (Lazarus, 1977). Among functional coping behaviors are reasoning, concentration, learning,

---

LEVELS OF DEFENSE MECHANISMS

Level 1 *Psychotic mechanisms* such as distortion, delusions, and extreme denial. These mechanisms are common in children up to five years of age and in the dreams and fantasies of adults. If the mechanisms intrude beyond these limits, they are inappropriate and dysfunctional.

Level 2 *Immature mechanisms* such as fantasy, projection, passive-aggressive behaviors, and hypochondria. These mechanisms are evident in children, in adolescents, and among adults experiencing depression, physical illness, or substance abuse disorders.

Level 3 *Neurotic mechanisms* such as intellectualization, repression, reaction formation, displacement, and dissociation. These are responses that often can be modified through counseling, introspection, and analysis of behavior.

Level 4 *Mature mechanisms* such as altruism, humor, suppression, and sublimation. These mechanisms expedite adaptation during the life cycle.

---

advance preparation, and accurate perception. Many motor activities, such as walking or running, are also functional coping mechanisms in that they reduce anxiety, discharge anger, or release tension without hurting the self or others. Emotional expression, in the form of tears, laughter, or verbalization, can also help individuals cope with difficult situations. Postponing immediate gratification, working toward a goal, establishing rewarding interpersonal relationships—all constitute methods of coping successfully.

Defense mechanisms are sometimes functional but are often dysfunctional means of dealing with life situations. In their functional forms, defense mechanisms effectively regulate instinctual drives and impulses that are unacceptable to the individual, family, or society (Freud, 1948). However, many defense mechanisms are dysfunctional because they prevent rather than promote adequate

Table 3-3. Social Readjustment Rating Scale

Rank	Life Event	Mean Value
1	Death of a spouse	100
2	Divorce	73
3	Marital separation	65
4	Jail term	63
5	Death of close family member	63
6	Personal injury or illness	53
7	Marriage	50
8	Fired from job	47
9	Marital reconciliation	45
10	Retirement	45
11	Change in health of family member	44
12	Pregnancy	40
13	Sexual problems	39
14	Addition of new family member	39
15	Business readjustments	39
16	Change in financial status	38
17	Death of a close friend	37
18	Change to a new line of work	36
19	Increased dissension with spouse	35
20	Mortgage disproportionate to income	31
21	Foreclosure of loan or mortgage	30
22	Change in responsibilities at work	29
23	Son or daughter leaving home	29
24	Trouble with in-laws	29
25	Outstanding personal achievement	28
26	Spouse begins or quits job	26
27	Beginning or ending school	26
28	Change in living conditions	25
29	Change in personal habits	24
30	Trouble with boss at work	23
31	Change in residence	20
32	Change of schools	20
33	Change in working hours or conditions	20
34	Change in recreation habits	19
35	Change in church activities	19
36	Change in social activities	19
37	Mortgage or loan over $10,000	19
38	Change in sleeping habits or eating habits	19
39	Change in number of family visits	19
40	Vacation	19
41	Christmas	19
42	Minor legal infractions	19

SOURCE: Holmes and Rahe (1967).

coping. Many persons cling to a few rigid defense mechanisms and do not try to expand or improve their coping skills. They may resort to such defenses as extreme regression or prolonged denial to avoid or distort a reality that is too difficult to endure. Vaillant (1977) categorized four levels of defense mechanisms, ranging from the extremely maladaptive to the extremely adaptive, depending on how and when the mechanisms are used. These levels are described in the accompanying box.

Adaptation to Life Changes

Every life change creates a new demand for adaptation, and each adaptational demand exacts a price that alters efficiency, consumes energy, and jeopardizes equilibrium to some extent. Ability to adapt to life change varies, but there is general agreement that frequent changes within a brief period of time predispose people to physical and psychological distress. It does not matter whether the change is positive, such as marriage or career advancement, or negative, such as divorce or unemployment. The crucial factor seems to be that any life change for which new responses are needed places people at risk.

Holmes and Rahe (1967) devised a way to assess the effects of life change by developing what they called the Social Readjustment Rating Scale. They assigned quantitative values, using "life change units," to various life changes, ranging from 100 units for the most stressful event, death of a spouse, to 19 units for such lesser events as vacations and minor legal infractions (see Table 3-3). The assumption made by Holmes and Rahe was that the higher a person's life change score, the greater the likelihood that physical or psychological illness would

follow within a year or two. Among subjects whose life change index exceeded 300 units in a year, 86 percent suffered adverse health effects in the following two years. Among subjects who scored from 150 to 300, 48 percent suffered adverse health effects in the same time frame.

The Social Readjustment Rating Scale is a useful assessment tool because it ranks specific life

58

changes according to the amount of adaptation needed to cope and it permits accumulated life changes to be identified and quantified. Because some life changes can be anticipated and regulated in advance, it is possible to help clients control the rate of change in their lives so that their adaptive capacities are not depleted. Helping clients monitor their rate of change is a form of primary prevention that helps clients avoid adverse reactions to a number of drastic changes occurring in rapid succession.

SYSTEMS THEORY APPROACHES

Holism implies interrelatedness among a host of variables operating at different levels. *Systems theory* is based on the idea of interrelatedness among components that are separated from the environment and from one another by boundaries. Thus, systems theory shares with holism the idea of interrelatedness but negates the notion of holism by introducing boundaries and substituting the less expansive concept of interdependent interaction.

Basic Concepts of Systems Theory

Adaptation to changes in the environment requires individuals, families, and groups to function as *systems* that can exchange material, information, and energy across system boundaries. There is usually a higher rate of transaction and interaction *within* the boundaries of a system than *across* the boundaries. Because the components and elements within a system are interrelated and interdependent, alteration in any part of the system produces alteration in other parts. Regardless of the extent of internal

---

SYSTEMS TERMINOLOGY

Structure. The organization or arrangement of various components within a system.

Function. The enactment of certain behaviors that permit the operations of the system to continue.

Process. An exchange of energy, information, or transactions within a system, between systems, or between a system and the surrounding environment.

Subsystem. A component or element within a system that carries out a particular function. In families, mother and father make up the parental subsystem; children make up the sibling subsystem.

Suprasystem. A larger system to which smaller systems relate or of which they form a part. The community is an example of a suprasystem to which families relate.

External variables. Conditions, influences, or factors outside the boundaries of a system.

Internal variables. Structural patterns and functional processes inside the boundaries of a system.

Feedback. A process that includes both input and output. Output discharged by a system is returned by external sources in the form of input to the system.

Negative feedback. Feedback that produces change in order to correct error.

Positive feedback. Feedback that maintains the status quo by validating or reinforcing current output from a system.

SOURCE: Anderson and Carter (1978).

---

alterations, the dual purpose of any system is to maintain a steady, balanced state and to continue functioning. When the system can no longer maintain this dual purpose, the result is malfunction of the whole system or some of its parts.

Open systems have boundaries that are easily penetrated, while *closed systems* permit only limited amounts of exchange across boundaries. This means that closed systems can operate with considerable predictability because their rate of transaction and change is relatively slow. The operations of open systems may be less predictable, since they permit the entry of large amounts of energy and information. Closed systems are less tolerant of change than open systems, are less accessible to

---

PRINCIPLES OF SYSTEMS THEORY

■ Systems theory differentiates functional and dysfunctional patterns, thereby facilitating identification of individual and family interactions for which corrective feedback is indicated.

■ Systems theory interprets human behavior as adjustment between social demands and personal needs. Developmental changes and situational stressors require ongoing adjustment within a system or between several systems.

■ Systems theory includes external factors (input) and internal responses (output) that affect social, psychological, and biological expressions of human behavior.

SOURCE: Anderson and Carter (1978).

---

input from outside, and are more susceptible to rising internal tension because of difficulty in discharging output across their boundaries.

One example of a relatively closed system is the traditional family that tries to preserve its values by isolating itself from mainstream society. This isolation is usually imposed by older members and may be resented by younger members who are eager to adapt to the dominant culture. The result may be conflict within the family system and tension among members that is dysfunctional and generates maladaptive behaviors. Conversely, a family system that is too open often lacks stability and is overly responsive to changes in the surrounding environment.

In order to discuss systems theory in a meaningful fashion, it is important to define some of the terms commonly used. Systems possess patterns of *structure* and *function*; specific terms used to describe these patterns and related phenomena are defined in the accompanying box.

Nursing Models

Nursing models are used by nurse theorists to define and conceptualize nursing practice. Nursing models are usually concerned with three major issues: (1) the client or consumer of nursing care, (2) the activities or interventions composing nursing care, and (3) the purpose or goals of nursing care.

Over the years changes have occurred in the way consumers of nursing care has been perceived by nurse theorists. Florence Nightingale saw the client as a passive recipient of care who responded to the same natural laws, whether sick or well. Thus, the early purpose of nursing activities was to improve the comfort, nutrition, and hygiene of the client in order to promote natural laws of healing. More recently, Henderson (1966) asserted that the purpose of nursing actions is to reduce deficiencies in the motivation and knowledge of clients so as to encourage their independence. It was Henderson who proposed that assessment, diagnosis, intervention, and evaluation are essential to nursing practice. Martha Rogers (1970) was concerned with the unity or wholeness of the individual and emphasized harmony between the individual and the environment. She asserted that the attainment of optimum health is the goal of nursing care and the criterion for evaluation. According to Rogers, nursing care plans deal with the "repatterning" of the total human being. Nurses endeavor to help people engage in adaptive living patterns that integrate rather than oppose environmental change.

A review of the work of nursing theorists shows that directions in nursing have moved from client as recipient of care to client as participant in care, and from environment as external and physical to environment as intrinsic and multidimensional (George, 1985). Thus, the thrust is toward the utilization of whatever social, cognitive, affective, psychomotor, and material resources are available to the client. This utilization of all available resources is, in effect, the essence of holistic nursing and it has particular implications for psychiatric mental health care.

The Roy Model

Sister Callista Roy (1970) has developed a nursing model based on systems theory. In this model, clients—whether individuals, families, or groups—are considered to be complex systems made up of interrelated and interacting components. Input from the external environment can generate tension and discomfort within the client. Therefore, nursing theory and practice must encompass the environment that surrounds the client. According to Roy (1976), nursing intervention promotes the selective modification or adaptation of aspects of the client or of aspects of the environment.

The other major assumptions of the Roy model are as follows:

1. Human beings are biopsychosocial organisms that constantly interact with their environment.
2. Health and illness are inevitable dimensions of human existence.
3. Coping requires inherent and acquired skills that are biopsychosocial in origin.
4. Adaptation is an essential response to environmental change and is influenced by life demands and by the adaptive capacity of the individual, family, or group.
5. Demands that are within the capacity of clients promote successful adjustment or adaptation.

MODES OF ADAPTATION According to Roy, human beings possess four modes or methods of adaptation: physiological needs, self-concept, role function, and interdependence. These four modes are in some ways similar to Maslow's hierarchy of human needs, as can be seen in Table 3-4.

An example of *physiological* adaptation is obtaining supplies from the environment in the form of food and shelter. Another example is the increase in white blood cells and inflammatory processes that occurs in response to infection. *Self-concept* is related to attachments and relationships, because attitudes and appraisals from others influence one's sense of self. One aspect of self-concept is self-esteem, which affects the ability to adapt or adjust to change in a functional way (Sullivan, 1953). *Role function* or *enactment* has a profound impact on the self-esteem

of most individuals. One's willingness and ability to enact assigned roles affect the way one is perceived by both family and community. Role function includes the concept of role status, which refers to roles assigned because of age and gender. The role status of parenthood, for example, is biologically determined. However, actual parenting behaviors (the role function) may not be carried out by the biological parents but rather by other family members. Sometimes parenting is delegated to a selected child or is taken over by a grandparent. This happens when family members occupying a particular role status are unwilling or unable to perform the responsibilities attached to the role (Miller, 1980).

Interdependence refers to the idea that individuals, families, and communities are dynamic systems in which every component is interrelated. For example, when a son or daughter marries, consequences follow in both families of origin and in the newly established family. Everyone concerned experiences complex changes in their ways of relating and interacting.

MODES OF HOLISTIC INTERACTION The purpose of nursing intervention is to facilitate functional interaction in the four modes. Although Roy's model is not the only one upon which to base a nursing care plan, it is sufficiently broad to provide a holistic perspective. For example, a community health nurse working with a pregnant woman thought to be a potential child abuser might develop goals, plan interventions, implement the plan, and evaluate the goals in terms of the four modes in the following manner:

Physiological mode
Provide information concerning prenatal nutrition.

Provide information about gestational changes.

Provide teaching regarding labor and delivery.

Self-concept mode
Offer explanation and emotional support concerning body image changes.

Help the client integrate motherhood into her self-concept.

Role-function mode
Utilize peer group interaction to facilitate role transition.

Help the client understand the role functions of motherhood.

Table 3-4. Comparison Between Maslow's Hierarchy of Needs and Roy's Modes of Adaptation

Hierarchical Needs	Adaptational Modes
Self-actualization needs (fulfillment)	Interdependence
Esteem needs (self-esteem)	Role function
Belongingness and love needs (relationships)	Self-concept
Safety needs (security) Physiologic needs (food, water, air)	Physiological

SOURCE: Adapted from Maslow (1970) and Roy (1970).

Interdependence mode

Involve the prospective father, if possible, in planning.

Involve the client's mother and other significant persons in advance planning and preparation.

ASSESSMENT GUIDELINES In addition to considering the four modes or methods of responding to change, Roy developed an assessment guide that looks at focal, contextual, and residual behaviors. *Focal behaviors* are those that receive initial attention because they seem to be the most obvious problems. *Contextual behaviors* are indicative of environmental factors; *residual behaviors* are those that involve complicated and long-standing issues.

In working with an obese client, the nurse might identify the focal behavior as the client's daily 5,000-calorie intake. The context might be the family home, where the client lives with his parents, both of whom are grossly overweight. As a residual behavior, the obesity might serve as a cohesive force in this family by isolating the three family members from other social interactions and holding them together. Mother, father, and son exist in a closed system into which the outside world seldom intrudes. Whatever emptiness they feel in their lives may be satisfied by food. In developing a care plan for this client, the nurse might begin with the focal behavior as the primary target. If the focal behavior is resistant to change, attention might then be directed to contextual and residual behaviors. The focal behavior might be approached on an individual basis or in a group setting where the client could receive help from peer interaction. Contextual and residual behaviors might be responsive to individual counseling for the son or to family intervention with all three members.

Sometimes a client's perception of what is needed differs from that of the nurse, and such discrepancies must be compared and reconciled. Sometimes a nurse cannot promote functional interaction or halt progressive decline. In such instances, the nurse may be able to provide only supportive measures, since functional interaction largely depends on the client's capacity and motivation.

CLINICAL TESTING AND ASSESSMENT

Nursing assessment is concerned with obtaining all available data pertaining to the client. By collecting as much information as possible, the nurse is better able to collaborate with the client and the health team. Many clients cannot explain themselves, and their behaviors, although meaningful to the clients, may be puzzling to the nurse. Although there is no substitute for attentiveness and careful observation, a number of testing and assessment methods have been designed to supplement the observations of nurses and other professionals in an effort to better understand client behaviors.

The terms *assessment*, *examination*, and *testing* are sometimes used interchangeably, but they are not synonymous. *Testing* is a rather limited activity that is usually carried out by a technician, whereas *assessment* requires the skills of a professional who relates to the client in a special way. A technician may perform blood tests or electrocardiograms, but only a professional can derive meaning from the data and safely use it. *Examination* is a broad term applied to testing or assessment, depending on the methods employed and the results obtained (Kaplan and Sadock, 1980). Although nurses are more concerned with assessing than with testing and examining, as professionals they should understand the relevance of information obtained from tests and examinations. It is therefore highly appropriate to describe the implications of several widely used testing and examining procedures. Here we shall focus on three main types of measures: intelligence testing, mental status assessment, and personality assessment.

Intelligence Testing

Intelligence is defined as the ability to solve new problems through reasoning and cognitive processes (Matarazzo, 1980). In the hands of competent professionals, measures of intelligence yield valuable information. However, when intelligence scores are considered in isolation or are used to label people, they have destructive potential. With this warning in mind, health care professionals will find that measures of intelligence may be helpful adjuncts to comprehensive assessment.

Intelligence tests are *standardized* by administering them to large representative groups of people. Those who achieve the median score on the test are assigned an IQ of 100 (see Figure 3-2). Because their test score exceeds that of 50 percent of other people, they are said to rank at the 50th percentile of the general population (Matarazzo, 1980). The higher the percentile rank, the higher the individual stands in the group. Thus, a person at the 90th percentile surpasses 90 percent of the group and is surpassed by 10 percent. Percentile rankings on IQ tests provides an indication of how the test taker performed in comparison to other test takers and unlike IQ scores do not stigmatize the individual.

Figure 3-2. *Normal curve for IQ test scores.*

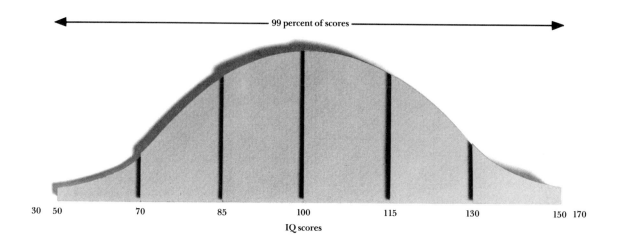

Reliability and validity are important concepts in testing of any kind. A test is *reliable* when repeated administration under similar conditions yields consistent results; a test is *valid* when the test measures what it is intended to measure. Intelligence scores indicate only what a person may be capable of achieving, and many persons do not perform up to their intellectual capacity. Persons of limited intelligence cannot achieve beyond their capacity, but their progress may be influenced by learning activities geared to their abilities.

Tests that measure intelligence are more reliable when administered individually, but for economic reasons they are often given to groups of subjects. The most commonly used individual tests are the Weschler Adult Intelligence Scales and the Weschler Intelligence Scales for Children. Individual testing allows the examiner to monitor the attitudes and behaviors of the subjects as they are tested. Most group tests are paper-and-pencil measures that reflect the reading skills of the subjects. Such tests rely on choices and short answers, making speed another intruding factor. In situations where subjects are emotionally unstable or unmotivated, group testing is not recommended. For subjects who are under stress, whatever the cause, individual testing, even when abbreviated, is always more valid and more reliable than group testing.

Mental Status Assessment

The mental status examination is an assessment tool used to obtain information with or without the client's active participation and cooperation. Because active client participation is not mandatory, nurses can readily make an informal mental status assessment of every client with whom they come in contact. A more formal mental status examination with active client participation is desirable at the beginning of a relationship with a client or whenever changes in the client's mental status are suspected. In many respects, mental status assessment is impressionistic rather than definitive. Even so, such assessment is important enough to be made a routine part of nursing practice.

There are many variations in the form of the mental status examination, but its purpose is uniform: (1) to note significant features in the appearance, manner, and behavior of the client, (2) to formulate impressions regarding problematic areas, and (3) to develop hypotheses concerning the client's strengths and weaknesses that will assist in setting realistic, mutual goals. The reason for recording mental status data is to give a precise description of the client's emotional and intellectual functioning at a specific point in time.

ASSESSMENT GUIDELINES Most forms of the mental status examination contain categories that provide organizational guidelines (MacKinnon, 1980). A typical mental status examination is likely to follow the format provided in the accompanying box. A narrative style is generally used in reporting mental status information, although some facilities or health care professionals may prefer a comparable checklist.

Appearance and General Behavior The mental status examination begins with a detailed description of the client's appearance and general behavior according to the categories listed in the box. In providing such descriptions, it is important to select words

```
┌─────────────────────────────────────────────┐
│              GUIDELINES FOR                   │
│         MENTAL STATUS ASSESSMENT              │
│         ▬▬▬▬▬▬▬▬▬▬▬▬▬▬▬▬                      │
│                                               │
│   I.  Appearance                              │
│       Age                                     │
│       Grooming                                │
│       Posture                                 │
│       Motor activity                          │
│       Stature (height and weight)             │
│       Voice                                   │
│                                               │
│  II.  General Behavior                        │
│       Cooperative      Compliant              │
│       Withdrawn        Histrionic             │
│       Apathetic        Anxious                │
│       Suspicious       Relaxed                │
│       Aggressive       Hostile                │
│                                               │
│ III.  Affect and Mood                         │
│       Appropriate      Sad                    │
│       Flat             Elated                 │
│       Labile           Angry                  │
│                                               │
│  IV.  Thought Processes                       │
│       Logical          Phobic                 │
│       Circumstantial   Suicidal               │
│       Dissociated      Flight of ideas        │
│       Obsessive        Ideas of reference     │
│                                               │
│   V.  Perception                              │
│       Illusions                               │
│       Hallucinations                          │
│       Delusions                               │
│                                               │
│  VI.  Cognitive Functions                     │
│       Level of awareness (orientation to      │
│       time, place, person)                    │
│       Attention and concentration             │
│       Memory (remote and recent)              │
│       Judgment                                │
│       Insight                                 │
│                                               │
│  SOURCE: Adapted from MacKinnon (1980).       │
└─────────────────────────────────────────────┘
```

that are exact and that do not convey value judgments. For example, the phrase "careless grooming" should be used only if it is followed by a precise description of the client's apparel and personal hygiene to support this evaluation. If general behavior is described as "withdrawn" or "hostile," examples of such behaviors should be provided. Motor activities are important, especially manifestations of restlessness, tremors, tics, or ataxia. Again, these characteristics should be described and not just labeled.

Affect and Mood   *Mood* is the inner emotional state of the client; *affect* is the outward expression of the internal mood. A client's mood can be assessed by the content of verbal communication, by voice tone, by facial expression, by posture, and by gestures. Affect is considered appropriate only if it is congruent with the subject matter being discussed. Thus, a client speaking of loss or deprivation in a laughing or jocular fashion would be described as showing inappropriate affect. Affect that is narrow or constricted in range may be described as *flat* or *blunted*. Affect that changes from moment to moment is usually termed *labile*.

When possible, affect and mood should be reported in the client's own words. If a client is not verbally responsive, the nurse should note signs and indications of subjective emotional reactions. Tearfulness, sweating, blushing, and rapid respirations are signs of emotional distress that deserve mention.

Thought Processes   Information about the client's thought processes can be obtained by asking questions or by allowing the client to talk at will. Ideas, vocabulary, and subject matter make up the content of the client's thought. Logic and clarity determine the client's coherence, regardless of the content (Cohen, 1981). Dissociated thinking is characterized by fragmentation and a lack of logical connections.

Perceptions   Perception refers to the client's awareness of events by means of the senses: tactile, olfactory, auditory, visual, and gustatory. Since perception is a subjective, internal experience, the perceptions of clients are difficult to comprehend fully. Verbal exploration and observation of behavior are two ways of investigating what the client perceives. Behavior, both verbal and nonverbal, is

63

> ### *POPULAR PERCEPTUAL DISTORTIONS*
>
> *Stereotype.* A widely held, oversimplified belief about an individual or group based on unscientific generalization.
>
> *Discrimination.* Behaving in a special way, usually negatively, toward members of a particular racial or ethnic group.
>
> *Prejudice.* An attitude held toward group members that results in prejudgment of their abilities and attributes.
>
> *Derogation:* Blaming victims for their own misfortunes, thus reducing one's belief in a just and moral world.

64

the client's outward response to what he perceives and is shaped by his perception of events (Guzetta, 1979).

Distortions of perception include illusions, hallucinations, and delusions. *Illusions* are misperceptions attached to external sensory stimuli in the environment. *Hallucinations* are sensory misperceptions that occur without external stimuli. *Delusions* are false, entrenched beliefs that do not respond to reason or reassurance.

Cognitive Functions A client who is oriented as to time, place, and person is functioning on at least minimal levels of awareness. Disorientation as to time, place, and person can result from functional problems, organic problems, social isolation, or sensory deprivation. Whatever the cause, disorientation is a significant factor in assessing the mental status of the client.

Other cognitive functions to assess include memory, concentration, judgment, and insight. The quality of recent memory can be ascertained simply by asking about events that occurred the day before, such as what the client had for dinner. A general estimate of concentration and recall ability may be made by asking questions that require a decision, such as how to dress on a wintry day. Even without asking direct questions, the nurse can collect information about the client's judgment merely by observing the safety and suitability of the client's behavior in ordinary situations. Insight is presumed to be present to some extent when the client is aware of not functioning well and is able to acknowledge this lack. Greater insight is evident when the client is aware of not functioning well, can

recognize some reasons for it, and begins moving toward altering maladaptive patterns (Freedman, Sadock, and Kaplan, 1973).

RELIABILITY OF MENTAL STATUS ASSESSMENT When assessing the mental status of a client, observations must be distinguished from inferences. An *observation* is made up of behaviors or events witnessed through the senses. An *inference*, on the other hand, is an interpretation of the observed behavior or event. The same observation may be interpreted differently by different observers because inferences are subjective. One way to determine the reliability of inferences is to compare those made by one person against those made by others about the same observation. Because mental status assessment has few objective standards, observations and inferences made about clients should be discussed and validated with colleagues. The more staff members who share observations and agree on inferences, the more accurate the assessment of the client is likely to be (Cohen, 1981).

Personality Assessment
Personality assessment is concerned with conscious and unconscious attitudes, behaviors, impulses, conflicts, and traits. Tests of personality include the MMPI and a variety of projective tests.

THE MINNESOTA MULTIPHASIC PERSONALITY INVENTORY (MMPI) The most extensively used personality test is the Minnesota Multiphasic Personality Inventory (MMPI). It is a paper-and-pencil test consisting of 399 to 550 statements, depending on the preference of the examiner. Subjects re-

MINNESOTA MULTIPHASIC PERSONALITY INVENTORY (MMPI)

The MMPI consists of 399 to 550 items dealing with multiple areas of functioning, both physical and psychological. Scores are obtained for nine different clinical scales, differentiated for males and females. Scoring is complex and requires each scale to be related to other scales in order to obtain an accurate profile. Computerized scoring is available but should be augmented with clinical judgment. It is important that examiners be proficient in administering, scoring, and interpreting this complex test. Social class, education, religion, and race are considered factors that may influence MMPI responses. Subjects answer test items with True, False, and Don't Know responses. The nine clinical scales are:

Hs Hypochondriasis Scale: 30 items dealing with bodily function.

D Depression Scale: 60 items dealing with discouragement, self-esteem, and worry.

Hy Hysteria Scale: 60 items dealing with specific somatic complaints and with the use of denial and repression.

Pd Psychopathic Deviate Scale: 50 items dealing with social maladjustment and deficient interpersonal bonds.

Mf Masculinity-Femininity Scale: 60 items dealing with aesthetic and vocational interests and with passive as opposed to active role preferences.

Pa Paranoia Scale: 40 items dealing with sensitivity, suspiciousness, rejection.

Pt Psychasthenia Scale: 40 items dealing with narcissism, magical thinking, sado-masochism, anxiety, and self-doubt.

Sc Schizophrenia Scale: 78 items dealing with social alienation, family dysfunction, delusional thinking, bizarre emotions, unusual somatic complaints, external influences.

Ma Hypomania Scale: 40 items dealing with expansiveness, excessive activity, flightiness, distractibility, irritability.

SOURCE: After Carr (1980).

spond to questions pertaining to general health, neurological and physiological factors, personal habits, family dynamics, sexual attitudes, religious beliefs, and political opinions. The subject is asked to label each statement as true or false; when the subject cannot decide, that item is not counted.

The MMPI test items are classified into nine clinical scales, each of which has been validated empirically by administering the test to various populations. These MMPI scales are listed in the accompanying box.

There are a number of disadvantages to using the MMPI. The test asks intimate questions that may seem threatening, and many of the items provoke anxiety, especially because they are written in the first person. Another problem with the test is that it tends to make subjects who can censor their responses appear better adjusted than they actually may be. It is possible for some subjects, for example, to anticipate what inferences may be drawn from certain questions and as a result to answer in a way they think will put them in the best light. The test does, however, discriminate well between depressed and nondepressed psychotic subjects and can therefore help identify suicidal behaviors (Freedman, Sadock, and Kaplan, 1973). The MMPI, like most tests, is an adjunct to but not a substitute for informed and ongoing observation.

PROJECTIVE TESTS Several tests of personality are called *projective tests* because subjects *project* aspects of their internal selves into their responses to ambiguous images or words. Subjects' patterns of reacting to projective tests vary not only from person to person but may vary for the same person

Figure 3-3. Inkblots similar to those used in the Rorschach test.

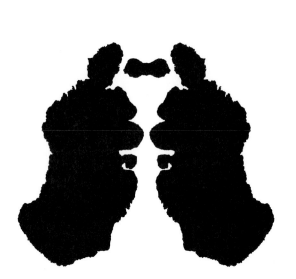
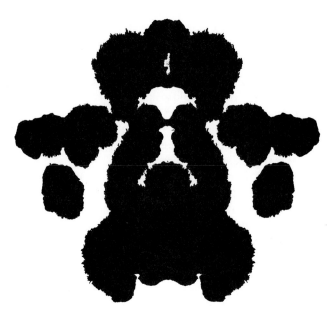

66

on successive tests. The most commonly used projective tests are the Rorschach, the TAT, and word association and completion tests.

The Rorschach Test The purpose of the Rorschach inkblot test is to identify personality attributes by analyzing a subject's responses to a series of ambiguous shapes. The subject is shown ten symmetrical inkblots printed on cards (see Figure 3-3). Five of the inkblots are black, gray, and white; two are red and gray; and three are multicolored. The subject is asked to hold the cards and describe the images formed by the inkblots. The examiner may then question the subject about descriptions for purposes of clarification. Subjects are free to elaborate on their descriptions, but the examiner makes no direct suggestions. Scores on the Rorschach test are divided into four groups:

1. *Area scores*. These indicate what portions of the image were described—the whole inkblot, a detail, or the white part of the card.
2. *Form scores*. These indicate what movements, colors, shadings, and shapes were described.
3. *Content scores*. These indicate what animate, inanimate, human, or animal figures were described.
4. *Accuracy scores*. These indicate the accuracy of descriptions applied to respective inkblots; the description is labeled good, poor, or indeterminate.

In addition to analyzing the responses themselves, the examiner records the manner in which

responses are made. Failures to respond, delays in responding, and recurrent themes are noted and interpreted by the examiner, who is usually a psychologist.

When properly administered, the test is considered valid and reliable. It can be used to identify and differentiate depressive and schizophrenic response patterns and can assist in making differential diagnoses of other psychiatric disorders (Carr, 1980).

Thematic Apperception Test (TAT) The Thematic Apperception Test (TAT) is a series of pictures showing men and women of various ages either alone or in groups. The subject is shown one picture card at a time and is asked to make up a story describing the experiences of the persons in the picture, their emotions, and the probable outcome of events. A similar test for children (the CAT) uses animals in the picture cards instead of people.

The TAT requires more than one session, and the number of pictures shown at a session is usually ten. Among the set of pictures is a blank card for which a story must be told. The blank card normally evokes wishes or fantasies about affection, affiliation, and security. If it provokes stories of fear, violence, or failure, this is considered an indicator of mood disturbances.

In interpreting the TAT, both the *content narrative* (the story that is told) and the *process narrative* (nonverbal behavior and gestures) are considered. Depressed subjects take a long time to react and are pessimistic in their content narrative. Obsessive subjects show indecision and inability to form definite opinions about the figures depicted on the cards.

THE THEMATIC
APPERCEPTION TEST (TAT)

The purpose of the TAT is to explore the dimensions of normal personality by means of a series of pictures. The subject is asked to make up a story about each picture that is shown, describing what led up to the event in the picture, the event itself, and the probable outcome. The test is thought to reveal feelings that subjects have about themselves and other people and to reveal interactional patterns that exist between subjects and significant persons in their life. Out of the available cards the examiner usually selects twenty or so pictures that seem likely to shed light on a subject's needs and conflicts. The following pictures are among those frequently selected:

Young boy looking at a violin.

Country scene showing a young woman carrying books, a man working, and an older woman watching.

Young boy with a downcast, bowed head.

Young woman covering her face with her right hand.

Elderly woman with her back turned toward a young man with a puzzled expression on his face.

Woman grasping the shoulders of a man who looks angry.

Gray-haired man looking at a younger man.

Older woman sitting on a sofa next to a young girl holding a doll.

Elderly man leaning over a young man on a sofa.

Young man standing and looking down at a partially undressed woman lying in bed.

Blank card.

SOURCE: After Carr (1980).

The TAT is less able to differentiate psychotic responses than is the Rorschach test (Carr, 1980).

Word Association and Completion Tests Information obtained from word association and sentence completion tests is apt to be questionable because norms for such tests are deficient. Interpretation is therefore dependent on the expertise of the examiner. Experienced clinicians are often able to correlate symptomatology with the responses of the client.

67

For some word association tests, norms are available that consist of lists of words most often associated. Several sentence completion tests also offer norms for certain age and gender groups.

SUMMARY

Holistic interaction is an approach to health that enables nurses to view human actions in their entirety and to consider the implications of human behavior, both functional and dysfunctional. A holistic approach requires the use of guidelines developed by nurse theorists and by members of other disciplines, many of whom have developed methods that facilitate data collection and assessment of client needs.

Adaptability, a quality possessed by all living systems, is related to the physiological, psychological, and social competence of individuals, families, and groups. Levels of adaptation range from dysfunctional defense mechanisms to functional coping mechanisms. Adaptive capacity is finite and limited. Therefore, prolonged or excessive demands for adaptive responses may deplete the resources of individuals, families, and communities.

The adaptation model conceptualized by Roy is a systems model that includes the client and the surrounding environment. According to Roy, people possess four modes of adaptation: physiological, self-concept, role function, and interdependence. The purpose of nursing intervention is to facilitate successful adaptation in one or more of the four modes. Roy also recommends the use of an assessment guide that looks at focal, contextual, and residual behaviors.

C L I N I C A L   E X A M P L E

ASSESSMENT OF HOLISTIC INTERACTION IN AN AMBULATORY CLIENT

Robert Bates is a sixty-year-old man who attends a community day treatment center three days each week. He has a long history of problem drinking but has been sober for the last three years. Mr. Bates lives in a modest home with his wife of forty years; his children are grown and have established families of their own. Before retiring on disability income, he had worked as a machinist. Some years ago Mr. Bates suffered several frightening episodes of delirium tremens that helped convince him that he must control his drinking.

The client's wife acts like a mother toward him. She takes care of his clothing, cooks for him, and supervises the routine activities of his life. His attendance at the day treatment center is partly due to his wife's need for relief from his presence. At the center he attends alcoholism and nutrition groups and engages in occupational activities. He is proud of the handcrafted articles that he makes and usually gives them to his wife or other family members.

At present Mr. Bates is in good physical health, but his years of excessive drinking have caused mental and emotional deficits that are thought to be organic in origin. Except for the episodes of delirium tremens, the organic brain damage has not produced psychotic reactions (loss of contact with reality). There are days when he seems confused and has trouble fully comprehending the interactions going on around him. When this happens, he turns to his friends in the day treatment center or to the staff for guidance. At home his wife is available to direct him and to clarify matters that are confusing.

Mrs. Bates realizes that her husband is very dependent on her but she accepts this situation. She says her husband has always looked to her for advice and assistance. She refers to herself as the "family manager" and has told her husband that she will no longer tolerate his drinking. Unless he maintains sobriety, either he or she will move out of the house. She is a religious woman and a regular churchgoer; her husband accompanies her to church irregularly.

Mr. Bates is frequently assessed by the staff of the day treatment center, all of whom are aware of the usual signs of organic brain damage. Staff members use the acronym *JOCAM* in observing and assessing his behavior, since organic brain deficits are often indicated by disturbances in judgment, orientation, comprehension, affect, and memory. The extent of functional impairment can sometimes be correlated with the extent of organic damage, but function is greatly influenced by environmental conditions (Dreyer, Bailey, and Doucet, 1979). New situations and demands tend to increase the client's confusion, whereas familiar surroundings and social support decrease his functional impairment.

The staff consider Mr. Bates to be in a stable condition. For the present he is controlling his drinking, and the circumstances in which he lives are acceptable to him and his wife. Considering the adverse effects of years of excessive drinking, Mr. Bates is handling his disability well. Ongoing assessment is needed, however, to help the client and his wife maintain their current level of adaptation.

It is an agency policy that all clients attending the day treatment center be assessed by designated staff members who try to recognize changes in their clients' physical, social, and emotional status. For clients like Mr. Bates who have chronic disorders, a weekly progress note is written. This is in addition to a monthly summary that includes a formal mental status assessment. Daily notes are recorded for clients who are unstable or in acute distress.

MENTAL STATUS EXAMINATION OF MR. BATES

Appearance

The client is a sixty-year-old white male who looks his stated age. He is smooth shaven and his hair is thin; skin, hair, and fingernails appear clean. His clothing is somewhat worn but adequate. He dresses appropriately for the weather but says, "My wife always tells me what to wear." When sitting or standing the client seems relaxed. His posture does not show tension or rigidity. Usually the client presents himself as affable and smiling. He rarely initiates conversation but responds pleasantly to conversational overtures by other people. His voice is of normal volume, and there is no discernible speech impairment.

Weight is within normal range at present. Client joined a nutrition group at the day treatment center and has lost a substantial amount of weight in the last three months. As a result, his clothing looks too large for him. Despite this, the client says he is pleased with the weight loss and so is his wife.

He moves about rather easily. There is no sign of ataxia, tremor, or restricted movement. However, he tends to move slowly. The same slowness is evident in his speech patterns and reaction time. It is the consensus of the staff that this retardation is due to the client's efforts to concentrate to avoid making mistakes.

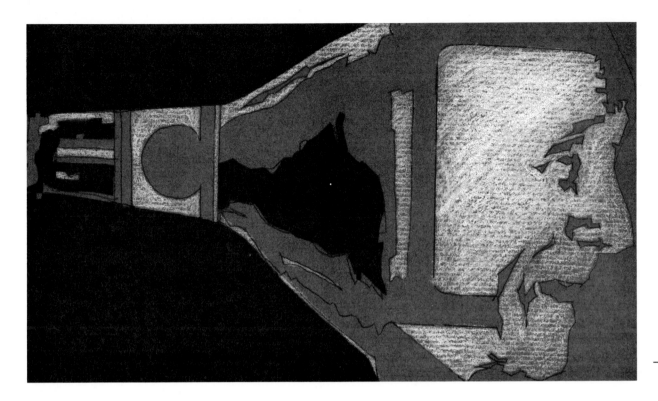

General Behavior

The client is congenial and cooperative in most interactions. He seems to fear giving offense and expresses himself in a self-effacing manner. When group decisions must be made, he is reluctant to vote or express an opinion. If projects are suggested, he is slow to join in. With encouragement he does participate and gives signs of enjoying himself. He has not been observed acting in a hostile or suspicious manner.

Affect and Mood

Mr. Bates's affect is somewhat flat; he seems neither euphoric nor depressed, and there are no extreme mood swings. The client seems responsive and eager to please, but he is more comfortable when discussing superficial topics. When interacting with some of the other members, he expresses anger indirectly through sarcasm. He does not show anger toward staff or toward day treatment members whom he considers to be his friends.

Thought Processes

There is no evidence of dissociated thinking, but the conversation of the client is sometimes tangential or circumstantial. Occasionally he can't find the word he wants and calls himself "stupid." Recent memory is somewhat impaired and he often must be reminded of the day treatment center schedule. He carries a small notebook and asks other people to write down reminders for him.

Perception

Mr. Bates shows no signs of perceptual disorders. Hallucinations and delusional thoughts are not apparent. His reality testing seems intact except for intervals of slight confusion.

Cognitive Functions

The client is oriented as to time, place, and person. Remote memory is good but recent recall is unreliable. Concentration is sufficient to permit him to work on crafts and to play cards. Judgment is sufficient to enable him to follow a schedule with help, attend group meetings, and assume minor responsibilities. His inability or unwillingness to deal with abstract thought makes it difficult to assess his capacity for insight, but he acknowledges that his past drinking has affected his memory.

PSYCHIATRIC AND NURSING DIAGNOSES

The following nursing and psychiatric diagnoses were made for Mr. Bates.

Nursing Diagnoses

Self-concept, disturbance in role performance (related to enforced retirement and dependence on others)

Thought processes, alterations in (related to confusion and difficulties in comprehension)

Multiaxial Psychiatric Diagnosis

Axis I   303.93   Alcohol dependence in remission
           310.10   Organic personality syndrome

Axis II   Dependent personality

Axis III   None

Axis IV   Code 2—Minimal severity

Axis V   Level 4—Moderate impairment in social and occupational functioning

Clinical assessment requires nurses to understand the relevance of data obtained through assessment, examination, and testing. The mental status examination that nurses use formally and informally provides general information about clients. Personality tests include the Minnesota Multiphasic Personality Inventory (MMPI), the Rorschach test, and the Thematic Apperception Test (TAT). Although personality tests are commonly administered by psychologists, data provided by these tests make a valuable contribution to client assessment, and the nature of these tests should be understood by nurses and other members of the health team.

Review Questions

1. What is holistic interaction? How does holistic interaction influence the practice of psychiatric mental health nursing?

2. What are the categories of adaptive and maladaptive defense mechanisms described by Vaillant?

3. What mechanisms do *you* employ in making adaptive responses to changing situations?

4. From your own experience or observation, give examples of successful adaptation to life demands.

5. From your own experience or observation, give examples of unsuccessful or questionable adaptation to life demands.

6. Describe the concepts of functional and dysfunctional patterns of adaptation.

7. Define the following terms as they are used in the Roy nursing model: role function; interdependence; focal behaviors; contextual behaviors; residual behaviors.

8. What is the major purpose of a mental status examination? What are the strengths and limitations of this assessment tool?

9. What are the purposes and implications of projective tests of personality?

References

Anderson, R. E., and Carter, I. 1978. *Human Behavior in the Social Environment: A Social Systems Approach*. Chicago: Aldine.

Carr, A. C. 1980. Psychological Testing of Personality. In *Comprehensive Textbook of Psychiatry*, 3rd ed., eds. H. I. Kaplan, A. M. Freedman, and B. J. Sadock. Baltimore: Williams & Wilkins.

Cohen, S. 1981. Mental Status Assessment. *American Journal of Nursing*, 81(8):1493–1518.

Cooper, C. L. 1981. *The Stress Check: Coping with Stresses of Life and Work*. Englewood Cliffs, N.J.: Prentice-Hall.

Dreyer, S.; Bailey, D.; and Doucet, W. 1979. *Guide to Nursing Management of Psychiatric Patients*. St. Louis: C. V. Mosby.

Dunn, H. 1959. High Level Wellness for Man and Society. *American Journal of Public Health*, 59:786–792.

Freedman, A. M.; Sadock, B. J.; and Kaplan, H. I. 1973. *Comprehensive Textbook of Psychiatry*. Baltimore: Williams & Wilkins.

Freud, A. 1948. *The Ego and Mechanisms of Defense*. London: Hogarth Press.

George, J. B. 1985. *Nursing Theories: The Base for Professional Nursing Practice*. Englewood Cliffs, N.J.: Prentice-Hall.

Goosen, G. M., and Bush, H. A. 1979. Adaptation: A Feedback Process. *Advances in Nursing Science*, 1(4): 51–65.

Guzetta, C. E. 1979. Relationship Between Stress and Learning. *Advances in Nursing Science*, 1(4):35–48.

Henderson, V. 1966. *The Nature of Nursing*. New York: Macmillan.

Holmes, T., and Rahe, R. 1967. The Social Readjustment Rating Scale. *Journal of Psychosomatic Research*, 11:213–218.

Horney, K. 1937. *The Neurotic Personality of Our Time*. New York: W. W. Norton.

Horney, K. 1950. *Neurosis and Human Growth*. New York: W. W. Norton.

Kaplan, H. I., and Sadock, M. D. 1980. Psychiatric Report, *and* Typical Signs and Symptoms of Psychiatric Illness. In *Comprehensive Textbook of Psychiatry*, 3rd ed., eds. H. I. Kaplan, A. M. Freedman, and B. J. Sadock. Baltimore: Williams & Wilkins.

Lazarus, P. 1977. Cognitive and Coping Process in Emotion. In *Stress and Coping: An Anthology*. New York: Columbia University Press.

MacKinnon, R. A. 1980. Psychiatric History and Mental Status Examination. In *Comprehensive Textbook of Psychiatry*, 3rd ed., eds. H. I. Kaplan, A. M. Freedman, and B. J. Sadock. Baltimore: Williams & Wilkins.

Maslow, A. H. 1968. *Toward a Psychology of Being*, 2nd ed. New York: Van Nostrand Reinhold.

Matarazzo, J. D. 1980. Psychological Assessment of Intelligence. In *Comprehensive Textbook of Psychiatry*, 3rd ed., eds. H. I. Kaplan, A. M. Freedman, and B. J. Sadock. Baltimore: Williams & Wilkins.

Mead, G. H. 1933. *Mind, Self, and Society*. Chicago: University of Chicago Press.

Mechanic, D. 1976. Stress, Illness, and Illness Behavior. *Journal of Human Stress*, 2(2):2–7.

Miller, J. R. 1980. Anticipatory Family Guidance. In *Family-Focused Care*, eds. J. R. Miller and E. H. Janosik. New York: McGraw-Hill.

Rogers, M. 1970. *The Theoretical Basis for Nursing*. Philadelphia: F. A. Davis.

Roy, C. 1970. Adaptation: A Conceptual Framework for Nursing. *Nursing Outlook*, 18(3):42–45.

Roy, C. 1974. The Roy Adaptation Model. In *Conceptual Models for Nursing Practice*, eds. C. Roy and J. P. Riehl. New York: Appleton-Century-Crofts.

Roy, C. ed. 1976. *Introduction to Nursing: An Adaptation Model*. Englewood Cliffs, N.J.: Prentice-Hall.

Roy, C. 1982. Historical Perspective of the Theoretical Framework for Classification of Nursing Diagnoses. In *Classification of Nursing Diagnoses: Proceedings of 3rd and 4th National Conferences*, eds. M. Kim, and D. Moritz. New York: McGraw-Hill.

Sullivan, H. S. 1953. *The Interpersonal Theory of Psychiatry*. New York: W. W. Norton.

Vaillant, G. 1977. *Adaptations to Life*. Boston: Little, Brown.

Supplementary Readings

Alston, J., and Levet, J. What's Happening? Practical Application of the Mental Status Exam. *Nurse Practitioner Journal* (1977):37–44.

Bower, F. L. *Distortions in Body Image in Illness and Disability*. New York: John Wiley & Sons, 1977.

Bower, F. L. *Normal Development of Body Image*. New York: John Wiley & Sons, 1977.

Cmich, D. E. Theoretical Perspectives of Holistic Health. *Journal of School Health*, 54(1984):30–32.

Dodd, J. Assessing Mental Status. *American Journal of Nursing*, 78(1978):1501–503.

Hagarty, B. M., and Packard, K. I. *Psychiatric Mental Health Assessment*. St. Louis: C. V. Mosby, 1984.

Kammerman, M. *Sensory Isolation and Personality Change*. Springfield, Ill.: Charles C Thomas, 1977.

Lamont, C. *The Philosophy of Humanism*. New York: Fredrick Ungar, 1967.

Rambo, B. J. *Adaptation Nursing: Assessment and Intervention*. Philadelphia: W. B. Saunders, 1984.

THEORETICAL BASES OF PSYCHIATRIC NURSING
Peplau's Theory
Leininger's Theory
Orem's Theory
Kinlein's Theory
Newman's Theory
Johnson's Theory
Aguilera's Theory
King's Theory

THE NURSING PROCESS
The Components of the Nursing Process
The Nursing Care Plan
Generic Nursing Care Plans

THE PRACTICE OF PSYCHIATRIC NURSING
The Anxious Client
The Delusional Client
The Demanding Client
The Hallucinating Client
The Angry Client
The Hypochondriacal Client
The Manipulative Client
The Regressed Client
The Ritualistic Client
The Suspicious Client
The Withdrawn Client

C H A P T E R

4

The Principles and Practice of Psychiatric Mental Health Nursing

Learning Objectives

After reading this chapter, the student should be able to:

1. Discuss the contributions of major nurse theorists to the field of psychiatric nursing.

2. Integrate concepts derived from major nursing theorists into the nursing process.

3. Use nursing care plan guidelines to develop plans that have a wide application in clinical practice.

4. Apply the nursing process to the care of clients with a variety of problem behaviors.

5. Determine which nursing interventions are appropriate for various problematic client behaviors.

Overview

The theoretical base of knowledge and therapeutic techniques used by psychiatric mental health nurses have evolved from several sources, including psychiatry, psychology, sociology, and, most recently, the work of nurse theorists. Some of the work of nurse theorists has been described in preceding chapters. The first section of this chapter provides a broader discussion of previously mentioned theorists and introduces the work of others who have provided guidelines for the psychiatric mental health nurse. The second section of this chapter describes components of the nursing process, a systematic method of identifying problems, planning and providing holistic care, and evaluating the effectiveness of the care provided. The final section of this chapter describes some problem behaviors and delineates the use of the nursing process in therapeutic relationships with clients who demonstrate these behaviors.

Canst thou not minister to a mind diseased
Pluck from the memory a rooted sorrow
Raze out the written troubles of the brain
And with some sweet oblivious antidote
Cleanse the stuffed bosom of that perilous stuff
Which weighs upon the heart.
WILLIAM SHAKESPEARE

75

During the 1960s and early 1970s, nursing therapy took place predominantly within inpatient settings. The nursing literature focused primarily on supportive therapy with dependent individuals. June Mellow (1969) was the first to advocate the role of the nurse as a major therapist rather than as an adjunct therapist to the psychiatrist. She used the term "nursing therapy" to refer to an approach to treatment that emphasized first meeting the immediate needs of the client, then conducting an investigative therapy based primarily on techniques borrowed from psychoanalysis.

Over the past two decades, nursing therapy has evolved as a specialized area of psychiatric nursing, and nurses have expanded their roles in outpatient settings as well. Psychiatric nurses now function as group and family therapists, as health educators, and as liaisons between inpatient and outpatient settings, between outpatient and other community facilities, and between psychiatric services and other services found in mental health facilities.

The practice of psychiatric nursing has its basis in psychiatry, psychology, sociology, and general nursing theory. Some theoretical approaches apply to all areas of nursing practice, while others are specific to care of the psychiatric client.

THEORETICAL BASES OF PSYCHIATRIC NURSING

Only in recent years have there been attempts to define nursing practice on a theoretical basis. This section presents some of the major theories that have been advanced to delineate the art and science of nursing and to provide guidelines for nursing practice and research.

Peplau's Theory

The model of nursing formulated by Hildegard Peplau stems from the interpersonal theorists, notably Sullivan, Horney, and Fromm. In this model, nursing is defined as an educative instrument, a maturing force that aims to promote forward movement of personality in the direction of creative, constructive, and productive personal and community living. According to Peplau, the core of nursing is the interpersonal relationship between the nurse and the client. This relationship serves as the mechanism within which nurses perform the many therapeutic tasks of their role (Peplau, 1965).

One characteristic of mental illness is the tendency for the person to repeat inappropriate or inept behavior and thus to perpetuate dysfunctional social interactions from which the behavior was derived. According to Peplau, nursing therapy, particularly that related to the *milieu*, or environment surrounding the client, should consist of recognizing these recurring problematic behavior patterns and disrupting them within the nurse-client relationship (Peplau, 1968). Nursing should be viewed as one way of *not* repeating, perpetuating, or reinforcing the cultural and interpersonal experiences that have already been damaging.

Peplau emphasized the utilization of *themes* in nursing situations. The first step in developing a therapeutic environment is for the nurse to become aware of how she feels about the client and then inquire into how the situation looks to the client. By finding out who and what interacts in a particular situation, the nurse can identify a broad pattern of themes of interaction that can then be used as guidelines for intervention. Examples of themes that may be present include respect and disrespect, safety and security, loneliness, and mutual withdrawal (Peplau, 1968).

Peplau suggested that the purpose of nursing care of psychiatric clients is to assist them in their struggle toward full development of their potential for productive living in the community. For a nursing strategy to be considered psychotherapeutic, it must have a demonstrable impact on the inappropriate or dysfunctional behavior of the client. The strategy must be used persistently and repeatedly in situations where a specific behavior is presented by the client and observed by the nurse.

Leininger's Theory

Madeleine Leininger's (1978) major contribution to nursing theory has been in the area of transcultural nursing. She has delineated several areas that need to be assessed if nurses are to make an impact on clients whose cultural background is different from their own. Leininger advocates making a broad, in-depth assessment of the client's patterns and lifestyles, with specific attention to cultural values, norms, and experiences regarding health and caring behaviors. The client's cultural taboos, myths, world view, and ethnocentric tendencies should also be noted. The nurse should have a clear understanding of both the folk customs and the professional health care system within the client's culture.

For Leininger, the essence of nursing is *caring,* and transcultural nursing demands the identification of caring nursing behaviors. Caring acts and decisions make the crucial difference in curing outcomes. In Leininger's view, caring is not only essential for effective therapy but also for self-actualization and, indeed, for human survival. Caring behaviors place heavy emphasis on supportive measures and helping activities extended to others in need. Caring behaviors also recognize the need to provide care to oneself. In some cultures, caring appears to be even more important than curing. Caring is a service that reflects concern, compassion, stress alleviation, nurturance, surveillance, and cultural considerations. Additional material on transcultural issues in nursing is presented in Chapter 19.

Orem's Theory

The model of nursing developed by Dorothy Orem (1971) delineates a framework for the nursing process that focuses primarily on assisting the individual toward health. This general theory of nursing has three components: (1) health self-care, or activities that individuals personally initiate on their own behalf based on their knowledge, attributes, and skills; (2) deficits in self-care or in caring for dependents, which create a need for nursing help; and (3) nursing systems that assist a person to exercise health self-care. These methods of assistance can include providing support, providing an environment that promotes personal development, and teaching.

Orem's general theory can be used to explain virtually all instances in which individuals and groups can benefit from nursing interventions. Orem's theory of self-care deficits is broad enough to express both the science and art of nursing.

Kinlein's Theory

Closely related to Orem's theoretical approach is the self-care concept of Lucille Kinlein (1977). For Kinlein, each client is an inexhaustible source of challenge, possessing unique knowledge, motivation, goals, understanding, ability, and perspective. The uniqueness of each client poses a challenge to the creativity of the professional nurse. When a client tells the nurse about a health need, the nurse must prescribe self-care measures based on a scientific body of knowledge, on an analysis of the nurse-client relationship, and on an appreciation of the client's individuality. These prescriptions should effect a change in the client's self-care priorities.

For Kinlein, the nurse-client relationship is an independent dyad that stands free of institutions and from other health professionals. The goal of the nurse-client interaction is to meet the client's needs to his or her own satisfaction.

Newman's Theory

According to Margaret Newman (1979), health is a synthesis of opposites: disease and nondisease. By this definition, health encompasses conditions that have traditionally been described as illness or pathology. In Newman's view, these pathological conditions can be considered as manifestations of the total pattern of the individual, and the pattern demonstrated by the disease can be regarded as a clue to what is going on in the person's life, the dynamics of which the person may not be able to communicate in any other way. Because this total pattern exists before the changes brought about by the disease are evident, removal of the pathology will not change the pattern.

In Newman's framework, disease is not something to be "gotten rid of" but something to be understood and experienced and regarded as a teacher. Rather than emphasizing the curing of an illness, Newman perceives illness as a factor that aids in the integration of the self and frees energy for an expanding consciousness. She sees health as the totality of life process that is evolving toward the expanded consciousness.

Expanded consciousness, according to Newman, involves awareness of movement, time, and space to facilitate the acquisition of a higher realm of understanding and feeling. The higher the level of consciousness, the more energy that is available. In Newman's view, the goal of nursing is not to make people well or to prevent illness but to assist people to use the power that is within them as they evolve toward higher levels of consciousness.

Johnson's Theory

Dorothy Johnson has created a behavioral systems model for nursing practice. In a systems theory context, Johnson has identified eight subsystems of behavior relating to social interaction. These include the affiliative, sexual, dependency, restorative, ingestive, eliminative, achievement, and aggressive protective subsystems. In Johnson's view, the nurse should use these components to assess the client's needs and to formulate nursing interventions. The success of nursing intervention can be measured in terms of the appropriateness of resulting behaviors.

Although this is a behavioral theory, the nurse must also have an in-depth understanding of interpersonal and developmental theories in order to make a complete assessment of the client's needs. The goals of Johnson's model are to make the client comfortable, to assist the client in adapting to an illness, to maintain the individual's developmental level of functioning, and to use behavior modification to help attain the client's expressed goals. Nursing interventions may include (1) repairing structural units (teaching new skills such as parenting), (2) temporarily imposing external regulatory or control measures (such as setting limits for behavior with manipulative clients), and (3) supplying essential environmental conditions or resources (providing contact between the young child and the mother in order to nurture the affiliative system) (Grubbs, 1974).

Aguilera's Theory

Donna Aguilera's (1982) contribution to nursing theory has been in the area of crisis intervention. In a period of crisis, three significant factors determine whether a state of *disequilibrium* replaces *equilibrium*: (1) realistic perception of the event, (2) adequate situational support, and (3) adequate coping skills. Assessment of the three balancing factors can provide direction and a basis for problem clarification and resolution.

King's Theory

Imogene King's (1971) model of nursing draws on both systems and interactional theory. She conceptualizes nursing as a process of action and reaction, interaction and transaction between individuals and groups in social systems. The perception and judgment of nurses leads to their actions; simultaneously, the perceptions and judgments of clients lead to

their actions. This continuous dynamic process is expressed by verbal and nonverbal behavior, resulting in reactions by both nurse and client and subsequent interactions. The goal of *transaction* is to assist individuals or groups to achieve health (defined as a continuous adaptation to stresses in the internal and external environment) or to adjust to health problems. Transaction occurs only when a reciprocal relationship is established with mutually defined health goals. Both parties must be active participants for a transaction to take place; at times transaction is impossible, as in caring for the comatose client.

According to King, there are three levels on which nurses perform their functions within social systems: the individual, the group, and society. The unifying element is human behavior. In assessing behavior, nurses make use of words, gestures, and actions to communicate information and establish relationships. Thus, analysis of verbal communication and of the natural situation provides a means for identifying underlying concepts that have meaning for the nurse and the client.

The eight nursing theories presented here are summarized in Table 4-1. It is the task of the individual nurse to study, evaluate, and incorporate those theoretical concepts that provide the best guidance for relationships with clients. This conceptual integration develops over time as the nurse gains experience in the mental health setting. It is not immediately acquired. Regardless of the theoretical framework being used, there are several interventions that are mandatory when working with psychiatric clients with particular presenting behaviors. The use of the nursing process with clients demonstrating problem behaviors is presented in the next section.

THE NURSING PROCESS

Because of the wide range of problems presented by clients, nurses are required to be adept at problem-solving techniques. Four barriers to efficient problem solving that nurses must overcome in order to deal effectively with client care and management include (Sorensen, 1979):

1. Failing to specify goals and purposes.
2. Jumping to conclusions about the cause of a problem and then proceeding on a course of action that may or may not solve the problem.
3. Plunging into action before considering relevant alternatives.
4. Failing to consider the probable consequences of a course of action.

Table 4-1.
Contributions of Major Nurse Theorists and the
Implications for Nursing Practice

Theorist	Major Element	Nursing Implications
Peplau	Interpersonal relationship	One-to-one relationship; observation of themes; disruption of problem behaviors
Leininger	Caring	Transcultural understanding; use of caring behaviors
Orem	Self-care	Identification of deficits in self-care; fostering of self-care abilities
Kinlein	Interaction	Focus on independent dyad of client and nurse; prescription of self-care measures that meet needs to client's satisfaction
Newman	Expansion of consciousness	Appreciation of person's total experience; assistance toward expansion of consciousness rather than prevention or curing
Johnson	Behavioral systems	Encouragement of appropriate adaptation to illness; use of behavior modification; provision of external structure and resources
Aguilera	Crisis resolution	Guidance toward accurate perception of events; provision of situational support; increase in coping skills
King	Interaction	Focus on action, reaction, interaction, and transaction to achieve goals of health and adjustment

78

The use of a systematic problem-solving process can help nurses overcome these barriers and make logical decisions concerning client care. The systematic process that facilitates problem solving is termed the *nursing process.*

The nursing process involves four sequential, interrelated, interdependent steps: (1) identifying the client's health problems (making nursing diagnoses), (2) formulating plans to solve the problem, (3) implementing the plans or delegating implementation to others, and (4) evaluating the effectiveness of the plans in resolving the problems that have been identified. Implicit in the nursing process is the need to involve the client and the family and the need to individualize the approach for each client's particular needs (Kozier and Erb, 1983).

The purpose of the nursing process is to provide direction and structure for the delivery of nursing care to meet the health needs of the individual, the family, and the community. The four steps of the process provide the organizational structure necessary to accomplish its purpose.

The nursing process model has several benefits. Its flexibility and versatility make it applicable to a wide variety of health care recipients. By being client-centered, the nursing process model addresses the individual needs of each client. It also creates a health data base, identifies actual or potential health problems, establishes priorities for nursing action, and defines specific nursing responsibility. Because care is planned and organized, the process encourages innovative nursing care and provides alternatives for nursing action. In addition, it develops nursing autonomy and fosters nursing accountability (Carlson, 1982).

The Components of the Nursing Process

The four steps of the nursing process can be identified as assessment, planning, implementation, and evaluation. These components are diagrammed in Figure 4-1.

ASSESSMENT An *assessment* is a deliberate, systematic, and logical collection of data. Data collection regarding the health status of the client begins with the initial contact. In addition to observing and interviewing the client, the nurse should acquire supplementary information from family members, from previous charts and records, and from participating members of the health team. The adequacy of an assessment is largely dependent on the data base collected. It is often necessary to accept the fact that early data collection may be less than complete. The compilation of information about any client must always be ongoing and continuous. The following categories of information are helpful to bear in mind when gathering data:

Figure 4-1. The nursing process is client-centered.

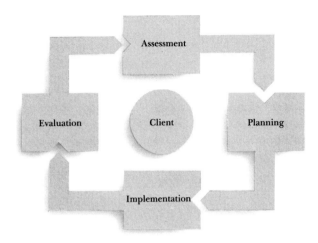

- Physical, psychological, and mental status of the client.
- Client's perception of the current situation.
- Impact of social, familial, and environmental variables on the client.
- Present habits, activities, and lifestyle of the client.
- Previous habits, activities, and lifestyle of the client.

After the assessment is completed, the nurse assigns meaning to the data by writing a statement about the client's problems—that is, the client's specific alteration or potential alteration in health status, which is called a *nursing diagnosis*. Nursing diagnoses are concise terms that accurately and effectively describe client needs, problems, and objectives. According to Neal et al. (1980), making a nursing diagnosis requires an interpretation of various data obtained concerning the client. Information about the client is clarified, validated, and categorized so that connecting relationships can be recognized.

Until recently "diagnosis" was a charged and forbidden word in nursing. A literal definition of the word, with no qualifier preceding it, conveys the idea that one is seeking knowledge or information about what needs to be corrected, what is causing difficulty, or what is interfering with normal functions. In this sense, the nurse can use the word "diagnosis" as effectively as can the physician or any other person who is trying to discover where efforts must be applied to perform a service for the benefit of the client. The difference lies in the purpose of the diagnosis. Whereas the physician is concerned with diagnosing the *cause* of illness so that he or she may treat the underlying pathological process, the nurse is more concerned with identifying the client's presenting problems.

The nursing diagnosis may be *descriptive*, as in "limited response to auditory and tactile stimuli"; it may be *etiologic,* as in "lessened intestinal sounds"; it may be primarily *physiological,* as in "inability to void"; or it may be *psychological,* as in "feelings of powerlessness."

PLANNING The purpose of *planning* client care is to develop guidelines for helping the client attain or maintain the state of optimal wellness. The plan is based on the nursing diagnoses and is designed to build on the client's strengths that have been identified in the assessment phase.

Planning includes consideration of various goals, objectives, and expected outcomes that may be long-term, short-term, or a combination of both. *Goals* are statements of the desired, achieveable outcomes to be attained within a predicted time span, given the presenting situation and available resources. Goals give direction and purpose for nursing action. Short-term goals are those whose focus is immediate achievement; they are probably the most concrete and tangible since they deal with expectations for the here and now. Long-term goals spell out the final desired outcome; they give the overall direction for care.

It is important to include the client in the process of establishing goals. Goals and objectives should be behaviorally stated in terms of what the client will be doing or of what the expected outcome will be for the client rather than for the nurse. The most usual way of expressing client-centered goals, objectives, or outcomes is to state simply that "The client will ———." It is important for nurses to realize that the terminology does not denote any degree of coercion but merely outlines identifiable, objective goals. As much as possible, the goals, objectives, and outcomes expected for the client should be specific. Whenever possible, a predetermined standard of measurement should be stated. For example, it might be noted that a socially isolated client will arrange to visit a friend once a week or attend a club meeting. Usually at least one goal, objective, or expected outcome should accompany every nursing diagnosis. These may be of a long- or short-term nature and should be so described.

IMPLEMENTATION *Implementation* involves putting into action the nursing interventions that have been planned. To *intervene* means to "come between." *Nursing intervention*, sometimes called nursing care, consists of actions taken by the nurse to assist a client. The nurse "comes between" a problem and its resolution by carrying out actions directed toward solving the problem.

Nursing interventions include all the nursing measures used to achieve the goals, objectives, and outcomes developed from the nursing diagnoses that in turn emerged from data collection and assessment. Some nursing interventions help clients achieve short-term goals. In turn, the achievement of short-term goals eventually facilitates the attainment of long-term objectives and outcomes.

Nursing interventions should be described simply and concisely in the care plan. A statement such as "encourage socialization" is less useful for other staff members than specific interventions such as "accompany client to morning meetings" or "invite client to go for daily walk." General instructions such as "Reward," "Discourage," and "Reinforce" are more apt to be clearly understood and consistently offered if they are fully described.

Involving the client to the greatest extent possible is an important part of nursing care. It is well documented in nursing literature that expressions of client satisfaction are directly proportional to clients' involvement in their care. Client involvement may entail more of the nurse's time, but in the long run the extra time expenditure is worthwhile and generally helps the client to become more independent.

To be helpful in assisting the client in meeting mutually established goals, nursing interventions should be (Sorenson and Luckman, 1979):

1. Consistent with the nursing care plan and the medical plan of care.

2. Designed to solve problems.

3. Therapeutically safe.

4. Specific to the nursing diagnosis.

5. Individualized to the client's needs, resources, and abilities.

6. Developed to use appropriate health facility resources.

7. Scheduled to coincide with the client's need for rest, exercise, food, sleep, recreation, and other activities.

8. Organized to allow both the client and the family to participate.

9. Used to teach the client self-care and avoidance of complications and setbacks.

10. Modified in accordance with changes in the client's condition and situation.

EVALUATION *Evaluation* is the process of determining to what extent the goals of nursing care have been attained. Sometimes it is possible to evaluate a client's response to a nursing measure after 24 hours. At other times longer periods of several days to several weeks may be needed. Evaluation of the client's response is essential for reassessment, reordering of priorities, and ongoing revision of the care plan.

If the client's problems and goals have been identified in precise terms, evaluation is relatively simple. There are a number of possible outcomes of the evaluation:

1. The patient has responded as expected.

2. Short-term goals have been achieved, but long-term goals have not yet been met.

3. No goals have been achieved.

4. New problems have arisen.

If some progress toward desired goals has been made, no major modification of the nursing care plan may be indicated. If little or no progress is discernible, there are salient questions to be asked. A basic question is whether major revision or merely a difference in emphasis is needed. Appropriate issues to be considered include:

■ Was the problem correctly identified?

■ Are the goals/objectives realistic for the client at this time?

■ What factors affected the attainment of the goals?

■ Is a reordering of priorities necessary?

■ Are there alternative measures that might be adopted to reach the goals or objectives?

■ Have the nursing measures emerged naturally and coherently, based on nursing assessment, diagnosis, and planning?

■ Based on evaluation of client responses, what aspects of the nursing care need reassessment and revision? What aspects do not need modification or revision?

The evaluation is carried out in a purposeful and organized way. It is an intellectual activity in which the client is assessed in terms of previously identified goals. Both the client and the nurse should participate whenever possible.

During the evaluation, the nurse may consider a number of questions: What factors affected the attainment of the goal? Was the problem correctly identified? If the problem was not resolved, why not? Was the nursing intervention directed toward the stated goals? What other nursing interventions would be more likely to assist the client to attain the stated goals?

The nursing process may seem complicated, and in some ways perhaps it is, since human behavior is complex. On the other hand, following the nursing process is less laborious than describing it and using the nursing process elevates problem solving to professional levels. Once the fundamental skills are learned, they can be carried out easily and confidently throughout each step in the process.

The Nursing Care Plan

The *nursing care plan* is a written statement that documents the evidence of the nursing process. The care plan has several purposes:

1. To indicate the objectives of nursing intervention. The objective of nursing care should include both short-term and long-term goals for the expected outcomes of client behavior. These are based on the nurse's assessment of the client and the nursing diagnosis. All objectives must also take into consideration the aim of any medical therapy.

2. To provide a guide to client-centered care. One purpose of making a nursing care plan is to provide a guide for client-centered, rather than task-centered, care. The plan provides information about the problems and needs of the client and suggestions about how to meet them. The client is always considered first. The disease is important only to the extent that it affects the physical and emotional aspects of nursing care.

3. To provide a means of communication. The written nursing care plan can be a valuable tool for everyone involved in client care because it provides consistent information concerning the ongoing

nursing interventions. In this way, the plan promotes a program of continuous individualized care.

4. To provide a guide for supervision. Because the plan gives information about what nursing care is needed and how it is to be given, it provides the supervisory nurse with a guide for making certain that the staff provides each client with proper nursing care.

5. To provide a basis for evaluating nursing care. Because the nursing profession does not yet agree on a specific definition of nursing care, nurses tend to evaluate their care on the basis of technical proficiency alone. Yet, the nurse should evaluate both the quality and quantity of nursing care provided by co-workers. A well-made nursing care plan defines the care for the individual client. By referring to this plan, the nurse can ask, "How well did we meet the needs of the client as identified in the nursing care plan?"

The following questions can be used as a guide for evaluating the nursing care plan:

1. Do the diagnoses reflect actual or potential alterations in the health status of the client?

2. Are the diagnoses logically derived from the data available?

3. Are the diagnoses stated in nursing terms, or are they medical diagnoses?

4. Are the diagnoses merely stating subjective and objective data, or do they reflect the client's basic needs?

5. Do the goals relate to the identified problem?

6. Is the short-term goal a required step in reaching the stated long-term goal?

7. Are the goal statements client-centered rather than nurse-centered?

8. Are the goals relevant, understandable, measurable, behaviorally stated, achievable, and attainable?

9. Are the interventions specific?

10. Are the interventions related to the identified goals?

11. Are the interventions clearly stated so that they are understood by team members?

12. Are the interventions written in nursing terms?

13. Is the plan of care individualized?

14. Does the plan provide for continuity of care?

15. Is the plan clearly and concisely stated so as to be understood by all team members?

16. Does the plan provide direction for those caring for the client?

Generic Nursing Care Plan: The Client Who Exhibits Delusional Thinking

Date	Assessment: Nursing Diagnosis	Planning: Goals/Outcomes	Implementation: Nursing Orders/Interventions	Evaluation
	Thought processes, alterations in	Client will maintain control and avoid behaviors upsetting to others.	Employ suicide precautions.	
	Sensory-perceptual alteration	Client will begin to verbalize feelings instead of enacting them.	Monitor eating and activity patterns.	
	Home maintenance management, impaired		Assess *general nature* of delusions.	
	Anxiety	Client will establish a trusting relationship with a care provider.	Note events preceding manifestations of delusional thinking.	
		Client will manifest improved orientation to reality.	Note and record behaviors indicative of delusional thinking.	
		Client will manifest lower levels of anxiety.	Note manifestations of sensory misperceptions.	
			Do not explore delusions in depth.	
			Offer empathy but reinforce reality.	
			Provide limits for inappropriate actions and discussions.	
			Interpret delusions as reactions to stress and anxiety.	
			Encourage family involvement to promote understanding and support for the client.	
			Explain medication regimen (rationale, therapeutic effects, precautions, side effects).	

Revised   Discontinued   Continued   Reviewed

17. Will the plan allow for evaluation of nursing strategies and interventions?

18. Is the plan realistic?

Generic nursing care plans that can be used as a basis for planning are provided next. These plans are designed to be used as guidelines only and must be individualized for each client.

Generic Nursing Care Plans

With the development of officially recognized nursing diagnoses, it has become possible to adopt a standard format for care plans. The specific care plan evolves from a comprehensive, ongoing assessment leading to nursing diagnoses that then become the basis for nursing interventions. The format of generic care plans may vary from one facility to another, but most plans have the following characteristics in common:

1. They use the four stages of the nursing process.

2. Goal setting arises from problems defined by the nursing diagnoses; desired outcomes proceed from the stated goals.

3. Problem-solving actions are presented as nursing orders or nursing interventions implemented on behalf of the client.

4. Implementation of nursing orders or interventions undergoes ongoing evaluation.

5. Evaluation of nursing orders or interventions results in a decision to continue, discontinue, or revise the specific nursing order or intervention.

The trend toward use of generic care plans is part of an attempt to provide clear, concise information that will facilitate the therapeutic nursing regimen. Generic care plans are not all-purpose guides, but when adopted by an agency or facility they can bring a high degree of consistency and professionalism to record keeping. Four examples of generic nursing care plans are provided here. They suggest some likely nursing diagnoses and appropriate nursing interventions for four types of behavioral manifestations displayed by clients. It should be remembered that any generic care plan must be tailored to the needs of the specific client and must adhere to the format approved by the facility providing care.

Generic Nursing Care Plan: The Client Who Exhibits Hypervigilance and Suspiciousness

Date	Assessment: Nursing Diagnosis	Planning: Goals/Outcomes	Implementation: Nursing Orders/Interventions	Evaluation
	Alteration in comfort Thought processes, alteration in Social isolation due to egocentricity and extreme distrust Anxiety	Client will be able to distinguish objective (external) from subjective (internal) reasons for suspiciousness. Client will manifest less hypervigilance and will show improved ability to interact with others. Client will establish a trusting relationship with one or more care providers.	Assess potential for aggressive or violent behavior. Avoid excessive friendliness or extreme aloofness. Avoid behavior such as whispering that suggests secrecy or concealment. Discourage competitive activities. Communicate clearly and simply; avoid confrontation or argument. Provide brief frequent contacts. Avoid physical contact with the client. Maintain a consistent, predictable schedule. Do not mix medication with food.	

Revised   Discontinued   Continued   Reviewed

Generic Nursing Care Plan: The Client Who Exhibits Hyperactivity

Date	Assessment: Nursing Diagnosis	Planning: Goals/Outcomes	Implementation: Nursing Orders/Interventions	Evaluation
	Health maintenance, alterations in Nutrition, alterations in: less than body requirements Fluid volume deficit, potential Self-care deficit: feeding, bathing, dressing Sleep pattern disturbance Home maintenance management, impaired	Client will maintain adequate physical health. Client will maintain reality orientation. Client will express recognition of the need for a protected environment. Client will express understanding of need for medication, side effects, and necessary precautions.	Set limits on intrusive or disruptive behavior. Present limit setting as protective for the client. Observe and monitor activity level. Observe nutritional habits. Monitor intake and output. Weigh daily; note signs of dehydration and weight loss. Decrease external stimuli. Negotiate and set regular bedtime. Offer moderate, noncompetitive physical activity. Make "finger foods" available. Encourage adequate fluid intake. Give simple, brief, clear messages. Seclude if necessary to reduce overstimulation and protect client from exhaustion. Involve the spouse in health teaching and anticipatory guidance.	

Revised   Discontinued   Continued   Reviewed

Generic Nursing Care Plan: The Client Who Exhibits Self-destructive Behavior

Date	Assessment: Nursing Diagnosis	Planning: Goals/Outcomes	Implementation: Nursing Orders/Interventions	Evaluation
	Injury, potential for Grieving, dysfunctional Sleep pattern disturbance Coping, ineffectual individual	Client's health and safety will be maintained. Client will not engage in self-destructive acts or gestures. Client will engage in active grieving. Client will begin to develop alternative coping behaviors. Client will recognize and utilize available support networks.	Assess suicide potential, present and past; assess lethality of plan. Initiate suicide precautions: Check every 15 minutes, place on 1:1 supervision p.r.n., seclude or restrain to ensure safety. Explore underlying sadness and client's perception of loss. Encourage verbalization of feeling. Help client realize that self-destructive actions only intensify feelings of frustration and depression. Help client realize the danger of impulsive behavior. Negotiate an agreement to seek help from specific sources of support whenever self-destructive impulses are activated. Assess response of significant others to client's self-destructive behavior. Observe for signs of physical injury: lacerations, burns, etc. Encourage problem solving and alternative means of coping.	

Revised   Discontinued   Continued   Reviewed

84

THE PRACTICE OF PSYCHIATRIC NURSING

The application of theoretical models and the nursing process to actual nursing care situations is the focus of the rest of this chapter. As each type of problem behavior is discussed, guidelines are provided for assessment, planning, implementation, and evaluation.

The Anxious Client

Anxiety is a subjective phenomenon that everyone experiences to a lesser or greater degree when confronted with situations that are perceived as threatening. It is an internal response to danger whose specific nature is unknown, and it can occur when people face circumstances that previously provoked anxiety or confront certain new situations or new roles. Anxiety may vary from mild feelings of uneasiness and nervousness to acute feelings of dread and apprehension. The degree of anxiety depends on the individual's evaluation of the severity of the threat. Intervention is indicated if the anxiety is of such a degree that the functioning of the individual is impaired. If not dealt with adequately in its early stages, anxiety tends to increase.

Normal anxiety is a reaction that is proportionate to the actual threat, that does not involve repression or other defensive indications of intrapsychic conflict, and that does not require dysfunctional behavior for its management. Normal anxiety can be dealt with on the level of conscious awareness or can be relieved if the situation is altered. Extreme, *dysfunctional anxiety* is a reaction that is disproportionate to the threat or danger. It may involve defense mechanisms such as repression, denial, projection, and displacement. In some instances, severe anxiety may be managed by such means as inhibitions or physiological and psychological symptoms.

ASSESSMENT A variety of behaviors are indicative of the anxious state. Clients may appear to be vague, uneasy, tense, nervous, or apprehensive. This may be apparent from the client's body language (sweating, pacing, jaw clenching) or from her verbal mannerisms (slow, rapid, or evasive speech). Anxious clients may complain of feeling helpless, alone, insecure, and rejected. At times they may act sarcastic, angry, irritable, or tearful or they may use derogatory or belittling remarks. Incessant talking, excessive demands on others' time and attention, and repeated questioning of the dependability and sincerity of others are also frequently seen in anxious clients.

Somatic symptoms of anxiety may include restlessness, increased muscular tension, breathlessness, chest pain, heart palpitations, tightness in the throat, sweating, headache, fatigue, and insomnia. Anxiety frequently affects the gastrointestinal tract, producing nausea, vomiting, diarrhea, and loss of appetite.

PLANNING Appropriate nursing goals for the anxious client should include the following:

1. To intervene when the client is unable to handle her anxiety.

2. To reduce anxiety in order to increase the client's comfort.

3. To help the client recognize that his behaviors are related to anxiety.

4. To assist the client in gaining insight into the reasons for her anxiety.

5. To help the client accept the fact that anxiety is an inevitable part of life and learn to tolerate and benefit from mild degrees of anxiety.

IMPLEMENTATION Clients' anxiety will only increase if they are urged to apply more insight to a situation than they can deal with at a given time. For insight to be possible, it is first necessary to reduce anxiety to manageable levels. After anxiety lessens, nurses can help clients make necessary connections between anxiety-producing situations, the feelings engendered by those situations, and the behaviors

Table 4-2.
Problems Associated with Anxiety and Suggested Nursing Interventions

Identified Problems	Nursing Interventions
Insecurity	1. Accept the client's anxiety without being provoked into sharing it. 2. Be willing to listen. Just talking may help the client alleviate his anxiety. 3. Recognize and acknowledge the client's distress and discomfort. 4. Provide control by a matter-of-fact attitude that combines structure with empathy. 5. Assess the situation from the client's point of view; avoid evaluating stress levels from personal standards.
Confusion	1. Identify behaviors that betray the anxiety the client is experiencing. 2. Help the client identify and describe her feelings and locate the source of distress. 3. Endeavor to help the client realize what she was thinking or doing before the anxious behaviors became apparent. 4. Explore what actually happened to the client and what she expected to happen. Discuss differences between expectations and reality. 5. List the sequence of other experiences that produced anxiety. 6. List the sequence of behaviors that have brought relief before.
Agitation	1. Provide outlets for expending energy by arranging activity or diversion. Suggest motor behaviors, such as walking and pacing. 2. Administer appropriate medication when needed, as prescribed. 3. Help the client talk when he is ready, do not force or probe. 4. Validate feelings the client has about his immediate situations.
Cognitive distortion	1. Offer feedback to correct thought distortions. 2. Relate new experiences to familiar ones to increase client's insight. 3. Help client discover relationships between feelings, thoughts, and actions. 4. Help client learn from experiences with difficult situations. Help client learn to tolerate some anxiety. Replace the concepts of self that cause anxiety with concepts of self that are realistic and functional. 5. Use anticipatory planning to prepare client for similar situation in the future.

85

prompted by the underlying feelings. Anxiety that is not recognized by nurses may be dealt with in ways that only increase clients' discomfort. Knowledge of the various ways that anxiety is expressed will guide nurses in helping clients cope with anxiety, find relief, and avoid deterioration. During the implementation phase it may also be necessary to seek the advice of other health professionals or to refer clients for more specialized help. Various problems associated with anxiety and suggested nursing interventions are described in Table 4-2.

*Now-a-days we can see as never before that the peril which threatens
all of us comes not from nature but from man and the psyches of the
individual and the mass. The psychic aberration of man is the danger.
Everything depends upon whether or not our psyche functions
properly. If certain persons lose their heads now-a-days, a hydrogen
bomb will go off.*
C. J. JUNG, MEMORIES, DREAMS, REFLECTIONS

86

EVALUATION A number of factors should be considered if an anxious client does not respond to nursing intervention. It may be that a nurse's own anxiety interfered with the ability to reduce the client's anxiety. A certain amount of anxiety and emotional insecurity is present in everyone, including nurses. An anxious client may heighten anxiety in a nurse. It is important for nurses to be aware of their own responses in order to remain effective in such situations.

Timing is also important in dealing with anxious clients. The failure to recognize anxiety in a client or the failure to intervene promptly and appropriately before anxiety escalates to panic may be other reasons why a client does not respond to nursing interventions.

The Delusional Client

Delusional individuals hold false, fixed beliefs that are maintained despite evidence to the contrary. Their delusions are attempts to deal with conflicts, problems, and stresses and may also be used as a symbolic means of communication or as a means of escaping reality. Confusion, misinterpretation, and distortion of reality help preserve delusions.

Delusions are thought to result from the displacement of unacceptable (ego-dystonic) feelings from the objects or individuals that caused them toward other, less-frightening objects or individuals. They are sometimes used to increase a person's self-esteem or to minimize the power the client thinks others possess.

Two layers of expression and belief characterize a delusion: the material or content that is verbalized and the material or content that the client actually believes. A delusion may be based on actual childhood experiences. Many delusions reflect the client's cultural orientation. For example, religious delusions are less common today than they were in times when religious beliefs were more strongly held. Many delusions today have a pseudoscientific flavor borrowed from notions of the space age. The delusion may also be an attempt at allegorical or symbolic communication of ideas.

Regardless of the question of truth, a belief that has its foundation in experience and expresses elements of the personality carries a strong sense of reality for the client. Such beliefs cannot be changed without first changing the client's external experience and making reality more acceptable to her.

ASSESSMENT Delusional clients often have difficulty in admitting their own errors, and they take pride in intellectualizing and in being considered correct. They are often adept at manipulating people and facts and tend to think in literal terms. They often resent being dominated, yet they themselves are often dominating and provocative, patronizing toward others, and inclined to misinterpret others' speech and actions. They are sensitive to minor injustices and are often resentful and hypercritical of health care personnel. Testing to determine others' trustworthiness may also occur within the context of a delusion.

PLANNING Appropriate nursing goals for assisting the delusional client should include the following:

1. To assist the client in recognizing the distortions of reality and to gain a realistic perception of himself.

Table 4-3.
Problems Associated with Delusional Thinking and Suggested Nursing Interventions

Identified Problems	Nursing Interventions
Insecurity	1. Demonstrate acceptance of the client as a worthwhile individual, without judgment. 2. Avoid demands for drastic change as long as behavior is not harmful or overtly distructive. 3. Respond to feelings indicated by the tone of the client's comments. 4. Allow expression of negative emotions without fear of punishment or rejection. 5. Contribute to security by being consistent. Let the client know what behavior is acceptable or unacceptable. 6. Make your identity and professional position clear. Describe your role to avoid becoming part of the delusional system. 7. Satisfy the client's need for control by allowing as many choices as possible over routines and activities.
Autistic communication	1. Ask the client to explain the meaning of his communication in order to understand what he is saying or experiencing. 2. Describe clearly and distinctly the reasons for hospitalization or treatment. 3. Reinforce the appropriate and non-threatening nature of reality. 4. Avoid debate or argument of any kind. Accept the client's right to feel as he does without necessarily approving. 5. Avoid exploring delusional content or displaying great interest in it. 6. Set an example of reality-based thinking and acting with clear and consistent communication. 7. Divert focus from delusions to discussion of reality. 8. Identify themes of client's delusions (e.g., persecution, grandiosity, religiosity, etc.). 9. Do not leave openings that permit encouragement of the delusion. 10. Search for underlying needs expressed by delusional thinking.
Inclusion of the nurse in delusional thinking	1. Take no action without the client's knowledge. 2. Contact no one about the client without her permission. 3. Do not make decisions about care without including the client. 4. If client believes substances are poisoned, permit her to watch others as they ingest or serve food or medicines. 5. Avoid tasting the client's food or medicines to convince her that substances are harmless. This does not reassure, but merely takes away client's defense mechanism and may cause her to include the nurse in the delusional pattern.

2. To help the client find more satisfactory ways of relating to others.

3. To accept the reality of the client's belief in the delusional ideation but to reject its reality.

4. To create an atmosphere in which the client may safely examine reality.

5. To provide opportunities for corrective experiences in emotional relationships.

IMPLEMENTATION Problems associated with delusional thinking and suggested nursing interventions are provided in Table 4-3.

EVALUATION Failure to help a client who is experiencing delusions is sometimes caused by inconsistency in approach by the staff. Once a care plan is formulated and agreed upon, it is necessary for all staff members to follow it. Lack of success in dealing with a delusional client may also be due to misunderstanding of the client's behavior or to feelings of inadequacy on the part of staff members. If nurses reinforce delusional beliefs or become incorporated in the clients' delusions, the delusions will strengthen and expand, and corrective measures must be taken.

The Demanding Client

When nurses label clients as "demanding," they may mean that the staff simply cannot give clients what they ask for. A large number of clients, inadequate staffing, and the pressures of other duties may contribute to the perception of demanding clients. If nurses allow their feelings, reactions, and perceptions to influence their responses to clients, then clients may indeed become demanding. Annoyance

and anger toward clients frequently exaggerate demands because the more frustrated and unfulfilled clients feel, the more demanding their behavior will become. On the other hand, if clients develop the conviction that the staff wants to help them and are interested in fulfilling their requests, they may become less demanding.

87

88

There may be several reasons for excessively demanding behavior. Many clients are demanding because of conflicting feelings about dependency. Some resent being dependent and react by giving orders in a bold, urgent way. Others seem to enjoy being dependent and regress to immature, cajoling behavior. Yet others act insecure and helpless and dread being abandoned. Whatever the outward behavior, it may mask feelings of anxiety, helplessness, inadequacy, hostility, fear of being deprived, or a need for attention. Demanding individuals wish to control others and direct attention to themselves.

ASSESSMENT Demanding clients usually make requests in an authoritative way, believing they have the right to have their demands met. These clients ask many questions, want a great deal of staff time, and seek constant attention. Others may be just as demanding but choose to adopt a whining, cajoling, "poor me" attitude. Still others act helpless and insecure.

PLANNING In dealing with the excessively demanding client, appropriate nursing goals should include the following:

1. To convey an attitude of concern for the client's needs and to meet realistic demands and requests.

2. To help the client derive satisfaction from relationships with others who are not staff members.

3. To assist the client in developing feelings of security and self-esteem that come from within, rather than from outside sources.

4. To encourage the client to look at interaction as

Table 4-4.
Problems Associated with Demanding Behavior and Suggested Nursing Interventions

Identified Problems	Nursing Interventions
Insecurity	1. Recognize your own reactions of anger at the client's incessant demands so that you can control the anger. 2. Show consideration for and sincere interest in trying to meet requests in a reasonable way. 3. Provide consistency when responding to requests. 4. Allow the client to verbalize irritation at necessary restrictions. 5. Avoid punishing or withdrawing from the client. 6. Reassure the client that essential needs are and will continue to be met.
Authoritative, hostile behavior	1. Clarify expectations for the client. 2. Determine what needs underlie the demanding, hostile behavior. 3. Set limits and keep within these limits without rejecting the client. 4. Let the client know what will be offered in terms of time and attention. Be sure to live up to this part of the contract. 5. Spend time with the client when she is not demanding, to reinforce appropriate behavior.
Regressive, placating behavior	1. Create an accepting climate in which it is safe to express needs openly. 2. Accept the client's right to think and feel as he does. 3. Provide a consistent relationship in order to build trust. 4. Identify any interests and talents of the client and reinforce abilities and skills to reduce regression. 5. Devise ways to redirect client's energy; reinforce and reward what is good, constructive, and useful in client's behavior.

---

a two-way process of giving and taking rather than as a one-way process of taking.

5. To help the client use more acceptable methods of getting needs met rather than demanding or whining.

6. To help the client understand and deal with underlying fears of being neglected or abandoned.

IMPLEMENTATION Reassurance and acceptance help demanding clients maintain contact with others and remain in touch with reality. Types of excessively demanding behaviors and suggested interventions are discussed in Table 4-4.

EVALUATION The usual reason for continued demanding behavior is an inconsistent approach in implementing the care plan. Staff members are often caught in a vicious cycle of overreacting to the client's demands with impatience or anger. Such reactions only increase the client's insecurity and demanding behavior. The nurse may not recognize

Life is not as orderly or well controlled as events in the laboratory . . . Suppose for example that an aspiring actor wears a blue shirt for his first audition and gets the part. At the next audition, which also results in a job, the actor is again wearing a blue shirt; the connection is coincidental but the actor may come to believe that one has caused the other and he will never attend an audition unless he is wearing his lucky blue shirt.

D. SCHULTZ, THEORIES OF PERSONALITY

her own feelings of anger and may fail to realize that the client's behavior is a protective mechanism for covering true feelings. When nurses react by physically and psychologically withdrawing from clients or by becoming punitive, retaliatory, or rejecting, they only aggravate the problem behavior.

The Hallucinating Client

Hallucinations are false or distorted perceptions of objects or events. They often carry a compelling sense of reality. Hallucinations tend to originate during periods of extreme emotional stress in which the individual is unable to cope successfully with the situation. The flight from reality represented by hallucinations is usually a way of expressing some phase of a troublesome problem in the inner life of the individual.

ASSESSMENT Clients with hallucinations are often introspective individuals who have not had satisfactory interpersonal relationships. These clients tend to withdraw from others and to discourage interpersonal approaches and communication. Their hallucinations are often used as substitutes for human relationships. They appear unaware of what is going on around them and have a low frustration tolerance to changes in their routine. Many assume a listening, watchful attitude and appear apprehensive without cause. They may follow "commands" of "voices," talk to themselves, or talk out of context while a conversation is going on around them. If a hallucination is threatening, the client may be terrified of the experience.

PLANNING Appropriate nursing goals in caring for clients experiencing hallucinations should include the following:

1. To interrupt the pattern of hallucination by helping the client interact with other people and establish satisfying relationships.

2. To involve the client in activities that reduce time for introspection.

3. To find alternative methods of working through or releasing anxiety so that hallucinations can be relinquished.

IMPLEMENTATION Correction of sensory distortion occurs not through arguing or confrontation but through concrete experience. A sincere interest in and honest response to clients often results in the disappearance of the hallucination. Problems associated with hallucinations and suggested interventions are provided in Table 4-5.

EVALUATION Failure to help clients who are hallucinating may be due to the staff's lack of knowledge about how to interrupt the hallucinations and replace them with more socially acceptable behavior. Sometimes staff members are intimidated by clients who are hallucinating. At times, staff may behave inappropriately around clients, not realizing that the hallucinating client remains acutely aware of her surroundings. It is also not therapeutic to react with annoyance to the client's incomprehensible behavior or to instruct her to stop hallucinating. Exhibiting surprise at her fantastic perceptions or imposing unnecessary security measures retards the establishment of a trusting relationship. The staff's anxiety may cause them to ignore the hallucinating client in an effort to increase their own comfort.

The Angry Client

Anger is a response to something that is perceived as a frustration or a threat, such as an illness, a change

Table 4-5.
Problems Associated with Hallucinations and Suggested Nursing Interventions

Identified Problems	Nursing Interventions
Insecurity	1. Provide a structured environment with a routine that has few changes. 2. Explain any changes before they are about to occur, so client knows what to expect. 3. Provide supervision to prevent injury to self or others. 4. Reassure client whose hallucinations are fearful or threatening.
Break with reality	1. Initiate interactions with the client for short periods of time, increasing time as tolerated. 2. Respond to any comments based in reality. 3. Avoid nonverbal approaches such as shaking your head or motioning with your hands; they may add to the hallucinations. 4. Ask client to let you know when hallucinations intrude into conversations and to tell you his reactions. 5. Validate the nature of the situation before making the assumption that the client is hallucinating. 6. Avoid conveying in any way that the hallucination is real. Let the client know that the "voices" are real for her but not for other people. Do not reinforce hallucinations by deep exploration. Be clear and specific in communication. 7. Help the client identify impersonal pronouns. If possible, use proper names in conversation.
Social withdrawal	1. Explore ways the client can relieve his anxiety in a more acceptable manner. 2. Help the client recognize his strengths and accomplishments. Reinforce healthy aspects of his personality. 3. Gradually increase interaction with others, widening the circle of people he trusts. 4. Help the client develop relationships with others so that interactions cause less fear. 5. Recognize that even though clients may appear remote and detached, consistent accepting approaches are probably having some influence.

in body image, a sense of inadequacy, a fear of loss, or an actual loss. It is an emotion that can range from mild irritation to uncontrollable rage. Every person feels anger on occasion. It can be healthy in some situations and pathological in others. A person will often become less angry when helped to identify the threat and when given alternative ways of dealing with the threat.

Anger is a derivative of anxiety, which in turn is usually the result of a feeling of powerlessness that may be rational or irrational. When anxiety is converted to anger, the underlying powerlessness and the irrationality are hidden. But suppression and repression do not eliminate anger; suppression forbids the expression of anger, while repression hides it from awareness.

ASSESSMENT Angry clients are inclined to do something harmful to themselves or others. The feelings surrounding anger include hate, rage, and aggression. Angry behaviors may take the form of gossiping, swearing, scapegoating, arguing, demanding, attacking, threatening, or abusing (physically or verbally). Less obvious expressions of anger include joking at the expense of others, deceptive sweetness, sarcasm or derision, suspiciousness, and lack of cooperation.

PLANNING Appropriate nursing goals in caring for angry clients should include the following:

1. To protect the client from harming himself or others until he can resume this responsibility himself.

2. To help the client express feelings of anger verbally, specifically, and in a safe, acceptable manner.

3. To facilitate the appropriate exploration and ventilation of anger without fear of judgment or retaliation.

4. To help the client recognize problems created by angry behavior.

5. To help the client cope with angry feelings in a way that will eliminate trauma to herself and others.

6. To facilitate the client's understanding of the cause of her anger.

IMPLEMENTATION Anger generally provokes anger in others. The first step in helping a client deal with anger is to be aware of one's own reactions to the client's anger so that they do not prevent therapeutic interactions. Working with angry clients requires a great deal of stamina and self-control. One should remember that anger protects the client from emotional states that are too powerful to face. Suggested nursing interventions for the angry client are listed in Table 4-6.

EVALUATION If the nursing intervention does not succeed with the angry client, it may be that the staff members were not aware of the factors likely to cause anger in him. If staff members tried to ignore the anger in the hope that it would fade away, the client learned nothing about handling his anger. Similarly, if the affective component of a statement was ignored and only the content heeded, there may have been no opportunity to explore the causes of an angry remark. If the staff became defensive or angry in response to the client's expression of anger, the client may only have become more angry. Avoiding the angry client or probing too deeply or prematurely into the causes of his anger may have made him confused or so antagonistic that a therapeutic relationship may have been impossible to establish or maintain.

The Hypochondriacal Client

Hypochondriasis is the persistent conviction that one is or is likely to become ill when illness is neither present nor likely. The hypochondriac is not a malingerer; her suffering and symptoms are very real. A physical disability, real or imagined, can serve as a method of escape from life's pressures or as an excuse for personal failure. Being physically ill provides a method of controlling others and monopolizing their attention.

The psychodynamics of hypochondriasis are extremely complex. Often this type of client has been raised in an environment that focused on

Table 4-6.
Problems Associated with Anger and Suggested Nursing Interventions

Identified Problems	Nursing Interventions
Insecurity	1. Recognize the client's feelings of anger. 2. Refrain from joking, laughing at, or teasing a client who is angry. 3. Use a matter-of-fact response when the client displays unacceptable, angry behavior. 4. Accept the client's anger without making value judgments. 5. Let the client know it is all right to feel angry. 6. Accept anger as legitimate but help client monitor the way she expresses anger. 7. Avoid close personal contact with the angry client except when protection of the client or others is needed.
Hostile behavior	1. Help the client become aware of the angry feelings causing his behavior. 2. Identify early clues or conditions that trigger feelings of anger. 3. Confront the client's unacceptable behavior and discuss alternative ways of reacting. 4. Find out what happened to cause the anger and what the client thinks about it. Reconstruct the events as the client experienced them. 5. Avoid coercing the client if she is not ready to face or deal with the problem of anger. 6. Withdraw attention when the client is acting in an unacceptable manner. 7. Do not intervene unless the anger is reaching dangerous proportions. 8. Encourage the client to assume responsibility for his own behavior and to exercise self-control.
Inappropriate outlets for anger	1. Help the client find constructive ways of expending physical energy and releasing anger, such as motor activities. 2. Help the client find healthy, competitive outlets for anger.

physical complaints and illness. Oversolicitous parents may have reinforced her concern about health. Perhaps a prolonged childhood illness may have caused her excessive preoccupation with the workings of her body.

ASSESSMENT Hypochondriacal clients exhibit a marked anxiety about health, an overconcern regarding body processes, and an exaggeration of any organic problems. Symptoms may relate to any body system, may range from mild to severe, and may be chronic or intermittent.

PLANNING Appropriate nursing goals in caring for the hypochondriacal client should include the following:

1. To assist the client in tolerating average discomfort without becoming an emotional cripple.

Table 4-7.
Problems Associated with Hypochondriasis
and Suggested Nursing Interventions

Identified Problems	Nursing Interventions
Insecurity	1. Accept the client as a person who is suffering and in need of help. 2. Show interest rather than impatience even though the symptoms are repeated frequently. 3. Refer all physical complaints to the attention of appropriate personnel. Some symptoms may indicate actual somatic disorders. 4. Recognize the negative feelings aroused in caregivers and others when dealing with hypochondriacal clients. 5. Reduce the client's interactions with those who reinforce his symptoms.
Preoccupation with physical symptoms	1. Listen attentively, but do not make symptoms the focus of the interaction. 2. Indicate awareness of physical complaints but guide conversation to other topics. 3. Help the client recognize how he uses symptoms to avoid dealing with life's problems. 4. Discourage the client from remaining unoccupied or inactive for long periods of time. 5. Plan activities in which the client can feel successful to enhance his self-esteem. 6. Help the client develop new interests and skills to reduce his preoccupation with somatic complaints.

2. To assist the client in finding other means of satisfaction and in developing healthy relationships with others.

3. To decrease the client's need for somatic symptoms as a means of control over others.

IMPLEMENTATION Reassurance is of only temporary value in the treatment of hypochondriacal clients because they often do not wish to be relieved of their symptoms. Legitimate medical issues should be addressed, but treatment should focus primarily on understanding the underlying conflict and assisting the client to find better ways of dealing with conflicts and meeting needs. Hypochondriacal clients who have some legitimate concerns can learn to live with their weakness and deficiencies and to mobilize available strengths. Suggested nursing interventions for the care of hypochondriacal clients are provided in Table 4-7.

EVALUATION If a client has used somatic symptoms as a way of relating to others for a long time, it may be extremely difficult to induce change. Frustration and an unaccepting attitude on the part of staff members may have been transmitted to the client and aggravated his behavior. Implying that the client should be able to control her symptoms may have made a therapeutic relationship difficult to establish. If symptoms were ignored or belittled the hypochondriacal client may have developed more severe complaints in order to retain the attention of staff members and others.

The Manipulative Client

Manipulation is an interpersonal process that occurs consciously and unconsciously in virtually all inter-personal behavior. If manipulation is used constructively, the individual's interpersonal capabilities and strengths are applied to promoting successful relations with others. Destructive manipulation, by contrast, is the exploitation of other people or the extraction of favors or behaviors from others for egotistical purposes that create difficulties in relationships and inhibit personal growth. Manipulation entails a series of interpersonal operations: one individual's needs are not met by another; therefore, anxiety levels rise. The needs of the other person are then disregarded, and manipulative adaptive maneuvers are tried. If these manuvers are successful, the person's initial needs are met, anxiety decreases, and the pattern of manipulation becomes entrenched.

Manipulation is usually learned in childhood. A common tactic is to induce sympathy or guilt in another person in order to make it impossible to refuse a request. Often the client does not trust others to fulfill her needs if she approaches them directly.

ASSESSMENT The manipulative client may bargain with, threaten, demand, flatter, or intimidate others. He is adept at finding others' weaknesses and using them to his own advantage. He may act as a helper, tale carrier, gift giver, or flatterer. Setting up one staff member or client against another

92

Table 4-8.
Problems Associated with Manipulative Behavior and Suggested Nursing Interventions

Identified Problems	Nursing Interventions
Insecurity	1. Provide consistent limits and reasonable expectations. 2. Allow reasonable freedom within the limits. 3. Communicate expectations and limits to all staff to prevent the manipulation of any one member. 4. Recognize the feelings, positive and negative, that the client arouses in the nurse and other caregivers.
Attempt to control others	1. Identify the client's attempts to manipulate staff and others. 2. Recognize the client's behavioral patterns and prevent her from using these patterns in an exploitive way. 3. Inform the client that you understand what she is trying to accomplish. 4. Help the client analyze what she is doing and why she needs to do it. 5. Refuse promises, gifts, and compliments from the client in return for favors or concessions. 6. Provide verbal reinforcement when the client functions within the established limits. 7. Encourage open and direct forms of communication.

through comparisons is common. The manipulative client can be charming and subservient when it serves his purpose. He may use tears and feign helplessness while making multiple demands and pressing unpleasant issues. The manipulator is attracted to staff members who unknowingly foster his behavior. Frequently he exploits caregivers' generosity and desire to be liked. He is indifferent to distinctions between truth and falsehood, feels little guilt, and has little capacity for insight.

PLANNING Appropriate nursing goals for the manipulative client should include the following:

1. To help the client become aware of her behavior in relation to others and find more appropriate ways to obtain what she needs.

2. To foster her ability to trust others to meet her needs without having to resort to manipulation and exploitation.

3. To mutually agree on consistent expectations and limits.

4. To teach the client the advantages of cooperation, compromise, and collaboration over manipulation.

IMPLEMENTATION If the manipulative client can learn to trust nurses in a therapeutic relationship and to employ direct methods of having his needs met, he may be able to generalize this experience to others and learn to interact in a more constructive manner. Setting reasonable limits allows a manipulative client to experiment with new behaviors, achieve self-control, and replace manipulative tactics with more constructive interactions. The pur-

pose of limit setting is not to control clients but to give them consistent expectations and guidance toward self-control. Suggested nursing interventions for care of the manipulative client are presented in Table 4-8.

EVALUATION The most common reason for failure to improve the behavior of manipulative clients is an inconsistent approach by staff members. These clients are adept at discovering those staff members who will be likely to respond to their efforts at manipulation. Often these clients are able to take advantage of staff members' own anxiety and need for approval. Hostility toward these clients is easily aroused, especially when staff members discover they have been manipulated. This hostility may cause staff to avoid manipulative clients or to respond in a punitive manner. Although this may protect staff members from further manipulation, it is not therapeutic for clients and may intensify their manipulative tendencies.

The Regressed Client
Regression is a defense mechanism that involves reversion to cognitive and behavioral patterns that were appropriate and brought pleasure at an earlier stage of development. Some regression is a normal and necessary part of life. Most people enjoy an

Table 4-9.
Problems Associated with Regressed Behavior and Suggested Nursing Interventions

Identified Problems	Nursing Interventions
Insecurity	1. Be direct, clear, and simple in all verbal communications. 2. Avoid punishment following periods of regression. 3. Explore the meaning of the regression if the client can tolerate it.
Dependency on others	1. Avoid taking over any tasks the client is able to perform herself. 2. Convey a partnership attitude by soliciting the client's contributions to planning and decision making. 3. Accept the client's present level; do not assign tasks that he is unable to accomplish. 4. Treat the client as an adult; do not use nicknames that detract from his dignity. 5. Avoid establishing a custodial environment. Permit maximum possible freedom. 6. Do not convey the impression of understanding what the client is talking about unless you really understand. 7. Indicate that the regressed behavior is unacceptable but only temporary. 8. Discuss plans for eventual discharge throughout hospitalization. 9. Do not reinforce or encourage regressed behavior. 10. Avoid the tendency to act like a disapproving parent.
Preoccupation with self	1. Involve clients in motor activities and verbal interactions. 2. Encourage group activities. 3. Emphasize talking and acting on a reality-oriented level. 4. Acknowledge the efforts of clients when they assume greater responsibility.
Regression due to a psychotic episode	1. Tolerate regression during acute stages. 2. Use minimal pressure to limit regression during acute psychosis or periods of extreme distress. 3. Emphasize contact, trust, and reality orientation, even when clients seem to be unresponsive. 4. Convey expectation that regression is only temporary and that the client's coping ability will improve. 5. Make provision for rest, food and fluid intake, exercise, and elimination.

occasional nap, shouting at football games, or going to costume parties. Society endorses regression in other circumstances, particularly during illness when persons are usually permitted to relinquish responsibilities. However, regression may become a fixed pattern that interferes with an individual's potential for growth.

By regressing, a person may retreat from responsibility for interpersonal conflicts, settle for lowered aspirations, and seek immediate gratification of his desires. Often regression is related to unmet dependency needs. Changes in relationships can result in regressive behaviors that lead to chronic dependency.

ASSESSMENT Regressed clients appear helpless and may be unable to take care of basic needs such as washing, feeding, or elimination. They often lack confidence in decision making and show evidence of clinging behavior. Severely regressed clients are preoccupied with themselves, have low aspirations, rebel against authority, and search for nurturing persons. Often they exhibit impaired reality testing and altered human relationships. Infantile behavior such as bedwetting, thumbsucking, and temper tantrums may be seen in extreme cases. In even more severe cases, the client may become autistic or mute and may even assume a fetal position.

PLANNING Appropriate nursing goals in caring for the regressed client should include the following:

1. To avoid fostering dependency and reinforcing childlike attitudes.
2. To expect the client to accept a partnership in the treatment.
3. To help the client tolerate unavoidable stress and anxiety without regressing further.
4. To help the client find gratification in the environment and in his accomplishments instead of dwelling on failures and inadequacies.

IMPLEMENTATION Problems associated with regression and associated nursing interventions are examined in Table 4-9.

As I follow the experience of many clients in the therapeutic relationship . . . it seems that each one is raising the same questions. Below the level of the problem situation—behind the trouble with studies, or wife, or employer, or with his own uncontrollable or bizarre behavior, lies one central search—each person is asking Who am I really? How can I get in touch with this real self underlying all my surface behavior?

CARL ROGERS, ON BECOMING A PERSON

EVALUATION Failure to achieve stated goals with regressed clients is frequently due to staff actions that foster dependency rather than encourage the acceptance of responsibilities. Hospitalization is a situation that requires some regressive behavior in any circumstances, but tolerance of consistently regressed behavior only promotes the possibility of the behavior becoming a pattern. Family attitudes may contribute to clients' regression by isolating them or by not permitting them to resume their previous roles after hospitalization.

The Ritualistic Client

Compulsive behavior is an irresistible impulse to perform a procedure repeatedly and in exactly the same way. Compulsive rituals are usually related to superstitious concepts and magical thinking. Fears and tensions are often discharged through ritualistic behavior, but the relief is only temporary. Ritualism also helps the person avoid making decisions yet maintain control over himself and others. The total body may be involved in the ritualistic behaviors, which may be physically exhausting or damaging to the individual.

ASSESSMENT The ritualistic client's behavior pattern may involve repeating an act in exactly the same manner each time or performing various seemingly meaningless acts. Examples of common ritualistic behaviors are continual handwashing, hoarding of unneeded items, and bizarre mannerisms. Ordinary precautions such as checking to see whether the lights are turned off or whether windows are locked may become ritualistic if the client must continually repeat the process.

PLANNING Ritualistic clients seldom ask for help because they have found their own methods of relieving anxiety and because they have a strong need for self-control. Appropriate nursing measures for the ritualistic client should include the following:

1. To intervene early in the anxiety-building process and endeavor to reduce the need for ritualism.

2. To help the client gain some insight into why the ritual is necessary.

3. To find alternative methods for dealing with anxiety.

4. To allow the client sufficient time to complete the anxiety-reducing ritual.

5. To encourage social interactions immediately after the ritual has been completed, when anxiety is at its lowest level.

IMPLEMENTATION Trying to prevent the ritualistic act may cause panic and terror in the clients. Although it is sometimes possible to substitute a less harmful ritual, it is not advisable to prohibit the ritualistic behavior entirely. Suggested nursing interventions for dealing with ritualistic clients are provided in Table 4-10.

EVALUATION The ritualistic client's failure to respond to nursing interventions may be a result of the failure of staff members to recognize the underlying cause of the ritualistic behavior. Critical reactions from nurses and others may have caused increased feelings of guilt and reinforced the need for ritual. The hospital environment itself often seems confusing and inconsistent to ritualistic clients, who

Table 4-10.
Problems Associated with Ritualistic Behavior and Suggested Nursing Interventions

Identified Problems	Nursing Interventions
Insecurity	1. Accept ritualism without scolding or ridicule. 2. Set consistent limits to prevent actual harm to the client or others. 3. Allow episodes of ritualism when the client finds this the only way to reduce anxiety. 4. Allow the client as much autonomy as possible.
Need for control	1. Establish routines for daily living and avoid anxiety-producing changes. 2. Provide activities that can lead to a sense of accomplishment and self-worth. 3. Provide assignments that the client can complete successfully. 4. Assign a living area that is as private as possible. 5. Encourage verbalization of feelings. 6. Substitute less harmful rituals, such as using an antiseptic hand lotion for excessive hand-washing. 7. Allow the client sufficient time to complete rituals. 8. Arrange activities just after ritual is completed and anxiety is relatively low. 9. Observe client for signs of mounting anxiety. 10. Observe the client's physical needs. Self-neglect is possible because of preoccupation with ritualism.

value order and uniformity. It requires a concerted effort on the part of the staff to provide a safe haven for these anxiety-prone clients so that they may improve.

The Suspicious Client

Trust and confidence in others are acquired throughout life as a result of experiences that do not result in harm. *Suspicious* clients have not learned to trust themselves, to trust others, and to test reality. They have not experienced feelings of adequacy and approval and thus tend to resort to the defense mechanism of projection. Projection is the attribution of one's own feelings, attitudes, or desires to others. Suspicious clients who feel inadequate and unworthy themselves project their feelings of inadequacy and unworthiness onto others.

ASSESSMENT Suspicious clients may appear aloof, mistrustful, irritable, quarrelsome, and extremely sensitive, with a tendency toward impulsive, destructive behavior. These clients are frequently hospitalized against their wishes and therefore see their environment as hostile and threatening. They blame others for their own discomfort and set un-

realistic goals for themselves and others. Frequently, suspicious clients attempt to set one person against another. They often search for evidence of error to prove their suspicions correct.

PLANNING Appropriate nursing goals for the suspicious client should include the following:

1. To assist the suspicious client in feeling secure and developing trust.
2. To divert excess energy into satisfying activities.
3. To provide an atmosphere that fosters feelings of acceptance and belonging and provides opportunities for success.

IMPLEMENTATION Demonstrations of genuine concern and interest may enhance trust and confidence in suspicious clients. Nurses working with suspicious clients must also realize the necessity of providing outlets for anger. Suspicious clients often have a limited capacity for coping with anger, and unexpressed or indirectly expressed anger inhibits their ability to relate to others. Behind the angry facade of the suspicious person is a lonely person who is terrorized by the thought of being exposed as inadequate. Verbalization of anger should be permitted without adverse consequences, but the client should also be encouraged to direct her anger at specific incidents and should be discouraged from expressing anger that is generalized to every situation and person she encounters. Suggested nursing interventions for the suspicious client are provided in Table 4-11.

Table 4-11.
Problems Associated with Suspicious Behavior
and Suggested Nursing Interventions

Identified Problems	Nursing Interventions
Insecurity	1. Keep contact with diverse staff at minimum; assign the same staff members if possible. 2. Watch for signs that the client is becoming more angry or vigilant. 3. Accept rebuffs and abusive language as symptoms and not as personal attacks. 4. Be scrupulously honest. Keep promises and maintain a consistent approach. 5. Be aware of negative feelings the client's behavior arouses in staff. 6. Be aware of the client's distrust of others and dissatisfaction with herself. 7. Allow verbalization of feelings without becoming defensive, angry, or punitive.
Distrustful behavior	1. Do not whisper or act secretively in the presence of the client. 2. Limit physical contact to that which is absolutely necessary. 3. Taste food only if requested to do so by the client. 4. Do not mix medication with food. 5. Allow the client to set extent of closeness and distance. 6. Start with solitary or one-on-one activities, then gradually advance to group activities. 7. Inform the client about schedules and what can be expected. 8. Avoid laughing or talking with others when the client can observe but not hear what is being said.
Sense of inadequacy	1. Provide meaningful tasks to encourage feelings of adequacy. 2. Avoid competitive activities. 3. Provide appropriate outlets for anger and aggression. Verbalization and motor activities may be helpful. 4. Provide opportunities for demonstrating skills. 5. Confer recognition for work well done. 6. Give the client the right to complain. Deal with the issues in a calm, rational manner.

EVALUATION Staff members may be ineffectual with suspicious clients because they fear working with a hostile person and are unwilling to become the targets of her hostility. Often nurses will avoid a suspicious person because they are uncomfortable with the client's mistrust. On the other hand, nurses may expect too much too soon from a suspicious client and attempt to establish a reciprocal trust prematurely. It is important to differentiate between the client who is merely suspicious and the client who is actively delusional, because the treatment approach for each is different. The merely suspicious client may slowly develop trust based on reality. The delusional client avoids the need to trust by creating a new reality that exists only for himself.

The Withdrawn Client

An individual's relationships are influenced by her self-concept and ability to cope with life situations. Repeated failures in relationships decrease self-esteem and cause a person to avoid others because of fear of failure. *Withdrawn clients* deny themselves the opportunity to share experiences and develop relationships. To replace the threatening world of reality, they may create a fantasy world that is free of stress, or they may remain in touch with reality and observe interactions around them carefully, even though they choose not to participate.

ASSESSMENT Clients who become withdrawn may be lonely, isolated, frightened, suspicious, and helpless. These clients often daydream, seem indifferent to others, sit alone, and stare into space. They seem to have a diminished capacity to tolerate the feelings that accompany interaction with others, and they cannot or will not invest in emotional attachments. They show a marked indifference to pursuing normal interests, a blunting of emotions, and a resistance to outside influences.

PLANNING Appropriate nursing goals for the withdrawn client should include the following:

1. Help the client modify her perception of her relationships to others.

2. Reduce the client's autistic and regressive tendencies.

3. Provide relationships that will foster the willingness to interact with others.

4. Help clients feel safe in a one-to-one relationship.

Table 4-12.
Problems Associated with Withdrawal
and Suggested Nursing Interventions

Identified Problems	Nursing Interventions
Insecurity	1. Provide a choice of activities that are neither monotonous nor excessively stimulating. 2. Avoid making demands that cannot be met by the client. 3. Avoid mutual withdrawal. 4. Observe for signs of physical consequences of apathy and inactivity. 5. Protect withdrawn client from being exploited by aggressive clients. 6. Avoid placing the client in situations where failure is inevitable.
Interpersonal and environmental withdrawal	1. Keep the client as active as possible in the hospital routine. 2. Recognize that the client is isolating himself as a protective maneuver. 3. Recognize the pattern of actions through which the client withdraws. 4. Seek out the client regularly without being intrusive. 5. Stay with the client, sitting in silence, if necessary. 6. Initiate nonthreatening conversations in which the client can give brief responses. 7. Use simple language and nonthreatening words. 8. Focus on everyday experiences. Comment on routine events. 9. Relieve client of decision making until he is able to make decisions. 10. Make consistent attempts to elicit a response but without demanding a response. 11. Indicate to the client that he may be less withdrawn at some later time and that the nurse will continue to be available.

98

IMPLEMENTATION Problems associated with withdrawal and suggested nursing interventions are discussed in Table 4-12.

EVALUATION Lack of success with withdrawn clients may be due to the staff's misunderstanding of their bizarre and seemingly illogical behavior. Frequently, nurses become impatient because of the large investment of time and energy expended on these clients and the slow progress made. Withdrawn clients tend to arouse anxiety in the staff, so the staff in turn may label them as "wanting to be alone" to justify paying less attention to them. With self-awareness and practice nurses can learn to become comfortable even with clients who remain silent or who continually rebuff efforts to interact or communicate. Another common problem is the tendency of staff members to become accustomed to the behavior of withdrawn clients and to not see their behavior as a problem. Since these clients make few demands on the staff it is important not to overlook their needs in the course of caring for other, more troublesome clients.

SUMMARY

As the profession of nursing has expanded its sphere of influence, nursing theory has been developed to guide practice, education, and research. Several theoretical approaches that can be adapted to a variety of settings have been postulated by nurse theorists, including Peplau's theory of inter-personal relationships, Leininger's theory of health care behaviors, Orem's theory of self-care deficits, Newman's theory of expansion of consciousness, and Johnson's theory of behavioral systems. Each nurse must learn to determine which guidelines will be the most helpful in each case when planning interventions within the nursing process.

The use of the nursing process in several problem behaviors has been presented in this chapter. One of the most important elements in working with clients with problem behaviors is providing a therapeutic atmosphere in which clients can find the security they need to begin to solve their problems and change their behavior. There is also no substitute for genuineness in relationships with clients, and it is imperative that nurses become aware of the feelings that certain clients can generate in them. Lack of success with clients can often be attributed to a lack of acceptance or understanding of their difficulties on the part of the nurse.

CLINICAL   EXAMPLE

AN ANXIOUS CLIENT

Ralph Smith is a fifty-four-year-old urban American male, who is married and the father of four children ranging in age from eighteen to thirty-four. Their family life has been one of continual bickering and stress. When the children were young, Ralph was able to maintain authority over them, but each child's adolescence and young adulthood brought family disruptions and periods of discouragement and frustration when Ralph's word was no longer accepted without question. His inability to tolerate some of their behaviors, such as refusing to help around the house and smoking marijuana, led to arguments with his wife, who seemed undisturbed by the children's behavior. When the children failed to become more obedient, Ralph withdrew from the family and blamed himself for not being able to influence them.

Although he is devoted to his wife and almost totally dependent on her for comfort and security, Ralph describes his relationship with her as less than happy. She is indifferent to him sexually, and although she consents to intercourse whenever he desires, he feels demeaned by her passive attitude and only approaches her when his needs become overwhelming.

Ralph has worked as an electronic technician for a large company for twenty years, a job that requires "troubleshooting" on a production line. Ralph is required to attend training programs to familiarize himself with new technologies. Although he is able to master the material in a reasonable period of time, he approaches these classes with severe apprehension because he learns less easily by reading and test taking than by hands-on experience. He is constantly afraid of being embarrassed by not knowing the correct answer in class.

Ralph has suffered from acute attacks of anxiety for several years. In some instances, such as during training classes, he is able to identify the cause of the anxiety, but at other times he cannot find a cause for his panic. He says these occasions cause his heart to beat "so fast I can feel it," and make him feel afraid of suffocating, dizzy, and unable to control or stop the panicky feeling. These episodes frequently occur shortly after he goes to bed at night, when he would like to reach out for his wife but feels afraid to do so. Occasionally he has felt an attack coming on at work, but he has been able to control his feelings long enough to leave the area and go for a walk to pull himself together. The panic attacks leave him exhausted and barely able to function the next day, although he does force himself to go back to work. His exhaustion leads to a variety of minor physical complaints, which he tries to explain to his wife, who responds only with impatience.

Ralph has been in and out of outpatient treatment for several years but has had little success in curbing his anxiety. On the latest occasion he presented for treatment because he was about to undergo surgery for an inguinal hernia and felt he would be unable to face hospitalization because he was "afraid of dying on the table" and didn't think he could stand to spend the nights away from his wife.

ASSESSMENT

In the first interview, Ralph presented as a neatly dressed man, small in stature, who sat rigidly in the chair and made very little eye contact with the nurse. He spoke rapidly in a monotone and frequently asked the nurse if he was "crazy" or if other people had similar problems. He was fully oriented to time, place, and person and the nurse estimated that he was of better-than-average intelligence. Based on the history and clinical picture, the following diagnoses were made:

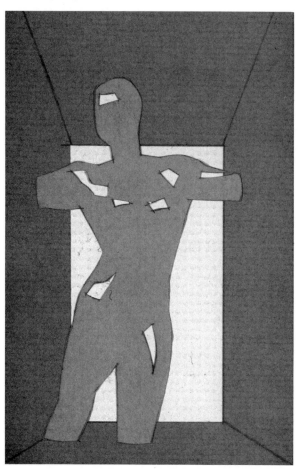

Nursing Diagnoses

Anxiety
(related to attacks ranging from mild to panic)

Coping, ineffective individual
(related to the ability to maintain the influence he deserved in the family)

Fear
(related to job performance and feelings of abandonment)

Knowledge deficit
(related to surgical procedure)

Self-concept, disturbance in
(related to dependence on wife and lack of confidence in his job)

Multiaxial Psychiatric Diagnoses

Axis I   300.01 Panic disorder

Axis II   301.60 Dependent personality

Axis III Inguinal hernia

Axis IV   Code 4—Moderate

Axis V   Level 4—Fair

PLANNING

The nurse used a number of nursing models in planning Ralph's care. Although the focus of each framework was different, each contributed to the formulation of appropriate interventions.

Peplau's Model: Engage Ralph in a one-on-one relationship in which he will be able to freely express his fears and explore the causes of his anxiety. The major themes are insecurity and fear of dying.

Leininger's Model: Convey interest and concern. Help Ralph feel that his problems are recognized as very real and worth listening to. An unjudgmental, interested attitude will let him know that the nurse does care, is willing to work with him, and will not reject him because his complaints are repetitive. Explore Ralph's values about how the head of the household ought to function. Determine how these differ from how he has been able to function.

Orem's Model: Help Ralph develop ways of nurturing and caring for himself in periods of stress. Support him through the surgery, and use his hospital experience as a period of learning and development. Promote anticipatory guidance by teaching about the surgery.

Kinlein's Model: Reinforce the job skills Ralph already possesses to increase his self-esteem. Help him recognize his achievements as husband, father, stepfather, and worker and persuade him to take pleasure in these accomplishments.

Newman's Model: Teach Ralph relaxation techniques. Refer him for self-hypnosis training to help him cope when he feels panic approaching, including during the impending hospitalization.

Johnson's Model: Teach Ralph new skills for coping with anxiety. Suggest the possibility of couple therapy to help his wife realize his need to be close to her and to help him decrease his dependency on her.

IMPLEMENTATION

The first task of the outpatient nurse was to establish a contract with Ralph for individual sessions whose initial focus was on preparation for surgery. Because there were only four weeks until the operation was scheduled, it was necessary to provide some external structure for Ralph. A decision was made and agreed to by Ralph for the nurse to explain Ralph's near-panic state to his surgeon because Ralph felt unable to talk to the surgeon himself. Plans were also made for a preoperative visit to the hospital and a "walking tour" through the procedure. During the period prior to hospitalization, Ralph was given the opportunity to transfer some of his dependency needs to the nurse. Subsequent sessions focused on helping Ralph to develop a sense of autonomy and self-confidence. The nurse began relaxation training sessions and referred Ralph to a consulting psychologist for training in self-hypnosis to begin after the surgery.

As Ralph became comfortable in his therapeutic relationship with the nurse and became able to talk about his fears freely, he acknowledged that he felt safe in the sessions. Although an effective nurse-client relationship had been built, it became apparent that Mrs. Smith should also be involved in the therapeutic plan.

Before Ralph's hospitalization, a session that included his wife was arranged. In this session, only Ralph's fears of separation from his wife and home were discussed. His feelings were interpreted to his wife not as deficiencies on her part but as his strong commitment to his home and family. During the session, the wife indicated some appreciation and recognition of Ralph's strengths and feelings. In this context, the nurse was able to help the wife realize that there were many areas in which Ralph depended on her and needed her support, such as during the impending hospitalization. With the help of the nurse and the increased participation of his wife, Ralph underwent surgery with only minor feelings of anxiety. Having seen the couple together, the nurse realized that future sessions should involve the wife so that she would have a better understanding of what Ralph's nonverbal behavior was actually communicating. Ralph's wife seemed to be somewhat insensitive but not a malevolent individual. Postoperative sessions had the general goal of helping the couple understand the unstated, behaviorally expressed needs each had for the other. Plans were made for a regular structured exercise schedule that Ralph could undertake whenever he felt his anxiety level begin to increase.

EVALUATION

With the help of the nurse, Ralph underwent surgery without an anxiety attack. As she became involved in counseling Ralph's wife began to become aware of Ralph's dependency needs. She acknowledged his contributions to the well-being of his family and his rudimentary self-esteem began to flourish. Ralph began to realize the benefits of physical contact with his wife and he became more comfortable with his dependency on her presence and approval. The wife's agreement to attend future sessions was an indication that the prehospital meetings were of value to her as well as to Ralph.

Review Questions

1. Describe the changes that have occurred over the last decade in the use of nursing therapy.

2. Describe the major elements of the eight nursing theories discussed in this chapter and their implications for nursing practice.

3. Compare and contrast the theories of Peplau and Leininger, Johnson and King, and Newman and Orem.

4. Define anxiety and describe its implications for the therapeutic relationship between nurse and client.

5. Explain the importance of remaining outside the clients' delusional system and ways that this can be accomplished.

6. Delineate the major elements of care for a demanding client. Explain the most common reasons for lack of success with this type of client and ways to prevent this failure.

7. Discuss healthy and pathologic means of manipulation and ways that nurses can recognize manipulation and avoid being manipulated by clients.

8. Describe the most important differences between caring for a client who has delusions and caring for a client who is suspicious.

9. Discuss the appropriate and inappropriate uses and expression of anger.

10. Discuss the importance of self-assessment for the psychiatric nurse.

References

Aguilera, D., and Messick, J. 1982. *Crisis Intervention: Theory and Methodology*, 4th ed. St. Louis: C. V. Mosby.

Carlson, J.; Craft, C.; and McGuire, A. 1982. *Nursing Diagnosis*. Philadelphia: W. B. Saunders.

Grubbs, J. 1974. The Johnson Behavioral System Model. In *Conceptual Models for Nursing Practice*, eds. J. P. Riehl and S. L. Ray. New York: Appleton-Century-Crofts.

King, I. 1971. *Toward a Theory for Nursing*. New York: John Wiley & Sons.

Kinlein, L. 1977. The Self-care Concept. *American Journal of Nursing*, 77:599–601.

Kozier, B., and Erb, G. 1983. *Fundamentals of Nursing: Concepts and Procedures*. Menlo Park, Calif.: Addison-Wesley.

Leininger, M. 1978. *Transcultural Nursing: Concepts, Theories and Practices*. New York: John Wiley & Sons.

Mellow, J. 1969. Professional Identity? Paper presented November 5 at the American Nurses' Association Regional Clinical Conferences at Atlanta, Georgia.

Neal, M. C.; Cohen, P. F.; Cooper, P. G.; and Reighley, J. 1980. *Nursing Care Planning Guides for Psychiatric and Mental Health Care*. Monterey, Calif.: Wadsworth Health Sciences.

Newman, M. A. 1979. *Theory Development in Nursing*. Philadelphia: F. A. Davis.

Orem, D. 1971. *Nursing: Concepts of Practice*. New York: McGraw-Hill.

Peplau, H. 1965. The Heart of Nursing: Interpersonal Relationships. *The Canadian Nurse*, 61:273–275.

Peplau, H. 1968. Psychotherapeutic Strategies. *Perspectives in Psychiatric Care*, 6:264–270.

Sorensen, K., and Luckmann, J. 1979. *Basic Nursing: A Psychophysiological Approach*. Philadelphia: W. B. Saunders.

Supplementary Readings

Chinn, P., ed. *Advances in Nursing Theory Development*. Rockville, Md.: Aspen Systems, 1982.

Chinn, P., and Jacobs, M. *Theory and Nursing: A Systematic Approach*. St. Louis: C. V. Mosby, 1983.

Clement, J. A. Actualizing Theory in Practice. *Perspectives in Psychiatric Care*, 20(1982)126–133.

Craig, H. M. Adaptation in Chronic Illness: An Eclectic Model for Nurses. *Journal of Advanced Nursing*, 8(1983):397–404.

Hoeffer, B. The Unfinished Task: Development of Nursing Theory for Psychiatric and Mental Health Nursing Practice. *Journal of Psychosocial Nursing and Mental Health Services*, 20(1982):8–14.

Iveson-Iveson, J. The Four-Dimensional Nurse in the Rogers Model. *Nursing Mirror*, 155(1982):52.

Iveson-Iveson, J. Standards of Behavior in the Johnson Model. *Nursing Mirror*, 155(1982):38.

Iveson-Iveson, J. Putting Ideas into Action: Orem's Model of Self-care. *Nursing Mirror*, 155(1982):49.

Iveson-Iveson, J. A Two-Way Process: Peplau's Nursing Model. *Nursing Mirror*, 155(1982):52.

Neuman, B. *The Neuman Systems Model: Application to Nursing Education and Practice*. New York: Appleton-Century-Crofts, 1982.

Perry, P. D. Conceptual Frameworks for Clinical Practice. *Journal of Neurosurgical Nursing*, 14(1982):316–321.

Peplau, H. *Interpersonal Relations in Nursing*. New York: G. P. Putnam and Sons, 1972.

Putt, A. M. *General Systems Theory Applied to Nursing*. Boston: Little, Brown, 1978.

Randell, B. *Adaptation Nursing: The Roy Conceptual Model Applied*. St. Louis: C. V. Mosby, 1982.

Rogers, M. *Theoretical Basis of Nursing*. Philadelphia: F. A. Davis, 1970.

Roy, C., and Roberts, S. *Theory Construction in Nursing: An Adaptation Model*. Englewood Cliffs, N. J.: Prentice-Hall, 1981.

Seigel, H. Misconceptions About Conceptual Frameworks: A Point of View. *Nursing and Health Care*, 4(1983):16–17.

101

ESTABLISHING A THERAPEUTIC RELATIONSHIP
ELEMENTS IN THE THERAPEUTIC
COMMUNICATION PROCESS
CHARACTERISTICS OF THERAPEUTIC
COMMUNICATION
Client-Centeredness
Goal-Directedness
Authenticity
Self-disclosure
Confidentiality
Acceptance

COLLABORATION
The Collaborative Continuum
The Therapeutic Contract

FACILITATING THERAPEUTIC COMMUNICATION
Affective Characteristics of Therapeutic Communication
Cognitive Processes in Therapeutic Communication
Therapeutic Communication and the Nursing Process

DOCUMENTATION OF CARE
The Health Status Profile
The Problem List
Progress Notes
Discharge Plans and Summary
Process Recording

C H A P T E R

5

Communication and Interaction in Psychiatric Mental Health Nursing

Learning Objectives

After reading this chapter, the student should be able to:

1. Analyze the essential components and characteristics of therapeutic communication.

2. Discuss goal setting and the therapeutic contract as a form of collaboration between nurse and client.

3. Apply therapeutic communication to the nursing process.

Overview

Therapeutic communication is the process by which the nurse and client collaborate to improve the client's health. The first three sections of this chapter describe methods for establishing a therapeutic relationship, elements in the therapeutic communication process, and characteristics of therapeutic communication. The next section explores the importance of collaboration and the use of the therapeutic contract to enhance collaboration. The final sections describe techniques for facilitating therapeutic communication and detail written methods of documenting clients' care.

Men must be taught as if you taught them naught
And things unknown proposed as things forgot.
ALEXANDER POPE

In mental health settings, communication takes many forms and is transmitted in many ways. Sometimes communication is only the flicker of an eyelash or the slight movement of an outstretched hand. Sometimes it is a quiet repeated muttering: "Oh no, no, no, no . . ." At other times it is a loud and angry shout: "Get away from me! Get away!" Sometimes the words come haltingly, hesitantly, painfully slow, after what has seemed to be interminable periods of silence. Sometimes the flow of words does not even seem to be in any known language: "Ya, pa, dee, may, may." At other times the words seem quite ordinary: "I'm hungry" or "I'm so tired." And sometimes the words seem to carry many messages: "I don't like what's going on around here" or "I don't understand what's happening."

Thus, an infinite variety of messages reach out to psychiatric nurses, sometimes eluding them, sometimes threatening them, sometimes discouraging them. But in all their infinite forms and varieties, the messages are the expressions of the clients' deep-seated needs. Just as varied are the responses made by the nurse. When nurses respond to clients, they choose their words carefully, selecting them to achieve specific purposes. Often the nursing response is nonverbal—reaching for a trembling hand, lightly touching a shoulder, leaning toward a client, or smiling quietly (Burnside, 1973). All these responses used by the psychiatric nurse are a part of *therapeutic communication*.

Therapeutic communication between client and nurse, regardless of the nature of the health care needs, is far more than the transmission of a message from sender to receiver. It is the reaching out of one human being for another. When a psychiatric nurse uses a simple phrase such as "I'll walk with you to breakfast now," she is offering her presence, support, guidance, strength, judgment, and protection to a client who may be feeling so overwhelmed, so weighed down by sadness, that motion seems impossible, or so anxious that the very appearance of the nurse arouses suspicion and fear. The communication that is developed and nurtured between nurse and client should be carefully planned and implemented so that the client feels protected, recognizes acceptance, and dares to attempt further communication, which in turn becomes the vehicle of progress and recovery.

ESTABLISHING A THERAPEUTIC RELATIONSHIP

Establishing a therapeutic relationship is a process that takes time. It must be carefully guided by the nurse and it must be predicated on *trust*. Trust between client and nurse occurs when the client is able to rely on the nurse's integrity, ability, character, and commitment to the client's well-being.

Creating a climate of trust begins with the *offering of self*, the reaching out of one person to another. A nurse reaches out to the client by offering his help: "I am Jim Williams. While you are here, I'll be your nurse. Please let me know if there is anything I can do to help you." Sometimes the nurse uses words that are less explicit but that are a clear statement of caring: "You seem upset; would you like me to stay with you for a while?" The nurse may also demonstrate caring without words, as by touching a hand or just staying with a client who is silent and withdrawn or anxious. Regardless of the specific way in which the nurse reaches out, the message

In some ways the word communication is similar to universal words such as freedom, love, or democracy. Although each of us intuitively knows what he or she means by such words, they can have different meanings for different people. Because communication has multiple meanings, it is important to identify a specific meaning and also to distinguish between different kinds of communication.

L. L. NORTHOUSE AND P. G. NORTHOUSE, HEALTH COMMUNICATION: A HANDBOOK FOR PROFESSIONALS

conveyed is the same: "I'm interested in you and I care about you." When a client entrusts herself to a nurse, she demonstrates confidence that she will be accepted, respected, and helped.

Another important step in establishing a therapeutic relationship is clarifying identities, roles, and expectations: "I am Beth Thomas, the nurse in charge on this unit. I will be helping the other nurses to help you. I'll be stopping by to see how you are at least once a day. If there's anything that concerns you about your care or your stay here on the floor, please let me know."

It is important to make clear not only what the client can expect of the nurse but also what the nurse expects of the client: "We eat together in a dining room at the end of the hall. I will expect to see you there each mealtime" or "We meet once a week for community meetings. We expect all residents to join us."

Making clear the expectations in relationships helps decrease anxiety and prevent misunderstandings. Clear expectations also create an atmosphere that feels safe because expectations that are clear can more easily be met. And feeling safe in the hospital environment may enable the client to adapt in more healthful and effective ways.

Above all else, trust in the nurse-client relationship depends on consistent behavior on the part of the nurse. This is particularly important because many persons seeking mental health care have not experienced positive, trusting relationships before. The nurse must ensure that his words and actions are congruent and that he keeps commitments to the client. A nurse who says he will return at a specified time or will pursue a particular question

demonstrates consistency and reliability when he does what he has promised to do. The nurse must also display congruence between verbal and nonverbal communication. The nurse who says that a behavior is acceptable but who nevertheless appears angry is giving the client an inconsistent and therefore confusing message.

A therapeutic relationship must be based on respect as well as trust. Respect means acknowledging the value of the client, accepting and valuing her individuality and recognizing her rights and needs. The nurse demonstrates respect for the client by listening to her viewpoint, respecting her preferences, giving her choices, and treating her with dignity.

Honesty is another prerequisite for trust. It is important that the client be able to believe what the nurse says. If a nurse says, "You can have your medicine in 30 minutes," it is essential that the client indeed receive the medicine on time. Even in setting limits the nurse must be honest, because honesty, like consistency, helps clients develop a sense of security.

ELEMENTS IN THE THERAPEUTIC COMMUNICATION PROCESS

Therapeutic communication is not a simple, unidirectional, one-dimensional transmission of a message but rather a multidimensional, complex interaction between two human beings. Each person must be viewed holistically and understood as a living system if communication is to be therapeutically effective. Both the nurse and the client bring to the

*Figure 5-1. Berlo's
communication model.*
SOURCE: After Berlo (1960).

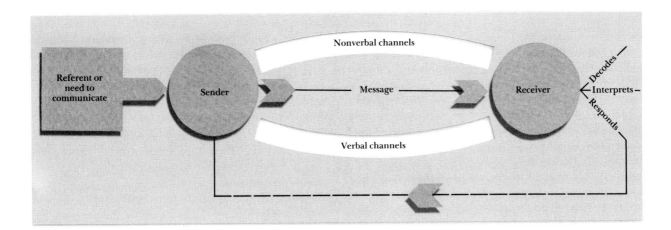

107

interaction their memories, feelings, fears, expectations, values, strengths, weaknesses, skills, and limitations. The overt message is only a clue to the full meaning of the interaction.

Berlo's (1960) classic model of the communication process describes the following components: A *referent*, a need that precipitates the original communication process, is transmitted by the *sender* in the form of the *message* through a *medium* (often referred to as the channel), until it is received by a *decoder/receiver*, who then interprets the meaning of the message. This process is diagrammed in Figure 5-1. Although such a model may not do justice to the complexity of human interaction, it can help us analyze the component parts of this complex phenomenon.

The nurse wishing to analyze any interaction should first ask, "What is the referent?" That is, what originally precipitated the interaction? Was it the return of the voices the client has been hearing, a sudden unexpected sound outside the client's door, the slow awakening into consciousness of a client who had been heavily medicated, the anticipation and anxiety that arise as visiting hours approach? What need prompted the client to initiate communication? Or, did the nurse initiate communication herself because she is trying to stimulate the client to greater activity and independence? Is the nurse perhaps trying to reassure a client who seems visibly distressed?

Once the nurse has identified what began the communication process, she should consider the perspectives of both the sender/encoder and the receiver/decoder. Sometimes the client is the sender and the nurse is the receiver who must decode and interpret the message. At other times the roles are reversed. In either case, certain questions can be asked: What past experiences, perceptual difficulties, beliefs, hopes, and fears have influenced the way in which the message has been sent and received?

Sometimes the medium or channel selected for the message gives a clue about the meaning the message has for either sender or receiver. The client who always whispers or who refuses to speak and insists on writing things down is indicating something about the personal meaning that the communication process holds for him. So, too, is the client whose feelings are so overwhelming that her only form of communication is with eyes that glance and quickly turn away. There are many different meanings for such silence. For example, a silent client may be trying to avoid anxiety or to control hostile impulses that are not acceptable to the client's value system. In either case the silence has a meaning that requires attention and interpretation by the nurse.

Sometimes the medium by which the message is sent seems to be in conflict with other messages being sent at the same time. One of the most important things to look for in analyzing communication is congruence between the verbal and nonverbal expressions of an individual. The nurse will often see clients whose nonverbal behavior seems not to correspond to their verbal behavior or whose nonverbal behavior seems somehow inappropriate for the message being sent. The client who says, "I really feel much better today; I feel much less nervous" but who continually paces and fidgets is displaying a lack of congruence that reveals her conflicting inner feelings.

The body language of both the client and the nurse also communicates a great deal of meaning. Messages of acceptance or rejection can be transmitted by posture, stance, and body movements. The amount of space maintained between two persons is also believed to convey a great deal of meaning about the amount of closeness desired in the interaction. Clients vary in the amount of personal space they need. Some indicate a preference for maintaining physical distance while others indicate an acceptance of physical closeness. It is important that nurses not violate a client's personal space by standing or sitting too close. Such a violation could cause extreme resentment and anger and could even precipitate panic in a severely anxious client. The nurse should be guided by the messages conveyed by the client, permitting the client to maintain whatever physical distance is comfortable. Sometimes a client will endeavor to reduce physical distance by moving close to the nurse. In such cases the nurse should react in a way that is role appropriate and professional. Nurses can use physical closeness to indicate caring, acceptance, and respect for the client, and they can gain clues about a client's desire for or fear of closeness by observing his use of space.

Another aspect to consider is the client's demands on the nurse's time. The client who attempts to monopolize all the nurse's time is indicating an urgent need for the nurse's attention. It is important to analyze why this is so important to the client. The nurse can control excessive demands in ways that communicate an important message to the client. Her willingness to commit certain amounts of time to the client reaffirms her valuing of and interest in him. But she must also set limits on time spent together to indicate to the client that she will help impose external controls when he is unable to set appropriate limits on his own behavior. Such limits also force the client to accept realities such as being alone at times.

CHARACTERISTICS OF THERAPEUTIC COMMUNICATION

The characteristics of therapeutic communication should not be entirely new to nurses studying psychiatric mental health nursing, for therapeutic communication is part of nursing practice in all settings. It is the central process in the nurse-client interaction system in any health care setting, regardless of the nature of the client's needs. However, certain characteristics of therapeutic communication are so essential to the psychiatric mental health setting that it is important to review them here. These characteristics include client-centered-

ness, goal-directedness, authenticity, self-disclosure, confidentiality, and acceptance.

Client-Centeredness

The purpose of a therapeutic relationship is to promote a client's health and well-being. It is therefore a *client-centered* relationship. All that the nurse says and does is designed to meet the client's health care needs. This is in sharp contrast to ordinary social communication, in which both parties expect to have their needs attended to and gratified. It is particularly important that nurses who are beginning to develop expertise in therapeutic communication keep this purpose in mind and avoid unknowingly using interactions with clients to meet their own needs. A nurse's needs for reassurance, self-esteem, affection, and belonging are, of course, quite legitimate and very important, but the skillful nurse will seek appropriate ways to meet personal needs, such as through interactions with instructors, peers, friends, and family members. Once personal needs are met, nurses can use their energy creatively to meet the client's needs.

Even a need as deceptively innocent as intellectual curiosity is an inappropriate intrusion into the therapeutic relationship. The nurse should seek information from the client only when it is needed to plan for and evaluate the client's care. Similarly, there should be little if any personal talk about the nurse, except perhaps as a way to establish trust or to achieve some specific goal in the client's plan of care.

The client-centered nature of the therapeutic interaction is important because it affirms the client's importance and value. Clients with mental health alterations suffer from poor self-esteem; therapeutic interaction serves to enhance that self-esteem.

At first therapeutic communication may seem awkward to the nurse, since she may become absorbed in techniques to the neglect of the client's needs. For example, when student nurses first learn the technique of reflection (discussed later in this chapter), they may find themselves so eager to try this technique in their interactions with others that they become oblivious to the effect it may have on the other parties. True therapeutic communication focuses not on technique but rather on the sensitivities, needs, comfort, and individuality of the client (Scheideman, 1979).

Goal-Directedness

The second critical characteristic of therapeutic communication is that it always be directed toward a goal. Each interaction between the client and the nurse should have a specific purpose related to the

Sometimes it is not enough to offer the patient a mirror in which to see himself: often he must be encouraged to open his eyes and be shown where to look. Very few patients are knowledgeable and mature enough to do all the work themselves.

K. K. LEWIN, BRIEF ENCOUNTERS: BRIEF PSYCHOTHERAPY

2. Within three days, the client will go to meals unaccompanied, meeting the nurse in the dining room.

3. By the end of the week, the client will also leave the room once in the morning and once in the afternoon for a walk around the unit, accompanied by the nurse.

Long-term goals might include:

4. The client will move about the unit freely, unaccompanied by the nurse, and will stay out of her room at least once during half of her waking hours.

A contract with this client might also include an agreement that, after each excursion outside the room, the nurse and client will spend a few minutes discussing the experience and the client's feelings about it. As progress is made toward achievement of the goals, the contract can be reviewed and revisions may be made.

Another example of a therapeutic contract might be one made with a severely depressed patient who has not been taking responsibility for hygiene and self-care. The nurse and client might discuss appropriate behavior in different areas of hygiene, such as mouth care, bathing, and grooming, and develop a plan whereby the client assumes increasing responsibility for these areas, with gradually decreasing amounts of assistance from the nurse. The nurse will want to verbally reinforce the client's progress while providing the amount of support and assistance that has been agreed upon. Sometimes a contract of this sort needs to be tied to certain requirements. For example, the contract may state that mouth care and dressing must be completed before breakfast may be eaten or that showering must be completed before television can be watched.

The types of agreements that may be made part of the therapeutic contract vary with client needs and with the ways in which clients express their needs. The nurse who devotes time and effort to developing a highly individualized contract with a client will find that considerable progress can be made within the terms of the contract.

Mutual agreement about contract terms is essential. For the contract to succeed, there must be mutual accountability and a sense of shared ownership. This makes both participants more committed to the designated goals and more aware of progress that is made. Once goals have been achieved, the contract should be revised so that the client assumes greater responsibility for his or her own well-being.

FACILITATING THERAPEUTIC COMMUNICATION

Facilitating therapeutic communication means creating a climate that will increase the likelihood that communication will be effective. A broad variety of factors are involved in facilitation of therapeutic communication. *Affective* factors—those related to attitudes, values, beliefs, and feelings—are reflected in the atmosphere in which nurse-client interaction occurs. They determine the emotional climate or "feeling tone" of the interaction. *Cognitive* factors—those related to thought processes—are reflected in the specific communication strategies or

*Besides helping the individual towards a new perspective, most
therapy situations also provide a protected setting in which he or she is
helped to practice new ways of feeling and acting, gradually
developing both the courage and ability to take responsibility for acting
in more effective and satisfying ways in the world.*

J. C. COLEMAN, J. N. BUTCHER, AND R. C. CARSON ABNORMAL PSYCHOLOGY
AND MODERN LIFE, 7TH ED.

techniques used to facilitate therapeutic communication (Hardiman, 1971).

Affective Characteristics of Therapeutic Communication

The emotional climate that facilitates therapeutic communication is determined by five main factors: acceptance, respect, introspection, self-awareness, and empathy. (A useful mnemonic device for helping to remember these five factors is the acronym ARISE.)

Perhaps the most important factor influencing the emotional climate of therapeutic communication is the nurse's *acceptance* of the client as she is, including whatever strengths, weaknesses, needs, and problems she possesses. Acceptance of the client often presents formidable challenges, for clients may display behavior that might be considered unacceptable or at least unappealing in social situations, such as whining, crying, moaning, drooling, pacing, staring, bluntness, anger, hostility, or excessive touching or avoidance of touching. The nurse's ability to accept these behaviors in a nonjudgmental way is critical to promoting therapeutic communication.

The nurse must also be able to convey a sense of *respect* for the client, regardless of how unpleasant his behavior may be. There are numerous ways to convey respect, including form of address, tone of voice, and degree of eye contact. Respect is also conveyed by a willingness to listen to the client's opinions, regardless of how much they may conflict with the nurse's own perceptions of the situation. Respect is shown by acceptance of the client's right to have attitudes, beliefs, and values that may differ markedly from those of the nurse.

Introspection refers to the inner examination of one's own behavior, thoughts, and feelings. Helping a client practice introspection and develop insight into his problems is often the key to successful outcomes in psychiatric mental health nursing. The nurse may help clients develop the capacity for introspection by suggesting means for expressing feelings. To the client who talks of feeling "lost" after the death of a friend, the nurse might suggest, "Sometimes people feel that way when they have lost something they care about a great deal." Another method of encouraging introspection is to ask the client to consider the thoughts and feelings that accompany certain behaviors: "What do you usually think about when you follow people in the halls? What are you feeling when you do that?" Or the nurse may make specific requests for the purpose of encouraging introspection: "Will you write down just how you feel at the times you ask for your medication?"

Introspection must in turn be based on *self-awareness*, or the recognition of one's own memories, ideas, feelings, fears, and wishes. The nurse can be instrumental in helping the client become more self-aware by pointing out significant behaviors: "I have noticed that you leave the room every time other patients come in" or "I see that you talk very little in group meetings, yet the rest of the time you talk a great deal." Sometimes the nurse can help the client become increasingly self-aware by asking questions that require him to consider his own behavior, feelings, and self-image: "How do you feel when people address you like that?" "How would you describe yourself?" "What do you usually do when you are angry?"

Empathy is the identification with and under-

COMMUNICATION SKILLS

I. Facilitating Client Expression
   A. Active listening
   B. Questioning
   C. General leads
   D. Silence

II. Understanding Client Expression
   A. Restatement
   B. Reflection
   C. Clarification
   D. Validation

III. Helping Clients Develop Self-awareness
   A. Focusing
   B. Interpreting
   C. Confronting
   D. Summarizing

IV. Helping Clients Control Behavior
   A. Limit setting
   B. Positive reinforcement

113

standing of another's situation, feelings, and motives. Empathy involves being able to perceive an experience as another person perceives it. Therefore, it involves figuratively stepping out of one's own shoes into another's in order to understand his or her attitudes, beliefs, values, feelings, thoughts, and circumstances. The nurse who is able to feel empathy for a client can understand that person's viewpoint (Hein and Leavitt, 1977).

Feeling and communicating empathy can greatly facilitate therapeutic communication. The empathic nurse creates an atmosphere in which a client feels safe, understood, accepted, and respected. This climate encourages clients to share their thoughts and feelings, which in turn facilitates further therapeutic communication. In this way a cycle of sharing and being understood is begun and maintained.

Cognitive Processes in Therapeutic Communication

Communication processes that encourage clients to express their needs and feelings include active listening, questioning, the use of general leads, and the use of silence. Strategies used to refine and pinpoint meanings include clarification, validation, restatement, and reflection. Additional strategies, such as focusing, interpreting, confronting, and summarizing, may also be used to help the client increase self-awareness and acquire insights into her thoughts and feelings. Communication techniques that help clients control certain behaviors or shape

behaviors into more socially acceptable ones include limit setting and positive reinforcement. All these various strategies are summarized in the accompanying box.

The nurse working with psychiatric clients needs to learn how to use these techniques to facilitate therapeutic communication. Because these strategies are useful in various settings, many nurses are already familiar with some of them and need only to learn how to use them effectively with psychiatric mental health clients.

FACILITATING CLIENT EXPRESSION Facilitating the client's verbal expression is one of the primary aims of the nurse. Hearing the client express what he or she is perceiving, feeling, and thinking provides the nurse with essential information that can be used to assess the client's needs and to develop a plan of care.

Active Listening One of the most effective ways of facilitating client expression is *active listening*. Active listening means attending closely to all that the client is communicating through verbal and nonverbal channels. Nurses should actively attend to what the client is saying, identifying themes in the client's communication. They should also observe the client's behavior, posture, facial expressions, gestures, mannerisms, use of space, and use of and reactions to touch. They should listen to the client's tone of voice, rate of speech, and choice of words to discern underlying feelings.

Such active listening is useful in two ways. First, it gives nurses the maximum amount of data with which to make assessments of the client's needs. Second, it indicates to the client that full attention is being paid to her, thereby indicating acceptance of and concern for her.

Questioning A second way in which the nurse may facilitate client expression is through *questioning*. By asking the client carefully formulated questions, the nurse elicits information about what the client feels, thinks, and perceives. Generally, the nurse should ask open-ended questions that encourage the client to respond with more than a few words and that allow the client to retain some control over the interaction. Such questions as "How are you feeling right now?" and "What brought you to the hospital?" invite the client to share as much information as he chooses.

Closed questions, in contrast, are those that can be answered by yes, no, or other limited responses. Examples of closed-ended questions include: "How many pills do you take each evening?" "Do you ever feel dizzy when you stand up?" and "Have you ever been in the hospital before?" Such questions can be useful for obtaining specific information and are particularly useful in crisis situations in which immediate intervention is imperative and specific information is required. They should be used sparingly, however, because they do limit client responses. Examples of closed questions that might be useful in a crisis include: "How many pills have you taken?" "Have you ever had chest pain before?" and "Do you know where you are?"

General Leads *General leads* are neutral expressions that encourage the client to continue talking, such as "I see," "Go on," and "Mmm hmm . . ." General leads let the client know that the nurse is actively listening, that she is interested in what the client is saying, and that she wishes to hear more.

General leads are used when the nurse wishes the client to continue, but they should not be used when the client is rambling in a way that does not contribute to assessment of needs or the achievement of goals. General leads should not be used when the client is using nonsense syllables or other forms of vocal behavior that the nurse cannot understand.

Silence The thoughtful and appropriate use of silence is another helpful communication strategy. This refers to the conscious and purposeful choice of letting silence occur or continue in order to achieve some specific purpose in an interaction. Silence can offer both the nurse and the client an opportunity to collect their thoughts, review what has been said, and determine the direction they would like the next part of the interaction to take. Silence can provide them with the opportunity to consider the meaning of what has been said. If the

interaction has aroused strong emotional responses in the client, silence offers him the opportunity to express these emotions, by crying for example, or to regain his composure. Silence also conveys the nurse's full acceptance, since the nurse is staying with the client regardless of whether he speaks or is silent.

Many people, including nurses, are intensely uncomfortable during periods of silence. Therefore, nurses need to develop the ability to tolerate silence comfortably. They need to learn how to sit quietly with a client without speaking, in spite of any discomfort they may feel, for gradually extended periods of time. To a novice, the period of silence may seem to last much longer than it actually does. It may therefore be helpful to time the silence, if this can be done unobtrusively. Periods of silence may initially be no longer than 15 to 30 seconds, but as the nurse becomes more comfortable, she will become able to remain silent for a full minute or even longer. It is also essential to assess the client's reaction to silence and to judge whether the client is benefiting from the technique or is feeling acutely uncomfortable.

UNDERSTANDING CLIENT EXPRESSION In addition to facilitating client expression, techniques of therapeutic communication can be used to gain an understanding of the meaning of the client's communications—that is, the client's perceptions, thoughts, and feelings. Strategies used to determine the meaning of the client's communication include restatement, reflection, clarification, and validation.

Restatement and Reflection *Restatement* and *reflection* are two of the most commonly used techniques of therapeutic communication, and most nurses become familiar with them in classroom and clinical settings. Both have the same purpose: to encourage the client to say more in order to make clear his intended meaning.

Restatement is a technique in which the nurse repeats to the client exactly what he just said, using the client's own words. This is usually done with the intonation of a question. Restatement has the dual effect of increasing the client's awareness of what he has said and of encouraging further explanation. Following is a dialogue that illustrates the use of restatement:

NURSE: Tell me what brought you to the hospital today.

CLIENT: I was so nervous I couldn't stand it. I felt like I was going to jump out of my skin. I was afraid I was going to do something terrible.

NURSE: You were afraid you were going to do something terrible?

CLIENT: Yes, like hit the baby or something. I felt like if she cried one more time I'd smash her into a million pieces.

In contrast to restatement, reflection is a technique in which the nurse repeats what she understands to be the essence of the client's message but rephrases it in her own words. For example, the nurse in the preceding example might have used reflection to continue the interaction: "You were afraid you were going to hurt the baby?"

Clarification It is not uncommon for the full meaning of a client's message to be somewhat obscure to the listener. In such cases the nurse may use *clarification* in order to reach a more precise understanding of what the client is trying to say. There are several ways in which the nurse can seek clarification, including questioning, use of examples, and contrast and comparison. For example, in the situation just cited, the nurse might ask, "What did you mean when you said you were afraid you might do something terrible?" In a different situation, the nurse might ask the client to provide examples to illustrate his meaning. For example:

CLIENT: I really feel uptight when people treat me like that.

NURSE: Can you give me an example of what you mean?

Sometimes clarification can best be achieved by the use of comparisons with other topics on which mutual understanding has already been reached. For example, a nurse might ask a client who is complaining of "feeling funny" to compare this feeling with feelings experienced at another time: "How do your feelings right now compare with the way you felt when you came into the hospital?" At other times clarification is best achieved by eliciting contrasting examples: "Do I understand you to be saying that your feelings now are much different from your feelings last night when Susan got angry?"

Once an understanding of a client's meaning has been achieved, it is important that the nurse verify the accuracy of his understanding through the technique called *validation*. A nurse using validation states his interpretation to the client and asks the client to verify whether it is correct. After an admission interview, for example, the nurse might validate his initial assessments with a statement such as "So the thing that bothers you the most is being alone?" or "So the thing that you feared the most

about coming to the hospital is what other people would think?"

HELPING CLIENTS DEVELOP SELF-AWARENESS A third major purpose of therapeutic interaction is to help clients develop greater self-awareness. Several specific communication strategies are used to accomplish this, including focusing, interpreting, confronting, and summarizing.

Focusing In *focusing*, the nurse selects portions of what the client has expressed and directs the client's attention to those areas in order to explore them more fully. The nurse makes her selection based on her judgment of what part of the message is most relevant to the client's health care needs. The nurse focuses the client's attention by a direct request:

"Let's talk more about what happened at breakfast today."

"I'd like to hear more about how you feel when your wife visits."

"It sounds like the relationship with your step-daughter is very stressful to you. Try to tell me more about what that is like."

Interpreting A second way in which the nurse can help the client develop self-awareness is through *interpretation* of his communication and behavior. The nurse can be helpful in this regard by first describing what seems to be happening: "I see that it is very hard for you to talk about this." Then the nurse suggests an interpretation for the behavior: "I wonder if it is hard to talk about the incident because you found it so frightening." At times the nurse may interpret the client's nonverbal behavior: "I notice that you become very restless when we discuss your marriage. You seem anxious and uncomfortable."

Confronting One of the most difficult yet important strategies available to the psychiatric mental health nurse is *confrontation*. To confront means to come face to face with, or to bring close together for comparison or examination. When the nurse confronts the client with something, she is making a demand that the client take note of a behavior and examine it. The nurse may elect to confront the client with a description of the particular behavior:

"You ask for your medicine an hour or more before it is scheduled each day."

"You say you want to lose weight, but I often see you eating candy and donuts."

"You never come to meals unless a staff member asks you to."

115

In this manner the nurse requires the client to acknowledge certain behaviors and expects to receive a response from the client.

Sometimes the client who is confronted in this way reacts in a defensive or angry manner. It is important that the nurse accept this type of response without becoming defensive in turn about why confrontation was used. The nurse must not deviate at this point but must repeat, if necessary, his confrontational statement. As long as the client feels that the nurse's acceptance has not been withdrawn, the client will usually be able to deal with the facts the nurse has presented.

Summarizing Another way in which the nurse can help the client gain self-awareness is through periodically *summarizing* what has been discussed. In summarizing, the nurse identifies and reiterates the main points of the total interaction. This helps the client review the interaction and hear how her communication has been perceived by others.

HELPING CLIENTS CONTROL BEHAVIOR The nurse can use two main techniques in helping clients control their behavior in appropriate ways: limit setting and positive reinforcement.

Limit Setting Limit setting is required when clients are not able to adapt in positive, constructive, appropriate ways to the stressors they are experiencing and therefore behave in ways considered socially unacceptable or potentially injurious to themselves or others. Limits must be set on such behaviors for the well-being of clients and of those around them.

In deciding whether limits should be set, the nurse should first assess the undesirable behavior, noting its nature and extent, the frequency with which it is used, and its actual and potential effects. For example, a client who frequently spits on the floor is creating a health hazard and is offending the aesthetic sensibilities of others. Another client who obsessively spits into tissues and throws them into a wastebasket may be behaving in a manner that is irritating, but he is not posing a threat to others' well-being. Thus, setting limits is more urgent in the former than the latter case. Whenever possible, the nurse should also assess the meaning the behavior has for the client and what actions might be appropriately instituted. For example, the client who spits on the floor may be responding to distorted thought processes that require psychotherapeutic intervention involving medical as well as nursing measures. The client using tissues may be trying to get rid of an irritation caused by certain medications and may respond to reassurance and the use of throat lozenges. In both instances, the meaning of the behavior must be investigated in order to set appropriate limits.

Limits should be set in a specific and direct manner, stating explicitly what aspect of the behavior is unacceptable: "Spitting on the floor is not acceptable, Mr. Smith. Tell me what makes you unwilling to use a tissue." Consequences of violating the limits should also be clearly stated: "Here are tissues to use when you spit. If you continue spitting on the floor, you may not remain in the TV room."

The type of communication that is most effective for setting limits consists of short declarative sentences delivered in a calm, quiet, courteous manner. It should always be clear to the client that the limits that are being set represent the nurse's unwillingness to accept certain behaviors but do not constitute a rejection of the client. Clients often test limits by repeatedly trying to break them. The nurse may have to communicate the same message repeatedly: "You may not spit on the floor, Mr. Smith. If you do, you must leave the TV room."

Occasionally it is necessary to use medications, seclusion, or physical restraints to assist clients in controlling their behavior when they have shown the inability to respond to limits communicated verbally. The careful use of medications and restraint with severely disturbed clients has value, but nurses should remember that medication, seclusion, and physical restraint are forms of communication that must be used carefully and without punitive intent in order to be therapeutic for clients with poor impulse control.

Positive Reinforcement Positive reinforcement involves rewarding clients for engaging in desirable behaviors. Such reinforcement may take the form of acknowledgment, recognition, or some other sign of approval of the behavior. Reinforcement should express an opinion or comment rather than a value judgment. It is not particularly useful to label behaviors as "good" or "bad." Instead of making such value judgments, it is often preferable to indicate a neutral reaction to the desirable behavior:

> "I see that you are up and dressed before breakfast time, Mary."
> "This is the first day I've found you waiting your turn for medication, Sam."

Sometimes positive reinforcement is used to convey actual rewards that have been agreed upon as the consequence of specific behaviors: "We agreed that if you ate your entire meal you could have a pass to the canteen. You ate all your lunch. Here is your pass."

When using positive reinforcement, the nurse should clearly indicate to the client which behavior is being rewarded, praised, or reinforced so that the client knows which behavior to repeat.

Therapeutic Communication and the Nursing Process

The concepts, principles, and techniques of therapeutic communication are inextricably interwoven with the nursing process at each stage of its application. The effectiveness with which the nurse uses the nursing process is highly dependent on his or her skill with therapeutic communication.

ASSESSMENT AND DIAGNOSIS The same factors that contribute to the development of therapeutic communication also contribute to effective data gathering during the assessment phase of the nursing process. The more comfortable the client feels in his relationship with the nurse, the more readily he will answer questions and share information.

The nurse may use a variety of communication strategies to collect data needed to develop a health assessment and plan of care. Open-ended questions and broad leads may be used to encourage the client to share information; closed questions may be used when necessary to elicit specific information. Through a client-centered, goal-directed approach, the nurse can collect data quickly, effectively, and efficiently by conserving the client's emotional energy without sacrificing completeness or accuracy.

The nurse may also need to gather data from secondary sources, such as the client's family, other health care providers, and past records. Because secondary data may be subject to inaccuracies, the nurse should be particularly careful to clarify and validate such information.

After collecting data about the client, the nurse should review and analyze the information in order to draw conclusions about its meaning. The process of data analysis leads to the formulation of nursing diagnoses that will serve as the basis for the client's plan of care. Validation of diagnoses is helpful with clients in all settings, but it is particularly critical in the mental health setting, for two reasons. First, nursing diagnoses of mental and emotional alterations may be more difficult to make than those of physical alterations and therefore may be more subject to error. Validation of the diagnosis with the client reduces or eliminates the likelihood of such error. Second, collaboration with the mental health client is crucial to the success of his therapy. Collaboration is in turn dependent on a mutual agreement about which problems are to be addressed.

The nurse can validate diagnoses with the client by sharing the assessments that have been made and by asking for feedback. Assessments may be worded a bit differently in discussions with the client than in documentation on the client's record. For example, a diagnosis recorded as "alteration in body image related to perceptual distortions" may be described to the client as "troubled feelings about your body because of the way things look to you." Similarly, "anxiety regarding interactions with other people related to poor self-esteem" might be described to the client as "nervousness about talking with other people because you think they will not find you interesting." In each case, the nurse would ask the client to validate the assessment: "Would you agree that this seems to be the problem?" or "Would you agree that this is one of the problems troubling you now?"

PLANNING Planning nursing care is highly dependent on collaboration among the nurse and client, the client's family, and various members of the health care team. Collaboration is in turn based on effective communication and on clear statements about roles and expectations. Whether collaboration is with the client, a family member, or other members of the health care team, clear, direct communication is essential. It enables both parties to agree on the problems to be addressed, to identify and consider possible interventions, and to select those interventions that will form the plan of care. During the planning phase, the nurse and client should reach agreement about priorities so that those areas considered most urgent will be dealt with first.

Once a plan of care has been developed, it should be available in writing to all members of the health care team. Nursing diagnoses should be stated clearly and concisely; short-term and long-term goals should be identified; and interventions should be stated as clear, precise nursing orders. A portion of a care plan might be stated as in Table 5-1.

IMPLEMENTATION The actual implementation of the nursing care plan is highly dependent on effective communication. In the case of the client referred to in Table 5-1, the establishment of a trusting, effective nurse-client relationship is a prerequisite to the implementation of the plan. Specific aspects of the plan will succeed only to the extent that communication is used effectively. The nurse accompanying the client to the dining room should indicate acceptance and empathy but also convey the clear expectation that the client will comply. "It is time to go to the dining room for lunch," the nurse might say. "I know it is hard for you to do that, but we have agreed that you will eat meals with the other residents. I am going to walk with you to the dining room and stay with you until you feel more comfortable."

EVALUATION As the nursing care plan is implemented, ongoing evaluation occurs. In the evaluation phase of the nursing process, the nurse

117

Table 5-1. Portion of a Nursing Care Plan

Nursing Diagnosis	Short-Term Goals	Long-Term Goals	Nursing Orders
Social isolation secondary to depression	The client will eat all meals in dining room beginning 11/21	The client will interact with others at mealtime by 11/25	1. Accompany client to dining room for all meals. 2. Seat client with others who are likely to interact with him. 3. Document interactions at meals.

118

should note the client's reactions to the care plan. For example, the nurse may invite the client to share her reactions and feelings about eating meals with others: "You seem less tense than you did at breakfast. Tell me how you feel now." The nurse may also help the client interpret her nonverbal messages: "You seem to be upset right now. Tell me what you are feeling."

Regardless of the nature of the client's problems or the interventions included in the individual care plan, exploration of the client's thoughts and feelings is central to care. There may, for example, be a goal for the client to verbalize feelings instead of expressing them behaviorally. Because the verbal expression of feelings is difficult to quantify and does not involve psychomotor skills such as those the nurse uses in other settings, its importance may sometimes be underestimated. Encouraging clients to verbalize their feelings is often the most critical intervention of all and can only be achieved through effective communication. The nurse caring for mental health clients must therefore develop genuine skill in the area of therapeutic communication, which will enable her to provide high-quality, meaningful nursing care.

DOCUMENTATION OF CARE

There are four ways to document the nursing process in the mental health setting; the nurse will probably be familiar with them from other settings: the health status profile, the problem list, progress notes, and the discharge plan and summary.

The Health Status Profile

The *health status profile* contains the data gathered when the client entered or reentered the health care system. A designated nurse usually conducts a thorough, systematic interview, called an *intake interview* or an *initial nursing assessment*. Typically, this interview deals with the client's present health status, the nature of the problems that brought the client to the health care system, the client's past health history, and the client's support systems, resources, and constraints.

It is helpful to note first the client's perception of what brought him to the health care setting and his description of the onset and characteristics of the current problem. The nurse might record a summary that indicates both the client's own words, referred to as the *subjective data*, and the nurse's observations of the client, or *objective data*, as follows:

Subjective:
"My husband brought me in. He said I had to come here because I wouldn't eat any more. He said I had to find out what is wrong."

Objective:
This thin, pale young woman was brought to the Emergency Department by her husband, who states client has not eaten for four days. Client speaks only when spoken to but responds to questions in a cooperative manner. Avoids eye contact. Affect is flat. Lies motionless in bed, seeming to stare at the wall.

During the initial assessment, the nurse should explore with the client the dimensions of the pres-

---

SAMPLE PROGRESS NOTES

PROBLEM: Anxiety related to marital difficulties

Subjective: "I dread hearing his car in the driveway. I just know he'll start yelling about something as soon as he comes in the door. I feel so scared I just pretend I am not there. I hope he won't even see me."

Objective: Client talks in quiet, hesitant manner, staring down at her hands, which she twists nervously. Makes no eye contact with nurse. Occasionally eyes well with tears, which she brushes away. Client appears pale and poorly groomed; smokes absentmindedly at intervals.

Assessment: Expressing feelings more readily today, but still visibly upset when discussing marriage. Smoking less than yesterday.

Plan: Continue daily periods of exploration of feelings about husband. Assist client in focusing on herself as a person and on her grooming and physical care. Develop contract regarding personal hygiene.

PROBLEM: Grief and suicidal ideation related to loss of pregnancy

Subjective: "If I can't have a baby there is nothing to live for." "Just leave me alone."

Objective: Client is crying hysterically, sitting in corner of room with arms drawn around flexed legs, rocking back and forth. Client was originally quite agitated when nurse entered room but quieted somewhat after a few minutes.

Assessment: Client continues to express feelings of hopelessness. Suicide risk still a possibility.

Plan: Continue suicide precautions. Discuss response to medications with physician. Continue supportive interactions with encouragement to express feelings about loss of pregnancy.

119

ent problem, including its onset and duration, the ways in which it is manifested, and anything that aggravates or relieves the problem.

The nurse should then take a complete health history, unless the client's condition precludes it. In addition to the client's own health history, the nurse should investigate the client's family history and social history, including the present living situation, major roles and responsibilities, and potential or actual support systems. The health history interview is usually accompanied by a physical health assessment of the client. The format for a comprehensive health assessment is the same for mental health clients as for all other clients. Particular attention should be paid to the mental status examination and assessment, as discussed in Chapter 3.

Once the initial assessment has been conducted by the nurse and by the other appropriate members of the health care team, all the data should be documented in an orderly fashion in the client's record, where it serves as the health status profile. The health status profile then provides the basis for diagnosing the client's health care problems and planning appropriate care.

The Problem List

The nursing diagnoses, as well as those made by other health care professionals, are listed on the client's *problem list* in the record. The problem list serves as a guide for all those participating in the client's care and also is used as the basis for organizing a record of the client's progress.

Progress Notes

The *progress notes* comprise the body of the client's record and describe the changing condition of the client. The frequency with which progress notes are written will depend on the rate at which the client's condition changes and the policies of the particular institution. All progress notes should be directed at a specific problem from the client's problem list and should contain subjective and objective data related to the problem, the nurse's assessment and evaluation of the meaning of the data, and the care plan revisions required by the assessment and evaluation. The progress notes make it possible for all those providing care to quickly review the client's progress and to use that knowledge as the basis for further work with the client. Accurate, concise progress notes are essential to comprehensive and

---

SAMPLE DISCHARGE PLAN

Problem	Status at Discharge	Plans for Follow-up
1. Anxiety	Client has good awareness of her own anxiety level; is using imaging and relaxation techniques with some benefit.	Dr. R. Jones to follow. First appointment Nov. 30.
	Adequately controlled on Valium 5 mg p.o. every 4 hr. p.r.n.	Client will continue to attend relaxation group on weekly basis.
2. Anorexia	Client has stabilized weight at 110 pounds. Goal now is maintenance. Was instructed to continue calorie count to maintain intake at 1500 calories per day.	Client to be weighed weekly after group meeting. Dietitian available p.r.n. Clinic nurses to evaluate weight and diet history weekly.
3. Concern regarding ability to carry pregnancy to term	Initial meeting with GYN consult went well; client is receptive to further workup.	Has appointment with Dr. B. Gunther on Dec. 1.
4. Lack of social supports	Client has acknowledged need for structured activities outside home; has made commitment to join weekly discussion group and to seek part-time employment.	Client has obtained information about discussion group meeting on 11/28. Plans to attend. To be referred to Bureau of Vocational Rehabilitation for intake interview and vocational testing if she expresses interest in this.

---

continuous nursing care and also serve as the legal record of the nursing care provided to the client. Sample progress notes are presented in the box on page 119.

Discharge Plans and Summary

When the client is ready to be discharged from the health care facility, the record should indicate the plans for discharge and for any follow-up care. Each of the client's identified problems should be addressed, and the plans for continued treatment of any unresolved problems should be indicated in the discharge summary. Specifically, the names of persons and agencies who have responsibility for the client's ongoing care should be noted.

In addition to the specific discharge plan, a brief summary should be written indicating the client's condition at discharge and summarizing the care provided. Examples of discharge plans and discharge summaries are provided in the accompanying boxes.

Process Recording

In addition to the written documentation that forms the client's record of care, the nurse may wish to use other forms of written communication to enhance understanding of the client or for the use of the interdisciplinary health care team. In psychiatric mental health settings, one form of written communication that is a commonly used and highly effective learning tool is the *process recording*. A process recording is merely a verbatim recording of what was said by each participant in the interaction, using alternating columns so that the communication of each person is clearly identified. A third column is then used to identify the meanings assigned to the interaction.

The purposes of a process note are:

1. To provide a mechanism for studying and analyzing the interaction by helping the nurse identify and understand the meaning of behavior, thoughts, and feelings exhibited by both the nurse and the client.

SAMPLE DISCHARGE SUMMARY

Mrs. Anderson is a 24-year-old married woman who was admitted on 10/4/83 following an attempted suicide with a Librium overdose. The attempt was apparently precipitated by the loss of a pregnancy by spontaneous abortion on 9/29/83, following which she had grown profoundly depressed, refused meals, suffered marked weight loss, withdrew from all social contact, and stayed secluded in her room. This is her third spontaneous abortion; she has no living children.

Mrs. Anderson has responded well to the plan of care, making rapid progress in acknowledging and dealing with her own problems. She has responded well to medication (Imipramine 100 mg q.d. at h.s.; Valium 5 mg p.o. every 4 hours p.r.n.), daily therapy with Dr. R. Jones, and supportive therapy from the nursing and activities staffs. She has par-ticipated in the relaxation group and community meetings. Her weight has stabilized at 110 pounds, and she has assumed responsibility for keeping her own calorie counts and planning her intake to meet a 1500 calorie per day goal. She has a realistic perception of her gynecologic difficulties and is aware of the options remaining to her for having a child. She has consented to further GYN workup.

Mrs. Anderson now recognizes the relationship between her anxiety and depression and her lack of social supports and is taking steps to make commitments outside her home, including a search for a part-time job and a commitment to join a discussion group.

She will be followed by Dr. Jones and by the outpatient staff of the mental health and GYN clinic.

121

FORMAT OF A PROCESS NOTE

Place where interaction occurred: _____

Time and date of interaction: _____

Purpose or goal of interaction: _____

Name of nurse: _____

Client initials: _____

Presenting problem(s): _____

Client Communication (verbal and nonverbal)	Nurse Communication (verbal and nonverbal, including thoughts, feelings, opinions)	Interpretation and Rationale
What does the client say? How does the client act? How does the client seem to the nurse? Tense? Anxious? Angry? Sad? Changeable or labile?	What is the emotional, cognitive, verbal, and nonverbal response of the nurse to the client, the environment, and the communication exchanged?	What is the client really communicating? Is verbal communication congruent with nonverbal communication? On what level does the client usually communicate? Behavioral? Cognitive? Emotional? Is the nurse communicating on the same level as the client? Does the client understand and accept what the nurse is trying to communicate? Was the communication of the nurse effective? If not, what alternative responses might have been made? Why might the alternatives have been more effective?

C L I N I C A L   E X A M P L E

STAFF-CLIENT DIFFICULTIES

Mrs. Murray is an alcoholic who has liver damage and neurologic changes due to excessive drinking. She is being treated in a 30-day residential rehabilitation program, and her stay is almost over. Before entering the program, she lived alone and had difficulty managing her daily activities. She has severe ataxia due to neuropathy of her legs. As a result, the staff doubt her ability to care for herself. They have suggested that she consider living in a proprietary residence where she can have an appropriate level of supervision and minimal responsibility for cooking, keeping house, and shopping for her personal needs. Mrs. Murray has been a cooperative client on every point except one: she insists that she is able to care for herself at home and refuses to heed staff members who urge her to view her situation realistically. The problem has not yet been resolved. The following nursing and psychiatric diagnoses were made:

Nursing Diagnoses

Coping, ineffectual individual

Home maintenance management, impaired

Physical mobility, impaired

Decision making, impaired

Social isolation

Multiaxial Psychiatric Diagnoses

Axis I   303.9x Alcohol dependence

Axis II   None

Axis III Alcoholic liver disease, periphreal neuro-
          pathy

Axis IV   Code 1—No apparent stressor

Axis V   Code 4—Fair, moderate impairment

The following process recording was made of an interaction between Mrs. Murray and her nurse:

Place: Client's room
Time and date: 2 P.M. July 23
Goal of the interview: To further explore the issues of discharge and aftercare.

Nurse: K. Winslow
Client initials: L.M.
Presenting problems: Impaired mobility, self-care deficits, social isolation

CLIENT	NURSE	INTERPRETATION AND RATIONALE
	Hello, Mrs. M. When we talked last week, you told me that you hoped to return to your home. I'd like to talk with you about this during our time together today. (Looks inquiringly at client. Nurse really wants to explore this issue and doesn't want client to say no.)	Stating purpose of interview.

Seeking collaboration and permission. |
| Are you going to help me get home? The social worker says I can't go home. | | Asking nurse to define her role. What can the nurse do for the client? |
| | No, I probably won't be able to help you get home. (Wishes she knew how to get client home.) I didn't know you had talked to the social worker. It must have been very discouraging to hear her say that! | Attempting to ascertain client's underlying feelings. |

I don't believe I won't be able to go home. I've had that home for twenty-five years. (Gestures angrily around room) I'm waiting.

You're waiting?
(Nurse wonders if client is waiting for something to happen. Is she using denial to cope with being here? Nurse wouldn't especially like living here, either. Doesn't know what to say.)

Client is angry but not discouraged because she doesn't believe she's not able to return home.

Reflection—nurse needs more information.

(Leans closer to nurse and drops her voice.) I keep myself busy, you know. I work my puzzles in the morning; then I have lunch; then I read a little in the afternoon, and sometimes I work on my knitting. I've done a lot of that. I know that I'll be able to take care of myself at home.

Communicating on behavioral level. Client has changed subject and is trying to show nurse how capable she is. Client derives satisfaction from handiwork skills.

You knit well. You certainly do a nice job! Have you sold some of your things? (Somewhat relieved that subject has changed to a safer topic.)

Nurse goes along with changed subject. [No evidence noted that client was getting anxious in talking about house, except for change of subject. Nurse could have said, "What are you thinking about while you keep yourself so busy?" If client answered, "I don't know," it might indicate she didn't want to talk about it. On the other hand, she had introduced the topic.]

123

I sold a lot of things at the sidewalk sale.

That's good. (Looks brightly at client.)

(Looks brightly back.)

(Realizing that client really doesn't want to talk about knitting or the sidewalk sale, nurse starts feeling a little anxious.)

(Leans back in chair, looks away from nurse and starts to work on the puzzle.)

Nonverbal. Client is not interested in this topic, either.

Well, I'll talk to you next week. Good-bye.

Responding to nonverbal communication from client. [Nurse does not achieve solution regarding the client's feelings about going home. Nurse is relieved when client talks about topics other than going home and allows the client to digress. The goal of the interaction has not been met fully.]

Good-bye Honey.

(Nurse leaves, wondering if there is any meaning to the client's use of the word "honey." She has an uneasy sense of being ineffective with the client.)

2. To provide a method of systematically observing and noting nonverbal and verbal communication.

3. To assist the nurse in examining and evaluating nursing interventions.

4. To offer a means by which the nurse can validate perceptions and interpretations.

5. To help the nurse collect, organize, interpret, analyze, and synthesize raw data gathered in the course of a nurse-client interaction.

6. To facilitate the application of theoretical concepts to clinical practice.

7. To promote ongoing assessment, planning, and evaluation of nursing intervention with a specific client.

The format for a process note is presented in the box on page 121.

124

SUMMARY

Therapeutic communication is the process that unites the nurse and the client in their collaborative search for improvement in the client's health status. The nurse-client interaction system is dependent on the therapeutic communication skills of the nurse through every phase of the nursing process.

By establishing trust, offering empathy, and communicating her acceptance of and respect for the client, the nurse begins the therapeutic relationship. Verbal and nonverbal messages are exchanged as the nurse guides the client-centered, goal-directed process that leads to growth and improved functioning.

Through a combination of authenticity and specific communication techniques, the nurse facilitates collaboration with the client and guides the establishment of a therapeutic contract. The nurse and client then use the communication process to pursue specific goals on the client's behalf. The nurse's ability to convey empathy and to facilitate increasing self-awareness and introspection on the part of the client helps the client move toward achieving the goals mutually set by client and nurse. A variety of communication strategies enable the nurse to deal effectively with the individual needs of different clients.

The nurse also uses the communication process to collaborate with other members of the health team and to document the assessment, planning, and implementation of nursing care and to evaluate the client's response to that care.

Review Questions

1. Describe four essential ingredients required for establishing therapeutic relationships.

2. Use the Berlo model of communication to analyze the elements of an interaction you recently experienced with a client.

3. Explain the role of each of these five essential qualities in the process of therapeutic communication: client-centeredness, goal-directedness, authenticity, self-disclosure, and confidentiality.

4. Define and describe the collaboration process.

5. Explain what is meant by a therapeutic contract.

6. Using the acronym ARISE, name, define, and describe five affective characteristics of therapeutic communication.

7. Give one example of each of the following specific communication strategies:
   a. open-ended questioning.
   b. general leads.
   c. clarification.
   d. validation.
   e. restatement.
   f. reflection.
   g. focusing.
   h. interpreting.
   i. confronting.

8. Explain how each of the following helps the client who has difficulty with emotional adaptation:
   a. active listening.
   b. use of silence.
   c. summarizing.

9. List and illustrate two ways in which communication can be used therapeutically to control behavior.

10. Name each step in the nursing process and list one way in which therapeutic communication contributes to the effective use of each stage of the process.

References

Almore, M. G. 1979. Dyadic Communication. *American Journal of Nursing*, 79:1076–1078.

Berlo, D. K. 1960. *The Process of Communication*. San Francisco: Rinehart Press.

Burnside, I. M. 1973. Touching Is Talking. *American Journal of Nursing*, 73:2060–2063.

Hardiman, M. 1971. Interviewing or Social Chit Chat? *American Journal of Nursing*, 71:1379–1381.

Hein, E. C. 1980. *Communication in Nursing Practice*, 2nd ed. Boston: Little, Brown.

Hein, E. and Leavitt, M. 1977. Providing Emotional Support to Patients. *Nursing 77*, 7:39–41.

Ramaekers, M. J. 1979. Communication Blocks Revisited. *American Journal of Nursing*, 79:1079–1081.

Scheideman, M. 1979. Problem Patients Do Not Exist. *American Journal of Nursing*, 79:1082–1084.

Truesdell, S. 1977. Communication: Key to Efficient Patient Care. *Nursing 77*, 7:52–53.

Supplementary Readings

Balzoni, N. Premature Reassurance: A Distancing Maneuver. *Nursing Outlook* 23(1975):49–51.

Barker, L. L. *Listening Behavior*. Englewood Cliffs, N.J.: Prentice-Hall, 1971.

Blondis, M. N., and Jackson, B. E. *Nonverbal Communication with Patients*. New York: John Wiley & Sons, 1977.

Brammer, L. M. *The Helping Relationship*. Englewood Cliffs, N. J.: Prentice-Hall, 1979.

Bromley, G. E. Confrontation in Individual Psychotherapy. *Journal of Psychiatric Nursing and Mental Health Services*, 19(1981):15–18.

Campbell, J. The Relationship of Nursing and Self-awareness. *Advances in Nursing Science* (1980):15–24.

Carr, J. B. *Communicating and Relating*. Reading, Mass.: Benjamin Cummings, 1979.

Davis, J. A. *Listening and Responding*. St. Louis: C. V. Mosby, 1984.

Fritz, P. *Interpersonal Communication in Nursing: An Interactionist Approach*. East Norwalk, Conn.: Appleton-Century-Crofts, 1983.

Geach, B., and White, J. Empathic Resonance: A Countertransference Phenomenon. *American Journal of Nursing*, 74(1974):1282–1285.

Hall, E. T. *The Silent Language*. New York: Fawcett World Library, 1959.

Haller, K. B., and Reynolds, M. A. *Mutual Goal Setting in Patient Care*. Orlando, Fla.: Grune & Stratton, 1982.

Hames, C. C., and Joseph, D. H. *Basic Concepts of Helping*. East Norwalk, Conn.: Appleton-Century-Crofts, 1980.

Hays, J., and Larson, K. *Interacting with Patients*. New York: Macmillan, 1965.

Heineken, J. Treating the Disconfirmed Psychiatric Client. *Journal of Psychosocial Nursing and Mental Health Services*, 21(1983):21–25.

Iveson-Iveson, J. The Art of Communication. *Nursing Mirror*, 156(1983):47–48.

Jones, E. Behind the Words. *Nursing Mirror*, 156(1983):33–34.

Kirk, W. G. A Brief Inservice Training Strategy to Increase Levels of Empathy of Psychiatric Nursing Personnel. *Journal of Psychiatric Treatment and Evaluation*, 4(1982):177–179.

Knapp, L. *Nonverbal Communication in Human Interaction*. New York: Holt, Rinehart and Winston, 1972.

Lamonica, E. L. Empathy in Nursing Practice. *Issues in Mental Health Nursing*, 2(1979):1–14.

McGaron, S. On Developing Empathy: Teaching Students Self-awareness. *American Journal of Nursing*, 78(1978):859–861.

O'Kern, B. F. Effective Helping: Interviewing and Counseling Techniques. North Scituate, Mass.: Duxbury Press, 1976.

Phickhan, M. L. *Human Communication. The Matrix of Nursing*. New York: McGraw-Hill, 1978.

Rosenthal, T. T. The Construction of a Relationship. *Health Values*, 6(1982):28–30.

Rudnick, S. Communicating Acceptance to the Psychotic Patient. *American Journal of Psychoanalysis*, 42(1982):265–269.

Ruesch, J. *Therapeutic Communication*. New York: W. W. Norton, 1961.

Seiger, P. Self-awareness and Nursing. *Journal of Psychiatric Nursing and Mental Health Services* (1979):24–26.

Sommer, R. *Personal Space: The Behavioral Basis of Design*. Englewood Cliffs, N. J.: Prentice-Hall, 1969.

Sundeen, S. J.; Stuart, G. W.; Rankin, E. D.; and Cohen, S. A. *Nurse-Client Interaction: Implementing the Nursing Process*. St. Louis: C. V. Mosby, 1984.

Walzlawick, P.; Beavin, J.; and Jackson, D. *The Pragmatics of Human Communication*. New York: W. W. Norton, 1967.

125

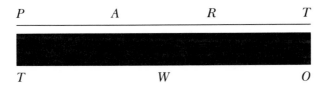
HOLISTIC
INTERACTIONAL
PATTERNS

ETIOLOGIC THEORIES OF THOUGHT DISTURBANCE
Genetic Theories
Biochemical Theories
Developmental Theories
Psychodynamic Theories

THE PROCESS OF THOUGHT DISTURBANCE
Types of Thought Disturbance
Primary Manifestations of Thought Disturbance
Secondary Manifestations of Thought Disturbance

THERAPEUTIC APPROACHES FOR CLIENTS
WITH THOUGHT DISTURBANCES
Psychotropic Drug Therapy
Relationship Therapy
Milieu Therapy
Family Therapy
Predictive Factors

C   H   A   P   T   E   R

6

Altered Patterns of Thought and Perception

Learning Objectives

After reading this chapter, the student should be able to:

1. Describe biochemical, genetic, psychodynamic, and developmental theories explaining the etiology of schizophrenia.

2. Identify various types of schizophrenia based on behavioral manifestations.

3. In terms of the nursing process, formulate appropriate nursing interventions based on altered thought and perceptions as expressed behaviorally.

4. Describe the functions and responsibilities of the nurse in the administration of antipsychotic medication.

5. Explain the principles of relationship therapy in caring for clients with alterations of thought and perception.

6. Describe the major components of milieu therapy as they relate to the nursing process.

Overview

In this chapter altered patterns of thought and perception are discussed, with special emphasis on those alterations that are manifested by persons with schizophrenia.

Schizophrenia refers to a group of disorders characterized by distortions of perception and thinking processes, often resulting in extensive withdrawal of the individual's interest from other people and the outside world and preoccupation with an inner world that is not based on reality. Genetic, biochemical, developmental, and psychodynamic theories about the etiology of thought and perceptual disorders are discussed in the first section of this chapter. Next, the types of thought and perceptual disorders known as schizophrenia are described behaviorally and their primary and secondary manifestations are discussed. The third section covers therapeutic approaches to helping the client with schizophrenia, including psychotropic drug therapy, relationship therapy, and milieu therapy. Nursing functions and responsibilities in utilizing these various approaches are emphasized. Factors influencing outcomes of therapy are discussed in the final section.

How weary, stale, flat, and unprofitable
Seem to me the uses of this world.
WILLIAM SHAKESPEARE

131

The relatively high prevalence of schizophrenic disorders and the lack of agreement regarding diagnosis, etiology, and treatment contribute to the challenges of dealing with the altered patterns of thought and perception known as schizophrenia. Because of differences in methodology and diagnostic criteria, statistics on the incidence and prevalence of schizophrenia vary considerably. Worldwide incidence rates have been estimated at between 1 and 2 percent, but it is impossible to make reliable comparisons from one culture to another. (*Prevalence* refers to the number of persons suffering from a disorder at the time of a survey; *incidence* refers to the number of new cases within a given period.)

In the United States, 2 million Americans can be expected to experience a disorder of thought and perception sometime during their life. Compounding the problem is the fact that initial episodes usually affect young adults, and a sizeable number of those affected tend to follow a pattern of gradual deterioration and chronic disability. This disorder therefore constitutes a major public health problem (Dunham, 1977).

Emil Kraepelin was the first to differentiate this disorder, to classify it according to observable behaviors, and to label it *dementia praecox*, which means "madness of the young" (Lehmann, 1980). The disorder was renamed "schizophrenia" by Eugene Bleuler in 1911, based on what Bleuler saw as a splitting of psychological functions. The person suffering from schizophrenia does not have a "split personality" but rather suffers a split, or departure, from reality. Another splitting aspect of schizophre-

nia is the separation between thought and affect that frequently develops. For instance, persons with this disorder may react to sad thoughts by laughing inappropriately.

For clinicians concerned with psychiatric classification, there are no unique identifying signs for schizophrenia, nor are there conclusive laboratory indicators. When there is lack of agreement regarding the psychiatric classification to which the client has been assigned, there are some general guidelines to consider. Most clients presumed to be experiencing schizophrenic alterations of thought and perception develop idiosyncratic interpretations of events that are revealed by inconsistent, confused, illogical statements or bizarre behaviors. Thoughts and ideas are randomly and incoherently comprehended and expressed, and learning abilities may be impaired. The person may withdraw from interaction with the external world and become preoccupied with subjective internal stimuli.

The clinical manifestations of schizophrenia have often been confused with those of organic brain syndrome, manic-depressive disorders, or drug abuse. Most organic brain disorders are accompanied by neurological changes, whereas schizophrenia is not. Another distinguishing feature is that organic brain disorders are more common in older persons and are characterized by deficits in memory and less dramatic signs of disorderly thinking. In manic-depressive illness and in severe states of depression, the emotional and behavioral state is dominated by excessive sadness or elation rather than confusion and disorganization. Certain hallucinogenic drugs precipitate thought distortions that may resemble a schizophrenic episode, and exploring previous drug use by a client may help in making an accurate assessment.

ETIOLOGIC THEORIES
OF THOUGHT DISTURBANCE

Etiologic explanations for the cluster of disorders classified as schizophrenia remain inconclusive, despite some progress in this regard. Current explanations are based on interactions among genetic, biochemical, psychological, and interpersonal factors that as yet are incompletely understood. These multifactorial interactive explanations suggest that a number of variables may be present, some of which remain unidentified. The most plausible theories to date suggest that the clinical manifestations of schizophrenia are mediated by neurotransmitters in the brain and central nervous system. Although considerable laboratory research points in the direction of biochemical causes, it is necessary to give attention to other etiologic explanations as well. Careful investigation of family and social factors is essential to understanding not only the etiology but also the nature of schizophrenia. Faulty communication patterns and inappropriate role enactment in families are considered significant in the development and prognosis of schizophrenic behaviors manifested by a family member. In this section genetic and developmental theories are presented in some detail because of the relevance of these theories to nursing process. Biochemical theories merit attention because of their primacy in research studies and because biochemical theories support and explain many aspects of pharmacologic treatment of schizophrenia.

Genetic Theories

Investigative studies indicate that genetic factors may influence the onset of schizophrenic disorders. It has been noted that the closer the biological relationship between an individual and a person considered to be schizophrenic, the greater the risk of that individual developing the disorder. Vulnerability seems to decrease as biological relationships become more distant. When one parent is identified as being schizophrenic, the probability of offspring becoming schizophrenic is 12 to 15 percent (Heston, 1977; Rosen, 1978). If both parents are diagnosed as schizophrenic, the probability of offspring developing the disorder increases to 35 percent.

In addition to statistical evidence that biological relatives of persons with schizophrenia are at greater risk, the following data are available to support theories of genetic transmission (Heston, 1977; Gottesman, 1978):

■ The incidence of schizophrenia in identical twins is three times greater than the incidence in fraternal twins and at least thirty times greater than in the general population.

■ The incidence of schizophrenia in identical twins reared apart is about the same as that in identical twins reared together.

■ The incidence of the disorder in children of schizophrenic parents placed early in life with other families is higher than that in the general population; data from some studies show incidence rates as high as if the children had been reared by their biological parents.

■ The incidence of schizophrenia is not greater in children adopted into homes where an adoptive parent develops schizophrenia.

■ In a study of monozygotic (identical) twin pairs where only one twin became schizophrenic, the incidence of schizophrenia in offspring of the unaffected twin equaled that in offspring of the affected twin.

From a genetic perspective, schizophrenia may be explained by either a *monogenic* or a *polygenic* theory. The monogenic theory holds that the disorder classified as schizophrenia is influenced by the transmission of a single gene that produces susceptibility to the disorder. The extent to which the gene is expressed behaviorally depends on environmental influences to which the susceptible person is exposed. Under stress, a genetically vulnerable person is likely to become schizophrenic, but under benign conditions this is less likely to occur. According to the polygenic theory, schizophrenia is caused by the inheritance of more than one gene. A person might inherit all the genes involved in schizophrenia and therefore be at high risk, or she might inherit only some of the genes involved and therefore be at less risk.

Whether of polygenic or monogenic etiology, precipitating factors in the appearance of schizophrenic behaviors seem to be related to social or environmental stresses. The high incidence of schizophrenia among relatives of persons with the disorder supports the possibility of inherited vulnerability. The extent to which inherited vulnerability leads to clinical manifestations of the disorder seems to depend on (1) the extent of inherited susceptibility, and (2) the amount of life stress encountered by the vulnerable individual (Goleman, 1984). What is less certain is the nature of the processes

Identification of high-risk groups currently points to inherited susceptibility to schizophrenia as an essential etiologic factor that is greatly intensified when combined with the following additional risk factors (Goleman, 1984):

■ Childbirth problems, including low birth weight and unusual birth position.

■ Poor maternal bonding in the first three years of life.

■ Poor motor coordination in infancy.

■ Separation from parents or multiple placements in early childhood.

■ Intellectual deficits, especially in verbal skills.

■ Cognitive deficits, especially in concentration and attention.

■ Social incompetence, especially contentiousness with peers and others.

■ Confusion in family communication patterns.

■ Hostility of parents toward the child.

and structures involved in a genetic predisposition to schizophrenia (Yahres, 1978; Barham, 1984).

Biochemical Theories

Biochemical explanations of the etiology of schizophrenia propose that the disorder is caused by physiological dysfunction. Biochemical investigations have not established the existence of a dominant causative factor, but in general, the evidence of biochemical research points to *bioamine* transmission as a likely factor, since bioamines act as neurotransmitters in the limbic system of the brain and mediate such functions as awareness, sleep, emotion, and sensations of pain and pleasure.

There are two broad categories of bioamines: the *catecholamines* (norepinephrine and dopamine) and the *indolamines* (serotonin and tryptamine). These bioamines are converted into metabolites that can be detected and measured in the urine. Studies of bioamine production and metabolism tend to confirm the idea that a relationship exists between the bioamines and schizophrenia. For example, urinalyses of schizophrenic persons have revealed abnormally high levels of indolamine metabolites. Researchers studying persons with schizophrenia found that one to five days before the onset of behavioral signs, levels of tryptamine increased in the urine. Levels remained high until the day before behavioral manifestations appeared, at which time the levels of tryptamine suddenly dropped. Additionally, when behavioral manifestations developed, urinary levels of catecholamine metabolites increased. Catecholamine levels in the urine began to rise prior to the appearance of behavioral signs and continued to increase as psychotic behavior became more pronounced. When the behavioral manifestations of schizophrenia escalated, urinary levels of indolamines and catecholamines both rose; when an individual showed signs of tension without behavioral manifestations of schizophrenia, only the catecholamine levels rose.

When the specific role of *serotonin* in the etiology of schizophrenia has been studied, it has been shown that administration of a monoamine oxidase (MAO) inhibitor is followed by increased levels of serotonin in the brain and the appearance of schizophrenic behaviors. Conversely, the phenothiazine group of drugs has been shown to block the action of dopamine and to reduce the behavioral signs of schizophrenia. Some investigators have therefore postulated that the schizophrenic process may be initiated and perpetuated by excesses of serotonin and dopamine (Rickelman, 1979).

Toxic substances in the blood of persons with schizophrenia have been linked to abnormal brain chemistry and aberrant behaviors. A substance known as *taraxine* has been found in the blood of persons with schizophrenia. When this substance is injected into animals and into humans who have had no previous psychiatric symptoms, schizophrenic-like reactions occur. Among schizophrenic persons receiving renal dialysis, improvement has sometimes followed, but since only 16 percent of such subjects in one study improved, it has been concluded that hemodialysis alone does not produce remission. However, it has also been noted that schizophrenic persons with normal renal systems who undergo dialysis experience a decrease in behavioral symptomatology (Rickelman, 1979). This is an area of research that deserves further study.

Developmental Theories

It is generally accepted by theorists and clinicians that all behavior has meaning and purpose, even if neither can immediately be discerned. It is also accepted that childhood experiences influence adult behaviors. Thus, developmental theories are considered a useful frame of reference for explaining the etiology of schizophrenia. Knowledge and

133

Table 6-1. Erikson's Psychosocial Theory

Developmental Stage	Time Frame	Developmental Task	Implication
Sensory	0 – 18 months	Trust vs. mistrust	Consistent loving care fosters trust; inconsistent harsh care fosters mistrust; some mistrust remains in every adult
Muscular	1 – 3 years	Autonomy vs. shame and doubt	Desire arises to control own thoughts and actions; success leads to sense of control over body and environment
Locomotor	3 – 6 years	Initiative vs. guilt	Child needs to explore world via senses, actions, imagination; conscience begins to develop, guiding initiative; negative relationships with parents promote a sense of guilt
Latency	6 – 12 years	Industry vs. inferiority	Child understands and accepts rules, engages in productive work, starts and completes tasks; excessive parental expectations induce feelings of inferiority
Adolescence	12 – 20 years	Identity vs. role diffusion	Adolescent attempts to rework problems of earlier stages; usually demonstrates interest in members of opposite sex; tries to integrate past and present experiences; copes with changing body image; searches for identity and a place in society
Young adulthood	18 – 25 years	Intimacy vs. isolation	Adult achieves sufficient identity to establish intimacy, accepts personal commitments, tries to understand others and to be understood by others; isolation results when intimacy is not attained

SOURCE: Adapted from Erikson (1968).

understanding of developmental stages enable nurses to assess behaviors in the context of the client's past experience. Two developmental theorists whose work has contributed to the conceptualization of interpersonal and psychosocial issues are Harry Stack Sullivan (1953) and Erik Erikson (1968). Their theories (introduced in Chapter 2) are summarized in Tables 6-1 and 6-2.

According to Erikson, the process of thought disturbance may start early in life when the relationship between the child and the primary caregiver is impaired or inadequate. As a result of deficient nurturing in infancy, the child has difficulty learning to interact with others. Erikson (1968) believes that if trust does not develop between the child and the caregiver during the first year of life, the child's ability to trust himself and others will be permanently impaired. According to Sullivan (1953), the person who has never experienced a secure, comforting relationship with another human being is at risk for developing mental disturbances. Such an individual is deprived of the kind of interpersonal relationships that promote self-esteem and establish a firm identity. The capacity to establish anxiety-free associations with other people fails to develop. As a consequence, such an individual

feels like a failure. Interpersonal relationships, regardless of their surface appearance, are menacing and potentially painful. Therefore, the individual feels that they must be avoided.

Both Erikson and Sullivan contend that maladjustment is more likely to occur when an individual has been neglected, rejected, and deprived of consistent nurture and affection in early life. Children who experience ridicule, abuse, or unpredictable actions at the hands of parents or other significant persons react by becoming insecure and anxious. The person or persons caring for the child may give mechanical attention or open rejection. Sometimes the child is treated as an inconvenience or nuisance by the parents and consequently feels inferior and devalued. An outside observer might not recognize the emotional trauma that is concealed by a semblance of appropriate family behavior. Disguised rejection is extremely detrimental to the child since it is often easier to deal with open rejection than with antagonism masked by apparent attention and concern. In this sort of situation, the child passes through the formative years constantly expecting pain and failure from interpersonal relationships, as significant persons have taught him to expect nothing else. Such a person perceives all aspects

Table 6-2. Sullivan's Interpersonal Theory

Stage of Development	Self System	Cognitive Experiences	Developmental Tasks	Relationships
Infancy: Birth to emergence of speech, about 1½ years	Barely emerging	Largely prototaxic	Learning to count on others to gratify needs and to satisfy wishes	During this period, an infant cannot be spoiled. Meeting an infant's needs lays a firm foundation for the development of trust.
Childhood: 1½ years to the emergence of the need to associate with peers, about 6 years	Sex-role recognition	Largely parataxic emerging to syntaxic	Learning to accept interference with wishes in relative comfort, to delay gratification	The child must have realistic limits set. The limits must be consistent if the child is to develop a sense of reality about the environment.
Juvenile period: 6 years to the beginning of capacity of love, about 9 years	Integrating needs—internal controls	Syntaxic most of the time; fascination with symbols	Learning to form satisfactory relationships with peers	The child learns to attend to peers' wishes in order to have needs met. Family rules may be ignored in deference to friends' ideas.
Preadolescence: 9 years to the first evidence of puberty, about 12 years	Somewhat stabilized	Syntaxic	Learning to relate to a friend of the same sex	More allegiance to friends than to family. The opposite sex is shunned and "best friend" shares secrets, dreams, and fantasies.
Early adolescence: 12 years to the completion of primary and secondary changes, about 14 years	Confused, but continuingly stabilized	Syntaxic (highly sexually oriented)	Learning to master independence and to establish satisfactory relationships with members of the opposite sex	Rebellion and dependence mark this era. Sexual relationships and peer values are more influential than family allegiance.
Late adolescence: 14 years to establishment of durable situations of intimacy, about 21 years	Integrated and stabilized	Fully syntaxic	Developing an enduring intimate relationship with a member of the opposite sex	During this period, a love relationship is established and marriage usually follows.

SOURCE: Adapted from Sullivan (1953).

135

of the social world as intimidating and tends to attribute these feelings of dread to deficiencies in himself.

Developmental theories concerning schizophrenia dwell on the child's need to receive and bestow love. What is traumatic for a child is not only a lack of maternal love but also unpredictable maternal love that is given and withheld suddenly and unexpectedly. When love is given and then withdrawn, the child who has responded with love is left with no one on whom to bestow that love. Seeking to obtain love, the child reacts by becoming overly involved with his mother and her problems. The mother and child thus become imprisoned in a symbiotic relationship that prevents the normal maturation of the child. The child cannot bear to endanger the symbiotic relationship by separating from his mother, for to do so would leave both of them helpless and alone (Searles, 1965).

Certain interactional patterns have been noted in the families of children who develop schizophrenia. Although, both parents are important to the psychological development of the child, the maternal relationship is considered crucial, especially in the early years. The mother whose attitudes and behaviors have been labeled "schizophrenogenic" has been described as overinvolved with the child yet anxious, ungiving, and unpredictable (Fromm-Reichmann, 1948; Lidz, 1958; Rosen, 1962). The "schizophrenogenic" father, on the other hand, has been described as a weak, ineffectual role model (Lidz, Fleck, and Cornelius, 1965), or as self-engrossed and seductive (Lidz, 1958; Wolman, 1976).

Additional theorists have studied the entire family system and explored dysfunctional interaction among all family members (Sullivan, 1929; Arieti, 1974; Wolman, 1976). In the schizophrenogenic family the relationships among all members are intricate and confusing. Longitudinal research undertaken in Europe and the United States validates some earlier work that attributed schizophrenia to flawed family interactional patterns. Researchers have discovered significant differences in

CONCEPTS FROM HARRY STACK SULLIVAN

■ The *one genus postulate:* No matter how much individuals differ from one another, differences between humans are far less than differences between humans and other species.

■ *Personality* is the result of the evolution of the self from recurrent patterns of interpersonal experience.

■ *Foresight* is the ability to choose actions appropriate to an experience; it helps maintain the integrity of the self.

■ *Instincts* are not predetermined but labile and are continuously modified by experience, maturation, and individual differences.

■ *Self-concept* is related to self-esteem. It evolves from the reflected appraisals of others. Evolution of the self-concept is gradual, but the need for self-esteem is present from birth.

■ The *good me* is the personification of experience in which the infant is rewarded by tenderness.

■ The *bad me* is the personification of experience in which satisfaction is withheld because the mother's tension and anxiety are transferred to the infant.

■ The *non-me* is the personification of the emotions of dread, fear, awe, loathing and horror that are dissociated or disowned as components of the self system.

■ *Anxiety* is related to the need for security. It is rooted in infantile dependency on the mother for survival and for the gratification of biological needs.

■ *Consensual validation* is the measuring of personal perceptions against the perceptions of others in order to correct distortion or validate accurate perceptions.

■ The *prototaxic mode* is the first experiential state of the infant. Experience at this time has a wholeness; before and after concepts are unknown. There is no connection between cause and consequences, no awareness of the self as separate from the rest of the world. Experience is undifferentiated, without limits, cosmic. The infant *is* the world.

■ In the *parataxic mode* the undifferentiated wholeness of experience is broken, but parts are not connected. Experiences are unrelated, illogical, fragmented.

■ In the *syntaxic mode*, experience is consensually validated; meaning is acquired from group, interpersonal, and social involvement.

■ *Selective inattention* operates to prevent consensual validation and preserve distortion by ignoring information that is unwanted or unacceptable.

the families of young people who become schizophrenic and those who do not. Among the habitual communication and interactional patterns noted in the families of schizophrenic persons were (Goleman, 1984):

1. Parents of schizophrenic children engaged in attacks on the characters of their children. Instead of criticizing a behavior, they assaulted the whole child himself, labeling the child as deficient or inferior.

2. Parents of schizophrenic children were very intrusive in the life of their children. Instead of acknowledging how their child thought or felt, the parents told her what to think or feel. For example, a child who wanted something was told that she did not really want it. As a result, the child became unsure of what she actually wanted, thought, or felt.

3. Parents of schizophrenic children employed an erratic communication style in which words were used inappropriately or ambiguously. Denial, distortion, and circumstantiality were employed in ways that caused the child to distrust his own perception of reality. From this communication distortion, the child learned chaotic, bizarre patterns of thinking and reasoning. As a result the child's cognitive and language abilities became deficient, unstable, and more likely to deteriorate during periods of stress.

Some of the specific dysfunctional patterns evident in the families of schizophrenics are described at length in Chapter 17, which discusses family theory and practice.

Sullivan believed that the frightening non-me experiences of early life (the sum of experiences that create such intense feelings of fear or dread that they have to be disowned—see Chapter 2) dominate some people's awareness and initiate schizophrenic episodes. According to Sullivan, the schizophrenic process is a withdrawal from interpersonal relationships into a timeless, spaceless world in which normal cause and effect cease to exist. The negative feelings about the world and the self originate in the bad me (the sum of experiences in which the infant's need for tenderness is not met) and non-me components of the self system and contribute to schizophrenic withdrawal from reality.

Sullivan believed that along with interpersonal withdrawal, the schizophrenic person discards the commonly understood or consensually validated words and meanings by which most people make themselves comprehensible to others. Language no longer is a means of reaching out and communicating with others but becomes a way of encapsulating and concealing the self. Shared meanings that can be consensually validated and understood by others become distorted as the schizophrenic person withdraws from reality and regresses to earlier developmental levels. Without language, the schizophrenic person loses the ability to preserve ways of thinking, acting, and feeling that make sense to other people. Consequently, the person with schizophrenia loses the ability to communicate and comprehend ordinary ideas, perceptions, and symbols. All these things are interpreted in a private, special way by the schizophrenic person. The consequence of interpersonal withdrawal, followed by loss of shared language and meanings, sets the stage for the appearance of internal experiences that take the form of hallucinations and delusions.

Psychodynamic Theories

Psychodynamic theories suggest that schizophrenic thought processes are largely the result of the formation of a fragile ego, which cannot withstand the demands of external reality. The individual with impaired ego development cannot cope with the stress of internal and external pressures that produce conflict. Conflict arises when there is a disparity between the psychological needs of an individual and sociocultural expectations. This disparity produces subjective discomfort, which is relieved by social withdrawal and other regressive behaviors.

According to traditional psychoanalytic theory, the relationship between mother and child normally contains opposing feelings of both love and hate on the part of the mother. The regressed behavior of the schizophrenic child represents a renunciation of normal separation and individuation; the child sacrifices emotional maturation for the sake of the mother. Frequently, the mother herself has inner feelings of emptiness and worthlessness that make her unable to tolerate the child's self-sacrificing love. As a result the mother acts in a way that makes it extremely difficult for the child to separate but then resents the child's inability to do so. Since any attempts on the part of the child to separate from his mother generate guilt and anxiety, the recourse of the child is to continue to exist in a state of psychological entrapment, anxiety, and conflict.

Arieti (1974) formulated the paradigm of *progressive teleological regression* to explain some of the manifestations of schizophrenia. In an attempt to deal with anxiety, the schizophrenic person regresses to a lower level of functioning for the purpose of maintaining some ego integration. Because the person with schizophrenia never achieved adequate ego integration to begin with, regression to a lower level of functioning rarely produces the hoped-for result. Therefore, the individual remains in a state of ego disintegration and fragmentation but now functions at more regressed levels. The regressed individual remains highly anxious and disorganized and makes continued efforts to dissipate anxiety by means of customary problem-solving methods. When customary methods fail, the person with schizophrenia resorts to trial-and-error behaviors. Trial-and-error methods lead to a reversed sequence or hierarchy of responses from the highest to the lowest level of functional, integrated behavior.

The regressive hierarchy of responses is called teleological because it has an ultimate purpose—namely, to avoid overwhelming feelings of tension and anxiety. It is progressive in that behaviors become more extreme, but the direction is toward lower and lower response levels. During the progressive teleological regression engaged in by the person with schizophrenia, three main processes are apparent: concretization, paleological thinking, and desymbolization and desocialization.

CONCRETIZATION In the process of *concretization* there is a loss of consensually validated words, symbols, and meanings. As a result of this loss, knowledge is not easily transferred from one experience to another, and each situation encountered by the schizophrenic person seems new and unique. The person resorts to a vigilant, watchful, listening attitude. As he tries to organize life experiences into meaningful patterns, abstract feelings are transformed into concrete ideas and sensations. Thus, an inner sense of being weak and vulnerable becomes a

137

Figure 6-1. Symbol substitutes for verbal messages. (a) Road sign for "falling rocks." (b) Shipping symbol for "keep frozen." (c) Hobo cat symbol for "kind lady lives here." (d) Navy signal flag for "I need assistance."

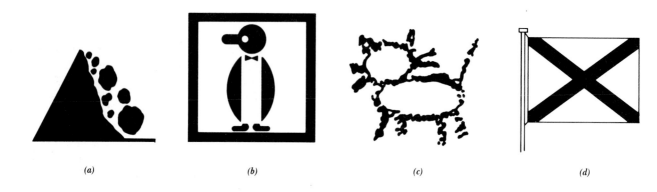

(a)   (b)   (c)   (d)

138

concrete idea that "someone is out to get me"; this concretization of an inner feeling of helplessness has been projected to the outside world. The next step is for the individual to reinforce the image of external enemies by means of visual and auditory experiences that take the form of hallucinations or false sensory experiences. When this happens, the essential ego function of *reality testing* is lost. Reality testing is the ability to differentiate between internal and external stimuli. What the individual sees, hears, feels, tastes, or smells in the form of a hallucination supports what is already believed—namely, that the individual is weak, helpless, and at the mercy of powerful forces.

PALEOLOGICAL THINKING *Paleological thinking* refers to thought patterns that are not those commonly used in everyday life and are therefore subject to misinterpretation by others. In expressing thoughts, the person with schizophrenia does not link subjects together, as most people do, but links predicates instead. Since coherent thinking and comprehensible communication are oriented to subjects or topics, the language of the schizophrenic client becomes individualistic, or *parataxic*, to use the terminology coined by Sullivan. An example of this incoherence is the following sentence: "Tall ships sail (sale) of people weep me a river flowing blood to the sea." In this sentence, the associations are not between the nouns but between the verbs or predicates. The rapid change of subject matter makes the meaning obscure until the message is seen as a form of communication based on predicate thinking. Only then can the association be understood by the listener. The time and energy

needed to decipher such paleological thought processes are enormous. In the meantime the person with schizophrenia manages to remain a riddle misunderstood by others and relatively inaccessible.

DESYMBOLIZATION AND DESOCIALIZATION   Symbols are a form of condensed language in which the symbol has meaning and implications far beyond its linguistic parameters. For example, a Red Cross has international significance recognized by millions. Gold medals and blue ribbons are other symbols, both of which convey recognition of excellence and achievement. Figure 6-1 shows the commonly understood meanings of various symbols encountered in everyday life. When an individual suffers a psychotic episode, the meanings commonly attached to symbols are replaced by more primitive connotations understood only by that individual. Since the acquisition of shared meaning occurs through socialization and communication, *desymbolization*—the loss of consensually understood symbolic meanings—results in *desocialization* and isolation (Arieti, 1974).

THE PROCESS OF THOUGHT DISTURBANCE

Schizophrenia is sometimes depicted not as a single disorder but as a group of disorders, each of which exhibits both similarities to and differences from the others (American Psychiatric Association, 1980). A common denominator among the schizophrenic disorders is thought and language distortion, which is manifested in various ways. The paradigm of tele-

Table 6-3. Sequential Steps of the Schizophrenic Process

Experiential State	Emotional Response	Behavioral Consequences
Inability to trust	Fearfulness, insecurity, ambivalence	Avoidance behaviors to decrease fear and insecurity and to handle ambivalence
Dissociation	Loneliness, isolation, unhappiness	Withdrawal from the social and physical environment
Displacement	Preoccupation with the self, narcissm, alienation	Replacement of attachments to others by self-attachment
Fantasy	Retreat from reality into a self-created world; excessive self-absorbtion and autism	Loss of contact with reality—the real world no longer exists, and only the fantasized world is real; behavior is shaped by events within the self-created world
Projection	Attribution of inner thoughts and feelings to people or objects in the external environment; thoughts and feelings are generated by conditions within the fantasized world	Denial of inner feelings; projection of inner feelings to others in order to avoid responsibility and self-determination

SOURCE: Adapted from Irving (1978).

ological regression described by Arieti is only one representation of the ways thought and language distortions are demonstrated by persons with schizophrenia. It is possible to describe the sequential manifestations of schizophrenia in a more general way. Table 6-3 identifies sequential steps of the schizophrenic process, the underlying emotions, and their behavioral consequences.

Types of Thought Disturbances

When Kraepelin identified and differentiated schizophrenia on the basis of systematic observation, his approach was descriptive, not etiologic. Interestingly, this early descriptive approach has been revived in DSM-III. One rationale for reviving descriptive classifications was the lack of agreement among researchers and clinicians on the issue of etiologic or causative factors.

The following excerpt from DSM-III describes the essential characteristics and manifestations of the disorders now termed schizophrenic:

The essential features of this group of disorders are: the presence of certain psychotic features during the active phase of the illness, characteristic symptoms involving multiple psychological processes, deterioration from a previous level of functioning, onset before age 45, and a duration of at least six months. The disturbance is not due to an affective or organic mental disorder. At some phase of the illness schizophrenia always involves delusions, hallucinations, or certain disturbances in the form of thought. (American Psychiatric Association, 1980, p. 101)

Table 6-4 presents the typology of schizophrenic disorders found in the DSM-III, along with the accompanying behaviors that are often present. Because this typology is based on behaviors that can be

identified and described, there is some overlap. The same person might demonstrate catatonic behavior in one acute episode but not in another; another individual may return to the same behavioral pattern during every psychotic episode. A wide range of diversity prevails in the clinical manifestations of schizophrenia. However, the use of a typology provides researchers and clinicians with a common language so that the manifestations can be identified and described.

Table 6-4. Typology of Schizophrenia Based on Behaviors

Type	Predominant Behaviors
Catatonic	Psychomotor disturbances, such as stupor, rigidity, posturing, negativism, excitement, alternating excitement and stupor, mutism, and waxy flexibility (retaining a position until the previous posture is gradually resumed)
Disorganized	Incoherence and/or flat, incongruous, inappropriate or silly affect; fragmented delusions and/or hallucinations; social eccentricity in the form of grimaces, mannerisms; hypochondriacal complaints; social withdrawal
Paranoid	Delusions and/or hallucinations that are persecutory or grandiose; demonstrations of anger, anxiety, argumentativeness, aggressiveness; doubts regarding gender identity
Residual	At least one previous episode of schizophrenia but no psychotic signs currently present; residual features persist in the form of illogical thinking, bizarre behavior, loose associations, blunt or unresponsive affect, social withdrawal
Undifferentiated	Obvious and prominent psychotic features that do not fit into other categories or that meet the criteria for more than one category

Primary Manifestations of Thought Disturbance
Bleuler (1950) described four primary indicators that are pervasive and identifiable in all persons with schizophrenia, regardless of typology. Each of the four primary indicators begins with the letter "A," which can serve as a mnemonic device: (1) associative looseness, (2) autism, (3) ambivalence, and (4) alterations of affect.

ASSOCIATIVE LOOSENESS The schizophrenic client exhibits alteration in normal modes of thinking. Instead of the logical thought patterns characteristic of adult thinking, the individual reverts to early, primitive modes of thinking. Unable to think or reason logically, the schizophrenic person cannot act in a rational manner. His irrational thinking is maintained because his thoughts and actions are based on personalized interpretations of reality that cannot be validated or understood by others.

Loose associations are thought and communication patterns characterized by unclear connections between one idea and the next. The individual has great difficulty in organizing thoughts, and her ideas are not followed to a logical conclusion. Consequently, her language is confusing and difficult to understand. An example of loose association is the statement of one schizophrenic client, "I like Tarzan, but the car doesn't eat bananas."

Magical thinking is another form of associative thought alteration. The person who engages in magical thinking believes that thoughts have the power to change events. As a result, the person is convinced that thoughts can bring about good or bad outcomes. If the client thinks negatively about someone and that person suffers misfortune, the client attributes this to the power of his thoughts. This also means that the individual believes that the thoughts of other people can be harmful and dangerous.

AUTISM Regression is a common phenomenon in schizophrenia that result in the individual's energies being directed inward toward the self. This defense mechanism enables the individual to return to an earlier stage of development regarding thoughts, feelings, and behaviors. As regression continues, she may return to infantile ways of relating to others. This causes deterioration in social relationships that depend on mutuality. The social environment is ignored, and a new environment is invented where customary ways of interacting can be abandoned and the client can become totally self-engrossed.

AMBIVALENCE The person with schizophrenia tends to have mixed feelings of love, hate, and fear toward persons he is expected to love. There are

similar feelings of ambivalence toward the self and toward objects, situations, events, and relationships. Ambivalence may be so great that the person is immobilized and can only cling to inactivity and apathy. Most people have ambivalent feelings about events and individuals in their lives. The difference between the normal ambivalence with which everyone must deal and the excessive ambivalence of schizophrenia is the degree to which ambivalence affects behavior. An example is the response of a client hospitalized on an inpatient unit who was given the privilege of leaving the unit unescorted for one hour. The client had been looking forward to this privilege but, when the time came to leave the unit, he decided not to go and expressed a desire to remain on the unit and play cards with a staff member instead.

Another way that ambivalence can be expressed is through negativism. The negativistic client refuses to participate in appropriate activities or to cooperate voluntarily. Repeated refusals indicate that she may be trying to handle ambivalent feelings that intensify anxiety. Such clients are equally likely either to refuse to begin doing something or to refuse to stop doing it. For example, a client may refuse to follow the routine of a treatment facility, resisting suggestions to get out of bed in the morning, to dress, to eat, or to participate in activities. Yet once the client becomes involved in an activity it may be equally difficult for staff members to persuade him to do anything else.

Some clients express ambivalence through repeated, ceaseless activity that appears to have no meaning. An example is the client who sits in a chair for a few minutes, gets up, looks out the window, returns to the chair, and repeats these maneuvers for hours if permitted to do so.

Other clients express their ambivalence by complying with everything that is asked of them but refusing to do anything unless asked specifically and told how to do it. Such clients must be told when to go to bed, when to get up, and what to wear, and they need detailed instructions about how these actions should be performed (Haber et al., 1982).

ALTERATIONS OF AFFECT When judged by ordinary standards, the emotions and outward affect of the individual with schizophrenia seem extraordinary. The terms "affect" and "emotion" are often used interchangeably, but it should be emphasized that *emotion* refers to the inner, somatic expression of feeling whereas *affect* refers to the outward behavior engendered by emotion (Kolb, 1982). Affective reactions permeate the psychic life of individuals, influencing their acceptance and rejection of events and experiences. The affective alterations noted in schizophrenic clients stem from their need to cope with intense feelings that might evoke unbearable anxiety if confronted directly. These affective alterations are distancing or protective actions taken to isolate or overcome painful emotions. Alterations of affect take the form of inappropriate affect, blunted affect, and apathy.

Inappropriate affect is an outward display of emotion that is not in harmony with reality. The client demonstrates a mood that is unsuited to the situation. An example is the client who breaks into boisterous laughter on being told that a faithful pet dog has been killed by a speeding car.

Blunted affect is an extreme decrease in the intensity of the client's response to any person, idea, or experience. For example, the loss of a month's stipend would be expected to arouse a strong negative response, but a schizophrenic individual might appear quite indifferent to the loss. People whose affect is blunted usually present themselves as unresponsive to events around them, whether pleasant or unpleasant. Their reactions are unemotional, flat, and dull, regardless of the nature of their experiences.

Apathy is a behaviorally demonstrated indifference to one's social and physical environment, characterized by a lack of commitment and involvement. For instance, a client's family might enter the dayroom of a psychiatric facility, carrying brightly wrapped packages and a cake aglow with candles, singing "Happy Birthday" to the client. Instead of responding with pleasure, the client might remain seated in a chair, ignoring the song, the cake, and the gifts, giving no outward sign or response to the celebration. In contrast, a person showing blunted affect would respond minimally to such an event but would be capable of acknowledging its occurrence. Often apathy and blunted affect appear in combination.

The client who is apathetic tends to be consistent in showing this affective state. Nursing records of such clients indicate little change in affect regardless of the client's situation. A graphic record of the affect of an apathetic client would consist simply of a straight line. The term *flatness of affect* is often used to describe the absence of emotional responsiveness characteristic of schizophrenic clients who display apathy and blunted affect (Kyes and Hofling, 1980).

Secondary Manifestations of Thought Disturbance

In addition to the primary features of schizophrenia identified by Bleuler, there are a number of secondary characteristics, which include alterations in language, alterations in perception, alterations in self-image, and alterations in thought.

ALTERATIONS IN LANGUAGE Verbal interaction depends on the ability to exchange thoughts and ideas, to express feeling, and to share perceptions. Schizophrenic alterations in language and communication reduce the ability of the individual to form relationships. Serious alterations or disruptions in thought patterns are reflected in the way that language is used. An alteration of language comes about for two reasons: (1) the individual cannot usually utilize language effectively and has thus developed a private language that no one else can understand (Beck, Rawlings, and Williams, 1984); (2) the person is unable to synthesize segments of thought into a whole and his language often identifies only fragments or part of an idea. As a result schizophrenic alterations in language frequently take the forms of echolalia, clang associations, neologisms, and word salad.

Echolalia is the purposeless repetition of a word or phrase that someone else has just spoken. For example, the nurse might say to the client, "In the next step blue yarn is used." The client would respond, "Yarn is used, yarn is used, yarn is used."

A *clang association* is a repetition of words or phrases having a similar sound but no other relationship. For example, when the client is asked, "What would you like to drink?" she responds by saying, "Drink, think, stink, blink."

A *neologism* is a private word or phrase that has special meaning for the client but that cannot be understood by others. For example, when a client is asked a question about a favorite television show, the response might be "Fodda sodda kor."

Word salad is a linking of words and phrases in a meaningless, disconnected way. As an example, a client seated at a dining table might say, "Coffee is innocent, and when the dog runs, the chair melts."

ALTERATIONS IN PERCEPTION *Perception* is the process of recognizing and interpreting stimuli. Perception is influenced by both cognitive and emotional processes. All people sometimes perceive stimuli accurately and sometimes distort or misinterpret them. An example of perceptual distortion with schizophrenia is provided in Figure 6-2. When distortion or misinterpretation of perceptions becomes habitual, the result may be the development of hallucinations.

Hallucinations are false sensory perceptions that have no basis in reality and that are generated by internal rather than external stimuli. They most often are auditory or visual misperceptions although olfactory, gustatory, and tactile hallucinations are also experienced. Tactile hallucinations are usually the result of an organic condition or drug or alcohol toxicity. There are five types of hallucinations:

1. *Auditory hallucinations* are sounds or voices heard only by the client. Often the voices berate and

Figure 6-2. Progressive perceptual distortions in altered patterns of thought and perception. These drawings were made by an artist with schizophrenia (Louis Wain, 1860—1939) over the course of his disorder.
SOURCE: © 1985 Aspect: Derek Bayes, CLICK/Chicago.

(a)

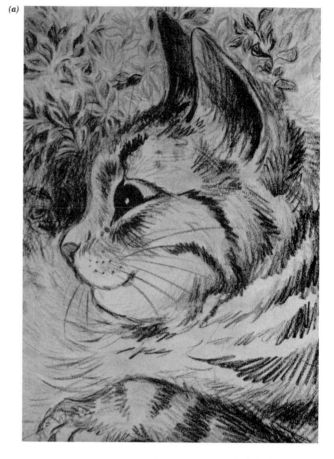

142

accuse the client; they are considered to be projections of the client's anxiety-producing thoughts and feelings, which must be disclaimed and attributed to external sources. An example of a person with an auditory hallucination is the client who hears voices telling her that her parents must not visit in the hospital. These messages may originate because the client fears parental disapproval of the hospitalization.

2. *Gustatory hallucinations* are sensations of tastes and flavors that reflect the internal experience of the client and have no basis in reality. An example of a gustatory hallucination is the experience of a client who learns of the death of her husband while drinking a particular soft drink and later experiences a bitter taste whenever she tries to drink this beverage.

3. *Olfactory hallucinations* are odors and aromas smelled only by the client that seem to emanate from specific or unknown sources. An example of an olfactory hallucination is the experience of a client who smells sulfurous fumes whenever a clergyman is present.

4. *Tactile hallucinations* are unusual somatic sensations that cannot be explained factually. An example of this type of hallucination is the experience of the client who believes that insects are crawling under his skin or that worms infest his vital organs.

5. *Visual hallucinations* are visual images that appear to the client in the absence of valid external stimuli. An example of visual hallucination is the experience of the client who sees deceased friends, historical figures, or threatening spectres. Another form of visual hallucination involves distortions in

(b)

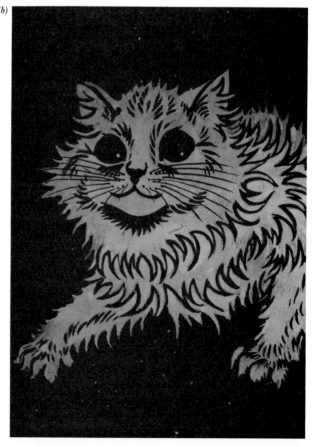

(c)

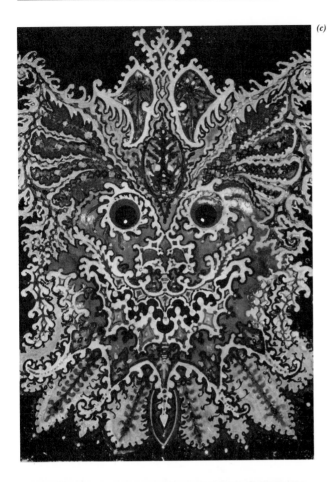

(d)

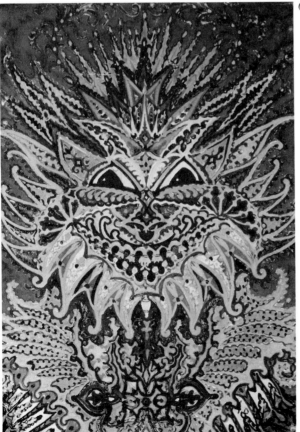

143

how things are perceived. For most people perceptual constancies act to promote accurate visual perception: size constancy, color constancy, shape constancy, and location constancy. In some visual hallucinations one or more perceptual constancies may be lost and objects seem to change unpredictably. Table 6-5 describes and gives examples of major perceptual constancies that may be lost during a visual hallucinatory experience.

ALTERATIONS IN SELF-IMAGE Often the client with schizophrenia experiences distortions in how the self is perceived. These distortions may affect body image, or they may affect ego boundaries. For many schizophrenic persons, body image is not a stable concept. Parts of the body are subject to imagined change, and the client may become preoccupied with changes not apparent to anyone else. When looking into a mirror, the client may believe that the reflected image really belongs to someone else or that her nose is becoming an eagle's beak.

Body image and ego boundaries are closely associated for the person with schizophrenia. The somatic and psychological boundaries that define the individual as a separate entity are sometimes so indistinct that the client is not able to maintain a sense of himself as an entity, distinct and separate from the environment. *Depersonalization* is the term used to define feelings of unreality and instability about the self. The result of depersonalization is a sense of living in a dream, an inability to discriminate between the inner and outer parts of one's body, and feelings of not being in control. When ego boundaries are indistinct, clients may believe that they have merged with the environment and are

Table 6-5. Definitions and Examples of Major Perceptual Constancies

Perceptual Constancy	Definition	Example
Size constancy	Objects are perceived as remaining the same size even though their visual images change at different distances	Approaching objects such as automobiles seem to get closer, while distant objects are perceived as distant
Color constancy	Objects are perceived as being of a stable color regardless of the amount of light in the environment	A white object appears white even in a dim light and a black object appears black even in a bright light
Shape constancy	Objects are perceived as having a stable shape even though their visual images change when they are seen at different angles	Round objects such as wheels are seen as circles even when the visual image is an ellipse; rectangular objects such as doors are seen as rectangular shapes even when their visual image is trapezoid
Location constancy	Objects are correctly perceived as stationary or moving despite movement of their visual images	Persons riding in an automobile see immobile objects being passed as stationary even though the images change with the car's movement

lost. For example, a client walking in the grass may feel that she has become part of Mother Nature. Feelings of depersonalization may render clients unable to reconcile body image with their assigned gender. Thus, a female client may believe that her body is masculine or a male client may feel that his mind is feminine.

ALTERATIONS IN THOUGHT The schizophrenic person may reveal gross or subtle alterations in normal modes of thought. Instead of the mature thought patterns characteristic of adult thinking, the schizophrenic person may return to the thought modes of childhood. When unable to think clearly or reason logically, the individual finds it difficult to act like other people. Thus, the altered thought modes produce individualistic interpretations that lead to puzzling, incomprehensible behaviors. Alterations that affect thinking and cognition may take various forms, including autistic thinking, concrete thinking, and delusions.

Autistic thinking is a form of thinking that endeavors to gratify unfulfilled desires and needs. Thoughts manifest themselves as daydreams, fantasies, and delusions. The unconscious level of mental awareness is the most active in autistic thinking.

Most people utilize stimuli and impressions gathered from the outside world to organize their experience in a meaningful way. The excessive anxiety of the schizophrenic person causes the self rather than the outside world to be used as a frame of reference in organizing experience. The outside world does not provide gratification, so the client looks inward for validation and satisfaction. Consequently, the client attaches personal and private meanings to experience to which no one else has access. Habitual autistic thought patterns in turn can lead to concrete thinking, delusions, loose associations, and magical thinking.

Concrete thinking is a primitive form of thinking in which thoughts are organized and coherent but generalizations and abstractions are deficient or absent. When engaging in concrete thinking, individuals can sort and classify cognitive material but cannot generalize from specific examples. Inductive reasoning powers are absent, as is the ability to understand logical implications surrounding events and experiences. For example, when a schizophrenic client is told by a laboratory technician, "I'm here to draw your blood," the client might reply, "You forgot your crayons and paper. How can you draw without them?"

Delusions are distorted thought processes in which the client's ability to evaluate and test reality is seriously impaired. A delusion is a false, fixed idea generated within the client in the absence of external stimuli. Delusions tend to repeat certain themes even though details may change over time. The forms that delusions often take and their content themes are presented in Table 6-6.

THERAPEUTIC APPROACHES FOR CLIENTS WITH THOUGHT DISTURBANCE

Schizophrenic disorders are multifactorial in origin and complex in their manifestations. For nurses and other health professionals caring for clients with schizophrenia, there is no precise set of rules or techniques that are uniformly applicable. Nurses

Table 6-6. Forms of Delusion and Content Themes

Form of Delusion	Content Themes
Delusions of persecution	False beliefs that one is being singled out for punishment or harassment. *Example:* A client may feel that co-workers are noisy because they want to interfere with work.
Delusions of grandeur	False beliefs about one's power or authority. *Example:* A client may believe that he is a reigning monarch and should be treated like royalty.
Delusions of control or undue influence	False beliefs that one is being controlled by others. *Example:* A client believes that beings from another planet control all the appliances in the kitchen.
Delusions of infidelity	False beliefs that a spouse or lover is unfaithful. *Example:* A husband is convinced that his wife is having an affair with the postman and that their letters are written in a secret code.
Somatic delusions	False beliefs about the body or a part of the body. *Example:* A client believes that the heart or kidneys are failing despite medical reassurance to the contrary.
Ideas of reference	False beliefs that certain statements or events have a special meaning for the client. *Example:* A panel of experts is discussing immorality on a television program and the client believes that she is being discussed.

need to respond to the behavioral signs of each client's internal experience and to avoid dealing with clients as psychiatric entities rather than as troubled human beings. Nursing intervention requires an encompassing perspective that considers all dimensions of a client's experience and formulates appropriate nursing interventions based on the client's individualized needs as they are manifested in his behaviors.

Psychotropic Drug Therapy

The discovery of antipsychotic medications has made it possible to control many extreme behavioral manifestations that accompany schizophrenic disorders. By means of appropriate medication, clients who might otherwise be unapproachable are now able to engage in human interactions that make rehabilitation possible.

ANTIPSYCHOTIC MEDICATIONS The first and most widely used antipsychotic drug, chlorpromazine (Thorazine), was discovered by chance. It was considered an antihistamine and was not used for antipsychotic purposes until 1952, when it was noted that the drug had profound effects on the thinking,

145

perception, affect, and behavior of schizophrenic persons. Antipsychotic medications, among which chlorpromazine is a prime example, cause the schizophrenic person to be less out of touch with reality, less withdrawn, less delusional, and less anxious (Kline and Davis, 1973).

Nurses usually do not prescribe medication, but they do administer medication and supervise clients who take medication on their own, and they frequently make recommendations based on their assessments of clients. The nurse is responsible for instructing clients, for noting the effects of the medication, and for monitoring and dealing with side effects. Most clients receiving an antipsychotic drug or any other psychotropic medication will be taking the drug for considerable periods of time and should know as much as possible about the action of the drug and any necessary precautions. Because nurses are closely involved in the aftercare of clients taking psychotropic medication, they should have accurate, up-to-date information regarding range of dosage, therapeutic action, and possible side effects (Boettcher, 1982).

The specific action of major tranquilizers administered to control manifestations of schizophrenia is not fully understood. One hypothesis is that in certain areas of the central nervous system there is excessive activity of the neurotransmitter dopamine, which is thought to precipitate the psychotic reaction. Antipsychotic drugs block dopamine receptors in the brain and central nervous system, thus reducing the severity of the psychotic reaction. The antipsychotic drugs used for schizophrenia differ only in their potency and side effects; the therapeutic effectiveness of most of the antipsychotic

Table 6-7. Antipsychotic Medications

Drugs by Category	Trade Name	Oral Dosage (mg/day)	Available Forms
Phenothiazines			
Chlorpromazine	Thorazine	50 – 1200	Tablet, liquid, injection, suppository
Promazine	Sparine	100 – 2400	Tablet, liquid, injection
Triflupromazine	Vesprin	30 – 150	Tablet, liquid, injection
Piperazines			
Acetophenazine	Tindal	40 – 120	Tablet
Butaperazine	Repoise	50 – 1000	Tablet
Carphenazine	Proketazine	25 – 40	Tablet, liquid
Fluphenazine	Prolixin	2 – 25	Tablet, liquid, injection
Perphenazine	Trilafon	12 – 64	Tablet, liquid, injection
Trifluoperazine	Stelazine	5 – 40	Tablet, liquid, injection
Piperidines			
Mesoridazine	Serentil	150 – 400	Tablet, liquid, injection
Piperacetazine	Quide	40 – 160	Tablet, injection
Thioridazine	Mellaril	50 – 800	Tablet, liquid
Butyrophenones			
Droperidol	Inapsine	None	Injection
Haloperidol	Haldol	2 – 100	Tablet, liquid, injection
Dibenzoxazepines			
Loxapine	Loxitane	15 – 100	Tablet
Oxoiodoles			
Molindone	Moban	15 – 225	Tablet
Thioxanthenes			
Chlorprothizene	Taractin	75 – 600	Tablet, liquid, injection
Thiothixene	Navane	5 – 60	Tablet, injection

SOURCES: Adapted from Harris (1981); Pasquale (1981).

drugs is similar, although their range of dosages is not equivalent.

Table 6-7 lists the generic and trade names of the most often used antipsychotic drugs, their dosage range, and the forms in which the drugs are available.

Antipsychotic medications are relatively safe for most clients, but there are a number of troublesome side effects. Truly dangerous side effects such as cardiac arrhythmias are rare, but there are more frequent side effects that prove uncomfortable and sometimes frightening for clients. Before antipsychotic medication is prescribed, the general health of the individual should be evaluated. Electrocardiograms should be done initially and at regular intervals thereafter. When side effects do occur, they should be identified promptly and measures should be instituted to restore the client's comfort. The common side effects of antipsychotic medications can be classified according to the physiological structures that are involved.

Allergic Reactions Blood dyscrasias are among the hypersensitive reactions that may develop. These include agranulocytosis, which often begins as a sore throat and fever, and eosinophilia, which is usually benign. Blood tests should be done regularly to monitor any blood changes. If a client has a history of blood dyscrasia, these side effects are more likely to appear, and when they do occur it is usually early in treatment.

Contact dermatitis is another reaction that is distressing to clients. Sometimes a skin reaction takes the form of urticaria, and the itching can be very uncomfortable. Pigment deposits in the skin cause darkened areas, especially if the client is taking chlorpromazine. Heightened sensitivity to sunlight is also a common side effect.

Autonomic Nervous System Reactions In some clients antipsychotic drugs cause dry mouth, constipation, and blurred vision. Persons with cerebrovascular insufficiency, renal insufficiency, or cardiac reserve insufficiency may be susceptible to hypotensive episodes and should be observed closely.

Choleostatic jaundice may appear during the first months of drug therapy; it is accompanied by yellowing of the sclera and skin and discoloration of urine and stools. Usually jaundice is preceded by flulike symptoms appearing in the first month of treatment. The medication should be discontinued if these conditions occur. Clients with a history of liver damage are at risk when taking antipsychotic medication, for they may not be able to detoxify the drugs.

The anticholinergic properties of the anti-

PRIAPISM

Priapism is persistent, abnormal erection of the penis, accompanied by considerable pain and tenderness. It sometimes is a side effect of psychotropic medication, but it also occurs in spinal cord injuries or diseases. It may also result from vesical calculus or trauma to the penis itself. The name is derived from Priaps, a king of ancient Greece who seduced a daughter of the gods. His punishment, according to legend, was to remain forever in a state of erection without ejaculation.

147

psychotic drugs may cause urinary retention or hesitancy. Men who have prostatic hypertrophy are at greater risk for these problems when taking an antipsychotic drug. Male clients may report inability to sustain an erection or to ejaculate. Occasionally males develop priapism, a painful condition in which the penis remains erect for long periods during which ability to ejaculate is inhibited.

Endocrine Reactions Side effects that involve the endocrine system can be particularly embarrassing for clients. Breast enlargement or lactation may occur in males and females and is especially upsetting to the male client. Female clients may suffer menstrual irregularities, such as amenorrhea, which can cause fears of pregnancy. Weight gain may be a source of concern for both male and female clients, especially if they are already troubled by body image changes.

Neurologic Reactions One-third of those taking an antipsychotic medication will experience extrapyramidal side effects. When extrapyramidal effects go unnoticed or untreated, the client may become frightened enough to refuse further medication. There are four general types of extrapyramidal symptoms: (1) parkinsonism, (2) akathisia, (3) dystonia, and (4) tardive dyskinesia.

Drug-induced parkinsonism is similar to Parkinson's disease and can appear after the first week of taking an antipsychotic drug. If it is to occur, it usually appears before eight weeks of drug administration. Akinesia (changes in posture, shuffling gait, muscular rigidity, and drooling) are manifestations of this drug reaction. Clients with akinesia also exhibit a lack of ambition and interest, fatigue, and slowed movements.

Akathisia is an uneasy feeling of restlessness and agitation. The client has great difficulty sitting still; when urged to do so the client will squirm, fidget, stand up, walk around, and sit down for only short periods. Akithisia appears after approximately two weeks of drug therapy and peaks at six to ten weeks. It is more common in women than men.

Dystonias are bizarre, uncoordinated movements of the neck, face, eyes, tongue, body, and arm and leg muscles. There may be a backward rolling of the eyes in their sockets (ocular gyration), sideways twisting of the neck (torticollis), spasms of the back muscles (opisthotonos), and protrusion of the tongue. The onset is sudden and dramatic, and as a result the client is usually very frightened. The spasms can be so severe that the client may suffer respiratory distress or be unable to swallow or talk. Dystonias may occur any time after the first dose of an antipsychotic drug, and each episode may last from a few minutes to two hours. Reassurance is often enough to calm the client as the reaction subsides. Diphenhydramine (Benadryl) injected intramuscularly is often administered to counteract this type of reaction.

Tardive dyskinesia is a disorder characterized by rhythmic, involuntary chewing, sucking, licking movements of the mouth, tongue, and lower jaw. Frowning, blinking, and tongue protrusion are often present. Two of the earliest indications of tardive dyskinesia are fine vermiform movements of the tongue and excessive blinking. Tardive dyskinesia is irreversible, and its manifestations tend to increase when the causative drug is discontinued.

Table 6-8. Antiparkinsonian Medications

Drug	Trade Name	Dose (mg/day) PO	IM	Available Forms
Diphenhydramine hydrochloride	Benadryl	25–50 Tid	10–100 Tid/Qid	Capsule, elixir, ampule
Biperiden hydrochloride	Akineton	1–2 Tid	1–15 Qid	Tablet, ampule
Procyclidine hydrochloride	Kemadrin	2–5 Tid		Tablet
Trihexyphenidyl hydrochloride	Artane	1–5 Tid		Tablet
Benztropine mesylate	Cogentin	1–4 Tid	1–2 Qid	Tablet, ampule

Because the condition is persistent once it develops, it is important to be alert to early signs. Occasional "drug holidays" are advisable if the client can manage to forgo medication for a short while. Another preventive measure is to change the antipsychotic drug the client is taking. Some clients can be maintained on a minor tranquilizer such as Librium, which has some antipsychotic properties.

The medications used to control parkinsonism and other extrapyramidal effects of antipsychotic drugs are referred to as *anticholinergic agents*. Sometimes these medications are given as soon as an antipsychotic medication is prescribed. At other times these medications are only administered when side effects become apparent. The most frequently used antiparkinsonian agents are outlined in Table 6-8.

The possible side effects of antipsychotic medications vary in severity as well as in form. The well-informed nurse can help clients deal with troublesome side effects and intervene if side effects are contributing to the client's distress. When teaching clients about the action and complicating factors of psychotropic medications, nurses should explore clients' emotional reactions to taking medication in addition to their physiologic reactions. Table 6-9 summarizes the side effects of antipsy-

chotic medications and outlines specific nursing interventions.

Relationship Therapy

The role of the primary therapist is usually enacted by a professional care provider with graduate preparation, but generalist nurses function as caregivers in many psychiatric settings in the hospital and the community. The care offered by the generalist nurse to clients with schizophrenic disorders is often based on principles of relationship therapy, which may be augmented by medication, group therapy, or individual therapy. Relationship therapy is the establishment of a one-to-one therapeutic relationship between nurse and client in which the nursing process is used to meet the client's needs.

The client's current level of functioning reflects the setting in which the nurse encounters the client. If, for example, the client is experiencing an acute psychotic episode, in all likelihood care will be provided in a hospital setting. If the client is living in the community, his behavioral symptoms are probably being controlled reasonably well by medication and supportive care.

Interpersonal communication and therapeutic relationships are areas in which schizophrenic

Table 6-9. Side Effects of Antipsychotic Medications and Nursing Interventions

Side Effects	Nursing Interventions
Allergic reactions Blood dyscrasias	1. Assess the client and note increased temperature, itching of the skin, sore throat, bruises, nosebleeds. 2. Withhold medication until the client can be evaluated further.
Contact dermatitis	1. Treat the symptoms and reassure the client. 2. Obtain a medical order for appropriate topical and oral medications. 3. Withhold antipsychotic medication until the client can be evaluated further.
Sunlight sensitivity	1. Advise client to wear sunglasses if necessary. 2. Advise client to use sunburn preventives when outdoors. 3. Advise client to avoid direct sunlight and to cover exposed skin with clothing when outdoors. 4. Remind clients with dark complexions that they may be sensitive to sunlight and are also at risk.

Table 6-9. Continued

Side Effects	Nursing Interventions
Autonomic nervous system reactions	
Arrythmias and T-wave abnormalities	1. Monitor pulse for irregularities. 2. Arrange for routine electrocardiogram. 3. Notify nursing and medical staff members.
Blurred vision	1. Arrange for periodic examination of client to determine whether retinitis pigmentosa is present. 2. Reassure client that visual disturbance is usually temporary and will probably subside in 2–6 weeks.
Constipation	1. Encourage client to maintain adequate fluid intake. Encourage greater intake of fresh fruits, prunes, and bran. 2. Offer stool softeners and mild laxatives if necessary. 3. Encourage more activity and physical exercise. 4. If condition is severe, withhold medication and notify physician so as to prevent paralytic ileus.
Dry mouth	1. Offer glycerine mouth swabs. 2. Encourage frequent sips of water. 3. Suggest sugarless gum or lozenges. 4. Examine for fungal infections.
Ejaculatory inhibition	1. Reassure client and explain probable cause. 2. Inform client that medication can be changed or dosage altered with approval of the physician. 3. Be sensitive to covert indications from client that this may be a problem. 4. Provide an open, permissive attitude so that the client feels able to discuss the problem freely. 5. Include information regarding the possibility of this problem when teaching the client about medication.
Jaundice	1. Observe client for yellowing of skin and sclera. 2. Assess for discoloration of urine and stools. 3. Withhold medication until client is evaluated further.
Hypotension or hypertensive crisis	1. Instruct the client to arise slowly from a supine to a sitting position, dangling the legs before standing. 2. Help client stand after rising if dizziness or disorientation occurs. 3. When antipsychotic medication is initiated, record sitting and standing blood pressure. If systolic reading drops more than 20 mm, withhold medication temporarily. Take blood pressure reading in 30 minutes. If unchanged, consult physician before administering medication.
Tachycardia	1. Monitor pulse rate. 2. Withhold medication and consult physician if resting pulse is 120 or more.
Urinary hesitancy or retention	1. Record intake and output to establish urinary baseline. 2. Observe client for signs of obstruction or infection. 3. Withhold medication if client continues to be unable to void and notify physician.
Endocrine system reactions	
Breast enlargement, lactation, amenorrhea, weight gain	1. Offer explanations of how the medication works, adapted to client's level of understanding. 2. Reassure client concerning the seriousness of side effects. 3. Inform female clients that amenorrhea does not indicate the absence of ovulation. 4. Encourage weight control through exercise and proper diet.
Neurological reaction	
Akathisia and akinesia	1. Reassure client that the condition is reversible. 2. Differentiate side effects from other features of client's condition, such as recurrence of psychosis. 3. Administer an antiparkinsonian agent as prescribed.
Dystonia	1. Obtain a p.r.n. order for an antiparkinsonian agent when an antipsychotic drug is prescribed, especially if client has a history of such side effects. 2. Teach the client to recognize the onset of side effects. 3. Remain with the client for the duration of an episode, offering reassurance. 4. Obtain help from other staff members in order to administer p.r.n. antiparkinsonian agent by IM or IV routes, since oral medication may be contraindicated during dystonic episode.
Tardive dyskinesia	1. Use antiparkinsonian agents concurrently with antipsychotic medication. 2. When necessary, use parenteral antiparkinsonian medication. 3. Use preventive measures such as "drug holidays." 4. Suggest reduced dosages or change of medication at first indications of tardive dyskinesia. 5. Assess all clients regularly who are receiving antipsychotic drugs. Report early signs of this complication immediately.

PRIMARY SYMPTOMS OF ALTERED PATTERNS OF THOUGHT AND PERCEPTION

- *Ambivalence.* Mixed, conflicted feelings about self, others, events, or relationships.
- *Autism.* Self-engrossment accompanied by regressed behaviors.
- *Altered affect.* Inappropriate, blunted, inconsistent emotional responses.
- *Loose associations.* Unclear connections between one thought and the next.

150

clients are likely to experience problems and in which nurses can be especially helpful. Initially, the nurse must try to understand the way that the client is experiencing the world. In beginning to establish a therapeutic relationship the nurse must convey a sincere wish to understand and to communicate, even if this is likely to be a slow process. Relationship therapy is effective only when trust is established and when the client experiences the feeling of being understood and accepted. Arnold (1976) proposed four principles of therapeutic interaction for these clients:

Acceptance The nurse's acceptance of the client requires that the client be met at the developmental and behavioral level at which he is functioning. Moreover, the nurse must recognize and accept the existence of her personal and private reactions to the client in order to foster self-awareness and preserve therapeutic objectivity.

Acknowledgment Whenever the client is not accepted as a unique human being and her communication efforts are not acknowledged in a caring and honest manner, she will feel that her legitimate needs have not been sufficiently acknowledged or fulfilled. The schizophrenic client needs to know that the nurse and other caregivers are attempting to understand the obscure messages that are being conveyed, verbally and behaviorally. It is important for the nurse to indicate to the client whether a message has been understood. For a nurse to pretend that a message has been comprehended when in fact it has not is a way of negating the client's self-worth and dignity.

Authenticity The nurse who works with schizophrenic clients should try not to engage in deception of any kind. Schizophrenic clients are highly sensitive to the emotional overtones of other people. Indeed, their extreme sensitivity probably contributed to the onset of their disorder. Every interaction between the nurse and the client should be honest and oriented to reality.

Awareness In order for the nurse and client to communicate effectively, the nurse must acknowledge and analyze the reactive feelings, thoughts, and actions that the client arouses in the nurse. Self-understanding on the part of the nurse, augmented by knowledge of verbal and nonverbal levels of communication, is essential to the establishment and continuation of a trusting relationship with the client.

Schizophrenia is a disturbance that includes cognitive and affective changes but eventually is expressed behaviorally. The nursing care plan must be tailored to the particular behaviors exhibited. Understanding the theoretical explanations for the client's behavior helps the nurse to realize that dysfunctional behaviors are part of the disorder rather than deliberate challenges. Table 6-10 enumerates some of the behavioral manifestations of schizophrenia and outlines some appropriate nursing interventions that can be adapted to individual client needs.

Schizophrenic clients who have been successfully treated with relationship therapy tend to see their caregivers as protective, friendly, and strong (Arieti, 1974), and they tend to recognize that efforts are being made to help but that excessive de-

Table 6-10. Behavioral Manifestations of Schizophrenic Clients

Behavioral Manifestations	Nursing Interventions
Withdrawal	Promote client's participation in grooming and personal hygiene by giving positive reinforcement for self-care activities. Protect the client's self-esteem by avoiding derogatory comments. Praise any efforts directed toward self-care or greater involvement: Encourage remotivation and resocialization group activities (Pasquale, 1981). Encourage and support the client as participation in structured activities is renewed.
Mutism	Recognize that mutism is a form of withdrawal. Exercise patience and communicate an attitude of hopefulness. Comment on nonverbal messages transmitted by the client. Communicate in a clear, simple fashion that does not require a verbal answer.
Immobility	Utilize nursing measures to prevent circulatory deficits, spasticity, or loss of muscle tone. Be attentive to general health needs. Exercise, diet, and adequate rest must be provided to clients whose coping skills consist of social isolation and self-neglect.
Excessive activity	Recognize that frenzied activity may be used to block out reality. Offer interventions directed to preserving physical well-being. Encourage activities and games that are not physically or mentally demanding.
Suspicion of others	Maintain a matter-of-fact attitude. Avoid close physical contact. Maintain eye contact judiciously. Maintain physical distance that is neither very close nor very distant. Do not put medication into food or liquids without the client's knowledge. Avoid power struggles with the client.
Communication deficits	Permit the client to make decisions when possible. Speak clearly and concisely. Avoid emotionally charged words. Speak in tones that are neither very loud nor very soft. Ask for clarification when the client's message is unclear. Let the client know when it is hard to understand autistic communication.
Inappropriate behavior	Protect the client from embarrassment. Protect others from anxiety-producing situations.
Delusions and hallucinations	Let the client know that the nurse does not consider the delusions and hallucinations to be real. Encourage the client not to discuss these issues with others. Do not argue with the client about the reality of delusions or hallucinations. Accept the fact that they are real for the client. Distract the client by encouraging a return to reality through activities or interpersonal involvement. For example, say to a client who is responding to internal stimuli, "You don't seem to be listening to what I am saying . . . try to concentrate on what is going on in this room."

mands are not being imposed on them (Wolman, 1976). The box on page 152 provides suggestions for therapeutic interaction between a schizophrenic client and a caregiver.

Milieu Therapy

Relationship therapy is an approach fully compatible with the nursing process and role. Milieu therapy is a variation of relationship therapy offered on a larger scale.

The basic principle of milieu therapy is that all of the client's surroundings, physical and interpersonal, constitute part of the therapeutic environment. The facility, whether an inpatient unit, a day treatment center, or a halfway house, should not be just a place where care is given but an actual component of the total treatment program. The concept of milieu therapy incorporates the idea of a therapeutic community devoted to holistic health care. The old-fashioned term "asylum" once implied a place of refuge, a safe retreat from the threats and dangers of the outside world. It is true that some emotionally disturbed people may indeed benefit from spending time in a safe, tranquil environment where they are not bombarded with excessive stimuli or subjected to stress. For people like this an asylum that lived up to its name might be quite helpful. However, the majority of clients with psychological problems already tend to withdraw from others and to avoid responsibility and involvement. Therefore, they need an atmosphere where they feel relatively secure but are encouraged to keep busy and to engage in positive social interactions. For schizophrenic clients, the inclination to regress and to become self-engrossed should be balanced by therapeutic programs that encourage outward rather than inward interests. Milieu therapy is a comprehensive approach that attempts to accomplish this goal.

The purpose of milieu therapy is to oppose regression and to foster in clients a sense of personal worth, to enhance their ability to interact with others, and to increase their social competence so that a return to a more rewarding lifestyle is possible. Milieu therapy is flexible enough to provide security and safety for some clients, limit setting for others, and remotivation and resocialization activities for all. Perhaps the most important function of milieu therapy is the restoration or maintenance of self-confidence and autonomy. This is done by providing an environment in which the individuality of each client is respected, where participation of staff

SUGGESTIONS FOR
THERAPEUTIC INTERACTIONS

1. Unconditional acceptance and support. The nurse accepts the client as an individual by treating the client with respect and dignity.

2. Flexibility of interaction. Interactions depend on circumstances and the situation. For example, a client with catatonic behaviors might be permitted to sit in a lotus position when alone but would be expected to sit in a chair like other clients when a community meeting is in session.

3. Individualization of treatment. Rules should not be enforced arbitrarily but rather adapted to the needs of each client. For some clients limit setting is necessary, while for others reassurance and support are more effective.

4. Reinforcement of reality testing. The client who appears to be listening to internal voices should be distracted or invited to participate in interactions in the real environment.

5. Parsimony of interpretation. The nurse may engage in an internal interpretation of the meaning of a client's behavior; however, interpretation need not always be shared immediately with the client.

Often an interpretation should be validated further before being shared; premature or inaccurate interpretations are counterproductive.

6. Management of transference. Schizophrenics often regress to infantile levels and become quite dependent on the caregiver. For this reason, nurses should maintain a professional attitude that protects the client but also promotes his eventual maturity to a point where protection and guidance are less necessary.

7. Management of countertransference. Self-awareness and introspection help the caregiver avoid inappropriate intimacy, which creates confusion and inhibits the emotional growth of the client.

8. Control of hostility. The schizophrenic client sometimes acts out hostile impulses. Physical expressions of violence are not acceptable. Not only are such expressions threatening to others, they are also damaging to the client's self-esteem. Clients should be reassured that hostile feelings are normal but that expressions of hostility must be limited to the verbalization of feelings.

and clients is cooperative rather than coercive, and where democratic policies guide the daily activities that compose the program.

Milieu therapy may be adapted for use in various types of facilities and modified according to the functioning level of the clients who are being served. Although milieu therapy may be offered in an acute care facility, the regressive behavior of clients will necessitate modifications in the way milieu therapy is implemented. In most instances, group activities in the form of community meetings and various collective enterprises are prominent in milieu therapy. As much as possible, clients are given freedom to make decisions for themselves, to discharge responsibilities, and to carry out commitments they have made. The clients and staff members of the facility share in developing and enforcing policies and rules. Clients and staff contribute to decision making and problem solving. If milieu therapy is to be successful, there must be a positive attitude on the part of everyone involved. This includes clients and personnel at all levels, including

professional, administrative, and housekeeping staff. Inservice education for staff members is essential so that new employees can become familiar with and accept the philosophy that underlies milieu therapy. Every individual with whom clients come in contact must have a constructive attitude and be a willing participant in establishing and preserving therapeutic interpersonal relationships.

The physical environment of the care facility is important to milieu therapy. Provision should be made for meeting the physical needs of the clients. Safety measures, cleanliness, harmonious colors, and comfortable furnishings all positively influence the behaviors of staff and clients. There should be rooms of different sizes so that large and small groups can meet. Provision should be made for occasional privacy and for the client who is upset or overwhelmed and needs to be alone or with one staff member for a while. Most clients with psychiatric disorders, especially schizophrenia, have difficulty trusting and relating to others. In a facility devoted to milieu therapy the staff members model

Our most malignantly regressed young people are in fact clearly possessed by general attitudes which represent something of a mistrust of time as such: every delay appears to be a deceit, every wait an experience of impotence, every hope a danger, every plan a catastrophe, every possible provider a potential traitor. Therefore, time must be made to stand still, if necessary by the magic means of catatonic immobility.

ERIK ERIKSON, IDENTITY, YOUTH, AND CRISIS

appropriate communication and behaviors. Self-control is encouraged, but some limit setting is inevitable. Ideally, limits are not imposed by the staff but are generated by the clients themselves. Limit setting may seem inconsistent with the democratic policies advocated in milieu therapy, but structure and respect for others reinforce the realities of living in a social world.

Group interaction is considered an effective way of modifying maladaptive behaviors. In group meetings clients learn to communicate with others, to become aware of how they appear to others, and to improve their communication skills. The emphasis is not on the past but on the present as clients begin to understand the impact of their own and others' behavioral patterns. Clients are permitted to know as much as possible about what is going on in the facility. They have a voice in decisions and their full participation is an important element of the program. Because staff and clients are actively involved in so many aspects of day-to-day activities, clients can be expected to begin to relinquish the passive behaviors that ensure safety but inhibit their progress.

The collaboration and role sharing in a therapeutic community can be intimidating for staff and clients alike. Professionals may be uncomfortable over their loss of authority over clients, while clients may search for staff members who will think and decide for them. When the search for a controlling, directive staff member is fruitless, clients may become angry for a time. Any nurse who chooses to practice milieu therapy must be willing to work in an egalitarian environment where staff and clients are engaged in a mutual process of shared responsibility and self-awareness.

One milieu that is appropriate for recovering schizophrenics is a halfway house. A halfway house is a community facility dedicated to tertiary prevention, or the prevention of further decompensation or impairment after an acute episode has been resolved. For clients with schizophrenia, tertiary prevention consists of a collaborative rehabilitative effort that involves client and family members in addition to health care providers. After the acute episode of schizophrenia has been dealt with, it is important to add structure and organization to the client's everyday existence. A halfway house that offers some freedom and some supervision can be a temporary home for the client whose family is less than wholehearted in its support.

A halfway house does not remove a client from society but instead places the client in a protected society. Clients recovering from an acute schizophrenic episode need follow-up care and a hiatus before returning to the everyday world. The halfway house may expose clients to the same pressures that are found elsewhere but more slowly and with better timing, so that the recovering client has an opportunity to modify behavior on the basis of insight into the nature of his problems.

Family Therapy

Family therapy is recommended and used by many caregivers in the treatment of clients with schizophrenia. The principles and use of family therapy are discussed in Chapter 18.

Predictive Factors

The prognosis for the client with schizophrenia is mixed. Predictive factors that may enhance a client's prognosis are abrupt onset of the condition, short

Generic Nursing Care Plan for Client with Thought and Perceptual Alterations

Identified Problem	Goal or Need	Specific Interventions	Rationale
Alterations in psychological comfort level resulting in increasing anxiety	Client will identify cause of anxiety; client will verbalize feelings of anxiety	1. Help client look at possible cause for anxiety and allow him to see if reasons are valid. 2. Explore ways to alleviate causes of anxiety. 3. Encourage client to talk out feelings of anxiety. 4. Explore actions that could be taken to alleviate anxiety. 5. Accept the client's anxiety without being provoked into reciprocal anxiety. 6. Avoid pushing the client ahead by probing into areas that he is not ready to explore. 7. Offer the client unconditional acceptance. 8. Encourage interest in activities outside of himself. 9. Provide reassurance and support.	To help client recognize and label anxiety. To allow the client to consider alternatives to master situation, learn new techniques for handling situations, and explore the realm of anxiety. To help the client describe feelings related to the source of distress, allowing the client to set the pace.
Decreased capacity for interpersonal contact resulting in emotional withdrawal	Client will take part in one group activity every day	1. Encourage socialization. 2. Encourage verbal expression of hurt and anger. 3. Help client recognize when he is isolating himself. 4. Respect client's body space. 5. Help client realize the destructiveness of withdrawal to him as a person. 6. Avoid making demands on him that he cannot meet. 7. Make consistent steady attempts to draw client into responding, but do not demand any response. 8. Use a warm, nonpressure approach.	To promote client's interaction with other people.
Alteration in level of cognitive functioning resulting in unrealistically based thinking	Client will verbally validate experiences with staff members	1. Identify the client's habitual mode of responding, and the maneuvers he uses to avoid closeness. 2. Help client to learn trust. 3. Be honest and consistent in interactions with client. 4. Be neutral, neither agreeing nor disagreeing with contents of the client's delusion. 5. Listen carefully to client's account and question any obscurities.	To understand general nature of the client's delusional system. To establish trust. To encourage development of a therapeutic relationship.

duration of the psychotic episode, and a stable and supportive social background. If there is an identifiable precipitating event, such as a loss or disappointment, the prognosis also seems to be enhanced. Other predictive factors that influence prognosis:

■ Prognosis seems to be best for those suffering catatonic schizophrenic episodes.

■ Prognosis seems to be poorest for those suffering from chronic and undifferentiated forms of schizophrenia. Prognosis is also poor for persons with paranoid delusions.

■ Prognosis seems to be related to age; the younger the person at time of onset, the poorer the prognosis.

Many persons with schizophrenia can recover from an acute psychotic episode but may experience recurrences. It has been estimated that one-third of clients will have a single episode followed by complete recovery. Another third will experience repeated episodes, followed by partial recovery each time. The remaining third seem to embark on a steady downward course following the first episode, with deterioration of social and mental functioning in spite of comprehensive therapeutic approaches (Rosen, 1978).

SUMMARY

Statistics on the incidence and prevalence of schizophrenia are unreliable because of disagreement about diagnosis and other factors, but the disorder is acknowledged to be a major public health problem. A comparatively large percentage of young people are affected, and a sizeable number of affected persons follow a pattern of gradual deterioration. There are no laboratory tests to indicate the presence of schizophrenia, and the disorder is often confused with organic brain syndrome, manic-depressive illness, or drug toxicity.

Etiologic explanations regarding the cause of the disorder remain inconclusive. Research indicates that genetic factors may play a role in the onset of schizophrenia. The closer the biological relationship between an individual and an identified person with schizophrenia, the greater is the risk of developing the disorder. Biochemical investigations suggest that the clinical signs of schizophrenia are associated with bioamines that act as neurotransmitters and mediate such functions as awareness, sleep, emotion, and sensations of pain and pleasure.

Developmental theories are a useful frame of reference for understanding the etiology of schizophrenia. Erikson and Sullivan believed that adverse experiences in early life cause a child to perceive the social world as frightening and to attribute these anxieties and fears to deficiencies in the self. Family relationships may play a role in the vulnerability of certain individuals. In the families of persons with schizophrenia, relationships between members are intricate and enmeshed, and relationships between the child and the mother seem particularly crucial to the development of the child's identity. Psychodynamic explanations of schizophrenia also emphasize the influence of the mother's inhibition of the child's progress toward individuation and separation.

Schizophrenia is sometimes considered not one disorder but a group of disorders with some common characteristics. All are characterized by thought and language distortion that can be expressed behaviorally in a number of ways. The types of schizophrenia are: catatonic, disorganized, paranoid, residual, and undifferentiated. An individual may demonstrate the same behaviors in every acute schizophrenic episode, or may demonstrate one kind of behavior in one episode and a different kind in another episode.

Although schizophrenia is a thought disorder, its behavioral manifestations are used as the bases for assessing the client and developing a comprehensive care plan.

The altered thought patterns of the schizophrenic client are accompanied by alterations in perception, which in turn may result in the development of hallucinations, or false sensory perceptions that have no basis in reality. Hallucinations may be auditory, visual, olfactory, gustatory, or tactile.

The schizophrenic client may also develop delusions, or false, fixed beliefs that have no basis in reality. The content of delusions varies, but usually a dominant theme can be identified, such as persecution, grandeur, control by others, or somatic distortions. Delusions are defenses used to avoid awareness of distressing thoughts or feelings. Therefore, they are persistent, and the client is reluctant to relinquish or modify them.

The discovery of antipsychotic medication has made it possible for clients with schizophrenia to engage in the human interactions that make rehabilitation possible. Most clients taking antipsychotic medication need to take the drugs for long periods and should know as much as possible about their action and possible side effects. Some side effects to antipsychotic medication are merely uncomfortable; others can be disfiguring or life threatening. Nurses need to have accurate, current information regarding dosage, action, side effects, and precautions relating to these drugs. Teaching and ongoing assessment of clients taking antipsychotic medication are important nursing responsibilities.

The therapeutic approach most suitable for generalist nurses working with schizophrenic clients is relationship therapy. The nurse must try to understand the way the client is experiencing the world and convey to the client a sincere wish to help. Relationship therapy is effective only after trust is established and the client experiences the feeling of being understood and accepted. Successfully treated schizophrenic clients tend to see the caregiver as protective, friendly, and strong. It seems to be important to them that caregivers make effort on their behalf without imposing excessive demands.

Milieu therapy is an approach compatible with the nursing process and role. It is a variation of relationship therapy on a larger scale. The purpose of milieu therapy is to oppose regression and to foster a sense of personal worth, social competence, and autonomy. In milieu therapy, as in most therapeutic approaches appropriate for clients with schizophrenia, the behavior of the client is used to assess needs and offer care. Some clients require support and reassurance while others respond to more structured intervention. Individualized nursing care is based on what the client's behavior expresses about his distortion of thought and perception.

155

CLINICAL EXAMPLE

ONSET OF AN ACUTE EPISODE OF
THOUGHT AND PERCEPTUAL
ALTERATIONS

Lance Walters is the oldest of three brothers. Shortly after the birth of his youngest brother, Lance's mother became indifferent to the needs of the children. Lance's father was an affable individual who had little sense of responsibility and worked only when he felt like it. He did not assume much responsibility for his wife and children. As a result, the children were marginally nourished and inadequately clothed. The family moved frequently and often lived in unsuitable places. Once they lived in a condemned building that had no heat and hot water and that was infested with rats. When Lance was about six years old, the family lived over a tavern where noise and violence occurred frequently. His father was out of the home for days at a time, and the children were so neglected that neighbors reported the situation to the local health department. An official investigation resulted in Lance's mother being committed to a community psychiatric hospital with the diagnosis of undifferentiated schizophrenia. The children became wards of the state.

Lance and his two younger brothers, who were four and two years old, went to live with a foster family that was willing to care for all three boys. The two younger boys adjusted fairly well and responded to the care and attention they received from their foster parents. The foster parents stated later that Lance was different from his brothers even when he first came to them. He was timid and turned often to his four-year-old brother for direction. He was afraid of the dark, and had trouble sleeping at night. He argued with his new foster mother and had temper tantrums whenever he was frustrated or even gently reprimanded.

As time passed Lance seemed to adjust to his new situation. He rarely asked questions about his mother but sometimes wondered aloud why his father never visited. He became very fond of his foster mother, helping her around the house so much that his brothers sometimes teased him about it. As Lance grew older it became apparent that he was gifted intellectually. He was conscientious and hard-working and therefore attracted favorable attention from his teachers. He preferred to keep to himself but often complained that children in the neighborhood disliked him. In high school he was a member of the school choir and the orchestra but was not interested in sports.

When he was a junior in high school, Lance began to neglect his schoolwork and lose interest in the choir and orchestra. His habits changed gradually. Instead of attending practice sessions after school, he began to go home to his room as soon as classes were over. He interacted less and less with his brothers and foster parents, spending most of his free time alone in his room listening to his records. At first his foster parents attributed the changed behavior to the fact that Lance was growing up. They became more concerned when Lance began to go out late at night and not return until early morning. When his foster mother questioned him, he became defiant although they had always had a close relationship.

Lance had worked after school but was fired when he stopped showing up. When this happened, his worried foster mother arranged for him to be seen by the family physician. The physician had known Lance for years and was concerned about his behavioral changes. The physician informed the foster parents that Lance was on the verge of a "nervous breakdown" and in need of help. He referred Lance to a community mental health clinic but it was three weeks before Lance could be seen. By this time Lance was hearing voices. He thought that his clothes were being worn by invisible people who watched him and called him filthy names.

Although it had never been discussed, Lance knew that his mother was in a mental institution. He told his foster mother, "I know what's wrong with me. I'm going crazy like my mother." Sometimes Lance talked sensibly, but often he seemed confused and unaware of his surroundings. When his brothers asked why he acted as he did, Lance said, "When these thoughts come to me, I don't understand anything or anybody." His brothers began to be afraid of Lance because he was so unpredictable. One night, during one of his nocturnal journeys, Lance was picked up by the police. He was confused, incoherent, and wandering aimlessly. His foster parents were notified, and Lance was hospitalized for a psychiatric evaluation.

ASSESSMENT

Lance was admitted to an inpatient facility for assessment. An interdisciplinary team observed him in a number of different situations, administered psychological tests, compiled a history, and most important, tried to get to know Lance and win his trust. The interdisciplinary team identified the following factors in their assessment:

A history of abuse and neglect before the age of six years.

An unstable mother figure with whom the client probably identified.

A distant, uncaring father figure with whom Lance could not identify.

Two younger brothers for whom Lance felt responsible.

Superior intellectual abilities that contributed to difficulties with peers.

Resurgence of early anxiety with the onset of adolescence.

It was the opinion of the persons assessing Lance that the factors that made him vulnerable—his superior mental ability, his affection for his foster mother, and his concern for his younger brothers—could become his sources of strength.

Nursing Diagnoses

Coping, ineffective individual
(related to inability to function at school, at home, or on the job)

Sensory perceptions, alterations in
(related to auditory hallucinations)

Social isolation
(related to inability to develop healthy peer relationships)

Thought processes, alterations in
(related to ideas of reference and delusions of persecution)

Multiaxial Psychiatric Diagnoses

Axis I   295.31 Schizophrenia, paranoid

Axis II   V71.09 No diagnosis

Axis III No diagnosis

Axis IV Code 5—Severe psychosocial stressors

Axis V   Level 5—Poor

PLANNING AND INTERVENTION

Lance was hospitalized for a period of about one month. During that time antipsychotic medication was used to reduce the thought and perceptual distortions that were adversely influencing his behavior. Because Lance had never had the opportunity to relate to a strong, caring male figure, arrangements were made for him to be cared for by male nurses during hospitalization and by a male therapist after discharge. The consensus of persons on the interdisciplinary health team was that the prognosis for Lance was quite good. Despite the deprivation of his early years, he remained a person who was able to show concern for others as well as for himself. His devotion to his foster mother and his affection for his younger brothers opposed his autistic tendencies and were considered sources of strength for him.

One strength that the health team hoped to mobilize on Lance's behalf was his impressive intellectual ability, which was a source of both anxiety and self-esteem for him.

The difficulties that caused Lance to be hospitalized originated many years before in his family of origin. His

problems seemed to stem from a resurgence of anxiety, often a characteristic of the adolescence period. Lance had maintained good adjustment for about ten years. After a brief hospitalization, augmented by good aftercare, Lance would probably return to his previous level of adjustment and perhaps be strengthened by his regressive psychotic behaviors, which drew attention to his inner turmoil. Although the prognosis for Lance was favorable, intervention would be of long duration also. In addition, Lance's problem was closely tied to the inadequacies of his biological parents and the needs of his younger brothers. A holistic approach would include Lance and his brothers as integral components of a family-focused approach and the foster parents as secondary influences.

EVALUATION

After a three-month hospitalization Lance was discharged to a community halfway house. He went to this facility because Lance and his foster parents decided that this was better for all concerned than returning home. Lance was discharged with an adequate supply of antipsychotic medication, about which he had been fully informed.

In the halfway house Lance was finally able to feel that he belonged. His natural parents had made him feel guilty for having been born, and his foster home was a place where he felt he had to adjust. In the halfway house Lance encountered people who were as lonely and as lost as himself. For the first time he was truly able to appreciate his intellectual gifts as he embarked on programs to improve his deficient interpersonal skills. In the halfway house a formal vocational assessment was done on Lance. This assessment, combined with a review of Lance's skills, interests, strengths, education, and intelligence, was enough to make his counselors optimistic about his future, and their enthusiasm was transmitted to Lance.

One of the rules of the halfway house was that residents must be involved in a daytime program. This rule gave Lance the impetus to return to high school even though he found the prospect frightening. On Sundays he frequently visited his former foster home; as his own problems became manageable he became better able to relate to his younger brothers who continued to look up to and admire him.

The prognosis for Lance was favorable in spite of the deprivation that characterized so much of his early life. His adjustment after being placed in a foster home had been good, due primarily to his superior intellectual gifts and the positive attitudes of his teachers. His concern for his younger brothers was an obligation but also a source of strength. Lance was wise enough to know that his success or failure would have a profound impact on his brothers. It would be too soon to predict outcomes with any degree of certainty, but there were a number of factors to indicate that Lance would be one of that fortunate 33 percent of persons who suffer a single schizophrenic episode, are rehabilitated, and experience no further relapses.

Review Questions

1. Describe three theories concerning the etiology of schizophrenia.

2. List the various types of schizophrenic disorders and describe their identifying characteristics.

3. Describe three alterations in affect manifested by clients with schizophrenia.

4. Relate the alterations and distortions of language to the behavioral manifestations of schizophrenia.

5. Differentiate delusions from hallucinations, giving examples of each.

6. Discuss the implications of body image and ego boundaries as they affect the client with schizophrenia.

7. Describe therapeutic approaches appropriate for generalist nurses caring for clients with schizophrenia.

8. Outline the major types of side effects associated with antipsychotic medications and appropriate nursing responses to each.

9. Identify the basic premise of relationship therapy and explain why it is compatible with the nursing role and process.

10. Describe the major principles of milieu therapy.

References

American Psychiatric Association. 1980. *Diagnostic and Statistical Manual of Mental Disorders*, 3rd ed. Washington, D. C.: The Association.

Arieti, S. 1974. *Interpretation of Schizophrenia*, 2nd ed. New York: Basic Books.

Arnold, H. M. 1976. Working with Schizophrenic Patients. *American Journal of Nursing*, 78:941–947.

Barham, P. 1984. *Schizophrenia and Human Value*. London: Blackwell Press.

Beck, C.; Rawlings, R. P.; and Williams, S. 1984. *Mental Health Psychiatric Nursing*. St. Louis: C. V. Mosby.

Bleuler, E. 1950. *Dementia Praecox on the Group of Schizophrenias*, tr. J. Zinki. New York: International Press.

Boettcher, E., and Alderson, S. 1982. Psychotropic Medications and Nursing Process. *Journal of Psychosocial Nursing and Mental Health Services*, 20(November): 12–16.

Dunham, H. W. 1977. The Impact of Sociocultural Factors. *Hospital Practice*, 12(June):61–68.

Erikson, E. 1968. *Childhood and Society*. New York: W. W. Norton.

Fromm-Reichmann, F. 1948. Notes on the Development of Treatment of Schizophrenia by Psychoanalytic Psychotherapy. *Psychiatry*, 11:263–273.

Goleman, D. 1984. Schizophrenia: Early Signs Found. *The New York Times*, December 11.

Gottesman, I. I. 1978. Schizophrenia and Genetics: Where Are We? Are You Sure? In *The Nature of Schizophrenia*, eds. L. C. Wynne, R. D. Cromwell, and S. Mathesses. New York: John Wiley & Sons.

Haber, J.; Leach, A. M.; Shudy, S. M.; and Sideleau, B. F. 1982. *Comprehensive Psychiatric Nursing*, 2nd ed. New York: McGraw-Hill.

Harris, E. 1981. Antipsychotic Medications. *American Journal of Nursing*, 81:1316–1328.

Heston, L. L. 1977. Genetic Factors. *Hospital Practice*, 12(June):43–49.

Kline, N., and Davis, J. 1973. Psychotropic Drugs. *American Journal of Nursing*, 73:54–62.

Kolb, L., and Brodie, K. 1982. *Modern Clinical Psychiatry*, 10th ed. Philadelphia: W. B. Saunders.

Kyes, J., and Hofling, C. 1980. *Basic Psychiatric Concepts in Nursing*. Philadelphia: J. B. Lippincott.

Lehman, H. 1980. History of Schizophrenia. In *Comprehensive Textbook of Psychiatry*, 3rd ed., eds. H. I. Kaplan, A. M. Freedman, and B. J. Sadock. Baltimore: Williams & Wilkins.

Lidz, T. 1958. Intrafamilial Environment of Schizophrenic Patients: Marital Schism and Marital Skew. *American Journal of Psychiatry*, 114:241–248.

Lidz, T.; Fleck, S.; and Cornelius, A. 1965. *Schizophrenia and the Family*. New York: International Universities Press.

Pasquale, E. 1981. *Mental Health Nursing: A Biopsychocultural Approach*. St. Louis: C. V. Mosby.

Rickelman, B. 1979. Brain Monoamines and Schizophrenia: A Summary of Research Findings and Implications for Nursing. *Journal of Psychiatric Nursing and Mental Health Services*, 17(September):28–34.

Rosen, J. N. 1962. *Direct Psychoanalytic Psychiatry*. New York: Grune & Stratton.

Rosen, H. 1978. *A Guide to Clinical Psychiatry*. Coral Gables, Fla.: Mnemosyne.

Searles, H. G. 1965. *Collected Papers on Schizophrenia and Related Subjects*. New York: International Universities Press.

Sullivan, H. S. 1953. *The Interpersonal Theory of Psychiatry*. New York: W. W. Norton.

Sullivan, H. S. 1929. Research in Schizophrenia. *American Journal of Psychiatry*, 9:533–567.

Wolman, B. B. 1976. *Manual of Child Psychopathology*. New York: McGraw-Hill.

Yahres, H. 1978. *Genes and Mental Health: The Mechanisms of Heredity in Major Mental Illnesses*. Rockville, Md.: National Institute of Mental Health, Publication 78–640.

Supplementary Readings

Adams, R. The Genetics of Schizophrenia: A Reassessment Using Modern Criteria. *American Journal of Psychiatry*, 140(1983):171–175.

Andreasen, N. C. Negative Versus Positive Schizophrenia: Definition and Validation. *Archives of General Psychiatry*, 39(1982):789–794.

158

Anthony, E. J. The Preventive Approach to Children at High Risk for Psychopathology and Psychosis. *Journal of Children in Contemporary Society*, 15(1982):67–72.

Bebbington, P. Social Management of Schizophrenia. *British Journal of Hospital Medicine*, 28(1982):396–403.

Bellak, L. *Disorders of the Schizophrenic Syndrome*. New York: Basic Books, 1979.

Bliss, E. L. Auditory Hallucinations and Schizophrenia. *Journal of Nervous and Mental Diseases*, 171(1983): 30–33.

Brown, M. A. Life Skills Training for Chronic Schizophrenics. *Journal of Nervous and Mental Diseases*, 171 (1983):466–470.

Crow, T. J. Is Schizophrenia an Infectious Disease? *Lancet*, 8317(1983):173–175.

Durel, S. H. Client Perception of Role in Psychotropic Drug Management. *Issues in Mental Health Nursing*, 4(1982):65–76.

Feinsilver, D. L. Antipsychotic Medications: Guidelines for Use in Emergencies. *Hospital Practitioner*, 17 (1982):92.

Galdi, J. The Causality of Depression in Schizophrenia. *British Journal of Psychiatry*, 142(1983):621–624.

Green, H. *I Never Promised You a Rose Garden*. New York: Signet Books, 1964.

Hartog, J.; Audy, R.; and Cohen, Y. A. *The Anatomy of Loneliness*. New York: International Universities Press, 1980.

Kanas, N. Homogeneous Group Therapy for Acutely Psychotic Schizophrenic Patients. *Hospital and Community Psychiatry*, 34(1983): 257–259.

Koontz, E. Schizophrenia: Current Diagnostic Concepts and Implications for Nursing Care. *Journal of Psychosocial Nursing and Mental Health Services*, 20(1982): 44–48.

Laing, R. D. *The Divided Self*. Baltimore: Penguin Books, 1965.

Lehrman, N. S. Effective Psychotherapy of Chronic Schizophrenics. *American Journal of Psychoanalysis*, 42 (1982):121–123.

Lidz, T. *The Origin and Treatment of Schizophrenic Disorders*. New York: Basic Books, 1973.

McGlashen, T. H. Intensive Individual Psychotherapy of Schizophrenics: A Review of Techniques. *Archives of General Psychiatry*, 40(1983):909–920.

Moran, M. G. Increased Psychotropic Side Effects in Geriatric Patients. *Hospital Formulary*, 17(1982): 1513–1517.

Muller, C. F. Economic Costs of Schizophrenia: A Post Discharge Study. *Medical Care*, 21(1983):92–104.

Nasrallah, H. A. L. Neurological Soft Signs in Manic Patients: A Comparison with Schizophrenic and Control Groups. *Journal of Affective Disorders*, 5(1983):45–50.

O'Brien, P. *The Disordered Mind*. Englewood Cliffs, N.J.: Prentice-Hall, 1978.

Pyke, J. M. Dependency Issues in Long-Term Treatment of Schizophrenia. *Issues in Mental Health Nursing*, 4(1982):77–85.

Rhoades, L. J. Psychosocial Intervention: A Way Out for Chronic Patients. *Hospital and Community Psychiatry*, 33(1982):709–710.

Roy, A. Depression in Chronic Schizophrenia. *British Journal of Psychiatry*, 142(1983):465-470.

Schwartzman, S. The Hallucinating Patient and Nursing Intervention. *Journal of Psychiatric Nursing and Mental Health Services*, 13(1975):23–36.

Shur, E. Family History and Schizophrenia. *Psychological Medicine*, 12(1982):591–594.

Szasz, T. *Schizophrenia: The Sacred Symbol of Psychiatry*. New York: Harper & Row, 1976.

Szymonski, H. V. Recovery for Schizophrenic Psychosis. *American Journal of Psychiatry*, 140(1983):335–338.

Travin, S. Mad or Bad? Some Clinical Considerations in the Misdiagnosis of Schizophrenia as Antisocial Personality. *American Journal of Psychiatry*, 139(1982): 1335–1338.

Tsuang, M. T. Physical Disease in Schizophrenia and Affective Disorders. *Journal of Clinical Psychiatry*, 44 (1983):42–46.

Wasow, M. Parental Perspectives in Chronic Schizophrenia. *Journal of Chronic Diseases*, 36(1983):337–340.

Whall, A. L. Development of a Screening Program for Tardive Dyskinesia: Feasibility Issues. *Nursing Research*, 32(1983):151–156.

Whileside, S. E. Patient Education: Effectiveness of Medication Programs for Psychiatric Patients. *Journal of Psychosocial Nursing and Mental Health Services*, 21 (1983):16–21.

Zigler, E. Hallucinations Versus Delusions: A Developmental Approach. *Journal of Nervous and Mental Diseases*, 171(1983):141–146.

159

DEPRESSION AS A MALADAPTIVE RESPONSE

CLASSIFICATION OF ALTERED PATTERNS OF
MOOD AND AFFECT

ETIOLOGY OF AFFECTIVE DISTURBANCE
Psychodynamic Factors
Biochemical Factors
Genetic Factors
Existential Factors

WORKING WITH DEPRESSED CLIENTS
Assessment
Planning
Implementation
Evaluation

WORKING WITH ELATED CLIENTS
Assessment
Planning
Implementation
Evaluation

SOMATIC TREATMENT MEASURES
Electroconvulsive Therapy
Antidepressant Medication
Lithium Therapy

GRIEF AND MOURNING
Adaptive and Maladaptive Grief
Phases of Grief
Anticipatory Grief
Helping the Grief Stricken

C H A P T E R

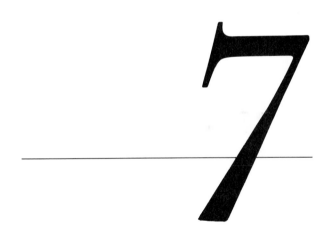

7

Altered Patterns of Mood and Affect

Learning Objectives

After reading this chapter, the student should be able to:

1. Discuss psychodynamic, biochemical, genetic, and existential factors contributing to altered patterns of mood and affect.

2. Compare various therapeutic approaches to working with depressed clients.

3. Compare various therapeutic approaches to working with elated clients.

4. Describe somatic interventions used with clients experiencing maladaptive alterations of mood and affect.

5. Recognize the responsibilities and contributions of the nurse in the administration of somatic interventions.

6. Identify nursing functions in preventing and alleviating maladaptive alterations of mood and affect.

7. Differentiate adaptive grief from maladaptive responses to loss.

Overview

Alterations of mood and affect are among the most common human responses to life changes and transitions. Altered mood and affect may range from mild, transitory states of sadness or joy to extreme prolonged states of depression or elation in which awareness of reality is impaired. This chapter discusses the nature of alterations of mood and affect, the risk factors involved, therapeutic approaches, and nursing strategies helpful in working with depressed and elated clients. The chapter closes with a discussion of grief and mourning as adaptive and maladaptive responses to loss.

I am mad north by northwest. When the wind is southerly,
I know a hawk from a handsaw.
WILLIAM SHAKESPEARE

Loss is an unavoidable experience to which most people manage to adjust. Although difficult, grief and mourning are adaptive responses that integrate the experience of loss into the pattern of life. *Depression*, on the other hand, is a frequent but less adaptive response to losses that are actual, anticipated, or symbolic. Depression is a complex response generated by the interaction of many factors, past and present, and also by anticipation of coming events.

DEPRESSION AS A MALADAPTIVE RESPONSE

Statistical reports of the altered affective state called depression underestimate its prevalence, partly because observable signs vary so much. This is particularly true of people who conceal their feelings of depression behind a facade of cheerfulness or who develop somatic complaints that serve to explain apathy or lack of pleasure (Dohrenwend, Dohrenwend, and Gould, 1980). In some respects depression is a universal phenomenon. Nevertheless, it has been found that certain people are more likely than others to become depressed. Such persons include the elderly, young people, alcoholics, and those who have suffered losses of some kind.

Increased longevity has contributed to the incidence of depression among elderly persons who no longer feel useful or productive. Many elderly people must deal with *transition overload*, and adaptive responses become more difficult for them with each additional life change. Among other transitions, the elderly encounter restricted relationships as loved ones die or move away and role reduction or rever-

sal as their vigor declines. Their resulting depressed moods are often attributed to the inevitable effects of aging and therefore receive little attention. To complicate matters, many elderly persons use drugs, either by prescription or by choice, that cause depressive reactions that are apt to go unrecognized.

Among children and adolescents, underlying depression may be expressed in rebellious or in withdrawn behavior. The aggressive child who is hyperactive, the passive-aggressive teenager who resists schooling, and the worried overachiever may each be exhibiting depression in his or her own way. Authority figures such as teachers, parents, or police officers who deal with these young people often interpret their behavior as delinquent rather than as depressed.

In very young children who can neither verbalize nor act out their feelings, depressed reactions are usually expressed physiologically. Spitz (1946) noted that infants deprived of mothering withdraw from their environment, and similar infantile responses were observed by Engel (1962). Somewhat older children may develop skin disorders, gastrointestinal disturbances, headaches, or anorexia. In meeting the needs of such children, nurses should recommend medical investigation and treatment for the focal symptoms, followed by family meetings to examine the context in which the maladaptive responses developed.

Alcoholism is a condition that can cause significant alterations of mood and affect. Despite its popularity as a relaxer and social lubricant, alcohol is a central nervous system depressant that acts to aggravate physical and mental depression. Alcoholics who suffer loss of control, family discord, and occupational difficulties tend to increase their

Table 7-1. Significant Factors in Depressive Reactions

Type of Loss or Change	Examples of Loss or Change
Loss of meaningful relationships	Alienation or estrangement from a loved one; death, divorce, separation from a loved one
Change in body image or self-image	Physical or functional change in self-concept due to disease, trauma, or aging
Loss of status or prestige	Career demotion or disappointment; social or interpersonal inadequacy
Loss of confidence and self-assurance	Lowered sense of competence, autonomy, and independence
Loss of security and safety	Economic or social reverses; loss of control; unpredictable future outcomes
Loss of dreams, fantasies	Unfulfilled hopes; unrealized and unreachable ambitions

164

consumption of alcohol, thereby adding to their problems.

Most people who develop depression have experienced a loss of some kind. The loss may be recent, in the past, or a combination of the two. Furthermore, the loss may be actual, anticipated, or symbolic. Whatever its characteristics, the loss is always perceived by the depressed persons as meaningful and excessive. Significant losses that are likely to provoke depressive reactions in vulnerable individuals are listed in Table 7-1.

The experience of loss is influenced by the perceived or symbolic meaning of the loss. For individuals whose self-esteem is linked to achievement and recognition, loss of status and prestige can promote depression. Individuals who rely more on internal awareness of competence may become depressed when their feelings of competence and self-assurance are threatened. Another type of individual may be more concerned with security than status and thus is more affected by threats to security. Loss of dreams and fantasies may produce a sense of loss leading to depression in individuals who come to believe that their life ambitions will not be realized. Loss of or separation from meaningful relationships is so significant and so prevalent that such losses will be discussed separately later in this chapter in the section on grief and mourning.

CLASSIFICATION OF ALTERED PATTERNS OF MOOD AND AFFECT

The term *affective disorders* includes those clinical entities in which alterations of mood and affect are expressed through psychological, physiological, and interpersonal channels. The words "mood" and "affect" are sometimes used interchangeably, but *mood* refers to an inner emotional state, while *affect* refers to outer responses to changing ideas or images (Klerman, 1980). Although human beings are capable of a wide range of emotions—fear, anger, anxiety, joy, amazement, and so on—the clinical manifestations of affective disorders take the form of depression and its opposite extreme, mania. The DSM-III categories for affective disorders are listed in the accompanying box.

Major depression is characterized by a history of one or more episodes of depression. Whenever a period of mania (elation and heightened activity) has occurred, with or without a history of depression, the category of *bipolar disorder* is used. *Cyclothymic disturbances* resemble bipolar disorders but are less severe. *Dysthymic disorders* resemble major depression but are shorter in duration and less severe, and they are not preceded or followed by manic episodes. *Atypical disorders* are affective alterations that do not fit bipolar or depressive classifications.

Many earlier categories of depression were made obsolete by DSM-III. At one time depression was classified as *neurotic* (mild in form and reactive to external events) or *psychotic* (severe in form and reactive to internal conditions). A similar typology classified depressive states as *endogenous* (arising from biological or physiological causes) or *exogenous* (arising from situational or environmental causes). Depressions that were considered endogenous were usually treated with somatic interventions such as electroconvulsive therapy and drugs. Depressions classified as exogenous were thought to be more responsive to psychotherapeutic intervention or environmental modification.

<table>
<tr><td>

**DSM-III CLASSIFICATION OF
AFFECTIVE DISORDERS**

Major Depression
   Single
   Recurrent
Bipolar Disorder
   Mixed
   Manic
   Depressed
Other Specific Affective Disorders
   Cyclothymic
   Dysthymic (depressive neurosis)
Atypical Affective Disorders
   Atypical bipolar
   Atypical depression

</td></tr>
</table>

165

At present, the differences between endogenous and exogenous depression are indistinct. Indeed, it is now believed that both internal and external changes accompany *all* alterations of mood and affect. External problems, such as marital conflict or occupational discontent, may follow depression or precede it. Thus, rather than trying to separate cause from effect, it is more useful to examine interrelated factors in the etiology of mood and affective disturbances.

ETIOLOGY OF AFFECTIVE DISTURBANCE

Alterations in mood and affect can be explained as the result of psychodynamic, biochemical, genetic, or existential factors. Although these factors are discussed separately here, it is their interdependence that is important in the development of affective disturbance. People function as systems whose efficiency is affected by input from many sources. Some of the input comes from genetic and biochemical sources; other input is derived from existential experiences of life and from the psychodynamic impact of these experiences on the individual.

Psychodynamic Factors

According to psychoanalytic theory, depressive tendencies can begin early. In the first year of life the dependency needs of the child are met by the mother or mother figure. Oral needs predominate, and if these needs are not sufficiently satisfied, the child develops a longing for love and security. The power of the mother either to withhold or to satisfy causes the child to both love and hate her. This ambivalence creates tension in the child; as a result, both the loving and the resented aspects of the mother become internalized or introjected by the child. The child comes to see the world as disorderly and unpredictable, and he feels confused and guilty because his surrounding world lacks meaning. Unable to rely on external sources of love or to establish order in the world, the child blames himself and feels angry and inferior. The result is a fragile sense of self-esteem and competence (Freud, 1957).

When nurturing is insufficient or inconsistent, children develop a wish or craving for affection and approval that lasts a lifetime. Two modes of behavior are apt to result. The individual may try to obtain what she needs from others by becoming openly dependent, or she may deny dependency needs by adopting high, unrealistic standards of performance (Cohen, 1975). Thus, the psychoanalytic explanation connects depressive tendencies with unmet dependency needs in early life. The findings of Bowlby (1973, 1980) that early experiences of loss threaten abilities of individuals to cope with later losses support this explanation.

Although traumatic experiences during the oral phase of life may generate excessive needs for affection and approval in later life, such vulnerability is not limited to the oral period. Bibring (1953) suggested that fixation or regression at any stage of psychosexual development may contribute to depressive personality traits. In his view, depression is associated with the lowering of self-esteem that occurs when the mastery of developmental tasks is impaired. Trauma in the toilet-training phase, for example, may incite life-long feelings of failure around issues of control. Similarly, difficulties during the phallic period may result in extreme com-

Figure 7-1. *Biochemical synaptic transmission.*

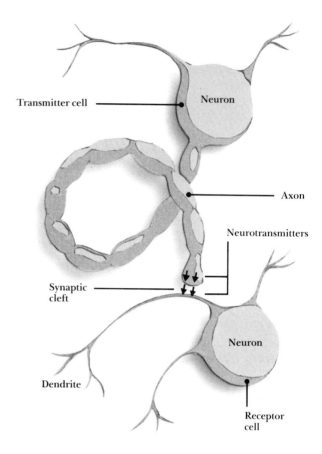

166

petitiveness or in an exaggerated fear of competing. Problems arising either in the stage of autonomy versus shame and doubt or in the stage of initiative versus guilt pose threats to the person's sense of competence and self-worth (Erikson, 1963).

Biochemical Factors

Alterations of mood and affect undoubtedly involve complex biochemical changes in the body. Among the identified changes are electrolyte imbalance of sodium and potassium and altered functioning of the thyroid, adrenocortex, gonads, and autonomic nervous system. In the last few decades belief has grown that affective disorders are related to the transmission of nerve impulses across the synaptic cleft (see Figure 7-1) by neurotransmitters, especially the biogenic amines. Both groups of biogenic amines seem to be involved: the catecholamines (dopamine and norepinephrine) and the indolamines (serotonin). Two altered neurotransmission patterns have been identified: norepinephrine deficiency in depression and serotonin deficiency in periodic mania and depression (bipolar disorder) (Wolpert, 1980). Although the results of biochemical investigation point to deficient amounts of norepinephrine as a major factor in depression, mania seems to be related to dopamine and serotonin function as well as to excess norepinephrine levels. Biochemical theories explaining mania and depression appear to be valid, but extensive investigation continues (Usdin, 1977; Wolpert, 1980).

The possibility that biochemical changes might contribute to mania and depression first came to light when it was observed that certain drugs can have major effects on mood and affect. It was noted, for example, that when certain drugs were pre-

scribed to reduce hypertension, the incidence of depression and suicide increased among persons taking these drugs. Subsequent research showed that the drugs used to alleviate hypertension depleted levels of norepinephrine, serotonin, and dopamine in the brain and neural synapses. About the same time it was noted that patients given monamine oxidase (MAO) inhibitors for treatment of tuberculosis experienced a state of elation or euphoria. When administered as antidepressants, these drugs proved to have the ability to elevate the mood of depressed persons. It was also discovered that these drugs *increased* the levels of norepinephrine, serotonin, and dopamine in the central nervous system. Currently it is thought that MAO inhibitors and another group of drugs called tricyclics produce their antidepressant effects by interfering with deamination of norepinephrine, thus increasing the availability of this biogenic neurotransmitter.

At present it is uncertain whether biochemical changes cause alterations of mood and affect, whether they are the results of alterations of mood and affect that reduce neurotransmission efficiency, or whether both factors interact in reciprocal ways (Hanin and Usdin, 1982). The fact that biochemical changes are associated with affective disturbances does not rule out psychological or situational influences in mania and depression. Human beings

ANACLITIC DEPRESSION

René Spitz, (1946) and John Bowlby (1969, 1982) were among the first to note that physical separation from the mother during infancy can cause apathy, withdrawal, and failure to thrive in the child. This condition, known as *anaclitic* separation or depression, is marked by conservation of energy and withdrawal from the social environment (Engel, 1962). In fact, many behaviors observed clinically in depressed children resemble the listlessness and inertia of some depressed adults who make no demands on the environment but wish only to be left alone.

167

adapt both physiologically and psychologically to internal and external conditions. For example, the fight or flight behaviors induced by anxiety are related to autonomic nervous system activity that influences the whole organism. In short, life experiences, past and present, can promote generalized and localized reactions that are both psychogenic and biogenic (Selye, 1956).

Genetic Factors

Some researchers are convinced that genetic factors play a significant role in mood and affective disorders, especially the bipolar types. Kallman (1953) considered manic-depressive disorders to be caused by a dominant gene with incomplete penetration and variable manifestation. That is, the gene is probably dominant but its behavior is unpredictable. It has indeed been found that close relatives of persons with bipolar disorder seem to be more susceptible to developing the disorder themselves than the general population, and susceptibility increases with the closeness of the relationship: The monozygotic twin of a person with bipolar disorder is more susceptible than a dizygotic twin, and a dizygotic twin is more susceptible than a regular sibling. Although current research supports the theory of a genetic factor in explaining the prevalence of bipolar disorder in some families, social factors in these families cannot be discounted (Juel-Nielson, 1980; Lumsden and Wilson, 1981).

Existential Factors

Existential factors in affective disturbances include accumulated or multiple life events that seem to predispose individuals to such problems. It is difficult, if not impossible, to separate life experiences from psychodynamic influences because personality traits, life experiences, and reactive behaviors are intertwined. Rejection by parents in childhood, poor marital adjustment, economic problems, and frustrated ambitions are only a few of the existential conditions that can influence mood and affect. In addition, some individuals spend their formative years in homes where there is a sustained atmosphere of hopelessness and a chronic expectation of failure. Such family depression can be contagious, and it is hard for any person living under such conditions to remain optimistic.

Individuals suffering bipolar disorder often come from families that are upwardly mobile, socially and economically, but somewhat isolated from the community (Gardner, 1982). The mother may have considerable authority in the family but is apt to be distant and unloving. The father is likely to be kinder but less powerful than the mother. The family member who develops bipolar disorder may have been the child expected to achieve high social and academic success, with parental approval conditional on the performance of the child.

During periods of depression, persons with bipolar disorder have feelings of failure and inferiority. During episodes of mania, their basic feelings are the same but are kept from conscious awareness by activity and energy that compensate for the underlying sense of inferiority. In periods of mania, as in depression, low self-esteem and fear of rejection persist but are disguised by grandiosity. Some theorists believe that manic behaviors are used to avoid reality, that sociability is compulsive rather than spontaneous, and that hyperactivity enables the individual to escape underlying fears and frustrations (Gardner, 1982).

INVOLUTIONAL MELANCHOLIA

Involutional melancholia is a form of depression that usually occurs in middle age. It appears in women near the time of menopause in their fourth decade, and in men about ten years later. In both men and women involutional melancholia tends to take the form of an agitated depressed mood. The disorder is more prevalent among women than men, but research on the link between involutional depression and hormonal changes related to menopause has been inconclusive. Although involutional melancholia may be linked to biological changes of late adulthood, existential factors cannot be ignored (Klerman, 1980; Wolpert, 1980).

In midlife, people have finished raising their families. Children have been launched and the nest is empty except for the parents, who are no longer young. They have achieved some life goals, but not others. Unachieved goals no longer seem close at hand but rather out of reach. Retirement nears, and with it comes the prospect of lowered income and additional role losses (Roy, 1981).

Usually people with involutional melancholia have been conforming, compulsive, and hard-working all their lives. Now they feel that they have been insufficiently rewarded and appreciated. Loss of youth and negative attitudes toward aging may contribute to their distress. Some are disappointed in themselves but project their disappointment onto others, becoming bitter and complaining.

In general, involutional melancholia is characterized by feelings of guilt, anger, and worry. In some cases delusions revolving around sin, poverty, and disease may be present. Some persons begin by thinking they have committed unpardonable sins but gradually project these sins onto others, becoming convinced that the sins have been committed against them. Delusions of persecution are therefore quite common.

Involutional melancholia is a serious condition: The risk of suicide may be quite high, and the suffering of clients and families can be extensive. It is no longer separated in DSM-III from other types of depression, but because of its prevalence and distressing manifestations, this form of depression merits particular attention from nurses and other caregivers. When individuals experience this form of depression, their agitation and the nature of their delusions can be very burdensome for family members, who need support and reassurance when dealing with a relative who has changed so much. The client and family members can truthfully be assured that the condition is self-limiting and that the eventual prognosis is hopeful, particularly when relief is provided in the form of psychotherapy and somatic measures such as antidepressant medication or electro-convulsive treatment.

WORKING WITH DEPRESSED CLIENTS

The clinical manifestations of depressed individuals offer a challenge to the nurse who recognizes that all behavior has meaning and purpose even when it seems self-defeating. In assessing a depressed client, it is important to go beyond outward behavior and consider every possible aspect. For example, many physical conditions manifest themselves as alterations of mood and affect, including carcinoma, cerebrovascular accidents (stroke), malnutrition, anemia, hypothyroidism, and multiple sclerosis. It is therefore unwise to assume that alterations of mood, whether depressive or manic, are primarily psychogenic until a full investigation of all factors has been made.

Assessment

Comprehensive assessment should include psychological, physiological, cognitive, and related factors.

PSYCHOLOGICAL MANIFESTATIONS Depressed people who are able to verbalize their feelings may describe themselves as helpless, worthless, hopeless, and despairing. They may feel guilty about deeds they imagine they have committed or resentful of misdeeds they believe have been committed against them. Psychoanalytic theory considers depressed people to be carriers of anger. This anger is explicit in the behavior of complaining, demanding clients who try to punish everyone in the vicinity because their needs are not being met, but it is less identifiable in depressed persons who make their de-

*Depressed . . . persons are always the center of attention in the family.
In them we see the power wielded by the inferiority complex. They
complain that they feel weak and are losing weight etc., but
nonetheless they are strongest of all. They dominate healthy persons.
This fact should not surprise us, for in our culture weakness can be
quite strong and powerful.*

ALFRED ADLER, THE SCIENCE OF LIVING

169

mands silently or indirectly. The nurse should remember that the behavior of a passive, withdrawn client may be just as directed toward winning attention as the behavior of the demanding client. Both behavioral expressions—aggressive and passive—tend to increase the power of the client over others.

In moderate to severe forms of depression, many individuals become indecisive and indifferent to their appearance or their surroundings. Others may engage obsessively in routine tasks and become preoccupied with unimportant details. Rumination (prolonged thinking about the same issue) is typical and is a factor in self-deprecation and indecisiveness. Attention span is often reduced to the extent that ordinary tasks require enormous amounts of energy and effort. Failure to accomplish or complete tasks then adds to feelings of guilt or worthlessness. Many depressed clients have distorted viewpoints and interpretations of reality that come to dominate their behavior. For example, some severely depressed individuals may develop somatic delusions, believing that their vital organs are diseased or decaying.

During depressive episodes, the whole quality of life seems to deteriorate. The person suffers from a poverty of ideas, restricted interests, loss of energy and spontaneity, and the belief that life is grim and unrewarding. *Anhedonia* (lack of pleasure) interferes with the individual's participation in activities that he or she once enjoyed. Anhedonia is accompanied by reduced sexual interest and desire, and by inhibited sexual excitement and orgasm in men and in women. Such sexual dysfunction may then jeopardize the individual's sexual relationships.

PHYSIOLOGICAL MANIFESTATIONS Depression is often accompanied by sleep disturbances, which may take the form of insomnia or hypersomnia, and by early morning awakening. Weight loss may occur in some persons as a result of anorexia, but other depressed people overeat as they try to relieve feelings of emptiness. Depressed clients express many somatic complaints, sometimes to the point of hypochondria. Because some complaints may have a realistic basis, it is essential to investigate and respond appropriately to any somatic problems, whether real or imaginary.

Psychomotor retardation may cause the client to move, think, and speak slowly. Constipation may become a problem, although it may be the expression of an emotional state rather than a direct result of physiological retardation. Not every depressed person exhibits psychomotor retardation; in fact, many engage in aimless, unproductive activity. When depression takes the form of agitation rather than psychomotor retardation, the individual becomes restless and fidgety, but the activity is often purposeless and undirected. Tasks are begun but rarely finished, further contributing to feelings of extreme inadequacy.

COGNITIVE MANIFESTATIONS The psychoanalytic explanation that depressed persons carry anger that has been internalized and turned against the self was questioned by Beck (1969, 1972), who has formulated a different explanation for depression. Beck began by analyzing the dreams of several hundred depressed and nondepressed subjects. He found that the dreams of depressed persons could be characterized by these common themes: (1) the dreamer tried to do or obtain something but was frustrated, (2) the dreamer lost an object or person

Figure 7-2. *Cognitive triad of depression.*

Negative view of self

Negative view of world

Negative view of future

Excessive demands by others

Constant frustration

Sense of inferiority

Moral, mental, physical defects

Burdens, obstacles, hardships

Failure, failure, failure

170

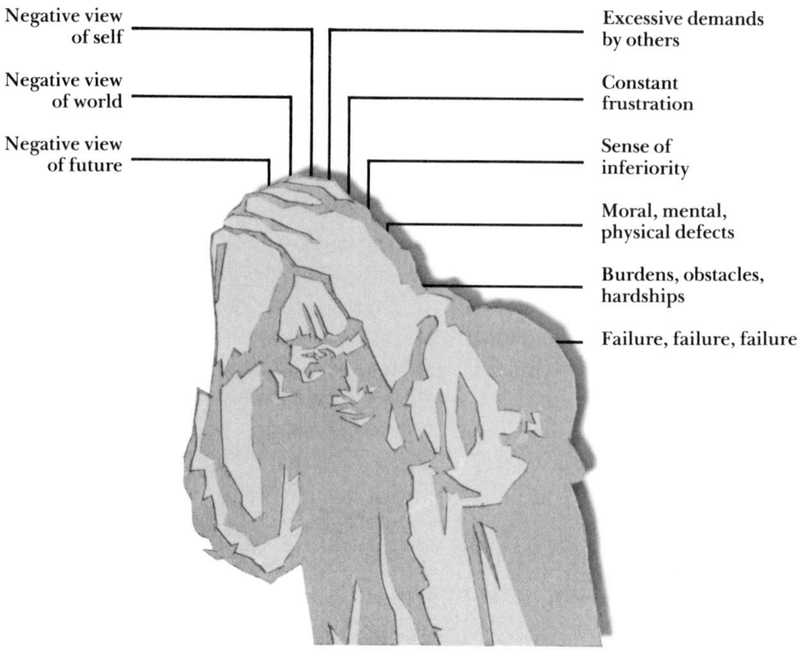

of value, or (3) the dreamer was deficient in health, appearance, or ability. Beck followed these dream studies with investigations of the thought content revealed by depressed clients. He found that depressed persons hold a number of negative attitudes toward themselves, their world, and their future. Beck labeled this group of negative attitudes the *cognitive triad of depression*; it is presented in the accompanying box and illustrated in Figure 7-2.

Having noted the distortions in the cognitive patterns of depressed persons, Beck tried to identify the mechanisms used to interpret situations negatively. He found that depressed persons overgeneralize by drawing global conclusions from a single, isolated event. A selective focus causes them to take details out of context, exaggerating negative features and ignoring positive ones. In addition, they reject pieces of evidence that contradict their negative interpretations. Errors in judgment are ignored or exaggerated, depending on which distortion is needed to support negative viewpoints.

When Beck's findings were applied clinically, it was apparent that depressed persons responded favorably to positive feedback given upon the successful completion of graded tasks. Rewards, in the form of praise and attention, had to be immediate to be effective, however. Exposure to consistent rewards and the experience of successful achievement contradicted the depressed client's conviction that success was impossible. Interventions that suggested that failure was not inevitable also seemed to reduce feelings of pessimism and ineffectiveness.

Planning

Nurses planning care for depressed clients should identify major problems, including the possibility of

a suicide attempt. Every depressed client is a suicide risk. When deeply depressed, a client may lack the energy or motivation to put a suicide plan into action. Thus, the danger of suicide is actually greatest just as the depression begins to lift. Not only does the client now have the energy to act on a suicide plan, but inexperienced staff members may be relaxing their vigilance.

In cases of potential suicide, hospitalization may be indicated unless social supports are reliable and available for the client. Suicide precautions are a routine procedure for depressed clients in psychiatric inpatient facilities and require staff members to know the exact whereabouts of the suicidal client at every moment. A discussion of the assessment of suicide risk, types of suicide, and nursing responsibility for suicidal clients is provided in Chapter 15, which deals with situational crises.

Many depressed clients suffer from sleep disturbances. Clients may be unable to fall asleep or may fall asleep readily but waken early. Some individuals sleep fitfully while others regress by sleeping day and night. When clients are wakeful, sedatives may promote sleep for a time, but they fail to solve the fundamental problems. Alert nurses have observed that administration of sedation to inpatients rises or falls depending on the staff assigned to evening or night rotations. Thus, at times sedation seems to be administered on the basis of staff needs rather than client needs.

Before deciding to administer sedation, the nurse should explore the possible causes of sleep disturbance. Many depressed clients behave in ways that encourage insomnia. They may sleep during the day or engage in activities such as watching television that are neither constructive nor rewarding.

THE COGNITIVE TRIAD OF DEPRESSION

Negative View of the Self
The depressed person generally perceives the self as deficient and inferior. Failure and frustration are attributed to physical, mental, or moral defects in the self. Therefore, the self is unlovable and unacceptable.

Negative View of the World
The depressed person believes that the world makes excessive demands and at the same time causes constant frustration. Actions meet with defeat; life is full of burdens, impediments, and disappointments.

Negative View of the Future
The depressed person assumes that the dismal conditions of the present will continue in the future. No relief can be seen; only a life of failure and hardship looms ahead.

171

When bedtime arrives, these clients cannot sleep because they are not tired or because the day has seemed wasted. Occasionally, family visits have been upsetting, making the client agitated and unable to sleep.

To address these causes, the nurse can plan activities for daytime hours so that tendencies to sleep all day and stay awake all night are discouraged. The nurse might also talk quietly with the client about unresolved incidents of the day or may attend to specific complaints that prevent the client from sleeping. Giving nonstimulating beverages or assisting with relaxing baths may be more effective in the long run than medication. Moreover, these measures assure the client that the nurse is concerned and wants to help.

Implementation
Many depressed clients are reluctant to engage in social interaction because of apathy and poor motivation. Their lack of confidence and feelings of worthlessness lead them to doubt their ability to converse or to inspire positive responses in anyone. Depressed clients may inadvertently cause staff members to withdraw and avoid them unless deliberate efforts are made by staff to prevent mutual withdrawal. Staff members should spend some portion of each day with hospitalized depressed clients, talking or listening in an accepting way or perhaps just sitting with them in order to communicate interest and a wish to help. Extreme cheerfulness on the part of caregivers is not helpful, as it conveys to the client that feelings of sadness are unacceptable.

Depressed clients seem to become resigned to their situation and want to give up. These feelings can be counteracted by using Beck's cognitive approach to correct distortions. When depressed clients express feelings of helplessness, it is appropriate to ask, "Are you really so helpless, or do you have some strengths you're not using?" If clients express feelings of hopelessness, suggest that "there are people available who want to help you begin to help yourself."

Feelings of worthlessness can be reduced by providing opportunities to succeed. Because the client's concentration and energy are limited, activities should be noncompetitive, undemanding, and of short duration. Indecisiveness in depressed clients is troublesome and intensifies their feelings of inadequacy. Therefore, a schedule or routine that eliminates some decisions can be helpful. When decisions must be made, the nurse can help the client reduce the number of alternatives so that confusion is lessened.

Consistency is needed from the nurse, as is the ability to tolerate anger without becoming angry in turn. When the client is angry, the nurse should be matter-of-fact rather than defensive. Motor activities such as walking and exercising can help to discharge anger and aggression without provoking additional guilt on the part of the client.

Because the clinical picture presented by depressed clients is not uniform, individual signs and behaviors must be considered in developing a care plan. Collaboration with the client is always an objective, but sometimes active collaboration must wait until the client becomes capable of participation.

Table 7-2. Planning Care for Depressed Clients

Client's Problem	Goal	Nursing Intervention
Feelings of inadequacy and helplessness	Client will experience a sense of acceptance	Active listening and honest reassurance
Rumination and indecision	Client will ruminate less and decide issues more easily	Clarification of issues so decision making and problem solving are simplified
Apathy and regression	Client will participate in appropriate activity and interaction	Encourage verbalization and social interaction
Direct and indirect expressions of anger	Client will be less afraid to express negative feelings	Accept expressions of anger without retaliating
Psychomotor retardation	Client will feel less inferior and incapable	Allow time for activities to be completed; encourage motor activities that client can tolerate
Somatic complaints	Client will realize that staff will respond realistically to somatic complaints	Work with health team to investigate and treat
Sleep disturbance: hypersomnia	Client will sleep an appropriate number of hours	Design schedule of activities with the help of the client
Sleep disturbance: insomnia	Client will sleep or rest an adequate number of hours	Promote relaxing bedtime routines: warm milk, bathing, quiet conversation

172

Clients who become troubled by a sleep problem may be told truthfully that this is not a permanent condition but rather a part of being depressed. In dealing with the problem the nurse and client should work together rather than at cross purposes. It is far easier to dispense medication than to establish routines that promote sleep, but only the latter is an independent nursing function. A number of interventions appropriate for sleep disturbance and other problems are listed in Table 7-2.

Evaluation

Making a nursing assessment, reaching a nursing diagnosis, identifying problems, and establishing priorities make clinical evaluation possible. One way to evaluate the progress of a depressed client is to note the client's increased involvement in self-care and decision making. Observations of the client's psychological, physiological, and cognitive responses in therapeutic interaction, accurate recording of observations, progress toward identified goals, and the abatement of subjective discomfort are used by the nurse to evaluate the effectiveness of the care plan and to modify specific treatment goals as needed.

WORKING WITH ELATED CLIENTS

Depression and mania represent two poles of the same continuum. Although the outward manifestations of the two affective states are diametrically opposed, their dynamics are similar. In fact, the manic state has been called the "mirror image" of depression. Whereas depression involves a devaluation of self in response to a loss, mania represents a denial of loss and a temporary restoration of self-esteem. Manic states may or may not be triggered by a precipitating event, and episodes of mania may be followed by periods of normalcy or of depression. Mania occurs more commonly before age thirty-five, while depression occurs more commonly after that age. In any form of bipolar disorder, little deterioration occurs between the maladaptive episodes, which may be separated by intervals of weeks, months, or years.

Assessment

Comprhrehensive assessment should include psychological, physiological, and cognitive factors.

PSYCHOLOGICAL MANIFESTATIONS Clients in a manic state are attempting to remove their doubts and conflicts by behaving in ways that free them from the restraints of logic and rationality. In *hypomania*, which is a less severe state than mania, hyperactive behavior may remain purposeful, goal directed, and productive. When full blown mania erupts, however, the client becomes elated, euphoric, and grandiose. To maintain the illusion of omnipotence, she may engage in reckless spending or may embark on impractical schemes to impress others. The defense mechanisms of denial and reaction formation are used to disguise feelings of dependence and insecurity. The manic client is demanding, exploitive, manipulative, and self-centered, but underneath she is uncertain and needs approval. The client may be easily angered because of her low tolerance for frustration.

Although the client seems eager for social interaction, she does not tolerate intimacy well and is quite sensitive to rejection. Because the client is

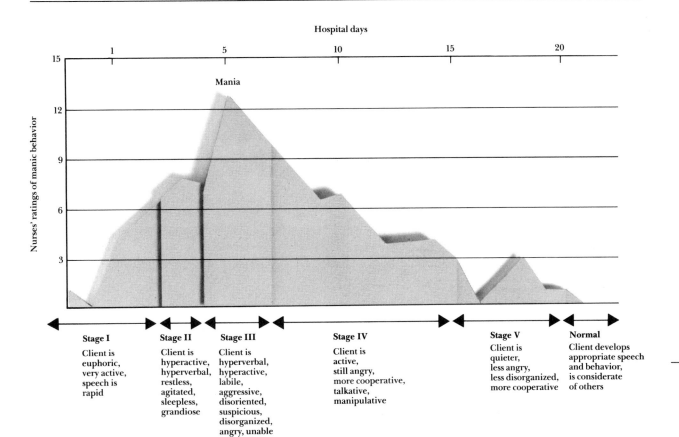

Figure 7-3. *Stages of a manic episode of a hospitalized patient over a three-week period.*

173

sensitive to and fears rejection, she constantly tests and manipulates others in an effort to achieve reassurance. The client expects much from others, is insensitive to their needs, and tries to control the social environment (Wolpert, 1980).

PHYSIOLOGICAL MANIFESTATIONS The client in a manic state engages in frenzied, unceasing activity that makes it possible for him to ignore reality-based messages from others. During the manic state, external stimuli are not screened adequately, and the client is easily distracted. His speech, thoughts, and actions are speeded to the point of incoherence. Singing, rhyming, dancing, dressing, and undressing proceed in rapid order until onlookers (but not the client) feel exhausted. The client's limitless energy and responsiveness to all stimuli make it difficult for him to maintain adequate nutrition or rest. Unless prompt measures are taken, he will suffer from total exhaustion and depletion of energy. The

stages of a typical manic episode are illustrated in Figure 7-3.

COGNITIVE MANIFESTATIONS Mania not only blocks out input from others but also enables the client to feel powerful. He has flights of ideas in which the content is somewhat related but is so fragmented that listeners find it hard to understand what he means.

The manic client has little awareness of experiencing impaired reality testing and is convinced of being superior to others. He adopts a cheerful, boisterous, conviviality to disperse anxiety and self-doubt. However, this facade is fragile and easily threatened. Whenever the manic client has cause to distrust his effectiveness, he may become angry, accusative, or hostile.

Nursing assessment of the manic client consists of analyzing the connections between the client's behavior and the contradictory feelings beneath. As

Table 7-3. Planning Care for Manic Clients

Client's Problem	Goal	Nursing Intervention
Inadequate nutrition	Client will maintain adequate food intake	Offer "finger foods" that may be eaten without sitting still
Inadequate sleep	Client will avoid total exhaustion	Encourage short rest periods if client cannot sleep longer
Poor personal hygiene	Client will comply with relaxed standards of dress and hygiene	Enforce minimal standards of dress and grooming
High energy expenditure	Client will accept a regimen that does not deplete energy	Suggest sedentary but interesting activities, such as drawing or painting; offer motor activities in moderation to relieve tension; avoid competitive games or activities
Excessive responsiveness to stimuli	Client will avoid unnecessary external stimuli	Remove client from situations that are highly stimulating; remove unnecessary objects from immediate environment; arrange for the same staff members to deal with client
Belief in personal omnipotence	Client will be protected from opportunity to test powers recklessly	Safeguard client from physical risks
Unrealistic attitudes toward financial and legal matters	Client will refrain from making purchases that prove detrimental to self or family; client will avoid adverse legal entanglements	Cooperate with family to discourage the client from making large expenditures or legal commitments
Demanding, manipulative behaviors	Client will understand what behaviors are acceptable; client will be treated consistently by staff; client will be diverted from unacceptable actions	Define and explain acceptable behaviors; negotiate limits with client; offer alternative activities; avoid frustrating the client unnecessarily; use diversion as a therapeutic tool

174

with depressed clients, assessment proceeds more easily if specific problems are identified and ranked in order of priority and if responsive interventions are formulated for the problems. Some of the typical problems resulting from the psychological, physiological, and cognitive manifestations of the manic client are described in Table 7-3.

Planning

A client in a manic state may be difficult to manage initially; usually medication in the form of a major tranquilizer or lithium carbonate is administered, but it may be several days before the medication takes effect. Two major considerations must be taken into account in planning the care of a manic client. One consideration is the maintenance of adequate food and rest until the manic behaviors are brought under control. The second consideration is the elimination of unnecessary sources of stimulation and distraction. Manic clients should be cared for by the same nurse or health care team during hospitalization. Even with this arrangement, the potential for manipulation of staff members remains. One way to avoid such manipulation is to include all staff members in explanations of the approaches to be used. As with any client, staff members who participate in planning are less likely to deviate from the agreed upon approach.

Implementation

The client who is in a manic state needs to know that staff members will help control unacceptable behaviors. Although the client may engage in grandiose schemes and manipulative tactics, she has underlying fears of losing control. She may interpret a permissive attitude on the part of staff members as a sign of indifference.

In setting limits, the staff should address specific behaviors and whenever possible suggest substitute behaviors so that the client cannot complain that "nothing" is allowed by the staff. For example, walking is a motor activity that is not too strenuous. Sketching and painting are other activities that help a manic client satisfy the need for action.

The grandiose behaviors of manic clients may annoy others and their outbreaks of anger may frighten others. It is thus important for everyone concerned that staff members clearly indicate the range of acceptable behaviors and institute procedures to modify unacceptable actions (Klerman, 1980). Establishing a regular schedule that alternates periods of rest and activity can help if all staff members are consistent in adhering to the regimen.

Therapeutic interventions should have a moderating effect on the client's disruptive, self-destructive behaviors. Suggested nursing interventions are provided in Table 7-3.

Evaluation

A problem-oriented care plan with specific interventions allows both nurse and client to determine whether expected outcomes have been reached.

During periods of mania, the client has little awareness of maladaptive behavior; thus, until symptoms subside the treatment plan should be largely supportive. After the acute phase of the manic episode has abated, it may be advisable to help the client explore feelings experienced before, during, and after the episode. The client with a bipolar disorder who learns to identify early symptoms is in a better position to seek help and to learn methods of coping.

SOMATIC TREATMENT MEASURES

Clients with severe alterations of mood and affect often require somatic intervention in the form of electroconvulsant therapy (ECT) or drug therapy. Drug therapy is important in treating clients experiencing mania or depression, and ECT, although controversial, has a place in the treatment of persons with moderate to severe depression who may be suicidal or for whom medication has proved ineffective. Nurses have an important part to play in the administration of such treatments and in preparing, supporting, and teaching clients, and should therefore understand the rationale and implications of such measures.

Electroconvulsive Therapy

Electroconvulsive therapy was introduced in the 1930s when it was noticed that psychiatric clients who had suffered spontaneous convulsions or seizures became less disturbed and that epileptic convulsions and schizophrenia were rarely present in the same individual. Two Italian psychiatrists, Cerletti and Bini, were the first to apply electrodes to the temporal region of psychiatric clients for the purpose of inducing therapeutic convulsions. The electrodes sent an alternating electric current through the head strong enough to cause the client to lose consciousness and to have a seizure of grande mal proportions.

A number of theories have attempted to explain the ability of ECT to alleviate depression. The behavioral explanation is that depression is a learned way of behaving and that the electrical charge interrupts neural pathways that may be maintaining the depressed responses. Interrupting these neural pathways is thought to permit a return to more adaptive responses. Another theory is that guilt, a major component of depression, is reduced by a treatment so unpleasant that it seems like a punishment. This punishment theory is indirectly supported by the reports of some clients who say that they fear ECT but "deserve" to undergo it (Salzman, 1975).

Since its introduction, ECT has been called barbarous by its critics, and with some justification. At first it was used indiscriminately for many types of psychiatric disorders and on people of all ages. It was also administered repeatedly without due regard for the possible consequences to the client. The convulsions induced were sufficiently severe to cause fractures and dislocations in some clients. Today the basic apparatus remains the same, but the techniques of administration have been greatly modified. Among the modifications is the use of atropine to reduce secretions and vagal stimulation. A muscle relaxant such as succinylcholine chloride (Anectine) is used to block the transmission of impulses to the skeletal muscles, thereby preventing muscle spasms. Because of precautions now taken, the convulsions are not severe and may be evident only in the involuntary movements of the client's toes as the current is applied.

A preliminary medical workup is necessary for every client receiving ECT, including a complete blood count, electrocardiograph, chest x-ray, urinalysis, and x-ray of the lateral aspects of the spine. Cardiac arrhythmias may develop during the seizures, and the potential for problems should be known in advance. As ECT is usually given in the morning, the client takes nothing by mouth after midnight. Dentures, metal hairpins, and shoes or slippers should be removed before treatment.

When ECT is administered, an anesthesiologist is present to inject a short-acting anesthetic such as thiopental (Pentothal) or methohexital intravenously. Before the electrical charge is administered, the client is oxygenated. An airway is inserted into the mouth, and the arms restrained at the sides of the body. Electrodes are placed on the temples at a point midway between the eyes and the top of the ears. Application of the electric current induces a tonic seizure lasting 5 to 15 seconds, followed by clonic seizures lasting 10 to 60 seconds. A single course of ECT consists of three treatments a week on alternate days over a period of three weeks, followed by a recess. Additional treatments may be given if indicated (Kalinowsky, 1980).

After several ECT treatments the client becomes confused and forgetful. As the treatments continue, the confusion and amnesia increase. These effects usually disappear in time, although some clients say that the forgetfulness never fully disappears. Immediately after a treatment the client is apt to be disoriented and must be reoriented to time, place, and person as he regains consciousness.

175

Table 7-4. Monamine Oxidase Inhibitors and Dosages

Generic Name	Trade Name	Range of Dosages
Isocarboxazid	Marplan	10−30 mg/day
Phenelzine	Nardil	15−30 or more mg/day
Tranylcypromine	Parnate	20−30 mg/day

SOURCE: Appleton and Davis (1980).

Vital signs are taken every 15 minutes as he recovers. When he becomes aware of his surroundings and can walk, a nurse accompanies him to his room, where he then sleeps for several hours.

Every state has its own laws regulating the administration of ECT, and there are legal and ethical dilemmas surrounding this treatment that nurses should understand. Before ECT is given a nurse may be asked to obtain written permission from the client or next of kin. Informed consent is the right of every client, but a severely depressed person may not be capable of making a rational choice. Families may then have to give written consent instead of the client. The procedure should be fully explained to families, including the limited information about how or why the procedure works. Providing information about the confusion and memory loss that follow ECT not only fulfills legal requirements but also reduces the concern of family members as they deal with the aftermath of the treatments.

Attitudes of nurses can greatly affect clients receiving ECT. If the nurse has ambivalent feelings about the treatment, he should keep these feelings under control to avoid giving negative messages to the client. Clients may be frightened by the confusion and amnesia that increase with each treatment and will want explanations. Support and reassurance should be based on the facts that the gross aftereffects do disappear and that depressed people who have not responded to other forms of treatment almost always improve as a result of ECT.

Antidepressant Medication

Drug therapy is often indicated for depressed persons, and clinicians may select from two groups of antidepressant drugs, the monamine oxidase inhibitors and the tricyclic antidepressants. A third group of drugs, the tetracyclates, are also available but are less commonly used. When using drug therapy it should be remembered that it constitutes but one aspect of the plan of care. Although biological and psychosocial approaches are concerned with different aspects of the client and employ different interventions, the approaches should be seen as complementary, not competitive or mutually exclusive (Wolpert, 1980).

MONAMINE OXIDASE INHIBITORS The therapeutic effect of *monamine oxidase* (MAO) *inhibitors* is to relieve depression and to act as psychic energizers. Because the MAO inhibitors are stimulants, some clients may experience euphoric, hypomanic, or manic reactions to them. Such reactions may occur at any time during the course of drug treatment. Furthermore, this group of drugs may intensify schizophrenic tendencies, making susceptible clients agitated or actively delusional.

MAO inhibitors act by blocking the metabolism of certain neurotransmitters, thereby increasing the amounts available. The drugs are long lasting and are thought to remain in the body for as long as two weeks after the last dose. Because their effects are cumulative, the antidepressant action of the MAO inhibitors are not apparent for one to two weeks after treatment is begun. Dosages of the MAO inhibitors must be regulated and clients carefully observed for undesirable side effects. The most widely used MAO inhibitors and their recommended dosages are shown in Table 7-4.

MAO inhibitors reduce the body's ability to metabolize epinephrine and thus should not be

DIETARY REGULATIONS FOR USERS OF MAO INHIBITORS

Forbidden Substances
Aged cheeses such as cheddar or Swiss
Sour cream
Yogurt
Brewer's yeast
Beer, sherry, ale, or wine
Raisins, canned figs
Bananas
Lima beans, kidney beans, bean pods, split peas
Pizza
Liver
Pickled herring

Permitted Substances
Cottage cheese, creamed cheese
Sanka (liberal amounts)
Coffee (small amounts)
Tea (small amounts)
Cola drinks (small amounts)
Chocolate (small amounts)
Licorice (small amounts)
Bread (liberal amounts)

Table 7-5. Tricyclic Antidepressants and Dosages

Generic Name	Trade Name	Range of Dosages
Amitriptyline	Elavil	50–300 mg/day
Imipramine	Tofranil	50–300 mg/day
Nortriptyline	Aventyl	20–200 mg/day
Dioxepin	Sinequan	25–300 mg/day
Protriptyline	Vivactyl	15–60 mg/day

given with certain medications containing ephredine. Because ephedrine is an ingredient of many nonprescription cold remedies, decongestants, and allergy preparations, clients taking an MAO inhibitor must be explicitly warned of the danger. In addition, the MAO inhibitors potentiate a number of other drugs such as morphine, meperidine, barbiturates, atropine derivatives, antihistamines, and some diuretics. Among the potential side effects of MAO inhibitors resulting from anticholinergic effects include blurred vision, constipation, dry mouth, and delayed micturition.

In addition to avoiding compounds containing ephedrine, persons taking an MAO inhibitor should avoid foods containing tryamine. When combined with an MAO inhibitor tryamine releases norepinephrine, and a hypertensive crisis results. Clients must be warned not to eat foods containing tryamine for several days prior to drug therapy, during drug therapy, and for two weeks after the drug is discontinued. If a client does eat foods on the restricted list while taking an MAO inhibitor, an emetic is usually given to induce vomiting. The accompanying box shows the major food substances to be avoided by persons taking an MAO inhibitor.

Contraindications for the use of MAO inhibi-

tors are glaucoma, liver disease, renal impairment, hyperthyroidism, hypertension, and cardiovascular disease. Because of the hazards in taking MAO inhibitors, they are usually prescribed only when tricyclic preparations prove ineffective. However, MAO inhibitors seem more effective for clients suffering fluctuating, atypical depression. For clients suffering severe depression with psychomotor retardation, the tricyclic drugs seem to produce greater improvement (Mansky, 1981; Gerald and O'Bannon, 1981).

TRICYCLIC ANTIDEPRESSANTS About 70 percent of individuals with depressive disorders of clinical proportions are relieved by antidepressants belonging to the *tricyclic* group (Kontos and Steinhilber, 1979). These antidepressants do not block neurotransmitter metabolism but rather prevent the reuptake of neurotransmitters into the presynaptic cleft, thus increasing the amounts of neurotransmitters available. Table 7-5 shows the generic and trade names of commonly used tricyclic antidepressants and their range of dosages.

As with MAO inhibitors, it takes two to three weeks for therapeutic effects to become noticeable. Although the drugs promote alertness in clients, they rarely cause excessive excitability or agitation. This is particularly true of Elavil and Sinequan, which have sedating and antianxiety properties that counteract stimulating effects. Tofranil, another drug in this group, does not have significant sedating or antianxiety properties and is often accompanied by antianxiety medications to avoid causing agitated behaviors. The tricyclic antidepressants are not cumulative in effect and seldom potentiate the action of other medications.

Table 7-6. Other Drugs Used as Antidepressants and Usual Dosages

Generic Name	Trade Name	Range of Dosages
Amoxapine	Asendin	150–400 mg/day
Maprotiline	Ludiomil	75–300 mg/day
Trazodone	Desyrel	150–500 mg/day
Trimipramine maleate*	Surmontil	75–300 mg/day
Dextroamphetamine*	Dexedrine	5–15 mg/day
Methamphetamine*	Me·hedrine	5–15 mg/day
Methylphenidate*	Ritalin	10–30 mg/day
Phenmetrazine*	Preludin	25–75 mg/day
Amphetamine sulfate*	Benzedrine	5–15 mg/day

*Psychomotor stimulants—used with caution for selected clients.

178

It is customary to give tricyclic antidepressants, particularly dioxepin (Sinequan) and amitriptyline (Elavil), in a single nighttime dose to reduce insomnia. This procedure reduces the need for additional sleep medication, which is often dangerous in the hands of a depressed client.

Like the MAO inhibitors, the tricyclic antidepressants are anticholinergic, so clients with cardiovascular problems should be carefully monitored by means of electrocardiograph. Tricyclics are contraindicated for clients with a history of glaucoma, urinary retention, benign prostatic hypertrophy, seizure disorder, or renal deficiency.

Most clinicians do not recommend the concurrent use of MAO inhibitors with tricyclic antidepressants. In fact, a washout period of at least a week is usually arranged before changing from an MAO inhibitor to a tricyclic antidepressant because of the danger of hypertension or hyperpyrexia if the drugs are both used within a brief time frame.

OTHER ANTIDEPRESSANTS Other antidepressants are available that are structurally unrelated to the MAO inhibitors and the tricyclic antidepressants (see Table 7-6). These include amoxapine (Asendin) and maprotiline (Ludiomil), which offer the advantage of more rapid improvement and less frequent occurrence of cardiovascular reactions. Little is known about their specified therapeutic action or their effect on neurotransmitters.

When a client is unresponsive to other antidepressant medications, a psychomotor stimulant is sometimes used to alleviate depression. These drugs stimulate the central nervous system, thereby increasing mental alertness and elevating the client's mood. However, the psychomotor stimulants are rarely effective when the client is severely depressed, so they are generally used only with mild to moderate states of depression when increased activity is desired. There are risks to the use of psychomotor stimulants for depressed clients because the energizing effects are short lived. When the effects of the drugs wear off, the client experiences a return of the depressed state or even a worsening of the symptoms. In addition, use of psychomotor stimulants may result in drug dependency and drug abuse. However, there are instances where psychomotor stimulants are used for relatively short periods and for selected clients.

NURSING MEASURES Nurses can do a great deal to prevent or relieve the troublesome side effects of antidepressant medications. Serious side effects such as cardiac arrhythmias can be avoided by teaching clients to note and report reactions promptly. Regular electrocardiogram evaluation should be part of the care plan for clients with a history of cardiac conduction problems. Dietary restriction and its rationale must be explained to persons using MAO inhibitors. Any client on antidepressant medications should avoid central nervous system depressants. Specific side effects of antidepressants are shown in Table 7-7, along with suggested nursing interventions.

Nurses working with depressed clients receiving antidepressant medication need to monitor compliance. It is possible, for instance, to commit suicide by taking an overdose of a prescribed antidepressant. Some deaths have been attributed to antidepressants at dosages as low as 700 to 1000 mg, especially when alcohol has been ingested at the same time. For this reason it is important to ques-

Table 7-7. Side Effects of Antidepressant Drugs

Effects	Nursing Interventions
Anxiety, agitation, excitement	Continue drug, but inform physician. Antidepressant with sedating action or antianxiety medication may be needed.
Disorientation, delusions, mania	Withhold drug and inform physician immediately. As depression lifts, a psychotic or bipolar episode may be revealed.
Fine tremor, ataxia	If severe, withhold medication and inform physician.
Convulsions	Withhold medication and inform physician immediately. Institute seizure precautions.
Tachycardia	Monitor vital signs, especially pulse. Withhold medication if pulse exceeds 120 beats. Notify physician.
Orthostatic hypotension	Record sitting and standing blood pressure. Withhold medication and inform physician if systolic pressure drops significantly.
Arrhythmias and T-wave abnormalities	Monitor pulse. Withhold medication and notify physician immediately. Suggest electrocardiograph if client has a history of conduction problems.
Drowsiness, slowed responses	Advise client not to drive or operate power tools. Administer most of medication at bedtime. Inform physician if symptoms persist.
Decreased or increased sexual desire; ejaculatory disturbance (premature or inhibited); failure to achieve or maintain erection	Reassure client that the problem may be temporary. Inform physician, since sexual dysfunction may cause client to stop taking medication. Explore with physician the possibility of altering dosage or using an alternative medication.
Dry mouth	Offer water frequently. Suggest sugarless hard candy or lubricating mouth swabs.
Constipation	Encourage fluid intake. Increase amounts of whole-grain cereals, fruits, and vegetables in diet. Observe client for signs of impaction or paralytic ileus.
Urinary retention or delayed micturition	Monitor intake and output. Note signs of abdominal distention. Notify physician if client cannot void. Suggest catheterization if client is uncomfortable.
Diaphoresis	Offer fluids to replace lost amounts. Monitor electrolyte balance.

tion clients about how and when the antidepressant is being taken, to check on the remaining quantity of the medication, and to make available only enough for a week or ten days (Irons, 1978).

Antidepressant drugs are often continued for several months after symptoms subside. When the medication is discontinued, clients and family members should be taught to recognize incipient indications of depression. Usually the same manifestations occur as in previous episodes.

Lithium Therapy

Until the early 1970s, people with bipolar disorders faced long years of disruptive mood changes for which no satisfactory treatment was available. This

situation changed with the discovery that *lithium carbonate* could be used to control episodes of mania and that, when offered on a long-term basis, it could prevent recurrences of both mania and depression.

Lithium carbonate is a salt that is readily absorbed in the gastrointestinal tract. It easily crosses cellular membranes and is therefore readily distributed throughout the body. The drug is not metabolized, is excreted by the kidneys, and has a serum half-life of 24 hours; that is, within 24 hours 50 percent of lithium in the body is eliminated. In acute manic episodes, symptom control requires 7 to 10 days. Because there is a delay in reaching therapeutic levels of lithium, antipsychotic medication in the form of a phenothiazine may be given concurrently for a time.

LITHIUM TOXICITY The range between therapeutic and toxic levels of lithium is narrow. Therefore, it is essential to regulate lithium levels frequently, particularly when the client is being stabilized on the drug. Initially, serum lithium levels may be taken twice weekly, then weekly, and later at monthly intervals. Once a client is stabilized on a maintenance dose, serum lithium levels should be taken every two to three months. Lithium levels between 0.8 and 1.5 mEq/l are considered within therapeutic range. Many clients show early signs of toxicity when serum lithium levels reach 1.5 mEq/l, and virtually all clients show severe signs of toxicity when serum lithium levels exceed 2.0 mEq/l (Fieve, 1980).

During the first few days of taking the drug, clients may complain of nausea and mild tremors, but these early reactions usually subside. Nausea developing after the first few days may be an indication of toxicity. The onset of lithium toxicity is

Table 7-8. Indications of Lithium Toxicity

Serum Lithium Levels	Early Signs	Later Signs
Therapeutic: 0.8 to 1.5 mEq/l	Thirst Nausea Dizziness Fine tremor Increased urine	Polyuria Polydipsia Edema Weight gain Goiter Hypothyroidism
Imminent toxicity: 1.5 to 2.0 mEq/l	Vomiting Diarrhea Vertigo Sluggishness Dysarthia	Slurred speech Tinnitus Twitching Increased tremor Increased muscle tone
Actual toxicity: 2.0 to 7.0 mEq/l	Hyperreflexia Nystagmus Seizures Oliguria Confusion Dyskinesia	Visual hallucinations Tactile hallucinations Anuria Coma Death

indicated by increased drowsiness, tremors that progress from fine to gross movements, nausea, vomiting, diarrhea, neurologic impairment leading to ataxia, visual difficulties, loss of consciousness, and coma (see Table 7-8). As a rule, mild to moderate lithium toxicity can be relieved by discontinuing or reducing the dosage of the drug.

LITHIUM MAINTENANCE When the client has regained a normal mood, lithium maintenance may be considered. This decision is made only after clients have undergone more than one cyclical episode of mania with or without depression. Once the symptoms of mania have subsided, tolerance for lithium subsides and toxicity may develop. Thus, the maintenance dosages of lithium are apt to be less than the amounts needed to control acute mania. Most clients who take lithium for long periods of time respond well; even those who continue to have mood swings will experience less-severe episodes. A maintenance lithium regimen seems to be most effective with clients diagnosed as having bipolar disorders. When clients experience recurrent episodes of depression without intervening periods of mania or hypomania, they may not respond well to the prophylactic use of lithium. For such clients either antidepressant or electroconvulsant therapy may be more effective.

NURSING MEASURES Lithium carbonate, whether used for remedial or preventive purposes, is a drug that requires considerable precautions. Before lithium therapy is begun, a complete medical examination is necessary, with special emphasis on cardiovascular, renal, and thyroid function. Lithium is rapidly absorbed and reaches its peak effect in 2 to 3 hours. Therefore, clients are usually instructed to take the drug in two or three divided doses daily.

Because lithium is a gastrointestinal irritant, the client should be instructed to take the drug with meals or just after eating. If a dose is forgotten, clients should be warned not to compensate by taking a double amount the next time, since this may cause a temporary reaction. Clients must be taught to maintain adequate sodium intake, because reduced sodium increases the possibility of a toxic reaction. Any unusual physical conditions such as fever or lowered food or fluid intake may predispose the client to dangerous lithium levels and should be reported to the person responsible for monitoring the drug regimen. Blood for monitoring of lithium levels should be drawn in the morning, 10 to 14 hours after the last dose. If the level is measured at any other time, particularly when the client has taken lithium a few hours before, the reading will not be accurate.

Women in the childbearing years who are taking lithium should be advised to practice contraception. If pregnancy is being considered, nurses should recommend preliminary consultation with a physician. Because lithium will cross the placental barrier, there may be some risk to the fetus, so the value of continuing lithium therapy must be weighed carefully. Nursing mothers who receive lithium should be warned that there may be traces in their milk. Again, there is a need for consultation that includes both psychiatric and physiological considerations.

Maintenance on lithium means that clients will be taking the drug for a number of years. The signs of lithium toxicity and the importance of regular

---

DRUGS INTERACTIONS WITH LITHIUM

Safe Drug Combinations

- *Antipsychotic drugs:* May be used during the time lag between initial administration of lithium and therapeutic effect. Chlorpromazine (Thorazine) and haldoperidol (Haldol) are commonly used in this way.

- *Antidepressants:* May be used to oppose the depressive reactions that occur at times even with lithium maintenance therapy. Both the MAO inhibitors and the tricyclics may be used with lithium.

- *Disulfiram* (Antabuse—used for adversive treatment of alcoholics): May be taken by lithium users.

Unsafe Drug Combinations

- *Diuretics:* May decrease lithium excretion and increase danger of toxicity.

- *Nephrotoxins:* The tetracyclines and spectinomycine may promote lithium toxicity.

- *Anti-inflammatory agents:* May cause lithium retention and possible toxicity; reported with indomethacin (Indocin) and phenylbutazone (Butazolidin).

- *Antihypertensives:* May cause temporary lithium retention.

- *Digoxin:* Decreased intracellular potassium resulting from lithium may lead to digoxin toxicity, nodal bradycardia, and atrial fibrillation. Combining lithium, digoxin, and a diuretic is especially hazardous.

- *Alcohol:* Intoxication in clients taking lithium produces more extreme confusion, uncoordination, and ataxia.

- *Narcotics:* May increase effects of morphine.

- *Muscle relaxants and anaesthetics:* Effects are prolonged in clients taking lithium. Lithium should be withheld for 48 to 72 hours before surgery.

181

need for various other medications may arise. Lithium is compatible with most antidepressants and major tranquilizers, but there are a number of drugs that are unsafe for persons taking lithium. The accompanying box lists a number of drugs that may be used concurrently with lithium and some that may not.

Somatic remedies in the form of electroconvulsive therapy and drug therapy enable psychiatric clients to escape the extremely disruptive effects of maladaptive mood alterations. For the vast majority of people, however, altered mood and affect do not result in a psychiatric diagnosis. Such milder alterations of mood and affect, particularly in the form of depression, are extremely prevalent in modern life. In fact, no matter what setting nurses choose for clinical practice, they will encounter depression and its disguised counterpart, mania or hypomania.

For clients who become depressed as a result of life stress, loss, or change, the intervention of a concerned nurse may reduce the suffering and disruption that mood alterations sometimes bring. Similarly, for the grief and sadness that are an inevitable part of the human experience, the intervention of another person who exhibits informed interest and empathy may be more appropriate than somatic treatments.

GRIEF AND MOURNING

Grief and mourning are normal responses to loss or separation from meaningful persons or objects. *Mourning* is the word generally applied to behavioral responses to loss, while *grief* is the inner subjective feeling. Although grief and mourning are often

testing should be emphasized to clients and their families (Fieve, 1980). Whenever a client is being maintained on lithium, all of the care providers involved with the client should be informed. Because of the prolonged nature of lithium therapy, the

182

associated with the death of a loved one, there are many other causes, including the loss of important relationships or the loss of certain possessions or surroundings. Homesickness is an example of this specific and common grief reaction. People who have lost something that was highly valued must allow themselves to feel grief and to mourn their loss before trying to resume normal life. In many respects active mourning, or *grief work*, is a painful but necessary response to loss (Engel, 1962; Jacoby, 1983).

Freud (1957) described the mourning process as a gradual withdrawal of attachment from whatever or whoever was lost, ultimately followed by readiness to make new attachments in the form of relationships and commitments. This means that people who feel grief are those who have learned to form attachments. Freud distinguished mourning from melancholia or depression, and Bibring (1953) pointed out that lowered self-esteem is a significant feature of depression that is not present in mourning.

Although it is necessary to withdraw attachment from a lost loved one in order to resolve grief, this withdrawal is not easy to accomplish. According to Schoenberg (1980), the activity of mourning is "carried out tediously and painfully, and at great expense in order to prolong the existence of the deceased" (p. 1349). Because many mourners feel that they cannot survive without the lost relationship, they seek to continue it, and the mourner may even adopt mannerisms once belonging to the deceased (Parks and Stevenson-Hinde, 1982). Such behaviors may indicate that attachment to or identification with the deceased has reached unhealthy proportions and that the mourner has refused to accept the

---

DEATH AND DYING

Dying may sometimes prove to be a long, slow process, and families need ongoing assistance as their needs change. Giacquinta (1977) formulated a four-stage guide for care providers working with families of terminal cancer patients. Recognizing the stage at which the family finds itself can help the nurse plan interventions that meet current needs.

- *Stage 1: Living with terminal illness.* At this point families learn the diagnosis and must deal with the immediate consequences of the illness. Nursing planning and interventions should be directed toward solving problems of daily living for the client and the family.

- *Stage 2: Restructuring in the living-dying period.* As the condition of the ill member worsens, the family reassigns roles and responsibilities. Families should now be encouraged to engage in retrospection that retains the dying person in the collective history of the family. This activity, called "framing memories," helps the dying person remain a living presence even as his strength fades.

- *Stage 3: Bereavement.* This is the stage of actual separation and loss. Only through active mourning can the death be accepted. Denial of loss or avoidance of grief is dysfunctional, for mourning is the only way to proceed to the next stage.

- *Stage 4: Reestablishment.* This is the period when the family begins to return to earlier routines and patterns of living and to reestablish activities given up during the time of impending loss.

---

reality of the loss. An effective intervention in such circumstances is to encourage the mourner to weep, to verbalize negative as well as positive emotions toward the deceased, and to engage in a life review by reminiscing about experiences in which the deceased person was a participant. This permits emotional and cognitive expression that emphasizes the loss of the relationship as well as its importance (Aneshensel and Stone, 1982).

Adaptive and Maladaptive Grief

Normal grief may be distinguished from pathologic grief by the functioning level of the bereaved and by

> *It has been said that because of his psychological constitution, man cannot live without attachment to some object which transcends and survives him, and that the reason for this necessity is a need we must have not to perish entirely. Life is said to be intolerable unless some reason for existing is involved, some purpose justifying life's trials. The individual alone is not a sufficient end for his activity.*
>
> EMILE DURKHEIM, SUICIDE: A STUDY IN SOCIOLOGY

the length of time that elapses before grief is overcome. Rubin (1981) found that acute grief lasts from three to twelve weeks, after which less extreme mourning may continue for a year or two.

The circumstances surrounding a death influence the mourning process. When death is untimely or unexpected, or when the mourner feels responsible in some way, the grief reaction may be more intense (Kirkley-Best and Kellner, 1982). The age of the mourner also influences how grief is expressed and its extent. Older people whose personal worlds have narrowed to a few cherished persons or objects may feel especially desolate. Adolescents mourn much as adults do, but younger children whose cognitive and language development are incomplete have difficulty comprehending or expressing feelings of grief (Smitherman, 1981).

In studying the behaviors of survivors of a nightclub fire that claimed many lives, Lindemann (1944) found that acute grief reactions could appear immediately after the loss, could be delayed, could take exaggerated forms, or could fail to appear. The implication was that losses are difficult for everyone to endure but that reaction to loss is less adaptive when the bereaved person is unwilling or unable to mourn. Severe or prolonged depression is more likely to develop in the absence of grief work and may even be a defense against the pain that active mourning brings (Lewis, 1982).

Phases of Grief

Many health professionals believe that grief is time limited and progresses in stages (Caplan, 1964; Parkes, 1972). Bowlby (1973, 1982) identified three phases of grief and mourning. Bowlby's phases of grief work are described in Table 7-9. In his view,

Table 7-9. Sequential Phases of Grief Work

Phase	Characteristics
Protest	Mourners are preoccupied with and attached to the deceased. All resources of the bereaved are used to prolong attachment and to protest loss. At this time mourners resent advice to accept the loss. Anger, tears, reproaches, and recriminations characterize the protest phase.
Despair	Efforts to continue the attachment give way to gradual acceptance of permanent loss. As the reality of loss is recognized, despair mounts. Behavior formerly devoted to preserving or regaining the lost relationship now becomes disorganized. Restlessness, anxiety, and sadness become apparent.
Detachment	This is the phase of reorganization, as the bereaved become resigned to the loss. As the permanency of loss is realized, acute grief begins to subside. When longing for the deceased does not lessen and hope of restoration is not discarded, the grief reaction may become pathologic, and depression follows.

SOURCE: Adapted from Bowlby (1969).

these three phases can be recognized in people of all ages, even children as young as six months.

The value of sequential models such as Bowlby's is that observed behaviors can be identified and understood more readily. Another well-known sequential model is that of Elisabeth Kübler-Ross (1969), who described five stages terminally ill persons undergo: denial, anger, bargaining, despair, and acceptance. Griffin (1980) warned that these stages vary and that for some persons the sequence may never be completed. For example, an individual who has reached the stage of acceptance may

BODY IMAGE CHANGE

Body image is one's mental picture of one's own body. Body image is determined in part by the appraisals of others and in part by the self-appraisal of the individual. Most people are dissatisfied with their body image, or at least parts of it. For example, a man may be proud of his physique but embarrassed by his thinning hair. A woman may take satisfaction in having a pretty face but dislike her size 10 feet. Such minor discontents with body image are shared by vast numbers of people.

Of greater consequence is the loss of any body part or function, for even the best-adjusted person will have difficulty dealing with such losses. Changing from a perception of oneself as whole to a perception of oneself as defective is comparable to grief felt at the death of a loved one. When a limb or breast is lost by surgery or trauma, phantom pain in the removed part lingers and is a bitter reminder of what was lost. Nurses and other care providers must permit expressions of protest and despair as the individual mourns for the intact person who no longer exists. Severe grief reactions also follow sensory losses, heart attacks, miscarriages, or any discovery of inadequacy or dysfunction in the body. Active mourning for what was lost is essential to eventual reorganization. Therefore, an extreme reaction to changed body image should be considered as being more adaptive than a failure to react at all.

184

revert to anger or bargaining, while another may never progress beyond denial.

More important than fixed sequences is awareness that different behaviors may arise at different times. According to one viewpoint, genuine grief is never fully resolved but is carried for a lifetime. This view may be valid, as evidenced by the phenomenon in which anniversaries of loss reactivate old grief.

Anticipatory Grief

For individuals and families facing the death of a loved one, *anticipatory grief work* is a form of primary prevention that can be helpful if used with caution. When grief work begins after the loss, the tendency is for grief to lessen over time. When grief work begins with the anticipation of loss, the pattern is for the intensity of grief to increase as the loss approaches. Anticipatory grief engaged in before the actual loss may cause some family members to detach prematurely from the dying person, which in turn can increase the isolation of the person who is terminally ill.

For families who are dealing with the expected death of a young person, anticipatory grief work may be impossible (Naylor, 1982). In some instances the anticipatory behaviors of family members are interpreted by young patients as withdrawal or abandonment. Vedeka-Sherman (1982) found that for parents the physical presence of a dying child prevented any anticipatory grief work. Other researchers reported both value and danger in promoting anticipatory grief (Gerber, 1974; Silverman, 1974; Parker and Brown, 1982).

Helping the Grief Stricken

Traditional care providers are not always sources of comfort for persons dealing with grief. In attempting to protect themselves, care providers may become highly task oriented and remote from families needing emotional support (Beardslee and De-Maso, 1982). As a rule, people who have already suffered similar losses are better able to understand the experience of the bereaved. Group support can be a valuable form of assistance when group members have confronted a similar loss. This is also true for professionals working with seriously ill clients, many of whom turn to co-workers for help when feeling overwhelmed by distressing events in the clinical setting (Hughes, 1982).

The therapeutic value of openly expressing grief has been documented (Martinson and Janosik, 1980), yet the bereaved are often prevented from doing so. Discouraging the expression of grief can take the form of inattention or restlessness on the

*For three days we waited—and I hoped while I could—oh—that
awful agony of three days! . . . I, who could not speak or shed a tear,
but lay for weeks and months half conscious, half unconscious, with
a wandering mind . . . The spring of life seemed to break
within me then.*

ELIZABETH BARRETT BROWNING, on the death of her favorite brother, who was drowned at sea

185

part of listeners. Professionals and well-meaning
friends may prematurely encourage mourners to
find new interests. Although this is a desirable future goal, detachment from the lost relationship
must precede new commitments.

Rituals can be used to ease grief reactions.
Funerals, wakes, and memorial services help resolve
grief by offering acceptable outlets for its expression. Informal rituals such as family reminiscing
or examining family albums are also productive. It
is necessary for the bereaved and for bystanders
to realize that grief is not something to avoid but to
be experienced, however difficult at the time.

Excessive solicitude and protectiveness on the
part of caregivers is rarely helpful, as it tends to
separate the bereaved from familiar routines that
may be reassuring. Persons dealing with loss should
be allowed to proceed at their own pace as much as
possible while receiving assurances that any feelings, even if negative, will be understood. If the
mourner's feelings toward the deceased were
ambivalent or inconsistent, grief is more difficult to
overcome because guilt becomes a prominent component. Even with losses where the relationship
with the deceased was a devoted one, the mourner
may be angry at the deceased for having abandoned
him or her. Expressions of anger toward nurses and
other professionals who did not perform life-saving
miracles are also to be expected, and this anger
should be interpreted as displacement used to defend against pain.

Those trying to comfort mourners have a
tendency to tell them that "it might have been
worse." One young widow whose husband was
killed in a car accident became enraged by loving
friends who said she was lucky her young son had

survived the accident. Months later she could acknowledge her initial reaction that her husband's
death was the worst possible loss for her to endure.
When asked what had helped most in her grief, she
replied that friends who simply listened brought
more comfort than friends who reassured.

Although friends and relatives may offer a
great deal of consolation and help immediately after
a death, as days and weeks pass their attention tends
to lessen and the bereaved find themselves alone
with their sorrow. This is a problem for those family
members who interpret reduced attentiveness as
another deprivation. To address this problem, a
program at St. Christopher's Hospice (near London, England) was organized to provide support to
survivors for extended periods after a death in the
family. A few days following the death, hospice staff
members made home visits and continued these
visits at weekly intervals for several months. It was
found that family members considered the lengthy
opportunity to express their feelings to the visitors
extremely helpful. Concrete assistance in the form
of referrals and consultation was given as families
began to resume their normal lives.

Assessment of suicide risk among survivors was
an important aspect of the work of the hospice visitors. They noted that even in the absence of suicide
risk the period of mourning was a time of vulnerability for surviving family members. There was a
significant increase of morbidity and mortality
among the bereaved, indicating a need for close
attention to somatic complaints even when they
seemed trivial at the time (Schoenberg, 1980).

For organizational purposes, grief and mourning, depression, and mania have been described
separately in this chapter, yet in many respects

Figure 7-4. Adaptive and maladaptive affective responses.

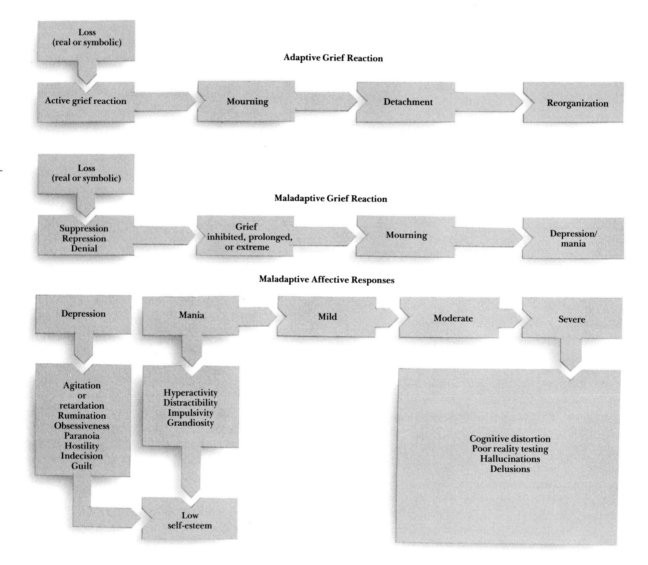

these alterations of mood and affect can be plotted on a continuum. Active grief work generally leads to reorganization and is adaptive in nature, but pathologic grief reactions can merge into mania or depression, both of which are maladaptive affective responses. Figure 7-4 illustrates the relationships existing among these adaptive and maladaptive affective alterations.

SUMMARY

Alterations of mood and affect are prevalent in modern life, but the symptoms are variable and are sometimes misinterpreted or unrecognized. Among psychiatric categories of affective disturbances are major depression and bipolar disorder.

CLINICAL EXAMPLE

DYSTHYMIC DISORDER IN A SINGLE PARENT

Joyce Howe is a thirty-three-year-old woman who has been divorced for three years and is the mother of a six-year-old boy and a nine-year-old girl. She is an assemblyline worker at a local factory and her job requires that she rotate shifts. When Joyce works the day shift, she picks up her children in the evening from a neighbor who babysits. Joyce and the children return home where she makes dinner. After dinner Joyce helps her daughter with homework, reads a story to her son, and oversees the children as they bathe and get ready for bed. Then Joyce reads the evening paper, does a few chores, gets ready for the next day, and is usually in bed by midnight.

When Joyce works the evening or night shift, she collects her children from the babysitter at midnight or at 7:30 in the morning. After she picks up the children at midnight, they are generally so sleepy that they can hardly remember being moved from one house to another. After she picks them up in the morning, Joyce takes them home for breakfast and sees that they start off for school. Although the babysitter is willing to prepare breakfast for the children, Joyce wants to do as much as possible for them. She has memories of her own mother working and of being unavailable. Joyce is determined not to let this happen to her children if she can help it.

Joyce's former husband has remarried and has a son by his second wife. The financial demands of his new family cause him to be delinquent in his child support payments. He rarely visits the children and they no longer ask about him. Joyce feels bitter toward him but tries not to reveal this to the children. She was very upset when he asked for a divorce and initially refused him. When he told her that his girlfriend was pregnant, she consented to the divorce. At the time he promised to assume full responsibility for the support of the children, but he has not lived up to his commitment. Until her divorce Joyce was a full-time housewife and mother.

Recently Joyce has been troubled by insomnia and by "nerves," complains of always feeling tired and has been having trouble meeting her production quota at work. She is well liked at work and it was her boss who suggested that Joyce see a physician. The physician performed some routine laboratory tests, discovered an anemic condition, and prescribed vitamin and mineral supplements. He also suggested that she go to a mental health center to talk about some of the current stresses in her life. When he saw that she was reluctant to seek psychiatric help, he made an appointment for Joyce at the mental health center. Reluctantly, she agreed to keep the appointment.

ASSESSMENT

The psychiatric nurse who interviewed Joyce saw a small, rather attractive woman who was dressed neatly but drably. Joyce wore a headscarf tied tightly under her chin and a pair of sunglasses concealing her eyes. She told the nurse that this was her first experience with a mental health facility and that she wasn't quite sure whether the visit was necessary. At times during the interview Joyce's voice trembled but did not break. She spoke slowly and her answers to questions were appropriate but brief. At times she seemed at a loss for words and would sigh deeply before answering. She denied any thoughts of suicide, stating that she had her children to live for and that they needed her. She added that she felt that she was living in a "black pit" that she would never be able to escape.

About a year earlier, Joyce had attended a club for divorced persons and single parents. There she had met Jerry, a salesman about five years younger than herself. Jerry's ex-wife and daughter were living in California. He missed his daughter and got along well with Joyce's children when he came to visit. Jerry was amusing and outgoing; Joyce enjoyed having him around in the evening and even during the day when she worked nights. She began to believe in herself again and in her ability to maintain a satisfying relationship with a man.

Approximately four months after meeting Jerry, Joyce was confronted with a new problem. Her little boy had several grande mal seizures in school, and the medical workup showed that the child had an idiopathic form of epilepsy. When this happened, Jerry was a source of strength for Joyce. She turned to him a great deal in those weeks and he never failed to offer support and understanding. Joyce was therefore unprepared for Jerry's announcement that he had found a single woman, a few years younger than himself, who had no problems or responsibilities. He told Joyce that he was fond of her but that her life was too complicated. As a result, Jerry had decided to move in with his new friend.

Losing Jerry sent Joyce into a state of extreme distress. Her job performance deteriorated greatly. Although she managed to adhere to her usual schedule, she found herself irritable and impatient with the children. As soon as possible she packed them off to bed so that she could sit alone in front of the television and drink enough beer to forget her worries and her loneliness. The house took on a neglected look because Joyce could barely manage to take care of herself and the children. The children missed Jerry almost as much as their mother did, and they also missed the loving attention that Joyce had provided. The little girl reacted by trying to take care of things for her mother. The little boy reacted by worrying about being a "bad boy" and by suffering more frequent seizures.

Based on the history supplied by Joyce and the clinical picture she presented, the intake team of the mental health center formulated the following nursing and psychiatric diagnoses:

Nursing Diagnoses

Coping, ineffectual individual

Coping, ineffective family

Grieving, dysfunctional

Home maintenance management, impaired

Knowledge deficit (regarding epilepsy)

Sleep pattern disturbance

Multiaxial Psychiatric Diagnosis

Axis I   300.43 Dysthymic disorder (or depressive neurosis) with melancholia

Axis II   Compulsive personality

Axis III   Secondary anemia

Axis IV   Code 5—Severe psychosocial stressors

Axis V   Level 5—Poor adaptive functioning

188

PLANNING

The intake team agreed that Joyce displayed signs of depression that were the result of a series of losses sustained in recent years but were not of psychotic proportions. Her everyday existence was stressful and demanding, but Joyce had coped well until she faced the problems of the past year. The chronic illness of her little boy had terrified her because she knew so little about epilepsy. All she knew was that she had lost her healthy vigorous child and now had to care for a sick child. Jerry's termination of their relationship had added to the price Joyce was paying for her son's illness. His leaving her for another woman also reactivated the sense of abandonment that she had suffered at the time of her divorce. Her fragile feelings of competence were further eroded by the recent events. The anemic condition added to her feelings of fatigue, and her psychological reserves were exhausted. Even though Joyce was not suicidal, she felt hopeless and helpless.

In planning Joyce's care, the intake team attributed her depression to situational stress that could be altered. It was important that she continue to be treated for anemia. She also needed help with domestic chores so that her leisure time was not always occupied with housework and child care. She needed help in expressing the bitterness and anger that she felt toward Jerry and her ex-husband but rarely voiced. Changes in her daily routine that offered opportunity for sports or exercise might be helpful in improving her sleep patterns.

IMPLEMENTATION

The nursing diagnosis was especially helpful in identifying the areas in which Joyce and her children needed help. Although the physical problems of her little boy were under treatment, Joyce needed to learn as much as possible about her son's disability so that she did not infect him with her feelings of desperation. She was there-

fore referred to a self-help group that combined education with psychosocial support for parents of epileptic children.

Joyce had not permitted herself to grieve adequately at the time of her divorce. She struggled to make up to the children for the loss of their father, but she had not worked through her own feelings of loss. Joyce accepted the suggestion that she enter time-limited individual therapy to help put her losses in perspective, to examine her conflicting feelings about her relationships with men, and to acknowledge her genuine strengths and accomplishments in recent years. The possibility of joining a therapeutic group for young adults at some future time was mentioned, pending the termination of individual counseling.

The team responsible for Joyce's care utilized the services of a psychiatric nurse and a community health nurse. The psychiatric nurse was primarily concerned with Joyce's psychological problems, especially the depression, while the community health nurse was primarily concerned with the health needs of the children. Both professionals worked together to coordinate care, maintain continuity and communication between various caregivers, and keep the team in the mental health center informed.

EVALUATION

The specific information contained in the nursing and psychiatric diagnoses was used to plan care for Joyce and to evaluate progress. In particular, the nursing assessment focused and guided therapeutic efforts and promoted a consistent approach by caregivers, each of whom was cognizant not only of his or her own responsibilities but of what was being done by other professionals working with Joyce and her children. Although Joyce's depression was the *focal* or target behavior, intervention was not limited to alleviating this problem. The *context* in which her depressive symptoms had developed was the single-parent household in which she functioned as mother, father, and sole provider. *Residual* issues included the divorce, the discovery of her son's illness, and the unexpected loss of an important adult relationship in her life. Her depression did not occur in isolation but was the result of accumulated disappointments and demands being made upon her. Concurrently, the depression further reduced her ability to cope. The realization that she was not functioning at her usual level of competence deepened her feelings of inadequacy and increased her depression. To be successful, the treatment plan needed to attend to all of these factors.

The comprehensive treatment plan alleviated much of Joyce's distress. As she learned more about her son's disorder, she grew less frightened about the future. With the help of the psychiatric nurse she began to deal with her feelings about her divorce. In time she joined a group program for single parents and began to see that her situation was not unique. Through the group program she developed friendships with several other women and established a network of social supports for herself and her children.

189

The notable feature of bipolar disorder is mania, with or without episodes of depression.

The etiology of depression involves the interaction of psychodynamic, biochemical, genetic, and existential factors. In dealing with depressed persons, nurses are advised to use an approach in which problems are identified and specific interventions planned. The use of problem identification and problem solving facilitates evaluation procedures, as outcomes can be measured against specific goals.

Mania appears to be the opposite of depression but in actuality shares many dynamics. Like the depressed individual, the manic client engages in psychological, physiological, and cognitive distortions. Nurses working with clients who display manic behaviors are guided by two major considerations: the protection of the clients from physical risk or exhaustion, and the protection of the client from excessive environmental stimulation.

A number of somatic measures are available for clients who experience drastic alterations of mood and affect. One somatic measure is electroconvulsive therapy, which is controversial but still has a place in the treatment of severely depressed individuals who are unresponsive to drug therapy. Among antidepressants available for depressed clients are the MAO inhibitors and the tricyclic antidepressants. Lithium carbonate is used to control symptoms of mania and to prevent recurrence of cyclical mood changes. Clients taking antidepressants or lithium need to be made aware of possible side effects in order to improve the likelihood of compliance.

Nursing responsibilities in administering somatic treatment to persons with affective and mood disorders are considerable. Careful observation is important, as is education of clients and families.

Because clients may be unaware of the recurrence of a mood swing, families need to be included in educational sessions. Somatic treatment is beneficial in the care of persons experiencing severe mood alterations, but the availability of these measures does not reduce the need for a psychotherapeutic approach.

The experience of loss is unavoidable for persons who have learned to form attachments and make commitments. Grief and mourning are normal, adaptive responses to loss, and depression is often experienced by those who are unable or unwilling to engage in the pain of grief work. Detachment from the lost person or object is necessary before the bereaved can resume normal activities.

Review Questions

1. Depression is sometimes described as a compensatory mechanism used to avoid the pain of grieving. Explain this statement.

2. Mania is sometimes described as a compensatory mechanism used to avoid depression. Explain this statement.

3. What precautions are essential in caring for a client in an acute manic state?

4. Under what circumstances is electroconvulsive therapy considered an appropriate treatment? What nursing responsibilities accompany the administration of electroconvulsive therapy before and after the procedure?

5. A depressed client is taking an MAO inhibitor. What information should be included in teaching the client about this group of antidepressants?

6. A client with a bipolar affective disorder is receiving lithium. What information should be included in teaching this client about lithium maintenance?

7. If a client of childbearing age is on a lithium maintenance regimen, what information should be included in teaching this client?

8. What aspects of grief and mourning promote adaptation to loss?

9. What types of loss are likely to produce grief reactions? Give an example of each type.

References

Aneshensel, C. S., and Stone, J. D. 1982. Stress and Depression. *Archives of General Psychiatry*, 39:1392–1396.

Appleton, W. S., and Davis, J. M. 1980. *Practical Clinical Pharmacology*, 2nd ed. Baltimore: Williams & Wilkins.

Beardslee, W. R., and DeMaso, D. R. 1982. Staff Groups in a Pediatric Hospital: Content and Coping. *American Journal of Orthopsychiatry*, 52:712–718.

Beck, A. T. 1969. *Cognition and Psychopathology in Depression: Clinical, Experimental, and Theoretical Aspects*. New York: Harper & Row.

Beck, A. T. 1972. *Depression: Causes and Treatment*. Philadelphia: University of Pennsylvania.

Bibring, E. 1953. The Mechanism of Depression. In *Affective Disorders*, ed. P. Greenacre. New York: International Universities Press.

Bowlby, J. 1969. *Attachment and Loss: Attachment*. New York: Basic Books.

Bowlby, J. 1973. *Attachment and Loss: Separation*. New York: Basic Books.

Bowlby, J. 1980. *Attachment and Loss: Loss*. New York: Basic Books.

Bowlby, J. 1982. Attachment and Loss: Retrospect and Prospect. *American Journal of Orthopsychiatry*, 52:644–678.

Caplan, G. 1964. *Principles of Preventive Psychiatry*. New York: Basic Books.

Cohen, R. A. 1975. Manic Depressive Illness. In *Comprehensive Textbook of Psychiatry*, 2nd ed., eds. A. M. Freedman, H. I. Kaplan, and B. J. Sadock. Baltimore: Williams & Wilkins.

Dohrenwend, B. P.; Dohrenwend, B. S.; and Gould, M. S. 1980. *Mental Illness in the United States: Epidemiological Estimates*. New York: Praeger.

Engel, G. 1962. *Psychological Development in Health and Disease*. Philadelphia: W. B. Saunders.

Erikson, E. H. 1963. *Childhood and Society*. New York: W. W. Norton.

Fieve, R. R. 1980. Lithium Therapy. In *Comprehensive Textbook of Psychiatry*, 3rd ed., eds. H. I. Kaplan, A. M. Freedman, and B. J. Sadock. Baltimore: Williams & Wilkins.

Freud, S. 1957. Mourning and Melancholia. In *Standard Edition of the Works of Sigmund Freud*, vol. 14. London: Hogarth.

Gardner, R. 1982. Mechanisms in Manic Depressive Disorder: An Evolutionary Model. *Archives of General Psychiatry*, 39:1436–1444.

Gerald, M. C., and O'Bannon, F. V. 1981. *Nursing Pharmacology and Therapeutics*. Englewood Cliffs, N.J.: Prentice-Hall.

Gerber, I. 1974. Anticipatory Bereavement. In *Anticipatory Grief*, eds. B. Schoenberg et al. New York: Columbia University.

Giacquinta, B. 1977. Helping Families Face the Crisis of Cancer. *American Journal of Nursing*, 77:1585–1588.

Griffin, J. Q. 1980. Physical Illness in the Family. In *Family-Focused Care*, eds. J. R. Miller and E. H. Janosik. New York: McGraw-Hill.

Hanin, I., and Usdin, E. 1982. *Markers in Psychiatry and Psychology*. New York: Pergamon Press.

Hughes, M. C. 1982. Chronically Ill Children: Recurrent Issues and Adaptations. *American Journal of Orthopsychiatry*, 52:704–711.

Irons, P. D. 1978. *Psychotropic Drugs and Nursing Interventions*. New York: McGraw-Hill.

Jacoby, S. 1983. Grief Should Be Allowed to Run Its Natural Course. *The New York Times*, April 21.

Juel-Nielson, J. 1980. *Individual and Environment: Monozygotic Twins Reared Apart*. New York: International Universities Press.

Kalinowsky, L. B. 1980. Convulsive Therapies. In *Comprehensive Textbook of Psychiatry*, 3rd ed., eds. H. I. Kaplan, A. M. Freedman, and B. J. Sadock. Baltimore: Williams & Wilkins.

Kallman, F. J. 1953. *Heredity in Health and Mental Disorders*. New York: W. W. Norton.

Kirkley-Best, E., and Kellner, K. R. 1982. The Forgotten Grief: A Review of the Psychology of Stillbirth. *American Journal of Orthopsychiatry*, 52:420–429.

Klerman, G. L. 1980. Overview of Affective Disorders. In *Comprehensive Textbook of Psychiatry*, 3rd ed., eds. H. I. Kaplan, A. M. Freedman, and B. J. Sadock. Baltimore: Williams & Wilkins.

Kontos, P. G., and Steinhilber, R. M. 1979. Using Antidepressants Effectively. *Postgraduate Medicine*, 64:55–56.

Kübler-Ross, E. 1969. *On Death and Dying*. New York: Macmillan.

Lewis, J. M. 1982. Dying with Friends. *American Journal of Psychiatry*, 139:261–266.

Lindemann, E. 1944. Symptomatology and Management of Acute Grief. In *American Journal of Psychiatry*, 101:141–148.

Lumsden, C. J., and Wilson, E. D. 1981. *Genes, Mind, and Culture: The Coevolutionary Process*. Cambridge, Mass.: Harvard University Press.

Mansky, P. A. 1981. Treatment of Depression. In *Psychiatric Medicine Update*, ed. T. C. Manschreck. New York: Elsevier.

Martinson, I. M., and Janosik, E. H. 1980. Family Crisis Intervention. In *Family-Focused Care*, eds. J. R. Miller and E. H. Janosik. New York: McGraw-Hill.

Naylor, A. 1982. Premature Mourning and Failure to Mourn: The Relationship to Conflict Between Mothers and Intellectually Normal Children. *American Journal of Orthopsychiatry*, 52:679–687.

Parker, G. B., and Brown, L. B. 1982. Coping Behaviors

190

That Mediate Life Events and Depression. *Archives of General Psychiatry*, 39:1386–1392.

Parkes, R. 1972. *Bereavement: Studies of Grief in Adult Life.* London: Tavistock.

Parks, C. M., and Stevenson-Hinde, J. 1982. *The Place of Attachment in Human Behavior.* New York: Basic Books.

Pincus, L. 1976. *Death and the Family: The Importance of Mourning.* New York: Vintage.

Roy, E. 1981. Specificity of Risk Factors for Depression. *American Journal of Psychiatry*, 138:959–964.

Rubin, S. 1981. A Two-Track Model of Bereavement. *American Journal of Orthopsychiatry*, 51:101–109.

Salzman, C. 1975. Electroconvulsive Therapy. In *Manual of Psychiatric Therapeutics*, ed. R. I. Shader. Boston: Little, Brown.

Schoenberg, B. 1980. Grief, Mourning, and Simple Bereavement. In *Comprehensive Textbook of Psychiatry*, 3rd ed., eds. H. I. Kaplan, A. M. Freedman, and B. J. Sadock. Baltimore: Williams & Wilkins.

Selye, H. 1956. *The Stress of Life.* New York: McGraw-Hill.

Smitherman, C. 1981. *Nursing Actions for Health Promotion.* Philadelphia: F. A. Davis.

Spitz, R. A. 1946. Anaclitic Depression. In *Psychoanalytic Study of the Child*, vol. 2, ed. P. Greenacre. New York: International Universities Press.

Thomas A.; Chess, S.; and Birch, H. G. 1969. *Temperament and Behavior Disorders in Children.* New York: New York University Press.

Usdin, G. 1977. *Depression: Clinical, Biological and Psychological Perspectives.* New York: Brunner/Mazel.

Wolpert, E. A. 1980. Major Affective Disorders. In *Comprehensive Textbook of Psychiatry*, 3rd ed., eds. H. I. Kaplan, A. M. Freedman, and B. J. Sadock. Baltimore: Williams & Wilkins.

Supplementary Readings

Anthony, E. J., and Benedek, T. *Depression and Human Existence.* Boston: Little, Brown, 1975.

Arieti, S., and Bemporad, S. *Severe and Mild Depression.* New York: Basic Books, 1979.

Beck, A. T.; Rush, A. J.; Shaw, B. F.; and Emery, G. *Cognitive Therapy of Depression.* New York: Guilford Press, 1979.

Belther, R. W. The Treatment of Depression in Brief Inpatient Group Psychotherapy. *International Journal of Group Psychotherapy*, 33(1983):365–385.

Bowder, C. L. Unipolar Depression: Commonsense Treatment That Really Helps Patients. *Consultant*, 22(1982):13–15.

Covi, L. Cognitive Group Psychotherapy of Depression: The Close-Ended Group. *American Journal of Psychotherapy*, 36(1982):459–469.

Frangos, E. Psychotic Depressive Disorder: A Separate Entity? *Journal of Affective Disorders*, 5(1983):259–265.

Friedman, R., and Datz, M. *The Psychology of Depression: Contemporary Theory and Research.* New York: John Wiley & Sons, 1974.

Gallant, D., and Simpson, G. *Depression: Behavioral, Biochemical, Diagnostic and Treatment Concepts.* New York: Spectrum, 1976.

Hirshfield, R. N. Personality and Depression. *Archives of General Psychiatry*, 40(1983):993–998.

Mathews, M. A. On the Psychology of the Aging Woman: Depression in Late Midlife—Change or Repetition? *Journal of Geriatric Psychiatry*, 12(1979):37–55.

Matussik, P. Personality Attributes of Depressed Patients. *Archives of General Psychiatry*, 40(1983):783–790.

McConville, B. J. The Causes and Treatment of Depression in Young Children. *Journal of Children in Contemporary Society*, 15(1982):61–68.

Nadelson, C. On the Psychology of the Aging Woman: Midlife Marital Issues—Renewal or Regression? *Journal of Geriatric Psychiatry*, 12(1979):57–70.

Ndetei, D. M. Schizophrenia with Depression: Causal or Coexistent? *British Journal of Psychiatry*, 141(1982):354–356.

Neff, J. A. Life Events, Drinking Patterns and Depressive Symptomatology: The Stress Buffering Role of Alcohol Consumption. *Journal of Studies on Alcohol*, 43(1982):301–308.

Pedder, J. R. Failure to Mourn and Melancholia. *British Journal of Psychiatry*, 141(1982):329–337.

Price, J. Changes in Hostility During the Course of Hypomanic Illness. *British Journal of Clinical Psychology*, 21(1982):103–110.

Pope, H. G. Distinguishing Bipolar Disorder from Schizophrenia in Clinical Practice. *Hospital and Community Psychiatry*, 34(1983):322–328.

Runck, B. ECT: Assuring Benefits and Minimizing Risks. *Hospital and Community Psychiatry*, 34(1983):409–410.

Rush, A. J. Cognitive Therapy of Depression: Rationale, Techniques, and Efficacy. *Psychiatric Clinics of North America*, 6(1983):105–127.

Swanson, A. Communicating with Depressed Persons. *Perspectives of Psychiatric Care*, 13(1975):63–67.

Wilson, D. R. Somatic Symptoms: A Major Feature of Depression in a Family Practice. *Journal of Affective Disorders*, 5(1983):199–207.

Wykes, T. Disordered Speech: Differences Between Manics and Schizophrenics. *Brain Language*, 15(1982):117–124.

Yudofsky, E. Electroconvulsive Therapy in the Eighties: Techniques and Technologies. *American Journal of Psychotherapy*, 36(1982):391–398.

COMPARISON OF HEALTHY AND
ALTERED SENSE OF SELF
The Healthy Self
The Altered Self
The Role of Anxiety and Fear

THEORETICAL FRAMEWORKS
Psychosexual or Psychodynamic Model
Psychosocial Model
Interpersonal Model

COMPARISON OF ALTERED PATTERNS
OF FUNCTIONING

ALTERED PATTERNS OF RELATEDNESS:
NEUROTIC PATTERNS
Anxiety Reactions
Obsessive-Compulsive Reactions

Posttraumatic Stress Syndrome
Phobic Reactions
Conversion Reactions
Dissociative Reactions
Hypochondriacal Reactions

ALTERED PATTERNS OF RELATEDNESS:
PERSONALITY DISORDERS
Schizoid Type
Compulsive Type
Histrionic Type
Antisocial Type
Passive-Aggressive/Passive-Dependent Type
Paranoid Type
General Nursing Approaches
Borderline Conditions

PHARMACOLOGICAL APPROACHES

C H A P T E R

8

Altered Patterns of Social Relatedness

Learning Objectives

After reading this chapter, the student should be able to:

1. Discuss the influence of anxiety on the development of maladaptive relatedness.

2. Trace the etiology of maladaptive relatedness by using psychosexual, psychosocial, and interpersonal frameworks.

3. Contrast the dynamics and manifestations of ego dystonic and ego syntonic alterations of relatedness.

4. Describe the clinical manifestations and underlying dynamics of the various alterations of relatedness.

5. Discuss therapeutic modalities and nursing activities appropriate for clients manifesting alterations of relatedness.

194

Overview

Altered patterns in relatedness are functional disturbances of the personality that arise when inner conflicts between drives and fears mainfest themselves in altered behavior patterns. These functional disturbances include neurotic disorders and personality disorders.

Neurotic disorders are psychological or behavioral alterations characterized primarily by anxiety. Defense mechanisms, in the form of maladaptive behaviors, are adopted by neurotic individuals in order to cope with their anxiety. The neurotic disorders include generalized anxiety states, phobia, obsessive-compulsive states, dissociative states, conversion disorder, posttraumatic stress syndrome, and hypochondriasis.

Personality disorders are syndromes in which individuals' inner difficulties are revealed by patterns of living that seek immediate gratification of impulses and instinctual needs without regard for society's laws, mores, and customs and without censorship of personal conscience. The personality disorders include schizoid type, compulsive type, histrionic type, antisocial type, passive-aggressive/passive-dependent type, and paranoid type.

The purpose of this chapter is to familiarize the student with various alterations of social relatedness and with the use of the nursing process as it is utilized to help clients manifesting disturbed social relatedness.

The mind is its own place and in itself
Can make a heaven of hell, a hell of heaven.
JOHN MILTON

195

In order to achieve and maintain successful inter-personal relationships, people must be able to perceive themselves and the manner in which they are perceived by others in an accurate way. When people relate to each other, they need to have a sense of who they are, who the other people are, and how they are seen by others. The ability to see both points of view is necessary for give-and-take relationships. People who have altered patterns of relatedness cannot maintain relationships that are reciprocal because they do not have the ability to see themselves as they are seen by others.

It has been stated that all people are "neurotic" to some extent, but this is not entirely true. Although everyone is likely to experience neurotic conflicts at times, most people have an extensive repertoire of defenses and coping mechanisms on which they can rely. On the other hand, a person who is suffering from a dysfunctional, altered pattern of relatedness clings to a few rigid, maladaptive behaviors that tend to be repetitive. Even when these patterned behaviors do not produce the desired results, the limited coping style of the individual causes him to use maladaptive behaviors again and again.

People who have *altered patterns of relatedness* show difficulty in certain areas of living but may be entirely competent in other areas. Despite their difficulties in coping with everyday life, they remain in touch with reality. Although they suffer a great deal, they are less disabled than individuals with psychotic alterations of thought or affect, who exhibit gross distortions of reality. Persons with *neurotic disorders* may have an intellectual grasp of their problems, but they remain trapped in conflict and are not comfortable with this pattern. These disorders are ego dystonic to the individual. Persons with *personality disorders* may also have an understanding of how their maladaptive behavior has caused difficulties in relationships, but they have become comfortable with the pattern; therefore the disorders are ego syntonic (see Chapter 2).

Both neurotic and personality disorders are functional rather than organic problems, but organic workups are always necessary to rule out any organic problems. An organic disorder is one in which there is a change in the structure of the body, for example, an infection, traumatic injury, or malformation of an anatomic structure. In a functional illness, there is no demonstrable change in structure; the symptoms are based on the unhealthy psychological responses of the individual. An example is conversion disorder, in which there is no physiological reason for a disability such as blindness or paralysis. Many clients assumed to have a neurotic or personality disorder have been found on later examination to have definite organic pathology. The psychological trauma to an individual who is aware of physical problems only to have them dismissed as "neurotic" can be considerable. Delay in receiving appropriate treatment can also result in more extensive debility and complications.

The prevalance of neurotic dysfunction is so great that nurses will inevitably encounter clients who display signs of disturbed relatedness. Greenberg (1977) believes that approximately 80 percent of Americans are, to some extent, impaired by neurotic disorders, many of which go undiagnosed and untreated.

COMPARISON OF HEALTHY AND ALTERED SENSE OF SELF

In order to understand the manifestations of neurotic and personality disorders, it is necessary to be aware of the differences between the person who has developed a healthy sense of self and the person who has an altered sense of self.

The Healthy Self

A healthy sense of self is possessed by people who have more or less fully developed their mental and physical faculties (Greenberg, 1977). Healthy people are basically courageous. Because they are not afraid, they are open and curious and can look calmly at the world around them. They are not afraid of new situations and can tolerate risks and uncertainty. They are not afraid to try new things, and they can learn from experiences that enable them to do better the next time.

Healthy people are realists who see things accurately and do not confuse what *is* with what *should be*. These people do not expect something for nothing and respect the limitations of time, energy, and money. Because they realize that they cannot do everything, they concentrate on what is most important to them. They do not seek the impossible; their best is good enough. They accept their own limitations and are not too uncomfortable with their shortcomings.

Healthy people are mature and disciplined. In the course of their development, they have worked out a set of values that are appropriate for them. They do not have to satisfy all their impulses and needs immediately; they are oriented toward growth and do not allow themselves to be diverted from their real goals by needs that clamor for immediate gratification. Healthy people are in control of their own lives; they listen to others but make up their own minds and take responsibility for their own actions.

Good judgment is another quality of healthy people. They can simplify problems and get down to essentials. They do not get lost in unimportant details and trivial issues. They do not look for perfect solutions but for the best available means of solving problems.

Healthy people have self-respect and self-esteem. They appreciate themselves and do not constantly seek approval from others. Healthy people are productive and creative; they take advantage of their abilities to experience the joys of living.

People who are healthy have good contact with their own feelings and can express them. They are also sensitive to the feelings of others. They are good observers of themselves and their circumstances. These people know who they are, what they want, and in what direction they are going.

Finally, healthy people have good relations with other people. They can be generous and helpful to others because they are not always preoccupied with their own problems. Healthy people are capable of experiencing both love and work to the fullest extent.

The Altered Self

People who have not developed a solid sense of self feel vulnerable, insecure, and inferior. They are too frightened to look at themselves realistically and are afraid to see their limitations and shortcomings. Instead, by distorting or ignoring reality, they create a picture of themselves that they believe will impress others and of which they can be proud. The creation of an idealized self-image has far-reaching consequences for every aspect of their life: it becomes more important to live up to the image than to appreciate and recognize their real needs.

People with an altered sense of self cannot function without their idealized image; it is needed to help them feel unique, superior, secure, and confident. This image furnishes a direction and shapes their interactions with others.

Frequently, the idealized self-image dictates standards that are so high that these people become engaged in a hopeless and never-ending struggle to mold themselves into their idea of a perfect being. Whereas healthy people live in reality and respect it, people with an altered sense of self live in an illusory world where nothing is impossible. Whatever enhances and glorifies the idealized image becomes desirable and important. Conversely, those qualities and tendencies that diminish or detract from this image are undesirable and must be avoided. This type of thinking leads to a set of standards in which all qualities and tendencies are considered either good or bad, to be proud of or ashamed of. These people do not do things that are in their own interests but rather things that maintain their self-image. They have lost control over their own lives and sacrificed their genuine needs in the pursuit of self-esteem according to the idealized image.

Whereas healthy people have an accurate picture of themselves based on a realistic evaluation of assets and liabilities, people with an altered sense of self are not realistic; they are too frightened to see themselves objectively. Their real interests and needs are sacrificed in the attempt to pursue an idealized image of themselves. Life is extremely difficult because they are tormented by the constant fear of failure.

A comparison of the healthy person and the person with an altered sense of self is provided in Table 8-1.

196

The Role of Anxiety and Fear

The central process in altered patterns of relatedness is anxiety and defense against anxiety. People suffering from these disorders do not consciously know what they are anxious about and are too frightened to look at their anxiety accurately and realistically.

Horney (1945) postulates that the basis of anxiety is the feeling of being isolated and helpless in a hostile world. It is the terror of being abandoned, of feeling impotent, inadequate, unlovable, and worthless. Anxiety is the prevailing experiential state of neurotic persons.

The common elements of anxiety are fear of exposure and fear of loss of control. Exposure of one's inner conflict and turmoil can lead to embarrassment, shame, ridicule, and feelings of inferiority. Many people harbor feelings that are unacceptable to them, and the fear that these feelings will become known to others creates intense anxiety. Feelings of anxiety usually mean that a person's methods of coping with stress are no longer functional—that an uncomfortable conflict is surfacing.

Both fear and anxiety are emotional reactions to danger. With fear the cause is obvious, but with anxiety it is not. Most people are afraid of fire and war, for example; they are real dangers. Because the threat is known, it is possible to be frightened yet deal with the problem. The individual who experiences anxiety, however, does not know the origin of her fear. The source is diffuse and nonspecific, arising from within the person rather than from external dangers.

Table 8-1. Comparison of the Healthy Self and the Altered Self

Healthy Self	Altered Self
Courageous	Fearful
Realistic	Given to wishful thinking
Disciplined	Impulsive
Good judgment	Given to extremes
Open-minded	Closed-minded
Spontaneous	Driven, compulsive
Flexible	Rigid
Assertive	Hostile, vindictive
Loving	Clinging, dependent
Zest for living	Apathetic, impoverished
Sincere	Self-deceiving
Deep feelings	Numb
Good relationships	Exploits or is exploited
Productive, creative	Wasteful
Oriented toward growth	Oriented toward fame, prestige
Sense of identity	Alienated, stranger to self

SOURCE: Adapted from Greenberg (1977).

A variety of events can trigger anxiety. If the anxiety is general, not associated with one particular thing, it is called a *free-floating* anxiety. Anxiety may also be triggered by specific objects or classes of objects, such as dogs, heights, or enclosed spaces. These objects are substitutes for the real cause of the anxiety. Since the real cause is not consciously recognized by the individual, anxiety creates feelings of helplessness, shame, and inferiority. The anxious person feels as though she has lost control over her life.

THEORETICAL FRAMEWORKS

Three conceptual frameworks are widely used in understanding the dynamics of neurotic and personality disorders. For additional information on these frameworks, see Chapter 2.

Psychosexual or Psychodynamic Model

According to psychodynamic theory, neurotic conflict represents a struggle between the *ego*—the part of the psyche that experiences the external world through the senses, organizes the thought processes rationally, and governs action—and the *id*—the part of the psyche that is the reservoir of instinctual drives and is dominated by the pleasure principle and irrational wishing. Freud believed that the ego mediates between the id and the *superego*—the part of the psyche that is critical of the self and enforces moral standards. The id contains two drives, libidinous and aggressive. The ego controls the free expression of these drives so that the behavior a person exhibits is acceptable to himself and others. The conflict between the id, which says "yes," and the superego, which says "no," persists throughout life. This endless conflict is particularly difficult for persons with neurotic tendencies.

A conflict usually represents the wish to behave in a certain way and a fear of the consequences of behaving in that way. For example, a student might wish to excel in class and win the approval of the instructors but fears that outstanding achievement might lead to being resented by classmates. The wish to excel is a manifestation of the aggressive drive; the wish to be accepted by classmates is a manifestation of the libidinous drive. Anxiety is the end product of these opposing urges.

Repression is one way of dealing with a conflict. Freud described the defense mechanism of repression as resulting from a traumatic experience, usually of a sexual nature, during childhood (Freedman, Kaplan, and Sadock, 1976). Because the experience was painful, it was forgotten or repressed. But the excitement elicited by the sexual stimulation was not extinguished and stayed in the unconscious

197

Table 8-2. Psychosexual Etiology of Neurotic Disorders

Developmental Stage	Objective	Pathologic Manifestation
Oral (birth to age one)	Establish trusting dependence, gratification of oral needs without conflict	Dependency, counter-dependency; dependence on others for maintenance of self-esteem; biting, sucking *Example:* depression, alcoholism
Anal (ages one to three)	Achieve autonomy and independence without shame or self-doubt from loss of control	Orderliness, abstinence, parsimony, defense against anal eroticism *Example:* obsessive-compulsive disorder
Phallic (ages three to five)	Focus erotic interest on genital area, lay foundation for gender identity	Unresolved Oedipal complex; lack of feelings of achievement, power *Example:* phobias

198

as repressed memories. Later, in response to another uncomfortable experience, the memory is revived, and the repressive mechanism fails. When the repression fails, anxiety increases. Because the memories are unacceptable to the person, the original sexual excitement is expressed by a new means—the neurotic symptom. The neurotic symptoms or behaviors are invoked to control the anxiety and protect the ego against forbidden impulses and memories.

Freud believed that neurotic conflict occurs because of traumatic childhood experiences before the age of five or six. He described three early stages of psychosexual development, each characterized by a specific conflict (see Table 8-2). Failure to resolve that conflict results in the person's becoming fixated at that level of psychosexual development. This view is no longer widely accepted. Other psychodynamic theorists have suggested that a person may develop neurotic patterns later in life when he experiences sufficient stress. The stress causes regression or fixation at immature levels, producing neurotic symptoms.

Identification of the basic conflict makes it possible to locate the psychosexual stage when the conflict originated, and it gives direction to nursing-process activities designed to facilitate conflict resolution. The use of the psychoanalytic framework dictates that treatment be long term and be aimed at the client's ultimate recognition of the nature of the conflict.

Psychosocial Model

Erik Erikson (1963), like Freud, proposed a sequential developmental model, but his model used a triad of forces or influences to explain the modification of experiences: biologic, psychologic, and cultural. In this framework, inborn sensitivity and temperament, parenting, and ethnic and cultural factors, in addition to psychological strengths and weaknesses, all affect the appearance or nonappearance of neurotic symptoms. Neurotic disorders may develop from critical tasks that are incompletely resolved. These tasks can best be resolved when physiological maturation, psychological aspirations, and cultural expectations converge. If critical tasks are resolved prematurely or belatedly, they may not be dealt with adequately, and incomplete resolution of early critical tasks has a detrimental effect on resolution of later tasks.

Interpersonal Model

Harry Stack Sullivan (1953), like Freud, looked for developmental fixation or regression to explain mental illness. But, unlike Freud, Sullivan believed that such developmental arrests are caused by inadequacies in personal relations in the home, school, and community. In addition, he thought that the personality structure of a person takes more than twenty years to develop rather than just the first five years of life. At any stage of development, favorable or unfavorable events can be influential.

Sullivan postulated two opposites: absolute euphoria and absolute tension. The level of tension, some of which is necessary for normal living, fluctuates daily. When a need is not satisfied, tension increases until satisfaction is obtained. When one's interpersonal security is threatened, usually as the result of the disapproval of a valued person, tension rises and anxiety develops. In order to cope with this

Table 8-3. Comparison of Neurotic Alterations and Psychotic Alterations

Factor	Neurotic Alteration	Psychotic Alteration
General behavior	Mild degree of personality decompensation; reality contact impaired, but client not incapacitated in social functioning	Severe degree of personality decompensation; reality contact markedly impaired; client incapacitated in social functioning
Nature of symptoms	Wide range of complaints but no hallucinations or other markedly deviant behavior	Wide range of complaints with delusions, hallucinations, and other severely deviant behavior
Orientation	Client rarely loses orientation to environment	Client frequently loses orientation to environment
Insight	Client often has some insight into nature of the behavior; feels suffering keenly, wishes to get well on a conscious level	Client rarely has insight into nature of the behavior; usually doesn't recognize that illness is present
Social aspects	Behavior usually not injurious or dangerous to client or society; social adjustment impaired but not prevented	Behavior frequently injurious or dangerous to client or society
Treatment	Client rarely needs institutional care; psychotherapy usually only treatment necessary	Client usually needs institutional care; shock and other somatic therapies in addition to psychotherapy frequently necessary
Thoughts	Delusions never present; thoughts, feelings, actions maintain normal relationships	Delusions common; thoughts, feelings, actions lose relationship to each other
Repression	Repression is maintained, but repressed matter finds expression in distorted form that is relatively acceptable to the ego	Repression may be destroyed; the ego is overwhelmed with unacceptable impulses

199

anxiety, one modifies the offending behavior to regain approval. Many individuals develop anxiety whenever they enact or even contemplate behavior that is likely to be rejected by others.

According to Sullivan, anxiety always pertains to interpersonal relations. This anxiety causes the person to focus on experiences that will meet with social approval. The person thus develops in relation to social norms and behavior patterns.

As a result of unpleasant past experiences, individuals can develop views and attitudes about themselves that are not validated by others (Freedman, Kaplan, and Sadock, 1976). These distorted views propel them into inappropriate situations and cause anxiety, which in turn leads to unclear thoughts, inaccurate perceptions, and inappropriate behavior. Dynamisms (processes used in everyday life in response to difficulties in living) help or hinder satisfactory interpersonal relationships. Dynamisms are processes of living acquired in earlier stages of development that, when wrongly applied, become self-defeating. Since they are frequently misused, they do not help an individual achieve satisfactory goals. An example of this process is the person who develops an obsessive-compulsive disorder, regressing to a stage in early childhood in which magical thinking and ritualistic behavior help preserve his interpersonal security. Although the obsessive-compulsive behavior reduces the person's anxiety, the problem is not resolved, and the conflict remains to be dealt with repeatedly.

COMPARISON OF ALTERED PATTERNS OF FUNCTIONING

As mentioned earlier, psychosis, neurosis, and personality disorder are different forms of altered patterns of functioning. In clinical practice, it is sometimes difficult to distinguish among these patterns with absolute accuracy. Tables 8-3 and 8-4 are presented as guides to help nurses differentiate

Table 8-4. Comparison of Neurotic and Personality Alterations

Factor	Neurotic Disorder	Personality Disorder
Conflict	Conflict continues, needs to be dealt with repeatedly	Conflict is resolved
Anxiety	Continually present	Not present
Feelings, thoughts, behaviors	Undesirable, distressing, irritating; are ego dystonic	Felt as part of the self; are ego syntonic

200

between neurotic and psychotic patterns of functioning and between neurotic and personality disorders.

The most distinguishing features of psychotic alterations are failure of reality testing and inability to differentiate between internal and external stimuli. Persons with neurotic disorders do not experience such a gross loss of contact with reality. The major differentiating factor of personality disorders is an acceptance of and comfort with the altered behavior and relatedness pattern. Persons with neurotic styles of relating, on the other hand, are not comfortable with their conflict and repeatedly try to resolve it.

ALTERED PATTERNS OF RELATEDNESS: NEUROTIC PATTERNS

In the second edition of the *Diagnostic and Statistical Manual* of the American Psychiatric Association (1968), disorders with the chief characteristic of anxiety were grouped as neuroses. One of the major objectives of the authors of the third edition was to avoid theoretical explanations regarding the etiology of the various conditions, because it was not possible to present all relevant theories for each entity. Because there is little consensus on the origin of neuroses (as evidenced by the three frameworks presented in this chapter), the content of DSM-III aims at description rather than explanation of processes. The term "neurotic disorder" is now used to describe specific conditions, rather than "neurosis," which implies a general neurotic process. *Neurotic disorder* refers to any mental disorder in which the

---

THE DSM-III CATEGORIES FOR NEUROTIC DISORDERS

Anxiety Disorders
Phobic disorders
  300.21 Agoraphobia with panic attacks
  300.22 Agoraphobia without panic attacks
  300.23 Social phobia
  300.29 Simple phobia
Anxiety states
  300.01 Panic disorders
  300.02 Generalized anxiety disorder
  300.30 Obsessive-compulsive disorder
Posttraumatic stress disorder
  308.30 Acute
  309.81 Chronic or delayed
  300.00 Atypical anxiety disorder

Somatoform Disorders
  300.81 Somatization disorder
  300.11 Conversion disorder (or hysterical disorder, conversion type)
  307.80 Psychogenic pain disorder
  300.70 Hypochondriasis
  300.71 Atypical somatoform disorder

Dissociative Disorders (or hysterical neuroses, dissociative type)
  300.12 Psychogenic amnesia
  300.13 Psychogenic fugue
  300.14 Multiple personality
  300.60 Depersonalization disorder
  300.15 Atypical dissociative disorder

Personality Disorders (coded on Axis II)
  301.00 Paranoid
  301.20 Schizoid
  301.22 Schizotypal
  301.50 Histrionic
  301.81 Narcissistic
  301.70 Antisocial
  301.83 Borderline
  301.82 Avoidant
  301.60 Dependent
  301.40 Compulsive
  301.84 Passive-aggressive
  301.89 Atypical, mixed

---

predominant symptom that is distressing to the individual is recognized by him or her as unacceptable and ego alien (ego dystonic). There is no implication of a special etiologic process. DSM-III categories and nursing diagnoses are presented in the accompanying boxes.

> ### NURSING DIAGNOSES APPLICABLE
> ### TO NEUROTIC PATTERNS
>
> Anxiety
>
> Coping, ineffectual individual
>
> Fear
>
> Health maintenance, alterations in
>
> Home maintenance management, impaired
>
> Noncompliance
>
> Self-concept, disturbance in
>
> Violence, potential for
>
> Powerlessness
>
> Social isolation

Although each neurotic disorder has its own manifestations, several characteristics are commonly displayed by all (Greenberg, 1977). For example, all neurotic persons develop some type of symptom to relieve their anxiety. According to psychoanalytic theory, the symptom is the result of a compromise between unacceptable impulses and the forces that operate to repress those impulses. The symptom contains elements of both; a compromise is more tolerable for the individual than the conflict and reduces anxiety. In addition, symptoms have another advantage: Whenever an individual suffers from an ailment, other people are sympathetic and not only offer assistance but excuse the person from customary responsibilities. These are secondary gains that may be of considerable benefit to the neurotic person. But since neurotic symptoms impair functioning and cause suffering, the benefit is only temporary.

Neurotic persons are frightened of the demands of everyday living. They would like to guarantee that unpleasant things will not happen to them. As a result, they construct a plan of defense that will protect them from dangers, assuming that if they do certain things in certain ways, they will always be safe from harm and get what they want. Such beliefs tend to be unrealistic and magical, with little regard for others. The defensive strategy is fixed and rigid. Consequently, the neurotic person is not prepared to meet difficult or novel situations when they present themselves. Neurotic individuals also expect too much from themselves. By setting up impossible standards, they give themselves a continued stream of orders to perform in a certain way without regard for conditions that exist at the time. Horney (1950) called this the "tyranny of the

'shoulds.'" The constant strain of responding to these inner dictates often leaves individuals tired, tense, and irritable. Spontaneity and zest for living are destroyed.

Externalization, or attributing one's own feelings, faults, and behaviors to others, is another manifestation of neurosis. By shifting the blame to others, neurotic persons can maintain the illusions they have created about themselves. A common method is blaming current difficulties on events that occurred in childhood. While it is certainly true that events of childhood influence adult perceptions, neurotic individuals refuse to take responsibility for their own contributions to their present difficulties. It is easier to blame everything on one's parents. Externalization also allows individuals to channel self-hatred and self-contempt to other targets and thereby reduce emotional intensity.

People suffering from neurotic disorders frequently try to solve their problems by logic and reason, or *intellectualization*. They suppress their natural emotions and, before making decisions, tend to consult all the authorities and read all the books available on a subject. Because they are guided mainly by intellect, some decisions are extremely difficult for them. Often feelings experienced by people are a better guide and may lead to better and happier decisions

Additional strategies used by individuals with neurotic patterns of relating are compartmentalization and rationalization. *Compartmentalization* is a means of trying to have it both ways. An example is the individual who engages in questionable business tactics during the week but is devout and religious on Sunday. *Rationalization* is devising a plausible excuse when behavior does not express the ideal self. An example is the father who engages in fore-play with a preadolescent daughter on the grounds that he is preparing her for mature sexual relationships in the future. Both compartmentalization and rationalization are self-deceptive.

Despite their problems, individuals with neurotic styles of functioning can manage fairly well for long periods of time. However, as the neurotic pattern increases in severity, it becomes more difficult to carry out the necessary functions of life. Because of the energy expended in maintaining a neurotic way of life, these individuals tend to be under-achievers, repeaters of mistakes, and subject to extremes of behavior and poor judgment. The most common reaction in neuroses is depression. Neurotic persons often feel alienated from themselves, which can lead to extreme self-hatred and self-destruction.

Although our discussion thus far has been based primarily on psychodynamic theory, the student should be aware that neurotic disorders can be understood from several other theoretical frameworks. Existential analysts, for example, view anxiety as a central feature of the human condition, and they attribute this anxiety to a fear of non-being, which is unrelated to conflict or to past experience. Learning theorists see anxiety or fear as an unconditioned, inherent response to dangerous external stimuli capable of providing a powerful motivating force for shaping learned behavioral patterns. Learning theory provides a useful model for understanding the formation of a number of neurotic symptoms and for treating certain disorders (Kaplan, Freedman, and Sadock, 1980).

In the rest of this section we shall examine the specific types of neurotic patterns. In general, neurotic reactions show a progression from primitive behavior, in which anxiety is discharged through direct somatic channels as a generalized *anxiety disorder*, to more sophisticated manifestations. *Conversion disorders* utilize sensory motor channels; *dissociative disorders* involve mental processes; and *obsessive-compulsive disorders* use both mental and behavioral channels for dealing with anxiety. *Phobias*, which are the highest level of neurotic behavior, use external methods by displacing or projecting the anxiety to specific external objects. Following the discussion of each of these disorders, appropriate nursing assessments and approaches are presented.

Anxiety Reactions

In generalized anxiety reactions, the threat to the consciousness of the individual arises from repressed emotions such as hostility and resentment (Mereness and Karnash, 1966). External events, such as loss of a job, divorce, or threats to personal

security, can be important causative factors. Since there are no elaborate symptoms, an anxiety reaction is considered to be the most primitive mechanism for handling conflict. The anxiety is neither focused nor displaced but rather involves the whole organism. It is usually experienced in the form of physical symptoms that center around the vital organs of the body (heart palpitations, upset stomach, constriction of the throat) but can involve other areas as well (numbness in extremities). These symptoms are frightening, and the person frequently becomes depressed, has difficulty concentrating and working, and dwells on fears about dying or becoming insane. Severe anxiety attacks may cause a person to fear being left alone, which results in clinging to familiar situations, avoiding crowds, and being unable to work because of the fear of impending doom.

Occasionally, anxiety attacks can reach panic proportions. *Panic attacks* can last from minutes to hours and are frightening and distressing to the individual. The cause of these attacks may or may not be known to the individual. For some persons, anxiety attacks may be mild enough to be noticeable only to the individual. For example, talking too much or not talking at all in stressful situations may indicate a mild form of anxiety attack.

The importance of a thorough physical workup cannot be overemphasized, as certain somatic conditions may simulate anxiety attacks. The most common organic causes are thyrotoxicosis, hypoglycemia, amphetamine usage, and synergistic or idiosyncratic drug reactions.

NURSING ASSESSMENT AND APPROACH The absence of systematic, repetitive defensive behaviors indicates a favorable prognosis. Spontaneous remission may occur without intervention, or chronic anxiety attacks may result. These attacks may be precursors of other forms of neuroses, such as phobias and obsessive-compulsive disorders. As with all neuroses, interventions should deal less with the real circumstances surrounding the attack and more with the client's perception of her inner experience. It is important to examine the context in which the symptoms occur but also to remember that extraneous factors may be crucial. Reassurance that the attack is not life threatening or permanent is appropriate. Supportive measures should be offered at first, but long-term treatment consists of helping the client to develop insight into the nature of the conflict causing the symptoms.

Proponents of psychodynamic theory advocate insight-oriented psychotherapy if the client has sufficient ego strength and demonstrates motivation and capacity for introspection. Supportive psychotherapy with reassurance and encouragement to face anxiety-producing situations may be helpful even if not curative. Relaxation techniques taught by hypnotists and behavioral therapists may also prove effective for some clients (Kaplan, Freedman, and Sadock, 1980). For further nursing interventions, see Chapter 4.

Obsessive-Compulsive Reactions

An obsessive-compulsive disorder is an emotional dysfunction in which certain ideas and behaviors occupy the client to such a degree that they interfere with normal work and social activity. In the obsessive-compulsive individual, conflicts are expressed in repetitious thoughts, words, and acts.

An *obsession* is a thought that occurs persistently despite the person's wish to avoid or ignore it. A *compulsion* is an act that is carried out, in some degree against the client's wishes, to avoid or control anxiety. The obsessive person may also be occupied with rumination, which involves not just single thoughts but large topics around which repetitive thoughts revolve without resolution or decision.

According to psychodynamic theory, obsessive-compulsive individuals are fixated or regressed to the anal stage of development. The underlying conflicts are related to cleanliness, authority, and control. Individuals may be very clean or very dirty. Behaviors are usually symbolic of holding on or letting go, for example, hoarding items or giving everything away. Ritualistic behaviors may be sadomasochistic. The abnormal fears of the obsessive-compulsive person usually develop out of disagreeable and socially unacceptable ideas. These ideas, with associated intense emotions, are repressed into the unconscious. The repressed energy attaches itself to an activity or idea that seemingly has no relationship to the original problem. A sense of relief from tension and anxiety is obtained when the ritual is performed, but the relief is only temporary, so the person is compelled to repeat the act.

The defense mechanisms used by obsessive-compulsive individuals include regression, isolation, reaction formation, and undoing (see Chapter 2). A well-structured obsessive-compulsive ritual protects against psychosis. Usually the obsessive-compulsive person who fears hurting others is in no danger of doing so—the idea of violence is frightening. An example of the interplay of defense mechanisms is illustrated by a woman who had ambivalent feelings about bearing a child and becoming a mother. When caring for her child, she developed a ritualistic behavior about keeping the baby clean, sterilizing all food or objects that the child came in contact with, and washing her hands continually. In this manner, she dealt with her hostile (and unacceptable) feelings toward her child through ritualized behavior. She repressed her hos-

tility and unconscious wish to harm the child and instead devoted all her energy to keeping the child and the environment impeccably clean (a reaction formation). Furthermore, the continual hand-washing (undoing) alleviated her guilt by making demands and causing discomfort.

An alternative approach is presented by learning theorists, who believe that obsession represents a conditioned stimulus to anxiety. Because of an association with an anxiety-producing stimulus, the obsessional thought gains the capacity to arouse anxiety. A compulsion is established when a person learns that certain actions reduce anxiety; these actions become fixed into a learned pattern.

NURSING ASSESSMENT AND APPROACH Obsessive-compulsive individuals rarely become suicidal, because their defenses protect them from acting out their impulses. They frequently engage in magical thinking and believe that thinking equals acting. It is important to negate this belief and reassure them that there are differences between thoughts and acts. Symptoms must be assessed in the context of the client's lifestyle and social supports. These clients usually have a chronic condition and show few prospects for growth. It is unrealistic to try to modify their behavior or personality radically. Often the symptoms increase as the client ages. It is usually more realistic to modify the external situation and to help the client cope with the demands of her ritualistic behaviors by reducing them or substituting less demanding behaviors, if possible. If long-term therapy is contemplated, the original source of the anxiety will need to be investigated, a task for the primary therapist.

The outlook for a client displaying an obsessive-compulsive reaction is related to the severity of his symptoms, including the rigidity in thinking and behaving, the quality of relationships with others, the tolerance for anxiety, the ability to tolerate introspection, and the capacity for insight. For specific nursing interventions, see Chapter 4.

Posttraumatic Stress Syndrome

Posttraumatic stress syndrome is a pattern of psychological symptoms brought about by the experience of a highly traumatic event (Ziarnowski, 1984). The syndrome involves such a severe stressor that almost anyone experiencing it could be subject to psychological distress. Victims of rape or assault, veterans of military combat, and survivors of natural or human-made disasters are all vulnerable to posttraumatic stress reactions and have the potential to manifest serious psychological impairment. Posttraumatic stress disorder was first identified in Viet Nam combat veterans, but it can be seen in the survivors of other traumatic situations as well.

203

When one is traumatized, the normal inclination is to withdraw and/or escape both physically and emotionally. Children who badly burn their hands on an oven door will put some distance between themselves and the stove, give it a wide berth in the future and may even develop a phobia toward the punishing object. People with post-traumatic stress disorder have been burned; but it is their psyches, not their flesh that is scarred. Like the burned child, they too would like to isolate themselves from the event and its emotional overlay; but the experience, with its many emotions and associations, is so complex that they cannot dissociate themselves from it without shutting down a good part of their emotional lives.

A. PETER ZIARNOWSKI (1984)

204

The indications of posttraumatic stress reactions are dramatic and compelling. First, there is a tendency to relive the event in some way: through nightmares, intrusive thoughts, or other obsessive ruminations. Flashbacks—the feeling of "being there again" set off by some seemingly neutral stimulus in the environment—are common. A second major indicator is the tendency to insulate oneself from one's emotions and feelings, known as "psychic numbing." Trauma involves a range of experiences and feelings that include fear, panic, guilt, anger, and physical and emotional pain. When one is traumatized, the normal inclination is to withdraw or escape both physically and emotionally. People with posttraumatic stress disorder have been psychologically scarred and try to isolate themselves from the event and its emotional overlay. However, the experience is so complex that they cannot dissociate themselves from the event and its emotional overlay without shutting down a good part of their emotional lives. By not feeling deeply, they can avoid being hurt again. Interpersonal relations can be profoundly affected. Things that were once enjoyable no longer hold any pleasure, and the client appears blunted, perhaps even schizophrenic in some cases.

In addition to reliving and psychic numbing, these clients may manifest hyperalertness, disturbances of sleep, survivor guilt, memory impairment, trouble concentrating, and avoidance of activities that are reminiscent of the trauma, or intensification of symptoms if such activities cannot be avoided. Anxiety and depression (often with suicidal ideation) are common, along with lowered stress tolerance and explosiveness.

Posttraumatic stress syndrome in Viet Nam veterans has been the subject of considerable attention in the media. Many of the men and women returning from Viet Nam have continued to relive war events and have suffered from flashbacks and nightmares. Many have been unable to resume the lives they had before combat. Because of their psychic numbing, they may no longer be able to relate to their families in a meaningful way. Many have turned to alcohol and drug abuse as a way of handling their conflict.

NURSING ASSESSMENT AND APPROACHES Sensitivity to the behavioral presentation of clients, especially those who may have experienced combat in Viet Nam, is crucial. Clients who appear angry, are hyperalert, and have sleep disorders may be suffering from the syndrome. The need for a careful and thorough history cannot be overemphasized, as most clients will not volunteer information about a traumatic event and, indeed, may not be aware of the relationship of an event to current feelings of distress. It is not uncommon to find alcohol and drug abuse among these clients, as these substances can be used to blot out traumatic memories. Because clients suffering from posttraumatic stress are at times misdiagnosed as schizophrenic, it is important for the nurse to be aware of the differences between the two conditions.

Phobic Reactions

A *phobia* is dread of an object that realistically is not dangerous but that has come to represent a danger and is specific enough to transform anxiety into fear. Phobias are sometimes called the normal

Her mind lives tidily apart,
From cold, and noise and pain,
And bolts the door against her heart
Out wailing in the rain.
DOROTHY PARKER

205

neuroses of childhood because they may result from inadequate parental protection or from fearfulness conveyed by a parent. Some common phobias are listed in Table 8-5.

According to psychoanalytic theory, a phobia may begin when a real threat causes fear and anx-

iety; the phobia then develops as a means of decreasing the anxiety. The particular phobic object symbolizes the conflict that is causing the anxiety. By replacing the anxiety with fear of the specific object, the person can reduce psychic discomfort by avoiding the feared object. For example, if one is afraid of heights, one avoids high places.

Some phobias involve the use of the defense mechanism of *displacement*. For example, a woman may wish to hurt her mother, but since these feelings are unacceptable to her, she displaces her feelings of hostility onto kitchen knives and becomes afraid of them because they represent her true feelings. Other phobias involve the use of both displacement and *projection*. In the story of Little Hans (Freud, 1955), the child had a wish to hurt his father, but because this wish was unacceptable to him, he projected his feelings onto his father, believing that his father wished to hurt him. Since this, too, was unacceptable, he displaced the fear of his father onto horses, developing a phobia about them.

Persons with phobic disorders have relatively mature ego structures. Since their fear is placed outside themselves, the mechanism is less punitive than in an anxiety or hysterical disorder. However, phobias can become generalized, causing discomfort and interfering with daily functioning. For example, a man may experience an accident or near-accident in an airplane, causing him to become afraid of flying; subsequently, his fear may become generalized to all moving vehicles and progress until he is afraid to leave his home for any reason.

A different explanation of phobias is offered by learning theorists, who use the traditional Pavlovian stimulus-response model of the conditioned reflex

Table 8-5. Common Phobias

Phobia	Fear of
Acrophobia	High places
Agoraphobia	Open places
Algophobia	Pain
Astraphobia	Thunder and lightning
Claustrophobia	Closed places
Coprophobia	Excreta
Hematophobia	Blood
Hydrophobia	Water
Lalophobia	Speaking
Mysophobia	Dirt, contamination
Necrophobia	Dead bodies
Nyctophobia	Night, darkness
Pathophobia	Disease
Peccatophobia	Sinning
Phonophobia	Speaking aloud
Photophobia	Strong light
Sitophobia	Eating
Taphophobia	Being buried alive
Thanatophobia	Death
Toxophobia	Being poisoned
Xenophobia	Strangers
Zoophobia	Animals

SOURCE: Adapted from Freedman, Kaplan, and Sadock (1976).

to account for the initial creation of a phobia. They suggest that fear becomes attached to an inappropriate object when anxiety is aroused by a frightening stimulus in the presence of that neutral object. Because of this association, the object acquires the ability to arouse anxiety on its own.

NURSING ASSESSMENT AND APPROACHES The prognosis for the client who is phobic is uncertain. Some phobic persons are stable and do not experience a major disruption in their lives because the object of their fear can easily be avoided. However, for others, fear may broaden to the point of incapacitation. The degree of impairment created by the phobia needs careful assessment because, in many cases, there is no need for treatment. If the phobia is incapacitating or if the client expresses a need to be rid of the phobia, several techniques may be successful. In *desensitization*, the client is repeatedly exposed to situations that cause progressively greater levels of anxiety until the client no longer feels great anxiety in the presence of the feared object. In *reciprocal inhibition*, an anxiety-producing stimulus is paired with an anxiety-suppressing stimulus until the anxiety is no longer uncomfortable. Reciprocal-inhibition techniques include meditation, yoga, and biofeedback. At times insight work is helpful. All these methods require special training and are to be used only after careful evaluation of the client's particular circumstances.

Recent research (Brody, 1983) has indicated that the cause of phobias and panic attacks may be biologic; thus, some new approaches to treatment involve the use of antidepressant medication combined with behavior modification. The drugs most frequently used are imipramine (Tofranil) and MAO inhibitors. Many clients respond to the three-phase approach of support, medication, and behavior modification. One advantage of this approach is that the client is helped to realize that the feared object is not the cause of the problem.

Conversion Reactions

In a *conversion reaction*, alterations in functioning of sensory systems or voluntary muscles are used to control anxiety (Hofling and Leininger, 1960). These alterations are never peripheral and are unrelated to the distribution of nerve pathways. Psychodynamically, conversions can be explained in terms of the ego's ability to control the sensory and motor apparatus by refusing to acknowledge incoming stimuli (as by blindness) or to carry out a particular motor function (as by paralysis of one hand). This control is always below the level of conscious awareness. In a conversion reaction, the conflict is not expressed in diffuse symptoms as it is in generalized anxiety. In fact, the symptoms have a specific meaning to the client. Neither is the anxiety displaced to an external object, as in a phobic reaction. Instead, it is expressed symbolically by altered functioning.

When considering the etiology of conversion reactions, the student should be aware of the sociological view that illnesses often reflect the expectations of valued persons and health care providers (see Chapter 2). According to Parsons (1951), the sick role is characterized by passivity—others are permitted to make all the decisions for the client. This enforced dependency diminishes the client's sense of autonomy and supports a state of helplessness.

People suffering from conversion reactions are sometimes misdiagnosed as malingerers. However, malingering is a conscious endeavor, whereas a conversion disorder is unconscious. The client with a conversion reaction has real symptoms and experiences discomfort from them; the malingerer does not. The person with a conversion disorder may be inconsistent in exhibiting symptoms because he or she does not fear detection; there is no feigning involved. The malingerer, on the other hand, will show considerable consistency; his symptoms and complaints are well thought through because he fears being exposed. People with conversion reactions cannot modify their disabilities of their own volition; malingerers can.

Repression is the fundamental defense mechanism in conversion reactions. The production of the symptom is dependent on keeping unacceptable thoughts and feelings in the unconscious. Since the symptom actually serves unconscious purposes, clients have a relative lack of distress toward their symptoms. The symptom binds the anxiety, thereby relieving distress. This has led to the use of the term *la belle indifference* to describe the casual attitude of the client.

Alleviation of anxiety is the primary gain of behaviors in all neurotic disorders—"primary" in the sense that the client receives advantages from the behaviors that are independent of the response of the environment. However, secondary gains may also be accrued from the environment. For example, a woman who has developed conversion blindness because she does not wish to "see" the evidence that her husband is having an affair with another woman also receives the secondary gain of increased attention from her family because of her disability. Secondary gain comes from the attention one receives; it is not part of the conversion reaction but is instead a complication. Removal of the secondary gain does not decrease the conversion reaction.

As in all instances where a functional disorder is suspected, it is important first to rule out the possibility of physiological pathology. For example, multiple sclerosis sometimes causes bizarre symptoms that are unrelated to nerve distribution.

NURSING ASSESSMENT AND APPROACHES Clients with a conversion reaction are usually suggestible and are fond of attention. Guilt is rarely a prominent feature. Conversion disorders are often associated with sexual repression and disapproval of sexual feelings in early life. Fewer cases are diagnosed than formerly, probably because of changing attitudes about sex and sexuality.

In the treatment of clients with a conversion reaction, therapists should not try to remove the symptom too quickly. If the symptom is suddenly removed but the conflict remains, emergency defenses such as depression or suicide may follow. Expressive, exploratory therapy that brings the conflict into conscious awareness can increase insight and decrease the need for repression. The symptom should never be the target; rather, the client should be allowed to retain the symptom while insight, self-understanding, and change take place. Because clients cannot make the cognitive connection between the way they feel and the cause of their symptoms, therapy should aim at achieving this cognitive connection.

Effective care of clients with conversion reactions is largely dependent on the attitudes and acceptance of health care professionals. It is at times difficult for caretakers to respond to the demands of these clients when there is no demonstrable physical cause of their symptoms. Treatment planning must be based on an acceptance of the symptoms as being real and on a search for the meaning of the symptoms.

Dissociative Reactions

In dissociative reactions, denial and ego splitting are used to decrease anxiety. The alteration is in mental functions rather than in sensory or motor functions. Portions of the ego are separated from the total personality and forced into the unconscious. The client still, however, possesses the majority of mental material, such as knowledge and skills related to work performance. Examples of dissociative reactions include amnesia and multiple personality. Modern literature has helped to create public interest in these conditions through such works as *The Three Faces of Eve* and *Sybil*. In these examples of brief amnesias with the emergence of new personalities and the alteration of two or more personalities, a portion of the person's psychic material was separated (dissociated) from other portions. However, genuine cases of multiple personality are relatively rare.

According to the psychoanalytic model, all hysterical neurotic reactions are related to the oral and phallic phases of development. The sexual seductiveness often displayed by the hysterical person indicates an Oedipal conflict, with a wish to regress to oral levels where love and security can be found.

NURSING ASSESSMENT AND APPROACHES In the past, dissociative ("hysterical") reactions were thought to occur only in women. However, recent research has shown that these reactions are at least as common, and perhaps more so, in men (Luisada, Peele, and Pillard, 1974). Both men and women initially seek treatment in their late teens or early twenties and both usually have a history of suicidal gestures. They are scholastic underachievers and rarely express having had sexual satisfaction. Misuse of alcohol and drugs is common, as are unreliability and lying.

Treatment should focus on the client rather than on the symptoms. Therapy should not become a long, self-rewarding process that reinforces the manipulative and dependent behavior commonly seen in these clients.

Hypochondriacal Reactions

Clients suffering from hypochondriacal reactions have a preoccupation with somatic symptoms as well as an erroneous belief that they are seriously ill. The condition differs from hysterical disorders in that there are no actual losses or distortions in function. Symptoms of the condition may appear in childhood but usually peak in the fourth decade for men and the fifth decade for women. The symptoms are diffuse and can involve many areas of the body.

NURSING ASSESSMENT AND APPROACHES A client with hypochondriasis will present his or her symptoms at length and in great detail. The content of the client's thoughts is entirely centered on bodily complaints and on unsuccessful attempts to achieve relief. In contrast to the indifference shown by clients with conversion reactions, these clients are frequently worried and anxious. They usually have a long history of repeated physician visits and multiple surgeries. Many show obsessive-compulsive traits such as defiance, obstinacy, miserliness, and egocentricity to the extent that they exclude any concern for others.

In the treatment of the hypochondriacal client, it is necessary to allow her to verbalize how she feels to help her decrease the need to demonstrate her feelings with body language. The client's physical symptoms should be accepted by the nurse but should not become the *focus* of the interaction. Honest and simple explanations for symptoms should be given without showing overconcern. Physical complaints should be discreetly brought to the attention

Nazi Field Marshal Hermann Goering "introduced the concentration camp and declared that it was not his duty to exercise justice but to anihilate and exterminate . . . Goering admitted that he had no conscience, his conscience was Adolf Hitler."

C. S. BLUEMEL, LAW, POLITICS AND INSANITY (1948)

of appropriate staff, as some may be legitimate and in need of further evaluation. The best therapy for a hypochondriacal client is an understanding and supportive relationship with sympathetic listening. The family should be included in the plan of care to assist them to understand the nature of the client's complaints.

ALTERED PATTERNS OF RELATEDNESS: PERSONALITY DISORDERS

Personality disorders are lifelong behavior patterns that are acceptable to the individual but that create conflict with others. Although the behaviors may resemble the patterns of some neurotic disorders, they are usually acceptable to the individual (ego-syntonic) and do not create anxiety because of their acceptability to the ego. Unlike neurotic persons, who must deal with their conflicts repeatedly, persons with a character disorder seem to have resolved their libidinous and aggressive conflicts once and for all. Latent anxiety may exist, but it does not usually surface unless the coping style is challenged or is no longer effective.

Usually, people with personality disorders do not see the problem as theirs but as that of others. Discontent is expressed only if their behavior pattern fails to obtain fulfillment of their needs. Their common complaint is that they are treated unfairly by others or by life in general. The ego structure of such persons causes them to react poorly to anxiety and depression. The behavior pattern is frequently a prolonged maladaptive way of interacting with others and usually becomes worse when a situation is stressful.

Little is known about the causes of specific personality disorders (Kaplan, Freedman, and Sadock, 1980). Genetic factors have been considered, since research has shown that monozygotic twins have a higher concordance of personality disorders than dizygotic twins (Pollin et al., 1969) and studies have indicated that children of parents with borderline schizophrenia raised by adoptive parents had a higher than average rate of schizotypal personalities (Wender, 1976).

Constitutional factors have been thought to play a role in personality disorders because some clients with emotionally unstable character disorders have shown an increase in neurologic deficits (Quitkin, Rifkin, and Klein, 1976). Other researchers have suggested that children with minimal brain dysfunction are predisposed to later development of personality disorders (Satterfield and Centwell, 1972). These factors have been useful in the explanation of personality disorders, but firm evidence has not been established.

Sociocultural aspects may also contribute to the etiology. Learning theorists suggest that persistent maladaptive social behavior is reinforced and maintained by rewards—usually social—that are present in the environment (Feldman, 1977).

The main types of dysfunctional personality patterns are termed schizoid, compulsive, histrionic, antisocial, passive-aggressive/passive-dependent, and paranoid.

Schizoid Type

People with schizoid personality disorders have problems with relationships, tend to withdraw from others, and are frequently seen as "loners." Despite this behavior pattern, such persons may be very

There's little in taking and giving
There's little in water or wine
This living, this living, this living
Was never a project of mine.
DOROTHY PARKER

aware of their intense need for others and may fear that if their needs are expressed they will overwhelm and hurt other people. They maintain a distance to protect themselves and others from being hurt. This style is often thought to be a way of avoiding homosexual impulses, as relations with the opposite sex are frightening. These clients often have a childhood history of poor relations with distant or cruel parents; they have essentially given up hope of love and caring.

Because of their hunger for a satisfactory relationship, these clients may be quick to form relationships with helping persons. They are frequently hypersensitive to rejection and have fragile defenses. The nurse must be aware of both their need for human contact and their need for distance from others. These clients should not be allowed to develop a dependency on one practitioner but should be exposed to a variety of clinicians. In some cases, group therapy may be most helpful.

Compulsive Type

Compulsive individuals are usually meticulous, conscientious, disciplined, and reliable. Because of the many pressures generated within, they tend to be relatively inflexible. If they are fortunate enough to have an appropriate job, they may function quite well, but adaptation to change is difficult. The conflict for these clients centers on control and aggression, which are dispelled by obsessive-compulsive activity. Often there are underlying fears of aggression, which the client is afraid of expressing. The childhood history may show authoritarian and rigid parents. Treatment should focus on helping clients to deal with their fears of closeness and aggression as well as to reduce some of the self-induced

stresses. In addition, clients should be assisted in regaining some control over their environment by appropriate verbal interaction.

Histrionic Type

Histrionic persons tend to be emotional and flamboyant with an appearance of seductiveness, which is actually competition with the opposite sex. In women, the origin may be a wish to have the power that men possess, and in men, there may be a wish to be cared for. These persons frequently have difficulty in mixed groups because they become competitive with persons of the same sex and seductive to persons of the opposite sex. The sexual behavior is usually deceptive, since it is actually a way of asking to be cared for.

Treatment should aim at reducing the self-destructive nature of the behavior and encouraging the development of the person's potential. Clients should be assisted to reduce the affective and emotional intensity of their behavior. Female nurses can help by providing nurturing responses in competitive situations, whereas male nurses can help by providing caring, nonsexual responses.

Antisocial Type

The person with an antisocial personality often manifests abnormal behavior that is in violation of laws, mores, and customs. Lacking a conscience, antisocial persons seek immediate gratification of their needs, are unable to tolerate delays or frustration, and are unable to postpone pleasure. Many of these people may appear quite charming in order to get their needs met. A comprehensive history often reveals ambivalent or inconsistent parenting in childhood.

210

Such people usually lack a sense of loyalty or concern for others and have little ability to maintain close and lasting relationships. Because they are without much anxiety or guilt feelings and do not learn from experience, punishment is rarely effective. The criminal who returns to prison again and again is an example of this personality style.

These persons frequently have poor school and work records because of their inability to conform to standards and relate to authority figures. Promiscuous sexual behavior with a variety of partners (who mean little to them), as well as socially unacceptable activities are frequently seen. In many instances, the problems are compounded by abuse of alcohol and drugs.

Treatment focuses on helping clients to take more responsibility for their own behavior and to realize that their problems come from within themselves.

Passive-Aggressive/Passive-Dependent Type

For individuals with passive-aggressive or passive-dependent personality disorders, the prominent trait may be either aggression or dependency that is expressed indirectly. Passive persons of either type are subject to depression if their needs are not met. The cause of these disorders may be inadequate mothering, as in schizoid disorders, but whereas the schizoid has given up hope of love, the passive-aggressive/passive-dependent person has not. He tends to search for the person who will meet all his needs, but since his needs are insatiable, the search is doomed to failure.

Masochism is often a factor in this personality structure. Masochists derive pleasure from being the victim and behave in ways that will increase the chances of their own exploitation. Many times they will hurt themselves in order to hurt others.

Treatment should be aimed at identifying underlying dependency needs and uncovering underlying aggression. Passive-dependent clients are unaware of their underlying anger and see themselves as good and kind. Therapy should focus on self-responsibility; group therapy is often the treatment of choice. Passive-aggressive individuals often have conflicts with authority. They need to be encouraged to express their needs directly to obtain what they want.

Paranoid Type

Persons with paranoid personality disorders are usually hypersensitive, rigid, suspicious, jealous, envious, and excessively self-important. They tend to project their inadequacies onto others and to blame them for their own difficulties. The interpersonal relationships of these individuals are extremely disturbed, and they are in constant conflict with friends, spouses, and people in positions of authority. The paranoid personality disorder may be a residual or latent schizophrenic process. People with paranoid personalities may be shy and reclusive or aggressive and outwardly hostile. They expend a great deal of energy in searching for clues to confirm their suspicions. They are extremely sensitive to slight rejections and inadvertent oversights.

Treatment should be aimed at strengthening self-confidence, improving reality testing, and increasing a sense of security. The client's sense of autonomy should be fostered whenever possible and freedom of choice given when feasible.

C L I N I C A L   E X A M P L E

██████████████████████████████

ALTERED PERSONALITY PATTERN

██████████████████████████████

Betty is a twenty-six-year-old white female, married for four years and currently majoring in mathematics at a local college. She also has a part-time job selling home products door-to-door or at arranged house parties.

Betty grew up in a rural area, the youngest of three children. Her mother was a quiet, nonassertive individual who disapproved of outside employment for women. Her father was a successful businessman who dominated the household. He had a closer relationship with his daughter than with his sons, whom he took for granted. Her mother was able to manipulate her father either by being quiet and seductive or by crying and dramatic behavior. Betty learned quickly that these techniques also worked for her with both her father and her brothers.

Betty's childhood was relatively uneventful, except for an incident that occurred when she was thirteen years old. On a camping trip, she was sexually molested by three strangers. Despite the emotional trauma involved, Betty confided in no one. Her parents were not aware of the rape until several years later.

After graduation from high school, Betty decided to spend the summer with some relatives in a distant state, despite the objections of her parents. It was there that she met David, who was to become her husband. David and Betty dated throughout the summer and decided to get married after the new year. The night before Betty was to return home, David attempted sexual relations with her. Although she consented at first, she screamed and blacked out for several minutes when he attempted penetration. After she regained consciousness, she tearfully explained that her reaction was due to her previous experience. David was understanding and sympathetic, and he assured her that he would be patient and kind in their marital relations.

After Betty returned home, she and David continued with their plans for marriage in spite of resistance from Betty's parents, who felt that she was too young for such a commitment. Her father was quite upset but refused to talk about the issue. He withdrew his support from Betty, and their relationship became strained.

After the marriage, Betty had less contact with her family because of the geographic distance, but telephone calls were frequent, and the couple did not make major decisions until they solicited her family's opinion. While David did not agree with these actions, he acquiesced to please his wife. All vacation time was spent in visits with Betty's family.

Despite David's vow to be patient and understanding in their sexual relations, difficulties continued. Betty was able to tolerate penetration only about 20 percent of the time intercourse was attempted, and there was no enjoyment for her and little for David, other than physical release. David was becoming irritable, and Betty was expressing feelings of depression. Finally, at David's insistence, Betty went to her local mental health center to seek assistance with her sexual problem.

ASSESSMENT

The nurse who interviewed Betty saw a mildly obese young woman who actually looked to be no more than sixteen or seventeen years old. This appearance was heightened by her hair, which was worn in pigtails, and by her youthful clothing style. She spoke in a quiet voice, almost a monotone, but she maintained good eye contact with the nurse. Although she verbalized feelings of depression, she giggled and smiled frequently during the interview. She stated that she would like to be able to have sexual intercourse on a regular basis to please her husband.

Based on the history and assessment interview, the following nursing and psychiatric diagnoses were made:

Nursing Diagnoses

Coping, ineffectual individual

Coping, ineffectual family

Fear

Rape trauma syndrome, silent reaction

Self-concept, disturbance in self-esteem

Sexuality, dysfunction of

Multiaxial Psychiatric Diagnoses

Axis I   306.51 Functional vaginismus

Axis II   301.50 Histrionic personality disorder

Axis III None

Axis IV   Code 4—Mild; beginning marital tension

Axis V   Level 2—Very good; functions well at school and on the job

PLANNING

The treatment team agreed that the plan for Betty should include several modalities. It was generally thought that her difficulties with sexual intercourse were related to the rape she had experienced and had never discussed or worked through, probably compounded by the rejection by her father. Even though several years had elapsed, it was felt that Betty might benefit from a women's support rape group to facilitate the expression

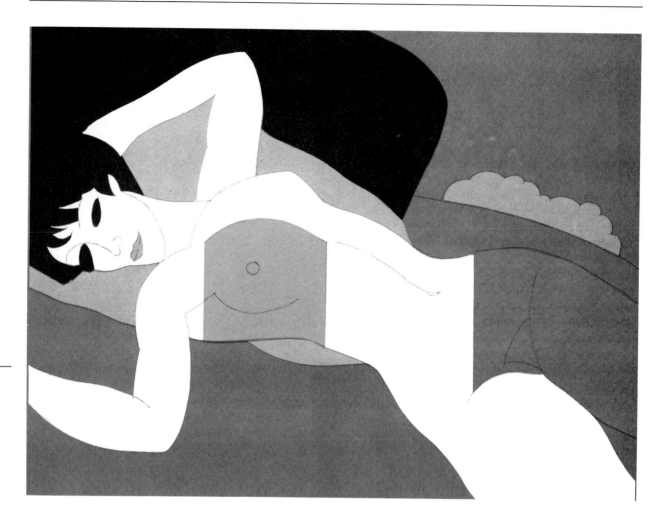

212

of feelings surrounding the incident. Relaxation techniques would also be of help. Plans were made for separate and conjoint interviews with David to evaluate progress in the relationship. A gynecologic workup was arranged to rule out any organic problems.

IMPLEMENTATION

Betty was assigned to a nurse clinician for weekly supportive sessions, relaxation training, and coordination of referrals to appropriate disciplines. The gynecologic examination was negative. Betty proved to be an avid student of relaxation techniques. However, in the group sessions, she was unable to do more than relate the facts of the rape as she remembered them. When speaking in the group, her affect was quite flat, and she never showed any emotion or dealt with the feelings surrounding the incident in other than an intellectual way. In the conjoint sessions, Betty and David reported that their sexual relationship was improving as Betty seemed able to relax more and penetration became easier.

After a few months, Betty began to complain that she periodically lost all feeling from her waist to her knee on the right side of her body and that at times one side of her pubic area was completely devoid of all sensation. At

this point, sexual intercourse again became difficult, not because of the penetration problem but because of her inability to perform because of the loss of sensation.

The treatment team met again to reconsider the plan and decided that Betty was in danger of developing a conversion disorder because the underlying problems were not being solved. She was again referred for a medical workup to rule out organic problems such as multiple sclerosis. An appointment was made for her to begin insight-oriented psychotherapy.

EVALUATION

The case of Betty highlights the difficulties of treating a client with a neurotic disturbance. In such a client, the basic personality configuration cannot be changed overnight. Premature eradication of a needed symptom frequently leads to the development of a replacement. In this case, Betty needed a symptom, any symptom, to handle her anxiety and so substituted one for another. The second chosen symptom, that of loss of sensation, was less dysfunctional than the vaginismus because at least now she could perform sexually. The aim of treatment should be to make symptoms less dysfunctional but still give the client the means to handle the anxiety.

General Nursing Approaches

Treatment of clients with personality disorders is difficult since they experience relatively little discomfort. Confrontation is necessary, but since interpersonal skills are poor, the confrontation must be carefully timed. It is difficult to get these clients to accept treatment, and they frequently drop out before any progress can be made. Group treatment is often effective.

Many clients instinctively resolve their own difficulties by choosing a mate who is complementary to them. For example, the passive-aggressive individual may choose a masochistic partner, or the obsessive-compulsive individual may find a hysterical partner.

It is often helpful to these clients to trace the course of their interpersonal difficulties rather than merely identifying the dysfunctional patterns.

Borderline Conditions

Persons with borderline conditions manifest episodic alterations of behavior patterns in times of stress—there is usually a prompt reorganization of the behavior when stress is removed. At times, the behavior of such persons may approach neurotic or psychotic proportions. They possess a global anger that helps them defend against closeness. They experience many interpersonal difficulties, lack self-identity, and have underlying depression and feelings of loneliness.

Regardless of overt manifestations, borderline clients have serious defects in their capacities to love and work (Masterson, 1976). Their capacity to love is hampered by the need to defend themselves against intimacy by either clinging or distancing. Their satisfaction at work is hampered by the need

to avoid spontaneous interaction. Often these two factors combine to form the common chief complaint of general discontent or dissatisfaction with life. They lack the essential capacities to enjoy their lives.

Treatment should be aimed at encouraging verbalization of feelings and thoughts. Because the needs of these clients tend to be excessive, their care requires consistency and structure. Difficulties must be conceptualized as the client's, not the caretaker's. Goal setting and limit setting are of primary importance.

PSYCHOPHARMACOLOGICAL APPROACHES

The most common drugs used in therapy for neurotic disorders are the antianxiety agents, sometimes known as minor tranquilizers. They are used to control moderate to severe daytime anxiety and tension without causing excessive sedation or drowsiness. The most commonly used agents are listed in Table 8-6.

The therapeutic actions of these drugs are thought to result from actions at subcortical sites, particularly depression of the limbic system (Eisenhauer and Gerald, 1984). High doses can also depress the cerebral cortex, producing sedation. Many antianxiety agents also possess anticonvulsant and skeletal muscle relaxant properties.

Antianxiety drugs are contraindicated with hypersensitive clients or those with a history of drug dependence. The most common side effects are drowsiness, lethargy, fainting, nausea, vomiting, and general gastrointestinal distress. At times, transient hypotension can be a problem. Blood pressure

Table 8-6. Commonly Used Antianxiety Agents

Generic Name	Trade Name	Usual Dose Range
Alprazolam	Xanax	0.25 – 0.5 mg tid
Chlordiazepoxide	Librium	5 – 10 mg tid
Chlorazepate	Tranxene	15 – 60 mg qd
Diazepam	Valium	2 – 10 mg tid
Flurazepam	Dalmane	15 – 30 mg qd hs
Halazepam	Paxipam	20 – 40 mg tid
Lorazepam	Ativan	2 – 6 mg qd
Oxazepam	Serax	15 – 30 mg tid
Prazepam	Centrax	20 – 60 mg qd
Temazepam	Restoril	30 mg qd
Trizaolam	Halcion	0.25 – 0.5 mg qd

should be monitored before and after administration of the medication. Because these drugs may impair physical and mental performance, clients should be warned not to operate a car or potentially dangerous machinery until the intensity of the drug response has been assessed. Clients should also be advised not to consume alcoholic beverages while receiving these drugs because of the combined depressant effects. Usual doses of these drugs should be reduced for elderly clients because they are more susceptible to drug-induced drowsiness, dizziness, and hypotension.

Sudden withdrawal of a drug after long periods of administration may worsen the neurotic state and precipitate withdrawal effects. Long-term administration may lead to the development of psychological dependence, tolerance, and possibly physical dependence.

SUMMARY

Conditions that cause altered patterns of relatedness include neurotic disorders and personality disorders. These alterations are usually the result of an altered sense of self in which the individual feels vulnerable, insecure, and inferior.

Clients suffering from neurotic patterns of relatedness have lost control of some aspect of their lives; they are frightened and prone to increasing anxiety. The anxiety is usually controlled by the development of behaviors that differ according to the type of neurotic reaction. The behaviors are the result of a compromise between unacceptable impulses and the forces that operate to repress those impulses. Neurotic conditions are classified as anxiety reactions, obsessive-compulsive reactions, post-traumatic stress reactions, phobic reactions, conversion reactions, dissociative reactions, and hypochondriacal reactions.

Personality disorders are lifelong behavior patterns that may be schizoid, compulsive, histrionic, antisocial, passive-aggressive/passive-dependent, or paranoid. Clients who suffer from altered personality patterns are comfortable with their altered relatedness and do not suffer from increased anxiety unless their particular style is threatened. Treatment for these conditions is difficult because clients rarely experience discomfort or a need for change.

Borderline clients have severe deficits in their capacities to love and to work. They are generally dissatisfied with life. Goal and limit setting are important aspects of treatment.

Review Questions

1. Contrast the clinical picture of client with a healthy sense of self with that of a client with an altered sense of self.

2. Explain the role of the unconscious and the ego in the development of anxiety disorders.

3. Compare and contrast neuroses and psychoses.

4. Identify the conflicts typical of the following types of disorders: anxiety disorders, obsessive-compulsive disorders, phobic disorders, conversion disorders, dissociative disorders.

5. Explain the influence of repression and conflict in the development of anxiety disorders.

6. What are the major nursing principles in the care of clients with anxiety disorders?

7. Describe two divergent approaches to helping clients with phobic disorders.

8. What are the major nursing principles in the care of clients with personality disorders?

9. Describe the major difference between anxiety disorders and personality disorders.

10. Discuss the personality deficits that are present in borderline clients.

References

American Psychiatric Association. 1981. *Diagnostic and Statistical Manual of Mental Disorders*, 3rd ed. Washington, D.C.: The Association.

Brody, J. E. 1983. Panic Attacks: The Terror Is Treatable. *The New York Times*, October 19.

Eisenhauer, L. A., and Gerald, M. D. 1984. *The Nurse's 1984–1985 Guide to Drug Therapy*. Englewood Cliffs, N.J.: Prentice-Hall.

Erikson, E. H. 1963. *Childhood and Society*. New York: W. W. Norton.

Feldman, M. P. 1977. *Criminal Behavior*. New York: John Wiley & Sons.

Freedman, A. M.; Kaplan, H. E.; and Sadock, B. J. 1976. *Modern Synopsis of Psychiatry II.* Baltimore: Williams & Wilkins.

Freud, S. 1955. Analysis of a Phobia in a Five-Year-Old Boy. In *Standard Edition of the Complete Psychological Works of Sigmund Freud,* vol. 10. London: Hogarth Press.

Greenberg, S. I. 1977. *Neurosis Is a Painful Style of Living.* New York: Signet Books.

Hofling, C. K., and Leininger, M. D. 1960. *Basic Psychiatric Concepts in Nursing.* Philadelphia: J. B. Lippincott.

Horney, K. 1945. *Our Inner Conflicts.* New York: W. W. Norton.

Horney, K. 1950. *Neuroses and Human Growth.* New York: W. W. Norton.

Kaplan, H. I.; Freedman, A. M.; and Sadock, B. J. 1980. *Comprehensive Textbook of Psychiatry III,* 3rd ed. Baltimore: Williams & Wilkins.

Luisada, P. V.; Peele, R.; and Pillard, E. A. 1974. The Hysterical Personality in Men. *American Journal of Psychiatry,* 131:518–522.

Masterson, J. F. 1976. *Psychotherapy of the Borderline Adult.* New York: Brunner/Mazel.

Mereness, D., and Karnosh, L. J. 1966. *Essentials of Psychiatric Nursing.* St. Louis: C. V. Mosby.

Parsons, T. 1951. *The Social System.* New York: Free Press.

Pollin, W. G.; Marlin, G.; Hoffer, A.; Stabeneau, J. R.; and Hrubee, Z. 1969. Psychopathology in 15,901 Pairs of Veteran Twins. *American Journal of Psychiatry,* 126:597.

Quitkin, F.; Rifkin, A.; and Klein, D. 1976. Neurologic Soft Signs in Schizophrenia and Character Disorders. *Archives of General Psychiatry,* 33:845.

Satterfield, J. H., and Centwell, D. P. 1972. Psychopharmacology in the Prevention of Antisocial and Delinquent Behaviors. *International Journal of Mental Health,* 1:227.

Sullivan, H. S. 1953. *The Interpersonal Theory of Psychiatry.* New York: W. W. Norton.

Wender, P. H.; Rosenthal, D.; Rainer, J. D.; Greenhill, L.; and Sarlin, M. B. 1976. Schizophrenics' Adoptive Parents. *Archives of General Psychiatry,* 33:845.

Ziarnowski, A. P. 1984. A Typical Crisis: Delayed Stress Reaction. In *Crisis Counseling,* ed. E. Janosik. Monterey, Calif.: Wadsworth.

Supplementary Readings

Adams, M. F. Posttraumatic Stress Disorder: An Inpatient Treatment Unit for Vietnam Veterans Who Had Traumatic Stress Disorder. *American Journal of Nursing,* 82 (1982):1704–1705.

Asarnow, J. R. Family Interaction and the Course of Adolescent Psychopathology. *Journal of Abnormal Child Psychology,* 10 (1982):427–441.

Barsky, A. J. Overview: Hypochondriasis, Bodily Complaints and Somatic Styles. *American Journal of Psychiatry,* 140 (1983):273–283.

Baskett, S. J. Differentiating Between Post Vietnam Syndrome and Preexisting Psychiatric Disorders. *Southern Medical Journal,* 76 (1983):988–990.

Beilman, B. D. Steps Toward Patient Acknowledgment of Psychosocial Factors. *Journal of Family Practice,* 15 (1982):1119–1126.

Berman, S. An Inpatient Program for Vietnam Combat Veterans in a VA Hospital. *Hospital and Community Psychiatry,* 33 (1982):919–922.

Blair, D. Neuroses and Character Disorders. *Journal of Geriatric Psychiatry,* 15 (1982):55–97.

xreen, H. J. Post Viet Nam Syndrome: A Critique. *Arizona Medicine,* 39 (1982):791–793.

Bursten, B. What If Antisocial Personality Is an Illness? *Bulletin of American Academy of Psychiatric Law,* 10 (1982):97–102.

Chambless, D. L., and Goldstein, A. J. *Agoraphobia. Multiple Perspectives on Theory and Treatment.* New York: John Wiley & Sons, 1982.

Charry, D. The Borderline Personality. *American Family Physician,* 27 (1983):195–202.

Chodoff, P. Therapy of Hysterical Personality Disorder. *Current Psychiatric Therapy,* 21 (1982):59–63.

Crook, T. Diagnosis and Treatment of Mixed Anxiety and Depression in the Elderly. *Journal of Clinical Psychiatry,* 43 (1982):35–43.

Deutsch, H. *Neuroses and Character Types.* New York: International Universities Press, 1965.

Drinka, G. F. *The Birth of Neurosis: Myth, Malady and the Victorians.* Philadelphia: W. B. Saunders, 1984.

Farberg, S. *The Magic Years.* New York: Charles Scribner's Sons, 1959.

Fenichel, O. *The Psychoanalytic Theory of Neuroses.* New York: W. W. Norton, 1943.

Friedman, D. Anxiety Disorders. *Journal of Family Practice,* 16 (1983):145–152.

Frosch, J. P. The Treatment of Antisocial and Borderline Personality Disorders. *Hospital and Community Psychiatry,* 34 (1983):243–248.

Furey, J. A. PTSD in Viet Nam Vets. *American Journal of Nursing,* 82 (1982):1694–1696.

Goldberg, R. L. Psychodynamics of Limit Setting with the Borderline Patient. *American Journal of Psychoanalysis,* 43 (1983):71–75.

Gossop, M. *Theories of Neuroses.* New York: Springer, 1981.

Gotti, R. Love and Neurotic Claims. *American Journal of Psychoanalysis,* 42 (1982):61–70.

Greenberg, W. C. The Multiple Personality. *Perspectives in Psychiatric Care,* 20 (1982):100–104.

Hagerty, B. K. Obsessive-Compulsive Behavior: An Overview of Four Psychological Frameworks. *Journal of Psychiatric Nursing* (1981):37–39.

Hickey, B. A. Transitional Relationships and Engaging the Regressed Borderline Client. *Journal of Psychosocial Nursing and Mental Health Services,* 21 (1983):26–30.

Johansen, K. H. The Patients with Chronic Character Pathology on a Hospital Inpatient Unit. *Hospital and Community Psychiatry,* 34 (1983):842–846.

Jorn, N. Repression in a Case of Multiple Personality Disorder. *Perspectives of Psychiatric Care,* 20 (1982): 105–110.

Kaminsky, M. J. Hysterical and Obsessional Features in Patients with Briquets Syndrome. *Psychological Medicine,* 13 (1983):111–120.

Kirk, J. W. Behavioral Treatment of Obsessional and Compulsive Patients in Routine Clinical Practice. *Behavior and Research Therapy*, 21 (1983):57–62.

Lesse, S. The Relationship of Anxiety to Depression. *American Journal of Psychotherapy*, 36 (1982):332–340.

May, R. *The Meaning of Anxiety*. New York: Ronald Press, 1950.

Modlin, H. C. The Antisocial Personality. *Bulletin of the Menninger Clinic*, 47 (1983):129–144.

Norman, E. M. PTSD: The Victims Who Survived. *American Journal of Nursing*, 82 (1982):1696–1698.

Papiasveli, E. Residential Therapeutic Community for Neurotics. *International Journal of Group Psychotherapy*, 33 (1983):387–395.

Plath, S. *The Bell Jar*. New York: Harper & Row, 1971.

Roy, R. E. Alcohol Misuse and PTSD. *Journal of Studies on Alcohol*, 44 (1983):198–202.

Runck, B. Research Is Changing Views on Obsessive-Compulsive Disorders. *Hospital and Community Psychiatry*, 34 (1983):597–598.

Russell, G. F. *The Neuroses and Personality Disorders*. Cambridge, Mass.: Cambridge University Press, 1984.

Sangal, R. Chronic Anxiety and Social Adjustment. *Comprehensive Psychiatry*, 24 (1983):75–78.

Sargent, J. The Family and Childhood Psychosomatic Disorders. *General Hospital Psychiatry*, 5 (1983):41–48.

Serban, G. *The Tyranny of Magical Thinking: The Child's World of Belief and Adult Neuroses*. New York: Dutton, 1982.

Shader, R. L. Panic Disorders: Current Perspectives. *Journal of Clinical Psychopharmacology*, 2 (1982):2–10.

Shapiro, D. *Neurotic Styles*. New York: Basic Books, 1965.

Sierles, F. S. PTSD and Concurrent Psychiatric Illness. *American Journal of Psychiatry*, 140 (1983):1177–1179.

Skeketee, G. Recent Advances in the Behavioral Treatment of Obsessive Compulsives. *Archives of General Psychiatry*, 39 (1982):1365–1371.

Stravynski, A. Social Skills Problems in Neurotic Outpatients. *Archives of General Psychiatry*, 39 (1982):1378–1385.

Sultana, M. Efficacy of Relaxation Therapy in the Treatment of Neurotic Adults. *Journal of Research in Social Health*, 103 (1983):97–98.

Summers, F. Neurotic Symptoms in the Post Acute Phase of Schizophrenia. *Journal of Nervous and Mental Disorders*, 171 (1983):216–221.

Tennant, C. Female Vulnerability to Neuroses: The Influence of Social Roles. *Australian New Zealand Journal of Psychiatry*, 16 (1982):135–140.

Tennant, C. The Relation of Childhood Separation Experiences to Adult Depressive and Anxiety States. *British Journal of Psychiatry*, 141 (1982):475–482.

Thigpen, C. H., and Cleckley, H. M. *The Three Faces of Eve*. New York: McGraw-Hill, 1957.

Tyrer, P. The Relationship Between Neuroses and Personality Disorders. *British Journal of Psychiatry*, 142 (1983):404–408.

Vanderkolk, B. A. Psychopharmacological Issues in PTSD. *Hospital and Community Psychiatry*, 34 (1983):683–684.

216

DRUG TERMINOLOGY
NURSING ATTITUDES
USE AND ABUSE OF ALCOHOL
CLASSIFICATION AND DIAGNOSIS OF ALCOHOLISM
CAUSES OF ALCOHOLISM
Physiological Theories
Psychological Theories
Sociocultural Theories
Learning Theory
PHYSIOLOGICAL CONSEQUENCES OF ALCOHOL
ABUSE
Alcohol and the Brain
Alcohol and the Liver
Alcohol and the Gastrointestinal Tract
Alcohol and the Heart
Alcohol and the Muscles
Alcohol and the Endocrine System
Alcohol and the Reproductive System
THE PROGRESSION OF ALCOHOLISM
ALCOHOLISM AND THE NURSING PROCESS
Acute Stage
Rehabilitation Stage

USE AND ABUSE OF DRUGS
COMMONLY ABUSED DRUGS
Stimulants
Opiates and Related Analgesics
Depressants
Cannabinols
Hallucinogens
Inhalants
CAUSES OF DRUG ABUSE
The Role of the Host
The Role of the Environment
The Role of the Agent
PHYSIOLOGICAL CONSEQUENCES OF DRUG ABUSE
Circulatory and Respiratory Complications
Hepatic Dysfunction
Gastrointestinal Disturbances
Skin Complications
Muscular Disorders
Miscellaneous Complications
DRUG ABUSE AND THE NURSING PROCESS
Acute Stage
Rehabilitation Stage

C H A P T E R

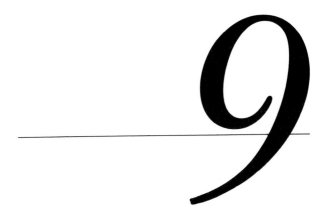

9

Altered Patterns of Societal Adjustment

Learning Objectives

After reading this chapter, the student should be able to:

1. Trace the psychological, physiological, and social variables affecting substance abuse.

2. Discuss the psychological, physiological, and social consequences of alcoholism and drug abuse.

3. Discuss approaches used in the acute toxic phases of alcoholism and drug abuse.

4. Discuss approaches used in long-term rehabilitative phases of maladaption caused by alcoholism and drug abuse.

5. Analyze the role of the professional nurse during various aspects of care for the substance abuser, stressing the importance of objectivity and consistency.

Overview

Throughout history, members of virtually every society have used drugs to change their mood, thought, and feeling. Within these societies, there have always been individuals who digressed from accepted social customs for use of these potent drugs, employing them as a means of coping with the stresses and problems of existence and rendering them at odds with society's norms and values. As a result, such individuals have developed altered patterns of societal adjustment.

Any drug, whether obtained legally or illegally, is subject to misuse. The term "substance abuse" is usually used in connection with drugs that dras-tically alter levels of consciousness. This chapter describes various factors relating to substance abuse and discusses its causes, treatment, and complications, as well as the application of nursing measures that alleviate substance abuse problems. Because of its widespread use and acceptability in society, alcohol is treated separately from other commonly abused drugs. However, it is important to remember that alcohol is indeed a drug that changes mood, feelings, and thoughts, despite the assertion of some alcoholic clients that they have never used "drugs" in their lives.

*Oh God! That men should put an enemy into their mouths
to steal away their brains; that we should with joy,
pleasure, revel, and applause transform
ourselves into beasts.*
WILLIAM SHAKESPEARE

219

DRUG TERMINOLOGY

The term *drug abuse* refers to the use of any drug in a manner that is different from the approved medical or social pattern in a given culture (Jaffee, 1983). Because this definition is largely a social one, it is not surprising that there are varying opinions of what constitutes abuse. For example, using a barbiturate to produce sleep is socially acceptable, but using the same drug to produce a feeling of tranquillity in a social situation is considered a form of abuse. Similarly, using opiates to relieve pain is acceptable but using them to produce euphoria is not.

Nonmedical drug use is a term that, although nonjudgmental, is so general that it includes everything from occasional drug use to compulsive drug use. Nonmedical use encompasses experimental drug use motivated by curiosity or by conformity to peer pressure, the casual or recreational use of a drug for its pleasurable effects, the circumstantial use of drugs (such as of amphetamines to stay awake while studying), and the intensive use of drugs to an extent commonly thought of as drug abuse.

Compulsive drug use usually results when individuals develop a dependence (psychological or physical) on a drug. Such individuals have less flexibility in their behavior toward a particular drug. Therefore, they continue to take the drug despite adverse medical and social consequences, and they behave as if they need the drug in order to continue to function. If their drug of choice is difficult to obtain, these users become preoccupied with ways to ensure their supply of the drug.

Compulsive drug use is commonly, but not necessarily, associated with the development of tolerance and physical dependence. *Tolerance* occurs when increasingly large doses must be taken to obtain the same effects experienced with original, smaller doses. *Physical dependence* refers to an altered physiological state produced by repeated use of the drug, necessitating continued use to prevent withdrawal effects. *Withdrawal symptoms* are physical disturbances that result when the person stops taking the drug. Withdrawal symptoms are characterized by rebound effects in the same physiological systems initially depressed by the drug. For example, amphetamines act to alleviate fatigue, suppress appetite, and elevate mood; thus, amphetamine withdrawal brings a reactive lack of energy, hyperphagia, and depression.

Psychological dependence can occur with all drugs of abuse. With psychological dependence, the user feels he needs the drug in order to reach a maximum level of functioning or well-being, regardless of whether he is physically dependent on the drug.

"Addiction" was previously associated almost exclusively with drug use but is now commonly applied to a variety of behaviors, from playing tennis to reading *The New York Times*. In this chapter, *addiction* refers to a behavioral pattern of drug use characterized by an overwhelming preoccupation with the compulsive use of a drug, the securing of a supply, and a tendency to readdiction after withdrawal. "Addiction" cannot be used interchangeably with "physical dependence" because it is possible to be physically dependent on a drug without being addicted. For example, it is possible to experience withdrawal symptoms after therapeutic doses of morphine given four times a day for as short a period as two to three days. Yet people in this situation are not addicted to the drug and have no

How solemn and beautiful is the thought that the earliest pioneer of civilization, the van-leader of civilization, is never the steamboat, never the railroad, never the newspaper, never the sabbath school teacher, never the missionary—but always whiskey.

MARK TWAIN

220

psychological craving once the physical condition that dictated the use of morphine is alleviated. Similarly, a large number of men who served in Viet Nam used heroin regularly, but only about half became addicted; the rest simply stopped using heroin without any special treatment.

Cross-addiction refers to the ability of one drug to suppress the manifestations of physical dependence produced by another drug and to maintain the physically dependent state. For example, alcohol can suppress the symptoms of barbiturate withdrawal and barbiturates can suppress the effects of alcohol withdrawal. Many alcoholics attempt to maintain sobriety by using marijuana, Librium, or Valium as a substitute for alcohol.

NURSING ATTITUDES

Nurses working with clients who are alcohol and drug abusers need to be aware of their own attitudes toward addiction and addicts. As the roles and functions of nurses expand, they will have increased exposure to such clients. Stereotyped pictures of the addict have influenced public attitudes for many years. Nurses, although they have chosen a helping profession, are not immune to such stereotypes. Clients are able to intuitively sense negative attitudes and an air of moral superiority on the part of nurses. A therapeutic atmosphere can be established only if nurses are nonjudgmental and accepting of clients. This accepting attitude is not possible unless nurses examine their own attitudes and values regarding drug abuse and drug abusers.

Alcohol and drug abusers are extremely difficult clients to work with. Several factors contribute

to this difficulty. Drug abusers tend to be skilled at manipulation, and they use flattery and ingenuity to get their needs met. The highly seductive tactics of the drug addict can be ego-enhancing for the nurse, who then becomes discouraged when seductiveness is withdrawn or demands become insatiable. Intermittent relapse may be a frustration for nurses working with a "revolving door" client who seems unable to change or to utilize treatment. Such behavior often causes nurses to become disappointed and angry. Although most nurses profess to believe that addiction is a disease, many still carry an underlying attitude that drug-abusing clients could stop their behavior if only they persevered. However, this attitude is as unrealistic as expecting clients to stop having diabetes or cancer if only they choose to do so.

Dealing with addictive clients can be a challenging and rewarding experience for caregivers who are able to monitor their own feelings and accept their clients as people in need of help. Frustration can be kept to a minimum by maintaining realistic expectations and by goal setting. The nurse must realize that the client may have been an abuser for years; expecting to reverse the process within a short time would not only be frustrating for the nurse but would also lead to inadequate treatment planning for the client.

USE AND ABUSE OF ALCOHOL

Alcohol has been around for a long time—evidence of wine and beer drinking has been found in archeologic records of the oldest civilizations. Early on, humans learned that fruits and grains could be

PREVALENCE OF ALCOHOL USE AND ABUSE

Alcoholism is a problem of enormous proportion. Over two-thirds of Americans drink more than just occasionally, with the male-female ratio approximately 4 to 3. The peak years of alcohol consumption are between the ages of sixteen and twenty-five, gradually decreasing thereafter. At any stage of life, the chances of being a drinker (not necessarily an alcoholic) are highest for people with greater education and higher socioeconomic status. The average American adult consumes 2.7 gallons of absolute alcohol per year, spending billions of dollars that represent almost 3 percent of total personal expenditures.

The highest rates of alcoholism are seen in men ages thirty to fifty and among those with lower socioeconomic status and the least education. However, it is important to recognize that alcoholism is prevalent in all socioeconomic classes, at all ages, in all religions, and among both sexes throughout the country (Schuckit, 1979).

fermented to become beverages with mood-changing effects. Alcohol soon became an integral part of religious rituals and offerings. It replaced fluids such as water or milk and honey because it was more suitable for evoking the moods of release, mystification, and ecstasy that were essential for communicating with invisible powers. The role of alcohol in religious ceremonies tended to give an aura of sanctity and solemnity to its use, and it became mandatory in worship, magic, and festivals.

The attitudes of Americans toward alcohol abuse have been ambiguous (Smithers Foundation, 1968). The alcoholic person has often been an object of scorn and derision. In religious thinking, the drinker has been considered a sinner; in social and economic thinking, the problem drinker has been considered useless and hopeless.

Even in the early days of the nation, widespread use of alcohol caused concern to civic leaders. In particular, Benjamin Rush, a signer of the Declaration of Independence and surgeon general of the Continental Army, was the first American to call the intemperate use of spirits a "disease." Worries about the effects of alcohol abuse laid the foundation for the temperance movement, which began around 1850 and was led by the Antisaloon League and the Women's Christian Temperance Union (WCTU).

221

Their campaign resulted in the 18th Amendment to the Constitution, adopted in 1919, which imposed nationwide Prohibition.

Paradoxically, the era of Prohibition made drinking fashionable. Speakeasies were open to men and women, and for the first time women could drink hard spirits in public places. After thirteen years of a national trial, Prohibition was repealed. One reason for the success of the repeal movement may have been a growing feeling among Americans that they had the right to choose their own behavior. In the years since Prohibition, the proportion of drinkers has steadily increased, but attitudes toward alcoholic individuals have been slow to change.

During the 1940s, a small group of alcoholics who openly admitted to their problem joined together in an effort to remain sober and to help others do so. This program, centering around the concept that alcoholism is a disease, became known as Alcoholics Anonymous (AA). Since then, AA has grown to include over 12,000 groups functioning in ninety countries (Smithers Foundation, 1968).

Also during the 1940s, medical and scientific articles dealing with the idea of alcoholism as a disease began to appear with regularity in newspapers and magazines. Local committees composed of private citizens and professional people were formed to discuss the problems of alcoholism. These committees later became the National Council on Alcoholism. By the 1960s the concept of alcoholism as an illness had been accepted by many professionals. E. M. Jellinek, coordinator of the Yale Center of Alcohol Studies, conducted extensive research on alcoholism and published his book *The Disease Concept of Alcoholism* (1960), which has become a classic

Thanks be to God, since my leaving the drinking of wine, I do find myself much better, and do mind my business better, and do spend less money, and less time lost in idle company.
SAMUEL PEPYS, JANUARY 26, 1662

reference in the field. His classification system for alcoholism is discussed in the following section.

CLASSIFICATION AND DIAGNOSIS OF ALCOHOLISM

Opinions about what constitutes the disease alcoholism are diverse. One of the most widely accepted definitions is that given by the National Institute of Mental Health (1968):

Alcoholism is a chronic disease, a disorder of behavior characterized by the repeated drinking of alcoholic beverages to an extent that exceeds customary dietary use or ordinary compliance with the social drinking customs of the community, and which interferes with the drinker's health, interpersonal relations, or economic functioning.

Jellinek (1960) divided people suffering from alcoholism into five major categories, using letters of the Greek alphabet for labeling purposes:

1. *Alpha alcoholism*—A purely psychological continual dependence or reliance on the effect of alcohol to relieve bodily or emotional pain. Undisciplined drinking—that which does not follow society's rules regarding time, place, and amount—occurs but does not lead to loss of control or inability to abstain. The damage caused by this type of alcoholism may be restricted to disturbance of interpersonal relationships, interference with family finances, absenteeism from work, and decreased productivity, but there are no signs of a progressive process or withdrawal symptoms. This type may develop into the more severe (gamma type) alcoholism, but frequently the drinker remains at the alpha

level for thirty to forty years without signs of progression. *Problem drinking* is another term applied to the alpha alcoholic. This category of alcoholic is the most likely to be cited for driving while intoxicated. His drinking is thought to be a symptom of another underlying disorder.

2. *Beta alcoholism*—A type of alcoholism in which complications such as polyneuropathy, gastritis, and cirrhosis may occur without either physical or psychological dependence upon alcohol. The incentive to drink is usually influenced by the customs of the social group or by peer pressure. Although withdrawal symptoms do not occur, nutritional deficiencies, financial difficulties, and lowered productivity are common.

3. *Gamma alcoholism*—Involves tissue tolerance to alcohol, adaptive cell metabolism, withdrawal symptoms and craving (physical dependence), and loss of control. There is a progression from psychological to physical dependence, and there are marked behavior changes. This type is recognized by some groups (AA included) as "true" alcoholism, since loss of control and craving are dominant criteria.

4. *Delta alcoholism*—Has all the characteristics of gamma alcoholism except loss of control. In its place is an inability to abstain. The ability to control the amount of intake on any given occasion remains intact, but the person cannot abstain for even a day without the beginnings of withdrawal.

5. *Epsilon alcoholism*—Periodic alcoholism, commonly known as "binge" drinking. Frequent periodic bouts can cause physical, psychological, and social damage.

In another type of classification, Freedman,

DSM-III AXIS I
DIAGNOSTIC CLASSIFICATION

305.0x Alcohol abuse

303.9x Alcohol dependence (alcoholism)

Code in fifth digit: 1 = continuous, 2 = episodic, 3 = in remission, 0 = unspecified.

Kaplan, and Sadock (1976) described alcoholics as either reactive or addictive. The *reactive alcoholic* becomes preoccupied with alcohol whenever he feels overwhelmed by external stress. In some cases, temporary relief is all that is needed, but in other cases depression deepens and greater amounts of alcohol are consumed. Physiological dependence may then occur, and the person continues to drink to prevent withdrawal symptoms. Premorbid adjustment of reactive persons has usually been satisfactory. In contrast, the *addictive alcoholic* shows gross personality disturbances prior to becoming alcoholic, manifested by inadequate and unsatisfactory interpersonal relationships. Such persons are often preoccupied with alcohol from the first experience; they drink without apparent reason and drink until they are unable to continue.

Other typologies, such as "problem drinker" versus "alcoholic" and "prealcoholic" versus "clinical alcoholic" (Barnes, 1980), have also been used, but those that we have described here are adequate to show the diversity involved in definition and classification of alcoholism. In this chapter the term "alcoholic" is used to describe those persons who have altered patterns of societal adjustment as a result of alcohol abuse. It should be kept in mind, however, that the label "alcoholic" should not be used pejoratively or as a means of stereotyping.

DSM-III classifies alcohol problems under substance abuse disorders. *Abuse* is defined as a pattern of pathologic use for at least one month *and* impairment in social or occupational functioning. Dependence indicates the presence of tolerance or withdrawal symptoms.

All five DSM-III axes are important in the nursing approach to the alcoholic client. Alcoholism causes clinical symptoms that are not attributable to any other psychiatric diagnosis. Personality disorders frequently accompany alcoholism. Axis V can be particularly useful in defining variations in functioning; for example, the client may currently be drinking heavily but has had long periods of sobriety during which she was functioning adequately.

CAUSES OF ALCOHOLISM

Physiological Theories

Alcoholism has long been known to be prevalent in certain families. The Greek philosopher Aristotle declared that drunken women brought forth children like themselves. During the so-called gin epidemic in eighteenth-century England, the notion that alcoholism is not only familial but hereditary enjoyed a sizeable acceptance, causing many people to denounce the consumption of spirits on the grounds that it engendered alcoholism in the offspring (Warner and Rosett, 1975). Later explanations favored the idea of genetic mutation—that exposure of the sperm or ovum to alcohol caused changes leading to the development of alcoholism in offspring. Eventually, the heredity and mutation theories were discarded in favor of the idea that alcoholism was the result of poor upbringing and crowded living conditions. In the past few years, however, the possibility of heredity as a factor in alcoholism has received renewed attention.

Family studies have consistently found a high prevalence of alcoholism among relatives of alcoholics. While surveys of the general population indicate that 3 to 5 percent of men and 0.1 to 1 percent of women are alcoholic, studies of families show a rate of 25 percent among male relatives of alcoholics and 5 to 10 percent among female relatives (Goodwin, 1979).

Twin studies have demonstrated that identical twins share a similar incidence of alcoholism more often than fraternal twins. Other research has focused on individuals separated from their alcoholic biological parents soon after birth and raised by nonalcoholic adoptive parents. Such studies have shown that sons of alcoholics are about four times more likely to suffer from alcoholism than sons of nonalcoholics, even when exposure to the parents' alcoholism is limited to the first few weeks of life (Goodwin, 1982). Although studies continue to indicate a familial relationship in alcoholism, more research is needed to isolate biological from environmental factors before the question of how alcoholism is transmitted can be addressed.

In some cases, biological factors are thought to protect individuals against the development of alcoholism (Mendelson and Mello, 1979). Many Orientals, for example, have an enhanced sensitivity to the effects of alcohol; that is, they experience flushing, abdominal discomfort, muscle weakness, dizziness, tachycardia, and decreased blood pressure with even small doses of alcohol. Such sensitivity may guard the individual from progressing to alcoholism because the uncomfortable effects are felt sooner, before physiological damage can be done. More research is needed to determine whether there really are physiological differences in reaction to alcohol and what these differences might be.

Alcoholism is more prevalent in certain racial and ethnic groups than in the general population; it has therefore been suggested that people in these groups metabolize alcohol differently (Mendelson and Mello, 1979). Results from various studies have been conflicting; varying rates of alcoholism have been found in all races and ethnic groups. What seems to be more important than ethnic variables is a past history of alcohol intake. Heavy drinkers have a significantly higher rate of alcohol metabolism than people who abstain or drink occasionally. Because alcohol consumption increases this metabolism, the pattern of alcohol ingestion appears to be more important than racial or ethnic characteristics in the regulation of alcohol metabolism.

Psychological Theories

Psychological approaches to alcoholism generally assume that it is a symptom of an underlying personality or emotional disorder.

PSYCHOANALYTIC THEORY Freud thought that al-cohol allowed the expression of repressed urges because of its ability to release inhibitions. He hypothesized that these repressed tendencies—including oral dependency and latent homosexuality—developed in childhood because of problems in the parent-child relationship (McCord and McCord, 1960). Otto Fenichel (1945) maintained that alcoholics were passive, dependent, narcissistic people who used their mouths as a primary means of achieving gratification. Karl Menninger (1938) placed greater emphasis on the self-destructive tendencies of alcohol abuse, asserting that people abused alcohol for oral gratification and self-punishment because of anger against their parents, thereby accomplishing a symbolic revenge. Others have postulated that alcoholism is a striving for power to compensate for feelings of inferiority and to bolster feelings of self-esteem (McCord and McCord, 1960). Psychoanalytic theories are difficult to test and are therefore inconclusive, but these ideas have continued to be used in the treatment of alcoholic clients, often with limited success.

PERSONALITY TRAIT THEORIES The search for an "alcoholic personality" has been the object of much research but has failed to find a single personality structure that can be described as *the* alcoholic personality. What has been identified instead are a variety of personality patterns or traits that have been associated with alcohol abuse. The most significant of these are (Burkhalter, 1975):

1. *Dependency-independency.* A predominant personality characteristic of the alcoholic is a conflict between the need to be dependent and the need to be independent, with dependency being most apparent. Because the alcoholic is unable to confront the conflict, he represses either his independent or his dependent needs to avoid the conflict. The desire to assert the repressed needs serves only to increase the desire for relief, which alcohol can provide. Since the conflict remains unresolved, a pattern becomes established and the need for alcohol is maintained.

2. *Anger and frustration.* Anger and frustration are often the result of strong dependency needs. Anger often arises from the inability to express feelings of worthlessness, failure, and inadequacy; alcohol allows the expression of this anger and serves as an excuse for the angry behavior. Also characteristic of many alcoholics is a low tolerance for frustration. The frustration caused by the inability to cope with daily stress is often the stimulus that leads to continued drinking.

3. *Feelings of omnipotence.* The desire to feel powerful and in control of one's destiny is expressed through the alcoholic's search for omnipotence.

The feelings of power that can be stimulated by alcohol help to momentarily ease feelings of frustration, guilt, and self-denigration. The basic need to feel important, valued, and respected is in conflict with the alcoholic's behavior; when she begins to sober up and realize this inconsistency, she experiences greater feelings of failure, which act as a motivator to resume drinking.

4. *Depression.* The depression experienced by many alcoholics can be viewed as an initial stimulus to drink (to self-medicate the depression), as the result of excessive drinking when the alcoholic realizes that his relationships with others are changing, or as a reason to continue drinking to decrease and mask the depression. Unfortunately, using alcohol for the relief of depression is self-reinforcing; it fosters the need for relief that alcohol brings, but drinking only increases the depression.

5. *Defense mechanisms.* Denial (and the rationalizations and projections associated with it) is a major defense mechanism used by alcoholics. Most deny that they have a problem controlling their alcohol intake, and many claim that they are not drinking at all. When they begin to suspect that their behavior is changing, they will invent reasons for the behavior and will project blame for their actions onto others who, in their minds, have driven them to drink. These mechanisms allow the alcoholic to continue to drink and to justify the drinking.

Various psychological tests that have been used in an attempt to isolate alcoholic personality traits have met with mixed results. The major difficulty with personality trait theories is that it is still unknown whether the personality traits predate the onset of alcoholism or are a consequence of the alcoholism.

Sociocultural Theories

The consumption of alcohol is a common occurrence in almost every culture and society. However, the *amount* used is determined by the basic security within each culture (Horton, 1959). Culture and social organization can influence rates of alcoholism in three ways: (1) the degree to which the culture operates to bring about tension, (2) the attitudes toward drinking that the culture produces, and (3) the degree to which that culture provides a substitute means of satisfaction (Bales, 1959).

Each culture establishes norms and regulations for the use of alcohol. Most cultural norms are based on the ideas that (1) alcohol is a drug that causes loss of control, (2) people are permitted to relax social and personal control under the influence of alcohol, and (3) alcohol abuse is associated with undesirable behavior (Jessor et al., 1968). Through a society's reactions to their drinking behavior, alcoholics be-

come publicly labeled as deviants and are forced by that society to live a deviant lifestyle. Merton (1957) proposed that the alcoholic's deviant behavior is brought about because of the discrepancy between prevalent goals in a society and the means of achieving these goals; for example, the American Dream of success and happiness is, in reality, far out of reach for many people. Failure to achieve this dream is a reality harsh enough to cause some individuals to escape by drinking to excess.

Learning Theory

From the social learning point of view, psychological functioning can be best understood in terms of a continuous, reciprocal interaction between behavior and the conditions of the environment. In this perspective, the behaviors of alcohol use and misuse are considered to be socially acquired through a variety of methods, including vicarious learning, peer and parental modeling, social reinforcement, and the anticipated effects of alcohol as a tension-reducing agent (Donovan and Marlatt, 1980). Learning theorists see alcohol ingestion as a reflex response aimed at reducing fear or anxiety. Drinking alcohol reduces tension and replaces this unpleasant feeling with sensations of well-being. Although the pain and discomfort experienced as the result of long-term drinking should appear to serve as punishment and as a deterrent to drinking, the immediate effect of drinking is pleasurable. The alcoholic goes for the short-term relief, not thinking of the long-term consequences.

Because finding a single cause for alcoholism appears to be unrealistic, most current practitioners use a multifaceted approach to this problem. More research is needed to gain a better understanding of the causes of alcoholism, so that better and more specific treatment interventions can be developed.

PHYSIOLOGICAL CONSEQUENCES OF ALCOHOL ABUSE

Heavy alcohol use has been implicated, either directly or indirectly, in a variety of illnesses. Alcoholics are subject to an exceptionally high rate of illness and death, with their life span being reduced by as much as ten to twelve years as compared with the general population. Not only do alcohol abuse and alcoholism contribute to many pathologic conditions, they complicate other illnesses that alcoholics may incur. Many of these alcohol-related conditions can be alleviated or reversed with appropriate treatment.

Alcohol and the Brain

Alcohol produces several syndromes that are the result of damage to brain cells or of the release of long-standing personality disturbances.

Blackouts occur frequently with excessive alcohol use and are an early sign of alcoholism. A person who experiences a blackout cannot remember his activities during a period of time, yet to those around him he appeared outwardly normal during the blackout period. Most frequently, the person cannot remember an evening of drinking the next day; however, blackouts can extend for longer periods of time. Some alcoholics have traveled across the country in a blackout state, not being able to recall any of the journey and finding themselves in a different place several weeks later. The mechanism of blackouts is unclear; explanations range from drug-induced amnesia, to a dissociative reaction, to a means of sustaining a psychological defense.

Pathologic intoxication is a state of agitation and altered consciousness that has a dramatic and sudden onset. Increasing anxiety, aggressiveness, and rage may be accompanied by confusion, disorientation, delusions, and hallucinations. Suicide attempts are common. This state may last from a few moments to a day or more and ends with a long period of sleep. Persons who experience such states may have a high level of anxiety and tension; alcohol provides loss of control and release of aggression.

Delirium tremens (DTs) is an acute psychotic state that follows cessation of drinking. The onset is usually 24 to 72 hours following the last drink. The delirium is usually preceded by restlessness, irritability, tremulousness, and disturbed sleep. Confusion and disorientation as to time and place are common. Other characteristics include visual hallucinations of spiders and snakes, severe agitation, fever, sweating, tachycardia, tachypnea, and seizure activity.

Acute alcoholic hallucinosis usually follows a long drinking bout. In contrast to the visual hallucinations of delirium tremens, this syndrome is characterized by auditory hallucinations, usually of a threatening nature. The alcoholic is still oriented to time and place and fits the hallucinations into her real environment, creating an elaborate delusional system. After recovery, the person can recall the events and feelings.

Wernicke's syndrome is characterized by clouding of consciousness and paralysis of eye nerves. It is associated with severe deficiency of Vitamin B_1, which occurs because the alcoholic is malnourished. Delirium, memory loss, confabulation, apathy, and ataxia result from neuronal and capillary lesions in the gray matter of the brain stem and in structures in the third and fourth ventricles.

Korsakoff's syndrome is characterized by amnesia, falsification of memory, disorientation to time and place, and peripheral neuropathy. It is mainly the result of a deficiency of thiamine and niacin. Memory loss is progressive. A superficial mood of light-heartedness is common.

Alcoholic paranoia is characterized by delusions of jealousy, suspicion, and distrust. Projection is intense. Because alcohol use weakens repression, forbidden impulses may arise that are defended against by an elaborate delusional system. Prognosis is guarded as symptoms frequently reoccur after treatment.

Alcohol and the Liver

Since the liver is the organ involved with processing alcohol in the body, it is often the most seriously affected by heavy alcohol use. Alcohol does not require digestion but passes directly into the bloodstream through the stomach or intestinal walls. As the alcohol travels through the liver, it is acted upon by enzymes that begin the process of changing alcohol into acetaldehyde. The acetaldehyde then breaks down into acetate (which can be used for energy), carbon dioxide, and water. A small part of the alcohol (10 percent) is eliminated by the kidneys, lungs, and sweat glands. Because the majority of alcohol is processed by the liver and there is no mechanism to adjust the rate of metabolism, the liver can be severely damaged by alcohol. Blood lactic acid is increased, which slows the excretion of uric acid by the kidneys and may give rise to symptoms of gout (Leiber et al., 1962). In addition, red blood cells in the capillaries tend to clump, which may result in inefficient oxygen transport to body cells (Moskow, Pennington, and Knisely, 1968).

Alcohol metabolism releases excess hydrogen in the liver, which inhibits certain metabolic functions important to producing energy. Energy is produced by burning hydrogen rather than fatty acids, and the unburned fats become deposited in the liver. This accumulation of fat ("fatty liver") is the first liver dysfunction caused by alcohol. It has few consequences and is usually reversible if alcohol intake stops.

Alcohol hepatitis is an inflammatory liver disorder that usually follows years of heavy alcohol abuse. It is characterized by fever, increased white blood cell count, pain in the upper abdomen, and jaundice. While it may recede if drinking stops, it often progresses to cirrhosis despite decreased intake.

Alcoholic cirrhosis, which occurs in about 10 percent of alcoholics, is a scarring of the liver. The scarring of the small veins in the liver causes narrowing and distortion of liver tissue by impairing circulation, which in turn leads to hypertension in the veins feeding the liver, often seen as esophageal varicies. If drinking continues, the person may die from hepatic failure or as the result of hemorrhage from portal hypertension. In some cases cancer of the liver may develop.

Alcohol and the Gastrointestinal Tract

The effects of alcohol on parts of the gastrointestinal system other than the liver have not been studied as extensively, but it is known that alcohol stimulates acid production in the stomach, which damages the stomach lining and causes gastritis and gastric ulcers. Malabsorption of vitamins such as thiamine, folic acid, and vitamin B_{12} may occur in the small intestine. Alcoholism is also associated with pancreatitis and pancreatic insufficiency.

Malnutrition is a common disorder in alcoholics because the alcohol itself represents a source of calories, reducing the appetite for food to fulfill caloric needs. Because alcoholic beverages provide "empty calories," the drinker has a deficient intake of protein, vitamins, minerals, and other nutrients. In addition, heavy alcohol intake can interfere with the process of food digestion and absorption.

Alcohol and the Heart

Long-term alcohol abuse can lead to *alcoholic cardiomyopathy*, with slow or sudden onset of left- and right-sided congestive failure. Manifestations include an enlarged heart, distended neck veins, narrow pulse pressure, elevated diastolic pressure, and peripheral edema. Significant EKG changes occur, tachycardia is common, and there may be episodes of atrial fibrillation.

Alcohol and the Muscles

Alcohol use affects the muscle system in three forms: subclinical myopathy, acute alcoholic myopathy, and clinical alcoholic myopathy. In the subclinical variety, there is an increase in the enzyme creatine phosphokinase (CPK) in the blood serum and a diminished rise of lactic acid in the blood after ischemic exercise. Acute myopathy is characterized by episodes of sudden muscle cramps in the extremities. The most severe form brings myoglobinuria, a concentration of muscle pigment in the urine; it is manifested by severe, painful swelling of involved muscles and by pronounced weakness. If alcohol use is discontinued, recovery usually follows, but the myoglobinuria may precipitate renal failure. With a history of prolonged alcoholism, chronic myopathy may develop, bringing weakness and atrophy, particularly to the muscles of the legs.

Alcohol and the Endocrine System

When alcohol is ingested repeatedly, the sensitive endocrine system is forced to adapt to maintain the body's internal balance. Although experimental data have been inconclusive, alcohol appears to affect the hypothalamic-pituitary-adrenal axis, causing adrenocortical insufficiency. It may also affect aldosterone, which induces retention of sodium, potassium, and chloride and increases the excretion of catecholamines. Alcohol affects urinary excretion by inhibiting the antidiuretic hormone of the pituitary gland.

Researchers have noted similarities between the symptoms of alcoholic patients and patients with endocrine disorders. It has therefore been suggested that failure of the endocrines may be a cause of alcoholism. However, cause and effect can be confused when studying people who already have alcoholism, and conflicting research results leave this theory open to question (U. S. Department of Heath, Education and Welfare).

Alcohol and the Reproductive System

The male alcoholic may experience erection problems that can become permanent if alcohol intake is excessive. Sexual functioning will usually return with abstinence.

Infants of alcoholic women are subject to various birth defects, now grouped as *fetal alcohol syndrome*. This syndrome is manifested by craniofacial, extremity, and cardiovascular defects that are associated with prenatal growth deficiencies and delayed development.

THE PROGRESSION OF ALCOHOLISM

Jellinek (1977) proposed the most widely accepted model of the progression of alcoholism, which is described in Table 9-1. More recently, researchers have begun to recognize the multifaceted aspects of alcoholism and have determined that not all alcoholic behavior follows this course. According to Albrecht (1973), drinking behavior is learned in the socialization process. Most people in the United States learn to drink, but not everyone learns to be a problem drinker. Problem drinking is a behavior that takes time to learn and needs to be supported by attitudes that permit drinking and an environment that supports heavy drinking. Attitudes and reinforcers in the environment are in turn affected by the drinker's cultural values, age, sex, socioeconomic status, and similar factors. Once an individual has learned a problem drinking pattern, the pattern becomes fixed because it is reinforced. When the effects of *not* drinking are highly aversive, the problem drinker continues to avoid that discomfort and his behavior persists. The need for fast re-

227

Table 9-1. The Phases of Alcoholism

Stage	Characteristics
Prealcoholic phase	Client confronts tension and anxiety by drinking, uses alcohol to relax, and begins to build a tolerance so that larger amounts are needed to achieve desirable effects.
Early alcoholic phase	Blackouts begin. Client sneaks drinks, hides bottles, becomes defensive, and denies the problem. A preoccupation with alcohol develops, with a need to assure a supply. Projection, rationalization, and denial are becoming clear.
Addiction phase	Client manifests loss of control over drinking and increased aggressive behavior. Relationships are altered and others are blamed. Withdrawal occurs if drinking ceases.
Chronic phase	Unplanned drinking sprees occur. Alcohol is consumed alone or with others. Physical complications of alcohol use begin to take place.

lief overshadows the knowledge that continued drinking will have long-term adverse effects.

Because the effects of alcohol can vary from person to person, research is continuing to determine how and why there are so many variations in the process of becoming or not becoming an alcoholic. Approaches and ideas that maintain a static, unidimensional model may be too simplistic. Pattison and his associates (1977) have proposed a multidimensional model for the progression of alcoholism that includes such ideas as:

■ There is no natural division between alcoholic and nonalcoholic drinking but rather a continuum of drinking that may result in various consequences.

■ Alcohol problems may develop gradually or rapidly. They do not necessarily proceed to severe fatal stages but may remain stable at any level of severity.

■ Because of the strong relationship between drinking behavior and environmental influences, treatment should be related to the person's drinking environment.

Nurses need to be aware of emerging concepts and changing ideas regarding the pattern of alcoholism.

ALCOHOLISM AND THE NURSING PROCESS

Application of the nursing process in dealing with alcoholic clients occurs in two stages: the acute phase and the rehabilitation phase.

Acute Stage

ASSESSMENT When clients are admitted for treatment in an intoxicated state, the nurse must make an assessment in several areas. At this point, the physical well-being to the client is of paramount importance, as acute intoxication can be a medical emergency.

A thorough assessment must include several aspects. The presence and severity of withdrawal symptoms must be determined by noting tremulousness, shaking, difficulties with coordination, short attention span, insomnia, hyperactivity, anorexia, and tachycardia. If the client is hallucinating, severe anxiety, disorientation, and DTs can be expected. Nutritional status must be determined by checking for loss of muscle tissue, underweight, and signs of vitamin deficiencies, such as gum disease. The fluid balance of the body is assessed by checking skin turgor and moisture, mucous membranes, and the specific gravity of the urine. Circulatory status can be checked by noting edema, pulse arrhythmias, respiratory status, the presence of congestion and purulent sputum, and the warmth and color of the extremities.

Since many people injure themselves easily under the influence of alcohol, the client should be checked for the presence of trauma, including scars, burns, and head injuries. The reaction of the pupils and the strength of the hand grasp should be noted. Mental status is determined by noting the client's orientation to person, place, and time and the stability of this orientation.

PLANNING AND IMPLEMENTATION Potential problems and nursing interventions for these problems are listed in Table 9-2. If the client is experiencing

Table 9-2. Interventions in the Acute Stage of Alcoholism

Client's Problems	Nursing Interventions
Withdrawal from alcohol	Monitor vital signs; observe closely for signs of convulsions and impending delirium tremens.
Inadequate food and fluid intake	Provide high-protein diet, vitamin and mineral supplements. Record intake and output. Test urine for specific gravity and the stool for blood. Encourage fluid intake. If client is not dehydrated, supply according to thirst.
Risk of self-injury	Provide adequate supervision while client is confused and disoriented. Remove potentially harmful items. Allow client to smoke (but not unattended) if this relieves anxiety.
Lack of self-care	Administer personal physical care if client is unable. Explain that this is a temporary measure. Delay unnecessary procedures.
Need for rest and relaxation	Use measures to induce sleep and rest, such as warm showers, darkened rooms. Avoid sudden approaches to client to prevent frightening him or contributing to hyperactivity.
Increased anxiety	Administer antianxiety drugs as ordered. Do not undersedate, as client has been accustomed to large amounts of alcohol. Explain reasons for all tests and procedures. Provide opportunities for ventilating fear and anger. Continually orient client to reality if confusion, delusions, or hallucinations are present.

delirium tremens, visitors should be banned, as they may add to the client's confusion and irritation. Siderails and restraints may be necessary to prevent injury. A light should be left on in the room to prevent distortions in perception. Unnecessary stimulation, such as a radio or TV, should be avoided.

It is of primary importance for the nurse to accept the alcoholic client as being worthy of his best possible efforts and to convey a kind, caring, accepting attitude while still maintaining objectivity.

EVALUATION When the client has been successfully detoxified, she will have regained her optimum physical health and will be free of all mood-altering drugs. Once this stage has been reached, the detoxification period has been completed and rehabilitation begins.

Rehabilitation Stage

ASSESSMENT After the client has been successfully detoxified, he needs to be assessed for the appropriateness of entering a rehabilitation program that will facilitate his return to the community. The client must be evaluated as to the degree of insight he has into his problem, his understanding of the disease, and his stage of denial. If the client is not yet

recognizing that he has a problem, support will be needed to facilitate this process.

Clients enter rehabilitation programs for a variety of reasons. The amount of motivation for change is a crucial component in the client's recovery. Clients who participate because of external pressure, such as a wife's insistence or a lawyer's encouragement in hopes of reducing a sentence, are usually less motivated to change their behavior.

A thorough drinking history should include: any experiences with blackouts, DTs or seizures; previous attempts at treatment and the client's understanding of reasons for failure; degree of depression and any suicidal ideation or suicide attempts; other acting out or violent behavior. Significant events in the past that the client has not yet resolved, such as divorce or death of a loved one, should be explored.

The nurse should assess the presence of support systems in the environment, the attitudes of significant others toward the drinking, the presence of a co-alcoholic or an enabler, and any problems with the law or the employer. It is important for the nurse to determine the role of alcohol in helping the alcoholic client cope. If alcohol abuse serves as an adaptive mechanism, it is easier to understand why the client drinks.

PLANNING AND IMPLEMENTATION Potential problems and suggested nursing interventions for these problems are listed in Table 9-3.

Intervention for rehabilitation of the alcoholic can take place on several levels and from a variety of approaches. Nurses need to be aware of different kinds of treatment not only to participate but to refer clients appropriately.

Table 9-3. Interventions in the Rehabilitation Stage of Alcoholism

Client's Problems	Nursing Interventions
Denial of illness	Guide client toward acceptance of fact that at least some of the difficulties in her life are due to drinking. Help her realize that her life must be managed without alcohol. Confront the use of denial and manipulation to satisfy needs and to avoid responsibility for her own behavior.
Lack of understanding of the disease	Educate the client about the disease of alcoholism and its influence, including the psychological, social, and economic effects of alcohol abuse.
Lack of self-esteem	Help the client regain self-respect and confidence by providing tasks that lead to success. Explore areas of competence and ways to broaden interests and complete projects. Verbalize the hope of arresting the alcoholism.
Loneliness	Provide experiences showing that satisfaction and support can be obtained from relating to others. Assist the client to directly verbalize needs and fear of change. Identify ways of preventing or alleviating feelings of loneliness.
Low frustration tolerance	Help the client find alternative methods of relieving tension and anxiety and develop constructive coping skills.
Possibility of relapse	Make appropriate discharge plans to facilitate return to the community. Determine feasibility of the plans for the particular client. Inform the client of available support systems.

Intrapsychic Approaches Many professionals treating alcoholics believe that the problem is a result of conscious or unconscious emotional factors. While this assumption is controversial, many experts agree that an important part of any treatment program is fostering trust. Individual therapy is the method of choice for some clients, but there are hazards in this approach. Because the therapeutic relationship tends to be prolonged and intense, the caregiver has to be wary of the client's developing an overwhelming dependency on the therapist. Group therapy is thus often the treatment of choice because it dilutes dependency and provides opportunities for confrontation of the alcoholic by his peers. In many instances, alcoholic clients will more readily accept the exposure of denial and game playing from another alcoholic than from a nonalcoholic therapist.

Aversion Therapy Aversion therapy, based on learning theory, is designed to associate a painful experience with alcohol use. The most commonly used technique is administration of the drug disulfiram (Antabuse), which interferes with the metabolism of alcohol and increases the amount of acetaldehyde (a toxic substance) in the blood. Drinking alcohol while taking Antabuse creates a physiological reaction that mimics severe shock, with deep flushing, a rise in blood pressure, difficulty in breathing, and violent vomiting. While the drug has few side effects when taken by abstainers, it can be lethal for clients with certain medical problems who drink while taking the drug. For this reason, Antabuse is not given to individuals with cardiac or kidney problems.

Interpersonal Approaches Interpersonal approaches focus on marital and family dysfunction and their influences on the alcoholic. In some marriages, the nonalcoholic spouse unconsciously resists the attempts of the alcoholic to recover because the family dynamics have come to be based on the illness. The spouse has been forced to assume most of the responsibility for the family, and it may be difficult for the spouse to give up some of these responsibilities as his or her partner gains sobriety.

Attention needs to be given to the life pattern of the alcoholic and to the role that the spouse plays in this pattern. Many partners find themselves contributing to the continuation of problem drinking by inadvertently rescuing the alcoholic and assuming responsibility for the alcoholic's actions. That is, they become "enablers." Others perpetuate the problem because they are more comfortable when the alcoholic is actively drinking—they are in control when the alcoholic is drunk.

Al-Anon and Ala-Teen are organizations available in most communities to help the spouse and children understand the problem and help themselves and the alcoholic person.

THE ROLE OF THE SPOUSE

Spouses who wish to be helpful to their alcoholic partners need to be aware of certain factors:

- Alcoholism is a family disease and each family member must be involved in treatment to facilitate change.

- Family members need to be educated about the disease of alcoholism.

- The spouse needs to stop protecting the alcoholic and allow him to take responsibility for his own behavior.

- Nagging and pouring out the alcohol will not stop the drinking.

- Developing a feeling of detachment and independence from the problem will help resolve the spouse's guilt and increase the spouse's sense of self-worth.

- It may be necessary to create a crisis to get the alcoholic to accept treatment.

Social Approaches The best example of social and small-group treatment for alcoholics is Alcoholics Anonymous. The aim of this organization is to help members maintain their sobriety. Their program is based on twelve steps designed to help the alcoholic recover. The organization is self-supporting and consists solely of lay people, not members of the helping professions (unless they, too, are alcoholic).

Another form of social therapy for the alcoholic is community halfway houses designed to fill the gap between hospitalization and independent living. These houses provide group therapy, a healthy environment with regular meals, and structure and peer support while residents job hunt or undertake vocational rehabilitation programs.

Alcoholism is a complex disorder, but it can be treated successfully. When the unique needs of each client are considered, the outlook is considerably optimistic. The nurse's role in the rehabilitation of the alcoholic extends from inpatient programs to outpatient care to involvement in community services. Whatever the modality, a kind, firm approach, based on knowledge and understanding, and a spirit of hopefulness will facilitate the client's progress and promote success.

EVALUATION Several factors should be considered in determining whether treatment has been successful. If the client has returned to drinking, his perception of events that may have precipitated this

231

relapse should be taken into account in planning future treatment. If the client has remained sober, there has been a measure of success.

Goals should be reevaluated for their appropriateness to the individual client. While complete abstinence is the ideal goal for most treatment, relapses seem to be a necessary part of the process. It is unrealistic to expect that all alcoholics who enter treatment will remain sober forever. Change takes time, and each attempt adds more insight and education. By keeping goals manageable, staff and clients are less subject to discouragement and feelings of failure.

When a client returns for additional treatment, the staff should reevaluate their attitudes regarding the client. Alcoholics can make the professional staff feel guilty if they don't get well or respond to treatment. Many times such clients are not "good" clients, which can lead to nontherapeutic responses from the staff—condescension, impatience, unwillingness to take time to listen, annoyance, resentment, and so on.

An additional area for evaluation is the role of support systems in a client's return to drinking. The previous treatment plan will need to be scrutinized to determine what areas should receive more consideration this time, such as greater family involvement, different housing arrangements, or more reliance on AA.

USE AND ABUSE OF DRUGS

Throughout recorded history, human beings have used drugs to alter their state of consciousness and

PREVALENCE OF DRUG ABUSE

It is estimated that there are about 300,000 heroin addicts nationwide, but the actual number may be two to three times that amount. About 1950, the typical heroin addict was a member of a minority group, lived in a large city, and was about thirty years old. Since that time, there has been a shift toward younger and younger addicts. New York City Addiction Services recently found that 42 percent of participants in drug abuse programs were black, 21 percent were Puerto Rican, and the rest were Caucasian. According to the Bureau of Narcotics and Dangerous Drugs, 51 percent of the addicts in the United States are white, with the average age being twenty-three (Freedman, Kaplan, and Sadock, 1976).

The prevalence of other widely used drugs has been reported by Schuckit (1979) as follows:

- Marijuana has been tried by some 36 million Americans, with over 50 percent of people ages eighteen to twenty-five reporting some use, 20 percent using it two or more times per week, and 8 percent using it daily. One in five adults report having used marijuana at some time.

- Hallucinogens are used on an occasional basis by 20 percent of the youth population.

- Solvents are usually taken intermittently by adolescents. About 20 percent of girls and 33 percent of boys have used solvents at least once.

- Depressants are prescribed in approximately 90 percent of hospitalized cases. More than 15 percent of American adults use these drugs during any one year. Psychological dependence is between 10 percent and 30 percent for individuals who have received these drugs for medical purposes, and physical dependence is between 5 percent and 10 percent.

232

to relieve the tension or monotony of existence. Over time, various mind-altering drugs have gained and lost popularity from culture to culture. Our contemporary society is highly drug oriented. We take pills to calm us or to excite us, to wake us up or to put us to sleep, to help us gain or lose weight.

The dividing line between "use" and "abuse" of drugs is often determined by social sanctions. For example, the teenage use of marijuana or stimulants to achieve a "high" is frequently considered abuse by the adult population, but youngsters claim their drug habits are no different from those of their parents who use alcohol or tobacco.

Often the legal system decides what constitutes use and abuse (Burkhalter, 1975). The Harrison Narcotics Act of 1914 was the first national attempt to control the flow of narcotics and opiates in particular. This act was aimed at regulating the supply available for persons dependent on these drugs. Although considered beneficial, this act led to the beginning of illegal drug traffic. Physicians could no longer legally prescribe narcotics to addicts to keep them comfortable by maintaining the accustomed use, forcing them to turn to illegal sources. The Harrison Act was challenged in 1925 when the guilty verdict for a physician who had prescribed a narcotic for a known addict was overturned by the Supreme Court. For the first time, narcotic abuse was described as an illness that could be legally treated.

In 1937, the Uniform Narcotics Law created a consistent method for record keeping at federal and state levels, but it left penalties for use, possession, and sale of narcotics up to the individual states. In 1956 the Federal Narcotics Control Act increased the penalties for narcotics and marijuana violations, imposing sentences that ranged from ten to forty years.

Society's perception of drug abuse has followed much the same course as that of alcohol abuse. In recent years, an effort has been made to treat drug abuse problems as illnesses rather than as criminal

Historically, there is ample evidence that drug abuse antedated drug therapy, just as toxicology paved the way for pharmacology. Primitive people seem to have been more interested in poisons than in medicines; even Hippocrates, although he recommended natural salicylates from willow trees for eye disease and childbirth, considered most drugs essentially useless. But when the Greeks wished to dispose of Socrates, they had a most effective herb . . . A number of therapeutic substances have been introduced with insufficient awareness of their potential for abuse.

L. GRINSPOON AND J. BAKALAR (1980)

or immoral acts. In 1962, a court case in California established that a person could not be punished as a criminal on the sole grounds of being a drug abuser. This decision helped emphasize the idea of drug dependence as an illness. In 1966, Congress established a policy for the treatment of narcotics abusers. Abusers found guilty of violating federal criminal law might be sentenced to prison or sent to a drug treatment center for detoxification and rehabilitation. But before confinement, it had to be determined whether the person could benefit from and respond to treatment efforts, which had the effect of screening out abusers judged to be potential failures.

The most recent legislation was the 1970 Compulsive Drug Abuse Control and Prevention Act. Penalties for violations were brought into greater accord with the danger and intended uses of the drugs. Under this law, a judge is free to arrive at alternative penalties, such as volunteer work for youthful offenders, rather than imprisonment.

COMMONLY ABUSED DRUGS

Drugs that are commonly abused fall into six major categories: (1) stimulants, (2) opiates, (3) depressants, (4) cannabinols, (5) hallucinogens, and (6) inhalants.

Stimulants

The *stimulants* comprise a variety of drugs that have the ability to stimulate the central nervous system at a number of levels. They include amphetamines, cocaine, and caffeine. As a group, they work by

causing the release of neurotransmitters such as norepinephrine. Common stimulants are listed in Table 9-4. These drugs act on the central and peripheral nervous systems and on the cardiovascular system, causing euphoria, a decrease in fatigue, a decrease in appetite, and an increase in energy. They may increase feelings of sexuality and may interfere with normal sleep patterns. In some cases they produce tremor of the hands, restlessness, and tachycardia.

Tolerance to stimulants develops within hours or days. Whether physical dependence occurs is still being debated by researchers and clinicians, but many feel that a physical syndrome does exist. There is no doubt, however, that psychological dependence can occur.

In the emergency room, any individual presenting with dilated pupils, increased heart rate, dry mouth, increased reflexes and temperature, sweating, and behavioral abnormalities should be considered a possible stimulant abuser. Panic reaction (fear of losing control or of going crazy) and am-

Table 9-4. Common Stimulants

Generic Name	Trade Name	Street Names
Amphetamine	Benzedrine	Bennies, greenies, footballs
Methamphetamine	Desoxyn	Speed, crystal, meth
Dextroamphetamine	Dexedrine	Dexies, hearts, oranges, Christmas trees
Cocaine		Snow, dust, "C," gold dust
Caffeine		

Opiate withdrawal occurs in the following pattern:

1. Within 12 hours—physical discomfort, tearing of the eyes, runny nose, sweating and yawning.

2. 12 to 14 hours—restless sleep.

3. 2 to 3 days—dilated pupils, loss of appetite, gooseflesh ("cold turkey"), back pain, and tremor.

4. 3 to 4 days—insomnia, incessant yawning, flulike symptoms, gastrointestinal upsets, chills, muscle spasms, and abdominal pain.

5. 5 days—symptoms decrease, usually disappearing in a week to 10 days.

234

phetamine psychosis (high level of suspiciousness and paranoid delusions) may develop. Because of the short action and rapid metabolism of these drugs, flashbacks rarely occur.

Opiates and Related Analgesics

The major *opiates* include natural substances such as opium, morphine, and codeine; semisynthetic drugs such as heroin, Percodan, and Dilaudid; and synthetic analgesics such as Darvon and Demerol (see Table 9-5). These drugs all produce analgesia, drowsiness, changes in mood, and, at high doses, clouding of mental functioning through depression of the central nervous system and of cardiac activity.

Opiate substances are highly addicting, and physical dependence develops with short-term use. Tolerance develops rapidly. Even therapeutic doses of morphine given four times a day for three days can result in mild withdrawal symptoms; clients re-

turning home after surgery often experience a runny nose, tearing, and yawning that they attribute to a cold contracted in the hospital.

Physical signs and symptoms of opiate use include increased pigmentation over the veins, thrombosed veins, skin lesions and abscesses, constricted pupils, swollen nasal mucosa (if drug has been snorted), enlarged liver, and swollen lymph glands. Panic reactions and flashbacks are rare.

An opiate overdose is a medical emergency; usual signs include decreased respiration, pale or cyanotic skin and lips, pinpoint pupils, pulmonary edema, shock, cardiac arrhythmias, and convulsions. Death may occur from the respiratory depression and pulmonary edema.

The withdrawal syndrome usually begins at the time of the next scheduled dose. The pattern of this syndrome is outlined in the accompanying box.

Depressants

Central nervous system *depressants* include a variety of medications such as hypnotics and antianxiety drugs (see Table 9-6). All have clinical usefulness and potential for abuse. The main effects are lethargy and sleepiness. Overdose can lead to death from respiratory and circulatory depression. Some depressant drugs can produce a paradoxical reaction, that of extreme excitement, when given to children and the elderly.

Tolerance occurs both metabolically and through adaptation of the CNS. If two depressant drugs, such as alcohol and barbiturates, are taken at the same time, they will compete for metabolism in the liver. Since the liver can only handle a certain amount at one time, neither drug will be metabolized properly, and the effects of one drug enhance

Table 9-5. Common Opiates and Related Analgesics

Generic (Trade) Name	Street Name
Heroin	Horse, smack, "H," junk
Morphine	Morf, monkey, white stuff
Codeine	Schoolboy
Hydromorphine (Dilaudid)	Lords, little D
Oxycodone (Percodan)	Perkies
Methadone (Dolophine)	Dollies
Meperidine (Demerol)	Demies
Diphenoxylate (Lomotil)	
Pentazocine (Talwin)	T's
Combination of heroin and cocaine taken intravenously	Hot shot

*A great deal of the literature tends to emphasize the differences
between alcoholism and other drug abuse. Yet the differences between
the games exist and the understanding of each kind of drug abuse
requires awareness of the specific differences between games. A
therapist who is successful with alcoholics can transfer a great deal of
knowledge from the treatment of alcoholics to the treatment of heroin
or methedrine addicts. Yet he cannot be effective until he acquaints
himself with the realities that characterize whatever new addiction he
investigates and attempts to treat . . . Alcohol addiction involves
gradual, long-term self-destruction of a socially acceptable sort.
Heroin use in the United States almost always involves speedy
psychosocial degeneration, and methedrine [a powerful amphetamine]
involves a fulminating "burn out." Thus, each drug is selected by the
addict with its specific properties in mind in a manner congruent
with the life script.*

C. STEINER (1974)

the effects of the other, because drugs remain in the blood longer.

All CNS depressants produce a withdrawal state when drug taking stops abruptly. Physical signs and symptoms of withdrawal include tremor, gastrointestinal upsets, muscle aches, increased pulse and respiration, fever, and grand mal seizures. These symptoms may last three to seven days for short-acting drugs but longer for drugs like Valium.

Panic reactions and flashbacks are rarely seen. A toxic reaction can develop in a matter of hours, occurring either unintentionally or as the result of suicidal overdose. Depressants can also produce a temporary psychosis, manifested by acute onset of auditory hallucinations and paranoid delusions.

Cannabinols (Marijuana)

Marijuana is the second most widely used mood-altering drug in America, after alcohol. Marijuana comes from the dried leaves of the marijuana plant, *Cannabis sativa*; hashish is made from the resins of the plant flowers. The active ingredient, tetrahydrocannabinol (THC), can cause panic reactions, toxic reactions, and generalized anxiety. Marijuana can be smoked, eaten, or injected intravenously.

Marijuana is primarily a hallucinogen, but at usual doses the dominant effects are euphoria and change in level of consciousness without hallucinations. Marijuana use increases the cardiac workload and causes fine tremors, decreased muscle strength, decreased coordination, and breathing problems with prolonged use. It may also precipitate seizures. High doses can produce short-term memory loss, paranoia, and, with toxic doses, confusion, disorientation, and panic. Tolerance and physical dependence do not appear to be a problem, but there is some debate as to whether withdrawal symptoms occur. Flashbacks—the recurrence of feelings and perceptions experienced in the intoxicated state—are commonly seen in marijuana users.

Of concern to nurses are recent findings associating marijuana use with a decrease in the body's responses, impairment of sperm production, and destruction of lung tissue (Weiten, 1983).

Hallucinogens

Hallucinogens (also called psychedelics) increase

Table 9-6. Common Depressants

Generic Name	Trade Name	Street Name
Hypnotics		
Thiopental	Pentothal	Barbs, sleepies
Methohexital	Brevital	
Pentobarbital	Nembutal	Yellow jackets
Secobarbital	Seconal	Red devils, red birds
Amobarbital	Amytal	Blues
Phenobarbital	Luminal	Phennies, pink lady
Methaqualone	Quaalude	Sopers, ludes, love drug
Ethchlorvynol	Placidyl	Dyls
Chloral hydrate	Noctec	
Antianxiety drugs		
Chlordiazepoxide	Librium	Libs
Diazepam	Valium	Blues (10 mg), yellows (5 mg)
Oxazepam	Serax	
Chlorazepate	Tranxene	
Meprobamate	Miltown, Equanil	

No single pattern explains all addiction, but there are certain factors
that produce or in some cases protect drug users from addiction:
1. Addiction associated with neural physiology, especially the still
undetermined role of endorphins as factors in addictive propensities.
2. Addiction associated with narcotics given for relief of pain, since
the majority of persons receiving narcotics for this purpose do not
become addicted unless a personality predisposition existed.
3. Addiction associated with psychopathology is supported by some
research studies, although it remains difficult to differentiate
preaddiction psychopathology from postaddiction psychopathology.
4. Addiction associated with sociocultural factors such as the appeal
of a deviant life style and alienation from the broader, more
traditional culture.

J. C. COLEMAN, J. N. BUTCHER, AND R. C. CARSON (1984)

236

awareness of sensory input, provide a feeling of enhanced mental activity and altered body image, and
decrease the ability to tell the difference between
oneself and one's surroundings. Common hallucinogens are listed in Table 9-7. Physical signs of use
include dilated pupils, flushing, tremors, increased
blood pressure, elevated blood sugar levels, and increased temperature. Tolerance develops rapidly
but decreases in about a week if drug use is discontinued. There do not appear to be any withdrawal
symptoms with these drugs. Flashbacks can occur,
lasting from several minutes to a few hours.

Some users experience "bad trips"—states of
high anxiety and fear. The individual is highly stimulated, frightened, hallucinating, and fearful of losing his mind. Hallucinogen-induced psychosis can
occur but usually clears within hours to days. In
cases where psychosis does not clear, a preexisting
psychotic problem, such as schizophrenia, is likely
to have been present.

Inhalants

Inhalants include glues, solvents, and aerosols (see

Table 9-7. Common Hallucinogens

Generic Name	Street Names
Lysergic acid diethylamide (LSD)	Acid, hawk, royal blue, sugar cubes, pearly gates, instant zen
Psilocybin	Magic mushrooms
Dimethyltryptamine	DMT
Mescaline (peyote)	Big chief, cactus, half moon
Phencyclidine	PCP, angel dust, hog, peace pill
Dimethoxymethyl amphetamine	DOM, STP ("serenity, tranquillity, peace")

Table 9-8. Commonly Abused Inhalants

Substance	Active Ingredients
Glues	Toluene, naphtha, benzene, chloroform
Cleaning solutions	Carbon tetrachloride
Nail polish remover	Acetone
Aerosols	Fluorinated hydrocarbons, nitrous oxide
Petroleum products	Gasoline, ether
Paint thinners	Toluene, methanol

Table 9-8). These substances can produce generalized CNS depression. They are popular because
they readily produce euphoria and are available,
cheap, and legal. Usually the high begins within
minutes and lasts about a half hour, with the person
feeling giddy and lightheaded. The person may
exprience a decrease in inhibitions, misperceptions
or illusions, clouding of thoughts, and drowsiness.
Acute intoxication causes irritation of the eyes, double vision, ringing in the ears, and irritation of the
mucous membranes of the nose and mouth.

Tolerance develops quickly, but withdrawal
symptoms do not develop. Overdose causes a life-
threatening syndrome, characterized by respiratory
depression, cardiac arrhythmias, loss of consciousness, and possibly death.

CAUSES OF DRUG ABUSE

In discussing the etiology of drug abuse and drug
dependence, it should be emphasized that there

DSM-III, AXIS I
DIAGNOSTIC CLASSIFICATION

Drug abuse is classified under substance use disorders in DSM-III, with *abuse* referring to a pattern of pathologic use for at least one month and impairment of social or occupational functioning. Dependence requires tolerance or withdrawal.

305.4x Barbiturate or similarly acting sedative or hypnotic abuse

304.1x Barbiturate or similarly acting sedative or hypnotic dependence

305.5x Opioid abuse

304.0x Opioid dependence

305.6x Cocaine abuse (No dependence because no withdrawal syndrome)

305.7x Amphetamine or similarly acting sympathomimetic abuse

304.4x Amphetamine or similarly acting sympathomimetic dependence

305.9x Phencyclidine (PCP) or similarly acting arylcyclohexylamine abuse (No dependence because no withdrawal syndrome)

305.3x Hallucinogen abuse (No dependence)

305.2x Cannabis abuse

304.3x Cannabis dependence

305.1x Tobacco dependence (No abuse because no clinically significant intoxication syndrome)

305.9x Other, mixed or unspecified substance abuse

304.6x Other specified substance dependence

304.9x Unspecified substance dependence

304.7x Dependence on combination of opioid and other nonalcoholic substance

304.8x Dependence on combination of substances, excluding opioids and alcohol

Code in fifth digit: 1 = continuous, 2 = episodic, 3 = remission, 0 = unspecified.

237

may be a difference between the factors that initially lead to abuse and those that tend to maintain the state of dependence once it has been established. The fear of symptoms caused by abstinence is, for the abuser, an important reason for staying on a drug. Many addicted persons resist hospitalization out of fear they will be asked to go "cold turkey." Others return to drugs after trying to withdraw themselves and suffering for several days.

While the exact causes of drug dependence are not known, it is possible to discuss the possible factors in three categories: the "host" (mental or personality makeup of the user), the environment, and the agent (the pharmacologic nature of the drug) (Glatt, 1974).

The Role of the Host
As with the alcoholic, a great deal of research has focused on trying to establish a personality makeup for the drug abuser. Some similarities have been found among abusers, with the major tendencies being (1) emotional immaturity, (2) a wish to ignore reality, (3) low tolerance for frustration, (4) an unwillingness to cope with tension, and (5) inability to persist at a task (Glatt, 1974). Certain emotionally vulnerable people have a tendency to look for ways to obtain relief from discomfort or to achieve a higher degree of satisfaction than previously experienced. For them, drugs are a means to these ends. Some drugs, such as alcohol, release aggressive impulses; others, such as heroin, weaken them. Therefore, the choice of drug may be somewhat determined by the individual's values and his ego ideal (the type of person he wishes to be and to portray to his peers).

As with alcohol abuse, genetic and environmental factors are difficult to separate. It is presently believed that genetic factors play less of a role in predisposition to drug dependence than to alcoholism. However, inherited factors may play a role in drug abusers who also suffer from schizophrenia or manic-depressive conditions (Glatt, 1974).

In Western culture, alcohol is widely accepted socially, but most other mind-altering drugs aren't. It is therefore likely that the proportion of immature and insecure personalities is much higher among abusers of other drugs than among alcohol abusers. Drugs are frequently taken as a rebellious act against authority. Since alcohol use is more accepted, it is not an acting-out method as much as other drug use is. Young people generally find drugs attractive for different reasons than alcohol. Curiosity, glamour, excitement, risk taking, a feeling of bravery, and the lure of the unknown may be factors in drug experimentation. It has been said that young people take drugs to rebel against their parents but take alcohol to emulate them (Glatt, 1974). In contrast, middle-aged drug abusers seem to have begun their abuse by a different route, self-medication. For example, a middle-aged woman who abuses amphetamines may have originally begun using them as a means of weight control.

The Role of the Environment

Drug-dependent individuals will often revert to drug taking long after the physical dependence has disappeared. This relapse mainly occurs when they resume contact with their former friends and subculture. They commonly return to their old neighborhoods because they have no place else to go, but in many cases, abusers return because of the need to belong and feel more comfortable in their old environments.

Environmental factors also play a role in the increasing use of drugs within the teenage population. Youngsters who engage in activities that are frowned on by authority figures become alienated from society's values, such as having a steady job, maintaining family ties, getting an education, and so on. Many sociologists suggest that the blame for drug abuse rests on our "sick" society rather than on the "weak personality" of the addict. Old social standards have largely disappeared without new guidelines to replace them. As a result, many young people feel insecure and bewildered. In this state of anxiety and insecurity, many reject society and look for new ways to gain satisfaction, including drugs (Glatt, 1974).

Another environmental factor that affects drug abuse is membership in a particular ethnic group or subculture. The low incidence of alcoholism among Jews, for example, is believed to exist because in Jewish culture drunkenness is frowned upon and holding one's liquor is not a status symbol. However, abuse of other drugs is more common among Jews, possibly because they have no clear-cut established attitudes against drug taking.

Easy access to certain drugs also appears to influence drug patterns. Thus, military personnel and businessmen, whose main access is to alcohol, may be more likely to abuse this drug, whereas doctors, pharmacists, and nurses have a greater access to opiates and other prescription drugs and are thus more likely to abuse these drugs.

The Role of the Agent

The pharmacologic properties of a drug may play a role in the process of addiction. Most people become physically dependent on opiates after using even small amounts, in a matter of a week or two. Barbiturate users, on the other hand, usually do not become addicted even after two to three months of administration slightly over therapeutic dose range. And it takes a long period of consuming large amounts for people using alcohol to develop a physical dependence. In general, drugs that can be injected produce dependence sooner than those taken by mouth.

Another factor in drug abuse is the drug's ability to serve as a reinforcer. The drug of choice gives a reward, whether the relief of tension or feelings of euphoria. With each use, the reward continues and drug usage is reinforced. Many times the pattern of drug use is begun with social reinforcement; then the desired effects take over as the reinforcement. Addicts also find that withdrawal symptoms provide *negative* reinforcement for continued drug use. Former heroin addicts have been known to experience withdrawal symptoms upon seeing drug equipment (syringe, needles) despite having been physically detoxified from the drug.

Drug abuse is a complex health problem whose causes are not completely understood. Research in this area is especially difficult because the main source of information is current users, who are highly defensive about their behavior. In addition, the reasons one person may choose a certain drug may be entirely different from the reasons another person chooses the same drug. Furthermore, people may abuse different drugs at different times in their lives. Nurses therefore need to be aware of the variety of factors that can contribute to beginning and maintaining drug abuse patterns.

PHYSIOLOGICAL CONSEQUENCES OF DRUG ABUSE

Long-term drug abuse is associated with a variety of complications.

Circulatory and Respiratory Complications

Bacterial endocarditis is a common complication of intravenous drug use. The infecting organism is usually *Staphylococcus aureus*. The left side of the heart and the aortic, mitral, and tricuspid valves are usually involved. Heroin addicts with bacterial endocarditis have a mortality rate of 28 to 75 percent.

Gangrene, caused by injection of drugs into an artery instead of a vein, can occur in the extremity distal to the arterial injection site. The damage is believed to be caused by chemical action on the intimal lining of the artery.

Vascular disorders such as acute and chronic thrombophlebitis and sclerosing of the veins are common. If contaminated drugs are injected, the result may be severe extremity lymphedema because of obstruction of veins and lymphatics. Intracranial hemorrhage has been reported with amphetamine use because of its hypertensive effect.

Pulmonary embolism occurs when foreign particles such as talc, cornstarch, and cotton are injected into the circulatory system. When emboli reach the lungs, granulomas or pulmonary fibrosis can result.

Respiratory infections occur with a high frequency in drug addicts because of general lack of health care, poor diet, and poor living conditions. Heroin addicts frequently develop pneumonia, tuberculosis, and pulmonary abscesses.

Hepatic Dysfunction

Acute and chronic hepatitis are common problems resulting from use of contaminated needles. Hepatitis is one of the most frequent medical complications of drug abuse, with 10 to 15 percent of heroin addicts showing signs of the acute process and another 60 to 75 percent showing signs of chronic hepatitis and liver disease.

Gastrointestinal Disturbances

Severe and rapid weight loss is common with amphetamine abuse. Long-term heroin users are troubled with vitamin deficiencies, severe constipation, and hemorrhoids.

Skin Complications

Skin problems develop at the site of drug injections and include scarring, abscesses, cellulitis, and ulcerations. When drugs are injected into surrounding tissue rather than the vein, necrotic ulcerating lesions appear. Such subcutaneous "skin popping" increases the potential for systemic infections.

Muscular Disorders

Long-term subcutaneous injection can cause a fibrosing myopathy, in which the veins become blocked, resulting in edema, and possibly leading to cellulitis and myositis, with chronic muscle damage.

Miscellaneous Complications

There is a high incidence of tetanus in the heroin-abusing population, as skin popping provides an excellent avenue of entry for infection. The mortality rate for tetanus among addicts is extremely high.

Eye emboli are caused by foreign substances, producing retinal hemorrhages with edema. In most cases, this problem is temporary.

Traumatic injury occurs because of decreased mental alertness, producing burns, fractures, lacerations, and contusions.

DRUG ABUSE AND THE NURSING PROCESS

Application of the nursing process in dealing with drug abusers occurs in two stages: the acute phase and the rehabilitation phase.

Acute Stage

ASSESSMENT The client with an acute drug reaction can present a medical emergency, especially if he has received an overdose. If the client is unable to respond, detective work is necessary to determine which drug was used. Comprehensive knowledge of the signs and symptoms of the various drugs will assist the nurse in this process. At times, verification can be made by someone accompanying the client.

A thorough physical assessment should include an inspection for scars, needle points, and abscesses. The possibility of overdose should be determined by assessing pupil size and reaction, reflex responses, vital signs, respiratory status, tremors, convulsions, and breath odor. Clothing should be inspected for signs of drugs and drug implements. Nutritional and hygiene status can be assessed by looking for signs of nutritional deficiencies and personal neglect. The assessment should also include determining the level of consciousness and looking for the presence of hallucinations or delusions, confusion, signs of complications, and physical injuries.

PLANNING AND IMPLEMENTATION As with alcohol treatment, the primary concern during the acute stage of drug detoxification is the physical well-being of the client, with attention to providing comfort and alleviating fear. Common problems and appropriate nursing interventions are presented in Table 9-9.

EVALUATION When the client is medically stable, referral for continued care can be made.

Rehabilitation Stage

ASSESSMENT Many of the assessments discussed for

239

Table 9-9. Interventions for Acute Drug Problems

Client's Problem	Nursing Interventions
Decreased circulatory and respiratory function	Monitor vital signs and neurologic reflex responses. Be prepared for emergencies, including CPR, keeping an airway open. Suction as necessary.
Impending withdrawal	Determine the stage of withdrawal. Medicate as ordered to alleviate discomfort. Approach the client calmly; avoid touching client without explanation. Limit visitors.
Potential for self-injury	Use restraints as necessary; remove all harmful objects. Monitor suicidal behavior.
Panic and flashback reactions	Have staff present as much as possible. Provide a caring presence and opportunity to ventilate feelings. Try to talk the client down. Reassure him through this difficult period. Orient him to person, time, and place. Do not support delusions and hallucinations. Let client know that these are very real for him but that you do not experience the same things.
Poor nutritional status, personal hygiene	Give conscientious skin care, being aware of the likelihood of skin breakdown. Record nutritional and fluid intake and output. Administer and monitor IV solutions until oral intake can be established. Provide small, frequent feedings when indicated.
Fear of "cold turkey," unavailability of treatment	Give honest reassurance about the client's condition. Begin education about drug abuse. Make plans for continued treatment. Discuss available treatment modalities. Have a recovered addict visit client.

240

the alcoholic client also apply to the rehabilitating drug abuser. Attention must be given to the motivation for treatment and the reasons for requesting treatment. Available support systems, including those that may encourage a return to drug abuse, need evaluation. Current living conditions may need to be included in the plan for change. It is especially important to assess the client's past treatment history, including types of programs attempted (such as abstinence and methadone maintenance), to determine the reasons for past failures and what might work better in the future.

PLANNING AND IMPLEMENTATION Whatever the chosen modality for continued treatment, certain problems will arise that need attention by nursing personnel. Such problems and suggested interventions are examined in Table 9-10.

The past decade has seen the development of a multitude of treatment possibilities for substance abuse, including maintenance, detoxification, use of antagonists, and drug-free communities. These types of treatment offer different approaches to drug abuse and may be most effectively used in combination at various points in rehabilitation. However, all too often proponents of one type of

therapy have attempted to compete with other types of therapy, thereby ignoring the potential benefits of each type and reducing the overall effectiveness of treatment by forcing an inappropriate approach on the client (O'Brien, Woody, and McLellan, 1983).

Maintenance Methadone maintenance is based on the assumption that basic addiction is a metabolic disease. The basic idea of this treatment is that if addicted clients are supplied with adequate quantities of opiate in the form of methadone, they will no longer have to engage in criminal activity to main-

Table 9-10. Interventions in Drug Rehabilitation

Client's Problem	Nursing Interventions
Denial of illness	Confront the client regarding his problem behavior. Help the client recognize his avoidance of responsibility. Identify projection of blame or defensiveness that prevent honesty.
Isolation	Encourage group participation, physical exercise, and new interests and activities. Help the client seek support from others.
Avoidance of responsibility	Encourage decision making and verbal expression of anger and depression. Provide a structured environment and planned routine. Prepare the client for a change in lifestyle after discharge.
Lack of knowledge about consequences of drug abuse	Provide education to help the client understand drug abuse as an illness.
Return to drug abuse	Encourage compliance with the planned treatment program. Explore goals for appropriateness and client resistance.

tain their supply. Oral doses of methadone do not produce euphoria but do satisfy the physiological desire for the drug and prevent onset of withdrawal symptoms. Although methadone maintenance programs have met with some success, they have also created medical, social, and legal problems, including sale on the illegal market and death from overdose. These difficulties have usually evolved when appropriate support services have been neglected (O'Brien, 1983).

An alternative approach, *heroin maintenance*, is highly controversial. Proponents believe that because heroin is the drug of choice for most addicted clients, providing a controlled supply of heroin keeps more addicts in treatment. Opponents of this program believe that it creates more problems than it solves because it makes addiction less costly and more socially acceptable, gives a free supply of heroin to potential addicts, and discourages other, more effective treatment plans.

Antagonists Narcotic antagonists block or antagonize the opiates, preventing them from acting. They do not provide the psychological effects of narcotics and are not addictive. Nalorphine (Nalline) has been used in the treatment of opiate overdose. Antagonists used for treatment have included cyclazocine, naloxone, and naltrexane. A problem with this approach is the lack of any mechanism to compel the addict to continue taking the antagonist. If he decides to eliminate the dose on one day, the effects of heroin can be experienced on the next day.

Drug-Free Communities Another treatment approach is drug-free therapeutic communities, usually with-

---

THE ROLE OF THE NURSE IN DRUG ABUSE TREATMENT

The following nursing approaches are applicable to inpatient programs, day hospital treatment, and less intensive outpatient care.

- Establish and maintain the therapeutic milieu by explaining policies and routines.
- Assess client's ability to handle stress and to participate in multidisciplinary team planning.
- Be alert for drug use, realizing that clients may try to smuggle in drugs or, if outpatients, continue to use drugs. Continuous assessment of physical and behavioral characteristics helps monitor abstinence.
- Teach new forms of interpersonal behavior by role modeling and confronting inappropriate behavior.
- Participate in group therapy and encourage client participation, being alert to client's expressed feelings and assisting her to become aware of them.
- Provide a full schedule of activities, encouraging new interests and development of potential abilities.
- Give medications as prescribed, being aware that clients may hoard medication to get a "high" later, may feign physical pain to obtain drugs, or may "cheek" medications to avoid effects.
- Evaluate the appropriateness of follow-up care and refer as indicated.

241

in a residential treatment facility. Former addicts live together and participate in group therapy sessions. Synanon, one of the first groups of this type, has stressed harsh group confrontation, reeducation, and hard work. The basic idea underlying such communities is that drug abuse is symptomatic of an underlying antisocial personality problem or behavior pattern.

Many treatment types can be combined effectively for subgroups of client populations. A client may begin on maintenance, progress to detoxification, then spend several months on an antagonist and eventually become drug-free. A variety of psychologic therapies have been found to add to the overall effectiveness of treatment by addressing the

242

particular group of problems often associated with drug involvement. Individual psychotherapy has been found to be effective with clients on methadone maintenance. A variety of behavior modification techniques, often used in conjunction with naltrexone, have been reported to have benefits in extinguishing drug-conditioned responses that may lead to relapse. Family therapy, vocational guidance, and legal counseling have also proved to be beneficial.

Psychotropic medication, particularly antidepressants, adds another dimension. When schizophrenia or affective disorders are present, neuroleptics or lithium may be combined with maintenance, drug-free, or antagonist programs. Even benzodiazepines, which themselves have a potential for abuse, may be used with naltrexone to reduce protracted withdrawal symptoms and to improve program compliance (O'Brien, Woody, and McLellan, 1983).

EVALUATION There are three major reasons why treatment fails to initiate change for a drug abuser. First, the original goals may have been unrealistic. Success for the drug abuser is often defined as being drug-free, being legally employed, and not engaging in crime. These are excellent goals, but for a drug program to adopt them as standards may be unfair to the client. It is unreasonable to expect that freedom from drugs will make other areas immediately improve. Employment, for example, is partly a function of skills and habits developed before drug involvement and is also related to economic conditions.

A second reason for failure is not taking into account the heterogeneity and complexity of problems found among drug-abusing clients. Not all drug abusers are alike. Unless the client's unique problems are assessed and incorporated into the plan, failure is likely.

The third main reason for failure is inappropriate choice of treatment program. The proper utilization of available modalities is a necessary component of treatment for the abuser. Only a few places presently provide all the available treatment approaches. The nurse can make a valuable contribution to the health care of the abuser by making accurate diagnoses and helping to match the client with the most appropriate program.

SUMMARY

Substance abuse has been a problem for centuries. Social perception of individuals who abuse drugs has varied over time; in recent years, knowledgeable members of the helping professions have come to see substance abusers as people suffering from an illness that is amenable to treatment. These clinicians are beginning to take an active role in research, case finding, and planning of treatment designed to assist clients who are unable to monitor or control their use of various substances.

Abuse of alcohol has resulted in problem drinking to the point of alcoholism for approximately 10 million Americans, and it affects the lives of 40 million others. The etiology of alcoholism has been explained by a variety of theories, ranging from physiological, to psychological, to sociocultural and learning theories. None explains the disease in its entirety, but each contributes to our understanding of the process of the illness. The excessive use of

C L I N I C A L   E X A M P L E

MULTIPLE SUBSTANCE ABUSE IN AN ADULT MALE

Hugh Peterson is a thirty-four-year-old white male, divorced for ten years and the father of a child whom he has never seen. He is currently unemployed because of physical disability and receives Social Security benefits. In 1975 he was walking along the side of a road and was hit by a car, suffering serious injuries. He was unconscious for two weeks and has neurologic deficits and a seizure disorder as a result of the accident. He has achieved a fairly normal gait but has residual problems from atrophied muscles and wrist drop in the left arm.

He attended college for two years but dropped out because he was "bored" and joined the Marines. While in the service in Viet Nam, he used heroin and contracted hepatitis, which has resulted in a chronic liver condition. His alcohol intake is currently one or two six packs of beer and a pint or more of whiskey per day. He no longer uses heroin but does smoke marijuana on a daily basis.

Hugh was married briefly after his discharge from the service but left his wife and their unborn child to join the drug scene in San Francisco. Because he felt the need to remain free of personal responsibility and anything that might tie him down, he spent several years "bumming" around the country. Currently he resides with his parents and describes the relationship with them as "good" when he is not drinking or using other drugs. Neither of his parents drink, but Hugh's friends are mostly other men about his age who all abuse drugs and alcohol. Their spare time is spent in playing cards, drinking, and getting high.

Hugh has attempted treatment at several facilities but has been unable to remain sober or abstain from marijuana use for longer than six months. He has developed cirrhosis of the liver and was recently hospitalized for emergency surgery because of ruptured esophageal varicies. He was told at that time that it was unlikely that he could survive another serious drinking binge. He has been referred for outpatient follow-up care.

ASSESSMENT

The nurse who interviewed Hugh saw a man who was casually dressed, wearing a variety of ornamental jewelry. Hugh was fully oriented, alert to his surroundings, and easily engaged in conversation. He tended to be rambling and long winded in recounting his past life. He was otherwise articulate, using words effectively to com-

municate ideas. The nurse estimated his verbal IQ to be within the bright average to superior range, although he did appear to have some cognitive deficits, showing up in abstract reasoning and some memory distortion. His affect was inappropriate. As he verbalized his concern over his behavioral and drinking problems, he was cheerful and laughed frequently. Throughout the interview, the nurse commented on these discrepancies, and Hugh was able to say that this was his way of handling his nervousness and that he was quite frightened over his poor physical condition but knew that this fear alone would not keep him abstinent. He said that he did not have any reason to believe that this attempt at treatment would be any more successful than previous ones.

Based on Hugh's history and clinical picture, the following nursing and psychiatric diagnoses were formulated:

Nursing Diagnoses

Anxiety: Moderate

Coping, ineffectual individual

Diversional activity deficit

Noncompliance with treatment

Self-concept, disturbance in

Multiaxial Psychiatric Diagnosis

Axis I   303.91 Alcohol dependence, continuous
         305.53 Opioid abuse, in remission
         304.31 Cannabis dependence, continuous

Axis II   301.20 Schizoid personality

Axis III Seizure disorder
          Poststatus esophageal repair
          Neurologic deficits

Axis IV   Code 0—Severity of stressors unknown

Axis V   Level 5—Poor adaptive functioning

PLANNING

The health team agreed that Hugh could achieve sobriety only with drastic changes in his lifestyle. Because of past failures at treatment, he needed a highly structured milieu and close contact with a counselor for support and guidance. Hugh's lack of constructive activity and continued contact with peers who abused drugs and alcohol were contributing to his return to drinking and marijuana use. Because of his physical disabilities, he had

243

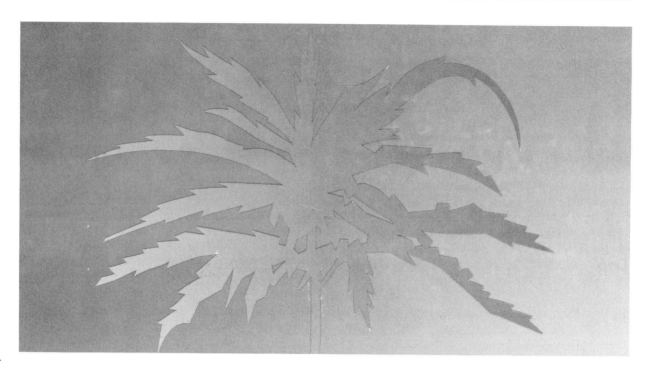

244

been content to exist on Social Security payments without making an effort to obtain some stability and direction to his life. Hugh's avoidance of work may have been caused by fear of failure or of public embarrassment because of his disability; thus the health team emphasized the need to set small, attainable goals. Hugh needed to experience some success. The team also noted the necessity of designing challenging and rewarding tasks for Hugh that would help him redefine his role as a person and as a functioning individual in society. In addition, it was necessary to plan individual counseling sessions to enable him to work through his conflicted feelings about his ex-wife and child. Because of his liver condition and poor physical health, Antabuse (disulfiram) was not considered an option. Contacts with Hugh's parents were initiated to determine the extent of their support or enabling of his behavior patterns.

IMPLEMENTATION

In order to maintain contact and establish the therapeutic relationship, Hugh's psychiatric nurse initiated a short-term contract with him for keeping appointments and beginning planned activities to structure his day. Since he had previously attended AA meetings in his neighborhood but had only participated superficially, it was arranged for him to take part in the care of the AA meeting place and to be responsible for the coffee hour. Although he was not stable enough to become a sponsor for others, his responsibilities in the center were designed to increase his involvement in a business-like, nonthreatening manner.

To achieve some sense of accomplishment and a feeling that he could become a contributing member of society, Hugh was placed in a community vocational evaluation program to assess his potential for either vocational training or constructive volunteer work. This program had the added benefit of providing a schedule and a task for each day. Hugh also accepted placement at a community halfway house to give him a new environment and a new, non-substance-abusing peer group.

EVALUATION

The goal of social rehabilitation for Hugh required the participation of caregivers representing a variety of disciplines and agencies. Medical follow-up was provided by physicians, placement and vocational rehabilitation was organized by the social worker, and the psychiatric nurse was responsible for the individual counseling, the family interview, coordination with AA, and the comprehensive planning. A primary responsibility of the psychiatric nurse was to coordinate these diverse efforts so that consistent goals were maintained and manipulation on Hugh's part was kept to a minimum. Coordination was not only an essential but a difficult activity that required preservation of the territoriality of the caregivers. In addition, it was necessary to ensure that the client did not receive mixed messages from the personnel involved.

As with all alcoholics, continuity of care was essential, and the presence of a primary stabilizing caregiver who maintained interest in the overall progress was paramount to beginning successful treatment. Most relationships had been transient and fleeting in Hugh's life. The progress Hugh made would have been impossible without the ongoing presence of one individual who made the rehabilitation program consistent with realistic goals that were acceptable to the client.

alcohol contributes to a variety of other illnesses and yields many severe complications, including damage to several of the body's systems, especially the brain and the liver.

Other drugs commonly abused fall into six major categories: (1) stimulants, (2) opiates, (3) depressants, (4) cannabinols, (5) hallucinogens, and (6) inhalants. Each of these drugs has particular presenting symptoms of misuse and varies in its ability to induce tolerance, withdrawal, and dependence. Physical complications, particularly from the use of opiates, can be severe and often life-threatening.

In the acute stage of drug intoxication, the physical well-being of the client is of paramount importance. Assessment of physical problems should lead to planning of measures to promote the client's comfort and medical stability. Interventions should be directed toward monitoring the client's physical condition and preventing additional complications. When medical stability has been attained, rehabilitation efforts can begin. The client's successful participation in a rehabilitation program depends on careful assessment of his motivation for change, his available support systems, and the resources in the community. Planning must include the client as well as all members of the health team to ensure the appropriateness of the treatment for the individual. Interventions can incorporate multiple modalities, including inpatient hospitalization, outpatient treatment, residential settings, and self-help groups. Evaluation of treatment efforts by the health team can lead to appropriate changes in care and to reassessment of goals, thereby ensuring realistic, attainable plans for each client.

Nurses who have contact with substance-abusing clients can find the work challenging and rewarding if they are able to examine their own attitudes toward substance abuse and the abuser, accept the clients for themselves, provide a caring and nonjudgmental relationship, and set realistic goals for themselves and their clients.

Review Questions

1. Describe your understanding of alcoholism and how this understanding will affect your plan of care for the alcoholic.

2. The client Hugh in the clinical example is suffering from alcoholism. Explain your understanding of the cause of his condition by using one or more of the proposed causal theories of alcoholism.

3. Describe alcohol's effect on the liver and the conditions that may result.

4. What are the important psychological factors that need to be taken into account when assessing a client's motivations for a rehabilitation program?

5. What precautions are essential in caring for a client who is experiencing an acute reaction to opiates?

6. Describe the interplay of the host, the environment, and the drug in determining substance addiction.

7. Describe the various treatment modalities available for the substance-abusing client and give your ideas about the timing and appropriateness of each.

8. Nursing attitudes toward the substance abuser can affect progress of treatment either favorably or unfavorably. Discuss this statement.

References

Albrecht, G. L. 1973. The Alcoholism Process: A Social Learning Point of View. In *Alcoholism: Progress in Research and Treatment*, eds. P. Bourne and R. Fox. New York: Academic Press.

Bales, R. F. 1959. Cultural Differences in Rate of Alcoholism. In *Drinking and Intoxication*, ed. R. McCarthy. New York: Free Press.

Barnes, G. E. 1980. Characteristics of the Clinical Alcoholic Personality. *Journal of Studies on Alcohol*, 41:894–910.

Burkhalter, P. 1975. *Nursing Care of the Alcoholic and Drug Abuser*. New York: McGraw-Hill.

Coleman, J. C.; Butcher, J. N.; and Carson, R. C. 1984. *Abnormal Psychology and Modern Life*. Glenview, Ill.: Scott, Foresman.

Donovan, D., and Marlatt, C. 1980. Assessment of Expectancies and Behavior Associated with Alcohol Consumption. *Journal of Studies on Alcohol*, 41:1153–1185.

Fenichel, O. 1945. *The Psychoanalytic Theory of Neuroses*. New York: W. W. Norton.

Freedman, P. M.; Kaplan, H. I.; and Sadock, B. 1976. *Modern Synopsis of Psychiatry II*. Baltimore: Williams & Wilkens.

Glatt, M. N. 1974. *A Guide to Addiction and Its Treatment*. New York: John Wiley & Sons.

Goodwin, D. 1979. Alcoholism and Heredity: A Review and Hypothesis. *Archives of General Psychiatry*, 36:57–61.

Goodwin, D. 1982. Genetic Aspects of Alcoholism. *Drug Therapy*, 57–66.

Grinspoon, L., and Bakalar, J. 1980. Drug Dependence: Non-narcotic Agents. In *Comprehensive Textbook of Psychiatry*, 2nd ed., eds. H. I. Kaplan, A. M. Freedman, and B. J. Sadock. Baltimore: Williams & Wilkins.

Horton, D. 1959. Primitive Societies. In *Drinking and Intoxication*, ed. R. McCarthy. New York: Free Press.

Jaffee, J. H. 1983. Drug Addiction and Drug Abuse. Paper presented at Northeast Regional Medical Education Center, Northport, N. Y.

Jellinek, E. M. 1960. *The Disease Concept of Alcoholism*. New Haven, Conn.: Hillhouse Press.

Jellinek, E. M. 1977. Phases of Alcohol Addiction. *Quarterly Journal of Studies on Alcohol*, 38:114–130.

Jessor, R.; Graves, T.; Hanson, R.; and Jessor, S. 1968. *Society, Personality and Deviant Behavior*. New York: Holt, Rinehart and Winston.

Leiber, C. S.; Jones, D. P.; Lasowsky, M.; and Davidson, C. 1962. Interrelations of Uric Acid and Ethanol Metabolism in Man. *Journal of Clinical Investigation*, 41:1863–1870.

McCord, W., and McCord, J. 1960. *Origins of Alcoholism*. Stanford, Calif.: Stanford University Press.

Mendelson, J., and Mello, N. 1979. Biologic Concomitants of Alcoholism. *New England Journal of Medicine*, 301:912–921.

Menninger, K. 1938. *Man Against Himself*. New York: Harcourt, Brace and Co.

Merton, R. 1957. *Social Theory and Social Structure*. New York: Free Press.

Mezey, E.; Jow, E.; Slaven, R.; and Tabon, F. 1970. Pancreatic Function and Intestinal Absorption in Chronic Alcoholism. *Gastroenterology*, 54:657–664.

Moskow, H.; Pennington, R.; and Knisely, M. 1968. Alcohol, Sludge and Hypoxic Areas of the Nervous System, Liver and Heart. *Microvascular Research*, 1:174–185.

National Institute of Mental Health, 1968. *Alcohol and Alcoholism*. Washington, D.C.: U.S. Public Health Service.

O'Brien, C. P.; Woody, G. E.; and McLellan, A. T. 1983. Modern Treatment of Substance Abuse. Paper presented at Northeast Regional Medical Education Center, Northport, N.Y.

Pattison, E. M.; Sobell, M. D.; and Sobell, L. C. 1977. *Emerging Concepts of Alcohol Dependence*. New York: Springer.

Schuckit, M. D. 1979. *Drug and Alcohol Abuse*. New York: Plenum.

Smithers Foundation. 1968. *Understanding Alcoholism*. New York: Charles Scribner's Sons.

Steiner, C. 1974. *Games Alcoholics Play*. New York: Ballantine.

U.S. Department of Health, Education, and Welfare. *Alcohol and Health*. New York: Charles Scribner's Sons.

Warner, R., and Rosett, H. 1975. The Effects of Drinking on Offspring: A Historical Survey of the American and British Literature. *Journal of Studies on Alcohol*, 36:1395–1420.

Weiten, W. 1983. *Psychology Applied to Modern Life*. Monterey, Calif.: Brooks/Cole.

Supplementary Readings

Alterman, A. I. The Transmission of Psychological Vulnerability: Implications for Alcoholism Etiology. *Journal of Nervous and Mental Diseases*, 171(1983):147–154.

Azrin, N. H. Alcoholism Treatment by Disulfiram and Community Reinforcement Therapy. *Journal of Behavioral Therapy and Experimental Psychiatry*, 13(1982):105–112.

Blechman, E. A. Conventional Wisdom About Familial Contributions to Substance Abuse. *American Journal of Drug and Alcohol Abuse*, 9(1982):35–53.

Blume, S. Alcohol Problems in Women. *New York State Journal of Medicine*, 82(1982):1222–1224.

Bry, B. H. Predicting Drug Abuse: Review and Reformulation. *International Journal of Addiction*, 18(1983):223–233.

Burtle, V. *Women Who Drink*. Springfield, Ill.: Charles C Thomas, 1979.

Cermak, T. L. Interactional Group Therapy with Adult Children of Alcoholics. *International Journal of Group Psychotherapy*, 32(1982):375–389.

Chapman, S. Can You Spot the Game Patients Play to Get Pills to Pop? *Legal Aspects of Medical Practice*, 7(1979):12–15.

Coleman, E. Family Intimacy and Chemical Abuse: The Connection. *Journal of Psychoactive Drugs*, 14(1982):153–158.

Estes, N. J. *Nursing Diagnosis of the Alcoholic Person*. St. Louis: C. V. Mosby, 1980.

Forrest, G. G. *Alcoholism, Narcissism, and Psychopathology*. Springfield, Ill.: Charles C Thomas, 1983.

246

Ghodse, A. H. Living with an Alcoholic. *Postgraduate Medical Journal*, 58(1982):636–640.

Hoor, C. H. Women Alcoholics: Are They Different from Other Women? *International Journal of Addiction*, 18(1983):251–270.

Kinney, J., and Leaton, G. *Understanding Alcohol*. St. Louis: C. V. Mosby, 1982.

Lister, G. R. Performance Impairment and Increased Anxiety Resulting from a Combination of Alcohol and Lorazepam. *Journal of Clinical Psychopharmacology*, 3 (1983):66–71.

Martin, R. L. Alcoholism and Female Criminality. *Journal of Clinical Psychiatry*, 43(1982):400–403.

Naegle, M. A. The Nurse and the Alcoholic: Redefining an Historically Ambivalent Relationship. *Journal of Psychosocial Nursing and Mental Health Services*, 21 (1983):17–24.

Nardi, P. M. Alcoholism and Homosexuality: A Theoretical Perspective. *Journal of Homosexuality*, 7(1982):3–7.

Nathan, P. E. Failures in Prevention: Why Can't We Prevent the Devastating Effect of Alcoholism and Drug Abuse? *American Psychologist*, 38(1983):459–467.

O'Brien, J. E. Behavioral Problems Due to Substance Abuse. *Topics in Emergency Medicine*, 4(1983):42–50.

Pallikkathayil, L. Substance Abuse: Alcohol and Drugs During Adolescence. *Nursing Clinics of North America*, 18(1983):313–321.

Peele, S. Love, Sex, Drugs and Other Magical Solutions to Life. *Journal of Psychoactive Drugs*, 14(1982):125–131.

Quayle, D. American Productivity: The Devastating Effect of Alcohol and Drug Abuse. *American Psychologist*, 38(1983):454–458.

Scherwerts, P. The Alcoholic Treatment Team. *American Journal of Nursing*, 82(1982):1878–1879.

Scoufis, P. Heavy Drinking and the Need for Power. *Journal of Studies on Alcohol*, 43(1982):1010–1019.

Selbert, M. H. Substance Abuse and Prostitution. *Journal of Psychoactive Drugs*, 14(1982):125–131.

Vanicelli, M. Family Problems Related to the Treatment and Outcome of Alcoholic Patients. *British Journal of Addiction*, 78(1983):193–204.

Wallace, J. After Hospitalization: Treatment Support of Alcoholics. *Bulletin of New York Academy of Medicine*, 59(1983):250–254.

Weist, J. K. The Hospitalized Alcoholic. *American Journal of Nursing*, 82(1982):1874–1877.

Wurmser, L. The Question of Specific Psychopathology in Compulsive Drug Use. *Annals of New York Academy of Science*, 398(1982):33–43.

ETIOLOGY OF ALTERED PATTERNS OF
CONGENITAL ORIGIN
Prenatal Factors
Perinatal Factors
Postnatal Factors

TYPES OF ALTERED PATTERNS OF
CONGENITAL ORIGIN
Mental Retardation
Down's Syndrome
Learning Disabilities: Attention Deficit Disorders
Phenylketonuria
Tay-Sachs Disease
Cystic Fibrosis
Hemophilia A
Sickle Cell Anemia
Cerebral Palsy
Spina Bifida
Klinefelter's Syndrome
Turner's Syndrome

THE IMPACT OF ALTERED PATTERNS OF
CONGENITAL ORIGIN
Changes in Family Roles
Stress and Coping
Adapting to Specific Disabilities
Genetic Counseling

THE NURSING PROCESS IN ALTERED PATTERNS OF
CONGENITAL ORIGIN
Assessment
Planning
Implementation
Evaluation

C H A P T E R

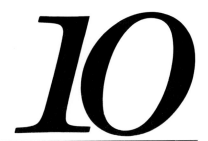

10

Altered Patterns of Congenital Origin

Learning Objectives

After reading this chapter, the student should be able to:

1. Discuss the influence of heredity in the etiology of altered patterns of congenital origin.

2. Contrast the effects of biological, social, and environmental factors in altered patterns of congenital origin.

3. Emphasize the importance of multidimensional data collection in formulating nursing approaches for clients and families confronting altered patterns of congenital origin.

4. Formulate principles of genetic counseling in response to the needs of clients, families, and groups at risk for altered patterns of congenital origin.

5. Utilize primary, secondary, and tertiary levels of prevention in nursing approaches to clients experiencing or at risk for altered patterns of congenital origin.

Overview

Years ago, the trend was to segregate persons with physical and mental disabilities from the mainstream of society and to limit their rights as individuals. Over the years, however, many positive changes have occurred in the treatment of the disabled. Trends such as normalization and mainstreaming have brought the disabled out of institutions and into their communities. As a result, greater numbers of health care providers are interfacing with these people, and nurses in all areas of specialization are being challenged in the care of this population.

It is essential for psychiatric nurses in particular to understand the various types of disabilities with congenital origins, including their etiology, impact on health and development, and complications, as well as current treatments and prevention. With this knowledge, the psychiatric nurse can appropriately assess client needs and plan nursing interventions, independently or in collaboration with others. The purpose of this chapter is to address these issues and prepare the psychiatric nurse to care for the disabled and chronically ill populations.

Everything in nature contains all the powers of nature.
Everything is made of one hidden stuff.
RALPH WALDO EMERSON

Each year, 250,000 infants are born and survive with significant defects. Indeed, 10 to 20 percent of all children under eighteen years of age have some type of chronic illness or sensory impairment (Pless and Roghmann, 1971), and it has been estimated that at least 15 million Americans alive today have an impairment of congenital origin, whether mild or severe (Darling and Darling, 1982).

Growing up with a physical or mental disability is a profound challenge for any child and his family. As the individual with an alteration of congenital origin enters adulthood, his physical and mental impairments can interfere with his ability to meet the expectations of society, putting him at great risk for psychosocial maladjustment. Often, it is the psychological impact of a chronic illness or disability rather than the physical complications that interferes with the person's ability to maintain health status and to function at the highest level of potential (Hamburg, 1983). For these reasons, psychiatric nursing can play a major role in the care of individuals with an alteration of congenital origin.

For the purposes of this chapter, "altered patterns of congenital origin" is used as a generic term to describe birth defects and disabilities. In caring for individuals with such problems, the psychiatric nurse should be familiar with the following definitions:

■ *Altered patterns of congenital origin* are abnormalities in growth, physical structure, and genetic makeup that result in cognitive and physical impairments.

■ *Developmental disability* is any severe, chronic disability attributable to a mental or physical impairment that is manifested before age twenty-two, that is likely to continue, and that will result in substantial functional limitations in self-care, language, mobility, self-direction and motivation, or the capacity for independent living (American Academy of Pediatrics, 1979).

■ *Chronic illness* is any illness with a protracted course that can be progressive and fatal or that is associated with a relatively normal life span despite impaired mental or physical functioning (Mattsson, 1972). It has also been defined as any illness that lasts for more than three months in any given year or that requires one month or more of continued hospitalization.

ETIOLOGY OF ALTERED PATTERNS OF CONGENITAL ORIGIN

Altered patterns of congenital origin vary greatly in their presentation and in their visibility, extent of involvement, potential for cure, and rate of occurrence. A wide range of factors are known to be involved in the etiology of these disorders. Genetic and environmental factors interact to produce the physical, mental, and biochemical characteristics of the developing child. Some defects are caused primarily by the genetic component, while others result primarily from environmental factors such as trauma or a serious infection. Many are the result of the interaction of both genetic and environmental factors.

Anomalies or insults can occur at any stage of fetal development; the timing of such occurrences is critical because it influences the presentation and involvement of the alteration. In particular, exposure to drugs or infections during the earliest stages of embryonic development can have the most profound consequences. A number of prenatal, perinatal, and postnatal factors have been identified in the etiology of alterations of congenital origin.

Prenatal Factors

Prenatally, genetic factors are a major source of altered patterns of congenital origin. Aberrations in the structure and number of chromosomes lead to defects such as Klinefelter's syndrome and Down's syndrome. Some disorders are inheritable through basic Mendelian patterns; examples are phenylketonuria and Tay-Sachs disease. Finally, a number of disorders, including spina bifida, result from the interaction of genetic and environmental factors (multifactorial inheritance).

Environmental factors that can have an adverse effect on the developing fetus include maternal infections, such as viruses, rubella, syphilis, and cytomegalovirus (CMV), and maternal exposures to radiation and industrial chemicals. Some drugs consumed during pregnancy are known to cause congenital malformations; see Table 10-1. Fetal alcohol syndrome is a recognizable pattern of multiple con-

Table 10-1. Drugs That May Affect the Fetus

Drugs	Effects on the Fetus

Antibiotics
  Streptomycin
  Terramycin
  Tetracycline
	Hearing loss; retarded skeletal growth; cataracts; staining of teeth.

Anticoagulants	Increased risk of fetal hemorrhage or death; mental retardation.
Alcohol	Small head; facial abnormalities; heart defects; low birth weight; mental retardation.
Aspirin and other salicylates	If used in large quantities, may cause neonatal bleeding and gastrointestinal discomfort.
Anticonvulsants	Heart defects; anomalies such as cleft lip; mental retardation.
Barbiturates	Digital and facial anomalies; heart lesions; hypocalcemia.
Hallucinogens	Suspected to cause chromosome damage; spontaneous abortion; behavioral abnormalities.
Narcotics	Maternal addiction increases risk of premature delivery; fetus often addicted to narcotic agent, which results in a number of complications.
Sex hormones	Cardiac defects; limb defects; masculinization of the female fetus; other anomalies.
Tranquilizers	Possible cardiovascular defects; may produce respiratory distress in newborns.
Nicotine	Growth retardation; increased risk of spontaneous abortion, stillbirth, infant mortality.

genital anomalies seen in infants of mothers with chronic alcoholism (Scheiner, 1980).

Extremes of maternal age also place the infant at great risk. Mothers under the age of seventeen are at risk for having a child with congenital or gestational problems (Scheiner, 1980). Mothers over the age of thirty-five have a significantly increased risk for having an infant with a chromosomal abnormality. Maternal malnutrition can result in intrauterine growth retardation. Mothers with a metabolic disorder such as diabetes also have a greater risk for prematurity and for congenital anomalies in their offspring.

Another major environmental factor that can affect prenatal development is maternal socioeconomic level. Women at lower socioeconomic levels are at greater risk for having poor obstetric care, inadequate nutrition, poorer health status, and pregnancies at an earlier age. All these factors may lead to complications during pregnancy and to congenital anomalies (Robinson and Robinson, 1976).

Perinatal Factors

During the perinatal period, obstetric complications and complications of the birth process may result in serious insults to the infant. Obstetric complications include premature labor, abruptio placentae, cord prolapse, multiple births, toxemia, and breech birth. Maternal factors that may place an infant at risk include a chronic history of abortions, births of infants with congenital defects, stillbirths, and premature labor.

During the birth process, an infant may suffer asphyxia or trauma, resulting in lack of oxygen to vital areas of the brain or in physical injury. Anoxia is a major pathologic mechanism in such disabling conditions as mental retardation and cerebral palsy. Gestational problems such as prematurity, low birth weight, and postmaturity have been associated with greater risk of developmental delay and physical impairments. Premature infants in particular are vulnerable to developing neonatal illnesses such as respiratory distress syndrome that may adversely affect their future development or even place them at risk for permanent impairments.

Postnatal Factors

A number of events occurring in the postnatal period can cause physical or mental impairment of the child. *Trauma*, one of the most common disabling conditions of childhood, can result in a physical impairment such as paraplegia or cerebral palsy. Traumatic injuries to the brain may lead to conditions such as seizure disorders and mental retardation. Serious infections such as bacterial meningitis and encephalitis have also been associated with residual impairments to the child; the extent of impairment may vary from a mild ataxia and learning deficit to severe mental retardation, cerebral palsy, blindness, and deafness.

Exposure to environmental toxins is another postnatal factor that can adversely affect a developing child. One of the most serious toxic problems today is lead poisoning. The clinical sequelae of lead poisoning include anemia, behavioral changes, and—in the severest degree—mental retardation, paralysis, blindness, and convulsions (Whaley and Wong, 1983).

Living in an impoverished environment can also have a significant impact on a child's ultimate health and development. Children in poor families may not receive adequate health care, nutrition, stimulation, or supervision from adults. In addition, children in such environments are less likely to be exposed to learning activities and parental attention that provide intellectual stimulation and help prepare them for school.

Chronically ill children may also suffer impairments that limit their functional abilities as a residue of their illness. For example, a child with a severe cardiac defect may have limited mobility and self-help skills because of circulatory compromise.

In the following discussion of types of altered patterns of congenital origin, the etiology will be addressed more specifically for certain disorders.

TYPES OF ALTERED PATTERNS OF CONGENITAL ORIGIN

This section of the chapter describes commonly occurring and serious altered patterns of congenital origin. Most of the defects presented here are apparent early in life or during the early developmental years. The disorders or disabilities are presented briefly to familiarize the psychiatric nurse with them and their treatments.

Mental Retardation

Mental retardation is one of the most prevalent and yet most misunderstood handicapping conditions in the United States today. In this country, individuals with mental retardation make up approximately 3 percent of the population. The majority of mentally retarded persons are classified as *mildly* retarded; this classification is approximately seven to eight times more common than any other degree of retardation (Whaley and Wong, 1983).

Tremendous changes have occurred in attitudes and philosophies regarding care for the mentally retarded. Years ago, mental retardation was treated as an illness, and individuals with this disability were segregated from society, institutionalized at an early age. Today the majority of mentally retarded individuals live in their homes and communities, and the care they receive is individually and developmentally focused. In recent years, federal legislation has been passed guaranteeing the rights of mentally retarded individuals to protection, treatment, and especially education. In addition, there has been growing awareness that mentally retarded children benefit from early intervention or teaching, especially in the home. Early intervention focuses on the teaching of basic life skills, language development, social skills, and fine and gross motor skills.

Changing attitudes toward care have major implications for all health care providers because they are likely to have increasing contact with mentally retarded individuals. Nursing can play a key role in the coordination of care, formulation of care plans, and management of problems associated with mental retardation. For this reason, it is crucial that nurses be knowledgeable in defining mental retardation and in managing its problems and be sensitive to the needs of the individual and his family.

DEFINING MENTAL RETARDATION According to the American Association on Mental Deficiency (AAMD), *mental retardation* is defined as "significantly subaverage general intellectual functioning existing concurrently with deficits in adaptive behavior and manifested during the developmental period" (Grossman, 1973, p. 3). It is important to realize that this definition emphasizes both intelligence and adaptive behavior as inclusive criteria for the diagnosis of mental retardation.

"Significant subaverage intellectual functioning" refers to an intelligence quotient (IQ) that is 2 standard deviations or more below the mean, or an IQ of approximately 70 or below. Most standard measures of IQ, such as the Stanford-Binet and WISC, are used to assess intellectual functioning. "Adaptive behavior" refers to the degree to which an individual meets the milestones or standards of personal independence and social responsibility expected for her age within a specific culture (Clifford, 1980). At different ages, different skills or tasks are expected for adequate adaptive function. Parents are often the first to notice signs of inadequate adaptive function, such as gross motor delays, delays in fine motor skills, delays in language acquisition, and poor judgment skills. In school-age children, measures of adaptive behavior are viewed in terms of academic performance. For adults, vocational skills, independent functioning, and social skills are used as indicators of adaptive functioning.

Five classifications are used to describe the degree of disability and educational potential of mentally retarded individuals. Table 10-2 lists the

Table 10-2. Classifications of Mental Retardation

Category	Preschool (birth to 5 years): Maturation and development	School age (6 to 21 years): Education and training	Adult (21 years and older): Social and vocational adequacy
Borderline IQ 68–83	Usually has minimal lags in all areas of development. May not be diagnosed until child enters school. Usually related to psychosocial causes.	Can achieve regular academic skills with special assistance (education).	Capable of social adequacy (marriage and child rearing). Capable of employment, but vocational choices may be limited to skilled labor. May need additional support during crisis.
Mild (educable) IQ 50–67	Develops normal skills at much slower rate (approximately half) than normal. May have impaired coordination.	Can acquire practical skills, purposeful reading and math skills to fourth grade level with special education. Achieves mental age of 8 to 12 years.	Functions primarily in sheltered workshop. Capable of vocational skills and independent living. May need much support during times of stress.
Moderate (trainable) IQ 35–49	Marked delays in development. Usually associated with disorders such as cerebral palsy, seizures.	Can learn necessary academic skills, manual skills, self-care skills to function in community with supervision. Achieves mental age of 3 to 7 years.	Can perform simple skills in sheltered environment. Is easily frightened and has limited judgment.
Severe IQ 20–34	Severe delays in infancy; little or no communication skills. Associated with other physical disorders or illnesses. Cause usually known.	Can respond to training in self-help skills, such as toileting. Achieves mental age of toddler.	Responds to daily routines and repetitive activities. Needs continuous supervision in protective environment; such as home, group home.
Profound IQ 0–20	Gross retardation, infantlike behavior. May walk but may not speak. Associated with other physical disorders or illnesses.	Obvious delays in all areas of development. Training is primarily in areas of developing sensory-motor skills. Achieves mental age of infant.	Needs complete custodial care, which may be provided outside of home.

various classifications according to range of IQ and expected skill level. In counseling parents, it is more important for the nurse to focus on the child's individual abilities, strengths, and skill level than on IQ numbers. Cases of moderate to profound degrees of mental retardation are often associated with other physical disabilities and with chronic illnesses such as seizure disorders. Individuals in this category are likely to have more acute illnesses and to need care for chronic problems and therefore will have greater contact with health care professionals.

The cause of mental retardation is known in only a small percentage of cases—approximately 6 percent. In the majority of cases, the cause is either unknown or not yet classified. The generally recognized sources of mental retardation were described earlier in this chapter.

PLAN OF CARE The goal of caring for a mentally retarded individual is to promote his optimum development and level of independence as a person within a family and community. In helping the individual achieve this goal, it is important for the nurse to understand the learning potential and deficits of the mentally retarded. With a knowledge of the learning problems associated with mental retardation, the nurse can use appropriate teaching methods to train retarded individuals.

The potential for a mentally retarded individual to learn self-help skills, vocational skills, and social skills depends on his functional level and on the appropriateness of the teaching techniques. Mentally retarded learners have marked deficits in their ability to discriminate between two or more stimuli and also have difficulty in areas of abstract thought. Such learners are best taught through concrete instruction and demonstration. Mentally retarded learners also have problems with short-term memory. Because of this, they learn best by simple step-by-step instruction. A teaching technique frequently used with the retarded is *task analysis*, in which a particular task is divided into progressive steps and the child is taught one step before moving on to the next. Because mentally retarded learners may lack motivation for learning a skill, motivation needs to be provided in the form of positive reinforcement. Techniques of behavior modification are frequently used to develop various skills in these individuals.

Several recent changes have made a significant impact on the habilitation of mentally retarded individuals. *Normalization* is a habilitation principle advocating that services be provided for handicapped individuals in the same manner as for nonhandicapped. The goal of normalization is to establish as normal a living pattern as possible for mentally retarded persons. An example of the impact of this principle is the movement of mentally retarded children and adults out of large segregated institutions into small community residences (group homes).

Children with Down's syndrome can live happy lives if they receive affection and encouragement from their companions.
SOURCE: Elizabeth Crews, Stock Boston, Inc.

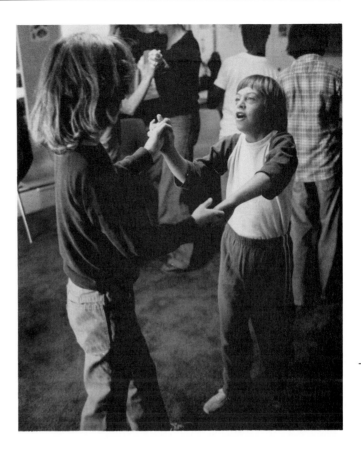

Another change that parallels normalization is the trend toward *mainstreaming*. The goal of mainstreaming is to place a disabled child in a community school that can provide the least restrictive environment to meet his educational needs. The trend toward mainstreaming has proven to be controversial when the educational programs do not provide the trained personnel and special assistance mentally retarded children may need. Many school programs have special classes (EMR class) with trained personnel and support services to best meet the mentally retarded child's needs.

Down's Syndrome

Down's syndrome, one of the most commonly known syndromes associated with a chromosomal abnormality, is actually a multiple system disability characterized by mental retardation and various physical manifestations. The syndrome is named for Dr. John Langdon Haydon Down, who first described it in 1866. The risk of occurrence for Down's syndrome is approximately 1 in 800 live births (Bergmsa, 1982).

In approximately 95 percent of all cases of Down's syndrome, an extra chromosome 21 produces the alterations in physical and mental development. The extra chromosome occurs as a result of faulty chromosome distribution in the egg or sperm or during division of the fertilized egg. Trisomy 21 is associated with increasing maternal age. The incidence of Down's syndrome increases strikingly as maternal age increases, especially over the age of thirty-five. In fact, 50 percent of all cases of Down's syndrome occur with maternal age greater than thirty-five. There is increasing evidence that paternal aging can contribute to Down's syndrome as well.

A small percentage of cases (approximately 4 percent) are caused by translocation of chromosomes 15 and 21. This type of genetic alteration is hereditary (a parent may be a balanced translocation carrier) and is not related to parental aging. With translocation there is a much greater risk of recurrence (10 to 15 percent) than with trisomy 21, which is a sporadic event with low recurrence. In cases of translocation, chromosomal analysis as well as sensitive, knowledgeable genetic counseling should be provided.

A third genetic alteration that has been associated with some cases of Down's syndrome is *mosaicism*. In mosaicism, the maldistribution comes at a later stage of the division of the fertilized egg, resulting in both normal and abnormal cells. Children with this type of Down's syndrome may have higher intellectual functioning and fewer physical problems than those with the other types of Down's syndrome.

CLINICAL MANIFESTATIONS The classic clinical manifestations of Down's syndrome include flat fa-

PHYSICAL CHARACTERISTICS OF DOWN'S SYNDROME

Hypotonia, especially in newborn period.

Flat facial features.

Flat nasal bulge.

Microcephaly.

Flat occiput.

Inner epicanthal folds.

Upward slant of palpebral fissures.

Speckling of iris (Brushfield's spots).

Small, malformed ears.

Narrow, high, arched palate.

Protruding tongue; may be fissured or furrowed.

Dental hypoplasia.

Short neck with redundant skin.

Short stature.

Hyperextensible joints.

Transverse palmar crease (simian crease).

Short, broad hands.

Incurved little finger (clinodactyly).

Characteristic dermal ridge pattern.

cial features, flat occiput, epicanthal folds, narrow palate, short broad hands with simian creases, and hypotonia. The accompanying box provides a more thorough list of the physical characteristics. Although the syndrome can be readily diagnosed by these clinical manifestations alone, chromosomal analysis is usually done to confirm the diagnosis.

A number of congenital anomalies and physical problems are associated with Down's syndrome. Approximately 40 percent of the infants born with the syndrome have a significant congenital heart defect. Less frequently occurring anomalies include intestinal atresias, seizures, strabismus, tracheoesophageal fistulas, and atlantoaxial subluxation due to hypoplasia of the odontoid process (Bartoshesky, 1980). Various types of leukemia also have increased incidence in children with Down's syndrome. Respiratory and ear infections are common and can be chronic. Because of chronic ear infections and potential middle ear malformations, Down's victims also have an increased risk of hearing impairment. Dental problems are common because of malformed teeth and gum disease. Delays in gross motor ability may occur because of hypotonia.

The most significant feature of Down's syndrome is mental retardation. The majority of affected individuals are mildly to moderately retarded, within the trainable average. Initially, infants with Down's syndrome appear to have normal mental development, but by age two there is a relative decline in performance, and a plateau is reached at about age four. Gross motor delays, visual impairments, and speech delays can all affect various aspects of the child's development. Individuals with Down's syndrome usually perform well on measures of social competence, but behavior disorders can occur.

PLAN OF CARE In recent years a great deal of research has been done on the care of individuals with Down's syndrome. Issues that have been investigated include institutional versus home care and the impact of early intervention. Home care provides many benefits for children with Down's syndrome. Early intervention programs have encouraged the earlier attainment of developmental milestones for these children.

The potential for the child with Down's syndrome is great if she has the care of a loving, supportive family, early appropriate stimulation and educational programs, and access to advanced medical technology. As with any disabled individual, the person with Down's syndrome has potential for growth and development. It is the responsibility of the health care provider to identify the needs, strengths, and weaknesses of the individual and to plan for appropriate comprehensive care to meet these needs.

Learning Disabilities: Attention Deficit Disorders

Learning disability, an alteration in cognitive pro-

> ### BEHAVIORAL MANIFESTATIONS OF
> ### ATTENTION DEFICIT DISORDERS
>
> Short attention span.
>
> Hyperactivity.
>
> Distractibility.
>
> Impulsivity.
>
> Difficulty reaching satisfaction.
>
> Difficulty with peer relations.
>
> Easily fatigued.
>
> Labile emotions.
>
> Sleep problems.
>
> Motor skill deficits.
>
> Impaired memory.
>
> Deficits in communication skills.
>
> Perceptual deficits (left/right confusion).

257

cesses, can be a severely handicapping condition with broad implications for the development of a child's self-esteem, educational achievement, and family life. A *learning disability* is an impairment in one or more cognitive processes such as attention, memory, visual perception, or written or spoken language (Levine, 1980). Manifestations of learning disabilities are seen in problems with reading, mathematics, spelling, or comprehension. Examples of learning disabilities include *dysgraphia* (difficulty writing), *dyslexia* (difficulty reading), and visual-perceptual disorders.

A number of etiologic factors have been known to place a child at risk for developing a learning disability. Such factors include familial patterns, early childhood illness, perinatal injury or stress, environmental deprivations, nutritional deficiencies, and stressful life events (Levine, 1980). A child from a lower socioeconomic background may be at greater risk for developing a learning disability because of danger of poor health care, poor nutrition, and lack of parental models to stimulate learning readiness skills.

The severity of learning disabilities may vary at different ages. For this reason, early identification and intervention is crucial for a learning disabled child to achieve academic success. Once a child is identified as having a learning disability, an appropriate school program with special education can be planned and provided.

Commonly associated with learning disabilities is a behavioral condition known as *attention deficit disorder* (also referred to as hyperactivity or minimal brain dysfunction). Attention deficit disorder is a behavioral problem characterized by chronic inattention, overactivity, and difficulty in dealing with

multiple stimuli. A number of manifestations have been associated with this disorder—see the accompanying box. For a particular child, the manifestations may be few or numerous, mild or severe, and they will vary at different developmental levels. For example, the behavioral manifestations may be apparent at an early age but the associated learning disabilities will not fully manifest themselves until the child enters school. Many of the characteristics of attention deficit disorder diminish by adolescence, but ongoing emotional difficulties may place the adolescent at risk for developing poor self-esteem, behavior problems, and sociopathic behavior. An individual with continual failures at home, in school, and in peer relationships will have a negative view of himself and of other people.

Because of varying definitions and descriptions of symptoms, it is difficult to estimate the incidence of attention deficit disorders. Some estimates place the incidence at 3 to 15 percent, and it is known that boys are ten times more frequently affected than girls (Whaley and Wong, 1983). The disorder is believed to be related to a lag in development of the central nervous system or to a maturational lag. Diagnosis is made from a pediatric exam, thorough history (including description of behavior at home and school), neurologic exams, and psychological and educational assessments.

There are multiple aspects to the management of children with an attention deficit disorder. Involved in such management are special education, family education and counseling, medication, and planned alterations in the environment. Individual psychotherapy may be necessary for a child to modify behavior problems or develop improved self-esteem. Medical research has shown that central nervous system stimulants are often effective in reducing the symptoms of affected children. The most commonly used stimulants are amphetamines, especially methylphenidate (Ritalin) and dextroamphetamine sulfate (Dexedrine).

Learning disabilities associated with attention deficit disorders are complex conditions that require early intervention, ongoing follow-up, and changes in management according to the individual child's needs.

Phenylketonuria

Phenylketonuria (PKU) is a relatively rare autosomal recessive disorder characterized by an alteration in the body's ability to metabolize the essential amino acid phenylalanine (Whaley and Wong, 1983). The basic defect is a deficiency in the liver enzyme phenylalanine hydroxylase. This enzyme deficiency results in an accumulation of phenylalanine in the bloodstream and in urinary excretion of an abnormal by-product, phenylpyruvic acid. The accumulation of phenylalanine can interfere with the normal growth and development of the brain and central nervous system. The term "phenylketonuria" comes from the presence of phenylpyruvic acid in the urine, which gives the urine a characteristic musty odor.

Normally, phenylalanine hydroxylase converts phenylalanine to *tyrosine*, which is essential for the formation of the pigment melanin. Because of the tyrosine deficiency that occurs with PKU, affected children have fair skin, blond hair, and blue eyes.

At birth, PKU infants appear perfectly normal. However, if the deficiency goes undetected and the

---

DSM-III CLASSIFICATION AND NURSING DIAGNOSES

Mental retardation and learning disabilities are classified in DSM-III as "Disorders First Evident in Infancy, Childhood, or Adolescence." Categories include:

317.0x Mild mental retardation

318.0x Moderate mental retardation

318.1x Severe mental retardation

318.2x Profound mental retardation

(Code in fifth digit: 1 = with other behavioral symptoms, 0 = without other behavioral symptoms)

Attention deficit disorder
314.01 with hyperactivity
314.00 without hyperactivity
314.80 residual type

Nursing diagnoses that may apply include:

Anxiety

Bowel elimination, alteration in: constipation, diarrhea

Comfort, alteration in

Communication, impaired verbal

Coping: ineffectual individual, family

Home maintenance management, impaired

Knowledge deficit (of parents)

Mobility, impaired physical

Parenting, alteration in

Self-care deficit

Sleep pattern disturbance

Social isolation

Urinary elimination, alterations in patterns of

---

infant ingests milk, increased blood and tissue levels of phenylalanine will develop. The accumulation of phenylalanine and its abnormal by-products will result in damaging effects on the nervous tissue and in such common clinical manifestations as developmental delay (mental retardation), failure to thrive, irritability, frequent vomiting, hyperactivity, and unpredictable, bizarre behavior. Seizure activity and abnormal EEGs are common in the severely retarded.

*Children sweeten labors; but they make misfortunes more bitter. They
increase the woes of life but they mitigate the remembrance of death.*

FRANCIS BACON

The need for early identification of PKU victims and immediate therapy is obviously paramount. If the condition is detected in the newborn, treatment can begin and the damaging effects can be prevented. The treatment of PKU is dietary regulation of phenylalanine. Because this amino acid is essential for tissue growth, the infant is placed on a low-phenylalanine diet—20 to 30 mg/kg of body weight of phenylalanine per day. The blood level of phenylalanine must be monitored closely; if the level is greater than 10 mg/dl, significant damage to the nervous system can result. If the phenylalanine level is too low (below 2 mg/dl), growth retardation can occur (Whaley and Wong, 1983).

Because all natural food proteins contain some amount of phenylalanine, dietary supplements must be provided in addition to the strict dietary regimen. Lofenalac, a formula low in phenylalanine, is substituted for milk and milk products. Most high-protein foods, such as milk products and meat, are eliminated from the diet or are restricted to minimal amounts. Other foods are monitored to allow for the prescribed amount of phenylalanine each day. Dietary restriction of phenylalanine should continue until the child is six to eight years of age.

For mentally retarded children with PKU, dietary restrictions of phenylalanine can limit the progression of the disorder and improve the child's behavior. Pregnant women with PKU are at risk of having an infant with congenital malformations if they have high levels of phenylalanine.

Primary prevention of mental retardation from PKU involves screening of newborns for abnormal levels of phenylalanine in the blood or of its by-products in the urine. The most commonly used test for screening newborns is the Guthrie blood test. For the test to be effective, the newborn must ingest a high-phenylalanine diet for at least 24 hours. This test is mandatory for all newborns in most states. If parents do have a child with PKU, genetic counseling should be made available to them. Since PKU is an autosomal recessive disorder, there is a 1 in 4 risk for each subsequent sibling having the disorder.

Tay-Sachs Disease

Tay-Sachs disease is an autosomal recessive disorder of relatively rare occurrence. This condition involves progressive neurologic deterioration and death before the age of four. Blindness and optic atrophy occur as the degeneration of the nervous system progresses. Varying degrees of mental retardation are associated with the disorder. The pathologic mechanism involved is a disorder of lipid metabolism, with a deficiency in the enzyme hexoaminidase.

Tay-Sachs disease occurs predominantly in Ashkenazic (Eastern European) Jews. Primary prevention of the disorder is possible with carrier screening.

Cystic Fibrosis

Cystic fibrosis is the most common fatal genetic disease among white children (Schwartz, 1978). Also known as mucoviscidosis, cystic fibrosis is a disease of generalized dysfunction of the exocrine (mucous-producing) glands. It is a complex disease affecting multiple organ systems in varying degrees of severity, but the majority of those affected have symptoms involving the respiratory system.

Cystic fibrosis is transmitted through an autosomal recessive mode of inheritance, and it has been

Cheated of features by dissembling nature.
Deformed, unfinished, sent before my time
Into this breathing world, scarce half made up.
And that so lamely and unfashionable
That dogs bark at me as I halt by them.
WILLIAM SHAKESPEARE, RICHARD III

260

estimated that 5 percent of the white population are carriers (Schwartz, 1978). The incidence of the disease is between 1 in 1600 and 1 in 2000 live births. It is hoped that future genetic research will produce methods for identifying carriers of the trait and for prenatal diagnosis.

The major clinical manifestations of the disease are gastrointestinal malabsorption related to pancreatic enzyme deficiency, progressive obstructive pulmonary disease, and elevated sweat concentrations of sodium and chloride. The primary mechanism causing these manifestations is a blockage of the organ passages by increased viscosity of mucous secretions. The mucous glands produce a thick mucoprotein that blocks the passages of the pancreas and bronchioles. The significant elevation of sweat electrolytes is related to malabsorption of sodium by the sweat glands.

The pancreatic enzyme deficiency results in impaired digestion and absorption of essential nutrients, especially fats and proteins. Thus, the child with cystic fibrosis has foul-smelling greasy stools and appears very thin (malnourished) despite a voracious appetite. The pulmonary complications are the most serious threat to survival. The obstruction of the bronchioles and the stasis of mucus in the lungs results in chronic respiratory infections, impaired oxygen–carbon dioxide exchange, and progressive pulmonary dysfunction.

The diagnosis of cystic fibrosis is suspected if one or all of the following are present: history of chronic respiratory disease, positive family history, and reported symptoms of gastrointestinal malabsorption (Larter, 1981). Confirmation of the disease occurs with a positive sweat chloride test.

The care of a child with cystic fibrosis is complex and primarily involves dietary management, the use of oral pancreatic enzyme replacements, treatment of respiratory infections, and good pulmonary therapy (postural drainage and cupping). Many advances in the management of individuals with cystic fibrosis have increased the life expectancy to young adulthood, but the prognosis still remains grim. The disease is characterized by continual acute exacerbations, chronic loss of function, and tremendous multiple stresses on the patient and family. The goal of caring for an individual with cystic fibrosis is to help the child reach the highest level of functioning at each stage of the disease. Care includes monitoring the individual's psychosocial adjustment, recognizing illness-related emotional problems, and providing the necessary psychosocial support.

Hemophilia A

Hemophilia is a generic term referring to a group of bleeding disorders that are due to a deficiency or an abnormality in one of the factors necessary for blood clotting. The two most common variants of this disorder are hemophilia A, or classic hemophilia (abnormal clotting factor VIII), and hemophilia B, or Christmas disease (factor IX deficiency). The symptoms are the same for all types of hemophilia, but specific factor deficiencies need to be identified to provide the appropriate replacement therapy.

Hemophilia A is an X-linked recessive disorder. In this type of inheritance, the mode of transmission is from a carrier female to her male offspring. Each son has a 50 percent chance of having the disorder, and each daughter has a 50 percent chance of

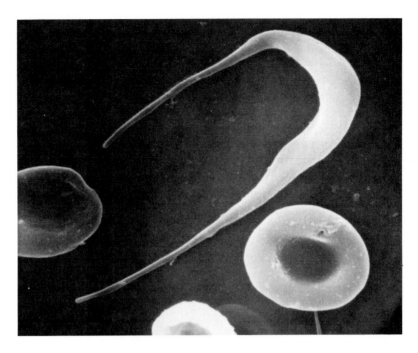

*Normal (*left and right*) and "sickled" (*center*) red blood cells from a person with sickle cell anemia.*
SOURCE: R. M. Zucker, B. F. Cameron, and R.C. Leif/BPS

261

becoming a carrier. The risk of occurrence for the disorder is 1 in 2500 live male births (Koerper and Diamond, 1982). A small number of cases are due to a genetic mutation.

The primary clinical manifestation of hemophilia is prolonged bleeding anywhere from or within the body. The degree of hemorrhage can vary from individual to individual. The first sign of the disorder can be bleeding from a minor surgical procedure such as circumcision or bruising from a slight injury such as a fall. Another warning sign may be bleeding from the loss of a deciduous tooth. The bleeding may also be internal, especially into a joint, which may result in physically disabling and painful deformities.

The disabling limitations of hemophilia may be minimized with properly administered replacement therapy. For hemophilia A, the treatment involves the administration of blood factor VIII. The frequency and dosage of the therapy will vary with the type of hemophilia and the degree of bleeding. Children and adults are usually taught to administer the replacement factors to themselves. Such home care has proven to be highly successful in the management of hemophilia. Treatment also includes local emergency therapy to control bleeding. Another aspect of treatment is the promotion of regular exercise programs to strengthen muscles and joints.

Children and adults with hemophilia must adjust their physical activity to prevent injury. Successful adjustment to this disorder results from an understanding of the illness, a strong support system, ability to cope with limitations, and a positive self-image.

Sickle Cell Anemia

Sickle cell anemia, an inherited disease, primarily afflicts blacks of African descent. Some 60,000 American blacks are estimated to have the disease, and there may be as many as 2 million carriers (Marx, 1978). Sickle cell anemia is named for the distorted shape of the red blood cells caused by an abnormal amino acid in the hemoglobin molecule. This shape causes the cells to clot and not to move smoothly through the tiny capillary beds of the body. As a result, oxygen is not distributed in adequate amounts.

Victims of this disease experience intense pain, often in the joints. The overall life span is greatly reduced by the damage resulting from the lack of oxygen to vital organs. Many victims die from heart or kidney failure in childhood or adolescence.

Cerebral Palsy

Cerebral palsy is one of the most common physical disabilities affecting children and adults. *Cerebral palsy* has been defined as a chronic nonprogressive disorder of the brain that results in alterations of motor function and coordination. The degree of impairment and involvement of other body systems varies from individual to individual, as does the etiology.

A number of prenatal, perinatal, and postnatal conditions have been known to cause cerebral palsy. Cerebral anoxia resulting from other conditions is the basic pathologic mechanism leading to brain damage and subsequent motor impairment. Prenatal factors known to contribute to cerebral palsy include intrauterine infections, brain anomalies, radiation, trauma, and maternal bleeding. Perinatal factors include prematurity, intracranial hemorrhage, birth trauma, cardiopulmonary problems, and hyperbilirubinemia. During childhood, conditions that may result in cerebral palsy include head trauma, cerebrovascular accident, and infections of the central nervous system (Abrams and Panagakos, 1980).

Cerebral palsy is usually classified according to the nature and manifestations of the neuromuscular dysfunction. The most common form, *spastic* cerebral palsy, is characterized by hypertonia, muscle weakness, persistent primitive reflexes, and delayed or absent postural control (Whaley and Wong, 1983). Spastic cerebral palsy is further classified according to the muscle groups involved; for example, hemiparesis involves one side of the body. Associated with spasticity are contractures of various joints, resulting in reduced functional ability and bony deformities.

A second type of cerebral palsy is *dyskinetic* or *athetoid*. The dyskinetic form is characterized by involuntary movements of all extremities and of the trunk, facial muscles, and tongue. These movements often decrease during rest and increase during times of stress. *Ataxic* types of cerebral palsy are the least common; they involve problems of imbalance and incoordination of the voluntary muscles of both the trunk and extremities. Some severely disabled children have a form of cerebral palsy described as mixed-type, which usually involves a combination of spasticity and dyskinesis.

CLINICAL MANIFESTATIONS A primary manifestation of the disorder is significant delays in gross motor development. An infant with cerebral palsy will show delays in all expected motor skills; this is particularly significant if the infant is normal in all other areas of development. Other manifestations of cerebral palsy include abnormal motor skills (abnormal crawling), muscle tone abnormalities, abnormal posture, and persistence of primitive infantile spasms (Whaley and Wong, 1983).

A number of other impairments may be associated with cerebral palsy. Half of the children with cerebral palsy are mentally retarded, and the greater the brain damage, the higher the likelihood of cognitive involvement (Abrams and Panagakos, 1980). Other commonly associated impairments include feeding difficulties, seizure disorders, hearing impairments, learning disabilities, attention deficit disorders, and strabismus. As with other disabled children and adults, cerebral palsy clients are at risk for developing poor self-esteem and psychosocial adjustment problems.

PLAN OF CARE The management of cerebral palsy is multiphasic and depends on the severity and in-

volvement of the disability. The goal in management of cerebral palsy is to help that individual reach his highest level of potential within the physical limitations of the disability. An important key to successful management is the early identification of involved infants and provision of necessary treatment. Treatment of cerebral palsy focuses primarily on orthopedic care, physical therapy, and occupational therapy. The treatment plans aim at encouraging mobility and self-help skills, correcting orthopedic deformities, and preventing additional deformities that may limit function.

An adult with cerebral palsy may seem more disabled than a child because of chronic contractures and bony deformities that limit function and because of the greater complexity of expected skills. The chronic treatment of cerebral palsy involves ongoing therapy, orthopedic follow-up, and the care of associated disabilities.

Spina Bifida

Spina bifida (meningomyelocele) is a major congenital malformation that affects multiple body systems. It is the second most common birth defect after Down's syndrome and its incidence in the United States is approximately 1 per 1,000 live births (Myers, 1984). It occurs more frequently in females, in families of lower socioeconomic status, and in groups from English, Irish, or Welsh background.

Meningomyelocele belongs to the group of neural tube defects that may include anencephaly, abnormalities of the head, and abnormalities of the spine. Meningomyelocele is characterized by a sac-like cyst, protruding through a vertebral defect, that contains the meninges, cerebral spinal fluid, and a part of the spinal cord and its nerve roots. Meningomyelocele results in damage to the underlying nervous tissue and associated neurologic impairment. The associated problems include partial or complete paralysis of the lower extremities, hydrocephalus, bony deformities, impaired lower extremity sensation, bladder incontinence, and bowel incontinence. The degree of involvement depends on the anatomic level of the defect and the size of the lesion.

ETIOLOGY The causes of spina bifida remain unknown, although it is believed to be the result of multifactorial inheritance. In multifactorial inheritance, a defect results from the interactions of genetic influences with factors in the fetal (maternal) environment. It is known that once a set of parents have had a child with spina bifida they have an increased risk (4 to 5 percent) of having a second child with the defect. An adult with spina bifida also has an increased risk of having a child with the defect.

A number of environmental factors have been proposed to cause meningomyelocele. Those include viral infections, maternal fever, and medications such as valproic acid (Myers, 1984). Vitamin deficiencies (especially folate) during the first trimester are also thought to contribute to the defect. A number of studies have been conducted to test the hypothesis that early vitamin supplementation may prevent meningomyelocele (Myers, 1984).

Although it is unknown what causes meningomyelocele, the pathologic mechanism resulting in the defect is known. Normally, formation of the neural tube begins by the twentieth day of gestation and the tube is fused or closed by the twenty-eighth day. In meningomyelocele, the neural tube fails to close and the surrounding tissues develop abnormally.

PLAN OF CARE When an infant is born with meningomyelocele, the initial care involves a multidisciplinary evaluation to assess the extent of the disability and the family's need for supportive care and education. Early surgical closure (within the first 24 to 48 hours) of the defect is recommended. Following closure, the infant is monitored closely for the development of hydrocephalus. In 75 percent of children with meningomyelocele, hydrocephalus occurs, usually the result of an Arnold Chiari malformation of the brain. Arnold Chiari malformation is a defect involving downward displacement of the brain stem and cerebellum through the foramen magnum. Surgical shunting procedures are performed to control the progression of hydrocephalus. The majority of children with meningomyelocele and shunted hydrocephalus are of normal intelligence but may experience learning disabilities.

Varying degrees of paralysis and bony deformities of the lower extremities occur as a result of the spinal defect. Because of imbalances between functioning and nonfunctioning muscle groups, clients are at risk for developing contractures and such problems as hip dislocation. The goals in orthopedic management are to reduce and prevent deformities of the lower extremities and to provide mobility. For children with flaccid paralysis, functional mobility is possible with a brace known as the Rochester parapodium. The parapodium allows the paraplegic to view the world from an upright position and to fully explore the environment. Orthopedic care also involves physical therapy and surgical interventions as necessary.

Meningomyelocele also results in impaired sensation in the lower extremities. Affected individuals are at risk for developing decubitus ulcers, burns, and abrasions that may be debilitating.

Urinary incontinence results from abnormal innervation of the bladder and bladder sphincter. Most children with meningomyelocele have a flaccid bladder, which leads to overflow incontinence. A small group have spastic bladders with small bladder capacities and incomplete emptying. In addition to urinary incontinence, bladder dysfunction can lead to recurrent urinary infections and such renal problems as reflux and hydronephrosis. These urologic problems can result in renal damage and renal failure. The goals in urologic management are preservation of renal function and promotion of socially acceptable continence. Today the major method of promoting continence is clean intermittent catheterization (CIC). Clean intermittent catheterization facilitates regular drainage of the bladder, thus reducing overflow incontinence and reflux. The success of CIC depends on compliance with the catheterization at scheduled intervals. Artificial sphincters have also been used to promote urinary continence, alone or with CIC.

Bowel incontinence results from abnormal innervation of the rectum, external anal sphincter, and abdominal muscles. With a dysfunctional anal sphincter, there is uncontrolled passage of stool. Children with a neurogenic bowel are at risk for chronic constipation and fecal impactions. The goals in management are to prevent constipation, manage constipation if it should occur, and promote stool continence (Henderson and Synhorst, 1977). Dietary changes (high fiber bran diets), regular toileting, and the use of stool softeners and laxatives are treatments utilized to address these goals.

Spinal cord dysfunction can also result in impaired sexual function. Males with meningomyelocele may be impotent or may have retrograde ejaculations with significantly reduced fertility. Females with this disability have decreased sensation but normal fertility.

Meningomyelocele is a complex disability that involves multiple body functions. The care of an individual with meningomyelocele requires long-term, comprehensive, coordinated management. The care provider must be sensitive to the ongoing psychosocial needs of the individual and her family and to the developmental needs of the individual. Recent advances in the medical care and habilitation of children with meningomyelocele have provided much hope for successful and satisfying growth through adulthood, although societal attitudes may limit a disabled adult's ability to achieve a satisfying lifestyle. Nursing can play a key role in advocacy for the disabled in the community.

Advances in genetic diagnostics have led to the availability of prenatal diagnosis for parents at risk for having a child with meningomyelocele. The most commonly used techniques are genetic counseling, ultrasound, and amniocentesis. These studies are usually done during the fourteenth to sixteenth week of pregnancy. Through amniocentesis, an elevation in alpha-fetoprotein levels may indicate the presence of meningomyelocele in the fetus. With open neural tube defects, alpha-fetoprotein is elevated in both the maternal serum and amniotic fluid. Prenatal evaluation for a neural tube defect allows the family to consider whether to continue the pregnancy. Much support is needed by a family going through this process.

Klinefelter's Syndrome

Klinefelter's syndrome is a congenital defect resulting from an alteration in the sex chromosome makeup of the male cells. In this syndrome, an extra (or possibly more) X chromosome joins to the normal XY pair to result in an abnormal karyotype of XXY. This defect occurs predominantly in white populations and has an incidence of approximately 1 per 600 live male births (Opitz, 1982).

The major impact of this disorder is an alteration in sexual development The syndrome may be detected in the newborn if significantly smaller than average testes are found, but it is usually not diagnosed until puberty. At that time, the primary manifestation of the disorder is delayed and immature male secondary sex characteristics. Individuals with this syndrome are usually significantly taller than normal males and are infertile. About 15 percent of those affected are mentally retarded (Opitz, 1982). Personality disorders, behavioral problems, psychosis, and alcoholism are also common. This syndrome is treated with the administration of male sex hormones, and psychological care is frequently needed. Secondary prevention includes diagnosis by amniocentesis and treatment of the clinical manifestations.

Turner's Syndrome

Turner's syndrome is a classic example of a defect in the sex chromosome makeup of female cells. Instead of the usual sex chromosome pattern of XX, the female with Turner's syndrome has only one X, producing a karyotype referred to as monosomy X. Turner's syndrome is rare, occurring in approximately 1 in 10,000 live female births (Summit, 19820).

The characteristics of the disorder include sexual infantilism, short stature, webbed neck, infertility, hearing impairments, and visual defects. Also associated with the syndrome are congenital heart defects that may shorten the life span. The usual treatment includes hormone therapy (estrogen) and administration of anabolic steroids to stimulate growth. Psychological counseling may be necessary to improve self-esteem and to deal with difficulties in body image.

THE IMPACT OF ALTERED PATTERNS OF CONGENITAL ORIGIN

A child with an altered pattern of congenital origin and his family are continually confronted with challenges in coping with the illness or disability. The child's disability affects not only his own but also his family's adaptation skills.

Alteration of congenital origin have an impact on all members of the nuclear family and on the extended family as well. The basis of the family, the marital couple, faces many stressors that are frequently aggravated by the child's disorder (Battle, 1975; Lawson, 1977). The birth of a disabled child or an initial diagnosis of disability precipitates profound feelings of grief for the parents (Drotar et al., 1975). The loss of the "perfect" child may lead to a state of chronic sorrow, but dealing openly with this sorrow can augment the parents' ability to raise their disabled child adequately (Olshansky, 1962). Difficulties with siblings often develop out of feelings of resentment, insecurity, and fear of being afflicted with similar condition (Battle, 1975; Lawson, 1977). Grandparents often suffer the same feelings of loss as the parents when an infant is born with a congenital defect.

The health services that provide care for families frequently segregate the mother and disabled child from the rest of the family, since services are usually available at times that are inconvenient for employed family members and school-age siblings (Doernberg, 1978). Overshadowing the everyday experiences of the disabled child may be parental uncertainties about the future because of complications associated with the disorder and a possible perception of the child as being vulnerable (Green and Solnit, 1964).

Changes in Family Roles

Any chronic illness or disability has a major impact on the family, and sacrifice may become a way of life for various family members. This is true regardless of the identity of the individual who is afflicted, but it is especially true for the congenitally disabled child who enters the family as a newcomer. In such cases, there is no shared experience of love or trust on which to build, for the disabled child is an unknown element who brings overwhelming problems into a family group that is often unprepared for the hardships and adjustments that lie ahead (Griffin, 1980).

A child with a congenital disability often becomes pivotal in the life of the family; major proportions of family time and activities tend to revolve around the special child. In some instances, the arrival of a child with a congenital disability may draw the parents closer as they endeavor to console each other. More often, however, a seriously disabled child represents a permanent challenge likely to test the strength of the marital bond and to impose complications on relationships between the parents and healthy children.

At the simplest level, someone has to care for the child around the clock. Thus, parents have less time to spend with each other and with healthy children and less time to pursue their own interests. Furthermore, medical expenses result in less disposable income for everyone. This means changed family habits and reduced amounts of money available for other purposes. Furthermore, the need to care for the disabled child may mean that the mother cannot work outside the home unless foster care can be arranged.

The financial burden of chronic illness is hardest on the middle-class family. Wealthy families can care for their child with minimal sacrifice, and poor families have access to public funds. But middle-income families may well be overcome by a disability of long duration.

A family with a disabled child requires help over the years, and the nature of this need changes as the child and family grow older. Friends and relatives cannot be expected to alter their lives permanently to help the family once the immediate crisis has been met. The parents may become so obsessed with their duties that they lose contact with friends and rarely escape from the pressures at home.

Some communities have established networks of parents whose children share the same disability. These groups are eager to help families with similar problems and to give practical advice, answer questions, and offer emotional support. Such groups are often living proof that parents can face problems that seem insoluble and still survive. Community groups may be affiliated with national organizations devoted to education and research concerning particular diseases or disabilities. These organizations provide additional resources for troubled parents. Many publish informative newsletters or journals that provide practical help to the parents and convey a feeling that they are not alone in their trouble.

A family with a chronically disabled child needs periodic reevaluation of its effectiveness. Adjustments that once strengthened the family may later become dysfunctional. In the first months after learning that an infant is seriously disabled, the mother may give all her time to caring for the child. At the same time, the father may take on more work to reduce family indebtedness. Healthy children are called upon for assistance and will respond to the best of their ability. These first adjustments are usually effective; the baby is cared for, income is increased, everyone is joined in a common goal. Over

time these same adjustments may become maladaptive, however. The mother may find she has become the sole caretaker of the child. Since she has been recognized as the expert, family members leave the child in her charge. She feels overburdened but is unwilling to allow her husband or the other children to take over her function. The father is deeply concerned about the child but his life is less dominated by the disability. As he sees his wife becoming more involved with the child he may become jealous and feel excluded. Rather than make more demands on his wife, he may withdraw further, spending more time at work or looking outside the home for companionship. At the same time, the mother may envy her husband's life outside the family. In their zeal to meet the needs of the disabled child, the parents may have caused their functions to be so separate that they have little in common with each other. Meanwhile, the healthy children in the family may be receiving insufficient attention, and their early willingness to cooperate may have deteriorated into indifference or rebellion.

Both father and mother may assign the disabled child the central role in the family. In these circumstances, family life revolves around the limitations of the disabled child and the needs of other members become secondary. Such overprotection inhibits the child's mental, physical, and psychological growth. The parents are so intent on coping with the disability that they lose sight of the real child. While single-minded attention to the sick child may create a strong partnership between the parents, it is unfair to the healthy children and may even prevent the disabled child from reaching her full potential.

A paradoxical form of the sick role develops when the family "scapegoats" the disabled child. In this situation, parents and siblings blame all adversity in family relationships on the ill child. This behavior relieves a family of the difficult task of finding out what is really wrong and trying to correct it. Since the child is unlikely to get better, family problems may never be resolved. Scapegoating the sick child allows all deficiencies to be rationalized. This may be the most pervasive distortion in families with chronically ill children.

A common secondary gain for families with a chronically disabled child is that family relationships are simplified by the routine task of caring for the child. Other gains result from friends' and neighbors' recognition of the family's strength and courage. The mother, in particular, may feel pride in having met and overcome such a challenge. It is not uncommon for a mother, after learning to care for her own disabled child, to return to school and become a specialist in caring for others with the

Wife, we scarcely thought us blessed
That God had lent us but this only child.
But now I see this one is one too much
And that we have a curse in having her.
WILLIAM SHAKESPEARE, ROMEO AND JULIET

same disability. The professionalization of the mother is worthwhile if she is willing and able to give her husband and her other children the attention they need. Otherwise, professionalization is only a sign of her total involvement with the disabled child and her inability to give to other members of her family (Griffin, 1980).

The guilt that occurs after the birth of a disabled child can take many forms. Some parents who have produced a defective child feel that they are being punished for their sins. Other parents may try to escape responsibility by blaming each other. Devoted parents may set unreachable standards for themselves, thereby increasing their feelings of guilt and inadequacy. As the child grows older, the parents may be ashamed to be seen with him in public, yet feel guilty for being ashamed. Siblings have similar feelings. They may be reluctant to bring friends home because of embarrassment and may feel guilty because their presence in the home diverts parental attention from the task of caring for the disabled child. Conflicting emotions complicate the lives of every family member.

It is difficult to predict the reaction of relatives to the birth of a disabled child. The disability may frighten relatives and cause them to seem cruel and distant. Some grandparents blame the disability on the in-laws and feel that their own child has been unfairly burdened. Other grandparents may feel guilty, suspecting that their genes may have caused the defect. Relatives may be upset by the birth of a congenitally disabled child, wondering if they, too, will have defective children. These understandable reactions may restrict the amount of help that the stricken family can expect from relatives.

Because of the chronicity of the illness, good relationships between health professionals and the family are important. In addition to a variety of health services, the family needs a primary professional who can coordinate treatment and engage in ongoing assessment and evaluation of the changing needs of the disabled child and other family members.

Stress and Coping

The family has rarely had time to prepare for raising a disabled child. Most families have little previous exposure to such situations to help them develop mechanisms for coping with the stressors they must face.

The stress experienced by a disabled child and her family is described by Sperling (1978) as having two phases: acute and chronic. The *acute* phase is dramatic and intense, occurring when the child is born, during hospitalization, or when there is an exacerbation in the condition. The *chronic* phase is associated with daily coping with the physical limitations caused by a disability.

Factors that may affect stress levels include the developmental stage of the child, the perception of the disability or illness, the support systems available to the family, and the family's coping abilities (Hymovich, 1976; Sperling, 1978).

MATURATIONAL CRISES Maturational crises occur throughout the development of a child, producing unique stressors for the disabled child and his family. Common maturational or developmental crises occur with entry into school, failure to meet developmental expectations for an age, and puberty.

"I have an overwhelming sense of guilt about Andy. This is always present and diminishes all my pleasures. I will never be able to forgive myself for the frustrations and restrictions of his life. To the extent that I am responsible for that life, his handicap does become my responsibility. Additionally, because the experts told us so often that guilt is destructive, I feel guilty about feeling guilty."

J. Q. GRIFFIN (1980)

For example, entry into school may present challenges in acquiring the appropriate services for the child and may emphasize the child's differences.

PERCEPTION OF THE DISABILITY The individual's and family's perception of a disability may affect the amount of stress it produces. If parents overestimate the extent of the disability, they may see the child as vulnerable and become overly protective. The family's socioeconomic level can be a significant factor in the perception of a disability. In higher social strata, for example, the birth of a mentally retarded child may be viewed as a tragic crisis that is frustrating to the aims of the family (Farber, 1968). In lower social classes, the birth of a mentally retarded child creates a crisis in role organization, as many parents are unable to meet the needs of the family because of disorganization.

SUPPORT SYSTEMS The amount of stress affecting a family with a disabled child may be reduced by the availability of support systems. Deep religious faith and a community of supportive relatives and friends have been identified as positive coping factors (Farber, 1968; Battle, 1975). Of particular adaptive value is a good relationship with the maternal grandmother (Farber, 1968; Battle, 1975; Lawson, 1977). Another helpful support system is a multidisciplinary health care team that provides high-quality, affordable care. A community with resources that are responsive to the needs of the disabled or chronically ill is also a valuable support system.

COPING ABILITIES Coping abilities are resources the person uses to adapt to stress. Personal qualities of the child that affect long-term adaptation include maturity, intelligence, and a sense of humor; adaptive family qualities include stability, flexibility, warmth, and commitment (Pless and Pinkerton, 1975). A strong marital relationship and financial stability also positively affect adaptation (Battle, 1975; Lawson, 1977). Another adaptive quality is a positive self-concept as a parent, which is essential for maternal attachment to a disabled infant. For this reason, parents tend to cope better if the disabled child is not their first. Another factor that can help the family adapt to disability is knowledge of the disorder and its expected changes or impact over time. Anticipatory guidance helps a family prepare for crises in the future.

Adapting to Specific Disabilities

The problems facing the child and her family often depend on the specific type of alterations of congenital origin present. Different coping mechanisms are needed for dealing with physical, behavioral, emotional, social, and cognitive alterations.

PHYSICAL ALTERATIONS A major goal in caring for individuals with physical impairments is to address their need for efficient mobility. Mobility is critical to the early development of the child, for through mobility she is able to explore her environment and learn from her interactions. Mobility is also vital for the older child to maintain interactions with her peers.

A physical alteration with major impact on a child's self-esteem is incontinence. As mentioned earlier, incontinence is a common problem with spina bifida. This problem needs to be thoroughly assessed, and interventions should be planned to improve the situation. Incontinence causes a child to be dependent on parents for a longer than normal time, and protective clothing infantilizes the older child. In adolescents, feelings of low self-esteem and anger may decrease compliance with suggested treatments, and the incontinence problem will be magnified. When a child gains control of his incontinence, he will have feelings of achievement and improved self-esteem.

BEHAVIORAL ALTERATIONS Individuals with an alteration of congenital origin are at risk for psychological maladjustment, which is often manifested in behavioral problems. Adolescents who realize the permanence of their disability may experience feelings of anger and denial. Those with attention deficit disorders may react to their feelings of anger and lower self-esteem by engaging in delinquent behavior. Because of negative feelings, compliance with medical treatments and self-care may falter. The vulnerable child who has been overprotected by her parents may become passive and dependent on adults for interactions. In light of these potential problems, it is important for disabled children's reactions and feelings to be continually monitored and to be addressed through supportive techniques.

EMOTIONAL ALTERATIONS A disability can have a major impact on the individual's self-esteem. Self-esteem is made up of one's self-image, the reactions of significant others, and the values placed on oneself. Disabled children and adolescents are at risk for low self-esteem because of negative views of themselves and their feelings of being different.

In emotionally abusive family situations, parents may downgrade the value of the disabled child and give him ambivalent messages. Such parents may not be able to separate their feelings about the child from those about the disability. Children who receive ambivalent messages are susceptible to feelings of low self-esteem. At the same time, parental reactions of overprotection and permissiveness can result in a dependent, demanding child. Such overprotectiveness is a consequence of guilt, anger, and ambivalent feelings. Parents do not give the child opportunities to develop feelings of initiative, independence, and self-esteem. Instead, the child learns to manipulate the adults in her life, and she interacts poorly with her peers.

SOCIAL ALTERATIONS The disabled or chronically ill child is likely to experience periods of loneliness, often as a result of repeated hospitalizations, social isolation, immobility, or limited peer interactions. Because the disabled child may have few opportuni-

ties to develop skills of social interaction with peers, the nurse should explore with the family methods and opportunities for increasing peer activities and other activities of interest.

Changes in societal attitudes and in the treatment of the disabled are making the community more accessible so that the disabled can participate in the mainstream of life. In addition, nursing interventions might include working with the family to improve accessibility in the home environment, such as the addition of ramps to provide greater independence for the disabled individual.

COGNITIVE ALTERATIONS Mental retardation and learning disabilities are primary manifestations of many alterations of congenital origin. In other disorders, however, learning problems may be secondary sequelae. Children who are chronically ill may have poor school attendance, leaving gaps in their learning and resulting in academic failures. Emotional and behavioral alterations can also limit a disabled child's ability to function optimally in school. Specific therapy directed at increasing the child's coping abilities can increase his success in educational and social situations.

Sensory and adaptive impairments will dictate special learning needs for disabled children. In those with spina bifida and shunted hydrocephalus, for example, visual-spatial and perceptual difficulties are common. For any child with an alteration of congenital origin, a thorough assessment of academic skills, intellectual functioning, adaptive skills, vision, hearing, and motor abilities should be performed prior to entry into school. Such evaluations should be tailored to meet the specific needs of the individual child. From the data gathered in a preschool assessment, an appropriate educational program can be coordinated.

Genetic Counseling

Hereditary and genetic alterations are significant factors in many alterations of congenital origin. It is therefore important to inform parents at risk or those who have already given birth to a defective child of the availability of *genetic counseling*. The goals of genetic counseling are (1) to inform parents of the risk of recurrence when a family member has a genetically influenced disorder and (2) to help prevent serious birth defects in children (Whaley and Wong, 1983). Genetic counseling and prenatal diagnostic techniques are recommended for parents who have had a child with a birth defect, who have a family history of a disorder, or who are at an age associated with increased risk. A genetic evaluation may be performed on an affected infant when the cause and diagnosis of a disorder are unclear.

Genetic counseling is usually performed by trained specialists who have a comprehensive understanding of genetics and of various inherited disorders, their occurrence, and their risk of recurrence. Teams of experts in genetics are often called upon in delivery of this service. The genetic counseling team usually consists of a nurse, a social worker, trained counselors, a medical geneticist (physician), and a pediatrician. This team may refer to consultants that include clergy, specialists in medical ethics, and psychologists.

A major step in the genetic counseling process is to obtain a complete, careful family history, which is recorded in a pedigree chart or family tree. The information necessary for an accurate pedigree chart includes data on the medical histories (diseases and disabilities), causes of death, abortions, stillbirths, and ethnic background for several generations. When the pedigree is completed, a particular problem may be identified and an estimation of risk may be given to the parents.

Prenatal diagnosis is conducted when a woman is already pregnant. It involves a family history, an ultrasound exam, and amniocentesis for chromosome analysis. If a positive diagnosis is made, intensive counseling regarding the nature of the disorder and available options is provided to the family.

A primary goal of genetic counselors is to establish a trusting relationship with clients through effective communication of positive regard and empathy (Muir, 1983). Most genetic counselors try to communicate facts in a nonjudgmental, neutral manner to better assist parents in their decision-making process.

Nurses who are involved in direct genetic counseling need to provide psychological support to families in the counseling program. It is essential that these nurses have a basic understanding of genetic problems and an awareness of services available to affected families. They especially need to be sensitive to the needs of families and to be available for support and listening to concerns.

THE NURSING PROCESS IN ALTERED PATTERNS OF CONGENITAL ORIGIN

Psychiatric nurses can play an essential role in the care of individuals with altered patterns of congenital origin. To care for these clients, the psychiatric nurse must be knowledgeable about the nature of disabilities, their etiology, their impact on the individual and his family, and appropriate interventions. In addition, nurses working with this population must be particularly sensitive to the needs and feelings of affected families (Tudor, 1978).

Nurses interact closely with a number of other health care professionals in planning coordinated, comprehensive care for disabled clients. Physical therapists intervene in areas of gross motor function, mobility, and development. Occupational therapists focus on the areas of adaptive function, fine motor skills, perceptual skills, and self-help skills. Furthermore, nurses from various areas of specialization may share in planning interventions. For example, a pediatric nurse may consult with a psychiatric mental health nurse regarding a hospitalized disabled adolescent who shows signs of depression.

In planning interventions, the care plan should be designed to meet the needs of the particular individual and his family. The client should not be considered alone but rather as a part of a family and community; a holistic approach to care of the client is essential.

Assessment

For disabled children to reach their highest potential of health and function, their health status should be monitored and their impairments assessed. Many children with altered patterns of congenital origin are at risk for secondary impairments and health problems that may result in reduced functional ability. Observing for complications necessitates an understanding of the child's baseline health status and an awareness of the potential complications for each disorder. For example, a child with hydrocephalus needs to be monitored for signs of shunt failure and progressive hydrocephalus. If the hydrocephalus is uncontrollled, sensory impairment, loss of cognitive ability, motor impairment, and even coma can result.

Psychological assessment is also important. Assessing a child's feelings and understanding may require special techniques, such as play therapy and drawing, based on the developmental level of the child.

It is also essential to assess the parents', child's, and siblings' knowledge of the disabling condition. During the period of initial diagnosis, the family may not hear all the information shared with them. Nurses often need to repeat information about the disorder, its treatments, and its potential complications. It is important that families feel comfortable enough with health care providers to ask their questions and express their concerns.

Another area for assessment is the support systems available to the family. If support systems are lacking, interventions can be planned to meet support needs. For example, the family may be referred to social service agencies, clergy, or parent support groups. Family assessment should occur in the home environment and, when needed, in the school environment.

269

Planning

Setting realistic goals for their disabled child may be a difficult task for parents. It is therefore important to help parents realize the strengths, potentials, and needs of their child. Realistic goal setting is influenced by the parents' perception of their child and by the child's degree of disability. Short- and long-term goals will be significantly different for a profoundly retarded two-year-old than for a school-aged child with mild motor impairment, for example. It is vital for parents to have hope for their child's future, but their expectations must be correlated with their child's actual potential. Providing parents with feedback regarding their child's abilities and impairments will help to reinforce a realistic perception of the child's future.

Parents of physically disabled children frequently look forward to their child reaching adulthood and independent living. But physically disabled adolescents are often ill prepared to meet the challenges of independent living. Preparation for independence should begin when a child is very young, and it needs continual reinforcement. A physically disabled child should be encouraged to be as independent as possible at each developmental age. As the child develops, his skills should be cultivated to reach his highest level of potential.

Implementation

Tudor (1978) has outlined goals for interventions with developmentally disabled infants, but these goals can be modified to meet the needs of any age child or adolescent:

1. In times of crisis the family must be sup- ported and provided with resources to adapt and meet the total needs of the family.

2. The individual child must be helped to reach the highest level of health, development, and independent function within her potential and degree of disability. Each child is an individual with unique strengths, abilities, potential, and needs. The family may need to be guided to identify these strengths and set realistic goals.

3. The disabled or chronically ill individual must become a loved, integrated member of the family and community.

A few major interventions are necessary to help meet these goals, including family intervention, realistic goal setting, coordination of comprehensive care, health assessment, and genetic counseling.

A nurse may interact with an affected family during any phase or stage of the disabling condition. Therefore, it is vital for the nurse to evaluate the individual family members' strengths, coping mechanisms, and reactions to the disabled member and to the disability. To understand the needs of a family and how they may respond to suggested interventions, the nurse must assess the impact of the disability on each family member, including parents, siblings, and extended family members. Fathers are often overlooked because mothers most frequently interact with the child's health care providers. It is essential for fathers to be included in all assessments and planning of interventions.

A major aspect of family intervention is being available, willing to listen, and sensitive to the particular needs of a family. Each family will respond differently to the stresses and crises associated with

C L I N I C A L   E X A M P L E

HELPING A CHILD WITH SPINA BIFIDA

Michelle is a fifteen-year-old who was born with spina bifida. At a spina bifida clinic visit, her parents recently reported major concerns about Michelle's affect, failure in school, and noncompliance with medical treatment. Said her mother: "Each day my daughter appears more and more depressed and she is so withdrawn. She used to be so active and happy."

Because of her defect, Michelle has complete paralysis of her lower extremities, bowel incontinence, bladder incontinence, and a surgically corrected spinal curvature. Over the past three years, she has had a total of nine hospitalizations for orthopedic, urologic, and skin problems. Her family has just been informed that she will need two more surgeries in the near future.

Three years ago Michelle had a surgical correction of her spinal curvature and for the following year was restricted to bedrest. Michelle now uses a wheelchair and is on clean intermittent catheterization for her incontinence. However, her parents report that she refuses to do her catheterizations and is continually incontinent. Recently Michelle has gained a considerable amount of weight, which has impaired her mobility and self-care and has affected her self-image.

Michelle lives with both parents and a younger brother on a farm in a remote rural area. She has been mainstreamed in her local high school, but her school grades have steadily declined over the last year.

ASSESSMENT

During an interview with the nurse clinician, Michelle appeared withdrawn and expressed little interest in school and any other activities. She reported having few friends who were not disabled. She did have a boyfriend who also had spina bifida but was no longer interested in seeing him.

When talking with the nurse, Michelle maintained little eye contact and answered questions as briefly as possible. She was moderately overweight, and despite parental efforts to create an attractive appearance she did not seem to be concerned about her grooming. The only time she became somewhat animated during the interview was when she talked about how she enjoyed swimming. However, the only available pool was architecturally inaccessible.

Based on the history and the clinical picture, the following diagnoses were made:

Nursing Diagnoses

Bowel elimination, alteration in

Coping, ineffective individual

Coping, ineffective family

Mobility, impaired

Urinary elimination, alteration in

Social isolation

Self-care deficit

Noncompliance

Multiaxial Psychiatric Diagnoses

Axis I   300.40 Dysthymic disorder
          V62.30 Academic problem
          V15.81 Noncompliance

Axis II   None

Axis III Spina bifida

Axis IV   Code 5—Severe stressor

Axis V   Level 5—Poor

PLANNING

During a team conference, Michelle's needs were discussed and interventions were planned to deal with her potential depression. Michelle and her family participated in the planning session. It was suggested that Michelle be referred for a thorough psychological evaluation to assess her emotional state and feelings of self-esteem. She seemed to be experiencing many of the difficulties of adolescence. She had a supportive family, but she needed interaction with disabled and nondisabled peers. Plans were made to find a disabled teen support group so that Michelle could benefit from sharing with others. It was also suggested that her home be evaluated for accessibility to promote her independence. Because participation in athletic activities might be highly beneficial for Michelle, the availability of wheelchair athletic groups in her area was to be investigated. If Michelle was interested, a referral to an adolescent weight control program would be made.

271

IMPLEMENTATION

Michelle was referred to a nurse practitioner associated with an outreach facility serving adolescents with a variety of problems. Under the auspices of the facility, group experiences were available that allowed Michelle to interact with young people her own age, some of whom were similarly disabled and some of whom had other problems relating with peers. It was thought that Michelle would benefit from learning that physical disability did not mean she was doomed to be lonely and frustrated and that physical health does not guarantee freedom from problems in living. In addition to the heterogeneous group, Michelle was introduced to other people near her own age who suffered from disorders that reduced their mobility.

The nurse practitioner filled several roles: as a coordinator of the treatment program, as a client advocate for Michelle when school personnel and others needed explanations regarding the physical and emotional ramifications of spina bifida, and as a mentor and teacher in helping Michelle deal with her disability, her changing body image, and her emotional needs. The nurse practitioner emphasized the fact that Michelle had the intelligence and capacity to become self-supporting and that in time she could drive her own car and become relatively mobile and independent.

To increase Michelle's confidence in her own potential, arrangements were made for her to answer the phone and take messages as a volunteer in the adolescent facility where her group met and her nurse practitioner was based.

EVALUATION

The interventions used were effective in achieving the following immediate nursing goals:

1. Helping Michelle increase her circle of peer group relationships so that she would feel less constricted and less different.

2. Arranging experiences that required Michelle to draw on the strengths she possessed, such as intelligence and reliability.

3. Focusing on the long-term goal of independence so that Michelle would find her future more promising and rewarding.

Although considerable progress was made in achieving the short-term goals, a flexible approach remained necessary so that long-term care could be modified and goals formulated in response to the progress and setbacks that Michelle would inevitably encounter as she reached young adulthood.

C L I N I C A L   E X A M P L E

HELPING A CHILD WITH CEREBRAL PALSY

The Smith family consists of Bob and Jane Smith, their four-year-old daughter Joanne, and their two-year-old son David, who was born with cerebral palsy. David has demonstrated several developmental lags and has required constant medical care and personal attention since birth. Most of the responsibility has fallen on Jane. Her husband helps with household chores but not with the care of his son. In the last two years Joanne has become his joy and solace. Father and daughter are very close; Bob spends most of his evenings reading to or playing games with his daughter. Joanne attends nursery school during the day, to provide her with playmates and to relieve the load on her overburdened mother.

ASSESSMENT

During the initial interview, it was noted that although the family had been coping, the distance between husband and wife had been widening. Jane had become increasingly resentful toward her husband. Bob, for his part, was repelled by the services his son needed and could not bear to observe the boy closely. Jane sensed this, although it was never discussed, and she became reluctant to ask Bob for assistance in caring for David. She also felt excluded from the happy times that Bob and Joanne shared in the evenings. In her loneliness, Jane began to feel that she and David were both rejects.

The following diagnoses were made:

Nursing Diagnoses

Coping, ineffective family

Family processes, alteration in

Parenting; alteration in

Multiaxial Psychiatric Diagnoses

Axis I   V61.10 Marital problem
         V61.20 Parent-child problem

Axis II None

Axis III Cerebral palsy

Axis IV Code 5—Severe stressor

Axis V   Level 5—Poor; marked impairment in
         functioning

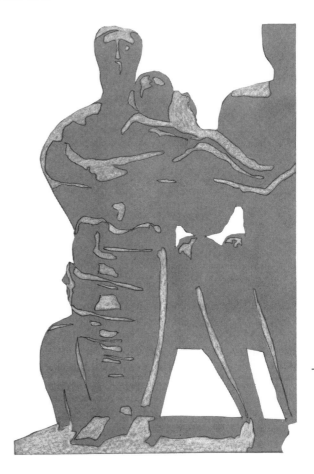

273

PLANNING

The family was visited regularly by a nurse practitioner from the local chapter of the Cerebral Palsy Association. It was to her that Jane turned for help. Although the nurse had been concerned primarily with helping Jane cope with David, she was aware of problems within the marital relationship. The first nursing goal was to reduce the excessive involvement between mother and son and to involve David's father to a greater extent. In this way, the nurse hoped to relieve the burden carried by Jane and to encourage a family structure that did not fragment parent and sibling relationships.

IMPLEMENTATION

The primary objectives for intervention were to reduce Jane's preoccupation with David and simplify his care, to modify the relationship between Bob and Joanne in order to include Jane, and to strengthen the marital partnership by encouraging communication and shared activity between husband and wife.

The first intervention the nurse made was to provide practical advice. As an expert in cerebral palsy, she was knowledgeable about special chairs, feeding aids, suction machines, and other labor-saving devices. Jane had some equipment, but David obviously could use more. By arranging to visit in the evening, the nurse was able to involve Bob in helping to simplify David's care.

The nurse commented on Jane's need for adult company and suggested that the couple plan some recreational activities together. She gave them a list of qualified babysitters endorsed by the local cerebral palsy chapter. Because Bob resisted the idea of joining a group of parents with children like David and needed more time to work through his feelings, the nurse put only Jane in touch with a parents' group. Even though Bob did not accompany her, Jane needed to meet with other parents who might alleviate her feelings of isolation.

EVALUATION

Because David's disability was permanent, evaluation, as with assessment and planning, was ongoing. Helping the

father adjust to his son's disability was likely to be a protracted process that might never be wholly successful. However, it was possible for the nurse to ascertain that the first primary objective had been accomplished. David's routine care was simplified and the demands made on his mother's time and energy were eased. Regular communication with parents experiencing similar problems helped reduce Jane's sense of isolation, even though her husband resisted the idea of participation. With more time at her disposal, Jane was able to devote additional attention to her daughter. The closeness between father and daughter continued, but Jane began to share in some of the games and activities from which she had previously been excluded.

Bob remained reluctant to undertake the physical care of his son, but he did agree to read to his son at bedtime and to stay with both children when Jane wished to attend meetings of the parents' group. Recruiting qualified babysitters allowed both parents to go out together occasionally, a welcome change for them. It allowed Bob to see Jane as a wife and companion rather than as a harassed, preoccupied caretaker. Jane began to realize that her narrow world could expand to include her husband and healthy daughter as well as her disabled son.

a disabling condition. Some families will progress rapidly in adapting to a new crisis; others will respond more slowly and need more time and intervention. In situations of maladjustment and major crisis, families may need intensive crisis intervention, individual therapy, or family therapy.

For a family to adjust and regain equilibrium, each family member must be supported and involved in the planning process. Supporting the disabled child may involve helping him reduce his feelings of being different. The child needs to understand the disability and realize his strengths and interests. He should be encouraged to share with disabled peers, to mobilize his coping abilities, and to verbalize his concerns. Allowing the child control of aspects of his life will also improve his feelings of self-esteem.

Child and parent education regarding the disability is an essential intervention in the maintenance of health status. The child and parents need to know the potential complications and necessary interventions, including therapies, medications, and special care needs.

Evaluation

Nurses can play a key role in the coordination of care of individuals with alterations of congenital origin because of their understanding of the medical care and the multiple disciplines that may be involved. It is the lack of coordination that frequently causes problems with treatment implementation. The role of the nurse as coordinator is a continuous evaluation process. Nurses are also involved in the day-to-day management of the problems facing a family with an affected child. With their knowledge of family needs, they have a unique perspective that is necessary to coordinate family-focused interventions. Coordination of care is essential to avoid gaps in service, miscommunications, and duplication of care. The health care team for a particular child may include the pediatrician, school nurse, teacher, specialty care providers, and therapists. Establishing lines of communication with all these providers and the family is an important function.

Modern care of the developmentally disabled often centers around established, coordinated, interdisciplinary teams. Some teams function primarily to diagnose needs and refer for services. Other multidisciplinary teams provide ongoing evaluation and treatment, such as spina bifida clinics, cystic fibrosis centers, and hemophilia centers. Each program should have the disciplines necessary to meet the needs of the population.

SUMMARY

The health care of a child with a physical or mental disability has experienced many changes over the years. Many such children are now treated in communities and in their homes rather than in institutions. This has resulted in greater numbers of nurses and other providers being involved with the care of these clients.

A number of prenatal, perinatal, and postnatal factors have been identified in the etiology of altered patterns of congenital origin. Genetic and environmental influences interact to produce the physical, mental, and behavioral characteristics of the developing child. The most common disorders of congenital origin include mental retardation, Down's syndrome, learning disabilities, phenylketonuria, Tay-Sachs disease, cystic fibrosis, hemophilia, sickle cell anemia, cerebral palsy, spina bifida, Klinefelter's syndrome, and Turner's syndrome.

It has been the goal of this chapter to help prepare psychiatric nurses for the care of individuals with altered patterns of congenital origin. The individual affected by a disability or chronic illness is at risk for maladaptation to the situation. Many challenges and stressors affect a disabled person and his family. Their understanding of the disorder, their social supports, and their coping abilities will influence their adaptation to the disability. Because psychiatric nurses may be called upon to intervene at various stages of a disability, they should be sensitive to the behavioral, emotional, social, and cognitive effects of the disability on the individual and his family. Armed with this sensitivity and a knowledge of disabilities, psychiatric nurses can serve as advocates for the disabled in their community. By being role models for others, they can help improve social attitudes toward the disabled and their acceptance in the community.

Review Questions

1. Compare and contrast genetic and environmental causes of alterations of congenital origin.

2. Discuss the impact of maternal age on alterations of congenital origin.

3. Describe the influence of the home environment on children with disabilities.

4. Describe the degrees of mental retardation and suggest appropriate nursing interventions for each.

5. A family with a child who has an alteration of congenital origin faces many problems throughout the development of the child. Discuss these problems and suggest nursing interventions.

6. What are the implications for both child and family if the child has both urinary and bowel incontinence?

274

7. How may the "normal" adolescent problems of growth and development be distinguished from those specifically attributable to a physical problem?

8. Discuss the critical components of family intervention.

9. Describe the process of realistic goal setting for a child with alterations of congenital origin.

10. Discuss available resources and the interaction of the treatment team in caring for the disabled child.

References

Abrams, I., and Panagakos, D. 1980. The Child with Significant Developmental Motor Disability. In *The Practical Management of the Developmentally Disabled*, eds. A. Scheiner and I. Abrams. St. Louis: C. V. Mosby.

American Academy of Pediatrics. 1979. Official Statement to the Committee on Children with Handicaps. Washington, D.C.: The Developmental Disability Council, U.S. Department of Health Education and Welfare.

Bartoshesky, L. E. 1980. Genetics and the Child with Developmental Disabilities. In *The Practical Management of the Developmentally Disabled Child*, eds. A. Scheiner and I. Abrams. St. Louis: C. V. Mosby.

Battle, C. 1975. Chronic Physical Disease: Behavioral Aspects. *Pediatric Clinics of North America*, 22:525–533.

Bergsma, D., ed. 1982. *March of Dimes Birth Defects Compendium*, 2nd ed. New York: Alan R. Liss.

Clifford, T. 1980. Cognitive Development of the School-Ager. In *The Process of Human Development: A Holistic Approach*, eds. C. J. Schuster and S. S. Ashburn. Boston: Little, Brown.

Darling, R. B., and Darling, J. 1982. *Children Who Are Different: Meeting the Challenges of Birth Defects in Society*. St. Louis: C. V. Mosby.

Doernberg, M. 1978. Some Neglect Effects on Family Integration of Health and Educational Services for Young Handicapped Children. *Rehabilitation Literature*, 39(4).

Drotar, D.; Baskiewicz, A.; Irvin, N.; Kennell, J.; and Klaus, M. 1975. The Adaptation of Parents to the Birth of an Infant with a Congenital Malformation: A Hypothetical Model. *Pediatrics*, 56:710–717.

Farber, B. 1968. *Mental Retardation: Its Social Context and Social Consequence*. Boston: Houghton Mifflin.

Green, M., and Solnit, A. 1964. Reactions to the Threatened Loss of a Child: A Vulnerable Child Syndrome. Pediatric management of the dying child, part 3. *Pediatrics*, 34:58–66.

Griffin, J. Q. 1980. Physical Illness in the Family. In *Family-Focused Care*, eds. J. R. Miller and E. H. Janosik. New York: McGraw-Hill. 1980.

Grossman, H. J. 1973. Manual on Terminology and Classification in Mental Retardation. *American Association on Mental Deficiency, Special Publication*, No. 2. Baltimore: Garamond Pridemark Press.

Hamburg, B. 1983. Chronic Illness. In *Developmental-Behavioral Pediatrics*, eds. M. Levine et al. Philadelphia: W. B. Saunders.

Henderson, M., and Synhorst, D. 1977. Bladder and Bowel Management in Child with Myelomeningocele. *Pediatric Nursing*, 3:24–31.

Hooks, E. B., and Chambers, G. M. 1977. Estimated Rates of Down's Syndrome in Live Births by One Year Maternal Age Intervals for Mothers Aged 20–49 in a New York State Study. *Birth Defects*, 13:127.

Hymovich, D. 1976. Parents of Sick Children, Their Needs and Tasks. *Pediatric Nursing*, September/October: 9–13.

Klaus, M., and Kennell, J. 1976. *Maternal Infant Bonding*. St. Louis: C. V. Mosby.

Koerper, M., and Diamond, L. 1982. Hemophilia A. *March of Dimes Birth Defects Compendium*, 2nd ed., ed. D. Bergsma. New York: Alan R. Liss.

Larter, N. 1981. Cystic Fibrosis. *American Journal of Nursing*, March:527–531.

Lawson, B. 1977. Chronic Illness in the School-Aged Child: Effects on the Total Family. *American Journal of Maternal Child Nursing*, 2:49–56.

Levine, M. 1980. The Child with Learning Disabilities. In *The Practical Management of the Developmentally Disabled*, eds. A. Scheiner and I. Abrams. St. Louis: C. V. Mosby.

Marx, J. L. 1978. Restriction Enzymes: Prenatal Diagnoses of Genetic Disease. *Science*, 202:1068–1069.

Mattsson, A. 1972. Long-Term Physical Illness in Childhood: A Challenge to Psychosocial Adaptation. *Pediatrics*, 50:801–811.

Muir, B. 1983. *Essentials of Genetics for Nurses*. New York: John Wiley & Sons.

Myers, G. 1984. Myelomeningocele: The Medical Aspects. *Pediatric Clinics of North America*, 31:165–175.

Olshansky, S. 1962. Chronic Sorrow: A Response to Having a Mentally Defective Child. *Social Casework*, 43:190.

Opitz, J. 1982. Klinefelter's Syndrome. In *March of Dimes Birth Defects Compendium*, 2nd ed., ed. D. Bergsma. New York: Alan R. Liss.

Pless, I., and Pinkerton, P. 1975. *Chronic Childhood Disorders: Promoting Patterns of Adjustment*. London: Henry Kimpton Publishers.

Pless, I., and Roghmann, K. J. 1971. Chronic Illness and Its Consequences: Observations Based on Three Epidemologic Surveys. *Journal of Pediatrics*, 79:351–359.

Robinson, N., and Robinson, H. 1976. *The Mentally Retarded Child*. New York: McGraw-Hill.

Scheiner, A. 1980. High-Risk Mother and Infant. In *The Practical Management of the Developmentally Disabled*, eds. A. Scheiner and I. Abrams. St. Louis: C. V. Mosby.

Schwartz, R. 1978. Cystic Fibrosis. In *Principles of Pediatrics: Health Care of the Young*, ed. R. A. Hoekelman. New York: McGraw-Hill.

Sperling, E. 1978. Psychological Issues in Chronic Illness and Handicap. In *Psychosocial Aspects of Pediatric Care*, ed. E. Gellert. New York: Grune & Stratton.

Summitt, R. 1982. Turner's Syndrome. In *March of Dimes Birth Defects Compendium*, 2nd ed., ed. D. Bergsma. New York: Alan R. Liss.

Tudor, M. 1978. Nursing Intervention with Developmentally Disabled Children. *American Journal of Maternal Child Nursing*, January/February: 25–31.

Whaley L., and Wong, D. 1983. *Nursing Care of Infants and Children*. St. Louis: C. V. Mosby.

Supplementary Readings

Arnold, L. E. *Helping Parents to Help Their Children*. New York: Brunner/Mazel, 1978.

Bennet, F. C. Cerebral Palsy: The Why and How of Early Diagnosis. *Consultant*, 24(1984):151–153.

Buckwalter, K. C. Musculoskeletal Conditions and Sexuality. *Sexuality and Disability*, 5(1982):131–142.

Coffman, S. P. Parents' Perception of Needs for Themselves and Their Children in a Cerebral Palsy Clinic. *Issues in Comprehensive Pediatric Nursing*, 6(1983):67–77.

Cowett, R. M. The Infant of the Diabetic Mother. *Pediatric Clinics of North America*, 29(1982):1213–1231.

Curry, J., and Peppe, K. *Mental Retardation: Nursing Approaches to Care*. St. Louis: C. V. Mosby, 1978.

Darling, R. B., and Darling, J. *Children Who Are Different: Meeting the Challenges of Birth Defects in Society*. St. Louis: C. V. Mosby, 1982.

Devine, P. Mental Retardation: An Early Subspecialty in Psychiatric Nursing. *Journal of Psychiatric Nursing and Mental Health Services*, 21(1983):21–30.

Fairchild, B. Parents Coping with Genetically Handicapped Children: Use of Early Recollections. *Exceptional Children*, 49(1983):411–415.

Farrell, H. M. Crisis Intervention Following the Birth of a Handicapped Child. *Journal of Psychiatric Nursing and Mental Health Services*, 15(1977):32–36.

Hayes, U. H. *Holistic Health Care for Children with Developmental Disabilities*. Baltimore: University Park Press, 1982.

Horon, M. L. Parental Reaction to the Birth of an Infant with a Defect: An Attributional Approach. *Advances in Nursing Science*, 5(1982):57–68.

Hourcade, J. Cerebral Palsy and Emotional Disturbance: A Review and Implications for Intervention. *Journal of Rehabilitation*, 50(1984):55–60.

Johnson, D. M. Sexuality and the Mentally Retarded Adolescent. *Pediatric Annals*, 11(1982):847–853.

Kalter, H. Congenital Malformations: Etiologic Factors and Their Role in Prevention. *New England Journal of Medicine*, 308(1983):424–431.

Krajicek, M. J. Developmental Disability and Human Sexuality. *Nursing Clinics of North America*, 17 (1982):377–386.

Lenzer, I. Relation Between Behavioral and Physical Abnormalities Associated with Prenatal Exposure to Alcohol: Present Speculations. *Perceptual Motor Skills*, 55(1982):903–912.

Lippman, L. D. *Attitudes Toward the Handicapped*. Springfield, Ill.: Charles C Thomas, 1972.

Llewelyn, S. Skills in Action: A Psychological Approach to the Setting of a Mental Handicapped Hospital. *Nursing Mirror*, 156(1983):34–35.

Loney, J. Hyperkineses Comes of Age: What Do We Know and Where Should We Go? *American Journal of Orthopsychiatry*, 50(1980):28–42.

Longo, L. D. Some Health Consequences of Maternal Smoking: Issues Without Answers. *Birth Defects*, 18 (1982):214.

Manella, K. J. Behavioral Treatment of Ambulatory Function in a Child with Myelomeningocele. *Physical Therapy*, 64(1984):1536–1539.

Milunsky, A. Fetal Malformations and Environmental Influences: A Perspective. *American Journal of Forensic Medical Pathology*, 3(1982):329–334.

Pennington, B. F. Learning Disabilities in Children with Sex Chromosome Anomalies. *Child Development*, 53(1982):1182–1192.

Rousso, H. Special Considerations in Counseling Clients with Cerebral Palsy: The Sexual Aspects of Their Lives. *Sexuality and Disability*, 5(1982):7–8.

Schild, S. Beyond Diagnosis: Issues in Recurrent Counseling of Parents of the Mentally Retarded. *Social Work Health Care*, 8(1982):81–93.

Sensky, T. Family Stigma in Congenital Physical Handicap. *British Medical Journal*, 285(1982):1033–1035.

Sharkey, P. L. Nursing Care of the Mentally Retarded: Communication Issues. *Issues in Mental Health Nursing*, 4(1982):191–198.

Shaw, M. Changes in Patterns of Care of the Mentally Handicapped: Implications for Nurses' Perceptions of Their Roles and Hospital Decision Making Processes. *Journal of Advanced Nursing*, 7(1982):555–563.

Slimmer, L. W. Helping Parents Cope with Their Child's Seizure Disorder. *Journal of Psychiatric Nursing and Mental Health Services*, 17(1979):30–33.

Suran, B. G., and Rizzo, J. V. *Special Children: An Integrative Approach*. Glenview, Ill.: Scott, Foresman, 1979.

Tervo, R. C. Cerebral Palsy: Functional Assessments. *Canadian Journal of Public Health*, 72(1981):191–194.

276

DEFINITIONS OF KEY TERMS

THE RELATIONSHIP BETWEEN AGING AND
ALTERED PATTERNS OF DEGENERATIVE ORIGIN

MAJOR DEGENERATIVE ALTERATIONS
Alzheimer's Disease
Parkinson's Disease
Huntington's Chorea

IMPACT OF DEGENERATIVE ALTERATIONS
ON THE CLIENT
Memory Impairment
Cognitive and Behavioral Alterations
Impaired Reality Testing

Impaired Judgment
Impaired Communication
Self-care Deficits
Social Alterations

IMPACT OF DEGENERATIVE ALTERATIONS
ON THE NURSE

THE NURSING PROCESS IN THE CARE OF
CLIENTS WITH ALTERED PATTERNS
OF DEGENERATIVE ORIGIN
Assessment
Planning
Implementation
Evaluation

C   H   A   P   T   E   R

11

Altered Patterns of Degenerative Origin

Learning Objectives

After reading this chapter, the student should be able to:

1. Differentiate between acute alterations in mental function and chronic alterations of degenerative origin.

2. Define the terms acute alterations, chronic alterations, organic brain syndrome, organic mental disorder, delirium, and dementia.

3. Discuss the etiologic theories for Alzheimer's disease, Parkinson's disease, and Huntington's chorea.

4. Describe clinical manifestations of alterations due to degenerative processes.

5. Examine nursing responsibilities and approaches in caring for clients experiencing alterations of degenerative origin.

6. Discuss nursing responsibilities toward families of clients with an alteration of degenerative origin.

278

Overview

Altered patterns of degenerative origin lead to changes in all spheres of an individual's life. A degenerative alteration has a profound impact physiologically on the client and psychologically and socially on the client, his family, and his social network. The earlier parts of this chapter deal with some of the major adaptive and maladaptive responses to altered patterns of degenerative origin exhibited by individuals. Nursing approaches that assist clients in coping with degenerative processes often make the difference between adaptive and maladaptive behaviors. They are outlined in a later part of this chapter. Because degenerative alterations usually rob the client of independence and the ability to think rationally, much of the nurse's work will involve the client's family, especially in the later stages of the disorder. Family-focused nursing interventions are therefore an important consideration in dealing with the client affected by a degenerative disorder.

Oh blessed health . . . thou art above all gold and treasure
. . . he that has thee has little more to wish for.
LAWRENCE STERNE

Until recent years, little was known about the etiologies, courses, treatment, or management of most alterations of degenerative origin. Because many of these degenerative disorders are primarily found in elderly individuals, they were regarded as inevitable outcomes of aging. As a consequence, degenerative alterations excited little research interest or clinical attention until demographic shifts toward larger numbers of older people (and, therefore, a higher incidence of such disorders) prompted scientific inquiry and societal concern. As Alex Comfort (1984) states, "Chronic brain syndromes are beginning to occupy the place filled in the nineteenth century by neurosyphilis, as the prime institutionalized mental disorder." Disorders of degenerative origin, particularly Alzheimer's disease, are coming to be considered major public health problems that, like neurosyphilis, are comprehensible and probably preventable (Comfort, 1984).

Nurses should have a clear understanding of degenerative disorders and their management. Of the 23 million persons over sixty-five in the United States, approximately 1 million have some degree of severe intellectual impairment due to degenerative disorders. Approximately 650,000 persons suffer from Alzheimer's dementia, with an expected 100,000 deaths a year resulting from this disease and related senile dementias. Taken as a whole, dementias constitute the fourth or fifth leading cause of death in the United States today (Brill, 1984).

In every field of clinical practice, nurses are called on to work with individuals suffering from degenerative disorders. General medical and surgical units are increasingly filled with older clients, and these individuals often present with cognitive disruptions of a short-term nature (delirium) superimposed on a degenerative disorder such as Alzheimer's disease. Acute disruptions are commonly due to electrolyte imbalance, dehydration, and the physiological and psychological stresses of trauma and surgery, medications, pain, and sleep deprivation. These same clients are often found in critical care units, where distinguishing the behavioral effects of delirium from those of the underlying degenerative alteration is a complex and important nursing function.

Degenerative alterations are the major invaliding problem of persons now occupying our country's 1.2 million nursing home beds (Plum, 1979). Nurses working in long·term care settings find that care of individuals with degenerative alterations constitutes a major part of their clinical practice. Contrary to popular mythology, the majority of individuals with a degenerative disorder are cared for at home by family members, and community health nurses are commonly involved in providing services to these families.

DEFINITIONS OF KEY TERMS

For purposes of this chapter, the term *alterations of degenerative origin* will be used to describe processes reflecting an underlying organic etiology that results in permanent disruption of central nervous system functioning. This distinguishes degenerative alterations from *functional alterations*, which result from either psychic conflict or psychological factors with no demonstrable brain damage or disturbance in brain tissue function (Pasquali et al.,

A popular theory—and one that makes a good deal of sense to many students—is the continuity theory. It postulates that the maturing adult develops certain habits, preferences, associations, commitments that become ingrained in the personality. As one ages, there is a continuity to that personality. The theory is reminiscent of the maxim: "In aging you are like you always were, only more so." It also allows for the various ways individuals adapt to aging. To study an individual's reaction to aging, one must study all of the complex interactions in the biological, psychological, personal, and situational experiences of the person.

IRENE BURNSIDE (1984)

1981; Wang, 1973). Here "degenerative alteration" and "degenerative disorder" will be used interchangeably.

Traditionally, imprecise and inconsistent use of terms relating to degenerative disorders has hampered rational and scientific communication regarding care of clients with these problems. Knowledge of the following terms will be useful to the nurse working with clients confronting alterations of degenerative origin.

DELIRIUM *Delirium* is a "transient organic mental disorder of acute onset, characterized by global cognitive dysfunction due to diffuse impairment of cerebral metabolism" (Liston, 1984). "Delirium" is often used interchangeably with *acute confusional state, acute brain syndrome, metabolic encephalopathy, toxic psychosis,* and *acute brain failure.* Considerable controversy surrounds the designation of delirium as always transient and reversible. It is now acknowledged that in some cases delirium may be persistent, and, if the course of the disorder is long enough, it may result in irreversible brain impairment (Liston, 1984).

ACUTE ALTERATIONS IN MENTAL FUNCTION VERSUS CHRONIC DEGENERATIVE ALTERATIONS *Acute* alterations in mental function (delirium) are generally reversible or amenable to curative intervention, and they usually have a sudden onset. *Degenerative* alterations tend to have a slow, insidious onset; their progression is not amenable to treatment and inevitably leads to death (Richardson and Adams, 1980). Degenerative alterations are characterized by permanent, irreversible damage to the central nervous system caused by a gradual, relentlessly pro-

gressive wasting away of neurons or disruption of neuronal function. Some common degenerative alterations include Alzheimer's disease, Parkinson's disease, and Huntington's chorea.

It is important to recognize that a person may suffer from both an acute alteration in mental function and a chronic degenerative alteration simultaneously, as in the case of a person with Alzheimer's disease (chronic degenerative alteration) who develops a delirium due to metabolic effects of pneumonia (acute alteration).

ORGANIC BRAIN SYNDROME *Organic brain syndrome* describes a "constellation of psychological or behavioral signs and symptoms without reference to etiology" (American Psychiatric Association, 1980). A diagnosis of organic brain syndrome is appropriate when the etiology of a brain disorder is unknown. Examples of organic brain syndrome include delirium of unspecified etiology, dementia of unknown etiology, and organic delusional syndrome.

ORGANIC MENTAL DISORDER   DSM-III defines *organic mental disorder* as "a particular organic brain syndrome in which etiology is either known or presumed" (American Psychiatric Association, 1980). The presence of a specific factor judged to be etiologically related to the abnormal mental state must be demonstrated by means of the history, physical examination, or laboratory tests. Examples of organic mental disorders are multi-infarct dementia, alcohol-withdrawal delirium, and primary degenerative dementia.

DEMENTIA   *Dementia* is defined by Cummings

Figure 11-1. *The neurobiology of aging.*

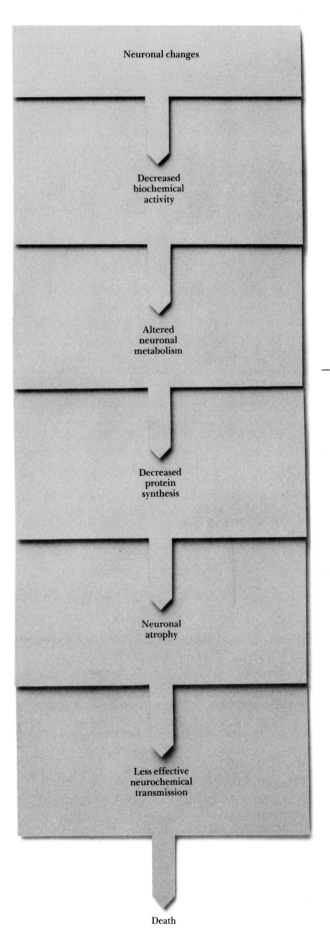

(1984) as an acquired, persistent compromise in intellectual function, with impairments in at least three of the following spheres of mental activity: language, memory, visuospatial skills, personality, and cognition (including abstraction, judgment, and mathematics).

THE RELATIONSHIP BETWEEN AGING AND ALTERED PATTERNS OF DEGENERATIVE ORIGIN

Although we have recently come to understand that aging itself is probably not the cause of degenerative disorders, the process of aging does result in neuronal changes in many individuals. These changes are the backdrop against which the cellular and biochemical pathology of degenerative alterations must be viewed. The neurobiology of aging begins with neuronal changes and results in decreased transmission of neurochemicals (see Figure 11-1). In addition to the neuronal alterations, senile plaques and neurofibrillary tangles develop during the aging process. *Senile plaques*, which consist of abnormal extracellular protein, are associated with decreased neuronal functioning. *Neurofibrillary tangles* (tiny nerve fibers tangled upon themselves and lying in the cytoplasmic space of nerve cells) lead to decreased functioning by interfering with intracellular transport; this results in permanent changes and impaired functioning. Both senile plaques and neurofibrillary tangles are thought to be implicated in some as yet unknown way in the development of Alzheimer's disease.

Wang (1973) has stated that aging is similar to a chronic illness in that it progresses with little remis-

---

THERAPEUTIC SUGGESTIONS FOR CAREGIVERS IN UTILIZING INTRINSIC AND EXTRINSIC SUPPORTS

Intrinsic Supports

- Analyze and accept your own feelings; self-awareness promotes self-control.

- Accept the fact that you are simply human, not Supernurse.

- Discard self-imposed performance standards that are unrealistic.

- Set sensible priorities.

- Acknowledge that you, like everyone else, have limits.

- Take pride in what you do accomplish.

Extrinsic Supports

- Share your feelings and problems with selected friends and colleagues.

- Actively participate in activities designed to improve working conditions.

- Learn to seek and accept help when necessary.

- Involve yourself in educational programs to improve your professional skills.

- Explore sources of group supports to insulate but not isolate yourself from the problems of clients receiving care.

282

sion until the final outcome of death. Successful adaptation to changes that accompany aging depends on the following:

1. Maintenance of identity and self-esteem.

2. Acceptance of inevitable losses and positive use of life experiences to compensate for losses.

3. A sense of satisfaction with life experiences.

Failure to adapt to inevitable situations exerts a strong influence on the development of degenerative disorders in the elderly. This psychological influence must not be overlooked when considering the physiological etiology of organic mental disorders.

MAJOR DEGENERATIVE ALTERATIONS

The three best-known degenerative alterations are Alzheimer's disease, Parkinson's disease, and Huntington's chorea.

Alzheimer's Disease

Alzheimer's disease is the most common of all degenerative alterations and is the diagnostic entity responsible for most of the cases of dementia found in the United States. Until recently, Alzheimer's disease was the label given to dementia-like syndromes occurring in the "presenile," or middle-aged population. Dementias occurring in the elderly were felt to constitute a distinct degenerative disorder and were commonly referred to as senile dementias. Most authorities now believe that this longstanding distinction between "presenile" and

"senile" dementias is no longer supportable, due to accumulating evidence that Alzheimer's disease and senile dementia are manifestations of the same underlying disease process (Comfort, 1984). It is now common to refer to both entities as "senile dementia, Alzheimer's type" (SDAT). The labeling of the dysfunction as either senile or presenile dementia is not as relevant to nursing care as are assessing client behaviors and level of functioning and planning appropriate interventions.

Alzheimer's disease was first described in 1907 by Alois Alzheimer, a German physician. The disease is characterized by certain neuropathologic changes: neurofibrillary tangles, granuovacuolar degeneration, neuritic plaques, and loss of dendritic spines (Cybyk, 1980; Albert, 1981). These neurologic changes are exaggerations of the degenerative changes seen in normal aging and are also similar to some neuropathologic features of Down's syndrome (Busse, 1973).

In Alzheimer's disease, the junctions between neurons develop deposits of amyloid, a starchlike protein (Charles, Truesdell, and Wood, 1982). This complex is referred to as a *neuritic plaque*. Plaque and neurofibrillary tangles interfere with transmission of electrochemical signals between neurons, leading eventually to disruption of intellect and memory, depending on the number, location, and size of the plaques and tangles (Palmer, 1983). Most of these lesions occur in the cerebral cortex and eventually lead to diminished brain mass. In the initial stages, atrophy is greatest in the frontal and temporal lobes. In advanced Alzheimer's disease, over half of the cerebral cortex may be atrophied (Charles, Truesdell, and Wood, 1982).

Another common finding in Alzheimer's dis-

DSM-III CLASSIFICATION AND NURSING DIAGNOSES

DSM-III classification of degenerative disorders is dependent on the identified cause of the disorder. Organic mental disorders of known etiology fall under the following diagnostic categories:

Primary degenerative dementia, senile onset:

    290.30 with delirium
    290.20 with delusions
    290.21 with depression
    290.00 uncomplicated

    290.1x Primary degenerative dementia, presenile onset
    290.4x Multi-infarct dementia

Substance induced:

    303.00 Alcohol intoxication
    305.40 Barbiturate intoxication
    305.50 Opioid intoxication
    305.60 Cocaine intoxication
    305.70 Amphetamine intoxication
    305.90 PCP intoxication
    305.30 Hallucinogen intoxication
    305.20 Cannabis intoxication
    305.90 Caffeine intoxication

Organic brain syndromes whose etiology or pathophysiologic process is either noted as an additional diagnosis from outside the mental disorders section or is unknown include:

    293.00 Delirium (acute brain syndrome)
    294.10 Dementia
    294.00 Amnestic syndrome
    293.81 Organic delusional syndrome
    293.82 Organic hallucinosis
    293.83 Organic affective syndrome
    310.10 Organic personality syndrome

Nursing diagnoses that may apply include:
    Anxiety
    Bowel elimination, alteration in:
        constipation, impaction
    Comfort, alteration in
    Coping, ineffectual individual
    Coping, ineffective family
    Family processes, alteration in
    Grieving
    Home maintenance management, impaired
    Knowledge deficit
    Mobility, impaired physical
    Nutrition, alteration in
    Powerlessness
    Self-care deficit
    Self-concept, disturbance in
    Sensory perceptual alteration
    Skin integrity, impairment of
    Sleep pattern disturbance
    Social isolation
    Thought processes, alteration in
    Urinary elimination, alteration in pattern of
    Violence, potential for

283

---

ease is a decline in the enzymes *choline acetyltransferase* and *acetylcholinesterase* in the cortex and the hippocampus, an area of the brain important to memory function (Palmer, 1983; Comfort, 1984). The result of these decreased enzyme levels is impaired utilization of the neurotransmitter *acetylcholine*. Several studies have attempted to determine a way to increase acetylcholine availability in the brains of Alzheimer's victims. Thus far, these studies have failed to show any appreciable effect in reversing or halting the dementing process.

ETIOLOGY Several etiologic theories of Alzheimer's disease have been advanced over the years, and research in this area has recently expanded exponentially. Some of these etiologic theories include:

1. *Heredity.* The incidence of Alzheimer's dis-

ease is increased in near relatives of affected individuals. There is also a significant association between Down's syndrome and Alzheimer's disease. Many persons with Down's syndrome eventually develop Alzheimer's disease, and the two diseases frequently occur in the same family (Wolanin and Phillips, 1981).

2. *Increased brain aluminum concentration.* Most people afflicted with Alzheimer's disease have a large increase in the amount of aluminum found in their brain tissue. At one time this was felt to be a promising lead in uncovering the cause of the disease. It is now felt that aluminum levels are high in the brains of most elderly persons, and levels probably correlate more strongly with age than with degree of dementia (Comfort, 1984).

3. *Slow virus infection.* Jakob-Creutzfeldt disease, a rare dementia similar to Alzheimer's disease,

Does any here know me? This is not Lear:
Does Lear walk thus? Speak thus? Where are his eyes?
Either his notion weakens, his discernings
Are lethargied. Ha! Waking? Indeed not so.
Who is it can tell me who I am?
WILLIAM SHAKESPEARE, KING LEAR

284

has been shown to be caused by the destructive effects of a slow-acting virus. Although research into this etiologic avenue continues, to date no conclusive evidence linking Alzheimer's disease and viral infection has been found.

4. *Autoimmune disorder.* This theory proposes that Alzheimer's disease may be due to a derangement of immune function that causes the production of antibodies targeted against the individual's own brain tissue. Research supporting this hypothesis has been disappointing to date (Wolanin and Phillips, 1981).

SYMPTOMS The characteristic behaviors of an individual with Alzheimer's disease are a result of the destruction of cerebral neurons. The cardinal symptom of early Alzheimer's disease is impairment of memory, particularly for recent events. Early in the disease, there is a gradual development of vague symptoms, including irritability and insomnia. The individual also begins to exhibit absentmindedness, lack of concentration, and emotional lability. These early symptoms, especially the initial memory loss, may be overlooked or considered a part of normal aging. Although an increase in forgetfulness accompanies normal aging, the degree of memory impairment is small in comparison to that exhibited by the Alzheimer's victim. The Alzheimer's individual may have a tendency to blame others for his increasing disabilities. Severe spatial disorientation may occur; the person may become lost in his own home or wander aimlessly around his neighborhood. Even with these symptoms, the client may be able to maintain an adequate facade (Cybyk, 1976; Dewis and Baumann, 1982). A unique characteristic associated with the early stage of Alzheimer's disease is that the client is often able to conceal his memory loss; his ability to think logically is not yet as impaired as his memory (Hayter, 1974).

As the dysfunction progresses, memory impairment becomes more noticeable. The individual may not remember close friends and relatives. The symptoms indicate progressive physiologic involvement of specific areas of the brain. Difficulties with attention, concentration, and comprehension increase. The person's speech may be impaired by such alterations as aphasia, echolalia, and logoclonia (repetition of last syllables). In addition, the client frequently demonstrates agnosia (inability to recognize shapes and sounds) and acalculia (difficulty in performing simple mathematic calculations). Muscular impairment is evidenced in apraxia and hypotonicity, and extrapyramidal symptoms of rigidity and altered gait usually appear. Epileptiform seizures are common; convulsions occur in 25 to 30 percent of all cases (Cybyk, 1976; Dewis and Baumann, 1982). Perseveration (repetitive movements), in the form of chewing, licking, tapping, or folding of hands, occurs. The client seems to be intent on mouthing all objects (hyperorality), putting everything in his mouth as if to examine it. The need of many clients to be in constant motion makes them seem goal-directed when they are actually performing meaningless activities (Hayter, 1974). Sleep disturbance is another common feature. Alzheimer's victims often sleep during the day and become active only at night, a situation known as day-night reversal.

The final stage of the illness is characterized by restlessness, irritability, and stereotyped movements. Emaciation, incontinence, and flexion contractures occur. The brain, muscles, and viscera

I don't know what's going to happen
and I'm afraid.
I might fall and break my hip and never walk again.
I might become senile and be a burden to everyone.
The money might run out.
I might have a stroke and wake up with one side of my face sagging.
I see these things happening all around me.
There seems to be no end to them.
And no end to the horror show that goes on behind my eyes if I let it.
Help me not to let it.
Help me not to look ahead but to this day, this hour, this minute.
If the present is difficult, help me cope with it.
If it is painful, help me bear it.
If it is empty, help me fill it.
If it is good, help me enjoy it.
Most of all, help me live it.

E. MACLAY, "I DON'T KNOW WHAT'S GOING TO HAPPEN," GREEN WINTER

285

atrophy with progression of the disease. In the final stages, the client appears to have wasted away. Cybyk (1976) describes this stage as "vegetative existence in the terminal phase" (p. 281).

Parkinson's Disease

Parkinson's disease is a progressive degenerative neurologic disorder first described by James Parkinson in 1817. Parkinsonism affects more than 1 percent of all persons over the age of fifty, which makes it one of the most common degenerative disorders of the nervous system (Gresh, 1980). Some 60,000 new cases per year are diagnosed in the United States alone.

Parkinson's disease first presents as a motor disorder in which clients gradually develop rigidity, tremor, slowness of movement, and problems maintaining balance (Strub and Black, 1981). The symptoms of bradykinesia or akinesia make the initiation of any movement difficult. The individual often exhibits a shuffling (fenestrating) gait and may "freeze" in place for several moments, unable to move her feet. There are also problems with fine motor movements of the fingers, which lead to difficulties with buttoning clothes and writing. Impaired muscle function eventually leads to development of the masklike facies of Parkinson's disease. The person's face appears dull and without expression even under conditions of considerable emotional arousal. Bradykinesia involving the muscles used in speech and swallowing results in dysarthria, dysphagia, and drooling. The client's voice becomes decreased in volume, high-pitched, monotonous, and often unintelligible.

Muscular rigidity, another manifestation of Parkinson's disease, may eventually cause muscular

aches and cramps and diffuse bone pain (Langan, 1976). The individual also develops a resting or "pill-rolling" tremor, most severely affecting the thumb and index fingers. Eventually the bradykinesia, rigidity, and tremor of the disease make even the most simple movement excruciatingly difficult to initiate or sustain.

Early studies of Parkinson's disease focused little attention on associated mental changes. Recently, there has been convincing documentation of the presence of a true dementing process in the later stages of the illness. It is important to remember that mental deterioration does not appear until the disease has been present for several years. It is often difficult to determine the extent of the dementia because the client's physical symptoms and deficits in communication make adequate testing of cognitive function problematical (Strub and Black, 1981). Despite these diagnostic obstacles, it is likely that a sizeable percentage of clients with parkinsonism (25 to 80 percent) develop a degenerative mental disorder as the disease progresses (Strub and Black, 1981). The manifestations of the degenerative disorder include a general lack of arousal that prevents normal cognition and social behavior, impairment of problem solving and concept formation, poor judgment, and apathy.

Parkinson's disease is thought to be due to a deficiency of the neurotransmitter dopamine in the corpus striatum, globus pallidus, and substantia nigra. These areas of the brain are responsible for the control of posture and voluntary muscular action. Diagnosis is difficult because there are no definitive tests for the disease, although urine samples may show a decreased excretion of dopamine. Therefore, diagnosis is based primarily on the

Figure 11-2. Inheritance pattern for Huntington's chorea, an autosomal dominant disorder. If one parent has the disorder, offspring have a 50–50 chance of developing the disorder.

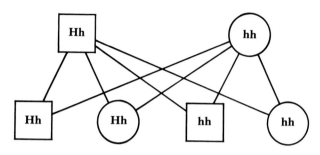

H = Gene for Huntington's chorea
h = Normal gene
Hh = Affected individual
hh = Nonaffected individual

□ = Male
○ = Female

286

client's history and motor symptoms (Langan, 1976).

Treatment for Parkinson's disease revolves around replacement of dopamine to near normal levels by use of levodopa, a precursor of dopamine. Unfortunately, levodopa may improve motor performance while actually precipitating confusional behavior (Strub and Black, 1981). To date, there is no known treatment that effectively reverses or even halts both the progressive motor and mental impairment accompanying the disorder.

Huntington's Chorea

Huntington's chorea is an autosomal dominant genetic disease that combines progressive dementia with bizarre involuntary movements (*chorea*) and odd postures. Autosomal dominant genetic transmission implies that the disease can be passed along to offspring by one parent, with each child having a 50 percent chance of eventually developing the disease (see Figure 11-2). The disorder usually becomes apparent between the ages of thirty and fifty; the remaining life expectancy is approximately fifteen years. Usually, symptoms do not occur until after the childbearing years, when potentially afflicted individuals may have already borne children likely to develop the disease in later life. Thus, much research is being focused on detecting the disease prior to the childbearing years (Wells, 1972; Richardson and Adams, 1980; Wilson and Carron, 1980).

The onset is insidious. Impairments slowly develop in problem solving, alertness, and concentration. Wilson and Carron (1980) report:

There are changes involving emotional states and emo-

tional lability including extremes such as euphoria, apathy, and irritability. Second, there are even more extreme changes involving inappropriate sexual behavior, preoccupation with the sexual misbehavior of others, delusions of persecution and/or grandiosity, and hallucinations. These manifestations often lead to diagnoses of mania, psychotic depressions, paranoia, or schizophrenia. (p. 13)

Impulsive behavior, a result of mental deterioration, may lead to such behaviors as alcoholism, drug addiction, and sexual promiscuity. As the intellectual losses progress, the individual is no longer able to care for himself and becomes totally dependent (Stipe, White, and Van Arsdale, 1979). Feelings of social isolation may be increased because the problems of intellect and communication inhibit the expression of fears and needs. As Stipe, White, and Van Arsdale (1979) have stated: "Emotional disturbances may result from distress over prognosis and difficulties in adjusting to a generally lower level of adaptive abilities" (p. 1428).

The neuropathologic changes of the disorder consist of cortical atrophy with ventricular dilatation. No specific cause of neuronal loss has been determined, but anatomic and pharmacologic discoveries indicate that the chorea that occurs in Huntington's disease is due to excess amounts of dopamine in relation to the acetylcholine and GABA within the caudate nucleus. Restoration of the balance among these three neurotransmitters may lessen choreiform movements (Stipe, White, and Van Arsdale, 1979).

The characteristic choreiform movements of Huntington's disease consist of uninhibited, involuntary writhing and twisting movements of the facial muscles and extremities. Psychological stress

Table 11-1. Comparison of Degenerative Alterations

	Alzheimer's Disease	Parkinson's Disease	Huntington's Chorea
Etiology	Unknown; suspected causes: trace minerals, virus, autoimmune, genetic	For idiopathic Parkinson's, unknown; may be drug-induced (by major tranquilizers)	Genetic
Neuropathology	Structural changes: neuritic plaques, neurofibrillary tangles, loss of dendritic spines, ventricular dilatation	Deficiency of dopamine in the corpus striatum, globus pallidus, and substantia nigra	Progressive atrophy of basal ganglia and cerebral cortex
Classical manifestations	Memory loss, disorientation, impaired judgment, decreased cognitive abilities	Bradykinesia, tremor, rigidity; mental impairment in later stages	Involuntary muscular movements, mental impairment, emotional changes
Medical treatment	None specific; tranquilizers, cortisones sometimes therapeutic	Dopamine replacement with precursor, levodopa; anticholinergic drugs	Palliative; dopamine antagonists

increases these movements. Because of involvement of facial and neck muscles, speech is impaired to the degree to which it is unintelligible, and swallowing becomes difficult. The later stages of the disease are characterized by physical helplessness with complete dementia and nearly constant writhing movements, leaving the client exhausted, emaciated, and often bedridden (Pinel, 1976). Huntington's chorea itself is not fatal, but death occurs from secondary complications, usually cardiac or respiratory in nature (Wells, 1972).

Table 11-1 compares the etiologies, neuropathology, manifestations, and treatment approaches for Alzheimer's, Parkinson's, and Huntington's diseases.

IMPACT OF DEGENERATIVE ALTERATIONS ON THE CLIENT

Common problems in the nursing care of clients with altered patterns of degenerative origin include memory impairment, cognitive impairment and behavioral alterations, impaired reality testing, impaired judgment, impaired communication, self-care deficits, and social alterations.

Memory Impairment

Memory deficits common to degenerative disorders interfere with the client's ability to learn new material and to recall previously learned information. At first, memory deficits have their greatest impact on complex activities such as reading, balancing a checkbook, finding directions, and engaging in complicated conversations. Eventually, even the most basic tasks involved in eating, dressing, bath-

ing, and toileting will become difficult for the client to perform independently because of his inability to remember the sequence of steps involved.

Early in the degenerative process, the client should be encouraged to continue as many normal activities as possible and to avoid situations that may prove too complex for him to handle. Routines should be established and followed as closely as possible. The client should be provided with an identification necklace or bracelet in case he becomes lost or disoriented (Mace and Rabins, 1981). Memory aids such as lists of tasks and prominently displayed clocks and calendars may be helpful. Familiar objects should be left in the same places after each use so that the client can easily locate them again. The client should not be expected to generalize knowledge from one situation to a similar one; each new situation will require direction and supervision, with tasks broken down into simple steps given one at a time. Hayter (1974) suggests that repetition of an activity will increase retention of the pattern of functioning. The client who does not respond to verbal direction may be capable of continuing an activity that another person has initiated for him.

Memory loss in the early stages of a degenerative disorder is often accompanied by a marked increase in anxiety as the client finds himself unable to fulfill social and occupational expectations. As memory loss progresses, the world becomes an unfamiliar and frightening place for the client, and he may respond with agitation, paranoia, delusions, and violence.

Assessing memory may sometimes be difficult. In the early stages of deterioration, a client may compensate for memory deficits. One of these coping behaviors is *confabulation*, the filling in of amnesic gaps with imaginary stories. *Circumstantiality*—avoiding a topic by talking around it—is also employed to cover memory losses. Both of these behaviors can be viewed as assets; they are attempts to adapt to a threatening situation (Pasquali et al., 1981). If not identified and dealt with, indications of memory deficits can also cause a client to become anxious and to question his competence (Mahoney, 1980).

Cognitive and Behavioral Alterations

The progressive dementia common to degenerative disorders leads to bizarre and irrational behaviors that may be difficult for the client, the family, and the nurse to understand and manage. Some of these behaviors include clinging to those with whom the client feels secure, hoarding, perseveration (repetition of behaviors and words), repeated fidgeting, and relocating and fondling of objects in the environment (Beam, 1984). The affected individual may follow trusted caregivers around continually but is often suspicious and demanding.

These odd behaviors lead to problems for both client and caregiver. Bizarre activity may cause caregivers to become exasperated, exhausted, or fearful of the client, and they may cope by withdrawing from her. For the community-resident client and family, these behaviors may lead to social isolation, as neighbors and friends find themselves unable to deal with the client's irrational acts and threatening physical alterations, such as incontinence, movement disorders, and inattention to personal hygiene and grooming.

The client with a degenerative disorder is at great risk for injury in any setting. Potential hazards include look-alike objects (a container of apple juice and a full urinal), forgotten cigarettes, lit stoves, and wandering outdoors in unfamiliar settings or inclement weather (Beam, 1984). For the client, coping with these hazards presents a constant frustration and challenge to her diminished physical and mental abilities. For the caregiver, the need for perpetual vigilance and foresight becomes burdensome and frightening.

Because of decreased cognitive ability, the client with a degenerative disorder has difficulty managing large amounts of stimulation. This inability to process incoming information may lead to a "catastrophic reaction," brought on by the client's fear of not reacting according to personal and social expectations. Wolanin (1981) describes catastrophic behavior as characterized by somatic and observable manifestations, such as sympathetic activation, apathy, anxiety, withdrawal, and confusion. If severe enough, the catastrophic reaction may lead the client to assaultive or self-destructive behavior.

In situations where behavioral alterations threaten the safety of the client and those around her, small doses of psychotropic medications may be indicated. Drug usage must be tailored to the client's disorder and her response to these medications. Most of the major tranquilizers are highly *lipidophilic*, meaning that most of the drug is bound to fat. Since the elderly have a higher body fat proportion than younger people, lower doses of these drugs should be used with older clients. The highest therapeutic success with the fewest side effects has been reported with thioridazine (Mellaril), haloperidol (Haldol), molindone (Moban), and loxapine (Loxitane) (Dellefield and Miller, 1982). For Parkinson's clients, it is essential to avoid drugs associated with extrapyramidal side effects, which mimic parkinsonian features of rigidity and tremor. These clients are likely to respond better to thioridazine and other drugs of the piperidine class (mesoridazine, piperacetazine) because they are relatively less likely to induce extrapyramidal side effects.

Impaired Reality Testing

The client with a degenerative disorder is apt to withdraw from reality, thus decreasing his awareness of the world around him. Confusion, which is increased by anxiety, interferes with the client's ability to test reality accurately. Disorientation may be increased at night by the lack of sensory stimulation and the client's diminished perceptual acuity. Placement in an unfamiliar environment may lead to prolonged disorientation to time, place, and person. Going along with the client's misperceptions to avoid upsetting him only adds to his insecurity and confusion, since he is then unable to trustingly test reality with those who represent security and sources of reliable feedback.

Reality can be reinforced by use of 24-hour reality orientation techniques, which incorporate environmental cues (such as reality orientation boards, signs, clocks, and calendars) and frequent reminders of time, place, and person. It is often helpful to reinforce time by associating reminders with daily activities such as breakfast, lunch, dinner, and bedtime. Reminiscing with the client about his past experiences helps to reaffirm his sense of past identity. Keeping some of the client's personal items, especially photographs, in his environment is also beneficial. According to Hirschfeld (1976), "Concrete symbols of one's past can offer the reassurance of continuity to the self now severely threatened by brain disease" (p. 1983).

The degree of reality orientation can be assessed by asking the client questions regarding time, place, and person. The client must be given enough time to respond to questioning. If he is hurried, his anxiety will increase and probably interfere with his response. In an institutional setting, responses to questions regarding orientation should be evaluated in light of the impact of the institution's milieu on the client's perception of time, place, and person. It may be unrealistic to expect even the mildly impaired client to know day, date, and clock time if he has limited access to newspapers, radio, television, watches, or windows with an outside view. In a similar vein, settings that allow for frequent changes of caregivers and other personnel make it difficult for the client to retain orientation to person.

Impaired Judgment

Another outcome of degenerative disorders is impaired judgment. The client becomes unable to objectively examine her behavior and its effects on herself and others, so she is likely to exhibit socially unacceptable behavior. One type of socially unacceptable behavior that commonly occurs is assaultiveness. The client may not purposefully be assaultive; however, she may be assaultive without knowing what she is doing. The client should always be approached slowly and within her line of vision in order to avoid startling her and perhaps provoking an assault. Touch should be used judiciously; some clients will become combative if touched, while others respond positively to touch that indicates genuine acceptance and support.

Impaired judgment may also lead to inappropriate displays of sexual behavior, such as public masturbation or exposure. Caregivers need to be aware that the client's sexual needs persist despite the disease process. Affection and caring are more effective than scolding and guilt inducement. The anticipation of needs and use of distraction may divert inappropriate sexual activity without provoking anger (Beam, 1984).

Impaired Communication

Most clients with degenerative disorders suffer from impaired communication. Communication problems may arise from impairment of facial and neck muscles (as in Huntington's chorea and Parkinson's disease) or from decreased intellect (as in Alzheimer's disease). As dementia progresses, comprehension may also be affected. It is impossible to accurately determine the exact degree of a client's comprehension. Therefore, caregivers must talk to a client as if he is capable of understanding. Relatives should be advised to continue to talk to the client as well. Every client has the ability to communicate, even if only on a limited, primitive level. Communication, both verbal and nonverbal, must be maintained. Caregivers should avoid administering physical care without talking to the client. Such behavior negates the client's existence and decreases his motivation to remain connected to real-

ity. Encouraging the client's efforts to communicate and praising his success will increase his ability and foster his self-esteem. If the client's communication problems are dealt with ineffectively, however, catastrophic reactions may result. Frustration over inability to communicate needs is a frequent precipitant of assaultive behavior, particularly in an institutional setting.

When communicating with the person whose mental abilities have deteriorated, it is important to pick out the client's meaningful comments. Often the meaning of the client's behavior is misunderstood. Teaching those caring for him about the problems associated with degenerative diseases is essential for improving the quality of client care. The family also needs adequate explanation of client behaviors to facilitate their adaptation (Hayter, 1974; Dewis and Baumann, 1982; Hayter, 1982).

Understanding the context of the client's communication may help the caregiver to interpret it. This is one of the most convincing arguments for consistent assignment of caregivers and routines. When the caregiver knows the client well, he or she can often "fill in the gaps" in the client's incomplete or incoherent messages.

When the client with a degenerative disorder is having difficulty with word finding (anomia), it may be helpful for the caregiver to supply the word for him or attempt to guess the content of his communication, while checking with the client for accuracy of interpretation. Referral to a speech therapist and utilization of common speech therapy techniques for enhancing communication may also be helpful.

When the client cannot communicate, it is necessary to establish a regular routine for checking on his comfort and safety (Mace and Rabins, 1981). Caregivers should systematically assure that the client's basic human needs for adequate nutrition, elimination, mobility, respiration, ambient temperature, and environmental stimulation are being met.

The diminished hearing and vision accompanying normal aging can compound the communication problems inherent in degenerative disorders. Referral to appropriate specialists for hearing and vision evaluations and prostheses may help to maintain adequate communication. In addition, communication techniques such as those in the box on page 290 should be consistently employed by those who interact with the client.

Self-care Deficits

As mentioned previously, the cognitive deterioration associated with degenerative alterations ultimately leads to either partial or complete inability to

COMMUNICATING WITH CLIENTS

When communicating with clients who have alterations of degenerative origin, use the following techniques (Mace and Rabins, 1981):

1. Eliminate distracting noises or activities. If possible, communicate with the client in a quiet, secure, well-lit environment.

2. Look directly at the client and be sure he is in a position to see your face and hands.

3. Lower the tone of your voice.

4. Use short words and short, simple sentences.

5. Ask only one question at a time.

6. Speak slowly and wait for the client to respond.

7. Use signals other than words to reinforce verbal information. Point, gesture, demonstrate, and guide the client with your own hands.

8. Physical demonstrations of caring may be understood when all else fails. Don't be afraid to hug, hold hands, or just sit companionably with the client if other methods of communication are no longer effective.

290

perform basic activities of daily living. Loss of these abilities acquired so early in life is extremely upsetting to the client, especially at the beginning of the disease process. It is important that these self-care deficits be handled sensitively and in a matter-of-fact manner to avoid further distressing the client with shame or performance anxiety.

Rehabilitation nursing texts are excellent sources of information on coping with self-care deficits. Referral to physical, occupational, and recreational therapists may also prove beneficial in determining ways to preserve maximum self-care ability. There is a growing availability of specially adapted tools for bathing, feeding, ambulation, and toileting; many of these items are now sold by nationally known mail-order catalogue firms.

Incontinence is a problem deserving special mention when considering the self-care deficits of the client with a degenerative disorder. Incontinence is one of the major precipitants for institutional placement of a person with a degenerative disorder. Because of our deeply ingrained ideas about the implications of inability to control one's bladder and bowels, many caregivers respond to the problem of incontinence with shame, disgust, or neglect. Any problem with incontinence requires thorough medical evaluation to rule out and correct treatable causes, such as infection, prostatic obstruction, cystocele, rectocele, and fecal impaction. Caregivers need to understand the reasons for incontinence and its management. In cases of incontinence for which no physical cause can be determined, it is important to develop consistent toileting schedules and to use incontinence management devices, such as a collecting apparatus and protective clothing, which minimize both embarrassment for the client and work for the caregiver. Above all, the caregiver must communicate to the client that her incontinence in no way diminishes her dignity or worth as a human being.

Social Alterations

The client with an altered pattern of degenerative origin and his family face a difficult and uncertain future clouded by the knowledge that the client's losses are progressive and irreversible. The client and family need help to begin the process of accepting the chronicity of the disorder. They also need to learn how best to manage the impact of the disorder so that it does not overwhelm and distort the workings of the entire family system and social network. The nursing goal in caring for the client and family is to assist with this adaptation.

Successful adaptation has been identified as the client's ability to live with himself and his condition. The client's acknowledgment of the disease and its limitations is evidence of the final stage of acceptance. According to Crate (1965), the nurses's role "is not to force, push, or try to change the client, but to develop a relationship in which he can use her as a guide as he makes the necessary changes within himself through the normal process of adaptation" (p. 76).

Science has not so far made a concentrated attack on the degenerative diseases, partly because it does not yet have the knowledge, and partly because it lacks the will. That is changing. In de Tocqueville's words, "The eveil which as suffered patiently as inevitable seems unendurable as soon as the idea of escaping from it crosses men's minds." That is happening now. Most of us are going to die of age-dependent diseases. These can only be picked off singly to a limited extent, and the best chance of improving our mileage lies in a medicine of rate control.

ALEX COMFORT (1976)

Families need a supportive person who is non-critical and nonjudgmental. Expressing their feelings reduces their psychological stress. As Hirschfeld (1976) has stated:

A nurse can help family members gradually face the unavoidable reality of the older member's mental decline, accept outbursts of anger and hostility, and examine guilt feelings together. (p. 1081)

According to Hayter (1982), families of relatives with irreversible degenerative disorders have many needs that are not being met adequately. Many need more information about the causes, treatment, and prognosis of the disorder. Families often state that they received comfort from knowing a specific diagnosis; the unknown is extremely frightening to them. The nurse must provide explanations in order to counter the myths and inaccurate information that abound about degenerative disorders.

One way to ensure that families obtain accurate and up-to-date information about degenerative disorders is to refer them to the Alzheimer's Disease and Related Disorders Association (ADRDA). Most metropolitan areas now have a local chapter of the ADRDA, which conducts self-help support groups for families of clients with degenerative disorders. Initially, the group provides the information crucial to coping with the diagnosis of the disorder. Many ADRDA groups promote networking of families who are in close proximity and in similar situations. These networks help with problems of anticipatory grief and isolation. They also offer practical and tested techniques for dealing with clients' problem behaviors (Gwyther and Matteson, 1983).

During the time that the individual with a degenerative disorder lives at home, the nurse needs

to be sensitive to threats to the client's self-esteem. The client should be encouraged to express what kind of care is acceptable to her (Dewis and Baumann, 1982). The family should also be involved in discussions of care, for they are often the primary caregivers in the early degenerative stages.

A major problem for the client may be that significant others cannot accept her current level of functioning. A client diagnosed with Alzheimer's disease wrote this in his journal:

I need understanding and support now and in the future to help me adjust to a new lifestyle during the next months and years. I need to know people accept me "as is." (Dewis and Baumann, 1982, p. 32)

Relatives often have negative feelings about the client's behavior. The disorder may necessitate role changes that are disruptive to the family. Relationships are altered as the client is transformed from an independent person to a dependent one. A husband may be forced to retire while the wife goes to work and becomes the major provider. A parent may become dependent on her child. Such changes result in family tension and resentment, particularly if some family members feel burdened by additional responsibilities. Ambivalent feelings about the client's impending death, role reversal, and competition and greed among siblings are all thorny family issues that may arise as the client's illness progresses (Lansky, 1984). The nurse needs to be sensitive to these issues while facilitating frank discussion and acknowledging that such painful feelings are to be expected.

Family members may employ many coping mechanisms, including projection, denial, and reaction formation (Hirschfeld, 1976). Utilization of reaction formation, that is, focusing on caring for the client in an attempt to negate the negative feelings that her behavior evokes, can be especially maladaptive. As Hayter (1982) points out, "The nurse can help the family find a balance between responsibility to themselves, their relative with Alzheimer's disease, and the remainder of the family" (p. 85).

As the degenerative alteration progresses, the client usually requires institutionalization. Often after the client has been institutionalized, the relatives experience feelings of relief mixed with guilt. This guilt may be alleviated somewhat by the nurse's acknowledgment of what the family members have done for the client. Also, the nurse can emphasize the unique role family members can play with an institutionalized relative. They can provide the client with love and affection (Hayter, 1982). The family may need to be encouraged to visit the client because his lack of response can alienate them.

IMPACT OF DEGENERATIVE ALTERATIONS ON THE NURSE

Caring for clients who are cognitively impaired is difficult and, at times, frustrating for the nurse. The nurse may become discouraged to see a client for whom he is caring continue to deteriorate. It is important for the nurse to remember that sometimes improvement in function is impossible. For the client who is unable to improve, it helps to remember that she remains a human being worthy of respect.

The caregiver must initially evaluate his own feelings about cognitive loss. Our society values intellectual achievement, and degenerative mental disease carries a social stigma (Hirschfeld, 1976). Through self-awareness, the nurse may realize that he is negatively biased toward an individual whose intellect is impaired. An increase in self-awareness can lead to empathy and greater understanding of what the client is experiencing.

The chronicity of degenerative disorders may also affect the nurse's reactions. As Butler (1977) has stated: "Chronicity is often used as an excuse for not doing anything when there may be many treatment techniques that could comfort, support, and even greatly increase the functioning of brain-damaged individuals" (p. 78). Once the brain damage has occurred, there is no return to a normal physical condition. However, functioning may be improved by treating some of the client's emotional and physical symptoms. The nurse working with the client with a degenerative disorder must be able to derive satisfaction from small improvements or even just maintenance in the client's functional abil-

ity. When this is no longer possible, she must realize the tremendous value of helping another human being face deterioration and, ultimately, death with as much dignity as possible.

THE NURSING PROCESS IN THE CARE OF CLIENTS WITH ALTERED PATTERNS OF DEGENERATIVE ORIGIN

Assessment

To help the client with a degenerative alteration reach or maintain his highest level of function, the nurse must be proficient in assessing both the client's deficits and his remaining strengths. Often, maximizing strengths helps the client to maintain feelings of adequacy and self-esteem despite ravaging losses in other abilities. For example, the client who can no longer remember what he ate for lunch may still be able to engage in meaningful social interaction by relating valuable experiences and insights gained over decades of living and coping successfully.

Assessment begins with gathering information about the life history of the client. How has the client coped with adversity in the past? What have been his sources of support and guidance? Who are the significant people in the client's life, and are they still available for support? Is his religious faith an asset? What losses has the client experienced, especially recently? When assessing losses, the nurse should include health factors as well as social and emotional losses (Wolanin, 1981).

The next area to be assessed is the client's environment. According to Wolanin (1981), environments should be assessed to answer two questions:

1. What in the client's environment facilitates his ability to function optimally?

2. What in his environment prevents this client from functioning optimally?

Both of these questions must be answered in terms of available human resources and the structure of the client's physical environment.

It is also important to assess how the client interacts with others. Here, it is necessary to observe how the client and family relate to one another. Does the family overprotect the client and inadvertently assign him the role of passive receiver of care? Or does the family expect too much of the client in view of his diminished capacities? Is the relationship between client and family warm and loving, or is it fraught with conflict from old, unresolved problems or new difficulties associated with the client's condition? Does the family understand the nature of the client's disorder and its long-term implications?

Thorough assessment of the client with a degenerative alteration mandates use of holistic nursing assessment techniques. Self-care deficits and abilities must be carefully determined by direct observation of the client's functioning in activities of daily living. Special attention should be given to the integrity of the client's sensoriperceptual abilities. A comprehensive mental status exam is of primary importance in planning care. It may be helpful to refer the client for psychological testing to determine functioning in attention, memory, orientation, constructional ability, judgment, and abstract reasoning (Strub and Black, 1981).

Planning

Realistic goals should be established on the basis of the client's known assets and liabilities. Planning care for the client with a degenerative disorder requires that the nurse have a good understanding of the expected course of the degenerative processes involved. This understanding must also be imparted to family members who serve as caregivers. Initially, planning focuses on the client's memory deficits and resulting anxiety. Caregivers need to help the client organize his activities so that there is consistency and predictability to daily events. Provision must also be made for the client's safety needs as her judgment and reality testing abilities decline.

Caregivers must plan for the reality of the client's increasing dependency on others for physical care. While the client is still a community resident, it may be useful to put families in touch with appropriate community health and service organizations. These agencies can help to arrange for personal care assistance, recreation, and transportation. It may also be possible to obtain respite care for families who need an occasional break from caregiving burdens.

As the degenerative disorder progresses, the issue of institutional care may become a major focus of planning. Nursing homes and other long-term care facilities are still viewed as negative options by many clients, families, and nurses. However, when the client reaches the later stages of a degenerative disorder, it may be impossible to continue to provide for his many needs at home. It is important for everyone involved in the placement decision to understand that not all long-term care facilities are the substandard places depicted in the media and that it is possible to find a facility where care is provided skillfully and compassionately. The nurse can provide an invaluable service at this time by assisting client and caregivers in carefully exploring placement alternatives. Most facilities welcome inquiries and will arrange nonobligatory interviews

and tours for interested parties. The client should be as involved in this exploratory process as his physical and mental capabilities will allow.

Ultimately, planning revolves around assuring a comfortable and dignified death for the affected client. This involves attention to planning for the client's physical comfort as well as his psychological ease. Throughout the long course of illness and disability, the client and caregiver should be supported in their decisions about the extent of treatment desired and the setting in which the client's final days will be lived.

Implementation

Throughout this chapter, interventions have been suggested for various problems associated with degenerative disorders. Table 11-2 summarizes many of these interventions and lists others that may be indicated in the care of clients with degenerative disorders.

Evaluation

Evaluation of the effectiveness of nursing interventions in the care of the client with a degenerative alteration is based on the degree to which established goals are attained. Since the degenerative process usually progresses over an extended period of time, periodic reassessments and adjustments of goals and interventions should be conducted. Sometimes a goal that was initially thought to be achievable may have to be revised because of unanticipated declines in the client's ability brought on by intercurrent acute illness or psychosocial stressors. In other instances, goals may need to be revised upward because the client responds more positively than expected to planned interventions.

In broad terms, evaluation of nursing care for the client with a degenerative disorder should be based on two parameters: the attainment of maximum functional ability and the achievement of the greatest possible comfort for the client and family. The nurse's evaluation of the effectiveness of care in promoting functional ability may be supplemented by evaluations from other professionals, such as occupational and physical therapists. Assessment of success in promoting both physical and emotional comfort is more difficult; the best sources of feedback are frequent observations of the client's behavior and regular, open discussions with his significant others.

SUMMARY

In nearly every arena of practice, nurses are increasingly challenged to provide knowledgeable

Table 11-2. The Nursing Process in Degenerative Alterations

Client's Problem	Goal	Nursing Interventions
Memory impairment	Provide safe environment; promote self-esteem	1. Maintain structured environment with a regular schedule of activities. 2. Provide memory aids (lists, frequent reminders). 3. Encourage reminiscing and ventilation of anxieties.
Cognitive impairment	Provide safe environment; maximize self-care ability	1. Encourage self-care in areas where client is capable of continued independence. 2. Teach families about anticipated problems with the client's cognitive function. 3. Minimize stimulus overload. 4. Remove potential hazards from the client's environment.
Behavioral alterations	Provide safe environment; prevent injury to client and others	1. Teach families about potential behavioral alterations. 2. Use psychotropic medications judiciously. 3. Use distraction instead of confrontation. 4. Break down tasks into simple steps.
Impaired reality testing	Maintain orientation to time, place, and person; provide safe environment; decrease anxiety	1. Use 24-hour reality techniques and teach them to the family. 2. Provide for consistent scheduling of caregivers. 3. Maintain consistent routine. 4. Keep client's treasured personal possessions in the environment.
Impaired judgment	Provide safe environment; decrease anxiety	1. Approach client cautiously and within her line of vision. 2. Avoid scolding and criticism for irrational behavior. 3. Positively reinforce desired behaviors. 4. Remove potential hazards from the environment.
Impaired communication	Meet client's basic physical and emotional needs	1. Provide consistent routines and caregiver assignments. 2. Refer client for speech and hearing evaluation. 3. Minimize distractions in the environment. 4. Use good communication techniques.
Self-care deficits	Promote maximum independence in ADL's; maintain client's self-esteem	1. Communicate about self-care problems in a matter-of-fact manner. 2. Obtain tools and products to maximize self-care ability. 3. Refer client to occupational therapy, physical therapy, or recreational therapy. 4. Provide family with information on personal care services and products.
Social alterations	Maintain client in community setting as long as possible; maintain client's relationship with family and friends	1. Care for the family as well as the client. 2. Encourage discussion of the effect the client's illness has on others in the family and social system. 3. Provide nonjudgmental support. 4. Educate the client and family regarding course of the disorder. 5. Refer family to self-help groups (such as ADRDA).
Deciding on institutional care	Maintain health of family members caring for client; meet client's needs for physical care; decrease family members' guilt feelings; decrease client's feelings of abandonment, relocation trauma	1. Facilitate discussion of institutional care, if appropriate. 2. Provide information about placement alternatives. 3. Support the family's decision. 4. Provide support for dealing with guilt, role reversal, and anticipatory grieving.

and effective care for the burgeoning number of clients with altered patterns of degenerative origin. Nurses are the primary caregivers for this population. If they are to adequately fulfill their role, they must increase their knowledge regarding the degenerative disorders and their management.

Degenerative alterations affect every sphere of client and family function. Physical alterations such

CLINICAL EXAMPLE

INDIVIDUAL AND FAMILY DISTRESS
RELATED TO HUNTINGTON'S CHOREA

Daniel Jackson was a sixty-three-year-old male who was becoming disabled because of Huntington's chorea. He was being cared for at home while he received outpatient care at a medical facility and was visited regularly by a community health nurse. Daniel lived with his wife, Mary, his twenty-five-year-old daughter, Diane, who worked as a secretary, and his twenty-year-old son, George, who attended a local college.

When he was simply sitting in a chair, Daniel gave little indication of his disability. However, when he attempted to move from one place to another, Daniel's gait was not purposeful but was characterized by wide, lurching movements that made it seem as if he was in imminent danger of falling. His arms and legs swung wildly as he moved in the general direction of his destination. Although others watched with apprehension, Daniel was usually able to navigate without colliding with objects or falling.

As his disease progressed, Daniel's problems gradually became even more apparent. His coordination was so impaired that eating could not be accomplished without smearing his hands and face and spilling food on his clothing and the floor. Daniel knew that family members found his eating habits repulsive, so he asked not so eat with the family.

The main burden of caring for Daniel fell on Mary, who became more frightened and resentful as the demands on her increased. Daniel felt himself in the grip of a great force that he could not control. He saw his family moving away from him, recognized the strain his wife was under, and saw the horror and dismay of his children as they witnessed his erratic behavior. Try as he might, Daniel was unable to control his movements and to reduce the amount of help he needed. His speech became more and more impaired. When he tried to talk with his wife and children, sometimes he could make no sound at all. At other times strange, animal-like noises came from his mouth. If people were patient enough, Daniel, with great effort, could form words that approximated human communication.

The atmosphere in the Jackson home was one of sadness. Diane, when home, spent most of her time in her room. George arranged to be out of the house as much as possible, except for meals. Mrs. Jackson felt isolated with only herself and her husband, although the community health nurse was a welcome visitor from the outside world.

Mary had a vague memory of her husband's father dying of a mysterious malady that seemed to resemble her husband's, but her father-in-law had died a few years before her marriage, and the details of his illness were unclear.

ASSESSMENT

Janice Wheeler, the community health nurse visiting the family, noted the devastating effects on family members as Daniel's chronic illness took its course. She saw the isolation of family members who had been close and loving not long before. As circumstances in the family changed, Janice decided that additional help was indicated. She saw that Diane and George were frightened young people using flight behavior in order to avoid dealing with their father's illness. They resisted any interaction with the nurse and did not acknowledge their father's plight or the burden on their mother. Janice realized that the children needed help in accepting the realities of the situation. Because of the genetic etiology of their father's illness, the children also needed to become aware of the implications for their own futures.

The following nursing and psychiatric diagnoses were made:

Nursing Diagnoses

Coping, ineffectual individual
(related to cognitive and communication losses)

Coping, ineffective family
(related to excessive responsibilities of the wife and flight behavior of the children)

Fear
(related to lack of knowledge and unexpressed anxiety concerning the father's illness and its implications for the whole family)

Mobility impaired
(related to impaired motor function)

Multiaxial Psychiatric Diagnosis

Axis I   290.21 Primary degenerative dementia with depression (Huntington's chorea)

Axis II   None

Axis III None

Axis IV   Code 5—Severe: Lack of support networks, loss of autonomy, depression

Axis V   Level 5—Poor: Impaired social functioning, impaired social relationships

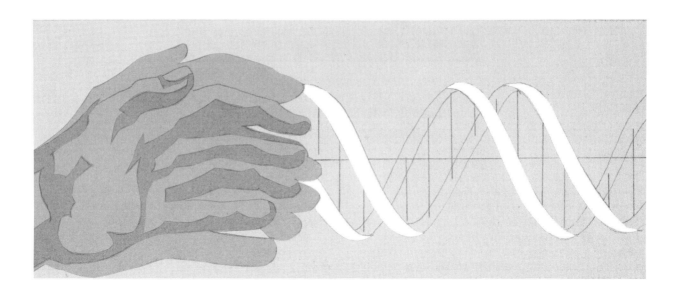

PLANNING

Janice explored Daniel's Social Security disability status and learned that he was eligible for care in a community day treatment center as long as he was ambulatory and had some capacity for self-care. She arranged a family meeting with the parents and children and explained to them that Daniel could apply for admission to the day treatment center and attend three days a week while continuing to live at home. A chairmobile could be provided by the supplementary Social Security funds to transport him.

At the meeting, the illness of Daniel's father was mentioned, and Janice asked for more information. Daniel was able to recall some facts, and for the first time Diane asked the question that had been troubling her for weeks, "Is this illness hereditary?" Janice gave an affirmative answer but disclaimed any special expertise in this matter. She suggested that George and Diane make an appointment to see a genetic counselor at the medical center where Daniel's care was being coordinated. Janice then began to guide the family toward a series of immediate goals. The goals to which the family agreed were:

1. Arrange an intake interview at the day treatment center to determine Daniel's suitability for admission to the day treatment program.

2. Divide the day-to-day responsibilities for Daniel's care among all three members of the family. Diane agreed to do the weekly shopping for groceries and to help with the laundry. George agreed to be available when his father needed help with bathing and shaving.

3. Accept Daniel's illness as a family problem and begin to learn more about the disorder that frightens all of them so much.

IMPLEMENTATION

With Daniel out of the house three days a week, his wife felt a sense of relief. She was able to visit friends occa-

sionally and to invite them to her home. Because she was experiencing some respite from her responsibilities, she was more patient with Daniel when he was at home. Attending the day treatment center gave Daniel a sense of social involvement. Staff members accepted his disability without making him feel rejected. The fact that he was still ambulatory enabled him to perform small services for other patients in wheelchairs and this, too, increased his feelings of self-worth.

The interview with the genetic counselor was difficult for Diane and George. They learned that Huntington's chorea was transmitted by a dominant gene, that one or both of them might develop the illness later in life, and that any children they had might be affected. Shock and dismay drew George and Diane closer. Neither was presently involved in a serious relationship, but both realized that difficult decisions lay ahead for both of them regarding marriage and children.

EVALUATION

Janice knew that Daniel's placement in the day treatment center was a temporary measure and that the time would come when hospitalization would be indicated. Fortunately, the family had access to a range of services to which Daniel's status as a disabled person entitled them. For the present, the family had adjusted as well as possible. Daniel was less depressed attending the day treatment center, where he felt like "one of the guys." He knew what the future held for him, but for the moment the quality of his life had improved. Mary now felt that her problems were manageable and that help would be forthcoming when the family required it. Diane and George were somewhat bitter, but their bitterness was not directed toward their parents. Several meetings with the genetic counselor and some independent reading had made them better informed. The realization of their situation was stark and frightening, but they gave each other mutual support. They also found that knowledge was better than ignorance and that working together as a family was better than being alone.

as movement disorders, sleep disturbances, and in-continence interact with the problems of memory and communication impairment, cognitive deterioration, behavioral alterations, impaired judgment, faulty reality testing, and social alterations. Nursing goals for clients with these disorders include promotion of self-esteem, provision of a safe environment, prevention of injury to self and others, maintenance of orientation and physical integrity, and reduction of anxiety. Goals involving the family include maintaining of the health of family caregivers, increasing the knowledge of family members regarding the causes and treatments of degenerative disorders, and reducing family members' frustration and guilt feelings.

The care of clients with degenerative disorders demands that the nurse use all of her skills in providing for both physical care needs and psychosocial requirements. Knowledgeable nursing care for the client with a degenerative disorder allows the client to function as well as he possibly can with as much comfort as he can possibly achieve.

Review Questions

1. Discuss the similarities and differences between delirium and dementia.

2. Compare and contrast acute and chronic degenerative alterations.

3. Describe the relationship between aging and altered patterns of degenerative origin.

4. Describe the pathological process of Alzheimer's disease.

5. Discuss the importance of genetic counseling for children of clients with Huntington's disease.

6. Compare the etiology, neuropathology, clinical manifestations, and treatment of Alzheimer's disease, Parkinson's disease, and Huntington's disease.

7. Design a nursing care plan for a client with memory impairment.

8. Discuss the use of psychotropic drugs for clients with degenerative alterations.

9. Explain why degenerative disorders are irreversible.

10. Describe three areas that the nurse must assess when caring for a client with an altered pattern of degenerative origin.

References

Albert, M. S. 1981. Geriatric Neuropsychiatry. *Journal of Consulting and Clinical Psychology*, 49(6):835, 850.

American Psychiatric Association. 1980. *Diagnostic and Statistical Manual of Mental Disorders*, 3rd ed. Washington, D.C.: The Association.

Beam, I. M. 1984. Helping Families Survive. *American Journal of Nursing*, 84(2):229–231.

Brill, N. Q. 1984. Alzheimer's Disease and Related Disorders: Introduction. *Psychiatric Annals*, 14(2):83–89.

Burnside, I. 1984. *Working with the Elderly: Group Process and Technique*, 2nd ed. Monterey, Calif.: Wadsworth Health Sciences.

Busse, E. W. 1973. Mental Disorders in Later Life. In *Mental Illness in Later Life*, eds. E. W. Busse and E. Pfeiffer. Washington, D.C.: American Psychological Association.

Butler, R. N., and Lewis, M. I. 1977. *Aging and Mental Health: Positive Psychosocial Approaches*, 2nd ed. St. Louis: C. V. Mosby.

Charles, R.; Truesdell, M.; and Wood, E. L. 1982. Alzheimer's Disease: Pathology, Progression and Nursing Process. *Journal of Gerontological Nursing*, 8(2): 69–73.

Comfort, A. 1976. *A Good Age*. New York: Simon & Schuster.

Comfort, A. 1984. Alzheimer's Disease or "Alzheimerism"? *Psychiatric Annals*, 14(2):130–132.

Crate, M. A. 1965. Nursing Functions in Adaptation to Chronic Illness. *American Journal of Nursing*, 65 (10):72–76.

Cummings, J. 1984. Dementia: Definition, Classification and Differential Diagnosis. *Psychiatric Annals*, 14: 85–92.

Cybyk, M. E. 1980. Alzheimer's Disease. *Nursing Times*, 76(7):280–282.

Dellefield, K., and Miller, J. 1982. Psychotropic Drugs and the Elderly Patient. *Nursing Clinics of North America*, 17(2):303–318.

Dewis, M. E., and Baumann, A. 1982. Alzheimer's Disease: The Silent Epidemic. *The Canadian Nurse*, July-August:32–35.

Gresh, C. 1980. Helpful Tips You Can Give Your Patients with Parkinson's Disease. *Nursing 80*, 10(1):26–33.

Gwyther, L., and Matteson, M. A. 1983. Care for the Caregivers. *Journal of Gerontological Nursing*, 9(2):92–95.

Hayter, J. 1974. Patients Who Have Alzheimer's Disease. *American Journal of Nursing*, 74:1460–1463.

Hayter, J. 1982. Helping Families of Patients with Alzheimer's Disease. *Journal of Gerontological Nursing*, 8(2):81–86.

Hirschfeld, M. H. 1976. The Cognitively Impaired Older Adult. *American Journal of Nursing*, 76:1981–1984.

Langan, R. 1976. Parkinson's Disease: Assessment Procedures and Guidelines for Counseling. *Nurse Practitioner*, (2)13–16.

Lansky, M. R. 1984. Family Psychotherapy of the Patient with Chronic Organic Brain Syndrome. *Psychiatric Annals*, 14(2):121–129.

Liston, E. H. 1984. Diagnosis and Management of Delirium in the Elderly Patient. *Psychiatric Annals*, 14(2):109–118.

Mace, N. L., and Rabins, P. V. 1981. *The 36-Hour Day*. Baltimore: Johns Hopkins University Press.

Mahoney, E. K. 1980. Alterations in Cognitive Functioning in the Brain-Damaged Patient. *Nursing Clinics of North America*, 15:283–292.

Palmer, M. H. 1983. Alzheimer's Disease and Critical Care: Interactions, Implications, Interventions. *Journal of Gerontological Nursing*, 9(2):86–90.

Pasquali, E. A.; Alesi, E. G.; Arnold, H. M.; and DeBasio, N. 1981. *Mental Health Nursing: A Biopsychocultural Approach*. St. Louis: C. V. Mosby.

Plum, F. 1979. Dementia: An Approaching Epidemic. *Nature*, 279:372–373.

Pinel, C. 1976. Huntington's Chorea. *Nursing Times*, 72:447–448.

Richardson, E. P., Jr., and Adams, R. D. 1980. Degenerative Disease of the Nervous System. In *Harrison's Principles of Internal Medicine*, 9th ed., eds. K. I. Isselbacher et al. New York: McGraw-Hill.

Stewert, C. M. 1982. Age-Related Changes in the Nervous System. *Journal of Neurosurgical Nursing*, 14(2):69–73.

Stipe, J.; White, D.; and Van Arsdale, E. 1979. Huntington's Disease. *American Journal of Nursing*, 79: 1428–1433.

Strub, R. L., and Black, F. W. 1981. *Organic Brain Syndromes: An Introduction to Neurobehavioral Disorders*. Philadelphia: F. A. Davis.

Wang, H. S. 1973. Special Diagnostic Procedures: The Evaluation of Brain Impairment. In *Mental Illness in Later Life*, eds. E. W. Busse and E. Pfeiffer. Washington, D.C.: American Psychological Association.

Wells, R. W. 1972. Huntington's Chorea: Seeing Beyond the Disease. *American Journal of Nursing*, 72:854–956.

Wilson, R. S., and Carron, D. C. 1980. Psychological Features of Huntington's Disease and the Problem of Early Detection. *Social Biology*, 27(1):11–19.

Wolanin, M. O., and Phillips, L. R. 1981. *Confusion: Prevention and Care*. St. Louis: C. V. Mosby.

Supplementary Readings

Beam, N. Helping Families Survive. *American Journal of Nursing*, 84(1984):228–232.

Boss, B. G. Acute Mood and Behavioral Disturbance of Neurological Origin: Acute Confusional States. *Journal of Neurosurgical Nursing*, 14(1982):61–68.

Burnside, I. Resource Materials on Dementia. *Journal of Gerontological Nursing*, 9(1983):108–109.

Coburn, M. Slow Steps to Memory. *Nursing Mirror*, 155(1982):48–49.

Cohen, G. D. The Mental Health Professional and the Alzheimer's Patient. *Hospital and Community Psychiatry*, 35(1984):115–116.

Cowie, V. Presenile Dementia: Old Before Your Time. *Nursing Mirror*, 152(1981):44–45.

Cross, J. N. Caring for a Demented Patient. *Nursing Times*, 79(1983):57–58.

Fischman, J. The Mystery of Alzheimer's. *Psychology Today*, 18(1984):27.

Footer, M. Alzheimer's: Aversive Disease of the Aged. *For Your Health*, 98(1983):14–15.

Foreman, M. Acute Confusional States in the Elderly: An Algorithm. *Dimensions of Critical Care Nursing*, 3(1984):208–215.

Gartz, C. M. Dementia: Easing the Anguish of the Elderly. *Consultant*, 22(1982):137–140.

Gibbard, F. B. Controlled Trial of Physiotherapy and Occupational Therapy for Parkinson's Disease. *British Medical Journal*, 282(1981):1196.

Gillis, L. S. Understanding and Handling Mental Disorders in the Aged. *Curatonis*, 3(1981):45–48.

Hamilton, H. L. Alzheimer's Disease: The New Epidemic. *Nursing Homes*, 32(1983):22–25.

Johnson, C. L. The Microanalysis of Senility: The Responses of the Family and the Health Professionals. *Culture, Medicine and Psychiatry*, 7(1983):77–96.

298

Kapust, L. R. Living with Dementia: The Ongoing Funeral. *Social Work and Health Care*, 7(1982):79–91.

Katzman, R. Early Detection of Senile Dementia. *Hospital Practice*, 16(1981):61–64.

LaPorte, H. J. Reversible Causes of Dementia: A Nursing Challenge. *Journal of Gerontological Nursing*, 8 (1982):74–80.

Langston, N. F. Reality Orientation and Effective Reinforcement for Treating the Confused Elderly. *Journal of Gerontological Nursing*, 7(1981):224–227.

Lincoln, B. What Do Nurses Know About Confusion in the Aged? *Journal of Gerontological Nursing*, 10 (1984):26–32.

Pajik, M. Alzheimer's Disease: Inpatient Care. *American Journal of Nursing*, 84(1984):215–222.

Pattison, E. M. Managing Agitated Persons in a Crisis. *Consultant*, 20(1980):143–146.

Powell, L. S., and Courtice, K. *Alzheimer's Disease: A Guide for Families*. Menlo Park, Calif.: Addison-Wesley, 1983.

Purdie, F. R. Acute Organic Brain Syndrome: A Review of 100 Cases. *Annals of Emergency Medicine*, 10 (1981):455–461.

Rader, J. Senility Isn't Normal Aging. It's a Physical Condition. *Oregon Nurse*, 49(1984):30–31.

Reisberg, B. Alzheimer's Disease: Stages of Cognitive Decline. *American Journal of Nursing*, 84(1984):225–228.

Reisberg, B. Diagnosis and Assessment of the Older Patient. *Hospital and Community Psychiatry*, 33 (1982): 104–110.

Ricci, M. All Out Support for an Alzheimer's Patient. *Geriatric Nursing*, 4(1983):369–371.

Richardson, K. Hope and Flexibility: Your Keys to Helping the OBS Patients. *Nursing 1982*, (1982):64–69.

Sands, R. G. Social Work and Victims of Huntington's Disease. *Social Work and Health Care*, 9(1984):63–71.

Schoenfeld, M. Attitudes Toward Marriage and Childbearing of Individuals at Risk for Huntington's Disease. *Social Work and Health Care*, 9(1984):73–81.

Selbst, R. Geriatrics: Evaluating the Confused Patient. *Consultant*, 24(1984):209–215.

Skolaski-Pellitteri, T. Environmental Adaptations Which Compensate for Dementia. *Physical and Occupational Therapy in Geriatrics*, 3(1983):31–44.

Shuman, J. E. Geriatric Patients with and Without Intellectual Dysfunction: Effectiveness of a Standard Rehabilitation Program. *Archives of Physical Medicine and Rehabilitation*, 62(1981):612–618.

Sloane, R. B. Treating Mental Disorders in the Elderly. *Consultant*, 20(1980):195–196.

Teusink, J. P. Helping Families Cope with Alzheimer's Disease. *Hospital and Community Psychiatry*, 35(1984): 152–156.

Toseland, R. W. Alzheimer's Disease and Related Disorders: Assessment and Intervention. *Social Work*, 9(1984):212–226.

HOLISTIC PERSPECTIVES

THEORIES OF STRESS AND ADAPTATION

DISORDERS OF ADAPTATION
Gastrointestinal Responses to Stress
Respiratory Responses to Stress
Cardiovascular Responses to Stress
Skeletomuscular Responses to Stress
Behavioral Responses to Stress
Psychogenic Pain Responses to Stress
Neoplastic Responses to Stress

C H A P T E R

12

Altered Patterns of Adaptational Origin

Learning Objectives

After reading this chapter, the student should be able to:

1. Describe Alexander's specific conflict theory and Dunbar's specific personality theory.

2. Explain the general adaptation syndrome described by Selye.

3. Discuss the role of the autonomic nervous system in activating the general adaptation syndrome.

4. Discuss the physiological and psychological factors present in gastrointestinal responses to stress.

5. Compare the behavioral traits of type A and type B personalities.

6. Discuss the physiological and psychological factors present in skeletomuscular responses to stress.

7. Identify the physiological, psychological, and cultural influences present in the behavior of the anorexia nervosa client.

8. Explain the value and limitations of visualization therapy as a therapeutic invervention with clients who have cancer.

9. Analyze the impact of aggression levels and control levels in clients exhibiting skeletomuscular, cardiovascular, and gastrointestinal stress responses.

10. Enumerate the major components of a holistic health care plan for clients with a stress-related disorder.

302

Overview

Virtually every disorder to which humans are susceptible can be affected, positively or negatively, by emotional states. Different views of the relationship between the mind and body are discussed in the first section of this chapter. Theories of stress and adaptation are the topic of the second section. The remainder of the chapter covers some representative alterations of structure and function that are related to stress and suggests nursing approaches that may well reduce stress levels and consequently help alleviate the client's physical and psychological distress.

*The best doctors in the world are Dr. Diet, Dr. Quiet,
and Dr. Merryman.*
JONATHAN SWIFT

HOLISTIC PERSPECTIVES

Relationships between mind and body have been viewed differently at different times in history (see Chapter 1). In tracing changes in the way mind-body relationships have been perceived, some paradoxes emerge. When the origins of human dysfunction were unknown, supernatural causes were often implicated and, as a result, therapeutic measures were brought to bear on the whole person: mind, body, and spirit. Ironically, this holistic approach narrowed as the frontiers of knowledge expanded. During the Renaissance, instruments were developed that revealed a previously invisible world. The Italian investigator Giovanni Morgagni (1682–1771), using microscopic lenses to study tissue samples from postmortem examinations, noted signs of disease in samples obtained from specific organs and linked these signs to observable dysfunctions previously noted in the deceased person. From such beginnings, altered cellular structures came to be associated with certain disorders. Theoretical explanations of the causes of dysfunction became more specific and more accurate, but their focus was almost entirely physiological.

Rapid expansion of knowledge about the physical world generated interest in the pursuit of learning. Scientific investigation was preoccupied with the objective or material world, which included the study of the body. Human beings gradually came to be considered triadic (three-part) entities consisting of body, mind, and spirit. The human spirit or soul became the concern of theologians, the mind became the concern of philosophers and teachers, and the body, or *soma*, became the concern

of scientists and physicians. Little attention was paid to spiritual influences on the physical self, and it became customary to deal with symptoms of illness rather than with the whole person. The division between mind, body, and spirit prevailed from the fifteenth through the nineteenth centuries (Kaplan, 1980).

One notable dissenter to the separatist movement was Thomas Huxley (1825–1895), who asserted that mental states are a consequence of physical processes. Another dissenter was Florence Nightingale, who was concerned for the welfare of the entire human organism and worked diligently to improve social and environmental conditions for her patients. However, it was not until the twentieth century that the interactive and holistic nature of human existence truly began to be accepted again.

The trend toward a holistic view of human dysfunction has accelerated in the past decade. It has become apparent that separating physical illness (the traditional domain of medicine) from psychological and social factors associated with dysfunction (the traditional domain of behavioral psychology and sociology) is untenable. Any dysfunction, whether apparently physiological, psychological, or social, represents a disorder of the whole person, not merely of the mind or the body. This comprehensive, holistic view of dysfunction is reflected in the modifications of the latest *Diagnostic and Statistical Manual* approved by the American Psychiatric Association (1980). The outdated term *psychosomatic*, which implies a duality of mind and body, was included in the standard nomenclature until 1968, when it was replaced by the term *psychophysiological*. DSM-III discards the category of psychophysiological disorders entirely in favor of the multiaxial

The word "stress," like "success," "failure," or "happiness," means different things to different people, so that defining it is extremely difficult although it has become part of our daily vocabulary. Is stress merely a synonym for distress? Is it effort, fatigue, pain, fear, the need for concentration, the humiliation of censure, the loss of blood, or even an unexpected great success which requires complete reformulation of one's entire life? The answer is yes and no. That is what makes the definition of stress so difficult. Every one of these conditions produces stress but none of them can be singled out as being "it," since the word applies equally to all the others.

HANS SELYE (1974)

304

coding system. All clients are now coded separately on different axes for psychiatric symptoms, developmental personality disorders, and accompanying physical conditions.

The classic definition of psychophysiological or psychosomatic disorders states that these conditions are physical illnesses that have been psychologically induced. Axis I now provides a category labeled "psychiatric factors affecting physical condition." This category is used when a physical disorder, coded on Axis III, indicates that psychological factors almost certainly played a part in the appearance of the physical disorder. This method of interactive classification permits the inclusion of psychological factors when considering any form of physical illness, even forms not previously considered to be psychosomatic or psychophysiological. In many respects, the holistic perspectives encouraged by the multiaxial classifications of DSM-III reinforce the use of nursing diagnoses, which, although specific, address physical, psychological, and social conditions affecting clients and families. The holistic perspective has been widely adapted by nurses providing primary, secondary, and tertiary levels of health care to individuals and families.

THEORIES OF STRESS AND ADAPTATION

Biopsychosocial research has demonstrated that emotional states can inhibit or accelerate the defenses of individuals against a wide range of disorders. Impressive numbers of research studies indicate that almost every disorder to which people are susceptible can be affected positively or nega-

tively by emotional factors (Collins, 1983). For example, Rahe (1974) found a correlation between health problems of a population sample and the life changes experienced in the period immediately preceding the onset of the problems. Jones (1977) found that positive emotions are associated with immunity or rapid recovery from certain physical disorders, while other researchers have found that negative emotional states induce or aggravate some physical disorders (Williams and Holmes, 1978; Coelho, Hamburg, and Adams, 1980). These and similar findings are important because they reinforce holistic approaches to health promotion, restoration, and maintenance (Smitherman, 1981).

Some theorists have tried to link specific disorders to particular conflicts or personality traits. Franz Alexander (1960) proposed that specific conflicts are likely to produce dysfunction or deterioration in particular organs or organ systems. For example, an individual who is conflicted between a wish for closeness and a fear of closeness might express the conflict somatically by developing a neurodermatitis, such as psoriasis or eczema. A related hypothesis was offered by Dunbar (1943, 1954), who compiled psychosocial data on over 1,600 individuals and developed personality profiles linked to specific disorders in which mind and body factors could be identified. Using individual and family data, behavior patterns, personality traits, living habits, and situational factors, Dunbar formulated a specific personality theory to explain the etiology of certain disorders. Persons with rheumatoid arthritis, for instance, were described as quiet, affable individuals whose pleasant exterior concealed considerable hostility.

CHRONOLOGICAL DEVELOPMENT OF ADAPTATIONAL CONCEPTS

Cannon (circa 1927)
- Demonstrated the physiological effects of emotion and the role of the autonomic nervous system.

Alexander (circa 1934)
- Discovered that symptoms occurred only in organs and organ systems activated by the autonomic nervous system.

- Found that symptoms resulted from prolonged physiological processes that were activated by psychological needs and that in turn acted on the autonomic nervous system.

Dunbar (circa 1936)
- Stated that a specific personality configuration is associated with specific adaptational disorders.

Selye (circa 1945)
- Believed that individuals respond to stress through the general adaptation syndrome. The general adaptation response is activated by the autonomic nervous system, and involves the endocrine system.

SOURCE: Adapted from Kaplan (1980).

Alexander's specific conflict theory and Dunbar's specific personality theory are now considered simplistic and reductionistic, but personality profiles still enjoy some credibility. Meyer Friedman and Ray Rosenman (1974) developed a classification of personalities to explain some of the etiologic factors of cardiac disorders. Their work was based on prospective as well as retrospective data; that is, their samples contained persons who had already suffered a myocardial infarction or coronary artery deficits as well as persons who had not at the time the study began. According to their typology, those with *type A* personalities are competitive, striving individuals, driven by a sense of urgency and a need to achieve.

Type A's are at greater risk for developing heart disease than those with *type B* personalities. Friedman and Rosenman described type B persons as less impatient, less competitive, and less easily angered than type A persons. Laboratory studies have shown that type A individuals have significantly higher levels than type B individuals of serum cholesterol, triglycerides, and abnormalities in lipoprotein ratios. In a prospective study, these three laboratory findings were significant predictors of heart disease, but the behavioral patterns of the subjects were the most important predictive factor. Some studies question the accuracy of this personality categorization and dispute the association between personality types and susceptibility to heart disease. Specific characteristics such as hostility and distrust have been cited as more accurate predictors of heart attacks than global personality generalizations. There is now considerable support for the idea that ambition and competitiveness in themselves may be less detrimental than was once supposed (Tierney, 1985).

Other theorists have taken a more general approach to the question of what role mind-body relationships play in the etiology of diseases. In the nineteenth century, long before the concept of stress was introduced, the French physiologist Claude Bernard noted that the internal environment of any living organism must remain constant despite external changes to which it might be exposed. About fifty years later an American physiologist, Walter Cannon (1932), applied the word *homeostasis* to the steady state that must be maintained within an organism if healthy functioning is to continue. It was Cannon who laid the foundation for a scientific analysis of the adaptive mechanisms that are necessary for the preservation of life.

While a medical student at McGill University in Canada, Hans Selye began searching for the answer to an intriguing question: Why do people with different physical problems share many of the same

> ## STAGES OF THE GENERAL ADAPTATION SYNDROME
>
> **Stage One: Alarm**
> The body is exposed to an adverse stimulus or stressor and immediately mobilizes to offer resistance in the form of compensatory behavior. For example, extreme cold produces shivering, which in turn increases body heat.
>
> **Stage Two: Resistance**
> Alarm and mobilization give way to resistance when the stimulus is excessive or prolonged. For example, in the presence of extreme cold, shivering may give way to fever or hypothermia.
>
> **Stage Three: Exhaustion**
> When exposure to the stressor continues, energy is depleted and the body becomes weakened amd exhausted. Exhaustion may be either reversible or irreversible. Selye differentiated *superficial energy*, which is accessible and renewable, from *deeper energy*, which is inaccessible to regeneration or restoration.

signs and symptoms? Selye had observed that a cluster of symptoms accompanied the sensation of feeling "sick," including loss of appetite, loss of strength, loss of interest, and loss of enjoyment. He undertook the task of analyzing the "sickness syndrome" and reducing it to its components. His search for the answer to this question led him to formulate a theory of adaptation that explains the etiology of psychophysiological illness in general terms.

In a series of animal experiments, Selye found that stimuli or irritants such as cold, heat, infection, trauma, noise, and overcrowding all produced the same kinds of physiological changes. He used the broad term *stressors* to encompass stimuli that precipitate similar physiological and psychological reactions, and he referred to the clusters of physiological responses to various stimuli as *local adaptation syndromes* and *general adaptation syndromes* (Selye, 1974, 1976).

When stressors produce a local injury that seems not to affect the whole organism or even an organ or organ system, a localized response is elicited. The endocrine glands, especially the pituitary and adrenal glands, produce hormones in order to contain the infection or trauma. The adaptive hormones present in local reactions may be anti-inflammatory or pro-inflammatory, but their purpose is to limit the damage to the organism. Perhaps the most important adaptive hormone is *adrenocorticotropic hormone* (ACTH), which is produced by the pituitary gland. ACTH stimulates the adrenal cortex to produce *corticoids*. The corticoids include glucocorticoids, such as cortisone, which decrease inflammatory processes, and mineralocorticoids, which promote inflammatory processes.

Sometimes deficient or excessive amounts of corticoids create *systemic reactions*. This might occur if excessive secretions of a pro-inflammatory hormone, produced in response to localized trauma, damaged tissues unrelated to the original injury. When this happens, the local adaptation syndrome gives way to general adaptation reactions that may initiate or aggravate disorders affecting organs or organ systems. A localized reaction to an insect bite might, for example, precipitate a systemic reaction in very sensitive individuals.

The general adaptation syndrome (GAS) identified by Selye (1976) consists of three stages of response to stressors: alarm, resistance, and exhaustion. In the first stage, the autonomic nervous system is called into action; in the second and third stages the endocrine system becomes involved. When stress is prolonged or extreme, the anterior portion of the pituitary gland, influenced by the hypothalamus, causes the adrenal cortex to release hormones into the bloodstream. One group of hormones, the glucocorticoids, are involved in sugar metabolism and have contradictory effects. They increase the amount of blood sugar available for energy and facilitate blood circulation, but they also reduce resistance to infection and reduce the ability of the body to repair tissue damage. The effects of the glucocorticoids include:

Figure 12-1. The physiological pathways of response to stressors.

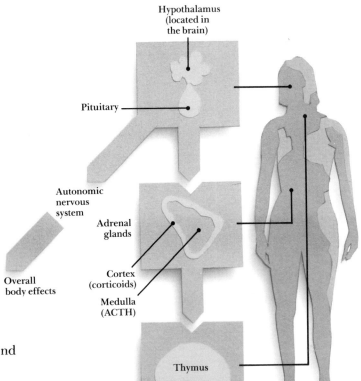

Hypothalamus (located in the brain)

Pituitary

Autonomic nervous system

Adrenal glands

Overall body effects

Cortex (corticoids)

Medulla (ACTH)

Thymus

307

Inhibition of new tissue formation around wounds.

Reduction in the formation of antibodies.

Reduction of the number of circulating white cells.

Depression of thyroid activity.

Reduction in production of reproductive and sexual hormones.

The accompanying box describes the three stages of the GAS.

A great many physiological processes are part of the general adaptation syndrome. The autonomic nervous system is the instigator of the reactive process and is involved throughout. Influenced by the hypothalamus, the emotional switchboard of the body, the pituitary gland stimulates hormonal production by the adrenal glands located just above the kidneys. Also involved is the thymus gland, a lymphatic organ in the chest, and lymph nodes in the cervical, axillary, pelvic, and other regions of the body (see Figure 12-1). The interaction of so many structures helps explain the importance of the general adaptation syndrome in the occurrence of dysfunctional alterations of organs and organ systems.

Once the general adaptation syndrome is activated, intervening factors help determine which organ or organ system is likely to be affected. Certain organs or organ systems seem more vulnerable than others, even though every part of the body is involved in the general adaptation response.

Another question Selye sought to answer was, why does the same amount of exposure to the same stimuli elicit responses of different intensity among different individuals? The explanation he offered was that different intrinsic and extrinsic factors in different people alter the intensity of their responses. Intrinsic factors might be related to genetics, age, or gender. Extrinsic factors might include environmental conditions, family or group influences, or personal habits. Any of these factors helps determine whether an individual can tolerate and overcome the effects of stressors or whether the stressors will lead to dysfunction.

Individual responses are also influenced by perceptions of events. One person's debilitating stress is another person's exciting challenge. In addition, some physiological reactions are the legacy of premodern times. Like our primitive ancestors, we react to perceived danger by stimulating the heart to send increased blood supply to the brain, legs, and trunk. In the physically dangerous world of our early ancestors, these and other changes activated by the autonomic nervous system were essential. Our forebears resorted to *flight* behavior to escape danger or *fight* behavior to overcome danger. Substances produced in the alarm state promoted vigorous activity and were dissipated. In present-day life, people often feel threatened but cannot resort to flight or fight behavior. Present-day stressors are likely to be symbolic rather than physical, yet the human body continues to respond as if the dangers of the modern world were primarily physical. The mobilization of the cardiovascular system,

Figure 12-2. The general adaptation response.

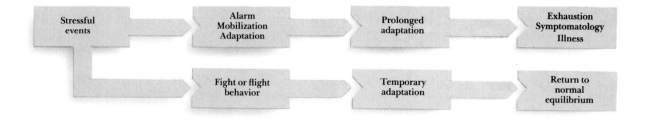

308

skeletomuscular system, and nervous system that was once so essential to survival now operates to predispose individuals to stress-related alterations (Miller, Ross, and Cohen, 1982; Day, 1984). Figure 12-2 illustrates the general adaptation response.

A prevailing belief is that stress is always an undesirable, uncomfortable condition. However, Selye (1974) explained that stress is not always painful. Some stressors, or *eustressors*, are rewarding and even pleasurable. The problem for most people is not the experience of stress but the management of it. Selye believed that it is possible to modify one's responses to stress in order to cope with the conditions of everyday life and to enjoy the eustress that accompanies satisfactory accomplishment.

To understand stress, it is necessary to accept the concept of *homeostasis*, or a dynamic steady state in which all systems of the body are working harmoniously. When stressors intrude, they upset the natural balance of the individual. Individuals are usually able to adjust only partially to stress; failing to adapt completely, they continue to exist in a subjective state of *distress* (Coyne and Holroyd, 1982).

It is difficult to measure the impact of a particular stressor in absolute terms, although Holmes and Rahe (1967) did assign numerical values to life change events (see Chapter 3). Although Holmes and Rahe posited that the higher the numerical value of a particular event, the greater the likelihood of developing an illness or sustaining an injury within a relatively short period of time, they established only correlations. Despite the assigned values given to life changes, no causal relationships were established.

There is no panacea for stress-related prob-

lems, but it is possible to identify stressors that are especially burdensome and to modify their effects. Stressors and the feelings they produce are cumulative. Life changes, work pressures, and family problems might be manageable if they arrived singly, but they become overwhelming if they occur within a brief period. It is helpful, then, to eliminate stressors that are avoidable and to learn to cope with those that are not. To accomplish this, a number of guidelines have been suggested as techniques to help people maintain a steady state as they adapt to conditions of the world they inhabit (Selye, 1974):

1. Ascertain your natural tolerance to stress. This is important because individuals vary in the amounts and kinds of stress they can manage. These individual differences are influenced by a variety of psychological, physiological, and social factors. Analyzing and accepting one's limitations is essential to the management of personal stress levels.

2. Learn to be both selfish and unselfish. Altruism, compassion, and desire for recognition may be sources of satisfaction and pride, provided your real needs are not sacrificed along the way.

3. Consider whether an objective is worth the struggle involved, in light of the situation in which you must function. Fight and flight behaviors are two extreme alternatives, but a middle course may be more advisable.

4. Confront problems promptly instead of procrastinating when a task is necessary but difficult. Delay due to procrastination tends to aggravate stress.

5. Contain or minimize stress by concentrating

All action takes place in some setting. The way a person behaves in a given environment pretty much determines how that environment reacts, particularly if it includes other people. A person who flouts all rules practiced in a community will evoke an aversive reaction from others. His position becomes socially untenable, and the reinforcement that normally comes from others is cut off; he becomes a social isolate and hence cannot function as a member of the community . . . No attitude, philosophy, feeling, belief, or habit pattern occurs de novo. All such states arise from interaction between the person and his environment. No human experience can be divorced from some environmental context. The importance and influence of the environment cannot be exaggerated.

FINLEY CARPENTER (1974)

on actions likely to improve conditions. Blaming yourself or others or ruminating about the painful aspects of a situation without engaging in active problem solving tends to increase stress.

DISORDERS OF ADAPTATION

Stress is a recurring theme in certain disorders believed to have a major psychological component. There are exceptions to this—some of the same disorders may occur in the absence of known stressors. However, emotions play a part in the onset and continuation of virtually all human dysfunction, especially alterations that are thought to be directly related to stress, hyperactivity of the autonomic nervous system, and the general adaptation response (Brody, 1983). Some stress-related disorders that affect organs and organ systems include:

Gastrointestinal responses to stress such as peptic ulcer and ulcerative colitis.

Respiratory responses to stress such as asthma.

Cardiovascular responses to stress such as hypertension and coronary artery disease.

Skeletomuscular responses to stress such as rheumatoid arthritis.

Behavioral responses to stress such as obesity, anorexia nervosa, and bulimia.

Psychogenic pain responses to stress such as migraine headache and tension headache.

Neoplastic responses to stress (cancer).

The remainder of this chapter is devoted to the role of stress in the development of various disorders that represent altered patterns of adaptation to stress. Sometimes the findings in this area are contradictory, but investigators continue to explore a multidimensional perspective of persons manifesting biopsychosocial alterations of organs and organ systems in response to stressors.

Gastrointestinal Responses to Stress

UNDERSTANDING THE CLIENT WITH PEPTIC ULCER

The term *peptic ulcer* includes both gastric ulcers and duodenal ulcers. Ulcers result from excessive production of acidic digestive juices, which erode the lining of the stomach and upper part of the small intestine, causing a lesion. Although multiple factors are involved, it is believed that worry, anger, anxiety, and other negative emotions tend to stimulate production of digestive secretions beyond normal levels, thus creating conditions likely to cause ulcers (Robinson, 1983).

Some studies support the idea that persons with unfulfilled dependency needs and difficulty in trusting or relying on others are especially prone to ulcer formation (Rosenbaum, 1980).

Engel and Schmale (1964) found it possible on the basis of psychological traits to identify which individuals produced high amounts of gastric secretions. They studied subjects who did not have ulcers and found that many of them had a physiological predisposition to ulcer formation based on high gastric secretion levels that were associated with a vulnerable psychological profile. From the data it was inferred that physiological predisposition and certain psychological traits, compounded by stressful life events, interact to generate ulcer formation.

Figure 12-3. Multiple factors that play a role in the etiology of ulcer formation.

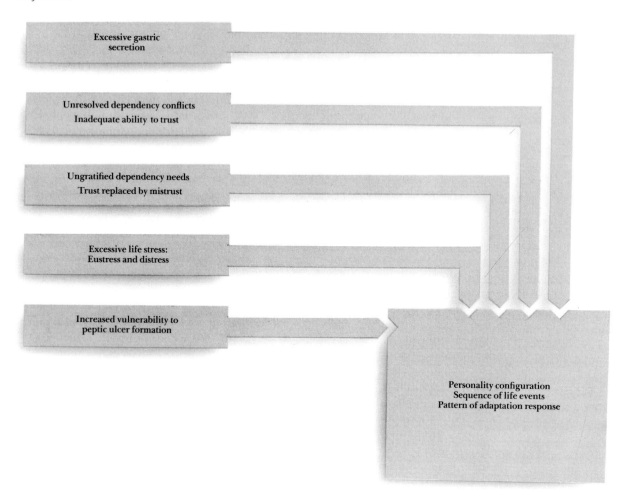

310

Figure 12-3 shows the hypothetical relationships between physiological tendencies, psychological traits, situational stress, and the formation of peptic ulcers.

Based on research concerning the needs of a client who has peptic ulcers, it is reasonable for nurses to assume that there may be an underlying problem of dependency, regardless of how the client behaves (Putt, 1970; Rosenbaum, 1980). If the defense mechanism of reaction formation is being used, clients may seem to reject assistance and will need reassurance that accepting help will not threaten their autonomy in any way. The person who has a peptic ulcer is suffering from a physical problem that requires attention, but nurses can do much to aid such persons besides monitoring medical treatments. The basic need is the establishment of a relationship that meets but does not reinforce dependency, and nurses are in a position to provide a therapeutic approach that enhances the client's sense of comfort and security. The client needs to learn that everyone must be dependent at times and that warm, caring relationships are important regardless of one's physical condition.

Nurses should encourage clients to share their thoughts and feelings verbally and directly, rather than behaviorally or covertly. Clients with a peptic ulcer may be either very demanding or very undemanding. Some of them are quiet and self-effacing, expecting nurses to guess their needs. They should be encouraged to state their requests, to have reasonable requests granted, and gradually to assume responsibility for their own care. Some of these clients, especially those who seem passive-dependent, exhibit regressive behavior. Tendencies to regress should be counteracted by fostering client participation in self-care activities. Some clients may resist taking responsibility for self-care because they are afraid of losing the attentions of staff and family members. It is useful to remind them that even well people need to depend on others, that dependency is acceptable in many situations, and that there are acceptable ways to be dependent besides enacting the sick role.

> ### NURSING PRINCIPLES IN
> ### THE CARE OF PEPTIC ULCER CLIENTS
>
> ■ Nursing interventions significantly influence the progress of clients hospitalized because of peptic ulcer.
>
> ■ Interactions with nurses significantly alter the client's perception of her problem.
>
> ■ Psychological support is an important addition to the care of the ulcer client but is not the only effective intervention.
>
> ■ Instructional programs that increase the client's cognitive understanding of the disorder may be more effective than psychological support alone.
>
> ■ An encompassing approach that includes cognitive learning as well as psychological support is beneficial in promoting healing, reducing discomfort, and preparing the client to cope with future as well as current demands.

311

In a nursing research project, Putt (1970) studied three groups of peptic ulcer clients who received different kinds of nursing care while hospitalized. One group of clients were offered psychological support in the form of unstructured interactions with nurses, which gave clients the opportunity to verbalize their feelings and to participate in self-evaluation and treatment. Minimum emphasis was given to diet or medication for this group. A second group of clients were involved in an instructional program about their disorder and its management. A third group received only the routine nursing care given to all persons with peptic ulcers.

Psychological testing, consisting of an anxiety scale and a semantic differential scale, was administered to all subjects. The anxiety scale showed no significant differences in the anxiety levels of the three groups. Semantic differential measures, used to test the subjects' conceptualizations of tension, food, dependency, and nursing, found no significant differences between the groups except in dependency. The group that was given psychological support by nurses reported a different perception of dependency than the other two groups.

After discharge, subjects were interviewed to learn the effects of the three types of nursing care. Those in the instructional group were more knowledgeable about their problem than those in the other two groups, and those in the psychological support group had learned more than those who had received routine nursing care. It was also found that the instructional approach was most effective in reducing discomfort after admission to the hospital, in improving the rate of healing, and in reducing the length of the hospitalization. The implications of the data were that the teaching activities of nurses are especially valuable for persons with a peptic ulcer and that health teaching should be part of the therapeutic regimen. The conclusion was that, for clients with a peptic ulcer, psychological support alone is less effective than a combination of instruction and psychological support, because the latter meets only the immediate needs of the client and does not encourage anticipatory planning. The proven success of the instructional program was attributed to teaching clients how to deal with future as well as with immediate problems.

This study included subjects between the ages of twenty-one and seventy-one, so the findings are applicable to many age groups. This is important because peptic ulcer is most common among adults in the third and fifth decades of life (Cheren and Knapp, 1980).

Hospitalization with an enforced period of respite from the daily routine is beneficial psychologically as well as physiologically because it permits the client to fulfill his desire to be dependent without producing excessive guilt. Diet, antacids, and surgery are frequently employed, but the care plan should also include cognitive instruction, psychological support, and environmental manipulation to reduce stressful conditions. The hospitalization experience can be crucial to outcomes for clients with peptic ulcer; after leaving the hospital, clients must draw on what they have learned about the disorder and about themselves as they reenter their usual environment. The accompanying box summarizes the principles underlying the care of persons with peptic ulcers.

Whether by chance, by insightful understanding, by scientific knowledge, by artistry in human relationships, or by a combination of all these elements, we have learned to initiate a describable process which appears to have a core of sequential, orderly events which tend to be similar from one client to another. We know something of the attitudinal conditions for getting this process under way. We know that if the therapist holds . . . attitudes of deep respect and full acceptance for the client as he is, and similar attitudes toward the client's potentialities for dealing with himself and his situations; if these attitudes are suffused with a sufficient warmth, which transforms them into . . . liking or affection for the core of the person; and if a level of communication is reached so that the client can begin to perceive that the therapist understands the feelings he is experiencing and accepts him at the full depth of that understanding, then we may be sure that the process is already initiated.

CARL R. ROGERS (1961)

312

UNDERSTANDING THE CLIENT WITH ULCERATIVE COLITIS Ulcerative colitis is an inflammatory disorder of the colon, primarily of the rectum and sigmoid colon. Clinical manifestations of the disorder include protracted diarrhea and bleeding that can be quite debilitating and even fatal. Diagnosis is sometimes difficult because other disturbances may simulate the disorder or coexist with it. Although the etiology is unclear and epidemiological data are inconclusive because of diagnostic difficulties, research has pointed to four areas of causation: infection, genetic factors, immunological factors, and psychological factors.

One unproven hypothesis is that the disorder may be caused by a viral agent. Genetic factors may play a part because the disorder is more common among Caucasians than among members of other racial groups and the incidence is higher among blood relatives than among conjugal or unrelated persons. Researchers who have noted a connection between periods of stress and the onset of severe symptoms allege that the attacks begin about three or four weeks after an unexpected threat to the safety and security of the individual (Kolb, 1973).

Some researchers postulate a consistent personality configuration typical of the persons with colitis, but replication of the studies and validation of the findings have not been very successful. Although methodological deficiencies may account for the confusing results, there is evidence for both opposing views about whether a typical ulcerative colitis personality does exist. Weiner (1977) found evidence to support the belief that a typical personality does exist but added that persons with ulcerative colitis differ from each other in degree

and possess a range of sensitivities that recede or emerge depending on life events and environmental conditions. The lack of agreement on this question indicates need for additional research performed by investigators with no previous bias.

Despite a lack of consensus and the need to consider multifactorial explanations, there are certain attributes that recur in the psychological profiles of persons with ulcerative colitis. Engel (1972), Bloom, Asher, and White (1978), and Stroebe and Stroebe (1983) looked at interpersonal rather than intrapsychic influences. Feldman et al. (1967) reported that persons with ulcerative colitis often have behaviors and attitudes indicative of conflict over control issues. Cheren and Knapp (1980) also cited data indicating that many persons with ulcerative colitis have characteristics revealing conflict about control issues. Conflict about control was expressed behaviorally through rumination, indecision, passive compliance, extreme conscientiousness, hypervigilance, and excessive self-restraint.

Other personality traits that have been associated with persons who have ulcerative colitis include obsessive-compulsive behaviors, perfectionism, and inflexibility combined with a strong desire for approval (Engel, 1954, 1972).

In meeting the needs of the client with ulcerative colitis, the nurse should give attention first to the physical discomfort of the individual. The struggle to control diarrhea and colonic bleeding is especially distressing for clients as fastidious and conscientious as are the majority of persons with ulcerative colitis. Nurses must monitor the amount and quality of the client's excreta in a matter-of-fact way that does not contribute to the client's feeling of

*Such character traits as ambitious behavior, which covers inadequacy,
or arrogance, which hides deep feelings of inadequacy, do indeed
protect the ego, but they have the serious defect that they are
maintained indiscriminately regardless of their appropriateness in a
given situation, and because they insulate the individual from external
stimuli, he becomes less susceptible to re-education.*

J.A.C. BROWN (1967)

self-disgust. Like the person with a peptic ulcer, the client who has ulcerative colitis needs a benevolent, accepting relationship that does not threaten his self-image and that allows him to control as much of the therapeutic regimen as possible.

Many clients with ulcerative colitis have little insight into their problems. The nursing care plan should include interventions that permit the client to feel in control while encouraging the client to establish nonthreatening relationships with helping persons and with others in the social environment. Table 12-1 lists some characteristics exhibited by this group of clients and appropriate interventions.

Table 12-1. Common Characteristics of Persons with Ulcerative Colitis and Suggested Nursing Interventions

Client Characteristics	Nursing Interventions
Perfectionism	Encourage lower self-imposed standards of behavior.
Rumination	Offer substitute activities to interrupt unproductive rumination.
Indecision	Simplify choices to facilitate decision making.
Inflexibility	Promote tolerance of alternative ways of thinking and acting.
Passive compliance	Encourage participation and self-care to increase the client's sense of control.
Vigilance	Reassure client by providing an interpersonal climate of trust and security.
Self-restraint	Reinforce verbal expression of thoughts and feelings, positive or negative.
Lack of insight	Encourage client to reflect on thoughts and feelings in an accepting way.

313

Respiratory Responses to Stress

UNDERSTANDING THE CLIENT WITH ASTHMA
Bronchial asthma is a recurrent disorder of the bronchial airways characterized by constriction of the airways, edema, and excessive secretion. Wheezing and apnea, the dominant manifestations of an asthma attack, result from physiological changes caused by infection, allergens, and psychological factors (Knapp, 1980; Knapp et al., 1976). Studies of persons with asthma have pointed to four major psychological precipitants: anger, excitement associated with pleasure, anxiety, and depression (Falliers, 1978).

Alexander, French, and Pollock (1968) tried to explain the interaction that leads from emotional disturbance to organic dysfunction. However, no psychological tests or research investigations have satisfactorily shown that asthma has an association with a specific conflict or personality configuration. This is true even though asthma has sometimes been attributed to deprivation of maternal love, and wheezing has been interpreted as a suppressed cry for the mother (Purcell, Weiss, and Hahn, 1970). The most credible hypothesis is that a variety of stressful stimuli, emotional states, and behavioral patterns are contributing factors. In most persons with asthma, especially children, there seems to be a fundamental allergic predisposition, and if the allergy potential is low, individuals are able to tolerate more stress without experiencing an attack (Knapp, 1980).

Another etiological hypothesis is that asthma represents learned ways of expressing distress. For example, infants or young children who receive little response from parents when they cry may learn

Figure 12-4. *Interactive model of etiology of asthma.*

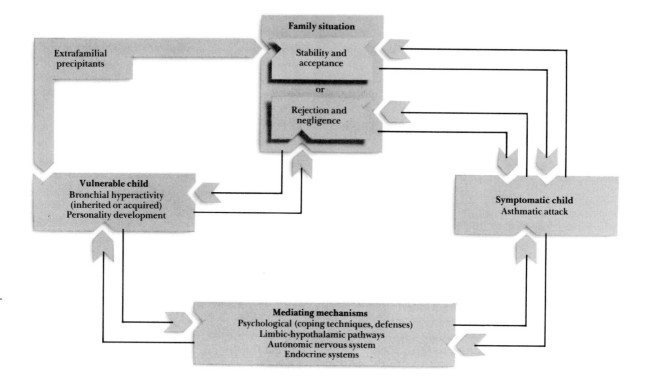

over a period of time that gasping, coughing, or wheezing behaviors elicit immediate attention. Even in these instances, however, a physiological predisposition is thought to exist. The multifactorial model developed by Mattson (1975) proposes that for asthmatics physiological vulnerability in the form of bronchial hyperactivity is present. Infectious, allergic, or psychological stimuli interact with physiological conditions to produce airway constriction. Unfortunately, recurrent asthma attacks often lead to repercussions within the family, which in turn aggravate the respiratory distress of the asthma sufferer and heighten the stress of other family members. Figure 12-4 illustrates the interactive explanation offered by Mattson for the etiology of asthma attacks, particularly among children.

In asthmatic children, excitement expressed by laughing or crying may be enough to cause constriction of the air passages and produce wheezing. During severe attacks, the child experiences fear of suffocating, which causes extreme anxiety that compounds the problem. Repeated interference with school attendance and activities of daily life place additional stress on the child. The attacks cause embarrassment and tend to lower self-esteem. The child's adjustment to the disorder is largely dependent on the family's attitude (Rambo, 1984; Cole-

man, Butcher, and Carson, 1984). Parents may be overprotective even when the child is asymptomatic; overprotection may increase the child's fears, erode her self-confidence, and create petulance that isolates her even more from the age-appropriate activities of her peers. Additionally, asthma may lead to sibling rivalry when the parents become preoccupied with the asthmatic child. Conversely, parents may harbor unconscious resentment and hostility toward the child who seems to threaten the stability of the family. Even apparently devoted parents may express covert feelings of hostility and believe that the illness is being used by the child to manipulate family members.

Two forms of asthma are thought to exist: intrinsic and extrinsic. The extrinsic form is characterized by reactions in response to such allergens as pollen, dust, and certain foods. Extrinsic asthma is more common in children and adolescents, many of whom seem to outgrow the disorder. Persons with intrinsic asthma are usually adults in whom sensitivity to allergens is less pronounced. This type of asthma often follows a pulmonary infection and is likely to be perennial rather than episodic. Adults who are severely affected may develop *status asthmaticus*. For these persons, medication is relatively ineffective and acute paroxysms continue. Frequent

It should be noted first that equilibrium is not an extrinsic or added
characteristic, but rather an intrinsic and constitutive property of
organic and mental life. A pebble may be in states of stable, unstable,
or indifferent equilibrium with respect to its surroundings and this
makes no difference to its nature. By contrast, an organism presents,
with respect to its milieu, multiple forms of equilibrium, from postures
to homeostasis. These forms are necessary to its life, hence are
intrinsic characteristics.

JEAN PIAGET (1968)

315

periods of *status asthmaticus* can lead to emphysema, resulting in dehabilitation that makes the individual highly dependent on significant people in the family or in the health care system.

Caring for an individual with asthma is a collaborative effort by all members of the health care team. Persons who have asthma often demonstrate one of two behavioral polarities:

Behaviors that indicate a strong wish for protection, security, and special privileges.

Behaviors that ignore or deny a wish for protection and security, substituting competitive actions and struggles to excel.

Asthmatic attacks may be major crises for clients and families until an adequate program can be initiated. To help control the condition, an individualized program that combines physical, environmental, and social factors should be made available. Medication, behavior modification, and hypnosis have been used with varying success. Systematic muscle relaxation techniques seem to result in lessening of constriction of the air passages and in lowered levels of anxiety. Intervention that includes family members is a useful approach. Improvement in family relationships and teaching family members to understand the physiological processes at work facilitate the adjustment of the individual with asthma. This is especially important if the person with asthma is a child or adolescent. When working with children who have asthma, health team members often seem quite willing to adopt a more holistic approach to care than when they work with adult clients. There is a tendency on the part of health professionals to dismiss adult clients once the most

urgent physical symptoms have been controlled. This is unfortunate, for persons with asthma need a multidimensional approach to care regardless of age (Knapp, Mathe, and Vachon, 1976; Robinson, 1984).

School nurses and community health nurses are often called upon to help persons with asthma maintain a normal existence. During acute episodes, oxygenation is a major need and medications are available for self-administration. Bronchodilators in the form of oral medication or inhalators are available for use on a selective basis. An understanding of the physiological processes involved can make an attack less frightening to the client.

In general, nurses caring for persons with asthma may be guided by the following facts and principles:

1. No typical personality configuration has been associated with this disorder.
2. Persons with asthma frequently seem to have a strong need for comfort, security, and protection (Alexander et al., 1968).
3. Although asthma has been attributed to separation anxiety, especially separation from the mother, no single pattern of mother-child interaction has been identified (Falliers, 1978).
4. Persons with asthma often engage in extreme behaviors; either they organize their lives around the disorder or they try to ignore its existence.
5. Caring for the client with asthma requires a careful balance between overprotectiveness on the one hand and neglect or denial on the other.

PRIMARY, SECONDARY, AND TERTIARY LEVELS OF INTERVENTION IN THE CARE OF ASTHMATIC CLIENTS

Primary Level of Nursing Intervention
Identify specific allergens.

Instruct the client and the family in avoiding food and environmental allergens.

Explore behaviors, events, and situations that precede an asthmatic attack.

Give permission to verbalize feelings, including doubts and fears.

Maintain a balance between overprotectiveness and denial of the disorder.

Secondary Level of Nursing Intervention
Provide relief for wheezing and apnea during the attack through prescribed measures.

Offer support and reassurance to reduce anxiety.

Involve family members in supportive and instructional interventions.

Tertiary Level of Nursing Intervention
Help families cope with problems arising from the chronic illness of a family member.

Explore the possibility of secondary gain derived by the asthmatic client or by a family member from the illness.

Encourage clear communication between all family members.

Introduce the client and family members to community resources, especially self-help groups.

Table 12-2. Common Behaviors of Persons with Asthma and Suggested Nursing Interventions

Client Behaviors	Nursing Interventions
Dependent, fearful, clinging	Offer support and reassurance without fostering dependency.
Helpless, hopeless	Instill hope by teaching.
Lack of confidence and self-esteem	Emphasize client's strengths, abilities, and accomplishments.
Noncompliance and denial of dysfunction or distress	Formulate with the client alternative activities and program modifications acceptable to her.
Rebellious or delinquent behavior	Encourage verbal rather than behavioral expression of feelings.

Primary, secondary, and tertiary levels of intervention in the care of clients with asthma are discussed in the accompanying box. Table 12-2 identifies behaviors frequently seen in clients with asthma and suggests appropriate nursing interventions.

Cardiovascular Responses to Stress

UNDERSTANDING THE CLIENT WITH HYPERTENSION Hypertension is one of the most prevalent health problems in modern life. Under normal conditions, the heart beats regularly and evenly; visceral organs are adequately nourished by blood circulation. Under adverse conditions, blood vessels supplying visceral organs contract. This contraction makes the heart beat more rapidly and more forcefully, thereby increasing diastolic and systolic blood pressure. For most people the increase is temporary; when conditions improve, blood pressure returns to normal levels. However, for some people the elevated blood pressure continues. Many persons with hypertension are not aware of their disorder because it produces discomfort only in severe cases. It is difficult to identify precise causes or preexisting factors; the term *essential hypertension* has been coined to indicate that the causes are unknown (Byassee, 1977; Day, 1984). The condition has been linked to emotional stress, job pressures, life changes, and diet. Essential hypertension is twice as

Figure 12-5. *Functional and dysfunctional hypertensive responses.*

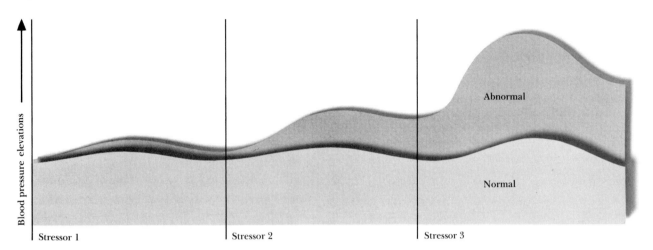

317

common among blacks as among whites, and is more common in lower socioeconomic groups (Eyer, 1979). Figure 12-5 compares normal and abnormal blood pressure responses to stimuli. The dysfunctional responses are characteristic of persons with essential hypertension.

The usual psychological explanation for hypertension is that it is related to unexpressed anger, but this is too simplistic. Some persons with hypertension seem to be type A personalities (competitive, hard-working achievers whose tension is evident in their behavior). There are, however, masked type A people whose outward behavior conceals inner tension and striving. Additional research is needed in order to identify the many psychological, physiological, and behavioral variations among the large number of persons with hypertension.

Thus far, the search for a specific personality or conflict associated with hypertension has been unrewarding. Some researchers allege that hypertensives are inwardly angry and outwardly pleasant, concealing hostility in order to be liked (Lipowski et al. 1977). No evidence of unexpressed hostility was found in a population sample whose hypertension was discovered in a routine screening. Correlations but not causal relationships have been found between hypertension and anxiety; no correlations have been established between hypertension and depression (Wheatley, 1977).

Nursing Interventions Nursing approaches to the control of hypertension are guided by four objectives:

■ Detecting essential hypertension as soon as possible.

■ Helping clients reduce and maintain lower blood pressure levels.

■ Helping clients modify habits contributing to hypertension.

■ Encouraging compliance with the total care plan.

Because many persons with hypertension have no symptoms, there is a tendency for them to discount the seriousness of the condition, leading to noncompliance. Pharmacological treatment is effective but is often complicated by undesirable side effects such as depression, loss of sexual desire, and sexual dysfunction. Nurses concerned with establishing a therapeutic relationship should endeavor to be supportive and informative without increasing anxiety in the client. Interpretations and confrontations are unlikely to be helpful since such interventions are likely to produce reactions that elevate blood pressure levels even more.

If drug therapy is instituted, nurses should be alert to the possibility of frequent or severe depressive reactions. Reserpine, methyldopa, and propanol are among the blood pressure regulatory agents that may cause depression. Ongoing assessment of hypertensive clients on medication is important; there have been reports of suicide attempts by persons suffering from unrecognized depression produced by antihypertensive medication.

The client who is hypertensive requires a comprehensive care plan that includes cognitive information, emotional reassurance, and support. For hypertensive clients a therapeutic relationship is not a substitute for but an adjunct to other methods of managing the disorder. Medication,

> ### INSTRUCTIONS FOR PROGRESSIVE RELAXATION
>
> Progressive relaxation involves all the major muscle groups of the body. Begin by tensing the entire body. Maintain a state of tension for five seconds. Then exhale slowly and silently. Command yourself to relax and let go. As you slowly exhale, try to experience a sense of calm and serenity as the whole body becomes slack and at ease. Next, tense one part of the body while leaving the other parts limp and relaxed. Keep one part of the body tense for a few seconds, then relax, breathing out slowly while allowing the tense part of the body to go limp. Follow this procedure for the head and neck, arms and hands, chest, back, stomach, legs, and feet.
>
> With sufficient practice, progressive relaxation techniques can become almost automatic in promoting tension reduction throughout the day without interfering with the daily routine. In fact, the sense of well-being that accompanies mastery of the technique is likely to enhance one's ability to cope with everyday life.

318

exercise, relaxation, biofeedback, modification of diet, and lifestyle are all important components of the care plan that can be coordinated by the generalist nurse. Because smoking constricts tiny blood vessels and exacerbates the problem, hypertensives should be made aware of the health risks posed by this habit.

Almost all individuals respond to frustration with elevated blood pressure and rapid heartbeat. If they are permitted to express their feelings verbally or through motor activity, there is usually a return to normal functioning. When no outlets for expressing frustration are available, there is far slower return to normal functioning. Therefore, in addition to other objectives, the nursing care plan should be designed to help hypertensive individuals express frustration and discharge tension through verbal and motor channels (Byassee, 1977).

Relaxation Techniques Management of responses to stress can help reduce discomfort due to tensions experienced in everyday life. Some mental health professionals advocate biofeedback training as part of stress management programs. *Biofeedback* is a technique by which bodily functions often thought to be involuntary, such as blood pressure and heartbeat, can be consciously regulated. Biofeedback equipment, which operates on the same principles as polygraph devices, measures various physical changes in the body that occur in response to greater or lesser amounts of accumulated tension. Individuals can use biofeedback methods to record and monitor blood pressure and to incrementally lower their blood pressure at each session. With biofeedback, lowering blood pressure becomes

much like losing weight; gradual, measured progress is made toward the client's goal.

Although helpful in many instances, biofeedback is not essential to learning relaxation techniques. *Progressive relaxation* is a technique that involves deliberate muscle relaxation as a means of reducing the discomfort caused by accumulated stress and tension. To relax muscles progressively one begins by tensing and then relaxing the major muscle groups of the body, concentrating on one group at a time. Consciously tensing and relaxing the muscle groups makes one aware of what happens in the body during states of tension and relaxation. Instructions for progressive relaxation are provided in the accompanying box. The muscle groups of the head, face, neck, and shoulders are primary sites of tension. Other muscle groups that are often involved are those of the arms, hands, chest, back, stomach, legs, and feet.

Relaxation simply means doing nothing with the muscles, neither assisting, resisting, or participating in any form of movement or gesture. Progressive relaxation is not difficult to learn, nor is the technique spectacular or dramatic. All that is required is awareness of what it feels like when a group of muscles is tensed or poised for action and when the same group of muscles is at rest.

Traditionally, men in American Society have been socialized from earliest youth to be strong, confident, and independent; to exhibit a capacity for daring and aggression; to display physical prowess and suppress tenderness, avoiding any behavior or traits that might be construed as effeminate. They have been expected to pursue success and status in the work world while demonstrating competence as breadwinners. Considerable pressure is exerted on men, then, to be action and achievement oriented. Dominance (power) characterizes their handling of interpersonal relations. However, they should be wise and "level headed" in their interactions with others, as well as in their management of themselves. One can already discern grounds for incipient role strain.

WINIFRED HUMPHREYS AND SUZANNE C. LEMA (1981)

319

It is possible to practice progressive relaxation at various times of the day whenever a few moments are available. Alternate states of tension and relaxation can be attained while waiting for an elevator or for a red light to change, typical situations that trigger tension in many individuals. Once an individual learns to recognize rising tension, he may use progressive relaxation to induce a less stressful internal environment. Stress is not eradicated by this technique, but its management can be improved (Charlesworth and Nathan, 1982).

UNDERSTANDING THE CLIENT WITH CORONARY ARTERY DISEASE Each year, more Americans succumb to heart disease than to any other disorder, even though such deaths have declined about 20 percent in recent decades. This decline in mortality rates is attributed to dietary changes, reduced smoking, and more emphasis on physical fitness.

Stressors such as job pressures, time urgency, frustration, and feelings of dissatisfaction with one's life have been associated with heart disease. For some persons, stress seems to be a natural way of life. They seem to transform everyday events into enormous ordeals and contests. This is certainly true of the type A personalities described by Friedman and Rosenman (1974). A prospective study by these investigators showed that type A persons were susceptible to coronary artery disease and were more likely to die after a heart attack. Autopsy examinations showed that type A heart attack victims had narrower arteries than other victims of fatal heart attacks. Studies consistently show that type A persons have a more extreme response to situations they perceive to be challenging. Current studies are aimed at identifying what aspects of type A behavior constitute the greatest risk. Early results indicate that persons with extreme amounts of hostility are most at risk. The kinds of challenges to which type A persons are exposed also seem to be influential. For example, type A personalities seem far more responsive than type B personalities in the way they handle cognitive tasks. On the other hand, little differences are found in the responses of type A and type B individuals to physical tasks (Turkington, 1984).

Physiological research indicates that it may be effects of the catecholamines, specifically epinephrine and norepinephrine, that are released during stressful situations that account for the vulnerability of type A individuals. Researchers have discovered no difference between the two personality types in baseline catecholamine levels, but stress produces an increase in the blood pressure and heart rate of type A subjects. Type B persons are relatively unaffected physiologically by stress. Researchers believe it is the rapid rise and fall of catecholamine levels in type A persons that is so damaging to the heart.

Although substantial evidence points to personality as a factor in heart disease, lifestyle and age remain important risk factors, as well. Males between the ages of thirty-nine and forty-nine are six times more likely to experience coronary artery disease than all the type A personalities in the general population (Matthews, 1982). Perhaps the heavy responsibility and the pursuit of success that characterize the fourth decade for most men heightens their vulnerability to heart disease.

Even though the impact of type A behaviors is

upheld by some theorists and discounted by others, psychological counseling remains an important adjunct to the care of anyone who has suffered a heart attack. Counseling should be directed toward curbing the sense of urgency, competitiveness, and easily aroused anger of type A individuals. In one three-year study, psychological counseling was found to be far more effective than any other intervention in preventing a second heart attack (Brody, 1983). Because type A behavior is viewed as a risk factor, efforts should be made to help such individuals modify their behavior. In this area behavioral approaches are often effective and may be attempted by generalist nurses. Behavior modification can be directed toward stress management and lifestyle modification. Stress management involves learning relaxation, identifying stressful situations, and moderating the impact of stressful situations. Nurses are in a position to advise these clients on nutritional regimens that are likely to reduce serum cholesterol levels and maintain normal weights. In addition, individuals should be encouraged to make changes in daily habits that are stressful and to reduce personal feelings of competitiveness, time urgency, performance standards, and hostility.

The client's and family's psychological distress should also be addressed. Croog and Levine (1977) found unnecessary psychological distress and invalidism in half the cardiac patients in a sample population and concluded that the distress of these individuals could have been avoided if reassurance, explanations, and advice had been provided by caregivers. The families of heart attack victims, especially the spouse, are subject to anxiety, fatigue, irritability, sleeplessness, and depression. Often their distress is overlooked by caregivers preoccupied with the client. Returning a recovering cardiac client to a living arrangement where the spouse is worried and dysfunctional is unlikely to promote recovery.

The nurse should offer support and information to the families of recovering cardiac clients, as well as to the client. Marital counseling may be especially needed in situations where the spouse is very attentive, even overprotective, yet resentful of the demands being made on her. Supportive nursing interventions combined with teaching help the client and the family plan for the future rather than dwell on the recent past. Sexual counseling for the recovering cardiac client and the spouse should be available routinely before discharge from a hospital. Many people have questions about when and how to resume sexual activity but hesitate to ask questions. Therefore, this topic should be introduced as a matter of course and should constitute an essential component of preparing clients for discharge.

The attitudes of health team members are also important factors in a client's recovery. A heart attack is a frightening experience, and clients are usually receptive to information and guidance. Vague or evasive statements by nurses and other health team members only increase the client's anxiety and lead to noncompliance. Communication between team members is just as important as communication with the client and the family. Health care teams composed of a cardiologist, a primary care nurse, a physical therapist, a dietitian, a mental health nurse, and a consulting psychiatrist, when indicated, can offer a coordinated approach to meeting the health needs of the cardiac client.

Skeletomuscular Responses to Stress

UNDERSTANDING THE CLIENT WITH RHEUMATOID ARTHRITIS Rheumatoid arthritis is a condition that has been associated with life stresses for many years. In the nineteenth century Sir William Osler, the renowned physician, identified worry, shock, and grief as precursors of rheumatoid arthritis (Garfield, 1979).

There is also evidence that rheumatoid arthritis may be an autoimmune disease. Current research suggests that an unspecified antigen probably stimulates the production of antibodies. The body then reacts to these antibodies as if they were foreign substances. The pathophysiological response of the immune system to the body's own antibodies, the *rheumatoid factor,* is present in some, but not all, persons with rheumatoid arthritis (Silverman, 1980). For some years the rheumatoid factor was thought to be the cause of the dysfunction, but this explanation has been discarded. The rheumatoid factor, when present, is now believed to perpetuate the problem but not to cause it. The rheumatoid factor consists of reactive antibodies that may be present in various other conditions, such as hypertension. It has been hypothesized that stress and distress activate the immunological system in nonspecific ways, one of which leads to the presence of the rheumatoid factor.

A number of investigators agree that persons with rheumatoid arthritis tend to overcontrol their aggressive impulses (Robinson, 1983; Coleman, Butcher, and Carson, 1984). Studies using different population samples have described persons with rheumatoid arthritis as self-sacrificing, hard-working, conforming, and, frequently, interested in physical activities until they are incapacitated. These studies are suggestive rather than definitive. The most likely explanation is that some personality traits combined with cumulative life stresses may contribute to the development of rheumatoid arthritis in persons with a genetic predisposition that involves the immune system.

One study attempted to identify specific stress responses in persons with essential hypertension and others with rheumatoid arthritis. Persons with rheumatoid arthritis reacted more to stress in their joints and muscles than did hypertensives. On the other hand, the blood pressures of persons with hypertension did not return to normal levels when stressors were removed as quickly as did the blood pressures of those with rheumatoid arthritis. These findings seem to support theories of specific response patterns that precipitate, perpetuate, or at least are present in certain disorders. The results are clouded by the fact that the population sample consisted of subjects identified as already having hypertension or rheumatoid arthritis; the presence of a certain form of dysfunction may intensify reactions in the organ system already affected (Silverman, 1980).

Rheumatoid arthritis runs a chronic course characterized by remission, alleviation, or progressive incapacitation. Assessment and planning must be flexible enough to adapt to the changing status of the client. The immediate goals are the management of pain and the enhancement of mobility. Long-range goals include the maintenance of a normal, fulfilling existence, the prevention of musculoskeletal deformity, and the fulfillment of psychological and social needs. The client and family members should understand the reason for certain procedures that may be uncomfortable, because they may tend to become discouraged when procedures are unsuccessful and relief does not come easily. The care of the client with rheumatoid arthritis often requires complex exercises and physiotherapy measures that are costly in terms of time and energy. A coordinator should oversee the various aspects of the plan and assume responsibility for continual assessment of the psychological and physical status of the client and family members who carry much of the burden of daily care. Depression and giving up are common in clients with this dysfunction. Such behaviors should be identified promptly so that relief can be provided through pharmacologic and supportive psychological intervention.

The emotional sensitivities of clients with rheumatoid arthritis require special consideration. Loss of mobility, loss of function, and body image changes are hard for clients to accept, especially if they previously thrived on activity. They may react with inward anger, which can worsen their discomfort. Supportive nursing interventions may be as valuable as physiotherapy or medication in relieving their physical and emotional distress. A structured, predictable, sustained relationship with a nurse can be helpful to the client striving to remain as independent as possible for as long as possible.

Persons who have rheumatoid arthritis tend to move less because of a natural wish to avoid pain. The desire to avoid pain is often coupled with a wish to regress, give up, and be cared for. These feelings are opposed by a desire to remain functional and independent. Awareness of these conflicting feelings in the client enables nurses to suggest compromises that can help the client cope with her contradictory feelings and alterations in structure and function.

Although there is no single personality configuration common to persons with rheumatoid arthritis, their families often describe them as having been vigorous, athletic, and competitive before the onset of dysfunction. Comparative psychological tests given to men with hypertension, rheumatoid arthritis, and peptic ulcer have shown that subjects with rheumatoid arthritis exhibit high levels of aggression and high levels of control, a combination very likely to induce anxiety and tension because the individual has aggressive impulses but feels that they must be strongly controlled. Table 12-3 summarizes levels of aggression and control in subjects with three types of stress-related disorders.

Any client with a chronic problem such as rheumatoid arthritis eventually becomes very familiar with the health care system and may lose faith in the system and in the benefits of therapeutic measures if her condition doesn't improve. She may feel anger toward family members and caregivers who have not fulfilled her expectations yet fear to express that anger toward those on whom she must depend. Usually the client can determine what kinds of physical efforts she is able to attempt. Unless the nurse encourages the client to indicate the extent of her abilities, the nurse may have a tendency to do things for the client or to neglect activities that exhaust the client unless she is helped. A meaningful dialogue between the client, family, and care providers will help ensure that the needs of the client will be perceived accurately and will be met (Robinson, 1984). Table 12-4 presents some basic needs of the client with rheumatoid arthritis and suggested nursing interventions.

Table 12-3. Psychological Features of Persons with Stress-Related Disorders

Type of Disorder	Level of Aggression	Level of Control
Rheumatoid arthritis	High	High
Hypertension	Low	High
Peptic ulcer	Low	Low

SOURCE: Adapted from Cobb et al. (1969).

Table 12-4. Needs of the Client with Rheumatoid Arthritis and Suggested Nursing Interventions

Client's Needs	Nursing Interventions
Reduced mobility	1. Allow the client time to adjust to loss of mobility without forcing the issue. 2. Encourage the client to be realistic in accepting methods and devices that will promote or maintain mobility. 3. Help the client enhance the quality of his life even though special arrangements may be needed for him to engage in such activities as seeing a film or eating in a restaurant.
Social isolation and feelings of alienation	1. Explore whether the isolation is self-imposed or caused by the indifference of friends and family members. 2. Help the client and the family plan activities that include one or two other people. 3. Introduce the client and the family to community groups and resources.
Pain and physical discomfort	1. Clients know more about their tolerance for pain than anyone else; permit the client to be the teacher in this area. 2. Respect the client's preferences for rituals and procedures that alleviate subjective discomfort.
Anger toward care providers (often displaced or suppressed)	1. Avoid being defensive. 2. Explain reasons for events and decisions; focus on specifics.
Anger toward family members (often displaced or suppressed)	1. Include family members in supportive and instructional nursing actions. 2. Try to change or moderate specific causes for anger, whether generated by family members or by professional care providers.
Preoccupation with oneself	1. Promote participation in self-care as much as possible; accept the occasional need of the client to regress and be dependent without fostering regression and dependency. 2. Accept and be attentive to verbal expressions of anger, pain, and discouragement.

322

Behavioral Responses to Stress

Behavioral responses to stress may take the form of eating disorders, such as obesity and anorexia nervosa.

UNDERSTANDING THE CLIENT WITH OBESITY
Obesity is popularly defined as an excessive accumulation of fat in the body. Usually obesity is said to exist when body weight exceeds 20 percent of the ratios given in standard height and weight tables, but it should be remembered that definitions of obesity and reactions to it are to a great extent culturally determined. In societies where food is scarce, fatness is a sign of status, whereas in affluent societies it is "in" to be thin. Social pressures in the United States encourage eating too much yet those who become obese are reproached. Youthfulness is highly valued in Western society, and slenderness is often equated with looking young (Bruch, 1973).

The first generation of American immigrants are likely to become overweight as they avail themselves of ample food. The second generation adopts the attitudes of mainstream America toward being overweight, and the prevalence of obesity drops drastically from the first to the second generation. Variables that affect the occurrence of obesity are listed in Table 12-5.

Obesity may result from an increase in fat cell size (*hypertrophic obesity*), an increase in fat cell number (*hyperplastic obesity*), or a combination of the two. Knowledge about clients' fat cell size and fat cell numbers would be valuable in assessing and treating obesity, but clinical use of these indicators is only beginning. Hyperplastic obesity seems to be a factor

in obesity among children, and the prognosis for weight loss is poor among persons who have been overweight since childhood. Such findings underscore the need for primary prevention to avoid an increase in fat cell number and a consequent lifelong weight problem. For youngsters already obese, weight control programs can help prevent social isolation and feelings of inadequacy caused by obesity.

Some obese persons report that they overeat when they are emotionally upset but also when they feel happy and well adjusted. Such eating patterns suggest that obese persons may be excessively responsive to any external stimulus that induces eating and quite unresponsive to internal feelings of hunger or satisfaction. Of those who consume abnormally large amounts of food, many are women whose food intake occurs at night. This nocturnal pattern may be due to stressful conditions encountered during the daytime. Nocturnal overeat-

Table 12-5. Demographic Variables Affecting Obesity Prevalence

Variable	Prevalence
Age	Obesity is most prevalent among those between twenty and fifty.
Gender	Obesity is more common among women in all age groups.
Socioeconomic status	Obesity is more prevalent in lower socioeconomic groups.
Social mobility	Obesity is more prevalent among the socially mobile (those moving from one social class to another).

BEHAVIOR MODIFICATION IN OBESITY

Advantages

- The dropout rate is low.
- Emotional reactions such as anxiety and depression are infrequent.
- Persons whose obesity began in childhood are more responsive to behavior modification than to traditional weight loss methods.

Disadvantages

- Weight losses obtained through behavior modification are modest, seldom exceeding 15 pounds.
- Weight lost as a result of behavior modification is regained just as easily as weight lost through customary methods.

---

ing differs from bulimia, or binge eating, in that the latter is more episodic whereas the former is ongoing. Both eating patterns are often followed by agitation and self-recrimination and both are attributable at least in part to stress.

Increased physical activity, combined with dietary measures, is essential to weight reduction. Physical activity should be taken up gradually by those who have been sedentary, and large amounts of weight loss should not be attempted except under carefully supervised conditions. Self-help groups for obese persons have proliferated in recent years. The best known are the nonprofit TOPS (Take Off Pounds Safely) and the profit-making Weight Watchers groups. Subjective reports indicate that the programs are helpful, but little objective data are available. The dropout rates are high, but so are the reentry rates. The programs do offer a rational approach to weight loss and for that reason merit attention.

Behavior modification is used often in the care of obese persons, but again there is little evidence of actual effectiveness. Although there is some disagreement on this issue, consensus has been reached on the points covered in the accompanying box.

One advantage of behavior modification in weight control is the fact that the procedures are clear and specific. Behavioral tasks can be assigned and forms given to help clients record their calorie intake and note their progress. When weight is lost, the client receives instant recognition and approval from the leader and from other members if the program involves a group. Group and individual behavioral approaches can be inaugurated by nurses working in schools, clinics, and health

maintenance organizations. These programs can be individualized and multidimensional as nurses apply their knowledge of physiological, psychological, and interpersonal processes to help the obese adult or child.

UNDERSTANDING THE CLIENT WITH ANOREXIA NERVOSA *Anorexia nervosa* is the extreme aversion to food, which results in life-threatening weight loss. The disorder is considered to be present if the client has lost 20 percent of her body weight, if there is no known reason for the weight loss, if she has a great fear of regaining weight, and if she has a gross distortion of body image. Until recently the disorder was presumed to be limited to adolescence and young adulthood. It is now realized that the disorder may extend into later years as women continue to be so obsessed with the need to be thin that they refuse to give up their starvation diets no matter how much weight they have lost. Indeed, for most anorectic persons reactions of joy rather than regret accompany the loss of pounds.

Anorexia nervosa is often accompanied by *bulimia*, a separate but related disorder in which the individual consumes enormous amounts of food and then deliberately vomits it. The bulimic person often resorts to harsh laxatives so that no nutritional value is obtained from whatever residual food is retained. Unlike the obese person, the bulimic individual is frequently able to maintain normal weight because binge eating is counteracted by vomiting and laxatives.

Statistics on the prevalence of anorexia and bulimia among different age groups are limited because the disorders are concealed as long as possible, especially by bulimic persons. A survey by the

Table 12-6. Nursing Interventions with Anorectic Clients

Nursing Interventions	Rationale
Have client weigh each morning after she has voided and before liquids are ingested.	To prevent the client from creating the illusion of weight gain by not emptying her bladder and drinking copious amounts of water.
Record daily intake of food and fluids and output of excreta; record quality and amounts.	To prevent dehydration, renal damage, and electrolyte imbalance.
Restrict bathroom privileges for two hours after meals unless client is supervised.	To control self-induced vomiting.
Prohibit laxatives; give stool softeners if needed.	To prevent misuse of laxatives (if diarrhea occurs, the client may be using laxatives secretly).
Offer small feedings about six times a day rather than three large meals.	To prevent stomach distention and circulatory overload after prolonged fasting.
Develop a comprehensive care plan to be followed consistently by all staff members.	To reduce tendencies of the client to control others through manipulation.

324

National Association of Anorexia Nervosa and Related Disorders indicated that among 1,400 respondents who admitted to being anorectic or bulimic or both, 1.8 percent were over fifty, 5 percent were over sixty, 2.7 percent were between forty and forty-nine, and 20.5 percent were between thirty and thirty-nine. Thus, 70 percent of the respondents were under thirty years old (Brozan, 1983).

Eating disorders are most prevalent among women, and their onset seems to coincide with physiological changes unique to women. When excess amounts of body weight are lost, the adolescent girl may feel more able to return to her carefree childhood years, especially if, as often occurs, weight loss is accompanied by cessation of menstrual periods. Bruch (1973) reported that pregnant women sometimes cannot tolerate the idea of having a large abdomen, and by means of fasting they manage to lose weight even during pregnancy. In some instances morning sickness was transformed into bulimia. For older women anorexia nervosa and bulimia seem to be connected with life stresses and transitions in work, marriage, or emotional relationships (Neuman and Halverson, 1984).

Control of one's life seems to be an important concern for anorectic persons. Eating is one area in which they can exert control, and food thus becomes a substance they fear and avoid. Initially, control of appetite takes the form of occasional dieting, such as is common among women. The anorectic, however, goes on to engage in a prolonged course of self-destruction that may end in death. Binge eating seems to represent temporary loss of control, and the vomiting that follows an effort to regain control. Among the intelligent, highly motivated achievers who are most prone to anorexia nervosa, emacia-

tion becomes a new achievement and an enormous source of satisfaction.

Eventually, during repeated fasting, the transmission of physiological messages signaling hunger seems to be lost. Anorectic behavior then moves beyond conscious control and becomes resistant to change. In some respects, the term anorexia is misleading; although anorectic persons deny themselves food, they do not actually lose their appetites until the condition has advanced to severe stages. In earlier stages the person is preoccupied with food, often collecting recipes and cooking for others but not ingesting food herself.

The immediate need of the client with anorexia nervosa is the restoration of nutrition and weight to a point where life can be sustained safely. When emaciation, dehydration, and electrolyte disturbance are severe enough to be life threatening, hospitalization may be needed to provide the client with a regulated environment. The nursing care of persons with severe anorexia nervosa begins with total bedrest, augmented with behavior modification programs that use reward and positive reinforcement to produce change. As the client begins to gain weight, total bedrest and other restrictions are gradually modified. Positive reinforcement might consist of increased physical activity, visiting privileges, and social outlets in return for gains of specified amounts of weight. At times, negative reinforcement in the form of isolation, tube feeding, and withdrawal of privileges may be necessary. Nursing interventions helpful in caring for anorectic clients are described in Table 12-6.

The physical care of a client with anorexia nervosa is only part of the therapeutic regimen. Family counseling is often necessary for younger clients

Diagnosis is dia: *through;* gnosis *is knowledge of. Diagnosis is appropriate . . . if one understands it as* seeing through the social scene. *Diagnosis begins as soon as one encounters a particular situation, and never ends. The way one sees through the situation changes the situation. As soon as we convey in any way (by a gesture, a handshake, a cough, a smile, an inflection of our voice) what we see or think we see, some change is occurring even in the most rigid situation.*

R.D. LAING (1971)

and marital counseling for older ones (Brozan, 1983). Clients with anorexia nervosa need help in realizing that control over their lives is possible without jeopardizing their existence through starvation. Depression is often a complicating factor when clients are very undernourished, and occasionally antidepressant medication may be used. Almost invariably, clients with anorexia nervosa require long-term psychological help, and the prognosis is better for younger than for older clients. The long-range goal is to enable these clients to stop judging themselves and the world in terms of pounds lost and calories not consumed.

Psychogenic Pain Responses to Stress

UNDERSTANDING THE CLIENT WITH HEADACHE
Headache is not an actual disorder but rather an uncomfortable syndrome that may result from many systemic conditions, some organic and some functional. Severe hypertension, for example, may cause a headache that is relieved only when the high blood pressure is identified and remedied. The majority of headaches, perhaps 90 percent of them, seem to be related to tension and to be accompanied by vascular constriction. It has been estimated that about 50 million Americans, the majority women, suffer from tension headache (Coleman, Butcher, and Carson, 1984).

Another form of headache is *migraine*, which is characterized by vascular dilation rather than constriction. In the 1940s it was discovered that the onset of migraine headaches was accompanied by the dilation of pain-sensitive cranial arteries. Migraine headaches usually involve only one side of the head at a time, although the headache may shift from one side to the other. Researchers have found that when migraine headaches are unilateral, only the cranial arteries on that side of the head are dilated. As soon as the attack subsides, the cranial arteries return to normal size. It has been demonstrated in laboratory studies that many stressors in the physical and social environment can bring about dilation of the cranial arteries in persons prone to migraine headaches, but not in others (Coleman, Butcher, and Carson, 1984).

Fromm-Reichmann (1937), in a classic paper on the psychogenic nature of migraine headaches, described the condition as the result of hostility that the individual will not or cannot express in other ways. According to this hypothesis, persons who suffer from migraine attacks are conscientious and conventional, loving and compliant, yet secretly hostile and ambivalent toward persons they think they should love. Because hostility is not compatible with their view of themselves, migraine sufferers deflect their hostility from others and direct it toward themselves as punishment. In support of this explanation, Fromm-Reichmann pointed to the symptoms of a migraine episode: constipation followed by diarrhea, continence followed by abundant voiding, pallor and chills followed by warmth and flushing, tension and spasticity followed by languor and relaxation.

Of the two types of headache, migraine is the more painful and less responsive to analgesic medication or procedures such as biofeedback that encourage relaxation. Pain is a subjective, individualistic experience, invisible and hard to describe to others. When the cause for pain is identified, it is easier for caregivers to offer relief. When the cause of pain cannot be demonstrated, there is a tendency to consider the pain insignificant and to label the

Figure 12-6. Mechanism of psychogenic pain in clients with recurrent headaches.

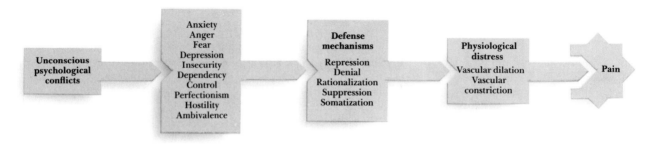

| Unconscious psychological conflicts | Anxiety Anger Fear Depression Insecurity Dependency Control Perfectionism Hostility Ambivalence | Defense mechanisms Repression Denial Rationalization Suppression Somatization | Physiological distress Vascular dilation Vascular constriction | Pain |

326

client as a malingerer or a hypochondriac. It is necessary to remember that psychogenic pain hurts just as much as organogenic pain. When no organic cause for pain can be discovered, nurses must draw upon their store of empathy, remaining receptive to the client's discomfort and willing to explore the nature of the problem in order to discover a solution. For clients with headaches who may have been dismissed as hypochondriacs, a nursing response that recognizes the validity of the client's experience is a promising start toward meeting the client's needs. Figure 12-6 depicts the mechanisms involved in psychogenic pain.

Headache may indeed be a sign of serious disorders, and extensive investigation is needed before organic causes are ruled out. If it is determined that the discomfort is primarily psychogenic, the care plan should include a range of nursing interventions aimed at control of physical discomfort, improvement of environmental conditions, identification and alleviation of stressors, and adoption of alternative coping methods. The first goal should be to explore the client's attitudes toward his family, himself, and his life situation. Caregivers can then begin to help the client modify behaviors that seem detrimental. In working with clients suffering from headaches, nurses should proceed slowly and deliberately. Many of these individuals already tend to be somewhat compulsive and perfectionistic. Supportive, empathetic caregivers allow clients freedom to express their concerns and fears. An accepting therapeutic relationship is all important in augmenting the medication, relaxation techniques, biofeedback, and hypnosis that may make up the total care plan.

Neoplastic Responses to Stress

UNDERSTANDING THE CLIENT WITH CANCER   A cancerous neoplasm is often envisioned as a sudden, unexpected eruption within the body whereby cells abandon normal, orderly restraints and reproduce madly and recklessly. Surgery, radiation, and chemotherapy are popularly thought to be the main weapons available against cancer. The cancer client is seen as a helpless witness to the turmoil that rages within her body. Cancer in many ways remains a mystery, but it is clear that the client with cancer could benefit from a holistic approach.

Some attempts have been made to enlist the cancer sufferer as a participant in his own care by integrating physiological and psychological methods. This approach to the care of cancer clients evolved from the documentation of spontaneous remissions of diagnosed cancer for which no explanations could be found. One explanation for spontaneous remissions, the *surveillance theory*, holds that aberrant or deviant cells are formed by everyone throughout life, but are usually promptly overcome by the immune system of the body. According to this theory, cancer develops only when the immune system fails. Therefore, any factors that influence the immune system affect an individual's ability to respond to deviant cell formation.

Supporting data for the surveillance theory have been provided by research studies (Abse, 1974; Garfield, 1979). Compared to subjects in control groups, cancer victims showed depression, energy loss, and suppression of emotional expressiveness. These emotional states correlated with impairment of the immune system. Psychological factors were even more influential on the course of illness. De-

Figure 12-7. Mind-body model of recovery.
SOURCE: Adapted from Simonton (1978).

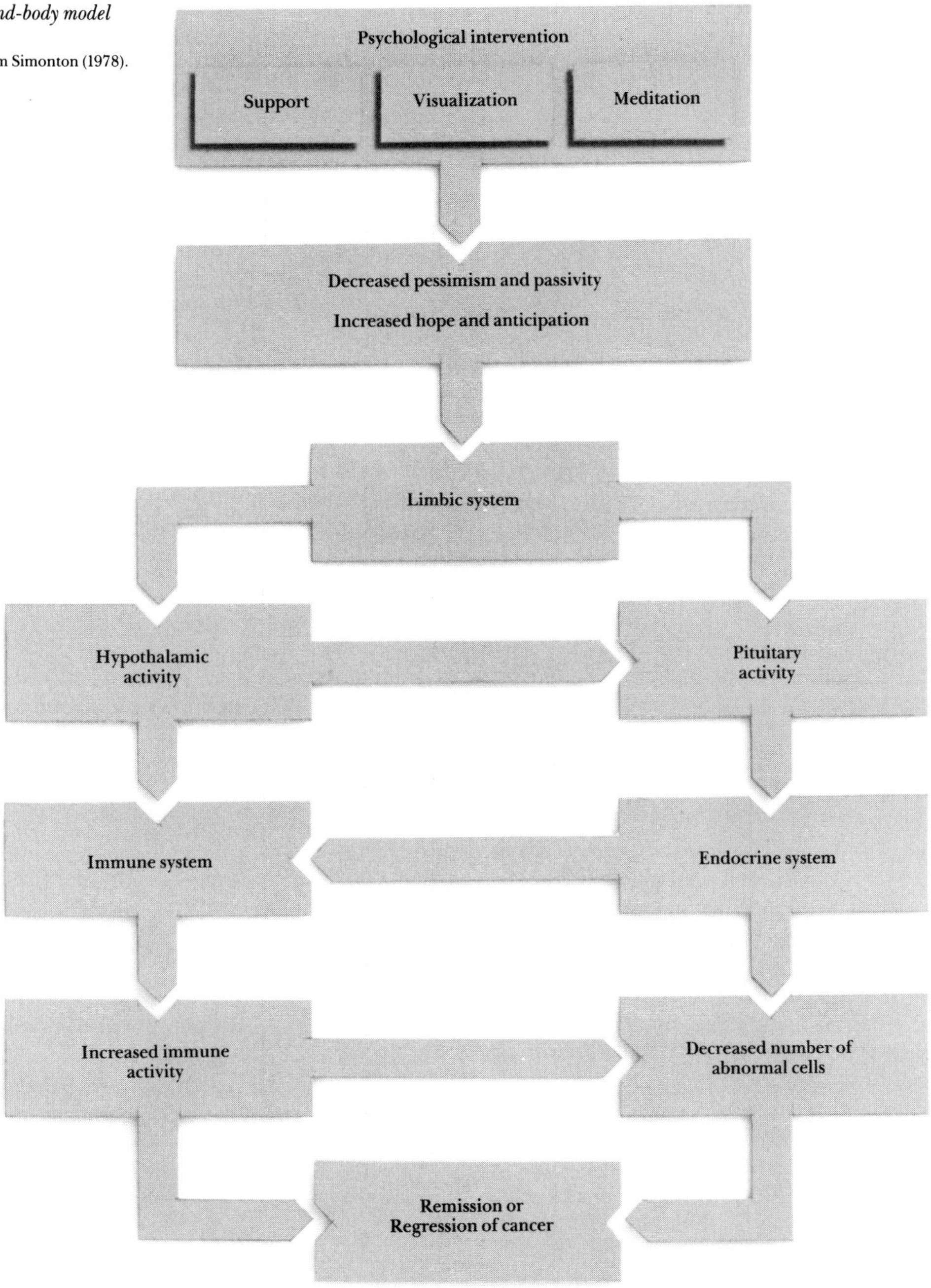

pression, anxiety, and hopelessness were associated with adverse outcomes. In another study the immunological responses of persons who developed cancer were found to be significantly depressed before the onset of the illness. Other research has shown that cancer victims react more strongly to life stresses than persons who do not have cancer. The same study also found that cancer subjects blame themselves for adverse events whereas subjects free of the disease do not engage in self-blame (Garfield, 1979). However, the presence of the cancer was an intervening variable that made the results of this study open to question.

Attempts are being made by an American radiologist and his social worker wife to help cancer sufferers achieve mental states that mobilize their immune systems. Group and individual methods are employed to persuade clients and their families that cancer may indeed be curable and that adopting a passive, hopeless attitude is counterproductive. Clients are taught to enter a meditative state three times a day, during which they visualize white warrior cells destroying cancer cells. Such meditation combined with imagery is called *visualization therapy* (Simonton, 1978). The mind-body model of recovery in cancer is shown in Figure 12-7.

CLINICAL EXAMPLE

DEVELOPING A HOLISTIC CARE PLAN FOR A CLIENT WITH RHEUMATOID ARTHRITIS

Neil Brown was a middle-aged, successful lawyer, prominent in community activities, and a good provider for his family. Neil and his wife, Bess, were devoted to each other and to their college-age son and daughter. During the Viet Nam War, Neil's son, Rick, was drafted into the Army immediately after his college graduation. This was a time when the anti-war demonstrations were at their peak. Rick and his parents discussed the possibility of his fleeing to Canada to evade the draft but eventually decided that this would not be an acceptable course of action. The only alternative was for Rick to allow himself to be inducted.

When Rick was sent to Viet Nam, his mother and sister were upset and worried, but his father was devastated. Neil had served with distinction in World War II and was proud of having served his country. However, he considered the Viet Nam conflict a very different matter. He saw it as an endless war that the United States showed no sign of winning. The reasons for the conflict were obscure to him. Battles were won or lost and nobody seemed to care. The daily body count was no more important to Neil's neighbors than the weather report. Neil was outraged that his only son was serving overseas while his friends' children evaded the draft or were not called upon to serve. He felt a special sense of responsibility because it was men of his generation who had allowed the Viet Nam War to escalate.

The family put up a brave front when Rick left. A number of parties were given in Rick's honor before his departure. Publicly, Neil was able to express pride and approval of his son's decision not to flee to Canada, saying that "We're not traitors in this family. If our country needs us, we are willing to fight. I'm not proud of the war, but I am proud of Rick." When it was time for Rick to leave, his mother and sister, Gail, dissolved in tears, but Neil was composed as he embraced his son. Rick's tour of duty was to last two years.

For several years Neil had been complaining of pain in his shoulder muscles. He was annoyed at times because the pain had caused his golf game to deteriorate. Cortisone injections relieved the pain temporarily, but physiotherapy had little effect. For some years the discomfort had remained at tolerable levels and sometimes even disappeared, but during the months after Rick's departure the pain became much worse. Even more worrisome was the fact that the pain was no longer confined to one area. Before long, other joints were affected; his hands and knees became inflamed, and he was constantly in pain. For a time Neil continued to play golf with his friends, but he soon felt that his disability robbed him of enjoyment of the game. He dropped out of the foursome that had played golf together over the years. As months passed Neil's range of motion became more and more restricted. His family physician diagnosed the condition as rheumatoid arthritis and referred Neil to a specialist when the discomfort proved unresponsive to conservative treatment.

Soon Neil was no longer able to drive his car or walk more than short distances. A whirlpool tub was installed in his home, and a community health nurse visited daily to help Bess with the complicated treatments that Neil required. The community health nurse helped simplify Neil's home care. He also helped Neil and Bess learn more about rheumatoid arthritis and offered them both emotional support. Although Neil received the best possible care, his condition continued to deteriorate.

The couple lived for the letters that came from their son and looked forward eagerly to Rick's return. Gail had her own apartment and was a frequent visitor. Both parents and Gail clung to the hope that the return of Rick would bring about Neil's recovery, although their physician and the community health nurse tried to help the family cope more realistically with his chronic disability.

ASSESSMENT

Neil exhibited some of the characteristics and lifestyle patterns seen in other persons with rheumatoid arthritis. He could not recall any close relative with the same disorder but knew that his father and grandfather had in their later years suffered from gout, a condition that also affects the joints. Neil was a loving father whose wife and children were the center of his life. Quiet spoken and hard-working, Neil was a man well respected in the community. Bess was effervescent and outgoing, a contrast to reliable, self-contained Neil.

Successful in his law practice, Neil was a disciplined, patriotic citizen who appreciated the fact that the United States government had helped him through law school by means of veterans' benefits. His personal value system was threatened when his only son was called upon to fight in a dangerous, controversial war. Yet his patriotism and sense of duty kept him from urging his son to avoid military service. Even before Rick was drafted Neil was experiencing localized arthritic discomfort but the disease process was exacerbated after his son left.

The following nursing and psychiatric diagnoses were made:

Nursing Diagnoses
Anxiety

Coping, ineffectual individual

Coping, ineffective family

Mobility, impaired physical (needs help from other people and equipment)

Home maintenance management, impaired

Self-care deficit

Diversional activity deficit

Comfort, alteration in: Pain

Self-concept: disturbance in body image, self-esteem, role performance, personal identity

Grieving, anticipatory

Multiaxial Psychiatric Diagnoses

Axis I   300.81 Somatization disorder

Axis II   None

Axis III Rheumatoid arthritis

Axis IV   Code 5—Severe

Axis V   Level 5—Seriously impaired

PLANNING

When it became apparent that Neil had rheumatoid arthritis, a great deal was done to keep him comfortable and help him retain a lifestyle close to normal. Neil had nevertheless become socially isolated, partly due to his refusal to make any demands on his friends. His self-imposed withdrawal from his friends increased the burdens on his wife and daughter, the only people on whom he depended. The community health nurse observed that Neil had unrealistic hopes that the return of his son would produce a remission, even though this was only a remote possibility.

The nurse voiced some doubts about sudden, miraculous cures but did not confront Neil and Bess directly, continuing instead to help the family manage Neil's care and live as normal a life as possible. With encouragement from the nurse and from Bess, Neil agreed to occasionally invite a few friends to his home for an evening of poker. It was difficult for Neil to hold the cards, so the nurse adapted a small music stand to serve the purpose. Neil jokingly remarked that he could only play poker with honest men who would not try to get a glimpse of the cards dealt to him.

The following goals were formulated for Neil and his family:

Neil will undertake the self-care tasks he is capable of performing.

Neil and Bess will practice the transfer from bed to chair or toilet with the assistance of a nurse.

Neil and Bess will become proficient in managing the transfer from bed to chair or toilet without additional assistance.

Neil and his family will attend at least three counseling/teaching sessions led by Neil's primary care nurse.

Neil and his family will participate in ongoing planning.

Neil and Bess will follow through on a referral to a family support group in the community.

Neil will accept home health services from a community health nurse.

IMPLEMENTATION

The care plan developed for Neil consisted of the following interventions either implemented or coordinated by the community health nurse who visited daily:

1. Assist Neil with bathing, dressing, and grooming, encouraging as much self-care as he seems capable of performing.

2. Teach Bess how to help Neil move from bed to chair to bathroom with minimum exertion for them both.

3. Provide honest answers and reading material to increase the couple's understanding of Neil's problems.

4. Watch for signs of discouragement in Neil and for signs of fatigue in Bess and respond supportively but realistically. Refer the couple for counseling if signs of depression or friction appear.

5. Inform the family of community agencies and self-help groups for arthritic clients and their families.

6. Coordinate the health care plan with the physician, physiotherapist, and mental health counselor, should one be needed.

7. Establish an ongoing relationship with the family as they await the return of their son, without encouraging or dismissing their hopes for a miraculous cure.

8. Encourage Neil to focus on the activities and diversions he is capable of enjoying rather than dwelling on his limitations.

EVALUATION

After serving his two-year tour of duty, Rick returned safely from Viet Nam. The family had chosen not to tell Rick of the extent of his father's disability until he returned home, so Rick was unprepared for what he found. He was shocked to see his vigorous, capable father now confined to a wheelchair and his attractive mother acting as a nurse. The only family member who had not changed greatly was Gail, and Rick derived comfort from the conversations with his sister. The reunion of the family was a happy event, but no recovery followed. Even though Neil did not improve much, the family was strengthened by Rick's return. His sister had someone near her own age in whom she could confide. His mother had someone on whom to lean when she was tired and discouraged. Neil was especially pleased when Rick indicated a desire to enter law school and eventually join his father's firm.

Even though Neil's condition was unchanged, the atmosphere in the family home was brighter. The momentum of Neil's disorder was slowed by competent medical treatment, good nursing care, and psychological support for the couple. The community health nurse continued to be involved with the family, teaching Neil and Bess, suggesting household arrangements that were more convenient, and offering supportive counseling.

329

INSTRUCTIONS FOR
VISUALIZATION THERAPY

1. Instruct the client to reach a state of relaxation by saying:
   a. My arms and hands feel heavy and warm.
   b. My legs and feet feel heavy and warm.
   c. My body, my neck, and my head feel heavy and warm.
2. Tell the client to close her eyes and imagine being in a place that is safe and comfortable. Then have the client imagine the following images, keeping her eyes closed.
   a. Visualize what is around you in this comfortable place. Imagine being surrounded by grass and flowers (or by sand and palm trees).
   b. Listen to the imaginary sounds around you. Is there silence, sounds of a waterfall or of waves breaking on the shore?
   c. Feel the currents of air around you. Is there a breeze? Does the sun shine on you, or are you resting in the shade?
3. Now direct the client to introduce into this tranquil scene an image of whatever is causing pain or distress:
   a. Headaches may be visualized as a savage, pounding drummer.
   b. Ulcers may be visualized as a jagged red line.

   c. Asthma may be visualized as a warm, sticky, gelatinous mass.
   d. Cancer may be visualized as a huge, rough stone.
4. Instruct the client to begin transforming the mental image in a positive direction:
   a. The imaginary drummer begins to beat more quietly, more gently, more slowly.
   b. The jagged red line becomes smooth and starts to fade.
   c. The gelatinous mass cools, lightens, and turns to ashes that blow away.
   d. The huge, rough stone begins to chip and flake, growing smaller.
   Reassure the client that transformation is a slow but sure process; it may take time but eventually will be accomplished because she controls the process.
5. Tell the client to continue visualizing the image for several minutes once the transformation is achieved. At this point the client may allow the images to fade and return to the place of comfort. Persuade the client that the place of comfort is always accessible and that the client may return whenever there is a desire to induce an internal atmosphere in which destructive processes can be reversed for a time.

SOURCE: Adapted from Pelletier (1979).

Neither Simonton nor any other reputable professional suggests that psychotherapeutic methods alone are sufficient treatment for cancer and statistical proof is inconclusive or lacking. Simonton continues traditional treatment, including radiation therapy for those clients who can withstand it. Some clients become too ill even to participate in visualization therapy. Nevertheless, some remissions have taken place, raising the possibility that psychological methods may have beneficial results for cancer clients, especially if their fears about treatment as well as cancer are honestly dealt with (Pelletier, 1979).

Visualization exercises, which can be beneficial to almost anyone wishing to induce a state of active relaxation, are described in the accompanying box.

Nurses working on oncology units are vulnerable to the same feelings of depression and futility that sometimes affect their clients. As a way of cop-

ing, some nurses take refuge behind a professional manner that helps remove them from the distress around them. Lengthy hospitalization and frequent visits to outpatient facilities tend to remove some of the barriers between nurses and clients. This can be a positive development for clients, but it may increase nurses' grief when clients fail to improve.

The inactive role assigned to clients in many treatment facilities can exacerbate nurses' low morale. The experience of nurses on one such unit illustrates how relatively minor changes in routine can improve the morale of both nurses and clients. In this account, nurses felt that physicians on their unit were distant and the clients too passive. The nurses felt frustrated and angry at the medical staff, who they felt left the psychological support of the clients and their families entirely to them. The nurses felt they had no guidelines on how to help their clients at various stages of their illnesses. The nursing staff consulted a psychiatrist to help them develop plans to meet the psychological needs of the clients and of the nurses. In group meetings with the psychiatrist, the nurses decided that since many of the clients did not require total bedrest, a communal dining room could be opened.

Being out of their rooms helped the clients to socialize with each other. Soon they began taking an interest in how the unit was run and began taking more active roles in their own care. At the clients' suggestion, some ward routines were eliminated or modified. With the introduction of these changes, the morale of both the clients and nurses improved. Turnover among the nursing staff decreased markedly. As the atmosphere on the unit changed, the physicians extended their visits and were more available to discuss care plans with the nursing staff. No miracles were reported, but clients and nurses alike felt more energetic and more involved in collaborative activities (Shlain, 1979).

SUMMARY

Almost a century after recognizing the influence of mind and spirit on physiological processes, health professionals are beginning to understand some of the mechanisms that influence the onset and course of human dysfunction. Researchers have established significant associations among emotions, the central and autonomic nervous systems, hormonal levels, and immunologic response systems. Early investigations between emotional states and physiological dysfunction tended to be simplistic. Dunbar's specific personality theory and Alexander's specific conflict theory have been replaced by multifactorial explanations for the etiology of various disorders.

Selye's general adaptation syndrome contributed to the popular acceptance of stress as a predisposing factor in various dysfunctional alterations of physiological processes. Human responses to stress are individualistic and greatly influenced by the meaning events hold for them. What one person perceives as overwhelming stress may be an exciting challenge for another. There is no panacea for stress-related problems, but it is possible to identify stressors that are especially harmful and to modify their effects.

Medical research has been devoted primarily to the understanding and treatment of physical illness, while social and behavioral research has been limited to the study of psychological and social factors. Both perspectives are inadequate, particularly for nurses who are concerned with providing holistic care. A number of physical disorders have traditionally been associated with stress and other psychological influences. Such disorders were orig-

inally categorized as psychosomatic, or later psychophysiological. In recent years, both terms have been discarded, as has the limited list of disorders considered to be psychologically induced. The current belief is that mind and body are inseparable and that the terms "psychosomatic" and "psychophysiological" imply a dichotomy that simply does not exist. Current research points to the fact that virtually every dysfunction to which human beings are susceptible can be influenced, positively or negatively, by psychological states. Therefore, the studies strongly suggest that teaching, counseling, and behavioral techniques should be included in any comprehensive nursing care plan. Most nurses are committed to holistic approaches to health care, and an understanding of the interactive nature of cognitive, emotional, and physiological processes is the point at which holism begins.

The review of disorders presented in this chapter is by no means complete and is merely representative of the vast array of conditions in health and illness that demand a multidimensional approach.

331

Review Questions

1. Explain how the development of scientific instruments contributed to a fragmented view of health and illness.

2. Differentiate the specific conflict theory from the specific personality theory of stress-related alterations.

3. Describe appropriate nursing interventions for the client categorized as a type A personality.

4. Select a representative disorder and explain the multifactorial theories concerning its etiology.

5. Name the principles that should form the basis of a nursing care plan for a client with peptic ulcer.

6. Explain the rationale for the following statement: "When psychological issues contribute to the clinical manifestations of dysfunction, psychological intervention will repair the dysfunction."

7. Trace the psychological, physiological, and cultural influences that contribute to the prevalence of anorexia nervosa.

8. Identify some common stressors in modern life and suggest ways in which nurses can help clients deal with these stressors.

9. Identify some common stressors confronted by nurses in their professional role, and suggest ways a nurse might effectively cope with these stressors.

10. Explain the following statement: "A holistic approach to health care requires a three-dimensional perspective."

References

Abse, D. W. 1974. Personality and Behavioral Characteristics of Lung Cancer Patients. *Journal of Psychosomatic Research*, 18:1–113.

Alexander, F. 1960. *Psychosomatic Medicine: Its Principles and Application*. New York: W. W. Norton.

Alexander, F.; French, T. M.; and Pollock, G. H. 1968. *Psychosomatic Specificity*. Chicago: University of Chicago Press.

American Psychiatric Association. 1980. *Diagnostic and Statistical Manual of Mental Disorders*, 3rd ed. Washington, D. C.: The Association.

Bloom, B. L.; Asher, S. J.; and White, S. W. 1978. Mental Disruption as a Stressor: A Review and Analysis. *Psychological Bulletin*, 85:867–894.

Brody, J. E. 1983. Emotions Found to Influence Every Human Ailment. *The New York Times*, May 24.

Brown, J. A. C. 1967. *Freud and the Post-Freudians*. Baltimore, Md.: Penguin.

Brozan, N. 1983. Anorexia: Not Just a Disease of the Young. *The New York Times*, July 18.

Bruch, H. 1973. *Eating Disorders: Obesity, Anorexia Nervosa, and the Patient Within*. New York: Basic Books.

Byassee, J. E. 1977. Essential Hypertension. In *Behavioral Approaches to Medical Treatment*, eds. R. B. Williams and W. D. Gentry. Cambridge, Mass.: Ballinger.

Cannon, W. B. 1932. *The Wisdom of the Body*. New York: W. W. Norton.

Carpenter, F. 1974. *The Skinner Primer*. New York: Free Press/Macmillan.

Charlesworth, E. A., and Nathan, R. G. 1982. *Stress Management: A Comprehensive Guide to Wellness*. Houston: Biobehavioral Publishers.

Cheren, S., and Knapp, P. H. 1980. Gastrointestinal Disorders. In *Comprehensive Textbook of Psychiatry*, 3rd ed., eds. H. I. Kaplan, A. M. Freedman, and B. J. Sadock. Baltimore: Williams & Wilkins.

Cobb, S.; Kasl, S.; Chen, E.; and Christenfeld, R. 1969. Some Psychological and Social Characteristics of Patients Hospitalized with Rheumatoid Arthritis, Hypertension, and Duodenal Ulcer. *Journal of Chronic Diseases*, 22:295–298.

Coelho, G. V.; Hamburg, D. A.; and Adams, J. E., eds. 1980. *Coping and Adaptation*. New York: Basic Books.

Coleman, J. C.; Butcher, J. N.; and Carson, R. C. 1984. *Abnormal Psychology and Modern Life*, 8th ed. Glenview, Ill.: Scott, Foresman.

Collins, G. 1983. A New Look at Anxiety's Many Faces. *The New York Times*, January 24.

Coyne, J. C., and Holroyd, K. 1982. Stress, Coping, and Illness: A Transactional Perspective. In *Handbook of Clinical Health Psychology*, eds. T. Millon, C. Greene, and R. Meagher. New York: Plenum.

Croog, S. H., and Levine, S. 1977. *The Heart Patient Recovers*. New York: Human Sciences Press.

Davidson, D. M. 1979. The Family and Cardiac Rehabilitation. *Journal of Family Practice*, 8:253–258.

Day, S. B. 1984. *Life Stress*. New York: Van Nostrand Reinhold.

Dunbar, F. 1943. *Psychosomatic Diagnosis*. New York: Harper & Row.

Dunbar, F. 1954. *Emotions and Body Changes*, 4th ed. New York: Columbia University.

Engel, G. 1954. Studies of Ulcerative Colitis: Clinical Data Bearing on the Nature of the Somatic Process. *Somatic Medicine*, 16(3):496–499.

Engel, G. 1972. *Psychological Development in Health and Disease*. Philadelphia: W. B. Saunders.

Engel, G., and Schmale, A. H. 1964. Psychoanalytic Theory of Somatic Disorder. *Journal of the American Psychoanalytic Association*, 15:344–365.

Eyer, T. 1979. Hypertension as a Disease of Modern Society. In *Stress and Survival*, ed. C. A. Garfield. St. Louis: C. V. Mosby.

Falliers, C. J. 1978. *Psychiatric Aspects of Asthma*. New York: Ciba-Geigy.

Feldman, F.; Cantor, D.; Soli, S.; and Bachrach, W. 1967. Psychiatric Study of a Series of 34 Patients with Ulcerative Colitis. *British Medical Journal*, 4:711–714.

Friedman, M., and Rosenman, R. 1974. *Type A Behavior and Your Heart*. New York: Knopf.

Fromm-Reichmann, F. 1937. Contribution to the Psychogenesis of Migraine. *Psychoanalytic Review*, 24(1):283–289.

Garfield, C. A. 1979. *Stress and Survival*. St. Louis: C. V. Mosby.

Jones, R. A. 1977. *Self-fulfilling Prophecies: Social and Psychological Effects of Expectancies*. Hillsdale, N.J.: Erlbaum.

Holmes, T. H., and Rahe, R. H. 1967. Social Readjustment Scale. *Journal of Psychosomatic Research*, 11:213–215.

Humphreys, W., and Lema, S. C. 1981. Sex Roles: Dilemmas for Women and Men. In *Understanding the Family*, eds. C. Getty and W. Humphreys. New York: Appleton-Century-Crofts.

Kaplan, H. I. 1980. History of Psychosomatic Medicine. In *Comprehensive Textbook of Psychiatry*, 3rd ed., eds. H. I. Kaplan, A. M. Freedman, and B. J. Sadock. Baltimore: Williams & Wilkins.

Knapp, P. H. 1980. Current Theoretical Concepts in Psychosomatic Medicine. In *Comprehensive Textbook of Psychiatry*, 3rd ed., eds. H. I. Kaplan, A. M. Freedman, and B. J. Sadock. Baltimore: Williams & Wilkins.

Knapp, P. H.; Mathe, A. A.; and Vachon, L. 1976. Psychosomatic Aspects of Bronchial Asthma. In *Bronchial Asthma: Mechanisms and Therapeutics*, eds. E. D. Weiss and M. Segal. Boston: Little, Brown.

Kolb, L. 1973. *Modern Clinical Psychiatry*, 8th ed. Philadelphia: W. B. Saunders.

Laing, R. D. 1971. *The Politics of the Family*. New York: Random House.

Lipowski, Z. J.; Lipsitt, D. R., and Whybrow, P. C. 1977. *Psychosomatic Medicine: Current Trends and Clinical Applications*. New York: Oxford.

Matthews, K. A. 1982. Psychological Perspectives on Type A Behavior Patterns. *Psychological Bulletin*, 91:293–323.

Mattson, A. 1975. Psychological Aspects of Childhood Asthma. *Pediatric Clinics of North America*, February.

Miller, L. H.; Ross, R.; and Cohen, S. I. 1982. Stress. *Bostonia Magazine*, 56(4):11–16.

332

Nelson, B. 1983. Examining Links Between Job Stress and Heart Disease. *The New York Times*, April 3.

Neuman, P. A., and Halverson, P. A. 1984. *Anorexia and Bulimia: Handbook for Counselors and Therapists*. New York: Van Nostrand Reinhold.

Pelletier, K. R. 1979. Adjunctive Biofeedback with Cancer Patients. In *Stress and Survival*, ed. C. A. Garfield. St. Louis: C. V. Mosby.

Piaget, J. 1968. *Six Psychological Studies*. New York: Random House.

Purcell, K.; Weiss, J.; and Hahn, W. 1970. Certain Psychosomatic Disorders. In *Manual of Child Psychopathology*, ed. B. Wolman, New York: McGraw-Hill.

Putt, A. 1970. One Experiment in Nursing Adults with Peptic Ulcer. *Nursing Research*, 19(6):484–494.

Rahe, R. H. 1974. Life Change and Subsequent Illness Reports. In *Life Stress and Illness*, eds. K. E. Gunderson and R. H. Rahe. Springfield, Ill: Charles C Thomas.

Rambo, B. 1984. *Adaptation Nursing: Assessment and Intervention*. Philadelphia: W. B. Saunders.

Robinson, L. 1983. *Psychiatric Nursing as a Human Experience*. Philadelphia: W. B. Saunders.

Robinson, L. 1984. *Psychiatric Aspects of the Care of Hospitalized Patients*. Philadelphia: W. B. Saunders.

Rogers, C. R. 1961. *On Becoming a Person*. Boston: Houghton Mifflin.

Rosenbaum, J. 1973. *The Mind Factor: How Emotions Affect Your Health*. Englewood Cliffs, N.J.: Prentice-Hall.

Rosenbaum, J. 1980. Peptic Ulcers. In *Comprehensive Textbook of Psychiatry*, 3rd ed., eds. H. I. Kaplan, A. M. Freedman, and B. J. Sadock. Baltimore: Williams & Wilkins.

Selye, H. 1974. *Stress Without Distress*. New York: McGraw-Hill.

Selye, H. 1976. *The Stress of Life*, 2nd ed. New York: McGraw-Hill.

Shlain, L. 1979. Cancer Is Not a Four Letter Word. In *Stress and Survival*, ed. C. A. Garfield. St. Louis: C. V. Mosby.

Silverman, A. J. 1980. Rheumatoid Arthritis. In *Comprehensive Textbook of Psychiatry*, 3rd ed., eds. H. I. Kaplan, A. M. Freedman, and B. J. Sadock. Baltimore: Williams & Wilkins.

Simonton, O. 1978. *Getting Well Again*. Los Angeles: J. P. Tarcher.

Smitherman, C. 1981. *Nursing Action for Health Promotion*. Philadelphia: F. A. Davis.

Stroebe, M. S., and Stroebe, W. 1983. Who Suffers More? Sex Differences in Health Risks of the Widowed. *Psychological Bulletin*, 93:279–301.

Tierney, J. 1985. Type A's, Maybe Now You Can Relax. *Science 85*, June 1985:12.

Turkington, C. 1984. Physical Factors Explored in Dieting, Type A Behavior. *Monitor*, February (1592):24.

Wheatley, D. 1977. *Stress and the Heart*. New York: Raven.

Williams, C. C., and Holmes, T. H. 1978. Life Change, Human Adaptation, and Onset of Illness. In *Clinical Practice in Psychosocial Nursing*, eds. D. Longo and R. Williams. New York: Appleton-Century-Crofts.

Weiner, H. 1977. *Psychobiology and Human Disease*. New York: Elsevier.

Supplementary Readings

Alpers, D. H. Functional Gastrointestinal Disorders. *Hospital Practitioner*, 18(1983):139–143.

Coleman, V. Identifying the Cause: Stress Induced Disorders in the Young and Elderly. *Nursing Mirror*, 155(1982):44.

Crown, S., and Crown, J. Personality in Early Rheumatoid Arthritis. *Journal of Psychosomatic Research*, 17(1980): 189–197.

Gottschalk, L. A. Vulnerability to Stress. *American Journal of Psychotherapy*, 37(1983):5–23.

Halden, C. Cancer and the Mind: How Are They Connected? *Science*, 200(1978):1363–1368.

Janis, I. L. The Role of Social Support in Adherence to Stressful Decisions. *American Psychologist*, 38(1983): 143–160.

Kozak, A. E. Stress, Coping and Life Change in the Single Parent Family. *American Journal of Community Psychology*, 11(1983):207–220.

Lachman, V. D. *Stress Management: A Manual for Nurses*. Orlando, Fla. Grune & Stratton, 1983.

Lazarus, R. S. Psychological Stress and Coping in Adaptation and Illness. *International Journal of Psychiatry in Medicine*, 5(1974):321–333.

Lazarus, R. S. Psychological Stress and Coping in Aging. *American Psychologist*, 38(1983):245–254.

Lynch, J. J., and Convey, W. H. Loneliness, Disease and Death: Alternative Approaches. *Psychosomatics*, 20 (1979):702–708.

Meissner, W. Family Process and Psychosomatic Disease. *International Journal of Psychiatry in Medicine*, 5(1974): 411–430.

Miller, R. S. Social Intimacy: An Important Moderation of Stressful Life Events. *American Journal of Community Psychology*, 11(1983):127–139.

Safranek, R. Coping with Stress: Does Humour Help? *Psychological Reports*, 51(1982):222.

Schill, T. Coping with Stress and Irrational Beliefs. *Psychological Reports*, 51(1982):1317–1318.

Schoeman, S. Z. Personality Variables in Coping with the Stress of a Spouse's Chronic Illness. *Journal of Clinical Psychology*, 39(1983):430–436.

Stone, M. H. Factitious Illness. *Bulletin of the Menninger Clinic*, 41(1977):239–254.

Turner, R. J. Class and Psychological Vulnerability Among Women: The Significance of Social Support and Personal Control. *Journal of Health and Social Behavior*, 24(1983):2–15.

Waring, E. M. Marriages of Patients with Psychosomatic Illnesses. *General Hospital Psychiatry*, 5(1983):49–53.

Weisman, A. D. *Coping with Cancer*. New York: McGraw-Hill, 1979.

PHYSIOLOGICAL ASPECTS OF HUMAN SEXUALITY
Anatomical Structures
Physiological Responses

INTRAPERSONAL AND INTERPERSONAL
DIMENSIONS
Socially Conditioned Sexual Expectations
Sexual Activity as a Coping Mechanism

ALTERNATIVE SEX ROLE ENACTMENT
Homosexuality
Bisexuality
Celibacy
Transvestism
Transsexualism

SEXUAL DYSFUNCTIONS
Decreased Sexual Interest
Increased Sexual Interest
Inhibitions
Orgasm Difficulties
Problems with Satisfaction

SEXUAL DEVIANCE
Fetishism
Zoophilia
Pedophilia
Exhibitionism
Voyeurism
Necrophilia

SEXUAL ABUSE
Sadomasochism
Incest
Sexual Harassment

COUNSELING
Premarital Counseling
Marital Counseling
Sexual Counseling

THE NURSING PROCESS IN SEXUAL HEALTH CARE

C H A P T E R

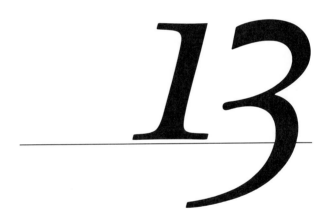

13

Altered Patterns of Sexuality

Learning Objectives

After reading this chapter, the student should be able to:

1. Delineate the physiological responses to sexual stimulation.

2. Examine the intrapersonal and interpersonal dimensions and cultural forces affecting sexual expression.

3. Differentiate between adaptive sexual expression, alternative sex role enactment, sexual abuse, and sexual dysfunctions.

4. Recognize the relationships between culture, sexual attitudes, and sexual behavior.

5. Formulate a nursing care plan for clients with sexual dysfunction.

336

Overview

Nurses have been leaders in advocating a holistic approach in health care, yet clients' sexuality has often been ignored by nurses. Some nurses are uncomfortable discussing sexual concerns with clients or do not have enough information about sexual physiology and psychology. Some believe common myths and misconceptions about sexuality. Fern H. Mims, professor of nursing at the University of Wisconsin, Madison, noted that many nurses believe only their own patterns of sexual behavior can be "right" and all other patterns must be "wrong." Such egocentricity does not promote sexual health. Mims suggests that a more ther-

apeutic approach is one that recognizes one's own value system while simultaneously accepting and withholding judgment of the values of others (Mims and Swenson, 1980). Nurses need to acquire accurate information and examine their own values and beliefs about sexuality before attempting to assist clients with their problems.

This chapter gives a brief overview of sexual anatomy and physiology, examines behavioral factors in sexuality, describes alternative styles of sexual expression, and discusses sexual dysfunction, deviance, and counseling.

I ne'er saw nectar on a lip
But where my own did hope to sip.
RICHARD BRINSLEY SHERIDAN

PHYSIOLOGICAL ASPECTS OF HUMAN SEXUALITY

Many people in our culture have received negative conditioning about the sexual parts of their bodies from earliest childhood. People learn to think of the genitals as something "down there" or the "privates," which are not to be looked at, touched, or discussed. Particularly for women in our culture, the genitals are a source of embarrassment; they are often considered shameful and dirty. This sense of shame may not remain limited to one's genitals but may extend to the whole body. One result of such negative attitudes about the body is that often people have little knowledge about their own anatomy and how it works. An important aspect of caring for clients with alterations of sexuality is to clear up any misconceptions they may have about their bodies and to provide them with information about sexual anatomy and physiology.

Anatomical Structures

The female external genitals, or *vulva*, consist of several structures (see Figure 13-1). The *mons veneris* is the fatty tissue over the pubic bone that is richly supplied with nerve endings; touch and pressure in this area can produce pleasurable sensations. The *labia majora* are the outer lips and the *labia minora* are the inner lips of the vulva. The labia minora join at the *clitoral hood* and can vary considerably in size, shape, and color from one woman to another. The *clitoris* consists of a *glans* and *shaft*, which contains two cavernous bodies called the crura (stalks) that extend internally. Although the clitoris is small, it has the same number of nerve

endings as the male penis and is highly sensitive to sexual stimulation. The remaining structures are the *urethral opening* and the *introitus* of the vagina.

The internal structures of the female consist of the ovaries, Fallopian tubes, uterus, cervix, and vagina (see Figure 13-2). The *vagina* has a very rich blood supply, and in a nonaroused state it is about three to five inches in length. During arousal, the vagina changes in size and shape and is capable of lubrication, which is related to the vasocongestion of the area. The existence of an area known as the *Grafenberg spot*, or *G-spot*, has been the subject of controversy in recent years. Advocates of this structure believe that it is located on the front wall of the vagina and surrounds the urethra midway between the cervix and the top of the pubic bone. This area is about the size of a dime in the unaroused state, but when a woman is sexually aroused it doubles in size. It is thought that this tissue is the female counterpart to the male prostate gland and arises from the same embryonic tissue. Some women find that direct stimulation of the G-spot is pleasurable and brings about a rapid orgasm. There have been some reports of a female ejaculation associated with G-spot stimulation, but it is not known how common a response this is (Barbach, 1982; Crooks and Baur, 1983).

The male sexual organs are more visible than the female genitals. The *penis* consists of the *glans*, which contains many nerve endings, and the *shaft*. In the shaft of the penis are spongy areas of erectile tissue called the *corpora cavernosa* and *corpus spongiosum*, which become engorged with blood during sexual arousal causing the penis to stiffen into an erection. Many men are concerned about the size of

Figure 13-1. *Female external genitals.*

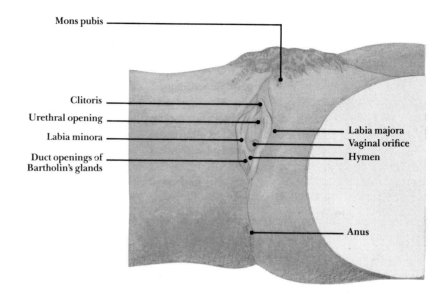

Mons pubis

Clitoris

Urethral opening

Labia minora

Duct openings of Bartholin's glands

Labia majora

Vaginal orifice

Hymen

Anus

338

Figure 13-2. *Female internal reproductive organs.*

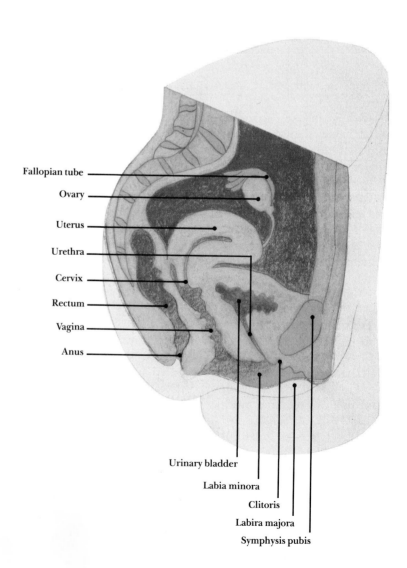

Fallopian tube

Ovary

Uterus

Urethra

Cervix

Rectum

Vagina

Anus

Urinary bladder

Labia minora

Clitoris

Labira majora

Symphysis pubis

Figure 13-3. *Male reproductive system.*

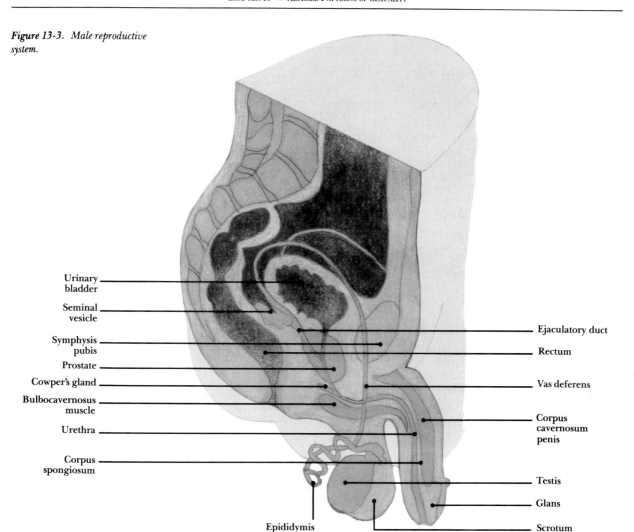

Urinary bladder

Seminal vesicle

Symphysis pubis

Prostate

Cowper's gland

Bulbocavernosus muscle

Urethra

Corpus spongiosum

Epididymis

Ejaculatory duct

Rectum

Vas deferens

Corpus cavernosum penis

Testis

Glans

Scrotum

339

their penis. There is a great deal of variation in penis length in the flaccid state, but erections in all men are about 5 to 7 inches long. Penis size is not related to body build, skin color, or sexual ability.

The two *testicles,* which are located in the *scrotum,* produce sperm (see Figure 13-3). From each testicle, the sperm travel through the *epididymis* and up through the *vas deferens,* whose terminal end forms a storage compartment called an *ampulla,* where sperm are held until ejaculation. The vas deferens and the *seminal vesicle* join to form the *ejaculatory duct,* which runs inside the *prostate gland* and joins with the urethra. The *seminal vesicles* are small glands that provide a fluid rich in fructose sugar, which activates the vigorous movement of sperm cells after ejaculation. The prostate gland contributes a thin, milky, alkaline fluid to the *semen.* The *Cowper's glands,* which are located below the prostate, secrete a clear, alkaline fluid into the urethra during sexual excitement. A small drop or two may be seen at the urethral orifice just before ejaculation

(Haeberle, 1981; Crooks and Baur, 1983). During ejaculation, the sperm, suspended in semen, are expelled through the urethral orifice. The smooth muscle sphincter at the base of the bladder is closed due to the higher pressure in the urethra caused by expansion of the corpus spongiosum, preventing the expulsion of urine during ejaculation.

Physiological Responses

Sexual arousal and response in humans is influenced by many factors and is a complex interaction of biological, psychological, and cultural components. Our understanding of the physiology of sexual arousal has been expanded by the work of William Masters and Virginia Johnson (1966). They used a variety of direct observation techniques in a laboratory setting to study human sexuality. According to Masters and Johnson, the human sexual response occurs in four phases: excitement, plateau, orgasmic, and resolution. The initial arousal is referred to as the *excitement phase,* during which

Table 13-1. The Sexual Response Cycle

Phase	Female Response	Male Response
Excitement	Myotonia (increased muscle tension) gradually increases. Moderate increase in pulse and blood pressure occurs. Clitoris becomes erect. Vaginal lubrication begins. Vagina increases in length and width and changes color to a deeper purple. Labia majora increase in size and flatten to expose vaginal opening. Labia minora enlarge to double or triple their size. Uterus pulls upward. Nipples become erect and entire breast begins to swell.	Myotonia gradually increases. Moderate increase in pulse and blood pressure occurs. Penis becomes erect. Scrotal tissue thickens and testicles pull upward toward abdomen by spermatic cord contraction. Nipples become erect.
Plateau	Myotonia, both voluntary and involuntary, becomes more pronounced. There may be facial grimaces. Pulse, blood pressure, and respiratory rate continue to increase. Sex flush may appear. Lubrication continues. The outer third of the vagina becomes congested with blood, which narrows it by about 33%. This is called the *orgasmic platform*. Labia minora continue to darken. Clitoris retracts under its hood. Breasts reach greatest expansion and nipple erection may subside.	Myotonia, both voluntary and involuntary, becomes more pronounced. There may be facial grimaces. Pulse, blood pressure, and respiratory rate continue to increase. Sex flush may appear. Testicles swell and continue to elevate. Cowper's glands secrete a few drops.
Orgasm	Muscular and nervous tension is suddenly released with involuntary muscle spasms. Sphincter muscles contract. Pulse, blood pressure, and respiration rate reach highest levels. Outer third of vagina contracts. Uterus contracts. Clitoris remains retracted under its hood.	Muscular and nervous tension is suddenly released with involuntary muscle spasms. Sphincter muscles contract. Pulse, blood pressure, and respiration rate reach highest levels. Ducts, urethra, and penis contract. About 1 teaspoon of semen is usually ejaculated. Orgasm and ejaculation are different processes and may occur independently of each other.
Resolution	Myotonia decreases. Pulse, blood pressure, and respiration rate return to normal. Nipples lose their erection. Sex flush disappears. Congestion in outer third of vagina disappears. Labia return to former shape and size. Clitoris reemerges from its hood. Uterus descends. No, or mild, refractory period, when no amount of stimulation will result in orgasm, occurs.	Myotonia decreases. Pulse, blood pressure, and respiration rate return to normal. Nipples lose their erection. Sex flush disappears. Penis loses erection. Testicles return to former shape and size. Refractory period occurs.

physiological changes tend to build rapidly. Muscle tension, respiration, heart rate, and blood pressure increase. Vasocongestion produces erection in the penis and swelling and hardening of the clitoris. Nipple erection occurs in both sexes. In the *plateau phase* (also called the *charge phase*), the physiological reactions continue, but at a less rapid rate. Sexual tension builds but may fluctuate. During the *orgasmic phase,* sexual tension is released in a spasmodic response centered in the pelvic region. Muscle spasms usually occur throughout the body, and a series of muscular contractions pulsate through the pelvic area. In males, orgasm is accompanied by ejaculation. Whether females experience a similar discharge during orgasm remains controversial. In the *resolution phase,* the body returns to the prearoused state. In males, there is a refractory period during which another orgasm is impossible. Table 13-1 summarizes the physiological changes that occur during the sexual response cycle.

INTRAPERSONAL AND INTERPERSONAL DIMENSIONS

Human sexuality is made up of a combination of biological, cultural, and psychological factors that are interwoven so intricately that it is almost impossible to isolate any one of them. The brain has been called the most important sex organ because it mediates the influence of these three elements. Physiologically, our five senses send messages to the brain, which then sends its neural messages via the spinal cord to produce the sexual responses of erection, lubrication, and orgasm. Our culture defines what is sexual or not sexual, so it thereby defines which incoming sensory messages the brain interprets as erotic. Sexual fantasies are a psychological process in the brain that stimulates a physiological response. Each of the three factors can be short-circuited by the brain itself. For example, feelings such as guilt, anger, anxiety, and fear will prevent the brain from sending the appropriate signals for sexual response.

It is important to recognize that sexuality is conditioned by an individual's cultural setting, or milieu. The social conditioning of sexual expectations and norms is very subtle, which often leads people to believe that their feelings and behaviors are innate. The range of acceptable sexual norms is very diverse. In some countries, such as the United States, there is a mix of acceptable norms; a single pattern of "American sexual behavior" does not exist.

Sexuality is an integral part of people's self-concept and as such is intrinsically related to body image and self-esteem. Thus, it is an important aspect of all feelings and behavior. Most people, regardless of sexual preferences, have a need for sexual self-validation—that is, validation of their masculinity or femininity. The sexual self, like other aspects of the self, needs to be constantly reinforced and supported. Sexuality is potentially a rich source of pleasure, but for many people it can also be a source of guilt, frustration, and conflict. They must resolve their sexual conflict and guilt in order for sex and sexuality to enhance their feelings about themselves and to help them relate more comfortably and positively to others.

Socially Conditioned Sexual Expectations

Each society dictates what is appropriate and inappropriate sexual behavior and thus strongly shapes its members' attitudes and expectations. Some of these socially conditioned expectations can interfere with people's sexual functioning and enjoyment because they rob sexual expression of freedom and spontaneity. Also, people may feel bewildered, hurt, or rejected when their partners are unable to meet their expectations. The socialization process is so subtle that many people are unaware of the impact of a number of unspoken expectations about sex. These expectations include (Kaplan, 1974; Siemens and Brandzel, 1982):

EXPECTATION 1 Sexual behavior should be instinctual. This assumption confuses sexual drive, which is innate, with sexual behavior, which is learned. Through the socialization process one learns what behavior is acceptable and what is unacceptable at each stage of life. Sexual drive changes throughout life as a person develops new sexual tastes and habits and experiences changes in sexual frequency needs. The belief that sexual behavior should be instinctual leaves little room for teaching and learning to occur within a relationship.

EXPECTATION 2 Sexual performance is all important. American culture is an achievement-oriented society, and people tend to evaluate themselves and each other by their sexual achievements. Sexual activity tends to become work if goals are set for intercourse and orgasm and little attention is paid to the process of lovemaking. Our language reflects such attitudes, for example, in the use of the word "foreplay." Such a term indicates that this activity is only meaningful when it is a preliminary to genital intercourse. Such expectations can contribute to anxiety, which in turn may block physiological responses. When a person becomes a spectator of his or her own sexual performance, the stage is set for sexual dysfunction. The high value some areas of our culture place on work and the low value placed on pleasure lead to the assumption that activities are important only if they are productive and that pleasure-oriented activities are selfish and unimportant. It is difficult for many people to set aside time for pleasure. Frequently, pleasurable activities such as sex are sacrificed in order that all other tasks for the day be accomplished.

EXPECTATION 3 Sex equals intercourse. This expectation minimizes the importance of all the touching, holding, and manual and oral stimulation that also compose sexual activity. Such an assumption allows people to consider themselves "virgins" even though they have participated in every sexual activity except intercourse. It can also lead to unrealistically high expectations about intercourse and to disappointment when it does occur. A couple's exclusive focus on the penis in the vagina may rob them of a great deal of pleasure and warmth. Such an exclusive focus also requires the attainment and maintenance of a penile erection for a long period, which is not always easy or possible.

EXPECTATION 4 Men are responsible for sexual activity. Men are expected to be more interested in sex, to initiate and direct the sexual act. Satisfaction for both partners is considered the man's responsibility. Women are expected to remain passive, innocent, and unknowledgeable. This expectation places an unfair burden on the man and discounts the woman's responsibility for satisfying herself and her partner. Because of this expectation it is difficult for many men to passively allow their partners to stimulate them and give them pleasure. Many men are also afraid to ask their partners about their sexual preferences for fear of being thought ignorant or unmanly. Women hesitate to tell men their preferences for fear of hurting their egos. They believe that if their partner loves them he will be able to divine their wishes. Thus both men and women are victims of this cultural conspiracy of silence.

EXPECTATION 5 Men are always ready for sex and should be able to get an erection with anyone, anywhere, at any time. This expectation dismisses the highly complex psychological and physiological processes that can short-circuit sex in both men and women. This misconception is often fueled by another—that men, by nature, have a stronger sex drive than women. Such unrealistic expectations frequently lead to disillusionment for both partners.

EXPECTATION 6 All physical contact should lead to sexual intercourse. Couples who hold this belief see touching and holding only as preliminaries to intercourse, not as acts valuable or pleasurable in their own right. Such couples may cease to touch and hold each other when sexual intercourse is neither desired nor feasible. They lose a valuable means of expressing warm, tender, and intimate feelings.

EXPECTATION 7 Intercourse should always end in orgasm for both partners. In reality, the orgasmic reflex can be triggered or inhibited by many physiological and psychological factors. While under most circumstances both partners may wish to achieve orgasm at some point during sex, it is possible for one or both partners to enjoy intercourse without orgasm. Some couples strive for simultaneous orgasm as the "right" way to have intercourse and thus are disappointed when it does not occur. Individuals vary widely in the amount of time and stimulation they need to achieve orgasm. It is unrealistic to expect simultaneous orgasm. Focusing on the orgasm tends to diminish pleasure in sex and to increase concern about performance. Other

aspects of sexual activity become neglected. Yet concentrating on the process of sexual interaction—touching, holding, caressing, meeting the partner's needs—is usually more rewarding than concentrating solely on having an orgasm.

EXPECTATION 8 Sexual activity requires an erection. This is closely related to the assumption that sex equals intercourse. Expecting an erection becomes another source of pressure and frequently results in a failure to maintain or achieve an erection. A couple needs to remember that the penis is not the only part of the man's body involved in lovemaking and that there are many other sexual activities they can try. It is unfortunate when couples forgo all pleasure when erectile difficulties occur.

EXPECTATION 9 Sexual activity should be spontaneous. This expectation rests on the belief that both partners should be in the mood for sex before any activity should be initiated. In reality, it is common for one partner to initiate sex and the other partner to get in the mood as lovemaking proceeds. With the busy schedules many people have, couples need to make "dates" with their partners to ensure they have enough intimate time together. Rather than a detriment to the mystique of sexual activity, planning can become a source of pleasurable anticipation that can enhance time together.

EXPECTATION 10 Women should have orgasms during intercourse and be able to achieve multiple orgasms. Expecting the woman to have frequent and multiple orgasms has become a measure of the liberation of the wife and of the sexual competence of the husband. Unfortunately, this obsession can interfere with sexual pleasure. Some women are unable to communicate their needs and preferences, particularly about other modes of stimulation besides genital intercourse. Research has shown that there is no "normal" orgasm and no "right" way to have orgasms (Masters and Johnson, 1966). The majority of women, in fact, have difficulty reaching orgasm solely by penetration of the penis.

Sexual Activity as a Coping Mechanism

Although the purposes of sexual activity are usually thought to be reproduction and the expression of affection, it may also be viewed as a coping mechanism. Whether it is an adaptive or maladaptive coping mechanism depends on two criteria: (1) how well an activity serves its intended purpose, and (2) whether it harms anyone.

Self-affirmation may be one of the greatest benefits of sexual activity. Feeling accepted and being able to give and receive pleasure are emotionally valuable consequences of sexual activity. They help

342

counterbalance the self-doubts and disappointments inherent in living. However, when the need for reassurance reaches such extremes that even frenetic sexual activity cannot fulfill it, then sexual activity can become a maladaptive response.

Sexual activity may also be used to relieve anxiety, since orgasm discharges tension fairly reliably. Many people use sexual activity as a kind of tranquilizer, especially during times of temporarily increased stress. However, extremes of anxiety can result in erectile failure or nonorgasmic response, consequently further increasing anxiety.

Although a decrease in sexual activity is usually associated with depression, an increase in activity may be seen in the milder depressions. This coping mechanism is an effort to counteract the depression through stimulation and personal contact.

Pleasure and excitement are human needs that must be met for optimal well-being, and sexual activity is one source of pleasure and emotional stimulation in people's lives. Sexual enjoyment can help people bear the difficult times that inevitably occur in life. But when sex becomes the sole source of excitement or cannot provide enough excitement to meet a person's needs, it can become a maladaptive response.

Some people view sex as a way to obtain love, but there is a great difference between sex as an expression of love and sex as a plea for love. The more manipulative a sexual activity is, the more maladaptive it becomes and the more painful its consequences can be. Some people may engage in sexual intercourse to obtain body contact and touching, but, again, the distinction must be made between sex as an expression of physical affection and sex as a plea for human contact.

The exercise of power over another person is another manipulative use of sex that is unlikely to have satisfactory consequences. People who feel dependent and helpless may believe their only means of wielding power is with sex. If an individual does not feel he has the power to gain what he wants directly, he may use sex as a reward or the withholding of sex as a punishment to get what he wants indirectly. Withholding sex can have a powerful effect. The partner not only ends up feeling inadequate as a lover but is also deprived of pleasure. Thus, what began as a coping mechanism may end up harming the couple's relationship.

ALTERNATIVE SEX ROLE ENACTMENT

Up until this point in the chapter, the assumption has been made that the partners in a sexual relationship are of different sexes. This assumption has been made as a matter of convenience because most

relationships do follow this pattern. Much of the material in the preceding sections also applies to homosexual couples. However, homosexual individuals and individuals who enact other sex roles deserve special mention because their needs and problems often differ from those of heterosexual individuals.

Homosexuality

The word *homosexual* is used to describe the sexual orientation of men and women who find their primary emotional and sexual fulfillment with people of the same sex. Homosexuality is only an aspect of personality, as is heterosexuality. Identifying people solely by their choice of sex partners tends to belittle them; it conveys the impression that homosexuals' only interest is in sex. Other aspects of an individual's personality tend to be ignored when sexual labels are applied, so such labels should be used carefully and with the understanding that the only basic difference between heterosexual and homosexual people is in their preference of sexual partners.

Our culture's negative attitude toward homosexuality has been strongly influenced by religious teachings that hold homosexuality to be sinful and by psychoanalytic theory, which has traditionally held that homosexuality is an emotional disorder caused by arrested psychosexual development. According to traditional psychoanalytic theory, homosexuality can be attributed to an unresolved masochistic attachment to the pre-Oedipal mother, a distant relationship with the father, a defense against castration anxiety, or an immature ego (Bell and Weinberg, 1978; Carrera, 1981). Other unproven theories about the causes of homosexuality include a fetal hormonal imbalance, peer pressure, and learning processes. (It is perhaps revealing that theorists have not tended to address the broader question of what causes *any* sexual orientation, whether homosexual or heterosexual. Until this broader question is answered, the causes of homosexuality cannot be fully understood.)

Homophobia, a strong, irrational fear of homosexuals or the fear of homosexual feelings within oneself, is so widespread in our society that many homosexuals are robbed or assaulted by people who feel they "deserve" to be punished. Homosexuals are often regarded as safe targets by criminals because they may be reluctant to press charges out of fear of exposure and publicity. In one study (Bell and Weinberg, 1978), one-third of homosexual men reported that they had been assaulted and robbed at least once in connection with their homosexuality. It was also found that 25 percent of homosexual men and women had been threatened with blackmail about their sexual preference.

343

MYTHS ABOUT HOMOSEXUALITY

Widespread ignorance about homosexuality in this country leads to the perpetuation of many myths. Nurses, as professionals, have a responsibility to counteract these myths with accurate information. The following are some of the common myths about gay people:

You can tell gay people just by looking at them.

Homosexual people are pretty much alike.

They could change if they really wanted to.

They make poor parents.

In a relationship, one plays the part of the woman and the other plays the part of the man.

Gay teachers will persuade young people to become gay.

Gays are sexually attracted to children.

Homosexual people are responsible for the majority of sexual violence.

344

In our culture, men appear to be more homophobic than women and more threatened by male than female homosexuals. Behaviors that demonstrate homophobia are making "queer" jokes, disparaging homosexuality, and verbally or physically assaulting homosexual people. Homophobic men tend to have rigid gender role stereotypes lest they be thought of as homosexuals. They avoid behavior that might be seen as homosexual by others, such as choosing "feminine" professions, hugging friends and relatives of the same sex, and engaging in oral-genital sex or manual-genital contact, even with their wives.

Homosexual behavior has been decriminalized in many countries, but most states in America still have laws against homosexual behavior. The sodomy laws make persons engaging in oral sex and anal intercourse subject to arrest and trial. Homosexuals are often also arrested for loitering to solicit and for disorderly conduct. Police officers at times use entrapment by posing as decoys soliciting sex. Homosexual people also have their civil rights infringed on in the area of housing and employment. They are discriminated against in the areas of credit, insurance coverage, divorce, child custody, and adoption. Because there cannot be a legal marriage, they have difficulties with tax benefits and property and inheritance rights.

A more liberal attitude toward homosexuality is beginning to emerge as churches reexamine their traditional attitudes and psychologists offer new studies and opinions. Alfred Kinsey's studies in 1948 and 1953 demonstrated that millions of Americans had engaged in homosexual behavior. His surveys showed that 50 percent of men and 28 percent of women had had some homosexual experience during their lives. These studies made it very clear that a person's sexual preference is not fixed and that sexual orientation can be seen as a continuum. Kinsey developed a six-point scale that rates people from "entirely heterosexual" to "entirely homosexual." He found that nearly half of people fell between these two end points. Kinsey's studies support the view that there is a natural variation of sexual expression among humans.

COMMON MISCONCEPTIONS A landmark study by Bell has also done much to dispel common misconceptions about homosexuality (Bell and Weinberg, 1978). Bell's study included 979 homosexual people matched to a control group of 477 heterosexual people. Such a volunteer group would be expected to be more open about their sexual orientation than a random sample of all homosexuals, but there has never been a true random sampling of American homosexual men and women because of the inherent difficulty of identifying such a population. Even so, the data in Bell's study do much to cast doubt on common assumptions about homosexuals.

Traditionally, therapists working with homosexual clients have tended to assume homosexual

HOMOSEXUALITY AND AIDS

AIDS—acquired immune deficiency syndrome—was first recognized in the gay community in 1980. AIDS is thought to be caused by a biological agent that is transmissible by a variety of routes, including sexual contact and intravenous injection. At the time of this writing there appears to be a link between the human T cell leukemia virus (HTLV) and AIDS. Studies suggest that the disease affects the thymus gland and breaks down the body's immune system. The AIDS victim has a decreased ratio of helper-to-suppressor T lymphocytes. Helper T cells activate the immune response, and suppressor T cells moderate or turn off the immune response. A decrease in helper T cells results in a profound suppression of a person's immune response (Marx, 1983). The syndrome is seen primarily in homosexual men (71 percent of AIDS sufferers), intravenous drug abusers (17 percent), Haitian immigrants (5 percent), and hemophiliacs who get blood transfusions (1 percent). The remaining 6 percent of AIDS sufferers are unclassified. The incidence of AIDS among Haitian immigrants is somewhat a puzzle because those victims have denied homosexual practices and drug use. The link may be with HTLV, which is more prevalent in the Caribbean area.

Currently, AIDS is incurable and usually fatal. Symptoms include fever, weight loss, diarrhea, oral thrush, lymphadenopathy, and blue or brown spots on the skin. The victims often suffer from a rare form of cancer called Kaposi's sarcoma or may die from a rare, highly fatal form of pneumonia known as *Pneumocystis carinii* pneumonia.

There is some concern whether heterosexual partners of AIDS victims are at risk for developing AIDS. In one study, seven female sexual partners of AIDS victims who were drug abusers were examined for signs of AIDS. The women denied any history of drug abuse and their only known risk factor was prolonged monogamous contact with a partner who had the disease. Of the seven women, one woman had AIDS, one had an illness like the prodrome of AIDS, and four women had clinical or laboratory abnormalities associated with AIDS. Only one woman had no abnormalities associated with AIDS (Harris et al., 1983).

The considerable public attention focused on AIDS has helped spur research, which is beginning to provide much needed information. The gay community has been very active in disseminating information about AIDS. It is cautioning gays against casual sexual encounters in order to limit the spread of the syndrome.

345

persons would like to relinquish their sexual orientation if they could. However, in Bell's study one-half of the homosexual men and two-thirds of the homosexual women had no regrets whatsoever about being homosexual. One-fourth of the men and one-fifth of the women had some regret related to being rejected by society. Less than one-fourth of the people agreed that homosexuality is an emotional disorder. In many other studies therapists have been unable to distinguish between homosexual and heterosexual persons on the basis of psychological adjustment, and both groups have scored the same for general health and happiness. Homosexual adults who have come to terms with their sexual orientation don't regret it; they can function sexually and socially and are no more distressed psychologically than heterosexual adults (Bell and Weinberg, 1978).

Another common assumption has been that the majority of homosexual people keep their orientation a secret from all but their homosexual acquaintances. Bell's study demonstrated that fewer people remain in the "closet" but that individuals differ in the extent to which they disclose their sexual preference. Fathers are the least likely to know that their adult children are homosexual, siblings are more likely to know than their fathers, and mothers are the most likely to know. Fifty percent of homosexual males reported that their employers either knew or suspected their sexual orientation, but only 32 percent of women believed that their employers knew or suspected. These data show that in spite of the gay liberation movement, the majority of homosexuals remain relatively covert about their sexual preference.

Homosexual people are generally thought to be very unstable in their work situations due to emotional instability. It is also thought that they run a risk of being fired if their orientation is discovered. Bell's study found that for homosexual males there was no evidence of greater job instability than for their heterosexual counterparts and that in fact homosexual men tended to like their jobs better. Homosexual women in the study had more frequent job changes than did the heterosexual women, but there was no difference in job satisfaction between the two groups.

It is not known how many homosexual men and women ever enter into a heterosexual marriage. Studies have indicated that married homosexuals are the most covert and the most fearful of having their sexual orientation exposed. Bell's data show that heterosexual-homosexual marriages are not customary, but neither are they extremely rare. Fewer than one-fifth of homosexual males had been married at some time while more than one-third of homosexual females had. Both groups had less frequent sexual activity with their spouses than did heterosexuals in the study, but many or most did have children. Usually, the heterosexual spouse was unaware of his or her partner's sexual orientation prior to the marriage. Almost all of the people in this sample were married only once (Bell and Weinberg, 1978).

Homosexual relationships are often thought to follow rigid patterns, but in reality they are as varied as heterosexual relationships, with the same joys, sorrows, commitments, and breakups. Researchers have identified five basic homosexual relationship styles to which 71 percent of the sample could be assigned. In a *close-couple* relationship the partners are closely bound and relate in a quasi-marital style. These couples seldom go out to gay bars or baths, report fewer sexual problems and have fewer partners than other homosexuals, and they report little regret over their sexual orientation. This group, which included 28 percent of the women and 10 percent of the men in Bell's sample, appear to be the happiest and most relaxed group.

Open-couple relationships are also quasi-marital, but individuals in these relationships tend to have more partners, to have more sexual problems, and to participate in more "cruising." (Cruising is the act of frequenting known gay establishments in hopes of finding new sexual partners.) Seventeen percent of the women and 18 percent of the men in Bell's sample shared an open-couple relationship.

Persons considered to have a functional style of homosexuality are "single" people who have a number of partners, a high level of sexual activity, little regret about their orientation, and few sexual problems. Functional homosexuals are more overt about their homosexuality and more energetic and optimistic. Ten percent of the women and 15 percent of the men in Bell's sample fit the functional style of homosexuality. The dysfunctional style of homosexuality (5 percent of women and 12 percent of men in Bell's sample) involves people who are not coupled and who have a number of partners, a high

level of sexual activity, and many sexual problems. They are more regretful of their partner preference and have the poorest psychological adjustment of all five groups.

The last type of homosexual behavior is asexual (11 percent of women and 16 percent of men in Bell's sample). These people are more covert than those in the other groups, are not coupled, have few partners, and describe themselves as lonely. They also have a lower level of sexual desire and activity than those in the other groups.

Stereotypes of homosexual men as being highly promiscuous and homosexual women as interested in a permanent "marriage" correspond with general sex stereotypes that men focus on sex and women on affection and commitment. It is true that men—straight or gay—are more easily able to separate sex from affection and that they tend to evaluate themselves by their sexual prowess. Therefore, it is no surprise that homosexual men tend to have more partners than homosexual women and are more apt to have sex with a stranger. About one-fourth of the men in Bell's sample were in a couple relationship, and almost one-half of the women were coupled.

Another myth is that homosexual couples take on sex roles in their relationships, one person being dominant ("the man") and the other submissive ("the woman"). Although this may happen at times, homosexual couples are actually less likely to embrace dominant and submissive roles than are heterosexual couples. The homosexual couple could well serve as a model of equality for heterosexuals.

Another common assumption is that certain sexual behaviors and practices are exclusively homosexual. In reality, homosexual people make love in much the same way as heterosexual people, except that they do not engage in penis-vagina intercourse. Homosexual couples kiss, caress, and stroke each other. In descending order of frequency, men use oral sex, hand-genital stimulation, and anal intercourse. Homosexual women use hand-genital contact most often, followed by oral sex and body rubbing. Contrary to popular belief, only 2 percent of homosexuals use dildos in their lovemaking. None of these practices is exclusive to the homosexual population (Bell and Weinberg, 1978; Crooks and Baur, 1983).

Homosexual people are often thought to be consumed by their uncontrollable desire for sexual activity. Some heterosexuals fear that homosexuals lie in wait to proposition them in public restrooms, movie theaters, or parks. But 40 percent of homosexual men do no cruising at all, and those who do usually do it in the safer setting of a gay bar or bath. Most homosexual activity takes place in the privacy of homes (Bell and Weinberg, 1978).

Homosexual men and women are also more likely to have more close friendships than heterosexual people. Perhaps this is because family commitments take priority over friendships among heterosexuals. Gay people tend to have both heterosexual and homosexual friends. Very few heterosexuals report that they have one or more friends of the same sex whom they know to be homosexual (Bell and Weinberg, 1978).

HOMOSEXUALITY AND PSYCHIATRY The psychiatry establishment's changing view of homosexuality was perhaps best characterized by the distinguished psychoanalyst J. Marmor (1973):

Surely the time has come for psychiatry to give up the archaic practice of classifying the millions of men and women who accept or prefer homosexual object choices as being, by virtue of that fact alone, mentally ill. The fact that their alternative life-style happens to be out of favor with current cultural conventions must not be a basis in itself for a diagnosis of pathology.

The official position of the American Psychiatric Association (1980) is that homosexuality in itself is not a disease. DSM-III does describe *ego-dystonic homosexuality* as a disorder. A person in this category is one who wishes to become heterosexual and whose homosexual arousal is a persistent source of distress. Factors that contribute to ego-dystonic homosexuality may be hostile societal attitudes and a desire for a socially approved family life. Homosexuality is not considered ego-dystonic if hatred of one's sexual orientation is merely a symptom of depression that disappears when the depression lifts.

Perhaps no other aspect of human sexual behavior is as controversial today as homosexuality. It is to be hoped that knowledge and understanding of homosexual behavior will help the public reach a more tolerant view.

Bisexuality

Many people fall on the continuum between exclusive heterosexual behavior and exclusive homosexual behavior. *Bisexuality* is defined as erotic attraction to and sexual fulfillment with people of both sexes. This definition excludes homosexual people who are married to maintain a pretense of heterosexuality or those who choose partners of other than the preferred sex when partners of the preferred sex are not available. Kinsey (1948, 1953) found that 18 percent of the men in his study and between 4 percent and 11 percent of the women had had as much homosexual as heterosexual experience. Bisexuality is as real an orientation as heterosexuality or homosexuality.

There are variations among the lifestyles of bisexual people just as there are among homosexual and heterosexual people. Bisexuality may be classified as transitional, historical, sequential, or concurrent. A *transitional* bisexual person is in movement from either heterosexual or homosexual preference to the opposite preference. During the time of transition, the person appears to be bisexual. The person who is *historically* bisexual had sexual experience in the past that was the opposite of his or her basic orientation. *Sequential* bisexuality occurs when a person is involved in heterosexual and same-sex relationships at different times. The number of such relationships varies among individuals (Klein, 1978). *Concurrent* bisexuality occurs when a person engages in simultaneous sexual relationships with both women and men.

Bisexuality has received less attention in the medical literature than homosexuality until very recently. The persistent belief that people are either heterosexual or homosexual and never in between has left this sexual orientation poorly researched and understood. It has been difficult for scientists and laymen alike to believe that people can feel desire, gratification, and delight with members of both sexes. Bisexuals are frequently viewed with contempt by both heterosexual and homosexual people. It is commonly thought that the bisexual person has not yet arrived at his or her true preference or that the bisexuality is a fearful compromise. Therefore it is quite common for the bisexual person to feel alienated and oppressed by both homosexual and heterosexual people. At the time of this writing there are very few support systems available for bisexual individuals, but as more "come out," support systems will emerge just as they have emerged for homosexuals.

Celibacy

Celibacy is a voluntary choice not to engage in sexual activity with other people. A person may choose celibacy either temporarily or permanently. There are many reasons a person may choose to be celibate, including dedication to a religious vocation, postponement of sex until marriage for moral or religious reasons, unavailability of one's partner, avoidance of sexually transmitted diseases, disappointment in past sexual relationships, or the protection of a newly developing relationship. For some people, celibacy may be a temporary necessity when other aspects of their lives assume precedence. Celibacy can be a beneficial choice for some people. It can enable them to conduct emotional self-exploration or regrouping apart from the conflicts of a sexual relationship. Sexual frustration need not occur during the time of celibacy because sexual pleasure through self-stroking and mas-

347

turbation often provides an acceptable alternative to the individual.

Transvestism

A *transvestite* is usually defined as a person who finds sexual stimulation in cross-dressing, or wearing clothing of the opposite sex. Most transvestites are male heterosexuals. A minority of male homosexuals also cross-dress, but primarily to parody women with misogynistic intent (Freedman, Kaplan, and Sadock, 1976). Female impersonators differ from transvestites in that they cross-dress to entertain rather than to express their female gender identity. The form of transvestism can vary from one individual to another. Cross-dressing may be limited to an article or two of women's underwear or may consist of an entire outfit, including makeup and a wig. Some transvestites cross-dress only occasionally and have no gender identity conflict. At the other end of the continuum are men who cross-dress as often as possible and who maintain their masculine identity with less conviction.

The transvestite cross-dresses to create the illusion of femininity—that is, "to pass" as a woman. Cross-dressing is not a vehicle for satire at women's expense; it is done primarily for sexual arousal. Some men move beyond the fetishistic stage and are no longer sexually excited by cross-dressing. These men go on to a more total form of female "passing" and take their aspirations to femininity seriously. They make genuine attempts to behave as well as to dress as women. The transvestite can live and work as a man without anyone knowing about his obsession. He is rarely effeminate in his male role (Ackroyd, 1979).

Cross-dressing is not harmful in itself, nor is it dangerous to other people. Its most distressing result may be the disapproval of family members. Some transvestites hide their cross-dressing from their wives in the fear that they may not understand or accept the behavior. Some wives who discover that their husbands are transvestites mistakenly assume that their husbands are homosexual. Other wives feel that their own sexuality and sexual identity are placed in doubt. After their initial surprise, many wives are able to eventually understand and accept their husbands' needs to cross-dress. Some transvestites are able to share this component of their personality with other family members, while others keep it hidden from them. There are societies for transvestites in many countries, and support groups are becoming active in this country. The Human Outreach and Achievement Institute in Boston is an educational group that offers informational programs for the helping professions and services for those concerned with gender issues.

Transsexualism

Gender is a person's biological maleness or femaleness; *gender identity* refers to a person's inner psychological conviction of feeling male or female. *Gender roles* are culturally determined rules about tasks, expectations, and feelings considered appropriate for each gender. Cultural rules determine what is considered "normal" and "abnormal" within a culture. *Transsexualism* is considered a disorder of gender identity: a person born as a biological male or female believes that he or she was born with a body that does not match his or her internal identity. Transsexualism is a life-long cross-gender identification that can be traced back as far as early childhood.

Chemical, family, and social factors have been proposed as the causes of transsexualism. The most likely cause appears to be hormonal. Transsexualism appears to be related to two syndromes of genital malformation. *Testicular feminization syndrome* occurs when a biochemical defect prevents testosterone from developing the genitals of a genetically male fetus; from birth the child is considered female. *Adrenogenital syndrome* occurs when a genetically female fetus produces large amounts of androgen so that it develops almost normal male genitals. It has been postulated that transsexualism is an incomplete testicular feminization or adrenogenital syndrome. In the male fetus, the genitals differentiate earlier. In a transsexual male, there may have been insufficient androgen to masculinize the sex-specific areas of the hypothalamus at the critical time. In a female transsexual, the androgenic influences may have been high at the critical time of hypothalamic development although not at the time of genital formation. This biological determinant theory is yet to be confirmed by research (Klein, 1978; Carrera, 1981).

Since transsexualism is a life-long characteristic, these people know that they are different very early in life. Some are fearful that they are "insane," and they do not discuss their feelings out of fear. Others may marry in hopes of adjusting to accepted standards of sexual behavior. Male transsexuals who desire relationships with heterosexual males do so not because they consider themselves homosexual but rather because they consider themselves female.

Because gender identity is fixed at a very early age for all people, the mind of the transsexual cannot be adjusted to the body; there is no evidence of cures by psychotherapy. It therefore seems appropriate to adjust the body to the mind with surgery. There are gender identity clinics at many major hospitals and universities where the transsexual can undergo medical tests to determine his health status and psychological tests to determine his emotional stability. For a period of one to two years the transsexual must live the life of the intended sex and prove that he can survive socially, financially, and emotionally in his new role. Hormone treatment is begun during this period. Anatomical males receive estrogen, which increases breast development, decreases erections and body hair, and softens the skin. Electrolysis may be used to remove unwanted facial hair, and the person may take voice training. Anatomical females receive androgen, which deepens the voice, coarsens the skin, increases body hair, causes hypertrophy of the clitoris, and stops menstruation. The transsexual continues in counseling during this phase of the treatment program.

The final phase of treatment is surgery, which merely confirms what has already occurred in the social and work life of the person. In the male-to-female transsexual, the penis is amputated and the testicles are removed. A vagina is created and is lined with skin from the penis. Breast augmentation is done, and the laryngeal cartilage may be reduced. In the female-to-male transsexual, the breasts are reduced and a hysterectomy and oophorectomy are performed. A penis is constructed using a tube flap of skin from the lower abdomen, and the clitoris is embedded in the new penis. A urinary conduit is run through the penis and a prosthesis may be implanted to allow for erections. The vaginal opening is closed, and a scrotum is fashioned from labial tissue with insertion of plastic testicles. Postoperative transsexuals are heterosexual in their orientation and are able to function sexually with partners. Both males and females maintain their orgasmic ability (Hogan, 1980). Although sex-change operations were initially greeted with enthusiasm, not all recipients of the surgery make good adjustments. Some become depressed, suicidal, or psychotic and have disruptions in their family lives (Lothestein, 1982).

After surgery the transsexual must apply to the courts for a name change and then follow through with changes in licenses, social security, and passports. Some states will issue a new birth certificate, but others will not. Insurance companies discriminate against transsexuals, and it is very difficult for them to obtain health and life insurance.

When the transsexual makes the decision to have sex-change surgery there may be a great deal of family distress. Spouses may feel bewildered, shamed, guilty, or angry. They may need counseling to work through the feelings aroused by their partner's decision. Likewise, children of the transsexual will need counseling and support, as it may be very difficult for them to comprehend the situa-

tion. It is hoped that a meaningful future relationship can be developed and that the transsexual is not castigated for his or her behavior.

SEXUAL DYSFUNCTIONS

Sexual problems can result from psychological, sociological, spiritual, or physical distress, or a combination of these sources. Sexual dysfunctions can take many forms, including decreased or increased sexual interest, inhibitions, orgasm difficulties, and problems with satisfaction.

Decreased Sexual Interest

A decrease in sexual interest can occur in one or both sexual partners. Unless there is interest in sexual activity, arousal usually will not occur even in situations of intense stimulation. However, a desire for sex can vary; it is not usually an all-or-none phenomenon. Most people can recall times of illness, fatigue, preoccupation, or anger when their interest in sex was reduced. If both partners are similarly uninterested, there is no problem in the relationship. The disparity of needs, not the frequency of sexual activity, determines whether a lack of interest is dysfunctional.

Decreased sexual interest is most frequently situational and acquired, but it may be generalized or inherent. A combination of factors may contribute to the problem. Sometimes a decrease in intimacy occurs in a long-standing relationship. People become so involved in work, childrearing, and household management that their communication often becomes shallow and goal oriented. A decrease in interdependency may lead to loss of feelings of closeness and a decreased interest in sexual interaction. A related complaint is that sex has simply become boring. Early in a relationship sexual activity involves discovery, novelty, and excitement. As relationships progress, some people feel they have explored all the alternatives and are bored with the same techniques and partner.

A change in self-perception may also precipitate decreased sexual interest. A person may believe that she has become less physically attractive with age and doesn't wish to "force herself" on her partner. The belief that older people lose interest in sex may also become a self-fulfilling prophecy. A person's self-image may be altered by illness or surgery and may produce feelings that are incompatible with sexual excitement. Likewise, a person who has been conditioned to consider the body dirty and shameful and sex as sinful may have difficulty in becoming interested in physical intimacy.

349

Situational disturbances may also interfere with sexual desire. These may include such things as loss of a job, financial worries, job dislike, or difficulties with children. The depression that often accompanies these disturbances is likely to lead to a significant decrease in sexual interest. Marital dissatisfaction is, of course, an obvious source of declining interest in sexual relations. Partners who are angry, bitter, or hurt are unlikely to want to share sexual intimacy. Any other type of sexual dysfunction may also reduce the interest of one or both partners. Since failure is emotionally painful, the person may begin to avoid activity in order to avoid failure.

Increased Sexual Interest

An increase in sexual activity and interest frequently accompanies manic episodes in persons who are subject to bipolar disorders. As the person's mood elevates, there is an increase in gregariousness and an inflation of self-esteem. The person begins to seek not only more sexual activity but also a variety of partners, with little regard for the results of this behavior. At the height of a manic episode, the person may actually experience a paradoxical decrease in sexual activity. This occurs because the person is so busy trying to seduce everyone he or she meets that there is no time to consummate any of the relationships. When the manic episode ends, the person's sexual interest and activity return to normal.

Poorly integrated sexual activity, a high number of sexual partners, and little concern for the consequences of such behavior may also occur in the person with antisocial personality disorder. It is thought by some that this type of person functions with a hypomanic mood level much of the time, which may explain the variety of partners and activities.

Inhibitions

Erectile inhibition, or the inability to achieve an erection, is caused by insufficient vasocongestion. It may be either primary (never able to maintain an erection) or secondary (presently unable) and can occur in either heterosexual or homosexual men. The term commonly applied to this condition is *impotence*, but that term is pejorative since it implies that the man is weak, powerless, and ineffectual. The term erectile inhibition is now preferred to describe erectile difficulty objectively.

Situational erectile failure is often related to fatigue, anxiety, anger, or too much alcohol. Such episodes can lead to secondary erectile failure if the man experiencing them does not accept them as normal occurrences.

Although physiological causes are uncommon, a man with erectile inhibition should be assessed for drug use, diabetes, endocrine problems, and vascular or cardiopulmonary disease. Psychological factors related to primary erectile failure may include a sexually repressed upbringing, life experiences that have decreased the man's ability to trust and love, or a traumatic failure during his first attempt at sexual intercourse. Performance anxiety and interpersonal problems may also contribute to erectile failure. A homosexual male in a heterosexual marriage may develop erectile difficulties because of the conflict between his homosexual desires and the heterosexual stipulations of marriage. Some argue that the women's liberation movement has increased the incidence of erectile failure. However, an emotionally healthy man is not threatened by a woman who is assertive and active in the lovemaking process. Most men delight in women who enjoy and accept some of the responsibility for sexual activity (Hogan, 1980).

Inhibition of vaginal lubrication, like erectile inhibition, is due to insufficient vasocongestion. Lubrication is the woman's first physiological response to sexual arousal. A variety of factors, including anger, fear, conflict, and decreased estrogen levels, may be the cause. Insufficient vaginal lubrication may cause aching, burning, and itching of the vagina during intercourse and may also cause pain for the male. It is important for women to know that vaginal lubrication naturally decreases during prolonged coitus. A water-soluble lubricant may be helpful in such cases.

Vaginismus is a strong, involuntary contraction of the muscles in the outer third of the vagina that makes penile penetration impossible. A woman does not consciously cause vaginismus. It is a conditioned, involuntary response to frightening, painful, or conflicting situations. A woman suffering from this dysfunction can learn to prevent these contractions through various relaxation techniques and behavior modification.

Orgasm Difficulties

In the past, nonorgasmic women were commonly referred to as *frigid*, but like "impotence," frigidity is an emotionally laden term that denigrates a woman's personality without specifically describing her difficulty with sexual response and enjoyment. Some women are *preorgasmic*, that is, they have never experienced orgasm by any means. Other women may be *secondarily nonorgasmic* in that they have experienced orgasm in the past or with a different partner. They may experience interest, arousal, lubrication, and enjoyment but their response stops before orgasm. Physiologically, the difficulty may be related to fatigue or to neurologic or vascular damage. A more common cause is psychogenic; it may be related to lack of knowledge, ineffective techniques, a negative attitude about sex, lack of feelings of intimacy, traumatic life events, fear of pregnancy, fear of losing control, or homosexual conflict (Hogan, 1980).

Rapid ejaculation may be defined in a variety of ways, but usually as ejaculation that is so quick that the man or his partner experience decreased enjoyment. This common male problem may be caused by anxiety, anger, or the tendency to hurry in early experiences, which has led to a conditioned response.

Ejaculatory inhibition is the inability to ejaculate during intercourse. This is a relatively rare problem and may be primary or secondary. Possible organic causes are drugs and neurologic conditions. Psychogenic explanations may be fear of causing pregnancy, guilt, interpersonal problems, or a compulsive personality that is afraid of losing control during orgasm.

Problems with Satisfaction

A person may be dissatisfied with sexual activity even though able to achieve arousal and orgasm. Disappointments about the length of time of lovemaking, the frequency of sexual activity, or the quality of satisfaction are common. The following conditions are important for a person to achieve fulfillment:

1. His or her personal rights should not be violated through the use of manipulation or force.
2. His or her experience should be compatible with his or her value system.
3. The relationship with his or her partner should be sensitive, caring, and tender rather than aggressive, competitive, or controlling.
4. He or she should be able to relate to his or her partner in a variety of ways.

Sexual health, then, is a process rather than a goal. It may be defined as the ability to relate responsibly with a partner in an intimate, fulfilling, and mutually pleasing manner that is compatible with one's chosen lifestyle.

SEXUAL DEVIANCE

In DSM-III, *paraphilia* is used to refer to deviant sexual behavior in which unusual acts or fantasies are required for sexual arousal or sexual satisfaction.

Sexual imagery often plays a part in sexual acts performed by consenting adults, but the term paraphilia is usually applied to fantasies that are acted out in some bizarre fashion. In order for sexual behaviors to be labeled deviant, psychological rather than physiological factors must play a major etiologic role. Disorders that have an organic cause may lead to psychological consequences, but they are not considered paraphilias. Transsexualism, for example, is not considered a paraphilia. The recognized forms of paraphilia include fetishism, zoophilia, pedophilia, exhibitionism, voyeurism, and necrophilia.

Fetishism

Fetishism is the achievement of sexual excitement by the substitution of an inanimate object, such as a glove or a shoe, or parts of the body, such as a lock of hair, for a sexual partner. Orgasm is achieved by fondling the fetish object, by looking at it, by masturbating onto it, or by having sexual intercourse with a partner in its presence. Usually the fetish object is associated with some childhood experience; the need for the fetish may begin in adolescence and continue into adulthood.

This extreme attachment to certain objects occurs more often in men than women, and it is possible that fears of mature genital expression may be alleviated by the symbolic meaning or reassurance conveyed by the fetish object. Many forms of fetishism are harmless; innumerable people find themselves aroused by a certain melody or aroma, for example. Other forms, however, require a nonconsenting donor who may be frightened even if not seriously harmed. Some behavioral modification programs may be helpful, and psychotherapy is sometimes recommended to explore the symbolic meaning of the fetish. The motivation of the fetishist and the possible victimization of others are crucial considerations in deciding whether treatment is indicated and what form it should take.

Zoophilia

Zoophilia is the use of animals as sexual objects or partners. It is probably more common in rural communities where people are isolated from human companionship for months at a time. Sometimes zoophilia stems from isolation and sexual frustration. When continued, the person practicing zoophilia may eventually respond sexually only to animals rather than humans. The custom is not always restricted to farm animals and their lonely keepers. Occasionally household pets may be trained to lick or rub against their human owners in a manner that generates sexual excitement and orgasm in the human partner.

352

Pedophilia

Pedophilia, or the use of children as sex objects and sex partners by adults, is quite common, although it is one of the least acceptable forms of deviance. A pedophile may be either heterosexual, bisexual, or homosexual. A bisexual or heterosexual pedophile is more likely to be attracted to prepubescent children, usually girls between the ages of eight and ten. Homosexuals usually choose older children of the same sex. It is possible for women to commit sexual abuse of male and female children, but the socialization of women for centuries has encouraged sublimation of female sexuality, which may explain why relatively few women make sexual advances to children. A number of lesbian groups have made official statements opposing the sexual exploitation of children by any adult, regardless of sexual preference (Finkelhor, 1979).

The sexual act may be limited to fondling, but penetration of a child by an adult male can be extremely traumatic, physically and psychologically, to the child. Current estimates show that ten times as many girls as boys are molested, but projected estimates indicate that if present trends continue, 25 percent of all girls born today will be molested before reaching age thirteen, and 10 percent of all boys born today will be molested in childhood by an adult (Rush, 1980).

Exhibitionism

Exhibitionism is the morbid compulsion to expose the genitals to a member of the opposite sex. Usually the exhibitionist is a male who wishes to affirm his manhood by startling the viewer. The exhibitionist rarely represents a genuine danger to others. This behavior is repetitive and compulsive; the exhibitionist frequently returns to the same neighborhood, exposes his genitals, and, by witnessing the fear of his audience, may become aroused and orgasmic. Exhibitionists are often apprehended because they repeat their behavior in the same vicinity.

Treatment is mandated by the courts. Often exhibitionists suffer from a deep sense of inadequacy. Their prognosis for change is only fair. As with most forms of sexual deviance, motivation to change is a significant factor in recovery.

Voyeurism

Voyeurism is the practice of obtaining sexual gratification by observing persons who are naked, disrobing, or engaging in sexual acts. A certain amount of voyeurism is present in almost everyone, and the books we read, the films we see, and the magazines we buy testify to this human tendency. Many voyeurs look but do not seek out sexual contact with the person or persons they observe. The voyeur may engage in masturbation while watching and derive satisfaction in this fashion. Sometimes the mere knowledge that the person being observed would feel humiliated if the presence of a "peeping Tom" were disclosed is in itself satisfying enough for the voyeur.

Necrophilia

There is a great deal of mythology surrounding *necrophilia*, or "love of the dead." Although no longer included in the list of paraphilias, this term is sometimes still used. For example, claims were made by both sides in the Viet Nam War that dead bodies were defiled sexually. It is also possible that necrophilia is a factor in crimes that involve murder and sexual mutilation, but it is difficult to find reliable, objective data.

SEXUAL ABUSE

Sexual abuse may be defined broadly as any act of a sexual nature that harms someone. The act can involve either verbal or physical mistreatment, and the person hurt may or may not consent to the abuse. Forms of sexual abuse include sadomasochism, incest, and sexual harassment.

Sadomasochism

The term *sadism* is derived from the name of the eighteenth-century French writer the Marquis de Sade, while the term *masochism* comes from the name of the nineteenth-century Austrian writer Leopold von Sacher-Masoch. DSM-III defines *sexual sadism* as the "infliction of physical or psychological suffering on another person in order to achieve sexual excitement." The behavior may occur with a consenting or nonconsenting partner. Sexual masochism is defined by DSM-III as "sexual excitement produced in an individual by his or her own suffering." *Sadomasochism* is a paradoxical combination of pain and pleasure. The pain may be verbal (abusive language, threatening, humiliation) or physical (hitting, slapping, whipping). Both sadism and masochism tend to be chronic behaviors. Some people stay at the same level of activity; others need to gradually escalate the behavior to achieve sexual excitement.

Sadomasochistic activity is not the same as the nibbling and biting that some couples do in the height of sexual excitement. Such acts are not deliberate attempts to create pain or humiliation. People who have sadomasochistic fantasies that they do not act out are not considered sadomasochists.

Sadomasochistic activity may range from mild inclinations to extreme forms. Bondage and discipline are usually mild forms that use various types of restraint and verbal humiliation. Bondage is frequently symbolic rather than real, and pain is not usually a component of the act. It may be playful and harmless if done carefully and with a consenting partner. Sadomasochism becomes a deviance when inflicting or experiencing pain becomes a substitute for or the main source of pleasure during sexual activity. It is the exclusive mode of sexual functioning for some people. At the extreme end of the continuum is the sexual sadist who inflicts extensive and possibly fatal injury on a nonconsenting person. A person with this severe disorder may rape, torture, and even kill victims.

It appears that there are fewer sadists than there are masochists, but generally one does not exclude the other and a person is likely to alternate between the two variations. Some sadomasochists believe that somehow it is better to be punished than to impose pain, and they are even willing to pay people to inflict pain on them. Both heterosexual and homosexual people engage in sadomasochism, although one study showed that 90 percent of sadomasochistic activity is among heterosexual persons (Carrera, 1981).

The causes of sadomasochism are not understood. One theory is that the sadistic person may have been taught as a child to loathe anything sexual. The guilt aroused during sexual activity is thought to be projected onto the partner so that the sadist is able to experience pleasure. The masochist is thought to believe that sex is sinful. To relieve guilt over any pleasure she may feel, she inflicts punishment on herself. Another theory is that the sadist suffers from feelings of inferiority that are alleviated by inflicting pain on others. The masochist may act out feelings of insignificance and dependency. Some theorists believe that sadomasochistic activity is a replaying of childhood trauma. Violent sexual activity may also be a way of indirectly acting out anger. For some, it tends to be an exaggeration of traditional sex roles and allows the person to give up responsibility for his acts during

353

sex. For others, it is a means of pretending to be a different person, for example, a powerful, successful man who can humiliate a "slave." Yet others may find sadomasochism alluring because it is unconventional.

Pain is not the main goal of sexual sadomasochism but rather a part of the drama, which may be structured or unstructured. The pain is usually controlled enough that it does not interfere with erotic feelings. It is believed that the muscle tension that accompanies the suspense increases sexual arousal. Most sadomasochistic people choose a trusted partner who will play the sadist's role within mutually agreed-upon limits. A partner who turns out to really enjoy sadistic acting out could become very dangerous. Some prostitutes offer sexual theater as a specialty. The drama includes not only a "script" but also various props such as blindfolds, restraints, handcuffs, collars, diapers, and whips. Sadomasochism is becoming more open, and there are special clubs, bars, and magazines available for interested people.

Incest

Incest, or sexual relations among family members, is the most common form of sexual abuse of children. It may occur between siblings, or with parents, grandparents, uncles, or aunts. Incestuous activity can range from caressing and fondling to masturbation, oral sex, and intercourse. Today, incest is an almost universal taboo, but in the past it was condoned among royal or rich families in some cultures as a way to conserve power and wealth. In the United States incest is illegal in every state.

It is difficult to determine the incidence of incest because fear of punishment, cultural inhibitions, and shame and guilt help hide the problem. It is also difficult for professionals to recognize the incestuous family. One study revealed that 7.7 percent of the women and 4.8 percent of the men queried had been involved in incest as children. Contrary to popular expectations, most of the boys had been molested by females, not by homosexual males (Crooks and Baur, 1983). Incest occurs in all socioeconomic classes and is usually ongoing rather than a one-time event. Father-daughter incest is most commonly reported and the best understood. Brother-sister incest is the most frequent type, but it is seldom discovered. Some professionals believe that brother-sister incest is the least damaging form because it is usually transitory and generally a form of experimentation rather than exploitation. Mother-son, father-son, and mother-daughter sexual interactions have not been well studied. The strongest cultural taboo is against mother-son relationships, and these are the least commonly reported (Schlesinger, 1982).

Incest between a father and daughter usually begins before the child understands the meaning of the acts. It may start with playful romping and progress to genital touching, oral or manual stimulation, and intercourse. The father tends to avoid emotional attachments with adults; he may abuse alcohol, and he may have been sexually molested as a child himself.

Sexual abuse of children is a symptom of a dysfunctional family (Janosik, 1984). It is a misguided attempt to preserve the continuity of the family. The family tends to be either a closed system with few outside relationships or a loosely organized system that has not accepted the taboo against incest. Five family factors promote the breakdown of the incest barrier:

1. A confused role development and distortion where the daughter replaces the mother as the central female figure and substitute wife.

2. Sexual dissatisfaction between the parents. This may be accompanied by severe marital conflict and spouse abuse.

3. The father doesn't seek a sexual partner outside of the home as a way of maintaining a stable family facade.

4. The entire family fears disintegration and is willing to go to extreme lengths to protect and maintain the family.

5. An unconscious sanction by the nonparticipant mother. She may not "notice" the incest or may deliberately go out and leave the father and daughter alone. This covert sanction is of key importance in the development of incest. The mother usually remains quiet because of shame, fear of reprisals by her husband, fear of her husband going to jail, or fear that she might have to resume sexual relations with her husband if the situation is discovered.

Various forms of coercion may be used against the child. The father may tell the daughter that he is teaching her, that he is doing something good for her, or that he is expressing his love for her. Bribery and pressure are other tactics to maintain secrecy. The child may be told that it will be her fault if other people find out and bad things happen to the family. Threats such as "Daddy would go to jail," "Mommy will get upset and sick," or "You will be taken away from us" may be used. With such pressure, the child feels isolated and afraid to tell anyone for fear of being blamed, punished, or disbelieved. Later, it may be difficult for the child to break a well-established pattern of incest with the father.

Incest is emotionally damaging to both parties according to all available data. It has a negative

354

effect on family relationships while binding the individual members together in a secret coalition that restricts other social relationships. Girls suffer from decreased self-image, guilt, shame, anger, and a sense of alienation from others. They may have difficulty in forming intimate adult relationships. Boys suffer from anxiety, guilt, and depression. Parents feel guilt and face criminal action, humiliation, and the risk of family disintegration (Carrera, 1981; Crooks and Baur, 1983).

The strong cultural taboo against incest does not prevent its occurrence but hinders its recognition and treatment. Treatment for incest should consist of an in-depth family evaluation and, if possible, family therapy from a systems perspective. Strong modeling of parental roles should also be a part of the therapy. The victims need education about sex and their own sexuality to alleviate their sense of guilt. A self-help group called Parents United has been established in some parts of the country for individuals and families who have experienced child sexual molestation in any form. A division of this group for children between the ages of five and eighteen is known as Daughters and Sons United.

Sexual Harassment

Sexual harassment is often a subtle but very real form of sexual abuse. A research and resource center, Working Women United Institute, defines it as any form of unwanted attention of a sexual nature from someone in the workplace that creates discomfort or interferes with the victim's job performance. It is a very common problem. One survey of 9,000 women reported a harassment rate of 88 percent. When 17,000 federal employees were questioned about sexual harassment, 42 percent of the women and 15 percent of the men said they had been victims of this abuse (Crooks and Baur, 1983).

Legally, harassment may be either verbal or physical. A person may be subjected to obscenities or made the target of sexual jokes. Some victims are expected to perform sexual acts for their superior or for customers. If the person does not comply she may risk losing a promotion, receiving a demotion, receiving a decrease in pay, having her vacation preferences denied, getting fired, or receiving poor references. Some people are too intimidated to reject unwanted advances, some try to ignore them, and some try to refuse politely. Those who cannot afford to risk losing their jobs, fear peer's responses, or fear being labeled a troublemaker may acquiesce. The emotional harm to the victim can be serious. She may feel embarrassed, degraded, helpless, humiliated, angry, and even guilty (if she feels somehow at fault). Stress-related illnesses may even develop (Strong and Reynolds, 1982).

Sexual harassment is a serious problem that is finally being brought out into the open and being dealt with in the courts (Strong and Reynolds, 1982). Companies can be held liable for sexual harassment that occurs at the workplace. Large monetary payments have been awarded through the judicial system for victims of sexual harassment (Crooks and Baur, 1983). A good initial stategy is for the victim to tell the abuser that his behavior is harassment and that it will not be tolerated. Usually there is an in-company protocol for filing a complaint. A complaint may also be filed with the Human Rights Commission or with the Equal Employment Opportunity Commission. If actual or attempted rape has occurred criminal charges may be filed.

COUNSELING

355

Whether sexual problems are the main reason for seeking the help of a psychiatric mental health nurse or whether such problems are discovered only in the course of therapy, premarital, marital, and sexual counseling often fall within the scope of a nurse's clinical practice.

Premarital Counseling

When couples marry they frequently experience a conflict in expectations about the "right" roles for men, women, husbands, wives, parents, and children. These expectations have been absorbed unconsciously in the family of origin and determine how people feel and behave and how they expect their mate to feel and behave. The greater the discrepancy between the expectations of the parties, the less likely each is to have his needs met, and the more likely the anger, frustration, and conflict between them will undermine their intimacy. One task of a couple who seeks premarital counseling is to integrate two designs for family living, two sets of expectations for the relationship, and two dreams for the future into a healthy marriage in which both people are able to cope constructively with their differences. If couples are unable to do so, each person will attempt to reform the other, an approach that is doomed to fail.

Modern life in this country requires that an adult be assertive, independent, and self-reliant, but the traditional concept of femininity has made many women unable to behave in these ways. On the other hand, an adult is also required to be able to relate to other people, to be sensitive to their needs and concerned about their welfare, and to be able to depend on them for emotional support. Frequently, the traditional concept of masculinity keeps men

Figure 13-4. *Role assessment tool.*

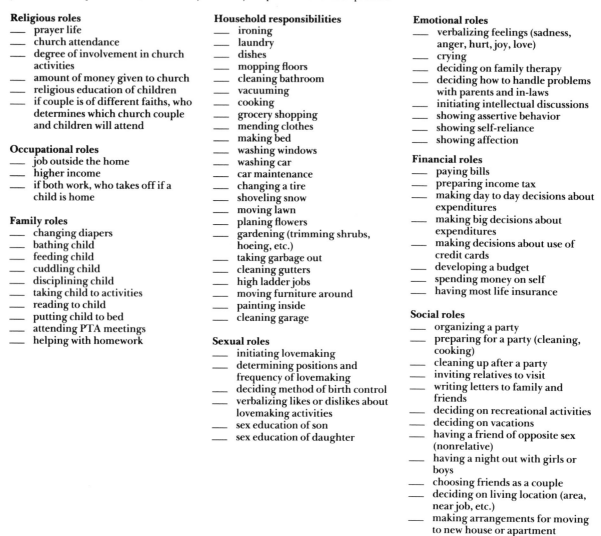

Please indicate on the line if you believe: the husband (H) should have the major responsibility for the area or job; the wife (W) should have the major responsibility for the area or job; or they both (B) should share the area or job equally. Please answer according to your beliefs and preferences, NOT what you think your partner believes or prefers.

Religious roles
___ prayer life
___ church attendance
___ degree of involvement in church activities
___ amount of money given to church
___ religious education of children
___ if couple is of different faiths, who determines which church couple and children will attend

Occupational roles
___ job outside the home
___ higher income
___ if both work, who takes off if a child is home

Family roles
___ changing diapers
___ bathing child
___ feeding child
___ cuddling child
___ disciplining child
___ taking child to activities
___ reading to child
___ putting child to bed
___ attending PTA meetings
___ helping with homework

Household responsibilities
___ ironing
___ laundry
___ dishes
___ mopping floors
___ cleaning bathroom
___ vacuuming
___ cooking
___ grocery shopping
___ mending clothes
___ making bed
___ washing windows
___ washing car
___ car maintenance
___ changing a tire
___ shoveling snow
___ moving lawn
___ planing flowers
___ gardening (trimming shrubs, hoeing, etc.)
___ taking garbage out
___ cleaning gutters
___ high ladder jobs
___ moving furniture around
___ painting inside
___ cleaning garage

Sexual roles
___ initiating lovemaking
___ determining positions and frequency of lovemaking
___ deciding method of birth control
___ verbalizing likes or dislikes about lovemaking activities
___ sex education of son
___ sex education of daughter

Emotional roles
___ verbalizing feelings (sadness, anger, hurt, joy, love)
___ crying
___ deciding on family therapy
___ deciding how to handle problems with parents and in-laws
___ initiating intellectual discussions
___ showing assertive behavior
___ showing self-reliance
___ showing affection

Financial roles
___ paying bills
___ preparing income tax
___ making day to day decisions about expenditures
___ making big decisions about expenditures
___ making decisions about use of credit cards
___ developing a budget
___ spending money on self
___ having most life insurance

Social roles
___ organizing a party
___ preparing for a party (cleaning, cooking)
___ cleaning up after a party
___ inviting relatives to visit
___ writing letters to family and friends
___ deciding on recreational activities
___ deciding on vacations
___ having a friend of opposite sex (nonrelative)
___ having a night out with girls or boys
___ choosing friends as a couple
___ deciding on living location (area, near job, etc.)
___ making arrangements for moving to new house or apartment

from responding in such "feminine" ways. Men are expected to be competent, aggressive, logical, emotionally unexpressive, insensitive to the feelings of others, interested in math and science, and not very talkative. Women are expected to be the opposite: helpless, unaggressive, intuitive, emotionally expressive, sensitive to others' feelings, uninterested in math and science, and talkative. These stereotypes limit both men and women. Couples may be constrained by roles that neither person really wants yet each has difficulty changing. Sex role stereotyping may make it difficult even in an intimate relationship to relate to a partner as a human being rather than as a role player. However, some couples find traditional sex roles comfortable and

useful because they allow the couple to avoid conflict.

Counseling may be needed in those cases where rigid gender role expectations block the couple's growth and their ability to be intimate with each other. In premarital counseling, *androgyny* is presented as flexibility in gender role and the acceptance of those positive human qualities that legitimately belong in the repertoire of both men and women. Karen Fontaine of Purdue University has developed a role assessment tool to be used during premarital counseling sessions (see Figure 13-4). Each partner receives a checklist and independently identifies who should be usually responsible for each behavior. Each person also stars those items that he or she would not be willing to do except under extraordinary circumstances. The partners then compare lists and discuss which expectations have been placed on them because of their gender, which they accept or defy, and which areas are likely to cause conflict between them. This tool is helpful in prompting discussion in areas that might cause problems later on. At six months and at one year after the marriage, the couple should be encouraged to recheck the lists and assess how the relationship has developed in terms of role expectations and identify any new problems that need to be solved.

Communication is a key factor in a successful, creative sexual relationship. Premarital counseling should include both sexual and nonsexual forms of communication. Many people find it difficult to reveal their inner feelings to others, especially concerning emotions and deeply held beliefs. For some it is not easy to verbally express love, intimacy, or even concern. In a sexual relationship such expressions count almost as much as physical contact. Whereas communication about sexuality has generally become more open over the past two or three decades, the intimate sexual communication of most couples has not followed suit.

Most couples develop nonverbal signals that indicate their interest in sexual activity. This is appropriate if the signals are clearly understood by each partner, but ambiguous signals can lead to hurt feelings and unmet expectations. An example of unclear signals is provided by a woman who was unable to tell her husband directly that she was interested in making love, so she would take a shower whenever she wanted sexual contact. Almost every time she took a shower her husband went into the bedroom expecting her to be sexually receptive, but discord arose whenever she took a shower for cleanliness. When the couple realized how ambiguous the signal was, they decided to state more clearly to each other their needs and expectations. It is equally important to establish clear signals when sexual activity is not desired. Many people interpret their partners' refusal to have sex as a personal rejection. They can easily accept their partners' refusal to eat out or go to a movie but not a refusal to have sex. Couples need to communicate openly and honestly so that a negative response is seen merely as a refusal at that particular time.

Many people also expect their partners to intuitively perceive their needs and desires, especially during sexual activity. This unrealistic expectation may be expressed in many ways: "If she doesn't know what I want, then she must be insensitive," "If he loved me, he would know what I want," and "If I have to ask for something, it detracts from my pleasure." Often a person does to his partner what he wishes to have done to him. Such means of indirect

communication usually fail. In premarital counseling couples can be taught how to diplomatically assert their needs. Couples should be taught to avoid "you" language, which evokes a defensive response and leads to arguments (Satir, 1967; Watzlawick, Beauvin, and Jackson, 1967). The recipient of a "you" statement feels accused, inadequate, and guilty. As she tries to defend herself the argument becomes a win-lose situation. Whoever wins the quarrel, the relationship always loses, and the power struggle escalates. To prevent such a situation, the couple should be advised to use "I" language, in which each person relates his or her own thoughts, feelings, and beliefs. The following are some examples of responsible "I" statements and accusatory "you" statements.

"I" language
"I am really too tired to make love tonight but I enjoy your interest in me."

"I miss all the little hugs and caresses we used to do spontaneously."

"I would like you to rub my clitoris more gently."

"I am unhappy with the way our sexual life is going."

"You" language
"You always wait until I'm too tired to approach me sexually."

"You only touch me when you want sex."

"You clumsy oaf—that hurts!"

"What you need is a sex therapist."

Learning to recognize and identify one's own feelings is not always an easy process. Individuals should assume responsibility for their own feelings and be supportive of each other as their communication skills improve. It takes time and practice before a person can satisfactorily express his or her sexual feelings and requests. If this process can begin early in the relationship, the couple will receive more pleasure and enjoyment throughout their sexual relationship.

Marital Counseling
Marital counseling focuses on promoting the growth of a relationship by broadening and deepening a couple's marital interaction. The counselor can help the couple define issues and establish goals in behavioral terms by asking questions such as: "What behaviors of yours and your partner's need to be changed in order for this relationship to work out?" or "Give me a word picture of what you will be like as a couple when your relationship has im-

357

proved." The goals, or expected outcomes, are written down and revised as assessment and intervention continue. The couple is viewed as a system and counseling as a joint effort to help them find meaningful, cooperative interdependence.

Part of the helping process consists of helping a couple clarify their attitudes toward each other and their problems. The counselor should identify any self-destructive attitudes, such as anxiety, anger, guilt, resentment, or fear of failure. At the same time, the counselor should identify positive attitudes such as good self-esteem, joy, creativity, and openness to change. Attitudes are learned in interactions with other people, and therefore they are open to modification.

As the counseling proceeds, past events should be analyzed in context. Individuals adapt in order to protect themselves. Couples should not be asked why they behaved as they did but rather where, with whom, under what circumstances an event occurred, and how it affected the other person. As each individual begins to understand the process of their interactions, he also begins to see how a situation is perceived by the other person. With this understanding a couple can seek alternative actions to solve relationship problems.

As in premarital counseling, marital counseling should address the questions of sex role stereotyping, unspoken expectations, and identification and expression of feelings. The couple may need to learn assertiveness techniques, such as the use of "No" and "I" language to express needs, wants, and feelings. Male-female co-therapy teams can be very effective in modeling the suggested behaviors.

Marital counseling is an opportunity for the growth of both the individuals and the relationship. It is not an easy cure but rather hard work for both persons. Their reward is the development of more effective relating skills, which will serve them in good stead when future difficulties arise.

Sexual Counseling

Sexual dysfunctions are considered shared disorders, and the relationship, not the individual presenting with the symptom, should be the focus of attention in sexual counseling. There are many possible causes of sexual problems, from merely an absence of sexual happiness to severe distress in the marital system. Some couples are able to get along sexually but not in any other context of their relationship.

Most typically, sexual counseling is done with a male-female therapy team, which enables the therapists to serve as models for effective and mutually satisfying relationships. Modeling is especially effective for people who grew up without marriage models or whose models were maladaptive. The ex-

amples of support and freedom the co-therapists demonstrate may teach a couple far more about interpersonal relations than what they actually say. A female-male team also permits the therapists to serve symbolically as gender role models for the couple.

The initial one or two sessions should consist of data collection and assessment of the identified problem. Complete sex histories and complete medical histories should be obtained. If an organic problem is suspected, the client should be referred to his or her physician for a complete physical examination. Frequently the counselor will recommend books from which clients can learn new sexual techniques. Couples should also be assured that masturbation and fantasy are normal sexual practices. The aim of counseling is not to change clients' value systems but rather to have clients explore the source and the validity of their value systems.

Sexual counseling should help promote both insight into behavior and behavioral change. Many people consider the ability to perform sexually as a mark of their manhood or womanhood and thus create a great deal of performance anxiety. One of the goals of counseling is to redefine the purpose of sexual activity as a way of giving and receiving pleasure. Negative attitudes toward sex, ambiguous methods of communication, and behaviors that are destructive to the sexual relationship should all be discussed. Couples should be encouraged to learn to recognize the positive rather than just focus on the negative in their interactions.

Homework may be assigned at each session to help the clients analyze their interactions, identify problem areas, and take responsibility for changing their own behavior outside the therapeutic relationship. Such assignments require that the couple cooperate and share their thoughts. Each should be instructed to seek to understand his or her partner's needs, preferences, and moods.

The homework usually consists of a process called *sensate focusing*, which helps the partners learn to give and receive pleasure by touching (Kaplan, 1974). In the beginning there is a ban on breast and genital touching and on intercourse. These restrictions free a couple from fear of failure and allow them to direct all their attention to the pleasure of touching. The exercise redefines the meaning of touching. It becomes not a demand for intercourse but an expression of affection and an opportunity to learn about oneself and one's partner.

The couple is instructed to spend 30 minutes a day doing the sensate focus homework at a time when they are not tired, angry, or anxious. During the first week many couples are surprised to discover that they seldom spend time alone together because of the many interruptions they allow to in-

Figure 13-5. Example of a homework sheet for recording sensate focusing activities.

Sensate Focus Homework Sheet

Name _____ Date _____ 1 2 3 4 5 6 7 week (circle one)

Make your comments in "I" language. Record your *own* reactions and observations about your spouse: negative, positive, questions, thoughts, etc. Be specific about the activity, for example, "touching face." Report each time sensate exchange took place.

Day	Activity done to me	Enjoyment on a scale of 1–10	Sexual arousal on a scale of 1–10	Comments	Day	Activity done to me	Enjoyment on a scale of 1–10	Sexual arousal on a scale of 1–10	Comments

trude. They are encouraged to make the time for each other, because the more frequently they practice, the more quickly their sexual relationship will improve. One partner gives and one receives pleasure for 15 minutes, and then they switch the roles for another 15 minutes. Giving and receiving simultaneously is discouraged because a person cannot fully enjoy either experience when he or she is trying to concentrate on both processes at the same time. Initially, some people are uncomfortable in the passive role, but as they learn that they have a right to pleasure, this discomfort eases.

The giver is instructed to hold, kiss, stroke, and massage the partner's entire body in order to learn what is pleasurable and arousing to the other person. He or she is asked to experiment with various types of touch and to focus on his or her own feelings during the touching. The receiver is instructed to relax and enjoy the experience and pay attention to his or her own feelings of pleasure and arousal. The receiver should tell the partner which kinds of touch are not enjoyed and which kinds he or she would like to have done during the exercise. Communication, through words and sounds, is ex-

tremely important because one's own arousal depends greatly on seeing and hearing one's partner becoming aroused. "I" language is encouraged as the preferred mode of communication.

The couple is also encouraged to experiment with massage oil, powder, lotions, or touching in the shower because these all give different sensations. It is important to "touch" the partner's mind by expressing caring and affection before touching the body in order to involve the whole person in lovemaking. The couple is encouraged to cultivate all five senses by using loving words, sensual whispers, music, the sound of a crackling fire in the fireplace, suggestive movements, sensual clothes, dim or colored lights, a favorite meal, a glass of wine, a favorite perfume. As couples experiment, they find that their sex life becomes less boring and more pleasurable.

Each person is directed to complete a homework sheet after the exercise and not to share the sheet with each other until the next counseling session. On these sheets they rate only their own enjoyment and arousal in both giving and receiving, not what they think their partner felt (see Figure 13-5).

The more specific they can be in their descriptions and comments, the more helpful the information will be to each partner and to the counselors in revealing strengths and identifying problems.

As the couple progresses, they move to breast and genital touching, and finally to sexual intercourse. Throughout each stage total body touching remains a part of lovemaking. About the third or fourth week, each partner is asked to choose a day when he or she will plan a surprise sensual or erotic evening for the partner. This could involve such things as moving the stereo into the bedroom, having the children out of the house, having a candlelight dinner, buying a vibrator, burning incense, going out for dinner and dancing, or whatever each thinks the other might enjoy.

Sexual therapy tends to be short-term therapy unless there is severe marital distress causing the sexual dysfunction. If that is the case, the marital issues need to be dealt with either first or concurrently with the sexual problems. Depending on the presenting dysfunction, other techniques are taught to the couple, such as squeezing the penis to prevent rapid ejaculation or self-stimulation to help the preorgasmic woman achieve climax. Detailed description of these methods can be found in many textbooks on sexual therapy.

THE NURSING PROCESS IN SEXUAL HEALTH CARE

Sexual health care is an important component of holistic nursing. As with other types of health care, the delivery of sexual health care should be based on the nursing process. First, the nurse must assess her (or his) own beliefs, values, and attitudes that affect how she deals with people. In particular, the nurse should assess her values and biases about human sexuality and make sure she does not project them onto her clients in her professional practice. She should remember that clients have the right to determine their own values and views.

Another aspect of self-assessment is the examination of one's professional practice. A question the nurse might ask is, "Do I deny, inhibit, or allow for the sexuality of my clients?" The nurse must consider whether the topic of sex is incorporated in the history taking and in client teaching. Even in the face of peer disapproval, has the nurse been able to function as a client advocate about sexual issues? Have appropriate referrals been made for clients suffering from sexual problems? In conjunction with this, it is important to develop an awareness of how one is perceived by others. If the nurse realizes that few or no clients discuss sexual concerns during nursing interactions, the next question is, "Do the clients I come in contact with have no or few sexual questions, or am I sending nonverbal messages that discourage people from discussing these issues with me?" The nurse should then evaluate how comfortable she is in discussing sexual concerns with clients. Most clients quickly perceive a nurse's discomfort and react accordingly. In order to confer with a client on the topic of sexuality the nurse must undergo a desensitization and resensitization process, discarding her own hangups and becoming sensitive to the client's feelings. This new sensitivity will help prevent hasty and judgmental responses to clients.

The nurse should appraise the extent of her knowledge of sexual physiology and psychology throughout the life cycle. Confidence in doing sexual counseling, as in all other kinds of counseling, is based on a thorough knowledge of the subject. It is very important that the nurse not convey incorrect information, misconceptions, and stereotypic values to her clients.

Interpersonal communication skills are important threads throughout the nursing process. Good interviewing skills and the ability to talk openly and nonjudgmentally about sex should be cultivated. Creating a comfortable atmosphere is essential; the nurse who is embarrassed or anxious only augments these reactions in the client. Managing one's own feelings and responding appropriately to those of the client are essential to good nursing practice.

The nursing process begins with the collection of data necessary for determining the sexual health status of a client. These data should include a physical assessment, a general sexual history, medical diagnosis, laboratory tests, and previous treatment regimens. A detailed sexual history is not appropriate unless it is indicated by the other data. The nurse needs to recognize that any alteration in a person's physical or emotional state may affect various aspects of his life pattern—including sexual activity. The nurse must refrain from making assumptions that will distort the process of gathering data, such as that all clients are heterosexual, that married clients are sexually active, and that single clients, especially older people, are sexually inactive.

The next step in the nursing process is the interpretation of the data to formulate a nursing diagnosis. Some of the possible nursing diagnoses are listed in the accompanying box.

Once the nursing diagnoses have been formulated, the nurse can help the couple formulate measurable expected outcomes or goals. This process should include the couple lest the nurse impose his own biases and expectations on the pair.

The nurse's role as teacher is very important

POSSIBLE NURSING DIAGNOSES FOR SEXUAL PROBLEMS

Fear related to returning to sexual activity after recent myocardial infarction or other medical problem.

Anxiety related to unrealistic performance expectations.

Knowledge deficit of sexual physiology.

Ineffective family coping related to unresolved anger between the couple.

Ineffective individual coping related to past history of incest.

Disturbance in self-concept or body image related to body and coital shame.

Disturbance in self-concept or self-esteem related to ego-dystonic homosexuality.

Disturbance in self-concept or role performance related to disparate gender role expectations of husband and wife.

Disturbance in self-concept or personal identity related to transsexualism.

Alterations in patterns of sexuality, such as organic erectile failure, related to colostomy or other surgical procedure.

Alterations in patterns of sexuality, such as retrograde ejaculations, related to neuropathy of diabetes or other chronic illness.

Alterations in patterns of sexuality, such as rapid ejaculation, related to a conditioned response.

Alterations in patterns of sexuality, such as nonorgasmic response, related to lack of knowledge of sexual anatomy and physiology.

---

when dealing with clients' sexual concerns and needs. Many problems can be solved simply with accurate information. The nurse should also be prepared to counsel the client in how to utilize new knowledge to develop a satisfactory and accountable life style. The sexual effects of medications and disease changes and alternate modes of sexual activity are among the most important in nurse teaching. The nurse must also be able to support the couple as they struggle with making adaptive changes. A nurse should have additional education and supervision in order to be able to intervene in the advanced level of sexual therapy. If a client is in need of sexual therapy and the nurse is not competent in

this area, she should refer him to an appropriate professional.

Nurses may also function at the primary level of prevention by teaching sex education in schools, in classes for adults, or with groups of adolescents who are struggling with sexual questions and values. Interventions may also take the form of client advocacy, such as removing the barriers to sexual expression in nursing homes and long-term care facilities.

Evaluations of nursing interventions in sexual health care should be based on how well the expected outcomes were achieved. If the outcomes were not met, the nurse must determine which step or steps of the nursing process must be modified in order to most effectively assist the client.

SUMMARY

Understanding and responding positively to human sexuality is essential to offering holistic health care, but there is no other aspect of human experience that is so subject to conflict. Through negative social conditioning, women are often taught to regard their sexual organs as unclean, while men often learn to equate sexual performance with competence and mastery in other areas of life. Nurses need to acquire accurate information about male and female sexuality in all its variations, to develop an awareness of their own values and to avoid making moralistic judgments of attitudes unlike their own.

Social and cultural variables have considerable influence in determining people's sexual expectations and in perpetuating myths about male and

CLINICAL EXAMPLE

SEXUAL DYSFUNCTION IN A MIDDLE-AGED COUPLE

Mary and Bill Wilson were referred for sexual therapy from an alcohol rehabilitation program, with the chief complaints of secondary erectile failure and disparity of sexual desire. They are a couple in their early fifties, married for twenty-four years, with five children ranging in age from fourteen to twenty-three. Both Bill and Mary are intellectual, articulate, and well-educated professionals. At the initiation of treatment, Bill, the alcoholic spouse, had been sober for four months and was active in Alcoholics Anonymous. Mary had been active in Alanon for two years. Bill's alcoholism had never seriously interfered with his work nor had he ever become abusive or neglectful with his family.

ASSESSMENT

When Mary was ten years old, her father deserted the family. Her mother took a job outside of the home, and Mary was left in charge of her two younger sisters. She described her home life as very happy in spite of the fact that she had to "grow up rapidly." Her family was both verbally and physically expressive, and sex was openly discussed. As an adult, Mary believed that she had to be the perfect wife and mother at the expense of meeting her own needs. She had difficulty in doing good things for herself and in expressing anger, as these did not fit her self-image as "super-wife/mother." She was able to express other emotions easily. One of her chief complaints was that she had had a greater interest in sex than Bill throughout the marriage and that she believed that she usually had to initiate sexual activity. She stated that she felt hurt and rejected when Bill refused sexual interaction.

Bill had three siblings, a younger brother and two younger sisters. His family of origin was not demonstrative either verbally or physically. Neither feelings nor sex were openly discussed. As an adult, Bill was emotionally stunted in his development. His intellectual capacities had served him well in most areas of life, but not in the relational area. He had compulsive traits, which were his way of defending himself against chaos and loss of control. Whenever he felt anger he suppressed it by telling himself, "It serves no good purpose to respond with anger. I would rather talk it out logically." Bill also did not recognize his dependency needs. He had always seen himself as the "rock of the family," a person who was strong and in control. Other than one time when he had decided to enter the alcohol treatment program, he stated that he could not remember ever having cried.

Both Mary and Bill used a great deal of "you" language during the initial session. Statements were made such as "You never initiate sex," "You are the one with the problem," "You think you don't have any problems," and "You read too much psychology stuff." Before entering therapy, both Bill and Mary were aware that the secondary erectile failure might have an organic basis related to the toxic effects of alcohol.

The following diagnoses were made:

Nursing Diagnoses
Knowledge deficit—Sexual physiology and psychology

Verbal communication, impaired

Coping, ineffective family

Anxiety (moderate, regarding performance expectations)

Self-concept, disturbance in (Bill's role performance)

Self-concept, disturbance in (Mary's self-esteem)

Sexual dysfunction

Multiaxial Psychiatric Diagnoses
Axis I   V61.10 Marital problem
          302.72 Inhibited sexual excitement

Axis II   None

Axis III None

Axis IV   Level 2—Minimal

Axis V   Code 2—Very good

PLANNING

Based on the clinical presentation of Bill and Mary, plans were made for couple counseling sessions to explore the issues of their sexual difficulties, with an emphasis on communications techniques. Both needed education about normal sexual response and a better awareness of their own sexual expectations. They needed assistance in expressing their thoughts and feelings about sexual issues and in learning to use "I" statements rather than "you" language.

IMPLEMENTATION

During the sessions, Bill and Mary were given reading assignments, and discussions were held about the physiology of sexual response. The counselor helped them to identify their own bodies' responses and to express their expectations about sex. With the help of the nurse, they analyzed the ways in which unspoken expectations led to disappointments and hurt feelings, and they were instructed to share one expectation a day with each other. The nurse expressed support of Bill and Mary's interest in changing the relationship.

The use of "I" instead of "you" language was taught in the sessions by the identification of "you" language and by the practice of restating expressions in "I" language. The nurse modeled both types of expression and discussed ways in which the pain caused by "you" language can lead to defensive behavior.

Some of the sessions were devoted to discussions of the importance of touch, particularly how touching was regarded in both their families of origin and how the expectation that touching would lead to intercourse increased anxiety and decreased the frequency of physical contact. Mary practiced asking Bill to simply hold her, using "I" language. Both of them were taught how to say "no" in an acceptable manner without feeling guilty.

Gradually, Bill and Mary were taught sensate focus and progressed through the various stages to help them redefine the purpose of their sexual activity as a way of giving and receiving pleasure. The nurse also helped them discuss their personal fears about the expression of angry feelings. They began to realize that avoiding con-

flict created a situation where anger might be expressed in other ways, such as erectile failure or alcohol abuse.

EVALUATION

Bill and Mary stated that the reading assignments were helpful in teaching them about sexual functioning and in prompting discussions about sexuality. Bill was able to articulate that his sexual desire decreased when there was a lot of stress at work. Mary was able to acknowledge that at such times her requests for sex must have felt like more work to Bill. At the end of therapy, they were continuing to seek alternative ways to meet both their needs.

At the beginning of therapy, both had expressed the belief that they spent a great deal of time together. By the second week, they had discovered that very little of this time was "private" time, and they decided to restructure some family activities and make "dates" with each other.

Bill and Mary were typical of many couples in that they had minimal communication about sexual activity at the beginning of therapy. They gradually learned to share their expectations prior to interacting sexually, and they learned to extend this skill to other areas of their lives, such as discussing expectations for leisure activities. They learned how to compromise on those issues and therefore experienced fewer hurt feelings related to unmet needs.

Bill and Mary were able to reframe the expression of their thoughts and feelings into "I" language, first during their sexual interactions and later in other areas of interaction.

Prior to therapy, Mary had been minimally verbal during lovemaking and Bill had been the silent partner. At first during sensate focus he was uncomfortable with talking and making pleasurable noises. He became more comfortable when he discovered that his communication was sexually stimulating to Mary. Mary was also able to increase her communication, which was stimulating to Bill.

After they agreed that it was acceptable to hug and touch without the expectation of intercourse, their physical contacts increased. Bill initiated more caring behavior. Bill and Mary completed the stages of sensate focus in seven weeks. They were able to experiment with various types of pleasurable activities that were satisfying to both of them. Bill was able to attain and maintain an erection with oral sex beginning in the fourth week of sensate focus. His erectile response continued throughout the therapy. Bill and Mary were relieved to know that Bill had no organic dysfunctions.

Many changes occurred for Bill and Mary that went far beyond their sexual life. They learned to share expectations, to use "I" language, and to identify angry feelings and deal appropriately with these feelings. Their children benefited from these changes in the sense that "I" language was now a model for them. They also received a more open sex education, and there was a decrease of tension in the home. The children also benefited from Bill's increased ability to demonstrate affection to them. The couple terminated treatment pleased that most of the expected outcomes had been achieved.

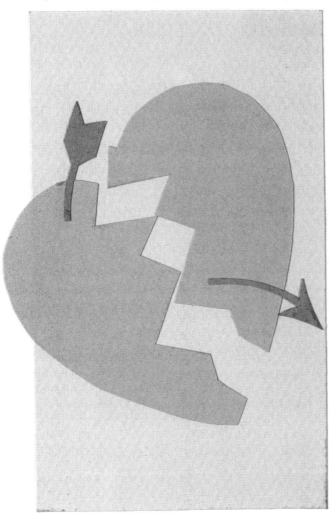

female sexual behavior. Nurses are in a unique position to dispel myths and to help individuals deal with their own sexual needs and limitations.

One type of alternative sex role enactment is homosexual activity, which may or may not be a source of distress to the individual. According to the DSM-III, only ego-dystonic, or anxiety-arousing, homosexuality should be considered a disorder. There is probably as much variation in the lifestyles of homosexuals as there is among heterosexuals, except that covert behavior is thrust upon many homosexuals because of social disapproval. Other alternative sex role enactments include bisexuality, celibacy, and transvestism. Most transvestites are heterosexual males who wear articles of female clothing as a means of sexual arousal.

Transsexuals are individuals who believe that their assigned gender is unnatural or erroneous. There are data to support the biological explanation for sexual ambiguity in some but not all transsexuals. Sex change procedures are possible but extremely complex surgically, medically, and legally.

Sexual dysfunctions include greatly increased or decreased sexual interest, the causes of which vary; erectile and ejaculatory problems in men; and vaginismus and orgasmic inhibition in women. Sexual deviance, or paraphilia, includes fetishism, zoophilia, pedophilia, exhibitionism, voyeurism, and necrophilia.

There are a number of forms of sexual abuse. Among them are sadomasochistic behaviors that range from mild to extreme. Incest is a common and reprehensible form of sexual abuse since it usually represents the exploitation of a weaker person. Incest is usually a seduction rather than a rape, but it is emotionally damaging to all family members. Although sexual harassment is a real problem, there remain many persons, male and female, who believe that women invite unwelcome sexual overtures by their dress and behavior.

Marital and sexual counseling is often within the scope of the nurse's clinical practice. In assessing a couple, their role expectations should be identified to determine what each partner seeks from the other. Teaching the partners to substitute an other-centered approach for a self-centered approach may reduce conflicts. Specific sexual counseling techniques and exercises have been well received. These techniques combine behavior modification principles with heightened interpersonal and sensual awareness.

Review Questions

1. Describe male and female sexual anatomy.

2. List the four phases of the human sexual response and the major characteristics of each phase.

3. Discuss ways in which sexuality is influenced by cultural settings.

4. List some of the unspoken expectations regarding sexual relationships and discuss the influence of these expectations on sexual response.

5. Discuss homophobia and its effect on the treatment of gay persons.

6. Explain the various aspects of bisexuality.

7. Discuss the many theories advanced to explain transsexualism. Which do you think offers the best insights? Why?

8. Discuss the role of self-perception and self-image in sexual response.

9. Describe the disorders of sexual deviance (paraphilias).

10. Explain the manifestations of sexual abuse, including sadism, masochism, incest, and sexual harassment.

References

Ackroyd, P. 1979. *Dressing Up*. New York: Simon & Schuster.

American Psychiatric Association. 1980. *Diagnostic and Statistical Manual of Mental Disorders*, 3rd ed. Washington D.C.: American Psychiatric Association.

Barbach, L. 1982. *For Each Other*. New York: Anchor Press/Doubleday.

Barbach, L. 1975. *For Yourself*. New York: Doubleday.

Bell, A., and Weinberg, M. 1978. *Homosexualities*. New York: Simon & Schuster.

Carrera, M. 1981. *Sex*. New York: Crown Publishers.

Crooks, R., and Baur, K. 1983. *Our Sexuality*. Menlo Park. Calif. Benjamin/Cummings.

Finkelhor, P. 1979. *Sexually Abused Children*. New York: Free Press.

Freedman, A. M.; Kaplan, H. I.; and Sadock, B. J., eds. 1976. *Modern Synopsis of Psychiatry*. Baltimore: Williams & Wilkins.

Friday, N. 1977. *My Mother/My Self*. New York: Delacorte Press.

Haeberle, E. 1981. *The Sex Atlas*. New York: Continuum.

Haley, J. 1963. *Strategies of Psychotherapy*. New York: Grune & Stratton.

Harris, C. et al. 1983. Immunodeficiency in Female Sexual Partners of Men with the Acquired Immunodeficiency Syndrome. *New England Journal of Medicine*, 308(20).

Hogan, R. 1980. *Human Sexuality: A Nursing Perspective*. New York: Appleton-Century-Crofts.

Janosik, E. H. 1984. *Crisis Counseling*. Monterey, Calif.: Wadsworth Health Sciences.

Kaplan, H. S. 1974. *The New Sex Therapy*. New York: Bruner/Mazel.

Kinsey, A., et al. 1948. *Sexual Behavior in the Human Male.* Philadelphia: W. B. Saunders.

Kinsey, A., et al. 1953. *Sexual Behavior in the Human Female.* Philadelphia: W. B. Saunders.

Klein, F. 1978. *The Bisexual Option.* New York: Arbor House.

Lothestein, L. M. 1982. Sex Reassignment Surgery: Historical, Bioethical, and Theoretical Issues. *American Journal of Psychiatry*, 139:417−426.

Marmor, J. 1973. Homosexuality and Cultural Value Systems. *American Journal of Psychiatry*, 130(11):1208−1209.

Marx, J. 1983. Human Cell Leukemia Virus Linked to AIDS. *Science*, 220(4599).

Masters, W. H., and Johnson, V. E. 1966. *Human Sexual Response.* Boston: Little, Brown.

Mims, F., and Swenson. M. 1980 *Sexuality: A Nursing Perspective.* New York: McGraw-Hill.

Money, J., and Ehrhardt, A. 1971. Fetal Hormones and the Brain. *Archives of Sexual Behavior*, 1.

Rush, F. 1980. *The Best Kept Secret: Sexual Abuse of Children.* Englewood Cliffs, N.J.: Prentice-Hall.

Satir, V. 1967. *Conjoint Family Therapy.* Palo Alto, Calif.: Behavior Books.

Schlesinger, B. 1982. *Sexual Abuse of Children.* Toronto: University of Toronto Press.

Siemens, S., and Brandzel, R. 1982. *Sexuality: Nursing Assessment and Intervention.* Philadelphia: J. B. Lippencott.

Strong, B., and Reynolds, R. 1982. *Understanding Our Sexuality.* St. Paul, Minn.; West Publishing.

Watzlawick, P.; Beavin, J.; and Jackson, D. 1967. *Pragmatics of Human Communication.* New York: W. W. Norton.

Zilbergeld, B. 1978. *Male Sexuality.* New York: Bantam Books.

Supplementary Readings

Barlow, D. H. Anxiety Increases Sexual Arousal. *Journal of Abnormal Psychology*, 92(1983):49−54.

Boyer, G. Sexuality and Aging. *Nursing Clinics of North America*, 17(1982):421−427.

Conine, T. A. Sexual Reactivation of Chronically Ill and Disabled Adults. *Journal of Allied Health*, 4(1982): 261−270.

DeLora, J. S., and Warren, C. A. *Understanding Sexual Interaction.* Boston: Houghton Mifflin, 1977.

Densen-Gerber, J. Sexuality of Chemically Dependent Women. *Journal of American Medical Women's Association*, 37(1982):207−210.

Fluker, J. L. The Perils of Promiscuity. *Journal of Psychosomatic Research*, 27(1983):153−156.

Fromer, M. J. *AIDS: Acquired Immune Deficiency Syndrome.* New York: Pinnacle Books, 1983.

Gagnon, J. H. *Human Sexualities.* Glenview, Ill: Scott, Foresman, 1977.

Gerrard, M. Sexual Experience, Sex, Guilt, and Sexual Moral Reasoning. *Journal of Personality*, 50(1982): 345−359.

Hartman, L. M. Relationship Factors in the Treatment of Sexual Dysfunction. *Behavioral Research Therapy*, 21(1983):153−160.

Hogan, R. M. Influence of Culture on Sexuality. *Nursing Clinics of North America*, 17(1982):365−376.

Hyde, J. S. *Understanding Human Sexuality.* New York: McGraw-Hill, 1979.

Jenkins, R. R. Adolescent Sexuality and the Family. *Pediatric Annals*, 11(1982):740−742.

Kaplan, H. S. *Disorders of Sexual Desire.* New York: Brunner/Mazel, 1979.

Keshusius, L. Sexuality, Intimacy and Persons We Label Mentally Retarded. *Mental Retardation*, 20(1982): 164−168.

Lion, E. M. *Human Sexuality in Nursing Process.* New York: John Wiley & Sons, 1982.

Lobsenz, N. M. *Sex After Sixty-five.* New York: Public Affairs Committee, 1975.

Mayer, K., and Pizer, H. *The AIDS Fact Book.* New York: Bantam Books, 1983.

Masters, W., and Johnson, V. *Human Sexual Response.* Boston: Little, Brown, 1966.

Masters, W., and Johnson, V. *Human Sexual Inadequacy.* Boston: Little, Brown, 1970.

Mims, F. A., Sexual Stress: Coping and Adaptation. *Nursing Clinics of North America*, 17(1982):395−405.

Mims, F. H. *Human Sexuality in Health and Illness.* St. Louis: C. V. Mosby, 1984.

Read, D. A. *Health Sexuality.* New York: Macmillan, 1979.

Safir, M. P. Psychological Androgyny and Sexual Adequacy. *Journal of Sexuality and Marital Therapy*, 8(1982):228−240.

Schusler, E. A. Nursing Practice in Human Sexuality. *Nursing Clinics of North America*, 17(1982):345−347.

Segraves, R. T. Psychosexual Adjustment After Penile Prosthesis Surgery. *Sexuality and Disability*, 5(1982): 222−229.

Tauer, K. M. Promoting Effective Decision Making in Sexually Active Adolescents. *Nursing Clinics of North America*, 18(1983):275−292.

Whitley, M. P., and Willingham, D. Adding a Sexual Assessment to the Health Interview. *Journal of Psychiatric Nursing and Mental Health Services*, (1978):17−27.

Winn, R. L. Sexuality in Aging. *Archives of Sexual Behavior*, 11(1982):283−298.

Woods, M. F. *Human Sexuality in Health and Illness*, 3rd ed. St. Louis: C. V. Mosby, 1984.

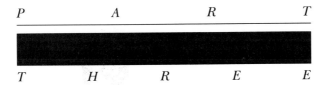
CRITICAL TASKS AND PATTERNS

DEVELOPMENTAL THEORIES
Erikson's Psychosocial Theory
Kohlberg's Theory of Moral Development
Piaget's Cognitive Development Theory
Duvall's Theory of Family Development
Nursing Implications of Developmental Theories

ALTERED MATURATIONAL PATTERNS OF
CHILDHOOD
Sleep Disturbances
Eating Disturbances
Urinary and Excretory Disturbances
Fears and Phobias
Working with Children

ALTERED MATURATIONAL PATTERNS OF
ADOLESCENCE
Identity Confusion
Antisocial Behavior
Body Image Distortion
Working with Adolescents

ALTERED MATURATIONAL PATTERNS OF
ADULTHOOD
Career Crises
Marital Crises
Parental Crises
Working with Adults

ALTERED MATURATIONAL PATTERNS OF OLD AGE
The Empty Nest Syndrome
Retirement Crises
Health-Related Crises
Terminal Crises
Working with the Elderly

C   H   A   P   T   E   R

14

Altered Maturational Patterns

Learning Objectives

After reading this chapter, the student should be able to:

1. Define the term "maturational crisis" and describe the importance of maturational crises in the life cycle of individuals and families.

2. Discuss the basic premise on which Kohlberg's theory of moral development is based.

3. Discuss the basic premise on which Piaget's theory of cognitive development is based.

4. Contrast adaptive and maladaptive maturational patterns in children.

5. Contrast adaptive and maladaptive maturational patterns in adolescents.

6. Contrast adaptive and maladaptive maturational patterns in adults.

7. Contrast adaptive and maladaptive maturational patterns in the elderly.

8. Integrate concepts of individual and family maturation in making a nursing assessment.

370

Overview

This chapter describes some important critical tasks confronted by individuals and families over the course of the life cycle and contrasts adaptive and maladaptive patterns of crisis resolution. It describes various factors influencing the accomplishment of critical tasks, along with the problems that may arise when critical tasks are not adequately resolved. The chapter also discusses the nursing implications of working with clients experiencing some type of maturational crisis.

To see a world in a grain of sand
And heaven in a wild flower
Hold infinity in the palm of your hand
And eternity in an hour.
WILLIAM BLAKE

DEVELOPMENTAL THEORIES

In the life of every human being, inevitable changes occur as one moves from childhood to old age. Some changes are predictable, while others are unexpected. The predictable changes that occur in the life of almost everyone are called *maturational crises* or *developmental crises*. These crises are accompanied by the emergence of transitional tasks that must be completed if the individual is to progress adaptively to the next stage of the life cycle. Because such tasks accompany each maturational crisis, they are known as *critical tasks*.

Many theorists have identified critical tasks specific to various periods of the life cycle including infancy, childhood, adolescence, adulthood, and old age. In this section four theories are presented that help explain some aspect of maturational crises. Each of the four theorists—Erik Erikson, Lawrence Kohlberg, Jean Piaget, and Evelyn Duvall—addresses particular aspects of human development. Erikson uses a broad perspective that includes many aspects of development, particularly the psychological and social. Kohlberg is interested in moral development, Piaget in cognitive development, and Duvall in family development. These theorists have been selected for discussion to help provide a multidimensional rather than unidimensional approach to development. The choice was based on the premise that holism requires a broad view of human development, one that includes family influences as well as individual ones.

Erikson's Psychosocial Theory

Erik Erikson (1963) divided the human life span into eight stages and suggested that each stage brings with it a specific critical task (see Chapter 2). Successful resolution of a maturational crisis means that the critical task for that stage has been accomplished. The achievement of the critical task results in the acquisition of desirable personality traits and in social adjustment, but failure to accomplish the task results in undesirable traits and maladjustment. However, if one fails to accomplish a critical task during the appropriate life stage, it is still possible to accomplish it later because subsequent events might present new opportunities. The box on page 372 summarizes the critical tasks that accompany maturational change.

Erikson's first three stages encompass early childhood. During the initial stage of *trust versus mistrust*, the infant learns that someone will meet her needs for food, warmth, shelter, and love. If the infant's needs are not met regularly and adequately, she will develop a mistrust of others that will continue into adult life. The second stage, that of *autonomy versus shame and doubt*, is characterized by demands for independence as the child begins to display qualities of willpower and self-direction. If the critical task of autonomy is not mastered, the child develops inhibitions that lead to diminished self-confidence and reluctance to develop new skills later in life.

Initiative, the critical task of stage 3, is concerned with the resolution of the child's ambivalent feelings of love and hate for his parents. During this stage, the child begins to imitate behaviors of authority figures. An inner sense of direction and purpose is the desirable outcome resulting from successful mastery of this stage. If the critical task of this stage is not successfully achieved, the result may be a lack of spontaneity and the appearance of a harsh and controlling conscience.

ERIKSON'S PSYCHOSOCIAL TASKS

Stage 1. Trust versus mistrust.
Stage 2. Autonomy versus shame and doubt.
Stage 3. Initiative versus guilt.
Stage 4. Industry versus inferiority.
Stage 5. Ego identity versus role diffusion.
Stage 6. Intimacy versus isolation.
Stage 7. Generativity versus stagnation.
Stage 8. Ego integrity versus despair.

372

The fourth stage, which occurs in middle childhood, is centered around the critical task of *industry versus inferiority*. During this stage, the child is actively involved in learning and practicing skills. As the child moves through this stage, she develops a sense of pride and accomplishment in completing tasks. In addition she develops the ability to set realistic goals for herself. The successful outcome of this stage is a sense of competence. Lack of success results in feelings of inadequacy and inferiority.

Stage 5 occurs during puberty and adolescence, from ages twelve to twenty. Termed the period of *ego identity versus role diffusion*, it is a time when the individual is confused about his identity and asks such existential questions as "Who am I?" It is also a time when sexual identity and sexual preferences are being expressed. Often the young person discovers and identifies with a role model. A positive self-image is the desired result of this stage, accompanied by the traits of devotion and fidelity. Problems with sexual identity and delayed selection of an occupation are common manifestations of failure to resolve the critical task of stage 5.

The sixth stage, lasting from ages twenty to forty, is the stage of *intimacy versus isolation*. The task of these years is to be able to commit oneself to meaningful, loving relationships with others. When intimacy is not achieved, the individual avoids or retreats from emotional commitments in various ways, such as being aloof, fleeing relationships as soon as they become intense, or being promiscuous so that no relationship is meaningful. Avoidance behaviors may take diverse forms, but they all have the effect of isolating the individual from closeness.

The task of the seventh stage, which lasts from ages forty to sixty, is the mastery of *generativity versus*

stagnation. In this period the individual shows concern for younger generations, usually by offering them guidance and support. Besides her own children, she may express a global concern for generations yet unborn. Although many adults experience a heightened sense of productivity and creativity at this time, those who have not accomplished the critical task may enter a period of stagnation, characterized by an inability to care for the needs of others. The stagnated person has an exaggerated self-interest, often manifested in preoccupation with somatic complaints or indifference to conditions except as they affect her.

The eighth and last stage, occurring after the age of sixty, is Erikson's period of *ego integrity versus despair*. The final developmental task is to accept one's life and its meaning. Wisdom, altruism, and solace are attributes acquired by the individual who is successful at this task of the life cycle. Those who cannot arrive at a state of satisfaction or contentment with themselves and their entire existence often desire to relive their lives in order to do things differently. These persons engage in wistful longing for the past, express deep regrets about the course their lives have taken, and frequently have a profound fear of death.

Kohlberg's Theory of Moral Development

Lawrence Kohlberg (1968) is a social scientist and educator who has proposed a theory of moral development that sees the individual going through a fixed series of states. This theory is based on a longitudinal study of males ranging in age from ten to twenty-eight. Data collection procedure consisted of reading the subjects stories that depicted moral dilemmas, then questioning them about their rea-

---

> ## KOHLBERG'S MORAL DEVELOPMENT STAGES
>
> ### Preconventional Level
>
> Stage 1. Punishment and obedience orientation.
>
> Stage 2. Instrumental relativist orientation.
>
> ### Conventional Level
>
> Stage 3. Interpersonal concordance or good boy/nice girl orientation.
>
> Stage 4. Law and order orientation.
>
> ### Postconventional Level
>
> Stage 5. Social contract legalistic orientation.
>
> Stage 6. Universal ethical principle orientation.

sons for arriving at particular solutions. Kohlberg's emphasis was on the subjects' reasoning processes in solving the moral dilemmas, not on the solutions themselves. A coding and scoring system was used that allowed researchers to classify and analyze the proposed solutions. As a result of this long-term investigation, Kohlberg identified three levels of moral development, each of which is further divided into two stages, making a total of six. The accompanying box outlines the stages and levels of moral development proposed by Kohlberg.

One of Kohlberg's basic assumptions was that the progression of moral development does not vary in any way. That is, each individual must proceed through each of the given stages in sequence and cannot omit a stage while advancing to higher levels of moral development.

Another underlying assumption was that individuals can comprehend (and then only vaguely) moral reasoning at one step beyond their present orientation. Each stage of moral development has its own particular orientation; ambiguity arises as individuals begin to question their present orientation stage. This questioning is resolved as individuals move to the next stage and find that the new orientation settles or reconciles their previous questions.

A third assumption was that individuals are intellectually attracted to the reasoning or orientation that is one stage above their present orientation. This assumption acknowledges that each successive stage resolves more questions. Kohlberg's fourth assumption was that ambiguity, or cognitive disequilibrium, is the impetus that challenges one to move through various stages. If a person finds that his present stage is not adequate to resolve a moral dilemma, he will gravitate toward the next highest stage.

These four assumptions underlying Kohlberg's theory should be kept in mind during the following discussion of Kohlberg's levels and stages of moral development.

THE PRECONVENTIONAL LEVEL   Kohlberg described the first, or *preconventional*, level as one at which the child is responsive to cultural labels of good and bad, right and wrong, but interprets these labels in terms either of the physical or psychological consequences of action (punishment, reward, exchange of favors) or of the physical power of those who enunciate the rules and labels. This level describes most children up to the age of early adolescence; however, some adults are fixated at this level, too. At this first level, actions are judged according to expected consequences. Rules per se do not have intrinsic value; they are merely indicative of anticipated pleasure or pain. Therefore, a preconventional person is self-centered and lacks feelings of group or societal identity. Kohlberg has suggested that a person must first develop the ability to role play or put herself in another's situation before she can fully understand what a society is and how it functions. At this stage, the individual is too egoistic to feel a part of society. Instead, she feels at the mercy of some greater force that sets rules and delivers punishment.

Fear governs the actions of a person at stage 1

of the preconventional level. Kohlberg's theory would explain the antisocial actions of criminals as behaviors of a stage 1, preconventional level. Kohlberg called stage 2 the instrumental relativist orientation. At this stage a person decides issues based on what satisfies her own needs and sometimes considers the needs of others. Persons operating at stage 2 of the preconventional level perceive society as made up of others like themselves, and they believe that if they extend help to others, they are likely to be helped in return. Because the person at this stage believes that all people are alike, she will begin to question why one person should have more rights than another. Thus, stage 2 marks the beginning of a sense of fairness. Nonetheless, self-interest remains important, and fear of authority is reduced. To obtain compliance from persons at this stage, it may be necessary to demonstrate what will be beneficial to them in a given situation or transaction.

THE CONVENTIONAL LEVEL The move from the preconventional level to the *conventional level* is accompanied by acceptance of group values and recognition of the importance of group rules and sanctions. The personal consequences of an action are no longer the only criteria by which to judge its goodness or morality. Instead, an action is judged by how well it meets the standards or expectations of others in a group or social order. When individuals identify with a group, the esteem and approval of others begins to displace tangible rewards as the dominant motivator of behavior. One aspect of the conventional level is *cohesiveness,* or the feeling of belonging to and valuing a group. People at the conventional level adopt standards of group conformity and loyalty to justify the group not only to others but to themselves.

Reference groups, or groups with which an individual identifies, become very important at this level because group norms and values often become the standards for judging what is right or wrong. Behavior that helps, pleases, or is approved of by others is usually considered to be good. Intent is often taken into account in judging an action as good or bad; self-sacrifice and altruism become acceptable reasons for winning group approval and are therefore labeled "good." Most teenagers operate at stage 3. Their concentration on heroes, idols, and fads is just one indication of the overwhelming importance they give to group identity and group approval. As a result, an appeal to group values is likely to have an impact on adolescents.

Once individuals become fully aware that society is composed of divergent groups with opposing value systems, the usefulness of broader laws, rules, and behavior codes becomes more apparent. It is at this point that individuals move on to stage 4, which

Kohlberg called the law and order orientation. Individuals at this stage believe they are acting correctly when they show respect for authority and comply with rules and laws. Because the law is considered to be the guardian of social order, no individual or group is thought to be above the law. It is Kohlberg's contention that the majority of adults remain permanently at this stage of moral development.

THE POSTCONVENTIONAL LEVEL With advancement to the *postconventional level* comes the first hint of independent or autonomous judgment. Prior to this level, behaviors are directed by fear of punishment (stage 1), expectation of pleasure or reward (stage 2), group norms (stage 3), or adherence to law (stage 4). Individuals who have progressed to stage 5 can make up their own minds about behaviors that are right or wrong. Instead of merely judging actions according to existing principles established or enforced by others, persons at the postconventional level consider what principles the individual and society *should* follow.

Those who have reached stage 5 (the social contract legalistic orientation), believe that individuals have a right to personal values, beliefs, opinions, and behaviors provided they do not harm others. The person at this stage makes a clear distinction between areas of personal freedom and areas of public welfare. In areas where individual actions may affect the lives of others, he recognizes the need for legislation and regulation. This viewpoint represents a radical departure from the belief that law is fixed and unchangeable.

A person functioning at stage 5 may be critical of the status quo, but this does not constitute a license to be arbitrary or anarchistic. He believes that existing and proposed legislation may be subjected to scrutiny and questioning but that laws cannot be discarded simply because they are personally objectionable. The official stance or posture of the government and Constitution of the United States is reflected in stage 5.

The sixth and highest stage of moral development is the universal ethical principle orientation. The individual at this advanced stage of moral development is guided not by fixed rules and regulations but by abstract principles compatible with internal values. These internalized standards include respect for the rights of everyone and devotion to principles of honor and justice. When the individual fails to live up to these principles, feelings of guilt and self-recrimination follow. Therefore, the individual will go to great lengths to avoid violating the self-imposed principles, even when adherence is followed by unpleasant consequences. A conscientious objector who refuses to bear arms and is willing to suffer imprisonment for his views exhibits behavior characteristic of this stage. Kohlberg believes that this stage represents an ideal that is often sought but seldom reached and thus discusses the stage in terms of potential rather than actual moral development.

It should be noted that the sample population of the longitudinal study on which Kohlberg's theory is based included no women and that a comprehensive moral development theory has yet to be formulated that gives a balanced consideration to both men and women. Comparative studies based on Kohlberg's premises tend to find the moral development of women "inferior" because it does not follow the fixed sequence outlined by Kohlberg. Carol Gilligan (1980) found two distinct modes of moral reasoning operating for boys and girls, one concerned with rights and justice and the other concerned with caring and relating. From her findings, Gilligan concluded that men are more likely to define themselves in terms of autonomy and achievement while women are more likely to define themselves in terms of relationships. Although there is need for additional research and reappraisal in this controversial area, there is merit in Gilligan's conclusion that priorities in moral development may be different for women than for men.

Piaget's Cognitive Development Theory

Jean Piaget was a Swiss psychologist who conducted extensive observational studies of children in an attempt to understand their stages of intellectual and cognitive development. On the basis of observation, interviews, and experiments, Piaget postulated four stages of cognitive development in children, lasting from birth to the beginning of adolescence. Although he gave normative ages to the stages, Piaget (1969) emphasized the range of individual differences in rates of development and therefore presented chronological ages simply as a guide (see Table 14-1).

SENSORIMOTOR STAGE Piaget termed the first stage of cognitive development the *sensorimotor stage*. Dur-

ing the first eighteen months of life, an infant uses her senses to learn about the world. By means of sight, hearing, taste, touch, and smell the infant explores her environment. Eventually she learns patterns of behaviors and looks for ways to test and replicate these patterns, and she gradually learns to predict actions based on the consequences of previous actions. For example, she may learn that dropping a bottle on the floor causes adults in the vicinity to retrieve the bottle and return it to her, an action that she finds gratifying. Such primitive sequences of cause and effect behavior are the foundation for future problem solving and lead to more complex intellectual development.

PREOPERATIONAL STAGE During the *preoperational stage*, the thinking of the young child is quite rigid and inflexible, partly because the child is *egocentric* and unable to appreciate ideas and viewpoints that are different from his own.

At this age, the child comes to realize that even though he cannot see a hidden object or a person who has left the room, the object or person continues to exist. Thus, he attains *object permanence*, the understanding that people and objects exist apart from the self. To the child in the sensorimotor stage, people or objects that are out of sight have disappeared permanently as far as he is concerned. Therefore, when a toy is taken away from him and concealed, he will not look for it. The child at the preoperational stage, on the other hand, will search for a concealed toy, demonstrating object permanence.

Another characteristic of the preoperational stage is the use of symbols in the child's thinking and communication. At this stage the child realizes that a single word or sign can represent more complex ideas and meanings. Bringing a ball to father is an invitation for father to play with the child; putting on a coat signifies a desire or readiness to go outdoors. Pumpkins signify Halloween and the flag signifies one's country. From such basic signs, the child learns the significance of symbols.

375

Table 14-1. Piaget's Cognitive Development Stages

Stage	Age	Characteristics
Sensorimotor	Birth–18 months	Child learns about self and surroundings through sensory and motor exploration and experience; learns through trial and error
Preoperational	18 months–7 years	Child develops language skills, acquires understanding of symbols, recognizes object permanence, learns to separate and classify
Concrete operational	8 years–11 years	Child uses and manipulates numbers, understands spatial relationships, learns to think logically and to reason
Formal operational	12 years–Adulthood	Adolescent understands abstract concepts, expands ability to think logically and to reason, formulates and tests hypotheses

Certain biologists define adaptation *simply as preservation and survival, that is to say, the equilibrium between the organism and the environment. But then the concept loses all interest because it becomes confused with that of life itself. There are degrees of survival, and adaptation involves the greatest and the least. It is therefore necessary to distinguish between the state of adaptation and the process of adaptation. In the state nothing is clear. In following the process, things are cleared up. There is adaptation when the organism is transformed by the environment and when this . . . results in an increase in the interchanges between the environment and itself which are favorable to its preservation.*

JEAN PIAGET (1969)

376

CONCRETE OPERATIONAL STAGE Between the ages of eight and eleven, the child is in the *concrete operational stage*. During this stage the child can use and manipulate numbers and begins to understand spatial relationships. These are the years when the concept of moral judgment begins to develop and when the cognitive skills of the child are burgeoning, although abstract thinking is not yet present. When asked to explain the meaning of the proverb "Never change horses in the middle of the stream," the child will give a literal interpretation, explaining that a rider changing horses in the middle of a stream would fall in and get wet. The child would be unlikely to generalize the meaning to other situations or to extract the message that anyone who starts a project and changes the original plan risks failure.

FORMAL OPERATIONAL STAGE The fourth stage of cognitive development, the *formal operational stage*, begins at about age twelve. This is the most sophisticated cognitive level. The individual becomes capable of abstract thinking and is able to formulate and test hypotheses. Problem solving at this stage is sequential and orderly, and reasoning processes are logical and usually consistent.

Duvall's Theory of Family Development

The developmental frameworks described thus far have been concerned primarily with individuals, although social considerations are sometimes mentioned. The developmental framework of Evelyn Duvall (1967, 1971) focuses on the family life cycle, dividing it into eight stages, each centered around specific tasks and based on the age of the oldest child

(see Figure 14-1). The eight tasks that determine the family's developmental stage are: (1) physical maintenance; (2) allocation of resources; (3) division of labor; (4) socialization of family members; (5) reproduction, recruitment, and release of family members; (6) maintenance of order; (7) placement of members in the larger society; and (8) maintenance of motivation and morale. Like the other developmental theorists, Duvall believes that specific tasks must be accomplished if the biological, psychological, and social needs of every family member are to be met. (For a more detailed discussion of critical family tasks, see Chapter 18.)

When children are quite young, the primary family task is to meet the children's needs for physical, emotional, and social nurture. At the same time, parents must also attend to their own needs for intimacy and privacy; the marital relationship must be sustained within the family relationship. As children enter school, parents must begin to concern themselves with the educational progress of their children and with the children's adjustment to the larger society, represented by school and community functions. When children become teenagers, parents must manage the delicate balance between being supportive and fostering independence. At the time when children leave home to launch their own lives, the parents must readjust to the contraction of family size. During the last stages of the family life cycle, parents must adjust to being a couple again as they adapt to retirement and aging.

In functional families, each individual member is supported in the accomplishment of individual critical tasks as the family as a whole adjusts to the changing needs of its members. The result is a sys-

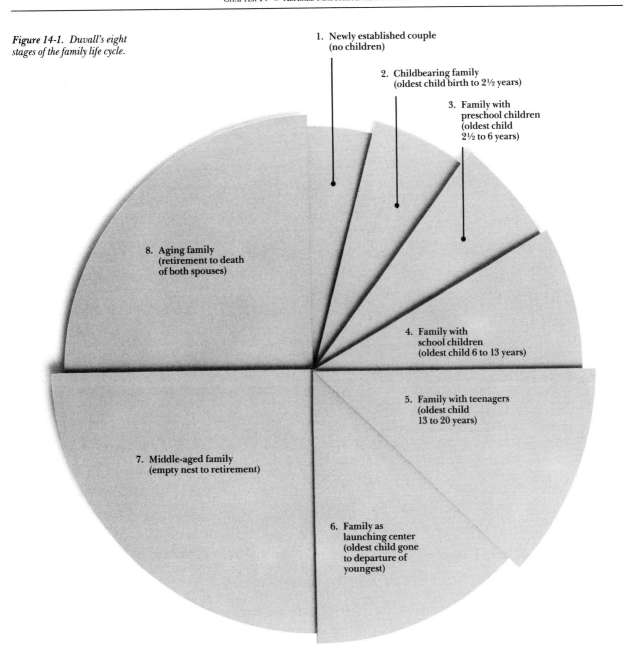

Figure 14-1. Duvall's eight stages of the family life cycle.

1. Newly established couple (no children)

2. Childbearing family (oldest child birth to 2½ years)

3. Family with preschool children (oldest child 2½ to 6 years)

4. Family with school children (oldest child 6 to 13 years)

5. Family with teenagers (oldest child 13 to 20 years)

6. Family as launching center (oldest child gone to departure of youngest)

7. Middle-aged family (empty nest to retirement)

8. Aging family (retirement to death of both spouses)

tem in which no member is unfairly exploited and in which the family continues to modify its operations in order to function adaptively.

STRESS AND ADAPTATION IN THE FAMILY Growth and maturational processes inevitably bring changes to individuals and families. These universal changes, even when predictable and anticipated, produce conditions of stress. Similar events can produce different reactions in different people (Barry, 1984). Thus, it is not the event itself that is the crucial factor but the response of the individual or the family. Most people are consistent in their manner of responding to stressful situations. Some usually respond with anger, while others use avoidance tactics. In addition, people vary in their ability to tolerate stress. Some people have little tolerance, while others appear to cope well (Selye, 1974, 1978). Nevertheless, everyone has a limit to the amount of stress he or she can handle at one time or within a brief time period. (For further discussion of the nature of stress and reactions to stress, see Chapter 12.)

Stress may be induced by factors generated within the self or by factors within the social environment. As the first social unit that molds personality, the family is a powerful influence on the young child. Family dynamics can be either constructive or destructive. For example, a mismatch between the temperament of a child and the expectations of the parents can be detrimental to the child's development. A highly organized, perfectionistic parent may be disappointed with the behavior of a child who is careless or indifferent about projects such as homework. Outgoing parents may become impatient with a shy retiring child, whereas quiet, reticent parents may feel overwhelmed by a boisterous, aggressive child. Such incongruity may inhibit the development of the child (Chess and Thomas, 1982).

In an ideal situation, the needs of the individual are compatible with the needs of the family; what seems beneficial for individual members coincides with what is deemed beneficial for the family. However, in the everyday world of real families there is frequent disagreement and incompatibility between what is good for the family and what is desired by individual members. The resulting conflict may be detrimental to the resolution of individual and family tasks. When a family member is working through a particular task, an optimal resolution would be to reconcile family needs and individual needs so that neither is achieved at the expense of the other. Unfortunately, this is not always easy to accomplish.

CULTURAL INFLUENCES ON THE FAMILY In a sense, maturational tasks are rites of passage that mark the transition from one phase of life to the next. These rites of passage are influenced by the values of the family, which in turn are shaped by the larger social order. Some families are fortunate enough to feel that they truly belong in the community in which they live, but other families feel that they have been transplanted from a familiar, more comfortable environment to a new community where they feel like strangers. In homogeneous societies virtually everyone shares a common language, customs, and goals. The United States, however, is not a homogeneous society but a vast pluralistic nation in which the orientation of any given family may differ greatly from that of the mainstream culture. When this happens, the family is perceived as deviant by others in the community, and this becomes a source of stress, especially for children and adolescents who feel strong pressure to conform to the norms of the larger society. Customs concerning childrearing, socialization, and parental expectations then become a source of contention among family members (Getty and Humphreys, 1981).

When the ways of the family are opposed to the ways of the larger society, the family may voluntarily withdraw from society and establish an isolated culture shared by other families with the same value system. The communities established by the Amish people and by Hasidic Jews are examples of societies that try to monitor family and individual behavior by reducing input from the mainstream culture. This option is not available to all "deviant" families, however. Since some transactions between such families and the community cannot be avoided, a way must be found to accommodate the values of traditionalist family members who are reluctant to adopt the values of the surrounding community.

Issues concerning independence and individuality must be settled by every family, but they often become problematic for families transplanted from one culture to another. Independence and individuality are highly regarded in American culture, but these attributes are often viewed with fear and suspicion by ethnic families who fear a drastic break with old customs (Feretta, Rivera, and Lucero, 1981).

Nursing Implications of Developmental Theories
Of the theoretical frameworks presented here, Erikson's psychosocial theory probably has received the greatest acceptance by nurses, perhaps because the contributions of Kohlberg and Piaget are more limited in focus. Nevertheless, these two theorists have a place in the assessment of human development. To illustrate, Kohlberg's identification of the search for group identity in adolescence helps nurses recognize the powerful impact of peer group influence. The nurse who can recognize the group standards of dress, diet, and conduct that influence the adolescent client is then able to use this information to devise interventions acceptable to the client. In the same way, a nurse who can determine whether a client is guided by fear of punishment, by a wish for social approval, or by an internalized value system will find it easier to collaborate with the client in setting mutually acceptable goals.

Piaget's theoretical framework can be useful to nurses trying to teach, reassure, and care for children of various ages, whatever the setting. Knowing that a young child cannot use or understand symbols will remind nurses to interact in a fashion appropriate to the child's age and cognitive abilities. The use of games, dolls, and puppets to explain various procedures to hospitalized children is one example of the application of Piaget's ideas. His framework is also helpful in understanding why separation from the mother is particularly distressing for children in the sensorimotor stage, who believe that absent persons and objects cease to exist.

There is no guarantee that every individual will proceed to the highest levels of cognitive and moral development. The capacity of individuals for growth is affected by innumerable factors; moral and cognitive growth are no exception. However, the frameworks independently determined by

Kohlberg and Piaget provide normative guidelines that are worthy of consideration.

In using Duvall's developmental framework to assess a family, a nurse might begin by asking questions designed to identify discordant areas in the operation of the family and the lives of its members. A nurse assessing the cause of maturational difficulties might well superimpose the individual tasks conceptualized by Erikson onto Duvall's framework. Formulating nursing interventions that help reconcile both individual and family critical tasks is one way of promoting adaptive functioning. The failure of any member to resolve maturational tasks may be a means of preserving family equilibrium, but the price is maladaptive behavior that neglects or exploits one or more family members. For example, a protective mother may be a necessity for young children but a detriment for older children as they begin to search for identity and intimacy outside the home.

When using a combined individual/family approach to assess maturational progress, the nurse might include the following points of investigation:

1. What is the developmental stage of the family?

2. What is the primary critical task of the family at this point?

3. What is the developmental stage of each family member?

4. What is the primary critical task of each family member?

5. What critical tasks of the family and of individual members are being achieved in an adaptive, compatible way?

6. What critical tasks of the family and of individual members are not being achieved in an adaptive, compatible way?

7. What are the sources of maladaptation and incompatibility?

8. How can incompatibility be reduced while attending to the needs of individual members and preserving the integrity of the family?

9. How have individual members and the family dealt with developmental issues in the past?

ALTERED MATURATIONAL PATTERNS OF CHILDHOOD

One of the first tasks of the infant is the formation of *attachment* to a parent, usually the mother. The process of attachment does not depend solely on the mother or on the child but rather is a mutual process influenced by what both mother and child bring to the relationship. If the mother's expectations for the child are reasonable, if she has an adequate support system, and if she does not feel overwhelmed by her responsibilities, the attachment process is likely to be successful. The temperament and responses of the child also play an important part in the attachment process. Children differ greatly in their behavior patterns, and the child who is demanding and difficult to care for will arouse negative emotions even in the most devoted parents.

Stresses in the life of the parents can greatly affect their ability to offer sustained affection and nurturing. Changes in the marital relationship, in the financial status of the family, or in the health of family members may have considerable impact on the parent-child relationship. Because young children have few channels other than crying to communicate distress, they tend to express anxiety, anger, and fear behaviorally in the form of sleep disturbances, eating problems, and excretory difficulties (Smitherman, 1981).

Sleep Disturbances

At birth the infant does not distinguish the self from the environment. In effect, the self is merged with the surroundings and the infant makes no distinctions between persons who give care. At about six to eight months of age, the infant begins to make distinctions between what is strange and what is familiar. Because the familiar is associated with mother, food, and security, what is familiar becomes welcome and what is strange becomes something to be avoided. Usually it is the mother's absence that produces the greatest fear, followed by the appearance of strangers (Bowlby, 1969, 1973, 1979). Prolonged separation from the mother can be highly traumatic during this crucial period.

Fear of separation from the mother (*separation anxiety*) is often manifested in sleep disturbances, such as refusal to sleep. When this happens the parents may be deprived of their own rest; fatigue then heightens the reactions of parents and fosters anxiety in them. In addition, when parents themselves are anxiety prone, their anxiety is sensed by the infant, who then becomes more anxious and less likely to sleep.

In infants, poor sleep patterns often have a physical cause, such as hunger, colic, itching, binding clothing, or a room temperature that is too hot or too cold. Treatment requires adjustment of the specific cause of the problem. Observant nurses who take the time to investigate can often discover the cause of the sleep difficulty. A formula may have to be changed, or the parents may need help in learning how and when to offer nourishment to the infant. Sometimes parents lack understanding of

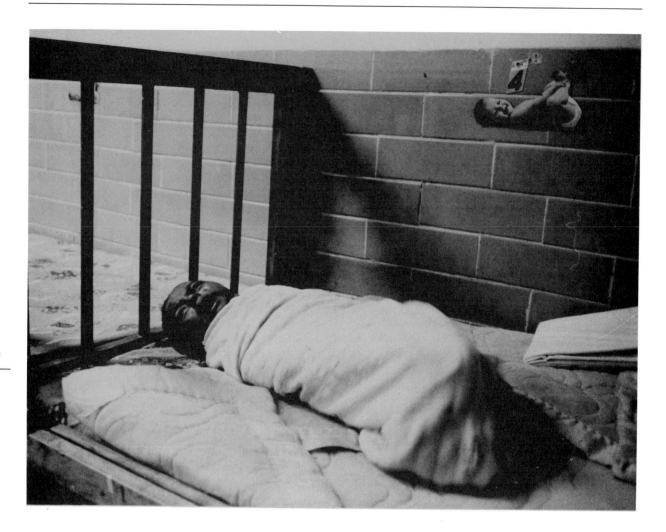

380

the sleep patterns of normal infants and need to be better informed about childhood patterns of growth and development.

The sleep disturbances common in childhood may take the form of resistance to sleep, restless sleep, nightmares, night terrors, sleepwalking, and wakefulness. These sleep disturbances are apt to have more varied etiology than the sleep disturbances of infancy. Parents who are inconsistent in the sleep routine they establish are the most likely to encounter sleep disturbances in their children. Although it is unwise for parents to permit the bedtime ritual to become too elaborate, a familiar routine can be reassuring to a child.

Fearfulness may keep a child awake or may contribute to restless sleep. Fear of the dark is a common phenomenon in young children. Their imagination can easily convert sounds and shadows into sinister agents, especially if they are alone in the dark. Unsuitable movies, violent television programs, and ghost stories told before bedtime can intensify what began as mild discomfort. A child may also be anxious and fearful about tangible problems either at home or in school. School wor-

ries may be related to peer acceptance or to academic performance.

Talking in one's sleep is a common occurrence among children, although their speech is usually mumbled and unintelligible. Occasionally, sleep talking is followed by screaming and crying. In contrast to sleep talking, sleepwalking is relatively uncommon in young children, occurring more frequently in adolescents. Many young people exhibit excellent coordination and balance when sleepwalking, but the practice can be dangerous. Sleepwalkers require protection in the form of parental vigilance and safeguards against open windows and stairways.

The response to sleep disturbances requires correction of any underlying physical cause and appropriate changes in bedtime routines. After an active or exciting day, children need a period of time to "wind down" before falling asleep. Bedtime stories and lullabies were invented for just this purpose. Children's fears and anxieties, however trivial, should not be ignored or carelessly dismissed but responded to in a caring, attentive manner. Another remedial approach is to explore the parents' attitudes toward the sleep patterns of their children. It is not useful for naptime or bedtime to amount to a state of warfare between parents and child. Equally inadvisable is the habit of sending children to bed as a punishment for unacceptable behavior.

Nurses can be of assistance to parents whose children have developed sleep disturbances. Warm baths and warm, nonstimulating beverages have been good inducers of sleep for many generations. A storytelling period when the child is lying in bed or a short interval when the child can talk in a relaxed way with a parent can be an enticement that helps prepare the child for sleep. It may also prove helpful to provide parents with information and education regarding the normal range of children's sleep behaviors and the individual differences in children that account for the wide variation in their sleep requirements. There are times when sleep problems prove resistant to the usual remedies. If a nurse suspects that the sleep problem is indicative of emotional disturbance, referral for more extensive evaluation is in order (Chapman, 1974; Meeks, 1975).

Eating Disturbances

Poor appetite in children is a complaint that frequently troubles parents. Although many infants exhibit a lessening of appetite toward the end of the first year, poor eating rarely becomes a problem before age two. During the first year, physical growth is dramatic; on the average, birth weight is tripled. After that the average weight gain from ages one to five is about five pounds annually. The rate of weight gain is sporadic, and months may pass without any appreciable gain. As a result, the need for food is correspondingly lower in the preschool years

and appetite is diminished. Parents who do not understand the reasons for this lessened appetite show their concern by pleading, coercing, or cajoling their child to eat. The discrepancy between parental expectations and the child's physiological needs may lead to eating disturbances during childhood and later (Bruch, 1973, 1978).

Between the ages of one and five, the child is in the process of developing independence. By resisting parental direction and by demanding to do things differently, the child is differentiating himself from others. Sometimes this means that the child refuses to eat when the parents want him to. By insisting that the child eat when and what they choose, parents lay the groundwork for an ongoing battle over food and eating. In such instances mealtime often signals the acting out of a struggle for dominance between parents and child (Sanger and Cassino, 1984).

Another parental behavior contributing to eating disturbances is continuing to feed a child who is capable of self-feeding. Although a mother may feel that it is neater and quicker to feed the child, her actions may frustrate the child and lead to a test of wills, resulting in refusal by the child to eat or to be fed. Parents who are rigid and inflexible about their child's diet may offer the child a way to annoy them merely by breaking or defying rules and schedules. Once established, patterns like this can become fixed and difficult to change.

Because many eating problems are either initiated or worsened by parental attitudes and behaviors, some primary prevention approaches are in order. From infancy onward, the surroundings for eating should be pleasant and free from irritating distractions. Schedules for mealtime should be regular without being excessively rigid. Children should be encouraged to feed themselves as soon as they show an interest in doing so and should be gently instructed in the proper use of eating utensils. Small portions of food should be served to the child, and parents would be wise not to insist that every morsel on the plate be eaten. If a child expresses a strong dislike for a certain food, it should be removed and reintroduced at a later time or in another form. Parents and other family members should avoid announcing their food biases, especially their dislikes, in the presence of a young child. By setting a tone of relaxation and anticipation about meals and by avoiding the temptation to bribe or reward children for eating, parents can do much to reduce the potential for conflict on this issue.

Urinary and Excretory Disturbances

Because the etiology of urinary and excretory disturbances in children may be physiological, this possibility must be investigated first so that proper corrective measures can be taken. A thorough physical examination of the child, accompanied by a family and social history, is essential before exploring the potential emotional sources of such problems. Common urinary and excretory disturbances include enuresis, constipation, and encopresis.

Enuresis is the involuntary discharge of urine, either during the day (diurnal) or at night (nocturnal), after the age of three. There are many possible physiological causes, including congenital abnormality of the urinary tract, diabetes mellitus, diabetes insipidus, and seizure disorders. All such possibilities must be thoroughly investigated.

Enuresis tends to be nocturnal and may occur every night with some children. For most children with this problem, nocturnal bladder control has never been achieved. When bedwetting takes place, the child rarely wakens even though the amount of urine voided may be quite large. It is estimated that 4 to 5 million children and young people in the United States suffer from enuresis (Coleman, Butcher, and Carson, 1984). An estimated 21.9 percent of boys and 15.5 percent of girls at age seven are enuretic; by age fourteen only 3 percent of boys and 1.5 percent of girls have the problem. Among young adults the incidence is 1 percent or less. There is no reliable way to identify the children who will remain enuretic as adults; thus, the consensus of experts is that the disturbance should receive attention in childhood (Coleman, Butcher, and Carson, 1984).

In some cases simple adjustments can alleviate nocturnal enuresis. Limiting or eliminating the amount of fluids ingested after the evening meal may have beneficial effects. Behavior modification procedures are sometimes effective. One procedure

is for the child to sleep on a mattress on which the first few drops of urine trigger an alarm bell that wakens the child and inhibits further voiding in bed. Such conditioning techniques inhibit reflex voiding but overlook emotional factors.

The emotional causes of eneuresis are multifactorial, ranging from family interactions characterized by anxiety and hostility, to insecurity and resentment engendered in the child by the birth of a new sibling, to developmental or maturational lags in the child due to emotional problems (Christie, 1981). When eneuresis is the response to a new baby in the home, it is often part of a generalized regression that includes petulance, whining, thumbsucking, temper tantrums, baby talk, and demands to drink from a bottle or to be diapered. Because these regressive behaviors indicate feelings of insecurity and resentment, solicitude and reassurance are needed. Extra attention, in the form of special time with mother and father, will help allay these feelings and encourage a return to age-appropriate behaviors.

Constipation is an excretory disturbance characterized by infrequent or difficult evacuation of feces. In an infant, the cause tends to be physiological, such as a redundant colon or a diet too low in roughage or too high in calcium. When constipation is habitual in older children, emotional factors deserve consideration. The attitude of the mother toward defecation and constipation may be a contributing factor. When the mother pays great attention to the time of evacuation and the appearance of stool, the child will sense the potential for conflict with and control over her mother. If enemas, suppositories, or cathartics are used to any great extent, habitual constipation is almost inevitable.

Encopresis is involuntary defecation after three years of age that is not related to dysfunction of the bowel. This condition is less common than enuresis and occurs more often in boys, especially between the ages of six and twelve. Initial intervention should include assessment for possible physiological causes, followed by a professional study of dietary habits in order to eliminate foods causing or exacerbating the condition. Because many children who are encopretic are also constipated, both conditions should be the object of study.

Treatment of encopresis requires physiological and psychological measures. When Levine and Bakow (1975) treated encopretic children using this dual approach, they found that 50 percent of the children had no episodes of encopresis within six months following treatment, while another 25 percent were improved. Another study of encopresis found that about one-third of the children in the study were also eneuretic (Levine, 1976). Many of the children soiled their clothing during stress, most

382

often in the late afternoon after school was over. Most of the children reported that they had no warning and did not know when they needed to have a bowel movement.

In dealing with the psychological aspects of encopresis and eneuresis, parents and professionals should be cautioned against employing rigid, compulsive actions that threaten the child's sense of confidence and self-control. Shame tactics should be strictly avoided. Shaming or humiliating the child is unlikely to be effective in curbing the behaviors and may in fact intensify emotional problems.

Fears and Phobias

Fear is a warning sign that a threat or danger is near. Because fear, especially realistic fear, is something of a necessity, it is not advisable to teach children that fear can be discarded; rather, they should be reminded that fear can sometimes be a protection against danger. Fears can be aroused by objective (external) or subjective (internal) stimuli. Examples of objective stimuli include things that can be seen, heard, or felt, such as loud explosions or growling dogs. Subjective stimuli are often affected by earlier experiences and by what an individual has been told or has imagined. Subjective fear-producing stimuli reflect the internal attitudes and responses of an individual and do not require the presence of the feared object or experience. Spiders, for example, are feared by a great many people regardless of whether they pose a real danger.

Between the ages of two and five, many children are afraid of anticipated and imagined dangers. Fear of the dark is common among preschoolers, many of whom also fear being left alone or abandoned by loved ones. Thus, separation anxiety may become linked with fear of the dark. When fearful children are called upon to endure darkness in isolation, a dread of imaginary creatures may also appear. Causal factors linked to fearfulness in children include (Jenkins, 1970; Kashani et al., 1981):

■ Unusual constitutional sensitivity to fear-producing stimuli.

■ Undermining of feelings of adequacy and security by an early trauma, such as accident, illness, or loss.

■ Exposure to unfamiliar surroundings such as a hospital or a new school.

■ Excessive warnings of the dangers of the world communicated to the child.

■ Repeated experiences with failure, reinforcing the child's feelings of inadequacy and inability to cope.

■ Inadequate interpersonal relationships extending beyond the family.

As children enter and progress through school, fear of failure and fear of the unknown may become joined in their mind. For some children the primary fear is of parental disapproval or of failure to attain satisfactory academic standards. Other children whose parents are less concerned with academic performance may fear not making friends or not being accepted by the group.

Childhood fears may continue into adolescence and adulthood, but this is not the prevailing outcome. As children become older and have more opportunities for social interaction, they are likely to encounter corrective experiences. Behavior modification procedures (including desensitization and assertiveness training) and experiences that promote autonomy and confidence help to eliminate childhood fears (Carstens, 1982).

In treating irrational fears, it is initially necessary to understand what the child fears. If the identified fear involves an imminent event, anticipatory guidance may be offered. The sequence of steps leading up to the feared event and the circumstances surrounding the event itself may be discussed with the child. This mental rehearsal, combined with reassurance and encouragement, does much to diminish fear of what might happen. If what the child fears is a repetition of a previous event that proved painful, the child can practice repeating the experience in a safe atmosphere. This technique would be appropriate for a shy child who is afraid of speaking or of being noticed in public.

It is important to distinguish between a fear and a phobia (see Chapter 8). A phobia has little or no basis in reality and therefore originates in subjective, internal stimuli. The identifying feature of a phobia is that the phobic person recognizes the irrationality of the feelings but cannot alter them. Thus, the unreasonable, unwarranted fears that surround the phobia continually intrude on conscious awareness. Perhaps the most common example of phobia in children is school phobia, also known as avoidant behavior about school, which is generally thought to be related to fear of separation from the mother. The restrictions that some phobias place on the life of any individual can be severe enough to require intensive measures. Behavior therapy may be used to help children and adults incapacitated by phobia, as may insight therapy that seeks to uncover the emotional basis of the problem. Sometimes both approaches are used in conjunction (Atkinson, Quarrington, and Cyr, 1983).

Working with Children

Childhood is often romanticized by adults. They like to think of children as living in a protected world where their needs are met, playtime is joyous, and happiness abounds. This is not wholly true, for

383

CLINICAL EXAMPLE

███████████████████████

ENCOPRESIS AND REGRESSION IN A CHILD

████████████████████

Mark Evans is six years old and the middle child in a family of three children. His sister, Connie, is eleven and he has a new nine-week-old brother. Connie had eagerly looked forward to the baby's arrival and is excited to have a new brother. She is old enough to realize that she is still the only girl in the family, and her mother reinforces this feeling by making Connie her unofficial helper as far as the boys are concerned.

Mark had reacted to the news of his mother's pregnancy by becoming more clinging, but he seemed to accept the situation as time went on. For the first two weeks after the birth of the baby, Mark was quiet but gave no serious indication of maladjustment. Then he began soiling himself at home after school. Realizing that Mark might be having problems accepting the new baby, his mother tried not to overreact to the episodes. She simply changed his clothing, gave him a hug and a cookie, and tried to overlook the incidents. It was more difficult for Mark's mother to remain casual when the soiling began to happen during the school day. Whenever Mark had an "accident," his teacher sent him to the school nurse, who made him as comfortable as possible until his mother arrived with a change of clothing. Because Mark seemed upset and reluctant to return to the classroom, his mother took him home. She usually left the baby with grandma or a neighbor, so the episodes of soiling gave Mark time to be with his mother without competing for her attention.

Within a week or two the "accidents" in school became more frequent while those at home subsided. Mark's teacher was annoyed by the disruptions to class routine, and the other children teased him constantly, but Mark did not seem overly distressed by the commotion. When the behavior showed no signs of improving, the school nurse suggested a physical examination and the possibility of getting psychological help if there was no physical explanation for Mark's problem. Mark's mother followed the nurse's recommendation and took him to the family pediatrician, who could find no physical explanation. Knowing that Mark had complete bowel and bladder control until his little brother was born, the pediatrician suggested an evaluation at a child guidance clinic.

ASSESSMENT

Mark's symptomatology accomplished a number of things. When he soiled himself in school, his mother left the new baby and came to the rescue. She then provided the care Mark had received and enjoyed as a much younger boy. Mark and his mother had always been extremely close, but when the new baby was born, she seemed preoccupied with him and Mark felt rejected. Assessment led to the following diagnoses being made:

Nursing Diagnoses

Anxiety: Severe

Coping, ineffectual individual

Fear

Self-concept: Disturbance in self-esteem

Multiaxial Psychiatric Diagnoses

Axis I 309.21 Separation anxiety disorder
307.70 Functional encopresis

Axis II None

Axis III None

Axis IV Code 4—Moderate

Axis V Level 4—Fair

PLANNING

Mark's encopresis was attributed to changes in the family caused by the entry of the new baby. Although Mark and Connie had been prepared for the arrival of a new brother or sister, there were safeguards for Connie that did not exist for Mark. Because of her age and gender, Connie was able to move into a new role as family helper without losing her special position as the only girl. Her closeness with her father was enhanced rather than threatened by the baby brother, and a new closeness was developing between Connie and her mother. Mark, on the other hand, had lost his special relationship with his mother and had found nothing to take its place. It was therefore considered important for Mark's father to build closer ties with the boy in order to compensate Mark for what he thought he had lost. When there were only two children, it was possible for the family to function with alliances between mother and Mark, father and Connie. The new baby changed the family balance. It became essential that the father form a new alliance that included both older children and that the mother reinforce Mark's important status as an older brother.

IMPLEMENTATION

Although Mark's encopresis was the presenting problem, this family had been divided for some time. Dysfunction was not evident because the division in the family was equitable and the alliances satisfied all family members. However, the alignment between mother and Mark and between Connie and her father meant that each child was uninvolved with one parent. The birth of the new baby allowed Connie to move closer to her mother without jeopardizing her special relationship with her father.

Mark, on the other hand, was ousted from his special position with his mother and yet continued to be excluded from closeness with his father. His soiling episodes at school were covert attempts to renew his previous relationship with his mother.

The counselor at the child guidance clinic assured Mark's mother than encopresis was unlikely to become chronic regardless of the emotional component but indicated that some family changes would be helpful. Since the changes required the father as well as the mother, both parents were asked to attend several sessions. The need for new family alliances was pointed out to Mark's father, and a strong recommendation was made that Mark be included in the closeness that existed between Connie and her father. This could be done by arranging activities that included both children, in addition to those that included only Mark and his father.

Mark's mother was advised to bring a change of clothing but not to take Mark out of school whenever he had an "accident." Mark's teacher and the school nurse were informed of this recommendation and agreed to cooperate. At home, Mark's mother began to rely on him to perform small services in order to encourage a sense of autonomy and self-esteem in him. This also had the effect of removing from Connie the role of the parenting child, a development that had further eroded Mark's self-esteem.

EVALUATION

Mark's episodes of encopresis gradually ceased over a six-month period. Mark's father made a conscious effort to establish a positive relationship with him and Mark proved receptive. Closeness with the father was facilitated because Connie continued to be involved with her mother and the baby. Both parents had learned the importance of including every child and excluding no child from parental attentiveness. Both had been devoted parents, but each had performed parenting functions as a solo act. Aware now of the reciprocal nature of parenting and of the importance of operating as a dyad, the parents were committed to the ideal of equitable treatment of all three children.

385

even in the best of environments, a child also lives in an inner world of uncertainty and apprehension, which may be aggravated by urgent maturational tasks. Because infants and young children must depend on parents or parent surrogates to meet their needs, teaching parents about maturational tasks and children's developmental progress can serve as primary prevention aimed at avoiding dysfunctional behavior patterns in children. Many altered maturational patterns are created or worsened by unrealistic parental expectations. When parents do not recognize the time frame of development and growth in children, they either hasten or impede processes that may already be within the normal range.

If behavior problems have already become apparent, a nurse can utilize principles of secondary prevention. If assessment indicates that a parent is the instigator of the problem, the nurse might arrange opportunities to model effective adult-child interactions. By explaining and demonstrating basic concepts of stimulus, response, and reward, the nurse can indicate those adult actions that initiate or reinforce undesirable behavior in children. The difference between discipline and punishment is a subtle one for parents who rely only on scoldings or spankings to alter the behavior of their children. Of prime importance is the need to show parents the effectiveness of positive reinforcement in bringing about improved behaviors. For some parents praise is more difficult to bestow than disapproval. Such parents need to be assured that approving gestures will not necessarily threaten discipline or erode their authority.

Most parents tend to repeat the kind of parenting practices they themselves experienced. A nurse who recognizes a generational cycle of parenting behavior that is contributing to dysfunction may have to begin by introducing alternative ways of talking to and interacting with the children. Often parents are resistant to the nurse's interventions until the nurse has gained their confidence and trust by acknowledging that parenting is a difficult, complicated task for which most people are not fully prepared.

ALTERED MATURATIONAL PATTERNS OF ADOLESCENCE

Adolescence is generally recognized as a turbulent period of life. The individual is maturing physically, intellectually, socially, and sexually at a rapid rate. In an interval of about seven years, the individual travels the territory between childhood and beginning adulthood. It is a strange and intense journey over an unknown terrain (Erikson, 1968). Most adolescents progress without undue difficulties, although the period is often stressful for parents as well as children. Perhaps the major task for adolescents is the establishment of identity as they move away from their family of origin. In the process of establishing a separate identity, they sometimes acquire problematic behaviors.

Identity Confusion

The task of creating a separate identity is complicated by the fact that most adolescents must accomplish it while continuing to live with their family of origin, on whom they are likely to be financially dependent. At this point the adolescent is asking him-

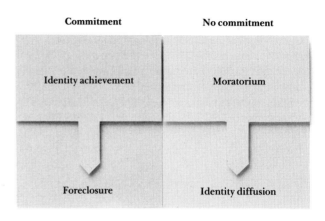

Figure 14-2. *Identity status of adolescents.*
SOURCE: Marcia (1966).

386

self such existential questions as "Who am I? What shall I do with my life? Where will I fit in?" While the adolescent is asking these questions and differentiating from his family, his peer group assumes a position of great importance. Fads, stereotyped activities, and group-approved behavior become highly influential, often moreso than parental viewpoints.

Marcia (1966) studied the commitment of adolescents to three issues considered important to the establishing of identity: religion, politics, and occupation. By combining the search for identity with these three issues, Marcia proposed four ways to assess adolescents in the identity stage of development (see Figure 14-2).

Adolescents who have examined parental attitudes on religion, politics, and occupation and then determined their own stand on the three issues have reached *identity achievement.* Adolescents who have reached this point (or *cell,* as Marcia calls it) may or may not agree with their parents but they have made a real choice and have arrived at their own opinions. Adolescents in the *foreclosure* cell have accepted parental positions on the three relevant issues without examining these positions. These teenagers do not seem to undergo an identity crisis and on the surface appear to have firm convictions. Yet they lack true ego identity because they have avoided confronting the three issues. Adopting parental attitudes without question may represent fear of parental disapproval or timidity in asserting one's own views.

Adolescents in the *moratorium* cell are indecisive. These teenagers are concerned with the three issues but have not yet made any decisions. For some young people the moratorium is merely a transitional phase during which decisions are deferred until late adolescence or early adulthood. Adolescents in the cell of *identity diffusion* are characterized by chronic indecision accompanied by lack of interest in the issues of religion, politics, and occupation.

Antisocial Behavior

There is a Chinese proverb that says, "A little child weighs on your knees, a big one on your heart." The truth of this statement is evident to parents who face the antisocial behavior of an adolescent son or daughter. The term "antisocial behavior" is subject to several interpretations, but here it is used to describe repeated acts of delinquency committed by a minor that would be considered criminal if committed by an adult.

A pattern of antisocial behavior can sometimes be discerned early in life. Between the ages of five and ten, the child begins to show signs of excessive defiance, temper tantrums, unruliness, and hostility (Smith, 1978). One of the consistent findings in the lives of delinquent adolescents is a constellation of unfavorable family characteristics. Parents of teenagers who display antisocial behaviors have a higher than average history of alcoholism, criminality, and marital conflict. The mothers frequently lack close emotional ties to their children and tend to ignore the delinquent behavior. The fathers tend to be strict and to use physical forms of punishment. Although disorganization is common in the families of delinquents, it is by no means a requirement. Antisocial behavior is expressed by adolescents from all socioeconomic levels, from intact nuclear families and one-parent families. In short, there is no clear-cut, simple formula to apply to delinquent-

Psychopathy is the one disorder which has its roots most firmly set in childhood with repeated and widespread antisocial behavior in early life often leading to later persisting disorders of personality. In spite of the persistence of the behavior from childhood to adult life, it appears that environmental factors are most important in its genesis.

M. RUTTER (1974)

387

producing families (Webster-Stratton, 1985).

When an adolescent engages in antisocial behavior, the entire family can probably benefit from counseling. Family issues are likely to be complex and to require the intervention of a skilled counselor. Just as no single cause precipitates antisocial behavior, so no single strategy is likely to rectify the situation (Szurek and Berlin, 1970). Approaches to intervention are varied. When facilities and staff are adequate, special schools, special programs, and specially prepared teachers can be of assistance. The major goals are to help adolescents learn about the world and themselves, to advance their education, and to teach them marketable skills. It is essential that peer group influences be directed toward resocialization rather than continuation of delinquent practices. Behavior techniques are usually part of programs designed to change maladaptive learned behaviors.

Residential institutions are dubious places for young people whose actions would not be considered criminal if committed by an adult. These would include such actions as running away from home and being sexually active. For this category of juvenile offenders, institutionalization might intensify rather than alleviate the problem. Institutionalizing juvenile status offenders along with persons who have committed violent antisocial acts places them under the influence of malevolent peers. However, failure to institutionalize young people who have committed violent crimes may be a disservice to society and to the young people themselves. A progressive step would be to remove felonies and misdemeanors committed by young people from the broad classification of juvenile delinquency and to formulate subgroups of offenses based on the

seriousness of the juvenile's action as well as the age of the offender (Fersch, 1980; Coleman, Butcher, and Carson, 1984).

Body Image Distortion

Most adolescents are intensely preoccupied and concerned with their body image. They monitor the somatic changes in themselves and make comparisons with the bodies of peers and with the physical ideals of society. In some adolescents, especially females, attention to one's body takes on compulsiveness that far exceeds the established limits of normalcy. One particular expression of body image distortion is the condition called *anorexia nervosa.*

Anorexia nervosa is a physiological disorder, psychogenic in origin, that is accompanied by voluntary, self-induced dieting that eventually exceeds the boundaries of conscious control and becomes compulsive. The syndrome includes episodes of fasting, gorging, vomiting, and purging (Potts, 1984; Sanger and Cassino, 1984). An early description by Dunton and Langford (1962) acknowledged the relationship between the anorectic and the environment, explaining that the anorectic has a compulsive preoccupation with food, weight, and dieting that is demonstrated in a never-ending struggle with the environment and with persons in the environment. Because the condition is sometimes a maladaptive reaction to stress, psychological or social, it is discussed from a different perspective in Chapter 12.

A behavior related to anorexia nervosa is bulimia, in which the person gorges on junk food followed by self-initiated vomiting and excessive use of laxatives. Bulimia may exist in conjunction with

Statistics on the frequency of eating disorders are almost nonexistent and the few that have been collected are limited. A survey conducted in 1981 by the National Association of Anorexia Nervosa and Associated Disorders . . . does indicate that the age range of victims is far broader than had been thought. Of some 1400 respondents who had diagnosed themselves as having anorexia or bulimia, 1.8% were 50 years or older; 2.7% were 40 to 49 years, and 20.5% were 30 to 39, making a total of 25% over 30 . . . There is also disagreement about which disorder strikes older women more often, though most authorities say that older bulimics outnumber anorectics in their age category. There is agreement that, no matter what the condition, the older the individual the more tenacious it will be.

NADINE BROZAN (1983)

388

anorexia nervosa or as a separate syndrome. Extreme weight loss is not usually a symptom of bulimia unless anorexia is also present (Sours, 1980).

Anorectics are usually intelligent, ambitious young women who are committed to high standards of control and perfectionism. Most of them are high achievers in school and display compulsive behaviors regarding academic achievement. The relationship between the anorectic young woman and her mother is thought to be highly significant. The mother of the victim is seen as a domineering perfectionist who is often dependent on her own mother yet displays controlling attitudes toward her daughter (Bruch, 1973). The anorectic young woman believes that there is little she can do to experience feelings of mastery so she looks for one area that she can control. Ultimately she discovers this mastery by controlling what she eats. As the disorder progresses she no longer experiences sensations of hunger yet continues to be preoccupied with preparing and discussing food (Halmi, Falk, and Schwartz, 1981).

Working with Adolescents

Erikson (1968) wrote that the adolescent engages in forms of fantasy and introspection that were suppressed in childhood and will again be suppressed in adulthood. He called adolescence a time of leaning over precipices and cautioned adults against overreacting to the role experimentation that adolescents engage in as they strive for identity. Whether or not the adolescent moves forward or regresses depends on the opportunities and rewards available in the family, in the peer group, and in society at large.

During adolescence, joys and sorrows are experienced intensely and turbulently. Occasionally, adults will take a casual attitude toward the intensity of adolescents, underestimating the pain and uncertainty of the adolescent experience. Because most teenagers are able to detect this attitude, they become less willing to share their feelings with adults. Professionals who belittle or misunderstand the seriousness with which adolescents view life are rarely given a second chance to be helpful.

In working with adolescents, nurses have the opportunity to offer primary prevention. Children and teenagers are accustomed to looking at nurses as experts and as sources of reliable information. Thus, one of the interventions nurses can provide is accurate information about the physical changes associated with adolescence and the normal range of changes. A nurse can reassure adolescents that the physical changes are natural and are part of becoming an adult. Nurses are also in a position to note when normal concern about the physical changes becomes maladaptive, as in the case of anorexia.

There is no need for a nurse to demonstrate to adolescents that it is possible to solve all their problems quickly and easily. Merely listening reflectively to a teenager's problems and to the solutions that have been attempted can be reassuring and can help the teenager trust the adult world.

Because peer groups are so influential with adolescents, group work can be highly effective. Meeting regularly with others of the same age who are experiencing the same difficulties is extremely beneficial for adolescents.

C L I N I C A L   V I G N E T T E

IDENTITY ACHIEVEMENT IN AN ADOLESCENT

Jenny was the oldest child in a conservative, devout, middle-class family. Her father was a prosperous corporate lawyer and her mother was an active club woman and avid golfer. Jenny did not question family values until she left home and became a college freshman. The college she chose was known for the liberal thinking of its faculty and students, many of whom were political activists. At college Jenny was influenced by the opinions of the people around her. Gradually she stopped attending church services because she no longer found them relevant. She became involved in a number of student organizations that took a strong stand on controversial issues, and she began marching in demonstrations, chanting, carrying signboards, and engaging in sit-ins. When she went home at vacation time, Jenny argued heatedly with her parents, who were shocked by most of the causes Jenny supported. She, in turn, criticized her parents for their affluence, their smugness, and their indifference to poverty and social injustice. Her school performance suffered because of her new interests, providing another source of contention between Jenny and her parents.

Relations between Jenny and her parents were strained until the beginning of her junior year, when she informed them that she had decided to go to law school after graduation. However, she warned her father that she was not at all interested in corporate law because

such lawyers were "social parasites." Instead, Jenny would become a lawyer who protected the rights of the poor and humble, even if this was less profitable than corporate law. Although her parents did not agree with their daughter's extremism, they were relieved that she had chosen an occupation that seemed acceptable.

Jenny herself was satisfied with her decision, and the family conflict abated. There were even times when she and her father could discuss legal matters without becoming enraged at each other. In effect, Jenny had resolved a maturational crisis, even though the resolution was a stormy, tumultuous time for the family. She had challenged her parents' outlook on politics, religion, and occupational choice. The sessions with her parents were difficult for everyone, but the questioning process undertaken by Jenny was important to her identity achievement as she identified and became committed to a value system of her own. The sequence Jenny followed in her search for identity can be summarized in six steps:

1. Group influences at college.
2. Challenge to family values.
3. Acquisition of new values.
4. Family crisis.
5. Commitment to individual values.
6. Achievement of individual identity.

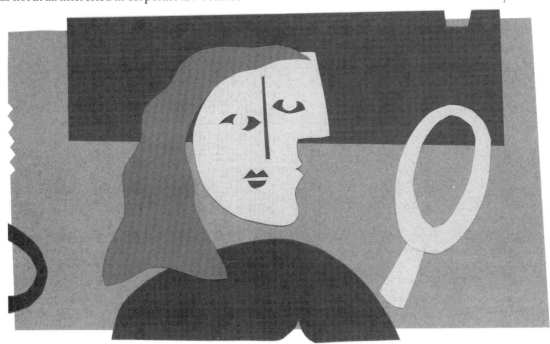

Periods of occupational stress are inevitable in any type of job.
SOURCE: Jackie Estrada.

390

ALTERED MATURATIONAL PATTERNS OF ADULTHOOD

Most persons reach adulthood after successfully negotiating the transitions of childhood and adolescence and make a commitment to career and family. This means that the maturational crises of adults are likely to revolve around career and family.

Career Crises

Children are asked so often what they want to be as adults that they soon learn that career choice is a serious matter. As they become teenagers they are pressured to choose an occupation compatible with the ambitions of their parents, even at the expense of their own preferences. Directly and indirectly, children are given the message that identity and status will largely depend on what they do for a living. Many young people believe they must select an occupation while they are still in high school. This means that some of them make a career choice based on a limited knowledge of opportunities and their own capabilities.

Even for individuals fortunate enough to have made a good career choice there are inevitable periods of occupational stress. This is true not only for persons performing menial jobs at minimum wages but for highly successful professionals as well. In the mind of the general public some occupations are considered more stressful than others. Among the workers believed subject to severe stress are air traffic controllers, policemen, and surgeons. However, an extensive study of the health records of 20,000 workers failed to show a correlation between specific occupations and stress-related disorders (McLean, 1980). In short, total avoidance of occupational stress is unrealistic and unattainable.

Although occupational stress cannot be wholly eradicated, there are ways of dealing with it. The first step is to recognize the existence of stress and to identify the cause. Many clerical, technical, service, and industrial workers suffer stress because of the repetitive monotonous nature of their work (McLean, 1980). Restrictive and regulated working conditions are also stressful, especially if production quotas are imposed. Workers' perceptions of themselves and their jobs can be a source of stress. Two factors are involved: quantitative and qualitative overload. *Quantitative overload* means having too much to do. Workers with this type of overload tend toward excessive drinking, low self-esteem, poor motivation, and high absenteeism. *Qualitative overload* means having tasks that are too difficult to do. Workers with this type of overload experience high levels of tension and job dissatisfaction, accompanied by a loss of confidence. Similar emotional reactions have been reported by workers who perceive that their abilities exceed the demands of the job (McLean, 1980).

Workers who experience occupational frustration have several available alternatives. Many workers are now asking that the conditions of their employment be less restrictive and more fulfilling. When workers are unable to obtain modification of undesirable working conditions, they may resort to retraining, additional education, early retirement, or passive resistance in the form of absenteeism or lowered efficiency. Occupational stress may be a contributing factor in psychophysiological dysfunction; the crucial issue is the interaction between the

In general, it is the inability to settle on an occupational identity which most disturbs young people. To keep themselves together they temporarily overidentify with the heroes of cliques and crowds to the point of an apparently complete loss of individuality . . . Young people can become remarkably clannish, intolerant, and cruel in their exclusion of others who are different in skin color or cultural background, in tastes and gifts, and often in entirely petty aspects of dress and gesture arbitrarily selected as signs of an in-grouper or an out-grouper. It is important to understand in principle . . . that such intolerance may be for a while a necessary defense against identity loss.

ERIK ERIKSON (1968)

391

worker's temperament and the work situation. Any job that is characterized by rapid change and unrealistic performance standards will be stressful for most workers, but the perception of conditions and reactions to conditions are highly individualized. In some instances, it is the worker who must endeavor to change, and counseling may be indicated. If the worker makes extreme demands on himself, the focus of counseling might be to encourage more realistic performance standards. However, if many workers share similar feelings of frustration, modification of company standards might be a group goal.

Marital Crises

At the time of selecting a mate or sexual partner, young adults are facing what Erikson (1968) calls the *intimacy crisis*. After progressing through prior stages of independence and identity, individuals begin to think of themselves as ready to form a meaningful union with another person in which there is space to regulate the activities of career, procreation, and recreation. Most individuals in Western society marry, even though there have been social changes in the last few decades that permit cohabitation without marriage, homosexual alliances, and communal living.

One of the contemporary changes in marriage is the increase in the number of dual-career marriages, in which both husband and wife work outside the home. With both partners committed to jobs or careers, there are heavy demands on the marriage. Job demands and homemaking responsibilities tend to absorb all available time, especially if there are children (Carter and Glick, 1976). The everyday demands of time and energy are sources of

stress in many dual-career marriages. In order for a marriage to weather the additional strains posed by two careers, both partners must make a conscious commitment to the relationship.

Even when a marriage does not involve dual careers, the marital relationship is vulnerable to the myriad demands placed on it. Conflicts over communication, sex, children, finances, fidelity, and changing personal interests are commonly cited causes of marital discord. Although the causes vary, the result is often alienation, separation, and divorce. In the past, social prohibitions against divorce were much stronger and many unhappy couples remained married. Today a great many marriages end in divorce, and as divorce becomes more common, less censure is applied. For many couples divorce seems the only solution to sustained marital crisis.

The dissolution of a marriage by divorce is an emotional experience that affects not only the marital partners but also their children, friends, and other relatives. In-laws who have come to care for a son-in-law or a daughter-in-law feel upset and confused. Married friends may see in the troubled marriage a reflection of their own problems and therefore feel threatened. Children feel frightened, angry, and guilty and frequently blame themselves.

The experience of divorce has been compared to death without the comfort of formalized mourning rituals (Weiss, 1979). Certainly, the painful aftermath of divorce must be endured without the social support given to those who have lost a husband or wife through death (Kitson, Moir, and Mason, 1982).

Within three to five years following divorce, 80 percent of persons remarry. This percentage in-

MATURATIONAL CRISIS IN A DUAL-CAREER MARRIAGE

Veronica and Archie were high school sweethearts who entered the same university, studied together, lived together, and were married in their senior year. Both were outstanding students whose grade point averages were rarely more than a half point apart. Archie majored in organic chemistry and Veronica was enrolled in a four-year nursing program. The couple had planned to begin graduate school together, but Veronica became pregnant the summer after graduation. Unwilling to undergo an abortion, she received permission from the university to defer her graduate school entry until the following year. Archie entered graduate school that fall as originally planned.

During the time that Veronica stayed at home to care for her baby daughter, she often felt envious of Archie, but she told herself that her turn would come. A year later, when her baby was six months old, Veronica resumed her nursing studies in a master's program. A friend of Veronica's who was the mother of two preschoolers and lived in an adjoining apartment agreed to care for the baby during the day. Her friend was conscientious and attentive to children, so Veronica envisioned no problems on that score.

When Veronica functioned as a full-time housewife and mother, she did all the housework in addition to caring for the baby. Although she and Archie had not discussed the mechanics of daily living after she returned to school, Veronica had assumed that she and her husband would revert to the task sharing of their undergraduate years. This was not exactly what Archie had in mind. While Veronica was at home with the baby, Archie had established the habit of studying with classmates and was reluctant to discontinue this practice. When talking to Veronica he minimized the requirements of her nursing program, telling her that his courses were more rigorous. Archie had agreed to share the shopping and cooking chores, but he did not become involved in the evening care of their baby, concentrating on his studies as Veronica hurried to feed the baby in order to get to her own academic work.

Sensing Veronica's impatience, the baby became increasingly fretful. This in turn annoyed Archie, who criticized Veronica and the baby and found excuses to study in the library with a friend. At home alone in the apartment, Veronica cared for her cranky baby and often did not get to her books until 10 P.M. or later. Not long

afterward, Archie would come home with his own assignments completed and promptly go to bed. By studying until 2 or 3 A.M. Veronica managed to keep up with her schoolwork. She worried about the baby and realized she was robotlike in her interactions with the child. Discussions with Archie about her predicament degenerated into shouting matches. On one occasion Veronica accused him of deliberately making her pregnant so he could be the superachiever of the family; he responded by saying it wouldn't help them if he flunked out of school. After repeated quarrels and barely passing her midterm exams, Veronica issued an ultimatum. Either they would see a marriage counselor or Veronica would leave Archie and move in with her friend who looked af-

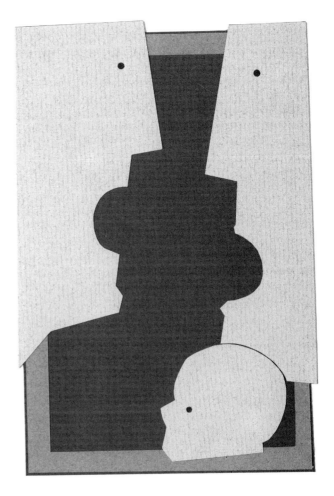

ter the baby during the day. After some hesitation, Archie agreed.

ASSESSMENT

Veronica made an appointment at a community mental health center serving the neighborhood in which they lived. She and Archie agreed that they did not want to seek help in an agency where they were known. After an intake interview at which they were seen together, the couple were assigned to a psychologist and a master's-prepared psychiatric nurse working in tandem. Because the couple's problems seemed to center around role enactment, it was thought that they would be served best by a male and female acting as co-counselors. It was obvious even in the intake interview that Archie and Veronica were equally committed to their careers but that Veronica had taken on full parenting responsibilities. There was some sharing of household tasks, but child care was not integrated into the pattern of family obligations. During pregnancy the wife had put aside her career ambitions, but her choice had not been carefully discussed at the time. Veronica had made the decision by default because it seemed the only choice open, and her husband failed to recognize that she had made a sacrifice that deserved future guarantees from him.

The following diagnoses were made:

Nursing Diagnoses
Coping, ineffective family

Family process, alteration in

Home maintenance management, impaired

Parenting, alteration in

Multiaxial Psychiatric Diagnosis
Axis I   309.28 Adjustment disorder with mixed emotional features

Axis II V71.09 No diagnosis

Axis III None

Axis IV Code 4—Moderate

Axis V   Level 4—Fair

PLANNING

Although the couple had been committed to equality in their relationship, parenthood shifted the balance in favor of the husband. Without meaning to, Archie had placed his wife in the position of sacrificing too much for too long. Preoccupied with his own goals, he overlooked the deprivation his wife was experiencing. Moreover, he considered her career obligations less demanding than his own.

Despite Archie's lack of concern about the daily demands of parenthood, he willingly accepted financial responsibility for his wife and child at some future time. Fear of not being able to provide well for his family was one of the reasons why he devoted so much attention to his academic work. His excessive attention to his studies, although perceived as selfish by his wife, was also moti-

vated by his wish to give his family financial security. What he failed to realize was that his wife wanted to share the role of provider and resented being relegated to the domestic sphere.

IMPLEMENTATION

Marital counseling focused on improving communication between partners. Even though Veronica and Archie knew each other as friends, students, lovers, and spouses, their parenting responsibilities were new. Veronica expected Archie to know intuitively when she needed help, just as he expected her to know intuitively that he appreciated her sacrifice in giving up school to have their child. Each needed to learn to express feelings, to ask directly, to acknowledge openly, and to compromise. Veronica was unwilling to give up her ambitions and was unaware that her husband had made her ambitions secondary because of his wish to provide well for her and their child. What remained was for these two intelligent young people to begin a process of negotiation and to begin rebuilding a relationship that had already proved its importance to them. With equitable and flexible role sharing the primary goal, the following problems were addressed:

393

1. Adequate support systems for child care and housework needed to be arranged. Evening help was necessary so Veronica could relax for an hour or so with her child before beginning to study. This period of relaxation should involve Archie as well.

2. Archie needed to share his study time with his wife as well as his classmates and to avoid comparing her educational program with his graduate program. Whatever the differences in the respective programs, the academic commitments of husband and wife merited equal consideration.

3. A competitive spirit had destroyed the cooperation that once existed between Archie and Veronica. If their individual ambitions could once again become shared ambitions, their relationship would be strengthened and their former pride in each other restored.

EVALUATION

Both partners had a threefold obligation: to each other, to their child, and to their careers. Role sharing was essential to the survival of the marriage, and traditional task allocation had to be modified if this family was to remain intact. There was no need for either of the partners to change drastically, but communication needed to be improved. The daily responsibilities of the couple were enormous, but energy was being dissipated in futile anger and resentment. It was pointed out to the couple that a return to their previous pattern of cooperation was essential if husband and wife were to achieve their career goals. Archie and Veronica were receptive to the idea of renewed collaboration. In addition, appealing to their genuine affection for each other was used effectively to help the couple maintain the necessary balance between marriage, parenthood, and dual careers.

cludes five out of six divorced males and three out of four divorced females. The intricate pattern of establishing a second marriage remains largely an unexplored area of research. Because most divorced persons are also parents, remarriage introduces tasks of blending the two families and enacting new roles as step-parents (Norton and Glick, 1976; Wallerstein, 1984). Forming a step-family is a challenging task for all concerned. Each individual comes to the new family with a different set of expectations and with memories that must be integrated into the new arrangements. A period of testing and uncertainty is almost inevitable. Three problems that may surface in second marriages have been identified (Janosik, 1984):

1. The new partner who has chosen to marry a single parent may be reluctant to accept the children as part of the package.

2. Former mates may accept the remarriage of a spouse but dislike the idea of their children having a step-parent.

3. Children may continue to entertain fantasies that their natural parents will reconcile in spite of the remarriages of the parents.

Stern (1978) found that one interactional pattern in step-families was likely to be more adaptive than other patterns. In this pattern the step-father was accepting of his wife's role as mother and of her preexisting relationships with her children. He began by making friends with the children of his new wife while carefully avoiding the role of rival. It was found that this interactional style encouraged all members of the new family to participate in the formulation and acceptance of revised family rules and norms.

Parental Crises

Although some couples are choosing not to have children, the majority of married couples become parents. In Eriksonian terms, the conscious choice to produce a child is an expression of creativity and generativity. Once children enter the family, the parents face years of hard work and sacrifice. Time, energy, and money must be expended to meet the physical and emotional needs of the children. New mothers speak of chronic fatigue, overwhelming domestic chores, and a decline in outside interests and activities. Mothers who gave up enjoyable employment to be home with their children frequently yearn for the stimulation of outside work, while mothers who must return to work feel guilty and unhappy at leaving their children. New fathers also report increased fatigue, greater worries over

money, and a decline in social activities. Both parents feel a loss of privacy and a decrease in sexual activity (Green, 1980).

As children grow older, parental time previously spent on the physical care of children is devoted to supervising and arranging school and community activities. The onset of adolescence brings new problems and concerns. The questioning of parental values that teenagers engage in as they pursue a separate identity is a cause of worry for many parents. The tendency of many teenagers to experiment with drugs, alcohol, and sex is another source of ongoing tension.

When adolescents continue their education in colleges or universities, they remain financially dependent on parents, and the costs of a college education can be extremely burdensome. At this time mothers who have never worked outside the home may have to look for paid employment. For some women this may prove a source of pride and accomplishment; for others it is an unpleasant reminder that the father is not adequately fulfilling the role of provider. In such instances additional strain may be brought to bear on the marriage.

Working with Adults

One approach a nurse can offer adults experiencing a maturational crisis is guidance in setting realistic, achievable goals. Many adults have an ideal of how they would like their lives to be, and most feel they have fallen short of that ideal. When adults feel disappointed in themselves or in their families, they need assistance in identifying the positive achievements in their lives. When they measure their achievements against impossible standards or set objectives that cannot be reached, they may need help in modifying or reordering their priorities. Thus, a man who is not promoted may need to be reminded of how far he has already advanced in rank and how much he is loved by his family and respected by the community. Such interventions represent a cognitive approach that counteracts the tendency of many adults to cling to impossible dreams.

Many well-adjusted people experience a temporary state of disequilibrium when they or a family member confronts a maturational crisis. For such individuals, referral to a *support group* may be helpful. Support groups are available for people dealing with various problems, maturational and situational. There are support groups for single parents, for the unemployed, and for the newly divorced or widowed, to name but a few. When there is no available group to meet specific needs, a nurse might use her skills to help individuals organize their own group. Support groups are widely used on a local and national level by persons with similar concerns.

They serve an important purpose in a mobile, transient society, offering acceptance and understanding to their members. Additionally, such groups present an opportunity for members to aid newer members, once their own problems have abated. This is a therapeutic aspect of the group experience, as was noted by Maslow (1970), who wrote that mature adults need to be needed. Support groups for adults in a maturational crisis are thus an avenue for the expression of generativity as well as a source of aid.

ALTERED MATURATIONAL PATTERNS OF OLD AGE

The maturational crises of the elderly are intensified by the way society regards old age. Youthfulness is highly valued in American society, and fear of aging is reinforced. Many individuals see in the elderly the prediction of their own future, fear their own aging, and try to avoid accepting the later stages of the life cycle until they must. This is unfortunate, because planning for the final life cycle stage can help avoid or ameliorate some of the problems.

Adjustment to recurrent loss is a prevailing theme in the lives of older people. In addition to the loss of youthful strength and vigor and of friends and loved ones, the elderly suffer role losses as their children become independent, and as retirement arrives.

The Empty Nest Syndrome

The *empty nest syndrome* refers to feelings of loneliness and depression experienced by many parents, especially mothers, after their last child has left home. Although the concept of the empty nest has been given considerable public attention, it is possible that the problem has been exaggerated and that it is experienced by a relatively small percentage of parents. The key factor in adjusting to the empty nest seems to be the number of options available to the parents. The absence of dependent children may be distressing to a woman who has treasured the role of mother beyond all else but not for the woman whose role as mother has already been supplemented by other roles. Some women work throughout the years that their children are dependent and suffer no great distress when all the children are gone. Even women who chose to be homemakers may see the empty nest period as an opportunity to enter the paid labor force, to continue their interrupted educations, or to become involved in community activities (Chenelly and Janosik, 1980).

The effect of the empty nest on fathers has received less attention than the effect on mothers. Farrell and Rosenberg (1981) did examine fathers' reactions to the departure of their children as part of a larger examination of men at midlife. They found a number of conflicting feelings among men whose children were in the process of leaving home. Further research is needed to address the effects of the empty nest on both parents.

Retirement Crises

Retirement has been defined as the socially sanctioned withdrawal from one's occupation in order to cope with changes in health or occupational status or to enjoy more leisure and freedom. Retirement includes the notion that the individual is entitled to stop working after being in the labor force for many years (Atchley, 1976). In many important respects, retirement represents a multiple loss. It is a loss of worker identity, a loss of power and privileges that accompanied the role of provider, and often a loss of income in absolute terms (Atchley, 1984).

Another loss associated with retirement is the disruption or severing of friendships or associations with colleagues and fellow workers. This can be a substantial loss that exacerbates feelings of loneliness and rejection. Reisman (1979) referred to friendships initiated and perpetuated in the workplace as *associative friendships*. Although the persons involved feel friendly toward one another, the friendship is dependent on the occupational association and on the roles they play. When the occupational roles change because of promotion, transfer, or retirement, the friendship attenuates or ceases to exist. Although promises may be exchanged to continue the friendship, this rarely happens when one of the participants leaves. Persons who remain employed generally replace the lost associates with others at the workplace.

The loss of associative friendships is keenly felt by retirees unless they have a network of more enduring relationships based on more than shared occupational interests. These friendships, called *friendships of reciprocity* (Reisman, 1979), help the retiree maintain social involvement after retirement as well as before. However, in order to sustain the same level of social involvement, a retired person must cultivate new friendships over the years to replace meaningful persons who move away or die. Given the circumstances of retirement, this may not be easy. After one has lost a number of beloved friends, the inclination is to retreat from new friendships to avoid the pain of further loss. This means that social contacts of older retirees may consist of depersonalized encounters with medical, nursing, or social agency personnel and of interactions with shopkeepers and other such service people.

395

Although reports on a variety of aspects of caring for the mentally impaired elderly have appeared in the literature, the "therapeutic nihilism" prevalent among health professionals about treating the aged is especially blatant in regard to the mentally impaired elderly . . . and little effort is made by staff members to prevent further slippage. The staff's ennui and lack of hope are soon picked up by family and friends, who sometimes cease to correspond with and/or visit the patient.

IRENE BURNSIDE (1984)

396

Atchley (1976) has described four paths to retirement and has associated adjustment with the reasons for retiring:

1. Planned and voluntary retirement. Those who follow this path are most likely to be satisfied with their lives after retirement.

2. Retirement imposed by the employer. This involuntary retirement is likely to be marked by dissatisfaction with the quality of life after retirement.

3. Retirement due to poor health. Parnes and Nestel (1981) report that persons on this path are the most dissatisfied with life after retirement, with their discontent encompassing their housing, leisure pursuits, and standard of living.

4. Gradual retirement, either by choice or as a consequence of unemployment. When the choice is voluntary and accompanied by a gradual reduction in working time, adjustment is relatively easy. When retirement is a decision made because of an extended period of unemployment, adjustment may be more difficult. However, the worker who realizes that there is little likelihood of obtaining another job can convert nonworking status into the more socially acceptable status of retiree. There are likely to be some residual feelings of anger or dissatisfaction if the decision is made reluctantly.

Adjustment to retirement is also affected by the extent of preretirement planning, but only a minority of the labor force has access to preretirement planning programs. These programs are often limited to an explanation of the employer's obligations and benefits extended to retirees (Silberstein, 1981). Such programs are likely to include information about pensions, Social Security payments, and simi-

lar matters. This is essential data, since adequate income has been identified as the single most essential element for successful retirement (Lamb and Duffy, 1979). Nevertheless, preretirement planning should not be limited to finances. Among other important issues to include in planning programs are use of leisure time, support networks and groups, and health-related matters.

Health-Related Crises

The inroads of physical decline represent another form of loss confronted by the elderly. Atchley (1980) defined *aging* as a gradual decrease in the viability and an increase in the vulnerability of the body. Although every system of the body ages, the rate of aging varies from person to person and from organ system to organ system. For example, an individual's gastrointestinal system may be healthy and resilient while her cardiovascular system may be degenerating. Therefore, chronological age is not a reliable predictor of the rate of aging, even though every individual undergoes the aging process over time.

With increasing age comes increased reaction times, and many actions take longer to complete. Botwinick (1978) attributes some of the changes in reaction time to cautiousness combined with a heightened desire to check oneself for accuracy. When older people feel hurried or under pressure, their anxiety further slows their reaction time and performance. One way to lessen this anxiety is to slow one's own movements and speech to match the pace of the elderly person. This relatively simple alteration in tempo will reduce the elderly person's anxiety and increase his comfort.

There are a number of ways in which an elderly

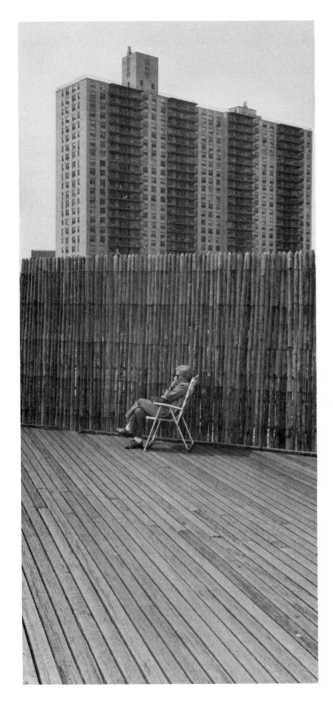

*For many people, old age is a
time of loneliness.*
SOURCE: Stephen Dunn.

397

fined grains, and cholesterol and too low in fiber, minerals, niacin, thiamine, and vitamins A and C (Weg, 1978). These deficiencies preclude optimal metabolism and promote physiological changes associated with aging. Improving the elderly person's diet is an area in which nurses can make a substantial contribution.

There is a strong social component in the eating habits of the elderly. People living alone, as many of the elderly do, often eat poorly or irregularly because there is no social impetus to prepare a meal or to eat. Few people, regardless of age, like to eat alone. Without the social exchange between individuals, much of the desire to eat abates. One of the most effective answers to the problem of persuading older people to eat well is the Title VII nutritional program available through County Offices on Aging. Meals are served at senior nutrition centers, which are located nationwide. There is a nominal fee for those who can afford it, but costs are suspended for those in need. This program meets socialization needs as well as nutritional needs and is one example of government response to the problems of aging Americans.

Terminal Crises

Death is repeatedly encountered by elderly people, who must deal with the loss of loved ones as well as the impending end of their own lives. The deaths of significant persons create crises that are difficult for the elderly to resolve. Each loss tends to reactivate memories of earlier losses and to remind the elderly of what lies ahead for them.

At the turn of the century, only 4 percent of the population lived to age sixty-five, compared with the current rate of 11 percent. At one time infec-

person's environment can be modified to accommodate his physical changes. Handrails near toilets and bathtubs compensate for impaired balance. Chairs with arms or with seats that lift or tilt compensate for a lack of muscle strength or coordination. Improved lighting arrangements can help remedy decreased visual acuity and poor night vision. Sensory losses can be offset in part by hearing aids, eyeglasses, large type, and the use of bright or contrasting colors for doors and stairways.

An important aspect of alleviating adverse changes associated with aging is the maintenance of proper nutrition. Studies show that the diets of older people are likely to be too high in sugar, re-

That evening she dies . . . the pain of irrevocable loss. A greater and deeper pain because there was no sense of unity, of fusion, of closeness and I had hoped to achieve this. The loss is greater and more terrible when closeness is not attained. All my life I had struggled to come closer to her, and now she was lost to me. It eluded me. Pain of remembrance. The lace unfinished. Her game of solitaire unfinished. That ordinary family last day, nothing to lift it from an ordinary family day, with family disharmonies stemming from childhood. Pain, her shrunken body in part dying, withering, but when she was very ill and I rubbed her body with alcohol her back was white, smooth, unwrinkled, shockingly smooth and not ready to die. Pain . . . as great as the stab of a knife. Pain not to have been there . . . Not only my mother had died, but my hope of fulfillment, of union with her, of an understanding penetrating love. I rebelled against death.

ANAIS NIN, THE DIARY, VOLUME V: 1947–1955

398

tious diseases, childbirth, accidents, and poor sanitation claimed the lives of people of all ages, so that death was not exclusively associated with old age (Atchley, 1980). Today, however, death is considered a concomitant of old age, and the death of a young person is considered an untimely tragedy. This thinking allows people to deny death until their own accumulated years force awareness upon them.

Death is denied in the way Americans treat and react to their dead. In previous generations, people died at home and adults knew how to treat a dead body (Feifel, 1973). Today the care of the deceased is almost the exclusive domain of professional morticians and undertakers. With fewer people dying at home there is less opportunity to see someone die or to view an unembalmed body. Such lack of contact with the physical remains helps people to keep death at arm's length.

One of the most painful encounters with death is the demise of a spouse, for this means the loss of a companion, confidant, friend, and lover. Because women tend to live longer than men and to marry men who are somewhat older, they are more likely than men to face widowhood. Atchley (1975) reported that among the population over age eighty, 85 percent of the women are widowed compared to 47 percent of the men. Of course, not all marriages are happy and not all partners find the role of husband or wife congenial or central to existence. Allowing for these variations, the dissolution of a marriage by death still brings strong feelings of grief and regret. Some widows and widowers may idealize the deceased, forgetting his or her faults and weaknesses. This may be disconcerting for those who have a more accurate recollection of the

deceased, but idealization is part of the grief process, and distortion need not be corrected (Fell, 1977). When the strengths and weaknesses of the deceased are accurately perceived by the mourner, it is likely that his or her grieving has been completed. (For additional discussion of grief and grieving, see Chapter 7.)

Working with the Elderly

One of the basic needs of all persons is recognition of their human dignity, and this need does not disappear with age. One way that human dignity finds expression is through the maintenance of activity and independence. It is therefore important to permit the elderly to feel useful and in control as much as possible. All too frequently, people live in progressively restrictive environments as they age. Although some restrictions may be necessary, the elderly should be allowed control over their possessions and should be given choices as long as they are able to make reasonable decisions. Until the moment of death, people need to feel that their wishes and preferences will be respected whenever possible. Although independence is valued by the aging person, interdependence is also a human need. To be interdependent means to be involved in a mutually rewarding exchange with one or more other people. Interdependence means giving and taking and sharing. Forming interdependent relationships is one way of preserving human dignity and maintaining the quality of life in old age.

One of the objectives of nurses working with elderly persons is to help them maintain their self-esteem despite the multiple losses that accompany old age. Self-esteem can be maintained in a number of ways. Some people are able to see themselves as

CLINICAL VIGNETTE

A CRISIS OF MANDATORY RETIREMENT

A few months after his sixty-second birthday, Eugene Willis suffered a myocardial infarction at the factory where he was plant foreman. Taken by ambulance to the nearest hospital, Eugene spent several weeks in intensive care before being transferred to a medical floor. After four weeks of hospitalization he was discharged with the stipulation that he return three times a week for cardiac rehabilitation. While he was in the hospital, Eugene was his customary jovial self. In the hospital and after discharge he complied with his regimen and stated firmly that he would be back on the job in a few weeks. In spite of his best efforts Eugene never completely recovered. When he tried to return to work, his application was rejected because his cardiologist recommended only limited exertion.

Even though he realized that retirement had been just around the corner, he became highly distressed when he found he was unable to return to work. Without advance warning or time to adjust, this outgoing man found himself a partially disabled retiree. Soon after his involuntary retirement, Eugene stopped attending the cardiac rehabilitation program. He began to stay away from home and spend his days at a local tavern. He was indifferent about his appearance and irritable with his wife, Diane. Disagreements and quarrels became more frequent, although Diane usually withdrew after saying that Eugene was a sick man who was destroying himself and his marriage.

Concerned because Eugene had dropped out of the rehabilitation program, the nurse in charge phoned to ask Eugene and Diane to drop in for a talk. After seeing the couple interact, the nurse realized how frightened Eugene was by his illness. Under his blustering behavior was a man who feared being dependent. Although surface harmony had existed between the couple for years, each had led separate lives. For Eugene, his job and the factory had been the hub of the world; for Diane, her home had been the hub. When Eugene was in the hospital, Diane was attentive and devoted, but when he was forced to retire, she was as unprepared as her husband. Accustomed to having her house to herself, she felt that her life had been disrupted, and she subtly indicated to Eugene that he was in the way. As a result of these hidden messages, Eugene left the house for the tavern, where he could find men who were willing to be his companions.

The nurse's initial purpose was to persuade Eugene to return to the cardiac rehabilitation program. After discussing the importance of the rehabilitation, she suggested that the couple join a spouses' group to discuss topics of interest to husbands and wives dealing with the aftermath of a heart attack. It was the nurse's hope that meeting other couples who had faced similar problems would help Eugene and his wife realize the need for communication and compromise in their home. The nurse did not become an advocate for either partner but tried to emphasize the importance of a stable marital relationship to Eugene's recovery.

After the couple began attending the spouses' group the nurse continued to see them occasionally. In the group and individual meetings, Diane was encouraged to look beyond Eugene's drinking and recognize his anxiety and depression. He, in turn, was encouraged to express his feelings verbally instead of through self-destructive tactics. Enforced retirement was a burden for both of them, and readjustment was essential. By focusing to some extent on Eugene's physiological needs, the nurse was able to induce him to resume the rehabilitation program. When Eugene became comfortable in the spouses' group, he was able to tell Diane that he went to the tavern in order to give her the freedom at home that she enjoyed. This indication of concern for her did much to convince Diane that she and Eugene were capable of dealing with their new lifestyle. After attending the group meetings for several months, the couple were looked upon as models who had much to offer other group members still struggling with adjustment to disability and forced retirement.

---

useful and competent individuals by means of positive self-affirmation of their own value. The person who believes in himself or herself can preserve self-esteem in the face of disappointment and reverses. Another way of maintaining self-esteem is to receive affirmation or validation from others, in the form of recognition, reinforcement, and reassurance. Even a person with good intrapsychic supplies can suffer a loss of self-esteem, especially after experiencing an illness or loss. Interventions from nurses and from others in the environment can be helpful in re-plenishing intrapsychic supplies. Lowered self-esteem that is not restored or replenished may lead to depression (Jacobsen, 1971; Mahler, 1974).

A nursing intervention that is often helpful for elderly persons is the *life review* process (Butler, 1963). Life review involves reflecting on past experiences and accepting the successes and failures of a lifetime. Sometimes the life review process may engender feelings of anxiety, depression, and even despair, but more often it is beneficial, particularly if the listener refutes destructive interpretations of events. By participating in the life review process as a sensitive listener, an empathic nurse can facilitate a therapeutic adjustment to aging and impending death. There may be times when a person engaged in a life review decides that her life has been useless. When this happens, nursing responses should be directed toward showing the client that this is an inaccurate perception that overlooks the client's strengths and accomplishments.

Much of the life review process may be a solitary pursuit that the individual chooses not to share. Butler (1963) noted that some elderly persons will engage in "mirror gazing"—staring into a mirror as if to see beyond the physical self, looking for a deeper image. The nurse should judiciously allow time for mirror gazing while monitoring it by making empathic verbal comments. By showing interest, acknowledgment, and respect, the nurse brings a realistic dimension to mirror gazing and signals a willingness to be available and to listen. Comments such as "You seem to be very interested in what you see in the mirror" and "What do you think of when you study the mirror so closely?" can be facilitative.

SUMMARY

Every person experiences predictable crises during the span of the life cycle. Each stage of the life cycle ushers in a maturational or developmental task that must be confronted and resolved. These critical tasks have been viewed in different ways by different theorists. Erikson has posited eight life cycle tasks in the context of a psychosocial developmental framework. Kohlberg formulated a theory of moral development that assumes individuals follow a fixed sequence as they move from simplistic to complex moral reasoning. Piaget contributed a framework of cognitive development that traces the thinking of children from early sensorimotor levels to formal operational levels. Duvall presented a sequence of family developmental tasks that, when combined with Erikson's individual tasks, permit the identification of conflict areas between the family and its individual members. A nurse familiar with the maturational tasks of individuals and families can assess whether progress is being impeded or prematurely hastened.

Sometimes maturational tasks are resolved adaptively, but often adaptive patterns are altered in various ways that may result in disturbances characteristic of a particular life stage. Among children these alterations may take the form of attachment disorders, sleeping and eating difficulties, excretory problems, fears, and phobias. In adolescence identity confusion, antisocial behavior, and body image distortions are among the manifestations of maladaptive maturational alteration.

Crises of adulthood most often involve problems with one's career, marriage, or parenting. Crises of occupational origin may be caused by premature career choices, by stressful conditions on the job, or by a combination of family- and job-related factors. The stresses caused by dual-career marriages are an example of the impact of combined family and occupational problems. In later adulthood the empty nest syndrome, retirement, physical decline, and death are among loss-related crises.

The nursing implications of maturational crises are multiple and diverse. Most of the predictable maturational crises cannot be evaded, but there are ways to help individuals and families respond adaptively. A nurse can provide primary prevention by assuring people of the universality of a particular maturational task and by encouraging them to engage in anticipatory planning, if possible. Many clients find solace in learning that they are neither alone nor unique in the worrisome situations they face. Simply explaining the normal, customary aspects of the task at hand helps people understand their reactions and examine possible outcomes. Advance knowledge of the possibilities inherent in a situation helps allay the anxiety generated by a maturational crisis. If an individual is already experiencing a maturational crisis, nurses can provide secondary prevention by offering intervention based on knowledge of the life cycle stage of the client, the probable critical task, the family life cycle stage, and family critical tasks and by being effective referral agents when the situation requires intervention beyond their own competence.

Review Questions

1. In what ways does Kohlberg's theory of moral development explain the decision-making process of adults?

2. In what respects do the developmental frameworks of Erikson and Duvall complement each other?

3. How does a teenager's reference group affect the resolution of the maturational tasks of adolescence?

4. What are some crucial issues to be considered when recommending institutionalization for an adolescent delinquent?

5. What are some of the problems likely to arise in step-families? How might these problems be avoided?

6. How does the entry of children into a family affect the marital relationship?

7. In what ways can the personality traits of a youngster influence parent-child relationships?

8. How does the departure of children from the family affect the marital relationship?

9. What aspects of retirement are likely to promote successful adjustment? What aspects are unlikely to promote successful adjustment?

10. How can Erikson's theory be used to explain the behavior of an elderly person who is in good health but is lonely, isolated, and friendless?

References

Atchley, R. 1975. Adjustment to Loss of a Job and Retirement. *Aging and Human Development*, 6:17–27.

Atchley, R. 1976. *Sociology of Retirement*. Cambridge, Mass.: Schenkman.

Atchley, R. 1980. *Social Forces in Later Life*, 3rd ed., Belmont, Calif.: Wadsworth.

Atchley, R. 1984. *Aging: Continuity and Change*. Belmont, Calif.: Wadsworth.

Atkinson, L.; Quarrington, B.; and Cyr, J. 1983. School Refusal: The Heterogeneity of a Concept. *American Journal of Orthopsychiatry*, 55(1)83–101.

Barry, P. 1984. *Psychosocial Nursing: Assessment and Intervention*. Philadelphia: J. B. Lippincott.

Botwinick, J. 1978. *Aging and Behavior*, 2nd ed. New York: Springer.

Bowlby, J. 1969. *Attachment*. New York: Basic Books.

Bowlby, J. 1973. *Separation*. New York: Basic Books.

Bowlby, J. 1979. *The Making and Breaking of Affectional Bonds*. London: Tavistock.

Brozan, N. 1983. Anorexia: Not Just a Disease of the Young. *The New York Times*, July 18.

Bruch, H. 1973. *Eating Disorders: Obesity, Anorexia Nervosa and the Person Within*. New York: Basic Books.

Bruch, H. 1978. *The Golden Cage: The Enigma of Anorexia Nervosa*. Cambridge, Mass.: Harvard University Press.

Burnside, I. 1984. *Working with the Elderly*. Monterey, Calif.: Wadsworth Health Sciences.

Butler, R. 1963. The Life Review: An Interpretation of Reminiscence in the Aged. *Psychiatry*, 26:50.

Carstens, C. 1982. Behavior Treatment of Functional Dysphagia in a Twelve Year Old Boy. *Psychosomatics*, 23:195–196.

Carter, H., and Glick, P. 1976. *Marriage and Divorce*. Cambridge, Mass.: Harvard University Press.

Chapman, A. 1974. *Management of Emotional Problems of Children and Adolescents*. Philadelphia: J. B. Lippincott.

Chenelly, S. A., and Janosik, E. H. 1980. Stresses of Postparental Couples. In *Family-Focused Care*, eds. J. R. Miller and E. H. Janosik. New York: McGraw-Hill.

Chess, S., and Thomas, A. 1982. Infant Bonding: Mystique and Reality. *American Journal of Orthopsychiatry*, 52:213–222.

Christie, B. L. 1981. Childhood Eneuresis: Current Thoughts on Causes and Cures. *Social Work Health Care*, 6(3):77–90.

Coleman, J. C.; Butcher, J. N.; and Carson, R. C. 1984. *Abnormal Psychology in Modern Life*, 7th ed. Glenview, Ill.: Scott, Foresman.

Dunton, H., and Langford, W. 1962. Psychodynamic Studies of Pubescent Girls with Anorexia Nervosa. *Bulletin of the Association of Psychoanalytic Medicine*, 1:51–56.

Duvall, E. 1967. *Marriage and Family Development*, 3rd ed. Philadelphia: J. B. Lippincott.

Duvall, E. 1971. *Marriage and Family Development*, 4th ed. Philadelphia: J. B. Lippincott.

Erikson, E. H. 1963. *Childhood and Society*. New York: W. W. Norton.

Erikson, E. H. 1968. *Identity, Youth, and Crisis*. New York: W. W. Norton.

Farrell, M., and Rosenberg, S. 1981. *Men at Midlife*. Boston: Auburn.

Feifel, H. 1973. *Dealing with Death*. Los Angeles: University of Southern California.

Fell, J. 1977. Grief Reaction in the Elderly Following Death of a Spouse: The Role of Crisis Intervention and Nursing. *Journal of Gerontological Nursing*, 33:17–20.

Feretta, F.; Rivera, G.; and Lucero, A. 1981. The Chicano Family: Myth and Reality. In *Understanding the Family: Stress and Change in American Life*, eds. C. Getty and W. Humphreys. New York: Appleton-Century-Crofts.

Fersch, E. A. 1980. *Psychology and Psychiatry in Courts and Corrections*. New York: John Wiley & Sons.

Getty, C., and Humphreys, W. 1981. *Understanding the Family: Stress and Change in American Life*. New York: Appleton-Century-Crofts.

Gilligan, C. 1980. *In Another Voice*. Cambridge, Mass.: Harvard University Press.

Green, E. 1980. Losses in the Family System. In *Family-Focused Care*, eds. J. R. Miller and E. H. Janosik. New York: McGraw-Hill.

Halmi, K. A.; Falk, J. R.; and Schwartz, E. 1981. Binge Eating and Vomiting: Survey of a College Population. *Psychological Medicine*, 11:697–706.

Jacobsen, E. 1971. *Depression: Comparative Studies of Normal, Neurotic, and Psychotic Children*. New York: International Universities Press.

Janosik, E. H. 1984. *Crisis Counseling: A Contemporary Approach*. Monterey, Calif.: Wadsworth Health Sciences.

Jenkins, R. L. 1970. Diagnostic Classification in Clinical Psychiatry. *American Journal of Psychiatry*, 127(5): 140–141.

Kashani, J. H.; Hiodges, K. K.; Simonds, J. F.; and Hilderband, E. 1981. Life Events and Hospitalization in Children: A Comparison with the General Population. *British Journal of Psychiatry*, 139(6):221–225.

Kitson, G. C.; Moir, R. N.; and Mason, P. R. 1982. Family Social Support in Crises: The Special Case of Divorce. *American Journal of Orthopsychiatry*, 52:161–165.

Kohlberg, L. 1968. Moral Development. In *International Encyclopedia of Social Science*. New York: Macmillan.

Lamb, T., and Duffy, D. 1979. *The Retirement Threat*. Los Angeles: J. P. Tarcher.

Levine, M. D. 1976. Children with Encopresis: A Descriptive Analysis. *Pediatrics*, 56:412.

Levine, M. D., and Bakow, H. 1975. Children with Encopresis: A Study of Treatment Outcomes. *Pediatrics*, 58:845–848.

Marcia, J. 1966. Development and Validation of Ego Identity States. *Journal of Social Psychology*, 3:551–558.

Mahler, M. 1974. Symbiosis and Individuation: The Psychological Birth of the Human Infant. *Psychoanalytic Study of the Child*, 29.

Maslow, A. H. 1970. *Motivation and Personality*, 2nd ed. New York: Harper & Row.

McLean, A. 1980. Occupational Psychiatry. In *Comprehensive Textbook of Psychiatry*, 3rd ed., eds. H. Kaplan, A. Freedman, and B. Sadock. Baltimore: Williams & Wilkins.

Meeks, J. 1975. Behavior Disorders of Childhood and Adolescence. In *Comprehensive Textbook of Psychiatry*, 2nd ed., eds. A. Freedman, H. Kaplan, and B. Sadock. Baltimore: Williams & Wilkins.

Norton, A., and Glick. P. 1976. Marital Instability, Past, Present, and Future. *Journal of Social Issues*, 37:5–20.

Parnes, H., and Nestel, G. 1981. The Retirement Experience. In *Work and Retirement: A Longitudinal Study of Men*. Cambridge, Mass.: MIT Press.

Piaget, J. 1969. *The Origins of Intelligence in Children*. New York: International Universities Press.

Potts, N. L. 1984. The Secret Pattern of Binge/Purge. *American Journal of Nursing*, 84(1)33–35.

Reisman, J. 1979. *Anatomy of Friendship*. Lexington, Mass.: Lewis.

Rutter, M. 1974. Relationships Between Child and Adult Psychiatric Disorders. In *Annual Progress in Child Psychiatry and Child Development*, eds. S. Chess and A. Thomas. New York: Bruner/Mazel.

Sanger, E., and Cassino, T. 1984. Eating Disorders: Avoiding the Power Struggle. *American Journal of Nursing*, 84(1):30–33.

Schulz, J. 1973. The Economic Impact of an Aging Population. *The Gerontologist*, 13:111–118.

Selye, H. 1974. *Stress Without Distress*, New York: McGraw-Hill.

Selye, H. 1978. *Stress of Life*. New York: McGraw-Hill.

Silberstein, C. 1981. Nursing Role in Occupational Health. In *Community Health Nursing: Keeping the Public Healthy*, ed. L. Jarvis. Philadelphia: F. A. Davis.

Smith, R. J. 1978. *The Psychopath in Society*. New York: Harcourt Brace Jovanovich.

Smitherman, C. 1981. *Nursing Actions for Health Promotion*. Philadelphia: F. A. Davis.

Sours, J. 1980. *Starving to Death in a Sea of Objects: The Anorexia Nervosa Syndrome*. New York: Aronson.

Stern, P. 1978. Stepfather Families: Integration Around Child Discipline. *Issues in Mental Health Nursing*, 1(2):50–56.

Szurek, S., and Berlin, I., eds. 1970. *The Antisocial Child: His Family and His Community*. Palo Alto, Calif.: Science and Behavior Press.

Wallerstein, J. S. 1984. Children of Divorce: A Preliminary Report of a Ten-Year Followup of Young Children. *American Journal of Orthopsychiatry*, 54:444–455.

Webster-Stratton, C. 1985. Comparison of Abusive and Non-Abusive Families with Conduct Disordered Children. *American Journal of Orthopsychiatry*, 55:59–69.

Weg, R. 1978. *Nutrition and the Later Years*. Los Angeles: University of Southern California, Andrus Gerontology Center.

Weiss, R. 1979. *Going It Alone: The Family Life and Social Life of Single Parents*. New York: Basic Books.

Supplementary Readings

Aten, M., and McAnarney, E. *A Behavioral Approach to the Care of Adolescents*. St. Louis: C. V. Mosby, 1981.

Blos, P. *The Adolescent Passage: Developmental Issues*. New York: International Universities Press, 1979.

Carino, C. M. Disorders of Eating in Adolescence: Anorexia and Bulimia. *Nursing Clinics of North America*, 18(1983):343–352.

Clarke-Stewart, A., and Koch, J. *Children: Development Through Adolescence*. New York: John Wiley & Sons, 1983.

Crosby, K. Self-Concept Development. *Journal of School Health*, 52(1982):432–436.

de Beauvoir, S. *The Second Sex*. New York: Vintage Books, 1974.

Ebersole, P., and Hess, P. *Toward Healthy Aging: Human Needs and Nursing Response*. St. Louis: C. V. Mosby, 1985.

Feinstein, S., and Giovacchini, P. *Adolescent Psychiatry*. Chicago: University of Chicago Press, 1981.

Fried, B. *The Middle Age Crisis*. New York: Harper & Row, 1976.

Furstenberg, F. *Unplanned Parenthood: The Social Consequences of Teenage Childbearing*. New York: Free Press, 1979.

Gress, L. D., and Bahr, T. R. *The Aging Person: A Holistic Perspective*. St. Louis: C. V. Mosby, 1984.

Lehmann, A. Anorexia Nervosa: Emancipation by Emaciation. *Canadian Nurse*, 78(1982):31–33.

Lidz, T. *The Person*. New York: Basic Books, 1968.

Muuss, R. E. *Theories of Adolescence*, 4th ed. New York: Random House, 1982.

Neugarten, B. *Middle Age and Aging*. Chicago: University of Chicago Press, 1968.

Piaget, J. *The Growth of Logical Thinking from Childhood to Adolescence*. New York: Basic Books, 1958.

Rosaldo, M., and Lamphere, L. *Women, Culture and Society*. Stanford, Calif.: Stanford University Press, 1974.

Rutter, M. *Changing Youth in a Changing Society: Patterns of Adolescent Development and Disorder*. Cambridge, Mass.: Harvard University Press, 1980.

Sandler, A. M. Psychoanalysis and Psychotherapy of the Older Patient. *Journal of Geriatric Psychiatry*, 15(1982):11–32.

Sheehy, G. *Passages*. New York: Dutton, 1976.

Stanwyck, D. J. Self-Esteem Through the Life Span. *Family and Community Health*, 6(1983):11–28.

Tackett, J. J., and Hunsberger, M. *Family-Centered Care of Children and Adolescents: Nursing Concepts in Child Health*. Philadelphia: W. B. Saunders, 1981.

Vanderzyl, S. V. Psychotherapy with the Elderly. *Journal of Psychosocial Nursing and Mental Health Services*, 21(1983):25–29.

THE CRISIS OF SUICIDE
Theoretical Approaches
Nursing Attitudes
The Nursing Process and the Suicidal Client

THE CRISIS OF THE VIOLENT INDIVIDUAL
Aggression, Alcohol, and Violence
The Violent Individual
The Nursing Process and the Violent Individual

THE CRISIS OF RAPE
Motivation to Rape
Reactions of Rape Victims
Attitudes Toward Rape
The Nursing Process and the Rape Victim

THE CRISIS OF THE VIOLENT FAMILY
Spouse Abuse
Child Abuse
Alcohol and Family Violence
Implications for Nursing
The Nursing Process and the Violent Family

C H A P T E R

15

Situational Alterations: The Crises of Suicide and Violence

Learning Objectives

After reading this chapter, the student should be able to:

1. Discuss the contributions of various theorists in the development of situational crisis concepts.

2. Discuss suicide as a response to crisis.

3. Describe characteristics of the perpetrator and victim of violence.

4. Formulate basic principles for assessing suicide and violence potential.

5. Determine the appropriate elements of the nursing process in response to suicide and violence.

Overview

Nurses often find themselves working with both the victim and the perpetrator of a situational crisis. This chapter contains the theoretical background, appropriate nursing responses, and nursing process approaches for four situational crises that nurses frequently encounter in their practice: the crisis of suicide, the crisis of violence, the crisis of rape, and the crisis of the violent family.

Situational crises occur in the lives of everyone, regardless of age, sex, race, and socioeconomic characteristics. The severity and intensity of reactions to such crises varies with the person's ability to adapt to and resolve the problem. Situational crises are often externally imposed, chance events that are unpredictable for the victim. These crises often demand solutions that the victim is unable to achieve and elicit an emotional strain that calls for additional resources or adaptive behavior. The individual's response depends on such factors as personality, perception of the event, social and cultural influences, and past experience dealing with stress. The situational crises with the greatest social ramifications are suicide, violence, and rape.

*Life's misfortunes, isolation, abandonment, poverty are
battlefields that have their heroes; obscure heroes are
sometimes greater than the illustrious heroes.*
VICTOR HUGO

405

THE CRISIS OF SUICIDE

Suicide is a denial of the human being's most urgent need: self-preservation; it is a contradiction of the value placed on human life that is implicit in social and democratic ethics. Yet there is recorded evidence that suicides occurred more than 4,000 years ago, and there is good reason to believe that people have been killing themselves since civilization began.

Although suicide is condoned in some cultures, most societies have condemned it. In ancient Greece and Rome, suicide was considered a crime against the state. In England during the Middle Ages, bodies of people who committed suicide were dragged through the streets and hung naked upside down in public view. The punishment was actually directed at the surviving family and was intended to be an example for others.

Suicide is considered a crime in several American states. Although legal action is not taken against the family, society's judgmental attitude is reflected in other ways. For example, the bodies of suicide victims may not be interred in the cemeteries of some churches, and it is difficult for families to collect insurance payments if the insured person committed suicide within two years of the inception of the policy.

Interest in the field of suicide and suicide prevention has shown a dramatic upsurge in recent times. The number of community suicide prevention centers has grown, and suicide research has expanded in new directions. During the past twenty years, the rate of suicide in the United States has been about 1 percent of all deaths each year, and suicide ranks as the tenth leading cause of death for all ages. These statistics are not totally reliable, however, as it is impossible to tell whether many "accidental" deaths, especially car accidents, may have been intentional. Also, because of persistent cultural taboos and financial pressures, some families and communities refuse to admit that a suicide has occurred.

Over the last twenty-five years, suicide has become the fourth leading cause of death among young people between the ages of ten and twenty-four. Most suicides occur in urban areas, and there is an upward trend in suicide among minority groups. Suicide most commonly occurs in April and May, with December having the lowest rate except around the Christmas holidays. Although one might expect that the autumn season with the coming of winter would be a more likely time for depression and discouragement, spring apparently brings feelings of rebirth and renewal that render some individuals unable to cope. Suicides are more likely to occur on Friday, Sunday, and Monday. People seem to feel loneliest at those times, and loneliness is one of the major causes of suicide.

Three times more women than men attempt suicide, but three times more men actually succeed. There are sex differences in the methods chosen: men are more likely to commit suicide with a gun, while women usually resort to barbiturates and other less violent methods. Some experts feel that women use these methods because they fear disfigurement or because society does not sanction violence on the part of females. People who attempt suicide also use the means most accessible to them. For example, while only 3 percent of all suicides on the national average are the result of jumping from

Suicide makes a clean sweep of the past and the present; worst of all, it repudiates love.
LEONARD UNGER

406

high places, the rate is 33 percent in New York City, where there are many tall buildings.

Some people destroy their lives in subtle, less deliberate ways. Examples include the man with a lung condition who continues to smoke, the diabetic who won't take insulin, and the alcoholic who won't seek help for her drinking problem. There are others whose actions might also be considered suicidal, including reckless drivers, stunt people, and racing car drivers who continually take unnecessary chances with their life.

People do not have to be mentally ill to commit suicide. Of course, some people who take their lives *are* mentally ill, and many are clinically depressed. Suicide occurs 500 times more often among people with serious depressive reactions than among the general population. Nurses who are working with depressed clients therefore need to be alert to the possibility of self-destructive acts on the part of these people.

Many suicide victims have feelings of loneliness, helplessness, and hopelessness that often have been aggravated by a loss. Suicides occur more frequently among divorced people than among single people and among single people more frequently than among married persons. For the survivors, suicide is a highly personal tragedy that produces feelings of pain, guilt, remorse, and bitterness.

Theoretical Approaches

Theorists from many disciplines have offered explanations for the phenomenon of suicide. The theories with the greatest implications for nursing care of the suicidal client are the sociological, psychological, communication, and social-psychological theories. None of these explanations should be considered alone, however; a multifaceted approach that draws from several theories is a preferable way to understand this complex problem.

SOCIOLOGICAL THEORIES Emile Durkheim (1897) believed that suicide could be explained only with reference to the social structure in which the individual exists. He proposed three categories of suicide: egoistic, altruistic, and anomic. *Egoistic* suicide results from the lack of integration of the individual into society. The more intensely individuals are forced to rely on their own resources in a society, the higher the suicide rate. Durkheim noted, for example, that the suicide rate was lowest among Catholics, whose religious beliefs closely integrated the individual into a collective life. Conversely, the rate of suicides among Protestants was high, which correlated with the tenet of individualism inherent in Protestant religions. Durkheim also found egoistic suicide in cases where individuals were not integrated into family life. The greater the concentration of families, the greater the immunity to suicide. In communities, the suicide rate fell in periods of crisis because society was more strongly integrated and the individual participated actively in social life.

Altruistic suicide occurs when the individual's life is rigorously governed by custom and habit. The individual takes his or her own life because of higher commandments, either religious sacrifice or unthinking political allegiance. Egoistic and altruistic suicides are symptomatic of the way in which the individual is structured into society—in the first case, inadequately, and in the second case, overadequately.

MYTHS CONCERNING SUICIDE

Over the years, a variety of myths have grown around the subject of suicide (Freedman, Kaplan, and Sadock, 1976). Nurses need to be aware of these myths and examine their own beliefs to provide adequate care of the potentially suicidal client.

- Myth 1. People who talk about suicide don't do it. *Fact*: Eight out of ten clients who kill themselves have given warnings about their intentions.

- Myth 2. Suicide happens without warning. *Fact*: The suicidal person gives many clues—they are just unrecognized or disgarded.

- Myth 3. Suicidal people wish to die. *Fact*: Most are ambivalent about dying and are gambling with death, hoping others will save them.

- Myth 4. Once a person is suicidal, he or she is always suicidal. *Fact*: Persons are suicidal only for short periods of time.

- Myth 5. Improvement after a crisis means the risk is over. *Fact*: Suicides commonly occur about three months after improvement, when people have the energy to put thoughts into actions.

- Myth 6. Suicide is inherited and runs in families. *Fact*: Suicide is an individual experience.

- Myth 7. Suicidal persons are mentally ill. *Fact*: Although suicidal persons are extremely unhappy, they are not necessarily mentally ill.

407

Anomic suicide, the third type, is due to the loss of the regulation imposed by the group to which the person has become accustomed. When horizons are suddenly broadened or contracted, anomic suicide increases. Sudden wealth, for example, can stimulate suicide, as the newly rich person is unable to cope with new opportunities. In the case of divorce, marriage no longer exercises its regulatory influence, and the likelihood of suicide increases. According to Durkheim, this anomic situation affects men more severely than women because men have profited more from the regulative influence of marriage.

Sociologists after Durkheim have included a multitude of variables in their attempts to isolate in-dicators of suicide. Suicide has been related to age, sex, marital status, socioeconomic status, occupation, and urban living (Bosselman, 1958; Wiele, 1960; Quinney, 1965). The inadequacy of these statistical explanations has been pointed out by many investigators. It has been noted that such correlations are somewhat simple and mechanical and that suicide is not a simple variable that can be compared directly with other single variables. To attempt a sociological explanation omits the basic internal struggle of the individual and fails to explain why only *some* individuals commit suicide (Beall, 1969). Psychological explanations are needed to provide additional insights.

PSYCHOLOGICAL THEORIES   Freud (1917) viewed suicide as a failure to externalize aggressive feelings, which are instead turned inward upon the self. He believed that suicide is a reaction to the loss of an ambivalently loved object. Menninger (1958) thought suicide represents the translation of a wish to kill into a wish to be killed and finally a wish to die. Zilboorg (1935) saw suicide as an attempt to thwart frustrating external forces, to gain immortality, and to maintain the ego rather than destroy it.

In psychoanalytic approaches, suicide has often been associated solely with depression and schizophrenia. Although suicide is frequently found with the affective disorders, it is not limited to depressive conditions, nor do all depressed persons commit suicide. Suicide has also been considered possible only in psychotic conditions (Stone, 1960). Others question this notion and suggest that schizophrenia may be a defense against suicide rather than a cause (Farberow and Shneidman, 1961).

The anguish that leads to suicide seems to follow no set path. But researchers believe they are making important progress toward understanding that painful process. They have identified a deficiency of a specific chemical—serotonin—in the brains of some people who are prone to take their own lives in the face of life's difficulties . . . and the hope now is that a drug could eventually be developed to correct the chemical deficiency and prevent at least some future suicides.

DANIEL GOLEMAN (1985)

408

Some theorists have seen suicide as an attempt to solve an identification conflict (Wahl, 1957). Litman (1964) considered suicide an attempt to restore lost identification with a symbiotic union. He suggested that suicide is likely to occur when there is a fusion of the self with the lost object.

Beall (1969) described two types of unsuccessful suicide attempts from a psychoanalytic viewpoint. One type is characterized by acting out with impulsivity, aggressiveness, and a lack of guilt feelings. This type of attempt is not usually very harmful and comes without advance warning. The other kind of attempt, more common in women, occurs with the hysterical personality style, where there is evidence that the person provokes guilt in a manipulative way. The method is dramatic and the attempt comes with clear warning, to allow rescue. According to Beall, a successful suicide most often occurs in an individual with internal conflict and an obsessive-compulsive personality that masks feelings of guilt caused by dependency needs. There is most likely an undramatic warning, and the method chosen is usually painful.

COMMUNICATION THEORIES In their book *The Cry for Help* (1961), Farberow and Shneidman called attention to the communication of messages in suicide. They suggested that all suicides represent an indirect form of communication. Meerloo (1962) described suicide as a form of mental blackmail in which the individual unconsciously attempts to punish a disappointing person. Karon (1964) also saw some forms of suicide as attempts to hurt someone else through the fantasy that killing oneself is an effective aggressive retaliation. Wahl (1957) considered suicide a magical attempt to solve a conflict and

achieve comfort by relieving one's own guilt and inducing it in others.

SOCIAL-PSYCHOLOGICAL THEORIES Social psychologists have been concerned with the precipitating role of unsatisfactory interpersonal relationships or the breakup of an adaptive relationship. According to social-psychological theories, suicide is the outcome of the process of social interaction rather than the result of a specific type of psychopathology. Suicide attempts and communication of intent are efforts to solve problems of living—they are pleas for help from others. Whether or not suicide is committed depends on the response from the environment (Hattem, 1964; Kobler and Stotland, 1964).

The four main types of theoretical approaches are summarized in Table 15-1. When working with a suicidal client, nurses should attend to all these theoretical approaches by assessing the social structure, the presence of psychopathology, the client's

Table 15-1. Comparison of Theoretical Approaches to Understanding Suicide

Type of Theory	Approach
Sociological	Suicide is related to position in and interaction with the social structure.
Psychological	Act is the result of aggression turned inward, loss of a love object, or loss of self-identity.
Communication	Act is a form of communication, a way of relieving guilt, a form of aggressive retaliation.
Social-psychological	Act is the result of unsatisfactory interpersonal relationships or breakup of adaptive relationships.

DSM-III CLASSIFICATIONS AND NURSING DIAGNOSES FOR THE SUICIDAL CLIENT

The suicidal client may receive various DSM-III diagnoses depending on the perceived etiology of the suicidal potential. Examples from Axis I are:

Major affective disorders

Adjustment disorders

Nursing diagnoses that may apply are more descriptive:

Coping, ineffectual individual

Fear

Grieving, dysfunctional

Self-concept, disturbance in

Family dynamics, alterations in

Social isolation

Role disturbance

need to convey a message to others, and the nature and quality of the client's interpersonal relationships. Any or all of these variables may be influencing an individual's suicidal expression.

Nursing Attitudes

Because working with suicidal clients can be taxing and draining, it is important for caregivers to examine their own feelings toward suicide and the suicidal person. Many caregivers believe that suicide is a justifiable act in some instances. Occasionally the terminally ill client who is suffering immensely is seen as having the right to end that painful existence. While such beliefs are subject to debate, it is the caregiver's duty to preserve life whenever possible. Therefore, interventions must be directed toward helping the client through difficult periods, after which the client's feelings may indeed change. Conversely, at times caregivers become overwhelmed by their own rescue fantasies and take personal responsibility for suicidal clients. Assuming such an inappropriate obligation can soon lead to discouragement and frustration.

During the crisis period, the client needs to be able to depend on the therapeutic relationship with the nurse. However, nurses need to be aware that this dependency can become overwhelming to them and destructive to clients if it is allowed to continue over an extended period of time. A gradual increase in clients' responsibility for their own decision making must be fostered with appropriate timing.

Because the clients' dependency needs tend to be difficult for the nurse, continual objectivity is of paramount importance. Many times the support of colleagues or a supervisor will help the nurse maintain this attitude.

The Nursing Process and the Suicidal Client

ASSESSMENT Nurses have extensive contact with a wide variety of clients and are in a primary position to assess people at risk for suicide. The following groups of clients are at higher risk of suicide than the general population:

1. Alcoholics and drug abusers. These clients frequently mix drugs, which can result in lethal doses. In addition, many clients are depressed and lack judgment when under the influence of a substance. Impulsive behavior becomes more likely at these times.

2. The elderly. Elderly clients have often experienced a multitude of losses, including changes in self-image, the empty nest syndrome, forced retirement, and loss of friends and spouses due to death. These clients are often at risk because of loneliness and feelings of uselessness. Some wish to commit suicide to spare their families an economic burden or the task of caring for them. Others may feel that prolonged life has little to offer. Low socioeconomic status or decreasing physical well-being may lead them to believe that suicide is the only rational solution.

3. Physicians. Psychiatrists in particular have a much higher rate of suicide than the general population. Perhaps this is a result of believing that they are the ones other people look to for solutions

and they cannot see anyone to help them with their own problems.

4. Adolescents. The teenage years are fraught with stormy interpersonal relationships and labile emotional periods. Problems that can be handled by adults often seem overwhelming to the adolescent. The many pressures from family and friends as well as the need to establish self-identity and life goals may seem too difficult to handle.

5. Previous attempters. Although it is commonly believed that clients who frequently attempt suicide will never actually complete the act, a previous attempt is actually one of the strongest indicators of potential suicide. For some, the aborted attempt is but another example of failure, increasing feelings of hopelessness and worthlessness.

In order to properly assess a client's potential for suicide, the nurse must be alert to several aspects of the client's presentation (Farberow and Shneidman, 1961).

The suicidal plan is probably the most significant of the criteria. Four main elements should be considered: the lethality of the planned method, the means to use the method, the thought and detail of the plan, and preparations for death. Planning to use a gun or hang oneself is more lethal than planning to take pills or slash one's wrists because the latter methods leave time for rescue. A threat of shooting oneself is more serious if the client has a gun than if no guns are available. If the client mentions specific details of the plan, such as when, where, and how, and if she has made preparations such as making a will and giving away cherished possessions, the seriousness of the plan rises markedly.

Current stressors must be evaluated, along with the client's ability to cope and adapt. Loss of a loved one, of a job, or of money, status, health, or body image can precipitate suicidal feelings. Impending surgery, with resultant fear and increased anxiety, can increase suicide potential.

Verbal clues to suicidal intent can be direct or indirect. Direct messages include "I want to die," and "I can't stand living any longer." Indirect statements are more subtle and take the form of "I won't be here when you get back," "This is the last time I will be here," or "I'm not worth much anymore." Behavioral clues can also be direct or indirect. The clearest example of direct behavioral communication is a suicide attempt, or "practice run."

The current psychological state of the client can also manifest suicidal tendencies. The most common suicidal states are depression, psychosis, and agitation. Evidence of severe depression can be elicited with questions about sleep, loss of appetite, weight loss, withdrawal, loss of interest, and apathy. Psychotic states characterized by delusions, hallu-

cinations, disorientation, and confusion can cause loss of control of suicidal tendencies. Agitated states are evidenced in tension, anxiety, guilt, shame, rage, hostility, and thoughts of revenge. Of most significance is the state of agitated depression, in which the client may feel unable to tolerate the pressure of feelings and anxieties and feels the need to act in some way to obtain relief.

The client's feelings about the suicidal thoughts are important to know. The client who is afraid of the thoughts (ego-dystonic) and wants to make them go away is at less risk than the client who is comfortable with the thoughts (ego-syntonic).

The client's environmental resources are often critical in determining whether he or she will live or die. Inquiry must be made into resources that can be used for support, such as family, relatives, friends, clergypersons, or social agencies.

The client's medical status may give additional information for evaluating suicidal potential. The client with a chronic debilitating illness that has caused considerable changes in self-image and self-concept may be at high risk. The client suffering from fears of a fatal illness may have a preoccupation with death and dying.

No single criterion for assessing suicide potential should be considered excessively alarming, with the exception of a lethal and specific plan for action. The assessment should be based on the general pattern of all the indicators related to the individual case. It is as important to assess the client's strengths and resources as it is to evaluate the negative aspects of the picture. Sometimes a client will present with alarming negative feelings and behaviors, but these negative aspects will be defused by a number of positive features within the situation.

PLANNING The goals of caring for the suicidal client are directed toward providing protection from self-destruction until the client is able to assume that responsibility himself. It will be necessary to assist the client to express feelings of aggression and hostility constructively and outwardly rather than focusing them destructively and inwardly. During this time, the client must be assisted to meet her physical needs, as she may be so preoccupied with self-destructive thoughts that she neglects other necessities. The long-range goal is to help the client achieve a more realistic and positive self-concept so that her feelings of self-esteem, self-respect, acceptance by others, and belonging are enhanced.

Clients with high suicidal potential who appear out of control will require hospitalization. In addition, clients without external support systems may need short-term hospitalization until supports can be established. The current laws permit commitment of clients who are a danger to themselves or others; nurses need to be familiar with the commitment proceedings of their particular state.

Most clients, however, can be treated on an outpatient basis, either by establishing a trusting relationship with close monitoring of the client's status or by referral to another suitable agency, depending on the need.

Several resources can be used in planning the client's care. The client should be encouraged to discuss his problems with the family if possible. If it is considered desirable for someone to be with the client during the crisis, a family member should be called and apprised of the situation even if the client may be reluctant to have this done. The family must be involved in accepting responsibilities for the emergency and in helping the client get the treatment that has been recommended. Close friends can often be utilized in the same way. If the client is involved in a church group, the clergyperson may be of assistance. The police should be used only in cases of clear and immediate emergency, such as when a suicide attempt is about to occur or has occurred. The client may need prompt medical attention, and the police are the ones who can procure that treatment most quickly.

IMPLEMENTATION Suicidal clients on an inpatient unit should be closely observed at all times, especially in the bathroom, where there are objects that can be harmful or where the client may attempt suicide by drowning. Some hospitals require that suicidal clients have someone with them on a one-to-one basis until the danger of suicide is believed to be past. During the period of close observation, the nurse has an excellent opportunity to assist the client to unburden himself and talk out his feelings. The need to be accepted, respected, and appreciated is paramount for such clients. Acceptance and respect penetrate even the most deeply depressed person if the communicating person is sincere. An attitude of hopefulness on the part of nursing personnel conveys reassurance of the client's worth.

It is important to determine what is meaningful to the client at the moment and to avoid imposing one's own feelings. Sensitive listening is important, but the client needs to be reminded that suicide is not the only choice and that there are other alternatives. The nurse can suggest alternative actions and work with the client to implement them. Disturbed thoughts cannot be forgotten until they are replaced with other thoughts. The client needs to know that seemingly insoluble problems can somehow be worked out. The client must be granted permission to make suicidal threats whenever there is a need. It is important not to argue with these threats and to take them seriously. The client needs to know

that it is permissible to discuss suicidal ideation or intent and that caregivers are committed to helping.

When suicidal clients are serious about their intent, they are going to become actively suicidal no matter what preventive measures are taken. The environment must therefore be checked for potential hazards. Anything sharp or potentially injurious, such as scissors, knives, razors, glass, neckties, sashes, and cleaning fluids, should be removed. Paper plates and plastic eating utensils are a good alternative to chinaware and metal utensils.

During the day, a therapeutic schedule should provide the client with tasks that will increase feelings of usefulness. Interaction with others should be encouraged. Adequate nourishment and physical care measures to induce rest and sleep are needed. Suggested nursing interventions are provided in Table 15-2. The nurse is the key person in providing liaison activities between the suicidal person and those who can give the continuing support and direction essential for the emotional recovery.

Because death is no easy escape from misery, the suicidal person approaches this finality with ambivalence. Even in deep despair and hopelessness, the depressed person longs to be rescued from his deadly inclination and usually communicates this longing to those around him. The prevention of

411

Table 15.2. Nursing Interventions for Suicidal Clients

Client's Problems	Nursing Interventions
Potential for self-destruction	1. Observe client closely at all times and reduce environmental hazards. 2. Supply nourishment and physical care as needed until client can assume responsibility for himself. 3. Take suicidal threats seriously; do not argue with client about them. 4. Use measures to induce sleep and rest. 5. Remind client that there are other alternatives to suicide. 6. Be alert for signs of acting-out behavior. 7. Observe client closely during recovery from depression, as danger of suicide may increase at this time.
Feelings of aggression toward self	1. Show interest in client and seek her out; encourage interaction with others. 2. Assist client to express feelings of aggression constructively and outwardly; help client to unburden himself and talk about feelings. 3. Provide a busy schedule; plan diversional activities. 4. Encourage client to make decisions for herself whenever possible.
Loss of self-esteem, self-respect	1. Listen to client to determine what is meaningful to him. 2. Be sincere and honest, making efforts to bolster client's confidence in himself. 3. Do not tell client she is getting better. Wait until she can make that observation for herself.

suicide consists of knowing the potential signs and responding when they appear. One of the most dangerous times is when a serious depression is lifting and the client now has the energy to mobilize his suicidal plan. The individual coming out of a depressed state may also commit suicide out of fear of having to reexperience such deep depression. Unfortunately, this may occur after the client has been discharged from the hospital. The early establishment of a trusting therapeutic relationship and supportive environment is therefore of extreme importance.

EVALUATION Nurses may not be helpful to clients unless they are able to perceive the clues to suicide and to recognize the implications of related behaviors and verbal communications. Remaining uninvolved and indifferent prevents nurses from responding to the client's cry for help. Telling the client that she seems better rather than waiting for her to discover that for herself will convey an attitude of not understanding the client's pain. Failing to convince a client that he really wants to live may be due to the nurse's refusal to accept the fact that the client wants to die. Another attitude on the part of the nurse that is nonproductive is interpreting suicide as a sinful or illegal act, which only adds distance to the nurse-client relationship and decreases its therapeutic effectiveness.

The reaction of others in the client's environment also needs evaluation. Significant others may be nonhelpful or even injurious. If they reject the client and deny the suicidal behavior, the client may withdraw physically and psychologically from continued communication. Sometimes significant others resent the client's increased demands and insistence on gratifying dependency needs. In other cases, they may act helpless and indecisive, giving the suicidal person the feeling that help is not available, thereby increasing his feelings of despair. To help the situation, treatment for the significant others may be indicated as well.

THE CRISIS OF THE VIOLENT INDIVIDUAL

Violence, whether between individuals or societies, has been present since the beginning of humankind. As a nation, the United States has used violence to attain its ends and has sanctioned the use of violence within certain contexts, such as war and civil control. The prevalence of violence in the media, especially on television and in motion pictures, provides exposure to violent acts for all age groups. Against this background of acceptable violence, it is little wonder that the management of vio-

lence between individuals and within families is one of the most difficult problems facing caregivers today. The remainder of this chapter deals with these aspects of violence: the violent individual, the rape victim, and the violent family. Because research has shown that alcohol use is frequently associated with violent behavior, the implications of alcohol use will be discussed for both the individual and the family.

Aggression, Alcohol, and Violence

Aggression, the precursor of violence, has been explained by means of several theories. Freud proposed that cruelty and a desire to hurt others is a prominent and inherent feature of the human psyche. Physiological theories have focused on chromosomal abnormalities, aggression centers in the central nervous system (Mark and Ervin, 1970), and the role of hormones (Connor and Levine, 1969). One popular theory states that aggressive behavior results from frustration. That is, when goal-directed behavior is blocked, frustration ensues, and an aggressive drive is induced that energizes behaviors against the perceived cause of the frustration (Dollard et al., 1939).

In contrast to these theories, social learning theory has been concerned with external rather than internal impellers to aggression—their origins, activation and provocation, reinforcement and maintenance (Lefkowitz et al., 1977). One line of research has focused on alcohol as an external impeller for aggression (Shuntick and Taylor, 1972; Zeichner and Pihl, 1979). This approach has produced three competing theoretical explanations of the relationship between alcohol and aggression:

1. Alcohol affects aggressive-related behavior through a physiologically based mechanism. Some proponents of this approach have stressed the "energizing" effects of alcohol absorption on general activity level, aggressive fantasies, and the need for power and dominance over others.

2. Alcohol does not elicit aggression directly but instead "disinhibits," thereby facilitating aggressive expression by reducing fear and anxiety and diminishing perceived impact of the physical and social consequences of aggression.

3. Alcohol use is mediated by a psychological expectancy set regarding the behavioral effects of alcohol consumption and by tendencies on the part of the drinker to attribute antisocial acts solely to the intoxicated state. According to this theory, drinking provides a socially acceptable reason for engaging in otherwise inappropriate behaviors, including aggression. These behaviors are frequently excused because the person is not held responsible for the behavior while under the influence of alcohol (Lang et al., 1975).

412

Although there continues to be a debate about the actual mechanism of releasing violent behavior, nurses need to be aware of the additional problems and implications for interventions when alcohol is involved in a violent or potentially violent situation. An individual who is highly intoxicated will be much less amenable to verbal interventions and may need more extreme measures of restraint. Such measures are described later in this chapter.

The Violent Individual

At times nurses find themselves working with clients who exhibit violent or acting-out behavior. This violence may be deliberate or may occur because the client has lost control. In order to function adequately, it is important for nurses to be aware of their own reactions to such clients. Knowledge and skill in working with violent clients will help to overcome fear reactions that may prevent the appropriate response. Being afraid of someone who can potentially cause harm is a natural human reaction. The recognition and acceptance of this fear is the first step toward actions that will benefit the client and safeguard the personnel.

According to Haber et al. (1982), several categories of clients may be prone to acting-out behavior. The client experiencing an acute attack of paranoia, either from a functional disorder or organic brain syndrome, sees his environment as hostile and threatening. Such distortions force the client to use destructive acts to protect himself. Clients suffering from organic brain syndrome may have distorted thinking and loss of reality testing, which can lead to a sudden onset of violent behavior with little warning for the staff. Often the client has had no history of assaultive behavior and has been unable to communicate his fears. Clients with temporal lobe epilepsy may have a history of rage reactions that result in violent fights with little or no provocation. Frequently such clients do not remember the incidents. Certain physiological conditions, such as metabolic or endocrine disorders, drug withdrawal, and space-occupying brain tumors, may increase the likelihood of acting-out behavior in clients who tend to react violently to uncomfortable situations.

Other clients who act out in a violent fashion may have personality disorders (see Chapter 8) or problems with impulse control. Such individuals tend to have a low tolerance for frustration and an impatience to get needs met; they lack guilt feelings for the results of their behavior—a lack that psychodynamic theorists attribute to inadequate superego development. This arrested development is thought to be due to inadequate or traumatic parenting, which has prevented the client's internalization of concepts of right and wrong. The ex-

plosive client, in contrast, does have a sense of guilt at having harmed others but lacks proper impulse control. This lack of control may be a result of inadequate socialization techniques or inappropriate role models during development. A wife beater, for example, may have learned this behavior by watching his father physically abuse his mother.

Whatever the cause, it is important for nurses to maintain a certain vigilance and awareness of possible violent behavior and to be able to intervene for their own protection and the safeguarding of the client. The best nursing interventions are directed toward reducing the rage and calming the client so that more extreme measures, such as the use of restraints, can be avoided.

The Nursing Process and the Violent Individual

ASSESSMENT Making an accurate assessment of a potentially violent client can enable the nurse to defuse the situation before the client becomes out of control. Taking an accurate history of past violent behavior and drug use will provide clues to a client's potential for violence. In addition, clients will often give a number of behavioral clues to accelerating anger. Any distinct behavior change should be regarded as an indication of a potential flare-up. A client who has been under control may begin to pace, bite his nails, and appear anxious and jumpy. The client may engage in verbal abuse and threatening gestures, such as throwing objects or pounding his fists into furniture. Conversely, a very active client may suddenly become quiet and withdrawn before an explosion. Nurses need to develop an observational ability about these clients that enables them to sense the acceleration and know at what point the client will strike out. The client who is actively hallucinating and who is confused and disoriented is also at high risk to act out.

PLANNING Once the potential for violent behavior has been determined, the nurse should plan the possible interventions. The short-term goals are to protect the client from self-harm and from acting out impulses until she is able to assume responsibility for herself. It will be necessary to help the client express her feelings of hostility in a safe and acceptable manner. To facilitate the exploration and ventilation of hostility, it is necessary to let the client know that she will not be judged or retaliated against. Initially, an effort should be made to talk calmly to decrease her anger. If this effort fails, plans must be made to restrain the client until she is able to regain control.

IMPLEMENTATION When the client shows threatening, angry behavior, it is necessary to remove other clients from the immediate area for their own pro-

413

> ### DSM-III CLASSIFICATIONS AND NURSING DIAGNOSES FOR THE VIOLENT CLIENT
>
> The physiological conditions resulting in violent behavior are classified according to individual syndrome—for example, organic mental disorders. The acting-out character disorder is classified as a personality disorder on Axis II. The explosive condition is classified under disorders of impulse control not elsewhere classified:
>
> 312.34 Intermittent explosive disorder (explosive personality)
>
> 312.35 Isolated explosive disorder (single violent act with a catastrophic impact on others, grossly out of proportion to any precipitating stressor)
>
> 312.39 Atypical impulse control disorder
>
> Nursing diagnoses that may apply include:
>
> Anxiety: severe, panic
> Consciousness, altered levels of
> Coping, ineffective individual
> Fear
> Self-concept, disturbance in
> Violence, potential for

414

tection and to reduce distractions. The nurse should keep a safe distance from the client, allowing him to remain in his present position without feeling pushed or attacked. The client needs space between himself and others. The next step is to help the client identify the anxiety that is causing the behavior and to reassure him that he will not be allowed to lose control. The client generally senses when he is about to lose control and needs to know this will not happen. At this point, an appropriate intervention would be "You seem really upset and I'm afraid you may injure someone if you throw that vase." The nurse should provide reassurance with statements such as "I want to help you control your behavior. I cannot allow you to lose control." The nurse can provide the client with alternatives with suggestions such as "Let's have a cup of coffee to talk this over." The nurse should also encourage verbalization of the anger rather than acting out: "Whatever happened to make you so angry?"

Many times this nursing approach will subdue the anger and relieve the situation. However, if this approach does not work, it may be necessary to restrain the client. The first step is to provide a show of strength or force, which consists of at least five people approaching the client from a side-front angle (not directly from the front, as this can be perceived as an attack). Such a show of force will usually subdue the client without having to actually restrain him.

If physical restraint is necessary, at least five people are needed; one to hold each limb and one to be available to administer intramuscular medication. Each member of the team must know what he is doing in order to prevent injury to himself. Eyeglasses and sharp objects should be removed before

approaching the client. Once the client is medicated and restraints have been applied, the client should have someone in attendance to provide physical care and an opportunity to talk about the episode whenever the client is ready. Restraints should be removed one at a time at intervals to massage the limb and to check skin condition. When the medication has taken effect and the client is calmer, restraints may be removed. Helping the client to return to the area with other clients must be handled with care, as the client will most likely be embarrassed and will need assistance to regain assurance. A summary of nursing interventions for the violent client is provided in Table 15-3.

EVALUATION After an incident of restraining a client, the staff should meet and discuss what happened and how the problem could have been prevented. A nursing staff that is insecure at functioning in such situations may have been part of the problem. Clients can sense fear in others, and this fear only accelerates their own misgivings that the episode will get out of control. The reaction of the

Table 15-3. Nursing Interventions for the Violent Client

Client's Problems	Nursing Interventions
Impending violent behavior	1. Allow client to remain in present physical position; give space and keep some distance. 2. Observe client while placing self between client and door; do not turn your back, and move slowly and deliberately. 3. Ask other clients to leave the area. 4. Identify the client's feeling of anxiety and encourage verbalization. 5. Offer alternatives, provide reassurance, and set limits.
Need for physical restraints	1. Assemble equipment and appropriate number of staff members. 2. Prepare a private room that is free of potentially dangerous items. 3. Explain to client that staff is going to help him control his behavior. 4. Approach the client slowly but deliberately, being careful to prevent injuries both to client and staff. 5. Once the client is restrained, have someone with the client at all times; medicate as ordered. 6. Take vital signs at least every half hour; observe extremities for lack of circulation or pressure. Offer snacks and fluids; give mouth care p.r.n. 7. Encourage client to express thoughts and feelings about the incident; explore the situation that caused the client to lose control. 8. Allow other clients who may have observed the incident to ventilate their feelings or concerns about the client or about their own potential for loss of control.
Loss of impulse control	1. Explore the violent episode and loss of control with the client; identify why this act was done at this time; was there a relief of tension and frustration? 2. Help client learn to identify the precipitating factors that led to the loss of control. 3. Validate the client's appropriate responses to anger and frustration; explore alternative modes of expression. 4. Work with family if possible so they may understand client and support new coping methods.

415

staff and their feelings during the restraining process need to be honestly explored to promote better performance and to decrease fear.

THE CRISIS OF RAPE

According to statistics, rape is the fastest growing crime of violence in the United States, but opinions differ as to whether rape is actually increasing or whether more rapes are simply being reported than in the past. It has been estimated that only one out of every ten rape offenses is actually reported (Rada, 1978).

Motivation to Rape
It is a widely accepted concept that rape is not a sexual act but an act of aggression (Sadock, 1972). The major motive of the rapist is a desire to control another person, and the means for gaining this control is the act of rape (Rada, 1978). In many instances, the intercourse itself is the least important part of the event. Emphasis is placed instead on the plan, the tension built up, and the apprehension of the victim. Although the sex act may be of secondary importance, the reason for assaulting in a sexual manner is that rape represents to the rapist a violation of the most sensitive personal control that a woman has. By forcing the victim to submit, he deprives the victim of control over her intimate privacy (Rada, 1978). Consequently, if the victim submits without a struggle, the rapist is left with a diminished sense of control and feelings of unfulfillment (Rada, 1978).

Reactions of Rape Victims
During the rape experience, the woman is in a state of panic in which she must make a quick decision on how much to resist. Her main concern is to stay alive. Since the rapist is usually physically stronger than she is, it is fairly easy for him to enforce submission. Regardless of how much resistance she offers, the aftermath of the rape finds the victim humiliated, confused, fearful, and enraged. These reactions do not abate quickly and may in fact persist in extreme form for several years, complicating the victim's interpersonal relationships.

Following the rape, the victim has a sense of living in a dangerous, unpredictable world, and she may become preoccupied with her own feelings of victimization and vulnerability. Some women are unable to resume normal sexual relationships with their chosen partners, either because of sexual revulsion or because of feelings of unworthiness. The ability of the victim to work through the trauma of rape and adapt to the changes in her life as the result of the rape depends to a large extent on the attitudes of caregivers, law enforcement officers, and the significant persons in her life.

Attitudes Toward Rape

The rape victim needs acceptance and empathy from health professionals and from the significant persons in her life. Hints by family members, friends, or professionals that the victim's own behaviors encouraged the rape will intimidate and prolong self-recrimination. The most detrimental attitude of all is for others to believe the myth that the rape victim is a seductive woman who has misled the unsuspecting male or that she is a manipulative female who is shouting "Rape!" in order to deny her culpability for a sexual encounter. The feminist movement has done much to eradicate such myths and to help ease the ordeal faced by victims who wish to bring charges against alleged rapists. The recruitment of policewomen as regulatory agents has also done much to assist rape victims and to raise the consciousness of other police personnel.

Nurses need to develop an awareness of their own feelings about the victim of a rape. If the nurse inwardly believes that the rape is the fault of the woman and that rape cannot happen to "nice women," the victim will sense this attitude and a therapeutic relationship cannot result. Overidentification with the victim can be equally detrimental. Nurses need to work through their own experiences and feelings about sex and rape in order to be helpful to rape victims.

Rape is a traumatic event with great potential for precipitating crises in victims and in their significant others. Because the reactions of family members and significant others are varied and unpredictable, it may not be advisable to notify anyone until the victim has given permission to do so. Many rape victims need time to deal with their own feelings before being intruded on by well-intentioned friends and relatives. The reaction of the victim's sexual partner is of particular importance. If the partner is concerned primarily with the emotional state of the victim and offers unquestioning support, a state of disequilibrium in the victim may be averted. But if he interprets the rape not as a crime against the victim but as a violation of his own rights, the needs of the victim will not be met.

Most towns and cities now have rape crisis centers or hotlines that function around the clock to provide services to victims. Professional staff working in hospital emergency departments collaborate with rape crisis teams and act as liaison agents when a rape victim is brought in for treatment. Close work relationships between rape crisis workers and hospital staff members prevent the destruction of important evidence during the postrape examination and provide continuity of care for victims.

The Nursing Process and the Rape Victim

ASSESSMENT The initial interview of the rape victim is of paramount importance in assessing the client's amount of psychological distress and in determining a plan of care. The purpose of the interview is to learn as much as possible about the incident and about the victim's reaction to it.

Attention needs to be given to the victim's nonverbal responses. Her general appearance tells how she feels about herself, which helps to assess the severity of the distress and the loss of coping skills. It is also important to determine whether any physical problems need attention. A medical and gynecological examination may be indicated as part of follow-up care.

The circumstances of the rape, the characteristics of the assailant, and the events that happened during the rape will all influence the victim's reaction. When and where was the victim approached? Where did the rape occur? Was the assailant known to her? Was she threatened? Did he have a weapon? Did she struggle? Guilt feelings about not resisting may add complications to the client's recovery process. What type of sex was demanded? For many women, the sexual aspect of the rape is highly distressing, especially if they have been forced to commit acts that are repulsive to them.

In order to provide appropriate treatment, it is necessary to determine the meaning of the sexual assault to the woman and her feelings about sex in general. The rape may create difficulties in the victim's present relationships and may stimulate doubt and fear about the possibility of future relationships.

The client's help-seeking behavior also needs to be explored. Where did the woman go for help? What was the encounter with the police like for her? How was she treated at the hospital? Is she considering pressing charges against the rapist? Who is available to help her? Who can she confide in? Who is she willing to tell about the experience? The social support systems of the victim can make the difference between successful resolution and continued fear and guilt.

PLANNING When planning care for the rape victim, the following goals need consideration:

1. To help her work through the experience and settle the crisis.

2. To help her resume her normal style of activity as soon as possible.

3. To assist her in making decisions about seeking someone to talk with, about informing friends and family, and about prosecuting the assailant.

4. To help her repair any estranged family and social relationships.

5. To attend to measures to regain her physical health.

6. To help her repair the emotional damage and overcome fear of future relationships.

IMPLEMENTATION Because of the severity of the crisis of rape, the victim should be encouraged to seek counseling to assist her in regaining control and in resolving the issue. Counseling should be directed toward suppressing anxiety and reestablishing the victim's sense of worth and value. The counseling sessions should help the victim talk about her fear that she may have unwittingly contributed to the rape. In order to proceed with her life, she must be helped to express her feelings. Talking about the rape helps to settle the experience. Depending on the reaction of significant others, couple or family counseling may be indicated.

Informing the victim of her legal rights, helping her talk about the experience, and enlisting her cooperation in apprehending and prosecuting the rapist are measures that reduce feelings of helplessness. Even when the rapist is not apprehended immediately, participating in the activities of law enforcement agencies distracts the victim from ruminating about the experience. A common fear is that the rapist will try to retaliate in some manner. The nurse should encourage the victim to work with the police on this issue to determine whether this fear is substantiated by concrete data.

The victim should be encouraged to resume her normal style of activity as soon as possible, since delays only lead to difficulties later on. The nurse should help the victim explore alternative actions and express her feelings about these alternatives. She needs to be assisted in making decisions about whom and when she is going to tell about the experience and who will make up her support system. By using available support systems, she can begin to regain the self-confidence needed to resume her normal lifestyle.

EVALUATION The victim has most likely come to terms with the rape when her memories are not as frequent and when the pain of the memories has decreased. A good sign is the resumption of a normal lifestyle. Not all women will be able to settle the crisis completely or to attain the same level of acceptance. If progress stagnates, it may be necessary to reevaluate the available support systems to determine some of the difficulties the woman is encountering.

THE CRISIS OF THE VIOLENT FAMILY

From 1939 to 1969, the *Journal of Marriage and the Family* did not contain any reference to family violence. Such violence was believed to be an isolated problem in disturbed couples that fulfilled the masochistic needs of the wife and was necessary for family equilibrium. Keeping family violence a private rather than a public problem enabled professionals to treat symptoms rather than to directly identify what was really happening (Hilberman, 1980).

But what was thought to be a relatively rare problem is actually one of epidemic proportions. Researchers such as Richard Gelles (1974) and Lenore Walker (1979) cite the incidence rate of violence between American couples to be as high as 60 percent. According to the Federation of Organizations for Professional Women (1977), 2 million Americans have used a lethal weapon against their spouse and an additional 2 million couples report beatings between husband and wife. In 1974, one out of every five policemen killed in the line of duty was killed while intervening in a family quarrel. In 1965, homicides among family members made up 31 percent of all murders in the United States, and half of these family murders were committed by one spouse upon another. By 1969, 25 percent of all U.S. murders were committed by one spouse against the other or were the result of lovers' quarrels (Gullatte, 1979).

The problem of family violence is obviously not a new one. What *is* new is that it is just beginning to be recognized as an important social problem. Violence in the family is a multifaceted phenomenon encompassing wives, husbands, children, and even pets. More recently, abuse of elderly parents has begun to receive attention as well.

Family violence is a widespread and complex phenomenon. As it becomes stripped of its pseudojustification, it is exposed and thereby accessible to study and to identification of possible intervention approaches. The increasing volume of literature attests to the researchable quality of the situation and the rising interest of many academic disciplines.

Spouse Abuse

Although family violence is often thought to be associated with lower socioeconomic groups, studies are showing that wife battering transcends all ethnic groups and social classes. DeLorto and LaViolette (1980), who operate a shelter for battered wives in Long Beach, California, found their clients to be 62 percent white, 20 percent black, 13 percent Chicano, 3 percent Asian, and 2 percent other and the husbands to represent almost every profession and occupation. It is currently believed that battering *appears* to be more prevalent in the lower socioeconomic classes because families at this level more often come to the attention of service organizations and law enforcement officials (DeLorto and LaViolette, 1980). When wealthy or middle-class husbands beat their wives, the behavior stays hidden because wives are often too embarrassed to let people know.

ADVOCACY FOR BATTERED WIVES

The organized movement against wife beating started in England in 1971, when Erin Pizzey opened a run-down house to which local women could flee from violent husbands. Within a few years, a network of refuges was developed throughout the United Kingdom, and a Parliamentary investigation of marital violence was begun.

In 1972, an organization called Women's Advocates, Inc. in St. Paul, Minnesota began a telephone information and referral service for women, and in 1974 it opened the first U.S. shelter for battered women. About this time, the first studies concerned with violence in the home began appearing in the sociological journals. It was not until 1976 that the first presentation of the problem was available to the general public through the book *Battered Wives*, by Del Martin of the National Organization for Women.

418

Wife abuse exacts a high physical, psychological, and social price. Abused wives frequently receive physical injuries requiring medical attention or hospitalization. Marital violence is frequently cited as grounds for divorce (Levinger, 1966; O'Brien, 1971) and is correlated with child abuse and child behavior problems (Hilberman and Munson, 1978; Rounsaville, 1978). Gaylord (1975a), in a study of 100 battered women in a shelter, found that 18 percent reported chronic physical illness related to the stress of abuse, 50 percent had been referred for psychiatric evaluation (21 percent were subsequently later diagnosed as depressed), 71 percent were taking tranquilizers or antidepressants, and 53 percent had attempted suicide at least once.

Why do husbands beat their wives? In recent years, a number of theoretical approaches have been advanced by various disciplines. Each emphasizes certain aspects as the most crucial for understanding spouse abuse. Nurses should use concepts from many theories to form their own basis of understanding and to develop a framework from which to plan their care of the battered wife.

INTRAPSYCHIC THEORIES   Traditional explanations of wife battering rested on Freud's (1959) theory of feminine masochism. According to Freud, the masochist wants to be treated like a little, helpless, dependent *naughty* child. The true masochist always holds out a cheek whenever there is a chance of receiving a blow. The maintenance of suffering is all that matters; punishment is used to try to erase feelings of guilt. In the Freudian view, this self-destructive behavior results from a failure to resolve the female version of the Oedipal complex. The girl is competitive with her mother for her father's

attention but fears loss of her mother's love. In order to show she is not interested in her father, she unconsciously provokes paternal aggression, which assures her that she has forsaken her father and thereby reduces the guilt feelings associated with her desire for her father. This pattern persists in adult relationships.

Shainness (1979) also saw battered wives as masochistic but incorporated sociocultural circumstances in her explanation. She postulated that violent men use violence as an ego-enhancing technique. Violent men play violent games because their nonviolent repertoire is restricted and limited. These are the kind of men to whom masochistic women relate. In this way, masochism can be considered in terms of developmental and cultural influences. The person has been influenced not only by persons who have become harsh but by significant adults who were harsh and cruel in earlier years.

According to psychoanalytic theorists, other factors, such as helplessness, plasticity, and long periods of dependency, make infants vulnerable to the masochistic process. The masochistic person is afraid to resist, refuse, offend, or insist on limits. In addition, sociocultural circumstances—awareness of superior masculine strength and lack of control in reproductive processes—have shaped submissiveness in women. Cultural acceptance of brutality to women has also caused women to play the role that will avoid the most conflicts.

The psychoanalytic stance has been attacked

In the violent landscape inhabited by primitive women and men, some woman somewhere had a prescient vision of her right to her own integrity . . . The dim perception that had entered prehistoric woman's consciousness must have had an equal but opposite reaction in the mind of her male assailant. For if the first rape was an unexpected battle founded on the first woman's refusal, the second rape was indubitably planned. Indeed, one of the earliest forms of male bonding must have been the gang rape of one woman be a band of marauding men. This accomplished, rape became not only a male perogative, but man's basic weapon of force against woman, the principal agent of his will and her fear. His forcible entry into her body, despite her physical protestations and struggle, became the vehicle of his victorious conquest over her being, the ultimate test of his superior strength, the triumph of his manhood.

SUSAN BROWNMILLER (1975)

419

from several perspectives. Based on clinical observations, Symonds (1979) has attacked the idea of the victim's masochism and attributes its popularity in part to society's need to reject and blame the victim. She and Martin Symonds (1978) suggest that violent marriages can be divided into two groups: those in which violence precedes the marriage and those in which the violence develops within the marriage.

In the first group, violence is brought into the marriage by a man with a history of violence. His violence-prone characteristics usually erupt early in the courtship and get progressively worse. He uses violence to handle any conflict and to express a pervasive feeling of powerlessness. His violence is ego syntonic and his aggression is poorly controlled. He has a history of early and prolonged exposure to family violence and was usually an abused child as well. Alcohol is frequently associated with his expression of violence. Why do wives stay with such husbands? According to Symonds and Symonds, women react to their situation in three phases: impact, traumatic psychological infantilism, and depression. The second phase is crucial to understanding the battered wife. In this phase, she is reduced to coping mechanisms from her early childhood; she becomes obedient and cooperative, doing anything her husband wishes in a desperate effort to save her life. Later, when she discovers there is no outside support system that can help her, isolation and hopelessness set in. The violence is not provoked by the wife; she is a convenient recipient of poorly controlled violent behavior.

In the second group of violent marriages, the violence comes as a last resort when all other attempts at communication have failed. These are

marriages with a neurotic interaction in which the behavior of one partner threatens the psychological defenses of the other, and each projects his or her feelings and shortcomings onto the other. The occurrence of violence makes both partners feel worse, not better. These relationships usually improve with therapy or marriage counseling.

After studying sixty battered women in a general medical clinic, Hilberman (1980) developed a theory of stress-response syndrome as another reaction to the psychoanalytic approach. She observed that battered wives exhibited a terror that was similar to women who had been raped except that the stress was unending and the threat of assault was ever present. These women were drained, fatigued, and numbed with a pervasive sense of hopelessness and despair. They saw themselves as incompetent, unworthy, and unlovable and felt powerless to make changes.

Susan Steinmetz (1978) also believes that psychoanalytical theories blame the victim for being abused. She points out that these theories suggest that certain types of women are prone to be victims because of their psychological defects or because they avoid taking steps to resolve their own problems. Research describing personality characteristics of battered wives often leaves the impression that these victims have permitted the violence to occur. The woman is seen as having few resources and as being fearful, isolated, dependent, helpless and trapped, overcome by anxiety, depressed, and full of guilt and shame. It is often suggested that violence can be reduced by changing the woman's social and economic resources, increasing her education and job skills, teaching her to be less submissive, and so on. These approaches tend to emphasize the

The distinction between formal and personal theories may not be as notable in the field of personality as in other disciplines. This does not mean that all personality theories are personal theories. Personality theories have some of the characteristics of formal theories. Some personality theories are based on the observation of a large number of and diverse kinds of people. The theories are tested against reality, either by the theorist who proposed the idea or by others, and the scientists try to be objective in their observations and analyses of data, which may or may not support the theory. Ultimately, the theories are as objective as the subject matter—the complex human personality—permits, but their principles owe much to the personalities and life experiences of the originators.

DUANE SCHULTZ *(1981)*

420

ability of a woman to control her environment, an ability many women lack. Thus, a profile emerges of a woman, who, by her own weakness, allows herself to be victimized.

Based on an examination of case studies of battered women, Steinmetz suggests that there is a need to reformulate this thinking about wife battering. Contrary to the notion that certain women are at risk to be beaten because of personality traits, she suggests that the dynamics of beatings are what produce these traits. She believes that the dynamics involved in severe chronic battering syndrome are analogous to those used in brainwashing. Brainwashing is made possible by isolating individuals from their usual supports and rewards. This isolation results in hypersuggestibility and increased receptivity to introduction and reinforcement of new values and behaviors. The only validation of the person's worth is that offered by the individuals enforcing the isolation. Inconsistent, confusing, threatening treatment, interspersed with kindness, produces the effects of brainwashing.

In another attempt to explain the psychology of battered women while rejecting the psychoanalytic approach, Lenore Walker (1979) has utilized Martin Seligman's theory of *learned helplessness*. According to Seligman (1975), people who are exposed to negative reinforcement unrelated to their actions learn that their voluntary behavior has no effect on controlling what happens to them. As a result, they learn to be helpless, their "survival" instincts are extinguished, and they become depressed. Walker believes that this sort of process occurs with battered wives.

Walker has also integrated the patriarchal nature of society into her theory. She believes that the very fact of being a woman automatically creates a situation of powerlessness. Women are systematically taught that their personal worth, survival, and autonomy do not depend on effective and creative responses to life situations but rather on their physical beauty and appeal to men. Having been trained to be second best, women begin marriage with a psychological disadvantage, since marriage in our patriarchal society does not offer equal power to men and women. The law seems to perpetuate the historical notion of male supremacy. Cultural values and beliefs, marriage laws, economic realities, and physical inferiority all teach women that they have no direct control over the circumstances of their lives.

SOCIOLOGICAL THEORIES In developing a sociological approach to family violence, Straus and Hotaling (1977) have noted the myth of family nonviolence, which is the culturally promulgated image of the family as a place of love and gentleness. Concurrently our culture maintains a set of norms that legitimize and at times encourage the use of violence between family members. The features of family life that contribute to intimacy also facilitate the occurrence of a high rate of family violence.

Adding to these variables is the widespread occurrence of violence in the United States as a society, which produces the norm that violence is an acceptable way of dealing with problems. The approval of violence in other spheres of life cannot help influence what goes on in the family. Indeed, there is evidence to show that it is a circular process: the violence occurring in the family is one of the things that makes for a violence-approving society in other spheres of life (Straus, 1974).

THE FEMINIST VIEWPOINT

In the last two decades the feminist movement has done a great deal to publicize the plight of the battered woman. Jane Roberts Chapman (1978) has written about the economic implications of the victimization of women. She believes that economic factors are an integral part of victimization and that limited resources are often a significant factor in the ability of a woman to extricate herself from a violent situation. Some victimization is thus made possible or prolonged by female economic dependency. The battered woman must consider not only the economic problems caused by the specific crisis but also how she will survive financially if she decides to leave her abuser. Many wives are ill-prepared to be breadwinners and remain in abusive situations because they cannot afford to do otherwise.

Even when women attempt to control their lives and maintain economic independence, Chapman maintains, they do not escape the prospect of victimization because they can be victimized by men in authority positions in the world outside their families. Sexual assault, sexual harassment, and medical exploitation are examples. Chapman mentions sexual advertising, pornography, and prostitution as methods used by society as a whole to promote and maintain the victimization of women.

Coming from an equally strong feminist viewpoint is Del Martin (1977), who states that every institution in our society is designed to keep marriages intact, regardless of the danger involved. Violent behavior is

excused by inaction committed to maintaining the status quo of male supremacy within the home and society. Women are described as too aggressive, too passive, too passive-aggressive, too masochistic, too assertive, too well educated, or "too" anything in order to justify the situation they are in. The husband is described as pathological as well, but the tone is different. He is under too much stress, he is unemployed, or he is drunk, and the behavior is excused.

Martin believes that men beat wives because they are permitted to do so and nobody stops them. She says women are beaten because they are trained, enforced, and maintained into dependence. Women are caught in a double bind. In a patriarchal society that depends on the subjugation and control of women, rules and roles are defined and enforced by male-dominated institutions. Marriage is a means by which women are routinely cast in the role of victim. They are taught from birth that their ultimate goal should be marriage and motherhood, or they forgo fulfillment. To catch a husband, she must be feminine and adopt the characteristics of a subordinate, passive, dependent, and permissive woman. She submerges her own personality to be "normal and well adjusted." Patriarchy then legitimizes the inequality. Her passivity makes her a doormat that provokes her husband's abuse. If she "steps out of line," she is again abused to put her "back in her place." She is in a "no win" situation.

Gelles (1974) has devised a structural theory of violence based on the assumption that deviance is unevenly distributed in the social structure, being more common among those occupying lower socioeconomic positions. He postulates that people in certain structural positions suffer greater frustrations and deprivations and that a common reaction to this situation is violence. This reaction is legitimized in some segments of society and is seen as an appropriate response to stress and frustration. Thus, violence may be more common in these social segments.

Gelles has listed several factors that play a role in the occurrence of family violence. They include: (1) the family of orientation, (2) forms of socialization, (3) family structure such as unwanted children

and religious differences, (4) structural stresses such as unemployment and health problems, (5) social isolation, (6) situational factors such as gambling and drinking, and (7) norms and values that regulate violent behavior.

Gelles emphasizes that "it takes two"; that is, acts of family violence are not sporadic outbursts of irrational violence. Rather, the role of the victim is an important and active one, with the victim commonly serving as verbal tormentor.

Straus (1973) has developed a general systems theory of family violence. This theory attempts to account for violence by viewing the family as a goal-seeking, purposive, adaptive system. Straus sees violence as a system product or output rather than as a product of individual pathology. He points out positive feedback processes that can produce an upward spiral of violence, such as sexual inequality and society's acceptance of violence, and negative feedback processes that serve to maintain or dampen the present level of violence, such as low community tolerance levels and diminished power of the aggressor relative to the victim. Straus's theory seeks to identify the processes that account for the *continuing* presence of a given level of family violence.

Pagelow (1976) called upon social learning theory in her explanation of wife battering. She has suggested that individuals raised in battering households are likely to learn to respond to frustration or stress with physical violence. If a man has been socialized in a society where physical aggression is approved, patriarchy is established, and male dominance over females is acceptable, the object of battering will be the female over whom he has dominance. If this female places strong emphasis on conforming to the socially approved sex roles, she is likely to make a heavy personal investment in her relationships with males and is unlikely to resist victimization.

At the macrosociological level, Dobash and Dobash (1979) provide a "context specific" explanation for spouse abuse. They suggest that wife battering cannot be understood in isolation but must be examined against the background of a society that is patriarchal. They argue that society has continually devised rules and regulations that are direct supports for a patriarchal society. Economic, religious, and legal institutions and processes have affected the status of women and have directly or indirectly affected the problem of violence against women. These institutions have emphasized the inferior and subordinate position of women, especially wives, and have supported patriarchal domination in general and the power of husbands in particular. They have emphasized strict obedience by subordinates, thus directly supporting male domination and indirectly supporting the use of various means, including violence, to achieve and maintain rightful control. The patriarchy is composed of two elements: its structure and its ideology. The structural element can be seen in the low status that women generally hold relative to men. The ideological element is reflected in values, beliefs, and norms regarding the legitimacy of male dominance in social spheres. Dobash and Dobash assert that the problem of wife abuse lies in the domination of women and the answer lies in the continuing struggle against this domination.

Maria Roy (1977), social worker and founder/ director of Abused Women's Aid in Crisis, New York City, has developed a broad perspective that encompasses historical, present-day, and future implications of wife abuse. She believes that the wife-beating phenomenon is cyclic—that it is passed from one generation to the next—and that it could be prevented by a gestalt approach involving societal, educational, and legislative changes. According to Roy, in a violent society all members are capable of violence against one another. Where violence is condoned and victims are blamed, all members tolerating the violence are potential perpetrators, and men, women, and children learn that physical aggression can be a useful tool. Roy asserts that city, state, and federal governments, organized religion, and the media must be held accountable and must respond to the problem with new programs, new laws, new interpretations of the marriage contract, and responsible television and radio programming.

The subject of wife battering is still in the early stages of research and understanding. More research is needed to isolate causal factors. Generally established treatment is not available, due in part to the fragmentation of the theoretical background. Most important have been the changes over the last ten years that have made spouse abuse a visible issue and its recognition as a dysfunction that requires help rather than punishment.

Child Abuse

For many centuries abuse of children was justified by the belief that severe physical punishment is necessary to maintain discipline and that parents, because their children are their property, have the right to inflict any action deemed necessary to enforce control (Helfer and Kempe, 1968). In various cultures, such practices as clitoridectomy, castration, and the ultimate abuse, infanticide, have been routine. Children have been misused in the workforce to the extent of slavery, and they have been abandoned in times of war and crises.

Concern about harmful treatment of children led to the founding of the Society for Prevention of Cruelty to Children in New York City in 1871. Other cities followed this example, and dedicated individuals began to force upon the public conscience the awareness of the plight of many children. In the early 1960s, Henry Kempe introduced the term "battered child syndrome" and conducted a well-attended symposium at the American Academy of Pediatrics in 1961 that was the stimulus for the beginning of present-day interest in the problem of child abuse.

Statistics on child abuse are unreliable, but it is estimated that about 3 million children are abused every year. In New York City alone, almost 30,000 cases of child abuse were reported in 1979, and twenty times that number of children were thought to suffer abuse within the confines of their family households (Robertson, 1979).

Many caregivers tend to believe that child abuse

occurs only among the disadvantaged and the poor. This is simply not true. Parents who abuse their children come from all socioeconomic strata. They live in large cities, in small towns, and in rural areas, their educational achievement ranges from grade school to advanced postgraduate degrees, and they represent a variety of religious affiliations and ethnic groups (Helfer and Kempe, 1968).

CONTRIBUTING FACTORS IN CHILD ABUSE A number of contributing factors are thought to play a role in child abuse, including characteristics of the abusing parent, of the nonabusing parent, and of the child.

Characteristics of the Abusing Parent Although abusing parents do not usually have overt psychopathology that distinguishes them from nonabusing parents, there are some characteristics they commonly display. These parents tend to be depressed at times and expect and demand a great deal from their children. Their expectations are usually beyond the ability of the child to comprehend and to react to appropriately. Abusive parents deal with their children as if they were older than they actually are, often feeling insecure and unloved themselves and looking to the children as a source of reassurance, comfort, and support. For the child abuser, infants and children exist primarily to satisfy parental needs, and the children's needs are unimportant. Kaufman (1966) has described these parents as projecting their own problems onto their children and feeling that the child is the cause of all their troubles. They attempt to relieve their anxiety by attacking the child instead of facing their own problems.

In many cases parents who abuse their children are re-creating the pattern of their own upbringing. They experienced abuse and a sense of intense and continuous demand from their own parents. Accompanying this demand was a sense of constant parental criticism, with their performance always seen as inadequate and inept. Everything was oriented toward the parent.

Helfer and Kempe (1968) suggested that abusing parents have not been able to develop the ability to adequately mother because they lacked a satisfying, confidence-producing relationship with their own mothers. This lack of a significant emotionally satisfying experience with their own mothers has created a disbelief in the possibility of a motherly relationship, which persists into adult life. Relationships for these persons tend to be distant, meager, and unfulfilling. Lack of confidence originating in inadequate mothering in infancy is reiterated in adult life experiences and plagues marriages and other relationships. Left with a conviction that needs can never be met by parents, spouse, or friends, the person looks toward his or her children as a last, desperate attempt to get comfort and care (Helfer and Kempe, 1968).

Contribution of the Nonabusing Parent Usually only one parent actually attacks the child, but the other parent contributes either by openly accepting the abuse or by ignoring it. If the nonabusing parent shows undue attention and interest toward the child, feelings of envy and resentment may lead to abusive behavior in the other parent. Any rejection from the nonabusing partner is a stimulus to attack, as the abusing parent's needs are neglected and rebuffed. In some cases, one parent is the active perpetrator and the other is the cooperator. These tendencies become obvious when one parent tries to change and the other one then becomes abusive. Sometimes the child is a scapegoat for conflict between the parents. Inability to solve frustrated dependency needs results in turning to the child for comfort that the child cannot give.

Contribution of the Child Although innocently and unwittingly, the child may contribute to his own abuse. Unwanted infants are common targets for abuse. So are infants who do not live up to their parents' idealized image of them. Parents who expected an active child may be disappointed when the child is placid, and vice versa. Children who are fussy and cry a lot may threaten the parents' self-esteem; they may feel that the baby is not responding normally because they are not parenting adequately. Other potential targets of abuse are children born with some type of congential defect that requires considerable attention and that may be a drain on the family finances.

CARE OF THE ABUSED CHILD The potential for encountering and identifying battered children is found in all areas of nursing practice, particularly in emergency rooms and in the community. Nurses should know whether the state in which they are practicing has permissive or mandatory legislation on reporting suspected abuse. Persons who report in good faith are granted immunity from court action. The failure to report suspected child abuse hurts not only the child but also the parents, who are in need of help.

Assessment The nurse can make observations that may lead to a diagnosis of child abuse. Children should be observed for unusual marks on the body, such as scars and unexplained bruises. Certain behavioral characteristics may also offer clues. These include a passive response to pain; fear and withdrawal, especially around the parent; flinching and withdrawal from touch; and violent and aggressive

423

play. Parents should be assessed for the presence of factors that may place them at risk for being abusers.

Planning Among goals that should be considered is protecting the child from further pain, fear, and neglect. The parents need support in adopting methods that will limit their potential for abusing the child. Appropriate referrals need to be made to groups or agencies that will assist the parents in adopting new coping mechanisms and that will provide the parents with support.

Implementation Suggested nursing interventions for helping abused children and their parents are provided in Table 15-4.

Evaluation If the child is to remain in the custody of the parents, it is important to establish support systems and to be sure that the parents are aware of how to contact helping persons when they are needed. Referrals should be made for family or individual therapy. Other problems, such as alcohol and drug abuse, must be attended to in the long-term planning.

In some instances, it may be necessary to remove the child to temporary placement in a foster home until the parents can receive the help they need. Nurses have a role in helping both the child and the parents to accept this plan, which is necessary for safety of the child.

Child abuse is a long-standing problem in many families and will, unfortunately, continue to be so.

Public recognition of and attention to the situation will help increase available facilities and services to aid abused children and to help parents develop their parenting potential and to stop the abuse. Rather than seeing these parents as uncaring and criminal, it is important for caregivers to see them as individuals in need of help and care. Without this help, abusive behavior will continue and may be passed on to their children, who may in turn become abusers.

Alcohol and Family Violence

As noted earlier in this chapter, violence is often associated with alcohol use, and family violence is no exception. Drinking accompanied the violence of 44 percent of the husbands in Gelles's (1974) sample of wife beaters and 93 percent of husbands in Hilberman's (1980) sample. Gaylord (1975b) described drunkenness as occurring regularly in 52 percent of wife abusers in his study and occasionally in an additional 22 percent. Roy (1977), reporting an even higher percentage of 95 percent, stated her belief that only a minority of husbands beat their wives when they are not drinking. Roy suggested that men do not beat their wives because they have been drinking, but rather they drink because they want to beat their wives. In this way the drunkenness is used as a "time out" period when they are not responsible for their actions.

Research findings about the role of alcohol in family violence are just beginning to emerge in the literature. Coleman, Weinberg, and Bartholomew (1980) studied factors affecting conjugal violence in

---

Table 15-4. Suggested Nursing Interventions for Child Abuse

Client's Problems	Nursing Interventions
Child's need for protection from injury	1. Monitor visitors. Note reaction of child when around significant others. 2. Make referrals to social service departments for continuous monitoring.
Child's difficulties in adjustment	1. Encourage child to talk about feelings; avoid judgmental comments. 2. Provide drawing materials, as children often depict their feelings through art. 3. Provide other play materials for expression of feelings. Do not probe. 4. Give comfort by holding and rocking, and make note of child's reactions.
Child's need for relationship with parents	1. Be aware of your own feelings and nonverbal messages. Maintain composure and refrain from implied criticism or rejection. 2. Consider asking parents to keep a daily diary of their feelings and situations in which they feel stress. Ask them to identify the triggers that set off a chain of events. 3. Help parents to talk through their feelings and start plans for family therapy. 4. Let parents know that you really care about them and that other parents share their feelings and frustrations.
Poor parent-child relationship	1. Help the parents to enjoy their child. 2. Point out lovable attributes of the child and introduce them to the pleasures of reading to and playing with their child. 3. Ask the parents to join you and the child in simple games. 4. Teach the parents about normal growth and development, giving them realistic expectations. 5. Demonstrate how limits can be set without harsh punishment. 6. Reinforce any attempts to nurture and express affection. 7. Reassure parents that they have rights and needs, too.

thirty couples who were seeking assistance for marital conflict. They found that the key variables identifying battered wives included frequent alcohol use by the husband, frequent marital arguments, low educational level, and frequent illegal drug use. These researchers contended that battered wives may inadvertently contribute to their physical abuse by complaining about the husband's drunkenness, which leads to an increase in alcohol consumption and subsequent violent behavior.

Coleman and Straus (1979) discovered a strong positive relationship between alcohol abuse and family violence except when alcohol abuse was extreme; that is, physical violence declined when drunkenness occurred "almost always." Alcohol abuse was more clearly associated with spouse abuse than with child abuse. They concluded that people have ample opportunity to learn that it is excusable to be violent when drunk. If the link between alcohol and violence were based on the physiological disinhibiting effects of alcohol, violence should have been greatest among those most often drunk. But the most severe alcoholics, rather than being disinhibited, were in effect anesthetized. They used alcohol to block out a world that was too painful to bear. On the other hand, those who got drunk only from time to time had a different subjective interpretation of inebriation. They were not seeking an escape but rather used alcohol as a means to engage in behavior that without the excuse of being drunk would be unacceptable to themselves and others.

Most researchers are convinced of the strong connection between alcohol and violence but are not sure that alcohol is a *cause* of spouse abuse. Straus, Gelles, and Steinmetz (1976), for example, pointed out that it is not clear whether people act violently because they are drunk or whether they get drunk in order to obtain the implicit social permission to act violently. Trying to resolve this question is difficult because the actors themselves are committed to attributing violent acts to temporary loss of control due to alcohol. Contributing to the confusion is the finding that some abusers are total abstainers because of firm religious beliefs or other moral convictions.

The reverse situation, that of the prevalence of violence in the alcoholic family, has received much less attention than the use of alcohol in violent families. In one survey of 100 wives of alcoholics, none of whom had been identified as victims of marital violence, Scott (1974) found that 72 percent of the women had been threatened, 45 percent had been beaten, and 27 percent had experienced potentially lethal assaults. Byles's (1978) study of violence, alcohol, and other problems in disintegrating families showed that although violence occurred in the absence of alcohol, it was more than twice as likely to occur in marriages where alcohol was abused. There has not been any investigation into the question of which alcoholics are at highest risk to be violent or on what characteristics are most prevalent in these individuals or families.

In summarizing the family research literature on the relationship between alcohol and domestic violence, Doucette and McCullah (1980) concluded that alcohol abuse, social isolation, parental history of abuse, abuse as a child, marital discord, life crises, lack of ability to utilize parental skills, lack of nurturing life experiences, and lack of support systems are some of the factors associated with abusive situations. Doucette and McCullah also found that the alcohol literature presented these same elements in the etiology and current behavior of alcohol abusers and their families. Personality characteristics apparently associated with the perpetrators of family violence were also similar to those of alcohol abusers. The domestic violence literature consistently reported that children of abusers became abusers, and the alcohol literature consistently reported that children of alcohol abusers became alcohol abusers.

The problem of alcohol within the violent situation keeps appearing again and again in the literature, yet its role and function are not understood. It may be that a subset of various population groups both misuse alcohol and are batterers while the majority of people do neither. The question of why some alcohol abusers are not violent has not been addressed.

Implications for Nursing

As awareness of the inequities between the sexes increases, as women enter the legal and health professions in greater numbers, and as feminist organizations identify problems common to women, family violence will be reported with greater frequency. It is an issue that demands social, legal, medical, and nursing intervention. As the problem of family violence comes out of the closet, the issue will become more prevalent for nurses. Awareness of the potential for violence in families must be part of case finding and identification of problems. Nurses in all settings need to be aware of the patterns of abuse so they can look for these patterns when assessing families.

Community health nurses are in perhaps the best position for case finding and recognition of the problem. These nurses have access to the setting in which the abuse is most likely to occur. The nurse in the emergency room needs to be aware of abusive injuries that may be presented as "accidents" for emergency treatment. Likewise, the nurse in the general hospital setting may be able to identify possible victims and to make the first steps of progress by assessing the problem, providing a safe environment, helping the client begin to trust the helping professions, and making the proper referrals. The pediatric nurse is in a position to detect child abuse, which may be an indication of generalized violence in the family. Psychiatric nurses, especially those involved in family therapy, will find family violence to be a prevalent presenting problem.

Nurses are in a unique position to be of assistance to the battered family. Unlike many of the other health services professions, nursing is concerned with the broad spectrum of physiological, social, and psychological aspects of patient care. In addition to having a substantial base of knowledge for understanding illness, nurses possess a holistic view that enables them to place needed emphasis on the psychosocial areas. Nursing is concerned with identifying what is right, whole, and functioning in clients, whether they are sick or well, and it attempts to maximize the clients' strengths, assets, and potentials for optimal levels of health, comfort, and self-fulfillment. By maximizing the client's existing strengths, nurses can provide comprehensive care in the battering situation.

The Nursing Process and the Violent Family

Nurses are greatly concerned with family dynamics, as the family is the context in which health is maintained or illness develops. Today, with the old psychoanalytical notions of female masochism falling by the wayside, nurses must develop an eclectic theoretical framework within which to formulate effective intervention stratagems. This framework should incorporate the approach that is unique to nursing—the advancement of health and the reinforcement of wholesome client attributes.

ASSESSMENT Several areas need to be examined to provide a baseline from which to plan and develop interventions.

What factors are present in the family of origin that would lead to violence? What does the use of physical violence symbolize within the family? Did the forms of socialization within the family include coercive tactics? If the family did indeed provide the training for violence as a means of problem solving, what factors are present that can be used to facilitate learning other ways? How strong is the parental influence, and can it be overcome?

Components of the family structure need to be evaluated. What are the family's financial resources? Were the children planned or unplanned? What stressors are currently acting on the family? Are religious differences or ideologies contributing to the justification of violence? Is there evidence of drinking, gambling, intense jealousy, or infidelity?

Are these factors amenable to change? Are other health problems evident? Are any family members emotionally isolated? What emotional demands are placed on the marriage? Total dependency of one spouse on the other provides fertile ground for dysfunctional relationships. How can this be changed? What other areas can be reinforced to provide relief? The norms and values in the family system are of primary importance. If the violence is justified and rationalized, the problem can take on different dimensions.

Assessment of the wife needs careful attention, especially if she has left home and is seeking assistance. Her coping style, strengths and weaknesses, and readiness for change and the availability of social supports need to be evaluated to plan appropriate courses of action.

The man who abuses his wife or children must, of course, receive attention in the assessment. If alcohol use is a problem, it may need to be treated before other interventions can be made. It is important to obtain an understanding of the man's point of view of the battering incidents and of the family situation as a whole. Making the assumption that he enjoys the results of his behavior can lead to inappropriate interventions. Many men are upset by their behavior and can be open to change. It is important to perceive the man as an individual who is also in pain rather than as one who only deserves punishment.

The influence of the child on the family needs attention. Does the child cry a lot? How do the parents manage the child's crying? Do the parents get upset when they are unable to comfort the child? Is the mother upset when she is left alone? Has she ever been afraid to be alone with her baby? Can she call someone for help at these times? Does she become anxious when someone watches her care for the baby? Does she feel others are critical of her parenting skills? When do the parents think that children are old enough to understand what is expected of them? How well do the parents feel their children understand expectations now?

During a family interview, the nurse should observe the body language of both parents and children. Do the parents hold their child at a distance? Does only one parent hold the child? Does the child cringe or show overt fear of a parent? Or is the interaction one of trust?

Obtaining a picture of the violence based on these factors will provide a baseline for planning interventions.

PLANNING In planning to institute change in the family, nurses need to utilize exchange theory. If the costs of violence continue to be less than the rewards, the violence will continue. The rewards for

426

nonviolent methods of problem solving must therefore be increased. The nurse can help by assisting the client to determine what is gained by the violence and to find other ways to reach the same ends. Goals must be reachable and realistic to the particular family setting.

Depending on the situation, individual, couple, family, or group therapy can be used. If the family is still intact, marital counseling may be the treatment of choice. Through this method, the communication problems and neurotic components of the marital relationship can be explored. Behavioral approaches can also be used, as they lend themselves readily to evaluation of effectiveness. In family therapy, emphasis must be placed on the relationship between the parents, as emphasis on the child may increase a parent's feelings of rejection and of having his needs cast aside in favor of the child's needs.

When planning action for battered wives, several factors need to be kept in mind. The abused woman should not be encouraged or urged to leave her partner until she is ready. She will not leave him until she has developed enough self-confidence and trust in the community at large to be able to do so. With opportunities now available for women to seek shelter from the abuse at battered women's centers, there are more alternatives that she can consider. Initially, the woman may need help recognizing that she has alternatives. After becoming involved in counseling, during which self-esteem is fostered, the woman may be more able to carry out structured plans.

Because the battered wife is usually ambivalent about her abusing spouse, it is important that the nurse not berate or deride him. There is a need to acknowledge the woman's ambivalence by recognizing the pain in being abused by a man who is at other times loving and sensitive to her needs. If the ambivalence is not dealt with openly and with support, she may feel further alienated and misunderstood.

Planning should take into account the woman's ability to face problems realistically. Factors to be aware of include (1) her sensible and concrete planning about income, shelter, and legal services, (2) her concern for herself as a person, and (3) her acceptance of the fact that the abuse is a long-standing pattern and not merely an isolated episode.

Group work with battered wives has the advantage of providing a support group in which women can, perhaps for the first time, realize that they are not alone. Their isolation is reduced because they now have the opportunity to share their traumatic experiences with sympathetic listeners. A supportive group network is also in a position to help with

such services as financial and legal advice and job counseling.

IMPLEMENTATION Interventions based on assessment and planning can be instituted by nurses at all levels of prevention. Suggested interventions are listed in Table 15-5.

Primary prevention can be done through early recognition of the signs of family violence as well as identification of couples at risk. In working with clients, nurses can use their knowledge to discern communication problems and to identify predisposing family backgrounds and existing structural elements that may act to increase the likelihood of violence. Early interventions can alter many of the existing problems to prevent further complications.

Of equal importance is the involvement of the nurse in premarital counseling to help clients explore their expectations of marriage and to identify potential problems shown by incongruencies in the plans and aspirations of the couple. Teaching appropriate ways of communicating can provide a better foundation for problem solving within the marriage.

Another area in which nursing can play a preventive role is in genetic counseling. Realization of risks and potential difficulties that can occur with a child who has a congenital alteration or illness can help reduce stress that could lead to violence.

Secondary prevention can involve crisis intervention for the violent family. Emphasis may be placed on helping the battered wife develop a realistic perception of her situation and decide whether

427

Table 15-5. Suggested Nursing Interventions for Helping a Battered Wife

Client's Problems	Nursing Interventions
Potential for injury	1. Provide clients with information concerning ways to obtain immediate help. 2. Help clients work through the need to leave the situation for safety if necessary.
Ambivalence toward abusing spouse	1. Encourage ventilation of feelings. 2. Allow expression of both the anger and the feelings of affection. 3. Respect the client's need to remain with the spouse until self-confidence allows different choices. 4. Be wary of alienating client by deriding her spouse. 5. Explore possibility of marital counseling to facilitate communication.
Isolation	1. Encourage group therapy to provide support.
Helplessness	1. Provide appropriate referrals for legal and financial aid. 2. Explore possibilities for job training, career counseling, continued education.

CLINICAL EXAMPLE

HELP FOR A POTENTIAL CHILD ABUSER

Patsy is an eighteen-year-old unmarried mother of a two-year-old boy. Paul, the boy's father, is a thirty-five-year-old construction worker who is married and the father of three daughters. Although he has no intention of leaving his wife, Paul is very fond of the little boy. He visits Patsy often and regularly contributes to the support of his only son.

The relationship between Patsy and Paul has been intense and stormy. He often accuses her of being unfaithful to him, and she is extremely jealous of the time Paul spends with his legitimate children. She shows her resentment by sending her son to stay with a girlfriend when Paul is likely to visit. She often leaves her son alone at night and goes to taverns, where she drinks and socializes. On occasion, she meets men and goes to their apartments or invites them home overnight. She taunts Paul about these episodes; he reacts with fury because of jealousy and worry over his son being left alone.

The battles between Paul and Patsy have been loud and violent. Often police officers have been called by neighbors hearing the uproar. The police have usually tried to soothe the couple and have treated the incidents as minor domestic squabbles, even when Patsy has obviously been bruised and Paul obviously intoxicated. When the little boy has been present, he has stared wide eyed and frightened at his battling parents.

On one occasion Paul came to the apartment in Patsy's absence. Finding his little boy alone, he took his son to the house of a neighbor woman, whom he paid to look after the child indefinitely. Meanwhile Patsy arrived home with a male companion. Both of them had been drinking and were engrossed in each other. It was not until her male companion left in the morning that Patsy realized her son was gone. Her first reaction was that kidnappers had snatched her son, and she was very upset.

When she called the police, the officers who arrived were already acquainted with the household situation. They phoned Paul, who promptly admitted having taken custody of his neglected child. The police left after telling Patsy there was little she could do except negotiate with Paul. After their departure she became hysterical. In a rage, she slashed the curtains, bedding, and clothing with a knife. She broke mirrors and windows and loudly threatened to throw herself out of a window. The police officers returned but were unable to calm Patsy, whose hands and feet were badly cut. Their recourse was to take her to a psychiatric facility for evaluation and treatment. She was admitted to an inpatient facility for a period of ten days in order to reduce her stress and implement plans for her and her son.

ASSESSMENT

During the initial interview with Patsy on the inpatient unit, the nurse saw a disheveled, wide-eyed, frightened-looking woman who used an abundance of makeup. She verbalized her intention not to talk with the nurse, stating that no one could help her anyhow, her life was a mess, and she wanted "out." She paced rapidly around the room; her speech became louder and her thoughts rambled. After waiting quietly until Patsy seemed to decrease her anxiety by expending physical energy, the nurse was able to calm her and to begin to take a history of the events leading to hospitalization.

During the interview, the nurse learned that Patsy had been an illegitimate child who was abandoned by her mother when she was three years old. She had been raised in a variety of foster homes with adults who had little interest in her and who at times had abused her. When she met Paul, she thought that she had at last found someone who would take care of her, despite the fact that he was already married. When her expectations were not met, she relived her childhood experiences of fear of loneliness and rejection. Although she was knowledgeable about birth control methods, she chose to get pregnant in hopes that this would cause Paul to leave his wife and marry her. Because of the pregnancy, Patsy had not completed high school and had no marketable skills. She was living on welfare and child support.

Based on the history that Patsy supplied and the clinical picture that she presented, the following diagnoses were made:

Nursing Diagnoses

Coping, ineffectual individual

Fear

Parenting, alteration in

Self-concept, disturbance in

Violence, potential for

Family dynamics, alteration in

Social isolation

Multiaxial Psychiatric Diagnoses

Axis I 309.4 Adjustment disorder of emotions and conduct

Axis II 301.5 Histrionic personality disorder

Axis III None

Axis IV Code 5—Severe psychosocial stressors

Axis V Level 5—Poor adaptive functioning

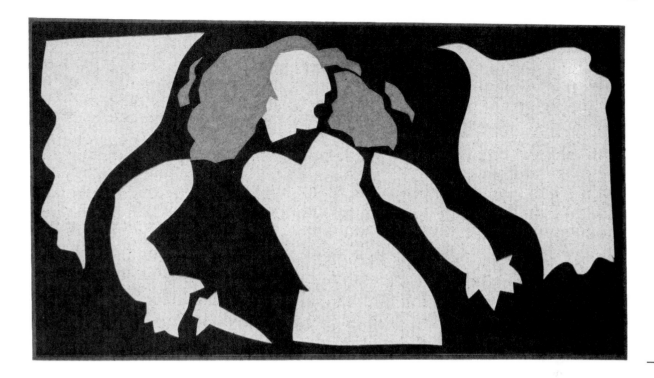

PLANNING

The mental health team decided that the primary focus for Patsy's treatment should be related to her loneliness, isolation, and unfulfilled dependency needs. Individual therapy that would emphasize building self-esteem was planned. Her suicidal gestures needed further evaluation, but the team felt that the need to act out in this manner would decrease as Patsy became more comfortable with herself. This acting-out behavior would be explored in the individual sessions. Attention was given to her lack of vocational skills and her inability to parent. In her isolated world, Patsy did not have any outlets for developing supportive, constructive relationships and was unable to see much hope for change in the future. Consequently, all her energy was directed toward obtaining the love and attention of someone to care for her rather than finding ways to care for herself.

The need to establish a peaceful, adult relationship with Paul was of paramount importance, for the safety of both her and her child and to provide for better communication between the two in order to arrive at a workable plan for the child's future contacts with them.

IMPLEMENTATION

The nursing diagnoses were helpful in identifying the areas in which Patsy needed the most help. Because of her inability to cope with her life situation and her feelings of being unloved, she was unable to give love and support to her child. She was encouraged to enroll in a parenting class, which was to be supplemented by supervisory visits by a community health nurse to assess Patsy's progress and give additional guidance. Because of Patsy's potential violence toward her son, the nurse's observations of the continued interaction would be used to determine whether the child should remain with Patsy.

In order to help Patsy begin to control her life, she was evaluated for vocational training and plans were made for her to finish her high school education. To facilitate this and to allow her time for herself and to develop new social outlets, her son was placed in a day care center for three days a week. This placement had the added advantage of a healthy environment where her son could be with other children.

Couple therapy was provided for Patsy and Paul to improve their communication and arrive at a mutually acceptable plan for visiting the child. This therapy complemented the individual sessions to enable Patsy to decrease her dependence on Paul while beginning to establish new patterns for her life. Paul contracted with the therapist not to see Patsy or her son outside the hospital until an agreement was reached.

EVALUATION

The complexity of Patsy's problems dictated coordination of efforts by multiple caregivers. Interventions could not be directed toward Patsy's problems alone; it was necessary to attend to her son's and Paul's needs as well. Once the safety of all involved was assured, emphasis could be placed on growth and change through vocational guidance and psychotherapy. Patsy needed to resolve the issues of her childhood and gain an understanding of their influence on her current behavior. Once her desperate need for love and attention was understood, further change could occur to build a more successful, independent life with less reliance on dramatic tactics to get needs met. By providing social outlets through schooling, Patsy had the opportunity to meet others and expand her contacts. This helped decrease her isolation and continued feelings of abandonment.

to leave the home, temporarily or permanently. Protection for the wife and her children needs to be considered. Current ways of coping with the violence need to be studied and new methods taught. During a crisis situation, the client's readiness for change will be enhanced and can be utilized to teach her new and more adaptive behaviors.

The family as a whole may be guided to seek professional help. When a history of violence has preceded the marriage, the focus of intervention may be placed on intrapsychic change. When violence has erupted as a result of conflict generated by the marriage, the focus of intervention may be on interpersonal issues.

In years past, the family was considered a unit of production. As the economic focus shifted to the husband/father being the individual wage earner, and as more goods became available for family use, the family became a unit of consumption. Currently, with the majority of wives working, the family is again returning to being a unit of production. Such change may be accompanied by economic pressures, role changes, separation, and individuation that create feelings of disenchantment and disillusionment among family members. Nursing interventions should be directed toward exploring such feelings. Communication therapy is indicated when meaningful exchanges and understanding of feelings are disintegrating. In dysfunctional families, abuse may be a substitute for or a method of communication.

Tertiary prevention for nurses involves encouragement of the family and referral to available resources. Nurses need to know what options are available to battered families, how to counsel them, and when and how to refer families to available community resources, including law enforcement agencies. Referrals are a vital part of preventing recurrence of injuries, as women and children need reassurance from professionals that they are victims of a crime, that others suffer similar abuse, and that they do not have to tolerate it and can get protection. Referral to such organizations as Alcoholics Anonymous and Parents Anonymous can supplement ongoing therapy to address issues that will assist families rebuild their lives.

EVALUATION Determining the effectiveness of nursing interventions can be done subjectively and objectively. Wives and families may feel they are getting better even if change is not evident to the observer. Likewise, nurses may be able to see changes occurring without the clients being able to identify them. For objective evaluation, realistic goals must be established as measures for determining whether desired changes have occurred. These goals are dependent on the nature and position of the individual family and on the use of violence within that family.

With the ability to utilize the nursing process, nurses are in a unique position to make a contribution to the understanding of alcoholism and of family violence. By using the holistic approach of integrating physical, psychological, and social aspects, nurses are able to examine the multidimensional problem of alcohol abuse and its interaction with spouse abuse. All levels of prevention can be instituted by nurses to treat this dual problem. Primary prevention is essential in stopping the pattern of alcohol use and its effects on rape, assault, and family violence. Secondary prevention aimed at stopping further emotional and social losses is important when working with the abused and the abuser. Tertiary prevention—rehabilitation of the alcoholic and of the battering family—will be improved as nurses are able to contribute to the knowledge base necessary to provide assistance to the battered family, especially one in which alcohol is abused.

SUMMARY

Clients in situational crises frequently come to the attention of mental health nurses because of the emotional strain imposed on these clients and their need to find additional resources to help them adapt. Four of these events likely to occur in people's lives are the crisis of suicide, the crisis of the violent individual, the crisis of rape, and the crisis of the violent family.

While certain populations are at higher risk for suicide than others, the phenomenon itself is very democratic, with little discrimination relative to race, color, creed, age, or sex. Various explanations of suicide have been offered, but the theories that have the greatest implications for nursing are the sociological, psychological, communication, and social-psychological. Nurses need to be acquainted with these approaches to formulate plans for accurate assessment and interventions.

Violence presents itself to caregivers in a variety of forms. One of the most frightening is the individual who is no longer in control of his behavior and threatens staff members, other clients, and himself. The ability to perceive the potential for violence and to defuse a situation before control is lost is an important role of nursing personnel. Of equal value is the ability to subdue an individual who is out of control in a therapeutic manner and to use that incident for learning, both for the client and for the nurse.

The victims of violence, particularly the rape victim, provide a different challenge to nurses.

Rape is a traumatic event that calls for a successful resolution of the emotional as well as the physical trauma involved.

The violent family, with its components of spouse abuse and child abuse, demands the ability of nurses to assess the complex interactions, determine contributing factors, and plan for change while safeguarding all family members. Because alcohol use has been associated with violence of both individuals and families, nurses need to be cognizant of this variable when implementing the nursing process.

Perhaps the most important aspect of working with clients who are in situational crises is nurses' insight into their own feelings and behaviors in relation to these clients. Self-assessment is a necessary prelude to successful therapeutic relationships.

Review Questions

1. Discuss factors that place individuals at high risk for suicide.

2. Explain your understanding of the interplay between sociological, psychological, communication, and social psychological variables that may culminate in suicide.

3. Explain the continuum of dependence and independence in nursing care for the suicidal client.

4. What is the influence of alcohol on aggressive behavior?

5. When confronted by a potentially violent client, what interventions should nursing personnel use to defuse or control the behavior?

6. What aspects need to be considered when helping a rape victim?

7. Based on the various theories of wife abuse, outline your own theory and understanding of the factors involved.

8. Explain the interaction of characteristics of the abusing parent, the nonabusing parent, and the child in child abuse.

9. Describe the elements that need to be considered in the assessment of the violent family.

10. How should nurses utilize the three levels of prevention when working with violent families?

References

Beall, L. 1969. The Dynamics of Suicide: A Review of the Literature, 1897–1965. *Bulletin of Suicidology*, March.

Benedek, T. 1959. Parenthood as a Developmental Phase. *Journal of the American Psychoanalytic Association*, 7: 389–417.

Bosselman, B. C. 1958. *Self-destruction—A Study of the Suicidal Impulse*. Springfield, Ill.: Charles C Thomas.

Brownmiller, S. 1975. *Against Our Will*. New York: Simon and Schuster.

Byles, J. A. 1978. Violence, Alcohol Problems and Other Problems in Disintegrating Families. *Journal of Studies on Alcohol*, 39:551–553.

Chapman, J. R. 1978. The Economics of Women's Victimization. In *The Victimization of Women*, eds. J. R. Chapman and M. Gates. Beverly Hills, Calif.: Sage Publications.

Coleman, D., and Straus, M. A. 1979. Alcohol Abuse and Family Violence. Paper presented at the American Sociological Association, Boston, August.

Coleman, K.; Weinberg, M.; and Bartholomew, H. 1980. Factors Affecting Conjugal Violence. *Journal of Psychology*, 105:197–202.

Connor, R., and Levine, L. 1969. Hormonal Influences in Aggressive Behavior. In *Aggressive Behavior*, ed. E. Segg. New York: John Wiley & Sons.

Davidson, T. 1978. *Conjugal Crime*. New York: Ballantine.

DeLorto, D., and LaViolette, A. 1980. Spouse Abuse. *Occupational Health Nursing*, 17–19.

Dobash, R. E., and Dobash, R. P. 1979. *Violence Against Wives: A Case Against Patriarchy*. New York: Free Press.

Dollard, J., et al. 1939. *Frustration and Aggression*. New Haven, Conn.: Yale University Press.

Doucette, S. R., and McCullah, R. D. 1980. Domestic Violence: The Alcohol Relationship. *U. S. Navy Medicine*, 71:4–8.

Durkheim, E. 1951. *Suicide: A Study in Sociology*. Glencoe, Ill.: Free Press. (Originally published 1897.)

Farberow, N. L., and Shneidman, E. S. 1961. *The Cry for Help*. New York: McGraw-Hill.

Federation of Organizations for Professional Women. 1977. *Women and Health Roundtable Report*, 10:1–4.

Freedman, A. M.; Kaplan, H. I.; and Sadock, B. J. 1976. *Modern Synopsis of Psychiatry II*. Baltimore: Williams & Wilkins.

Freud, S. 1948. Mourning and Melancholia. In *Collected Papers*, vol. IV. London: Hogarth Press. (Originally published 1917.)

Freud, S. 1959. The Economic Problem of Masochism. In *Collected Papers*. New York: Basic Books.

Gaylord, J. J. 1975a. Wife Battering: A Preliminary Survey of 100 Cases. *British Medical Journal*, 1:194–197.

Gaylord, J. J. 1975b. Battered Wives. *Medical Science Law*, 15:237–245.

Gelles, R. J. 1974. *The Violent Home*. Beverly Hills, Calif.: Sage Publications.

Goleman, D. 1985. Clues To Suicide: A Brain Chemical Is Implicated. *The New York Times*, October 8.

Gullatte, A. C. 1979. Spousal Abuse. *Journal of the National Medical Association*, 71:335–340.

Haber, J.; Leach, A.; Schudy, S.; and Sideleau, B. 1982. *Comprehensive Psychiatric Nursing*. New York: McGraw-Hill.

Hattem, J. V. 1964. The Precipitating Role of Discordant Interpersonal Relationships on Suicidal Behavior. *Assertation Abstracts*, 25:1335–1336.

Helfer, R. E., and Kempe, C. H. 1968. *The Battered Child*. Chicago: University of Chicago Press.

Helfer, R. E., and Kempe, C. H., eds. 1976. *Child Abuse and Neglect: The Family and the Community.* Cambridge: Ballinger.

Hilberman, E. 1980. Overview: The Wifebeater's Wife Reconsidered. *American Journal of Psychiatry,* 137: 1336–1347.

Hilberman, E., and Munson, R. 1978. Sixty Battered Women. *Victimology: An International Journal,* 2: 460–470.

Karon, B. 1964. Suicidal Tendency as the Wish to Hurt Someone Else and Resulting Treatment Techniques. *Journal of Individual Psychology,* 20:206–212.

Kaufman, I. 1966. Psychiatric Implications of Physical Abuse of Children. In *Protecting the Battered Child.* Denver: American Humane Association.

Kobler, A. L., and Stotland, E. 1964. *The End of Hope: A Social Clinical Study of Suicide.* New York: Free Press.

Lang, A.; Goechner, D.; Adesso, V.; and Marlatt, G. 1975. Effects of Alcohol on Aggression in Male Social Drinkers. *Journal of Abnormal Psychology,* 84:508–518.

Lefkowitz, M.; Eron, L.; Walder, L.; and Huesmann, L. 1977. *Growing Up to Be Violent: A Longitudinal Study of the Development of Aggression.* New York: Pergamon Press.

Levinger, G. 1966. Sources of Marital Dissatisfaction Among Applicants for Divorce. *American Journal of Orthopsychiatry,* 26:803–807.

Litman, R. E. 1964. Immobilization Response to Suicidal Behavior. *Archives of General Psychiatry,* 11:282–285.

Mark, V., and Ervin, F. 1970. *Violence and the Brain.* New York: Harper & Row.

Martin, D. 1977. Society's Vindication of the Wife Beater. *Bulletin of the American Academy of Psychiatry and the Law,* 5:391–410.

Meerloo, J. A. 1962. *Suicide & Mass Suicide.* New York: Grune & Stratton.

Menninger, K. A. 1958. *Man Against Himself.* New York: Harcourt Brace.

O'Brien, J. E. 1971. Violence in Divorce Prone Families. *Journal of Marriage and the Family,* 33:692–698.

Pagelow, M. 1976. Preliminary Report on Battered Women. Paper presented at the Second International Symposium on Victimology. Boston, September.

Quinney, R. 1965. Suicide, Homicide, and Economic Development. *Social Forces,* 43:401–406.

Rada, R. T. 1978. *Clinical Aspects of the Rapist.* New York: Grune & Stratton.

Robertson, N. 1979. A Preventive Approach to Child Abuse. *The New York Times,* December 24.

Rounsaville, B. J. 1978. Battered Wives: Barriers to Identification and Treatment. *American Journal of Orthopsychiatry,* 48:487–494.

Roy, M. ed. 1977. *Battered Women.* New York: Van Nostrand Reinhold.

Sadock, V. A. 1972. Special Areas of Interest. In *Comprehensive Textbook of Psychiatry,* 2nd ed., eds. H. E. Kaplan, A. M. Freedman, and B. J. Sadock. Baltimore: Williams & Wilkens.

Schultz, D. 1981. *Theories of Personality,* 2nd ed. Monterey, Calif.: Brooks/Cole.

Scott, P. D. 1974. Battered Wives. *British Journal of Psychiatry,* 125:433–441.

Seligman, M. E. 1975. *Helplessness: On Depression, Development and Death.* San Francisco: W. H. Freeman.

Shainness, N. 1979. Vulnerability of Violence: Masochism as a Process. *American Journal of Psychotherapy,* 33:174–188.

Shuntick, R., and Taylor, P. 1972. The Effects of Alcohol on Human Physical Aggression. *Journal of Experimental Research in Personality,* 6:34–38.

Speigel, J. 1955. Emotional Reactions to Catastrophe. In *Stress Situations,* ed. S. Liebman. Philadelphia: J. B. Lippincott.

Steinmetz, S. 1978. Wife Beating: A Critique and Reformulation of Existing Theory. *Bulletin of American Academy of Psychiatry and the Law,* 6:322–334.

Stone, A. A. 1960. A Syndrome of Serious Suicidal Intent. *Archives of General Psychiatry,* 3:331–339.

Straus, M. A. 1973. A General Systems Theory Approach to a Theory of Violence Between Family Members. *Social Science Information,* 12:105–125.

Straus, M. A. 1974. Cultural and Social Organizational Influences on Violence Between Family Members. In *Configurations: Biological and Cultural Factors in Sexual and Family Life.* New York: Lexington Books.

Straus, M. A.; Gelles, R.; and Steinmetz, S. 1976. Violence in the Family: An Assessment of Knowledge and Research Needs. Paper presented for the American Association for the Advancement of Science, Boston.

Straus, M. A., and Hotaling, G. 1977. *The Social Causes of Husband-Wife Violence.* Minneapolis: University of Minnesota Press.

Symonds, A. 1979. The Myth of Masochism. *American Journal of Psychotherapy,* 33:161–173.

Symonds, M. 1978. The Psychodynamics of Violence Prone Marriages. *American Journal of Psychoanalysis,* 38:213–222.

Wahl, C. W. 1957. Suicide as a Magical Act. *Bulletin of the Menninger Clinic,* 21:91–98.

Walker, L. 1979. *The Battered Woman.* New York: Harper & Row.

Wiele, E. F. 1960. On Social Psychological Questions in Suicide Personalities. *Psychological Research,* 11:37–44.

Zeichner, A., and Pihl, O. 1979. Effects of Alcohol and Behavior Contingencies on Human Aggression. *Journal of Abnormal Psychology,* 88:153–160.

Zilboorg, G. 1935. Suicide Among Civilized and Primitive Races. *American Journal of Psychiatry,* 92:1347–1369.

Supplementary Readings

Barile, L. A. A Model for Teaching Management of Disturbed Behavior. *Journal of Psychosocial Nursing and Mental Health Services,* 20(1982):9–11.

Boettcher, E. G. Preventing Violent Behavior: An Integrated Theoretical Model for Nursing. *Perspectives of Psychiatric Care,* 21(1983):54–58.

Campbell, J. C., and Humphreys, J. C. *Nursing Care of Victims of Family Violence.* Reston, Va.: Reston Publishing, 1983.

Campbell, W. The Use of Seclusion in a Psychiatric Hospital. *Nursing Times*, 78(1982):1821–1825.

Claerhout, S. Problem Solving Skills of Rural Battered Women. *American Journal of Community Psychology*, 10(1982):605–614.

Cotton, P. G. Dealing with Suicide on a Psychiatric Inpatient Unit. *Hospital and Community Psychiatry*, 34 (1983):55–59.

Davis, P. A. *Suicidal Adolescents*. Springfield, Ill.: Charles C Thomas, 1983.

Foley, T. S., and Davies, M. A. *Rape: Nursing Care of Victims*. St. Louis: C. V. Mosby, 1983.

Fromm, E. *Anatomy of Human Destructiveness*. New York: Fawcett, 1978.

Gemmiel, F. B. A Family Approach to Battered Women. *Journal of Psychosocial Nursing and Mental Health Services*, 20(1982):22–39.

Gentry, T. The Solution for Child Abuse Rests with the Community. *Child Today*, 11(1982):22–24.

Gerlock, A. Factors Associated with the Seclusion of Psychiatric Patients. *Perspectives of Psychiatric Care*, 21(1983):46–53.

Hilbery, J. L. Documentation in Child Abuse. *American Journal of Nursing*, 83(1983):236–239.

Keith, C. R. *The Aggressive Adolescent: A Clinical Perspective*. New York: Free Press, 1984.

Kinard, E. M. Child Abuse and Depression: Cause or Consequence. *Child Welfare*, 61(1982):403–423.

Kroloski, P. C. Child Abuse and Violence Against the Family. *Child Welfare*, 61(1982):435–444.

Lanza, M. L. Origins of Aggression. *Journal of Psychosocial Nursing and Mental Health Services*, 21(1983):11–16.

Long, C. Geriatric Abuse. *Issues in Mental Health Nursing*, 3(1981):123–135.

Marohn, R. C. Adolescent Violence: Causes and Treatment. *Journal of the American Academy of Child Psychiatry*, 21(1982):354–360.

Maadenberg, A. M. The Violent Patient. *American Journal of Nursing*, 83(1983):402–403.

McCoy, S. M. Seclusion: The Process of Intervening. *Journal of Psychosocial Nursing and Mental Health Services*, 21(1983):8–15.

Miller, M. *Suicide Intervention by Nurses*. New York: Springer, 1982.

Turkat, D. The Relationship Between Family Violence and Hospital Recidivism. *Hospital and Community Psychiatry*, 34(1983):552–553.

Turpin, J. P. The Violent Patient: A Strategy for Management and Diagnosis. *Hospital and Community Psychiatry*, 34(1983):37–40.

Waswleski, M. Spousal Violence in Military Homes. *Military Medicine*, 147(1982):760–765.

Williams, J. O. Restraints: When and How. *Ohio Nurses Review*, 58(1983):6.

433

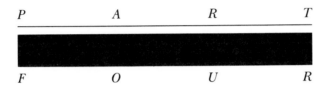

P A R T

F O U R

THEORY AND PRACTICE OF PSYCHIATRIC MENTAL HEALTH NURSING

CHARACTERISTICS OF CRISIS
Opportunities in Crisis
Crisis and Emergency
Duration of Crisis

PATTERNS OF CRISIS BEHAVIOR

CRISIS ASSESSMENT AND INTERVENTION
Crisis Counseling
Types of Crisis Work

TYPOLOGY OF CRISES
Dispositional Crisis
Transitional Crisis
Traumatic Crisis
Developmental Crisis
Psychopathological Crisis
Psychiatric Emergency

STAFF BURNOUT AS CRISIS

C H A P T E R

16

Crisis Theory and Practice

Learning Objectives

After reading this chapter, the student should be able to:

1. Describe the role of anxiety, stress, and grief in crisis.

2. Differentiate anxiety-provoking and anxiety-suppressing approaches to crisis intervention.

3. Identify criteria for the selection of clients for particular treatment approaches.

4. Classify various types of crisis based on the relative impact of external and internal forces on persons in crisis.

5. Formulate appropriate assessment and intervention strategies applicable to crisis work.

Overview

Crisis is a human response to conditions that are perceived as health threats or problems by individuals, families, and communities. There is no doubt that crisis theory and practice is relevant to nursing, especially in light of the American Nurses' Association's definition of nursing as the "diagnosis and treatment of human responses to actual or potential health problems."

This chapter begins by defining what constitutes crises and describes response patterns used by clients as they react to crisis. The chapter discusses the origins and characteristics of crises and functional and dysfunctional responses to crisis situations. It also examines appropriate assessment and intervention strategies for various types of crises.

Panics in some cases have their uses; they produce as much good as they hurt. Their duration is always short; the mind soon grows through them and acquires a firmer habit than before . . . they bring things to light which might otherwise have lain forever undiscovered.

THOMAS PAINE

439

For a crisis to be present, a problem or threat, real or perceived, must exist. People respond to crises in a variety of ways, expressing themselves through biological, psychological, and social channels. They try to deal with the threat by employing methods that have worked for them in the past. When customary coping techniques fail, disorganization, or disequilibrium, follows. Disorganization is an internal, subjective experience that, in effect, constitutes a state of crisis.

Two nurse authors, Loomis and Wood (1983), developed a classification of actual or potential health problems, any of which may precipitate a crisis. The categories of health problems they identified are:

- Developmental life changes.
- Acute health deviations.
- Chronic health deviations.
- Culturally induced stressors.
- Environmentally induced stressors.

There is no actual or potential health problem that cannot be assigned to one of these five categories. In reacting to such health problems, individuals, families, and communities may use more than one response system. Acute or chronic illness, for instance, may elicit biological, psychological, and social responses. Culturally induced stressors, on the other hand, may evoke psychological and social responses primarily.

A broader categorization of crises differentiates developmental crises from situational crises. These two categories were discussed at length in Chapters 14 and 15. Every individual experiences developmental crises periodically during the life cycle. Even for those fortunate individuals who are able to move tranquilly through life, every new experience, whether developmental or situational, contains the potential for crisis if customary coping methods prove inadequate and alternative methods are not found.

Interpreting crisis as a human response to actual or potential life problems helps to reduce the mystery surrounding crisis theory and practice. Identifying the response systems being used by clients and assessing the usefulness of the responses helps nurses construct a multifactorial assessment model that recognizes the nature of the crisis and identifies the response systems that are involved. Such an assessment model leads to the problem-solving activities that are the core of crisis intervention (deChesnay, 1983).

CHARACTERISTICS OF CRISIS

A pioneer in the development of crisis theory was Gerald Caplan (1964), whose work contributed greatly to the community mental health movement and validated the concepts of primary, secondary, and tertiary prevention described in Chapter 1. Caplan described crisis as the result of frustration caused by impediments to the attainment of life goals. Preceding any crisis is an event or hazard that is perceived as a threat to one's fulfillment, aspirations, or even existence. The threat may not be real or seem important in the eyes of others, but it is very real and very distressing to the person or persons in-

Table 16-1. Characteristic Behavioral Patterns in Disequilibrium

Behavior Pattern	Characteristics
Fight-flight behavior	Blaming others (fight) or avoiding responsibility (flight)
Conflicted behavior	Accomplishing tasks partially but not fully; behaving inconsistently; showing indecision
Helpless behavior	Placing responsibility on other people; showing childish, incompetent behavior
Hopeless behavior	Surrendering all autonomy; becoming passive, apathetic, and unresponsive

440

volved. It may take the form of the loss of a significant person (Engel, 1964), or of a challenge to competence, growth, or self-esteem (Parks, 1977; Glazer, 1981). The type of threat often influences the response that follows. Losses are likely to produce grief reactions or depression. Threats to security are likely to cause anxiety. Challenges to maturity or self-esteem may result in feelings of inferiority unless the challenges can be overcome (Adler, 1954, 1969).

Several factors must be present for a crisis to develop. First, a precipitating or hazardous event must intrude on the life of an individual, family, or group, causing an inner state of tension that is uncomfortable. Second, the person experiencing the tension tries to deal with the event or hazard by using customary coping measures. If the coping measures successfully relieve tension, an internal state of equilibrium is preserved and crisis is avoided. If the coping measures are not successful in reducing tension, the person is propelled into the state of disequilibrium known as crisis.

During the disequilibrium of crisis, people do not behave in their usual fashion. Their internal discomfort increases to the extent that there is disorganization and distortion—emotional, cognitive, and behavioral. The disorganization, confusion, and distortion further reduce their problem-solving abilities and coping skills. At this point they feel overwhelmed and may turn to friends or professionals for assistance.

Opportunities in Crisis

Crisis is a phenomenon that combines danger with the possibility of growth. The disequilibrium of crisis provides opportunity for growth and for expanding one's repertoire of coping skills. This is a time when the person initially tries to search for solutions, either alone or with help from others. The search is impeded by the distortions and disorganization that accompany crisis. Sometimes the solutions that are tried are functional and sometimes they are not. Dysfunctional solutions include denying or avoiding the hazardous event, being indecisive, ruminating endlessly, or becoming depressed and angry. In such cases the danger surrounding crisis outweighs the opportunities for growth. Inability to cope in a functional way not only hinders current problem solving but also has an adverse effect on future problem solving.

In dealing with a crisis, people tend to cling to preferred or accustomed ways of behaving. Some individuals will experiment with one solution after another, trying new ways of coping as soon as an earlier one fails. Other individuals procrastinate and do little or nothing to deal with the crisis. Often the person is angry and projects personal feelings of inadequacy onto the crisis worker, who is then labeled inept or unhelpful. Others in crisis suffer a sense of personal failure and blame themselves for events, even when they are beyond their power to control. Self-blame is counterproductive because it intensifies feeling of helplessness and hopelessness.

During the disequilibrium of crisis, dysfunctional behaviors often are variations on one of four patterns: fight-flight behavior, conflicted behavior, helpless behavior, and hopeless behavior. Table 16-1 shows how these patterns of behavior might be expressed during a period of crisis.

Many persons in crisis, however, are able to seek

Life is an adventure in a world where nothing is static; where unpredictable and ill-understood events constitute dangers that must be overcome, often blindly and at great cost; where man himself, like the sorcerer's apprentice, has set in motion forces that are potentially destructive and may someday escape his control. Every manifestation of existence is a response to stimuli and challenges, each of which constitutes a threat if not adequately dealt with.

RENÉ DUBOS (1959)

441

Table 16-2. Alternative Outcomes in a Family Crisis

Type of Solution	Coping Strategy	Outcome
Functional	Relocation of the mother is discussed by the daughter, her husband, and the children. Agreement is made that family life will go on as usual, with all members taking some responsibility for Grandma. The daughter and husband share results of the family conference with the elderly mother. Common expectations are discussed.	*Improved coping skills:* Preliminary agreement and planning prepare the family for change. Future turmoil and dissension are avoided.
Questionable	Daughter tries to interact with family as if nothing has changed. She does this by placating her mother, her husband, and her children, as she has always done. Her motto is "Peace at any price" even if this requires considerable self-sacrifice on her part.	*Unchanged coping skills:* Family equilibrium is preserved. The family and elderly mother are comfortable. Daughter feels entrapped by her mother's demands and her family's needs, as she often has since her marriage.
Dysfunctional	Daughter aligns herself with her mother and against her family. She struggles to satisfy all her mother's whims and argues constantly with her husband. Eventually her husband moves out of the house; the marriage is in serious trouble. The family is in crisis.	*Impaired coping skills:* Family is in a state of disequilibrium. The children are enraged, and the husband is estranged. Grandma is content, but her daughter is unhappy.

help and to engage in a search for alternative behaviors that bring the crisis to a successful resolution. In the process of responding to the crisis, individuals learn new ways of coping that will be available to them in the future. The new coping methods may enable them to avoid future crises or to respond more effectively in crisis situations if and when they recur. Table 16-2 illustrates the three possible outcomes of crisis resolution in the situation of a demanding elderly woman, unable to continue living alone, who moves in with her married daughter.

Crisis and Emergency

Everyday annoyances are commonly but inaccurately referred to as crises. There is a tendency, for example, to confuse a *crisis* with an *emergency*, but it is not difficult to distinguish between the two (Parad and Resnik, 1975). A working mother whose babysitter suddenly becomes unavailable and must make other arrangements might call this a "crisis." Actually, what the mother must deal with if she wants to get to work that day is an emergency. If the situation occurs repeatedly and the mother is unable to find a reliable babysitter, she may lose the job she needs so

Figure 16-1. *Progression of an emergency condition to a crisis condition.*
SOURCE: Adapted from Lindemann (1944) and Caplan (1964).

CRISIS AND STRESS

The term *stress* is sometimes used as a synonym for crisis, but the two are quite different. Stress is an interactive process in which people must adjust or adapt to conditions shaped by themselves or others (see Chapter 12). It is a complex stimulus-response situation that is influenced by a number of intervening variables. One variable in stress situations is individuals' evaluation of their own performance and of whether the rewards are worth the efforts that must be made to adapt to the situation (Garfield, 1979). For example, nurses working on a children's oncology unit may be able to adapt to the stressful conditions and to take vigorous measures to meet the demands made on them. The nurses may feel that they are sufficiently rewarded when they see extremely ill children improve. If, however, the physical and emotional demands made on them are excessive or prolonged, some of them may become exhausted, or "burned out." (Such burnout is discussed in detail at the end of this chapter.) When excessive demands are not alleviated in some way, burnout can take on proportions severe enough to be considered a crisis. Therefore, stress alone does not constitute a crisis, but it may be a precipitating or hazardous event that leads to crisis (Cassel, 1979; Haack and Jones, 1983).

Figure 16-1. *Progression of an emergency condition to a crisis condition.*
SOURCE: Adapted from Lindemann (1944) and Caplan (1964).

badly. If this should happen, the mother may then find herself facing a genuine crisis. On the other hand, if the mother can make arrangements that permit her to get to work regularly and on time, she has dealt with the emergency and has avoided crisis. Only if the mother cannot locate a reliable babysitter despite her best efforts and loses the job she needs to support her child has the emergency situation deteriorated into a crisis.

Emergencies are sudden, distressing events in which prompt action is needed. The persons involved may or may not take steps to help themselves, but unless some remedial action is taken quickly, an emergency may have serious, even life and death, consequences. Nevertheless, most emergencies respond to almost any active intervention, such as reassurance, explanation, distraction, control, or rescue.

A *crisis* is often less immediate and less urgent than an emergency. Entering school, relocating,

and marrying are not emergencies, but circumstances surrounding these events may introduce hazards that can lead to either emergencies or crises, depending on conditions and the responses of the persons involved. Some theorists believe that an emergency exists if immediate intervention is warranted. If the persons in distress can wait 24 hours for help, a crisis rather than an emergency is present (Caplan, 1964).

Figure 16-1 shows the progression of an emergency condition to a crisis condition and the stages involved. An emergency situation is apt to induce reactions of shock, disbelief, distress, and anxiety. Intervention at the time of an emergency may result in relief or rescue so that the emergency situation does not assume the proportions of a crisis. However, an emergency situation often deteriorates into a crisis if the immediate intervention produces only temporary or questionable relief.

Duration of Crisis

All crises are of limited duration, usually lasting up to six or eight weeks; at the end of this time the subjective distress and disequilibrium lessen. Whether or not there has been effective problem solving, the state of crisis abates. It is thought that crisis has a natural termination regardless of outcomes because it is impossible for people to tolerate the subjective distress and disequilibrium of crisis for very long. In other words, the severe disorganization of crisis must eventually diminish in order for people to endure and survive.

Although the state of crisis may be time limited, the manner in which the crisis has been handled has long-term consequences, in that coping skills may

442

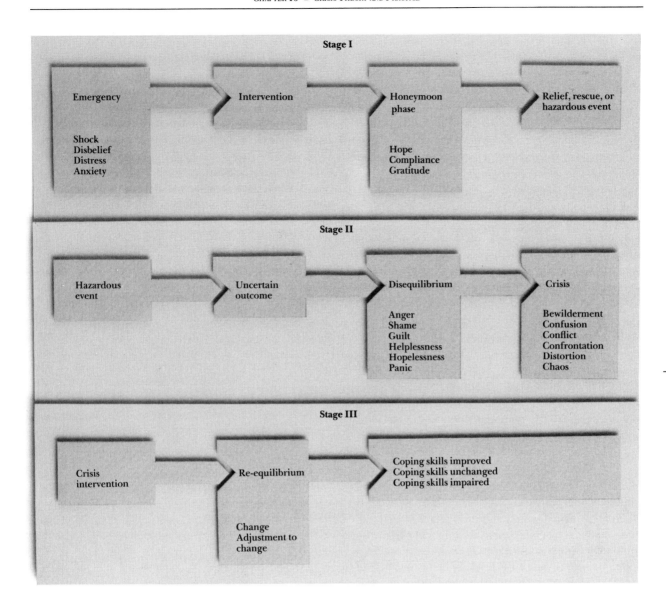

have improved or deteriorated. Such changes in coping skills in turn influence the way in which crises will be responded to in the future.

PATTERNS OF CRISIS BEHAVIOR

Knowledge of how people react in crises has been enhanced by the work of Lindemann (1944), who studied the grief responses by survivors of events in which loved ones were lost. Lindemann found both similarities and differences in the way people reacted to the loss of a loved one. When survivors were able to grieve or mourn for the one who was lost, they proved eventually able to accept the loss, to disengage from the lost person, and to begin to form new relationships. However, such losses became crises for people who were unwilling or unable to proceed with grief work or mourning.

Belief that the process of grieving has a beginning and an end is prevalent among theorists and clinicians in the health field (Engel, 1964; Parks, 1977; Searl, 1978; Lindy, Grace, and Green, 1981). A variation of this viewpoint is that the crisis of grief is rarely resolved once and for all but is only partially resolved or is reactivated periodically in ways that may even generate another crisis (Caplan, 1974). For many survivors the period of grieving may last for years, but most of them learn to live with the burden of loss as they try to integrate the experience into their lives and readjust.

People who have suffered the loss of a loved one are not the only ones entitled to be called survivors. Individuals who have undergone major surgery or have recovered from a serious illness may be regarded as survivors, as may those people who have lived through disasters such as fire or flood or experiences such as war or internment in a prison

---

POPULAR MYTHS ABOUT CRISIS INTERVENTION

■ *Myth One:* Crisis intervention is appropriate only for psychiatric emergencies.

■ *Myth Two:* Crisis intervention is limited to a single therapeutic session.

■ *Myth Three:* Crisis therapy is practiced only by paraprofessionals.

■ *Myth Four:* Crisis intervention offers only temporary stabilization until more lasting help can be given.

■ *Myth Five:* Crisis intervention can be considered only a primary prevention method.

■ *Myth Six:* Crisis intervention requires no special knowledge or expertise if the clinician is experienced in more traditional therapeutic approaches.

SOURCE: Adapted from Ann W. Burgess and Bruce A. Baldwin, *Crisis Intervention Theory and Practice* (Englewood Cliffs, N.J.: Prentice-Hall, 1981).

---

camp. By understanding the effects of a survival experience, nurses can help people use the experience as a way of expanding rather than restricting coping skills (Fell, 1977; Smith, 1979).

When the experiences of people who have recovered from a serious illness are compared with those of people who have survived a common disaster, certain differences emerge. Whenever a shared disaster occurs, there is considerable social support in the form of external rescue efforts and internal common interests. This is not generally the case with severe illness, where support networks may not extend beyond the family. Even so, the survivors of serious illness and shared disasters exhibit some similar reactions. Both types of survivors seem to experience a transformation of values. Personal relationships in particular seem to become more precious to them. Smith (1979) found that after any critical life experience, individuals spoke of a heightened awareness of the beauty to be found in life. Many persons expressed determination to exercise more control over events in their lives, but still others became more tolerant of change and were resolved not to be overwhelmed by whatever happened but to "roll with the punches."

In their desire to relieve the physical and psychological discomfort of survivors, nurses should not overlook the growth potential inherent in having survived a life-threatening illness or disaster. In caring for survivors, Smith (1979) recommends the following nursing interventions:

1. Encourage people to talk about their experience and about any changes in their personal values, without suggesting what those changes should be.

2. Encourage people to realize that others have had similar experiences, although the dimensions of the experience are unique for each individual. Speak of the whole range of human experience without belittling the individual experience in any way. Recognizing the universality of the experience may help people to live through it without feeling so overwhelmed by it.

3. Encourage survivors to talk with others who have had similar experiences, especially with others who are at various stages of distress or recovery. This is particularly important for survivors whose experience has been solitary rather than shared.

CRISIS ASSESSMENT AND INTERVENTION

One of the first steps in crisis work is to explore the meaning of the crisis to the person or persons involved. Often the client perceives the significance of events as far greater than outsiders perceive it. The nurse or other crisis worker begins by accepting the reality of the client's distress, inasmuch as the situation may have a symbolic meaning to the client that is not immediately apparent. For example, an ambitious man passed over for promotion may in his disappointment discount his impressive accomplishments and may become discouraged and depressed so that he is no longer able to function well at work. The same man, if promoted to a position he has sought, may feel doubtful of his ability to meet the new demands made on him. He may become anxious, unable to concentrate, unable to sleep, and

---

CRISIS ASSESSMENT TOOL

Initial Steps

1. Collect data that indicate the dimensions of the problem, using various sources of information.
2. Formulate a dynamic hypothesis concerning the problem and the coping responses of the client.
3. Assess the problem in terms of intrinsic and extrinsic factors and determine a therapeutic approach.
4. Involve the client in problem-solving activities.
5. Negotiate a contract that sets clear, reachable goals.
6. Explain that treatment will be terminated according to the terms of the contract.

General Procedures

1. Obtain demographic data.
2. Define the problem in realistic terms.
3. Assess the mental status of the client(s).
4. Assess the physical status of the client(s).
5. Assess the psychosocial status of the client(s).
6. Assess coping skills of the client(s).

Coping Skills Assessment

1. How does the client deal with anxiety, tension, or depression?
2. Has the client used customary coping methods in the current situation?
3. What were the results of using customary coping methods?
4. Have there been recent life changes that interfered with customary coping methods?

5. Are significant persons contributing to continuation of the problem?
6. Is the client considering suicide or homicide as a way of coping? If so, how? When?
7. Has the client attempted suicide or homicide in the past? Under what conditions?
8. Assess the extent of suicidal or homicidal risk presented by the client. Hospitalization may be necessary as a protective measure.

Planning and Problem Solving

1. Is the present crisis new or a reenactment of similar events that occurred in the past?
2. What alternative methods might have been used to avoid development of the present crisis?
3. What new methods might be used to resolve the present crisis?
4. What supports are available to strengthen new problem-solving methods?

Anticipatory Guidance

1. What sources of stress remain for the client?
2. How might the client deal with problematic issues in the future, based on the current repertoire of coping skills?
3. How might the current repertoire of coping skills be maintained or expanded?
4. With termination of the contract for crisis intervention, is further referral or follow-up care necessary?

445

---

unable to function well at work. In the first instance, failure to attain a goal has created a crisis; in the second instance, success in attaining a goal has created a crisis. The common aspect of both examples is *change*, which creates inner turmoil, leading to disequilibrium.

After accepting the authenticity of the client's feelings, the nurse should explore the actual extent of the crisis. Initial assessment includes acceptance of the subjective experience of the client followed by exploration of the objective proportions of the cri-

sis. The basic steps in crisis assessment are outlined in the accompanying box.

Crisis Counseling
Crisis intervention is directed toward mobilizing and channeling the client's own problem-solving and coping skills. Because people in crisis are in a state of disequilibrium, reducing the inner turmoil is a prerequisite for problem solving. Services that are provided should be flexible, and the nurse or other crisis worker should arrange to be accessible

to the client by phone or in person whenever needed.

The essential element of crisis work is that it represents a shift in emphasis from the intrapsychic life of the individual to interaction of the individual with others or with the environment (Morgan and Moreno, 1973). Every crisis involves an individual, a family, or a community responding in a particular way to particular circumstances. During the crisis contract, the nurse, in words and actions, acknowledges the existence of a compelling problem that is causing distress. The focus of crisis work is on the search for a solution to the immediate problem.

The contract for crisis counseling is usually short term, lasting for the six- to eight-week duration of acute crisis. The counseling sessions may vary in length from 15 minutes to an hour. Frequency of meetings is a decision reached jointly by the client and the nurse. If distress is extreme, if the client has poor impulse control and may be destructive to himself or others, daily meetings may be necessary. The nurse may consider it appropriate to give the client a phone number where she can be easily reached. If the client has a reliable support network, weekly or bi-weekly meetings may be sufficient. During the sessions, the crisis caregiver is actively involved but does nothing for the client that the client is able to handle himself. Some clients may become dependent on the nurse or other crisis worker, but the dependency is not too worrisome because crisis intervention and the period of the therapeutic contract are brief (Sifneos, 1980).

Sometimes nurses working on a long-term basis with a family or individual will observe that a crisis situation has developed. It may be necessary for the nurse to alter the approach being used and to become more active in order to facilitate resolution of the crisis. Then the nurse may have to resume her previous approach in which involvement was less intense. One way to accomplish this is to introduce other professionals into the care plan, so that any dependency on the nurse can be gradually reduced.

For nurses engaged in helping clients in a crisis, a primary rule is not to make decisions *for* them but to become involved in making decisions *with* them. Restoration of equilibrium through improved coping behavior is the maximal goal of crisis work. A minimal goal is to help the clients return to at least precrisis levels of functioning, but there are occasions when even this lesser goal is not achieved.

DEALING WITH DISTORTIONS In dealing with persons in crisis, the nurse should use an approach that considers three major forms of distortion that may be present. After exploring the nature of the crisis and its meaning to the client, the nurse should endeavor to identify and encourage correction of *cognitive, emotional,* and *behavioral* distortions.

People in crisis find it difficult, if not impossible, to think clearly and rationally. This means that their ability to deal realistically with events, to plan, and to make decisions is greatly reduced. Often these individuals are easily distracted, incoherent, and tangential. Because of their cognitive distortions, they are overreactive emotionally. The emotional distress they experience may lead to such somatic symptoms as insomnia or anorexia. Behaviors are not goal directed but may take the form of apathy or of pointless, unproductive activity.

An early task of the nurse engaged in crisis intervention is to go over with the client the sequence of events that led to the crisis, asking questions about what happened, when, and to whom. It is also necessary to ask what efforts were made to cope with the crisis. The exploration yields important information and also helps the client begin to put events into perspective. Often, people in crisis cannot make a cognitive connection between the hazardous event, unsuccessful efforts to deal with the event, and the eventual disequilibrium. Therefore, tracing the sequence of events clarifies the situation for the client and sometimes leads to a more realistic view of what actually happened. In discussions with the client about what led to the crisis, the nurse should convey confidence in the ability of both of them to find a solution together.

Emotional or affective distortions are also present. The cognitive exploration is often helpful in reducing emotional reactivity to manageable proportions, but some people in crisis need to be allowed a period of emotional ventilation, or catharsis. In the first sessions, free emotional expression should be permitted and even encouraged. It is advisable, however, to call attention to extreme emotional reactions as soon as possible, since prolonged outbursts are likely to impede problem solving. The nurse may offer empathy by making statements about how difficult things must seem to the client but should add that the situation will not always seem as overwhelming as it does now. In other words, the nurse should offer hope and set limits, along with providing empathy.

Behavioral distortions should also be confronted—not only distortions in the client's own behavior but also in the client's interpretation of the behavior of others. Blaming oneself or others is dysfunctional; emphasis should be placed not on past errors or misjudgments but on making the future better.

Emphasis on cognitive processes should continue throughout the duration of the therapeutic contract. Behavioral and emotional distortions can be modified by introducing additional social or professional resource people into the picture. Persons in crisis are reassured by the contributions of an expanded support network. These other contributions not only reduce dependency on the nurse but also convince the client that others care and will help.

DEALING WITH ANXIETY Anxiety has the ability to generate energy, but when levels of anxiety are high, energy becomes undirected and disintegrative (Freud, 1936; Peplau, 1952). Sullivan (1953) used the word "euphoria" to describe the absence of anxiety and described anxiety as perhaps the most unpleasant human experience. *Mild* anxiety releases energy that can be used for problem solving. *Moderate* anxiety usually decreases efficiency, while *severe* anxiety leads to frustration and distortion. When anxiety rises to panic levels, available energy is directed toward escape. In the disequilibrium of crisis, anxiety hovers between severe and panic levels. The nurse who is dealing with a client in crisis must assess the level of anxiety being experienced and endeavor to reduce anxiety so that coherent communication between nurse and client can take place. Table 16-3 shows the various levels, characteristics, and appropriate interventions for anxiety.

For persons in crisis, anxiety is pervasive and retards the restoration of equilibrium. Therefore, the nurse should offer enough reassurance to foster a sense of safety and hopefulness. Such general statements as "I think it was wise for you to come for help" indicate to clients that their disorganization is not total. Excessive solicitude is apt to foster regression, but clients will respond to a nurse who seems confident that a solution can be found. Fostering an attitude of hopefulness increases the client's motivation and problem-solving skills. Delineating the outlines of the crisis and exploring problem-solving efforts of the past help the client to reduce anxiety to manageable levels. Because mild levels of anxiety are facilitative, a central challenge for the crisis worker is to help the client tolerate mild anxiety and direct it into constructive, problem-solving behaviors.

DEALING WITH VIOLENCE During the entire course of crisis counseling but especially in the first sessions, any homicidal or suicidal thoughts should be appraised. Clients should be asked if they are thinking about suicide or if they have any urge to harm others. If the answer to either question is affirmative, additional questions should probe the seriousness of the thought, the details of any plan, and the availability of the means to carry out the plan. There is a popular myth that bringing up the topic of suicide or violence toward others may put ideas in the client's head. This myth attributes more power to the clinician than actually exists. If a clinician is reluctant to ask such questions and to discuss them openly, the client will tend to conceal intentions.

If the client has a well-thought-out plan and available means, hospitalization may be indicated unless the client has reliable social supports. Suicidal persons who seek professional help are likely to be ambivalent about carrying out an attempt. This means that they are likely to respond to a caring, concerned nurse who is accessible to the client at any time during the acute phase of suicide intention.

Crisis intervention is effective for suicidal persons who are ordinarily stable but who have been thrown into disequilibrium by sudden, stressful events. The end of a romantic relationship or failure to pass final examinations may induce suicidal feelings that will not be acted on if other people are available who care and want to help. Chronically depressed persons, alcoholics, psychotic clients, and

447

Table 16-3. Levels, Characteristics, and Interventions for Anxiety

Level of Anxiety	Characteristics	Nursing Interventions
Mild anxiety	Alertness and vigilance	1. Reconcile demands of the situation and the expectations and perceptions of the individual.
Moderate anxiety	Reduced perception and attention; subjective distress	2. Trace connections between the causes and symptoms of anxiety.
Severe anxiety	Selective perception and attention; subjective distress	1. Encourage motor activity. 2. Promote cognitive expression (talking, thinking). 3. Permit emotional expression (crying, talking).
Panic	Gross perceptual distortion; inability to communicate; inability to function	1. Offer firm structure and direction until panic recedes.

SOURCES: Adapted from Peplau (1952) and Sullivan (1953).

withdrawn, socially isolated individuals are not good candidates for crisis intervention because they usually require help for longer periods of time (see Chapter 15). Many suicidal persons require a long-term relationship with a supportive clinician. Such persons may regard the short-term crisis contract as another abandonment.

Violent and assaultive individuals are usually brought to emergency departments by the police. Staff members may be more comfortable when police or security guards are present, but there is reason to exclude them as soon as trust has been established between staff members and the client (Joel and Collins, 1978). If, however, there are grounds for believing that the client cannot remain in control, the presence of police or security guards is warranted. Some persons verbalize a wish to harm others but have not previously carried out their threats and seem unlikely to do so. As with suicidal clients, the presence of a detailed plan for violence plus access to the means of activating the plan is a significant sign of actual intent. Occasionally clients will lose control without warning, but it is likely that a crisis of violence has been foreshadowed by previous behaviors.

Persons experiencing delusional or hallucinatory thoughts are often capable of unpredictable actions and therefore require vigilant supervision. If a client has a history of committing violent acts, or if the current situation is complicated by addiction, antisocial behavior, or severe neurological or psychiatric disorders, crisis intervention is not appropriate. As a rule, violent, assaultive persons need emergency treatment followed by long-term treatment. Prolonged assessment is necessary in order to discover whether assaultive behaviors are directed toward a specific target, are generated by particular events, or are global in nature. Disposition and follow-up care are guided by the client's history and prognosis, the wishes of the family, and the safety of the community (Janosik, 1984).

Types of Crisis Work

Although crisis work is not considered psychotherapy, some principles of brief psychotherapy may be applied to crisis intervention. Sifneos (1967, 1972, 1980) described two kinds of brief psychotherapy: (1) *anxiety-provoking*, or exploratory, psychotherapy and (2) *anxiety-suppressive*, or supportive, psychotherapy. The standards used to select clients for the two types of treatment and their interventions and goals are quite different.

ANXIETY-PROVOKING INTERVENTION The basic premise of short-term anxiety-provoking psychotherapy is that a certain level of anxiety is needed to motivate clients to examine the underlying causes that lead them to act in dysfunctional ways. In this approach the clinician carefully monitors anxiety to make sure that the client is not overwhelmed. At the same time the clinician uses interpretation and confrontation to help the client identify resemblances between the current problem and earlier problems. The client is encouraged to use introspection and self-awareness in order to make connections between problematic events and her contribution to the problem.

Certain requirements must be met before brief anxiety-provoking psychotherapy is attempted. First, the clinician must have extensive knowledge of psychodynamic theories. This type of treatment should only be undertaken by qualified individuals with advanced preparation in their discipline who also have access to adequate supervision or consultation (Peplau, 1982). Second, candidates for anxiety-provoking therapy must have sufficient psychological strength to tolerate increased levels of anxiety, since anxiety is deliberately increased in order to persuade them to alter dysfunctional interactions and behaviors. According to Sifneos (1967, 1972), clients selected for anxiety-provoking treatment should meet the following standards:

1. They must have at least average intelligence.
2. They must have at least one meaningful relationship.
3. They must have an identifiable problem.
4. They must be motivated to solve the problem.
5. They must be able to verbalize their emotions.

Anxiety-provoking crisis intervention (sometimes called exploratory crisis work) follows much the same format as short-term exploratory psychotherapy, except that crisis work is usually of shorter duration than brief psychotherapy, which may last from a few months to a year. In anxiety-provoking crisis work the same criteria are used in the selection of clients. The goal of the nurse or other crisis counselor is to maintain or improve the client's coping skills, and the following issues are addressed:

■ Establish trust and rapport between client and nurse.

■ Review sequence of events leading to the crisis.

■ Analyze the coping behaviors the client has used.

■ Analyze the coping skills the client is capable of using.

■ Introduce alternative coping measures for the client to consider.

■ Engage in anticipatory guidance for future critical events.

During the period of anticipatory guidance, the current problem is linked to earlier problems and to similar problems that may occur in the future. Opportunities are provided to discuss and rehearse new behaviors that may avert future crises or facilitate future crisis resolution. Like brief anxiety-provoking psychotherapy, crisis intervention that provokes anxiety is used to bring about limited amounts of change in a context that considers more than the present crisis situation. Both variations of anxiety-provoking treatment employ a *review* of previous problems and a *preview* of future problems, using the current situation as a learning as well as a problem-solving process.

ANXIETY-SUPPRESSING INTERVENTION   Supportive, or anxiety-suppressive, brief psychotherapy may last from a few months to a year, while anxiety-suppressive crisis intervention lasts only six to eight weeks. Supportive approaches, whether they consist of brief psychotherapy or crisis intervention, are the treatments most appropriate for persons with a history of poor adjustment and inadequate social relationships. Such persons are likely to respond poorly to any increase in their anxiety levels. They require prompt relief of subjective discomfort, which is best accomplished by means of offering supportive strategies. In these instances the nurse or other counselor tries to alleviate the elements that are causing the client so much distress. Emotional support, environmental manipulation, and reassurance are essential if the anxiety of the client is to be diminished. Although previous difficulties may be touched on, more attention is paid to the current situation and to the remediation of the presenting crisis. Table 16-4 contrasts various aspects of anxiety-provoking and anxiety-suppressive treatment approaches.

GENERIC AND INDIVIDUAL CRISIS INTERVENTION
The decision to offer anxiety-provoking or anxiety-suppressive treatment depends primarily on the characteristics of the client and on the client's potential for insight and growth. Another methodological choice is available based on the nature of the crisis and the qualifications of the care provider. If the crisis is of a developmental nature and if the care provider is not an expert in psychodynamic theory, a generic form of crisis intervention may be advisable. In *generic* crisis work, attention is paid only to the crisis episode, and similar interventions may be used with most persons facing similar crises. An example of generic crisis work is the encouragement of active grieving in persons who have suffered the loss of a loved one. Lindemann (1944) showed that avoiding or discouraging active expressions of grief often leads to pathological states later on.

The *individual* approach to crisis work demands an extensive assessment of the unique needs of each client; therefore, the interventions in individual crisis work do not have universal applicability. An example of a person requiring an individualized type of crisis work might be a parent who has left a toddler unattended for a few moments during which the child has wandered into the street and been seriously injured by an automobile. In such a case normal grieving would be impeded by guilt, remorse, family involvement, and a host of other factors that necessitate an individualized rather than a generic approach.

TYPOLOGY OF CRISES

Baldwin (1978) formulated a classification system for crises that is helpful in assessing clients and plan-

449

Table 16-4. Anxiety-Provoking and Anxiety-Suppressing Therapeutic Approaches

Type of Treatment	Duration	Goals	Client Selection Criteria
Anxiety-provoking brief therapy	2 months to 1 year	Problem solving; exploration; psychological growth; behavioral change; anticipatory guidance	Psychological stability; social resources; average intelligence or more; emotional expressiveness
Anxiety-provoking crisis work	6 to 8 weeks	Problem solving; situational change; exploration; behavioral change; anticipatory guidance	Psychological stability; social resources; average intelligence or more; emotional expressiveness; crisis disequilibrium
Anxiety-suppressing brief therapy	2 months to 1 year	Support; reassurance; symptom relief; problem solving; behavioral change; anticipatory guidance	Psychological vulnerability; potential for deterioration
Anxiety-suppressing crisis work	6 to 8 weeks	Support; reassurance; symptom relief; situational manipulation; problem solving; anticipatory guidance	Psychological vulnerability; crisis disequilibrium; imminent deterioration

ning care. He identified six types of crises, moving from lesser to greater degrees of psychopathology:

1. Dispositional crises.
2. Transitional crises.
3. Traumatic crises.
4. Developmental crises.
5. Psychopathological crises.
6. Psychiatric emergencies.

As the gravity of the psychiatric disability increases, the causes of crises become internal rather than external, and the approach of the crisis worker must be modified accordingly. In devising his classifications Baldwin considered internal and external causation, estimated relative degrees of psychopathology, and suggested corresponding interventions. Clinical examples for the six types of crises follow. Although it is difficult to state arbitrary rules, the last two types of crises should be handled largely by mental health specialists.

Dispositional Crisis

Grace was a young nurse who had expected to get married a month after her graduation. Two weeks before her wedding date, her fiance married another girl. In the following weeks Grace alternated between hysterical weeping and depression. She lost her appetite and was unable to sleep. Her performance at work was so erratic that her head nurse insisted that Grace see a mental health counselor. In her first interview with the counselor, Grace denied serious thoughts of committing suicide but admitted that she wanted to make her former fiancé feel guilty. She frequently drove past the apartment where he lived with his new wife. At times she nearly slashed the tires of his car when it was parked at the curbside but restrained the impulse with difficulty.

Category: Class 1.

Causation: The crisis was caused by external situational factors. It was an acute episode of distress of a temporary nature.

Plan:
1. Clarify and define the situation with Grace.
2. Permit ventilation of feelings of anger and humiliation.
3. Offer support and guidance.
4. Suggest peer interaction.
5. Reinforce social networks.

Transitional Crisis

Bob and Barbara recently retired from running the restaurant where both had worked for many years. After a brief vacation Barbara settled down to enjoy her new leisure. She played bridge with old friends, visited her grandchildren, and adjusted easily to retirement. Bob was restless and discontent. He visited the restaurant every day and criticized the decisions of his son-in-law, who was managing the business. At home he was irritable and surly. He stopped attending his lodge meetings, lost his appetite, and had trouble sleeping. He began to insist that Barbara give up her social activities in order to stay home with him. In desperation, Barbara persuaded him to seek counseling.

Category: Class 2.

Causation: The crisis was caused by a predictable life change that could have been anticipated and prepared for in advance. Retirement meant a positive change for the wife but not for the husband.

Plan:
1. Discuss and clarify the life transition.
2. Contrast role changes of the spouses.
3. Encourage some shared and some independent activities.
4. Involve both husband and wife in counseling.

Traumatic Crisis

The Jones family, consisting of husband, wife, and two children, occupied a trailer on the outskirts of town. One winter night a kerosene heater ignited. Awakened by smoke, Mr. Jones led his wife and children to safety. When he returned for the family dog, he became trapped inside. The dog escaped through a window, but Mr. Jones died in the fire. His wife did not express her grief openly, but after the fire she refused to let her children out of her sight. They slept in her bed, and she withdrew them from nursery school. Two months after the tragedy she showed no signs of working through her grief. A community nurse who had supervised the health of the children was asked by Mrs. Jones's mother to resume visiting.

Category: Class 3.

Causation: The crisis was caused by a sudden, unanticipated event. Mrs. Jones withdrew from all social interactions and increased her emotional ties to her children, thus impairing their development.

Plan:

1. Encourage grieving and help Mrs. Jones detach from her dead husband.

2. Encourage reminiscing.

3. Permit expression of feelings of guilt.

4. Expand social interactions.

5. Promote healthy disengagement from the children.

6. Offer anticipatory guidance.

Developmental Crisis

When Bill was a college freshman, his father died suddenly. His mother was a homemaker who had never worked outside the home and who had depended on her husband to make decisions for her. Bill's college was about 500 miles from his home town. He was shocked and grief stricken by his father's death but was even more dismayed when his mother begged him to move back home and attend a local college. Bill had adjusted well at school and resented the prospect of becoming "the man of the house" for his mother. Yet he found it difficult to say no to her. He was able to return to school to finish the semester, but the idea of returning home was so disturbing that his academic standing was affected. He confided in one of his professors, who suggested that Bill make an appointment with the counseling service. Bill's dilemma was especially difficult because the college he was attending was his father's alma mater. His father had been proud of Bill's college record and had been instrumental in convincing Bill's mother that their son would benefit from not being too close to home. Bill's mother had no real financial worries; other family members, including Bill's married sisters, lived close to her.

Category: Class 4.

Causation: Bill was making progress in his developmental task of separating from his family of origin until the death of his father. This meant that Bill had lost an ally and a role model. His mother had other resources on which to rely but was determined that Bill would fill the place of her deceased husband. Thus, Bill's developmental task was impeded, and his mother was able to avoid coming to terms with her loss.

Plan:

1. Encourage a sibling alliance between Bill and his two sisters.

2. Help Bill's mother to accept the death of her husband, to grieve, and to gradually begin making new attachments.

3. Encourage Bill to continue his present task of making his own way in the world and establishing an identity.

4. Help all the siblings to be involved in comforting their mother so that Bill will not be the only child to whom she turns for solace.

Psychopathological Crisis

John was brought into the emergency department of a hospital by police, who had found him standing on the steel railing of a bridge. A forty-year-old male, John was disheveled and incoherent on admission. In response to questions, he kept repeating, "It's over. It's over." Identification cards found in his wallet showed him to be the resident of a halfway house for chronic psychiatric clients living in the community. Emergency room nurses learned that John had been in a rehabilitation program for several months.

The morning that John was found on the bridge had been stressful for him. Another client enrolled in the program had accused John of stealing his tools. The same morning John had been assigned new tasks that were more complicated than those he had just mastered. One of the counselors told John that as soon as he learned the new assignment, he would complete the training program and be ready for a real job.

The various incidents of the morning had made John anxious and confused. He left the training program without telling anyone and walked aimlessly for a while. Then he decided that too much was being expected of him and that he couldn't go on. He climbed the bridge railing and balanced himself precariously, scared to jump into space but afraid to climb back into a world that asked more of him than he could easily accomplish. The reassuring instructions and outstretched arms of policemen persuaded him not to jump. The suicide gesture had successfully communicated to others his desperate state of mind.

Category: Class 5.

Causation: The crisis was caused by internal psychopathology. A minor dispute and excessive demands created high anxiety. For John, fear of failure was linked to fear of success. This created conflict engendered by ambivalence between achievement and security.

Plan:

1. Acknowledge John's preexisting instability. Limit crisis intervention to stabilizing or restoring functioning.

451

2. Discontinue current efforts to push client to achieve.

3. Discourage John's tendencies to regress further.

4. Coordinate crisis work with the long-term treatment plan. Make referrals for further treatment as needed. Maintain communication with staff of the halfway house.

Psychiatric Emergency

Ben was a city employee who had lost his job when public funds were cut. He had never been an outgoing man and had difficulty getting along with other workers. He accused them of going through his desk, disarranging his files, and talking about him. After losing his job Ben became more irrational. He began drinking heavily; sometimes he was verbally abusive, and at other times he was mute and unresponsive. He believed that his phone was tapped and that FBI agents followed him whenever he left the house. Because he had always been suspicious of others, his wife thought that his normal behavior patterns were exaggerated because he had lost his job. She was taken by surprise one day when he grabbed a loaded hunting rifle and ran from the house, shouting that he was going to take care of the FBI and his enemies in city hall. His frightened wife notified the police, who took Ben into custody near city hall, where his bizarre stalking movements and rifle had attracted attention. A police officer trained in crisis work was able to disarm Ben and take him to a medical center for psychiatric evaluation and disposition. Ben's wife was notified, and she was present while Ben was evaluated.

Category: Class 6.

Causation: The crisis was caused by paranoid thinking, loss of control, and feelings of incompetence. Ben's problems were made worse by heavy drinking and by aggressive impulses toward others.

Plan:

1. Assess the situation promptly.

2. Intervene to protect Ben and others. Obtain medical, psychiatric, and security backup; take Ben into custody, and hospitalize if necessary.

3. Work with the family in arranging for follow-up and continuity of care.

4. Remain mindful of the rights of Ben while considering the safety of the family and the community.

STAFF BURNOUT AS CRISIS

Burnout has been described as a state of physical and emotional exhaustion that produces a poor self-concept, poor job attitudes, and deficient concern for clients (Pines and Kanner, 1982). Burnout may manifest itself in somatic complaints, such as headache, backache, and general malaise, and in such behaviors as neglecting one's assigned tasks, becoming angry over minor matters, and coming to work late and leaving early. It may also be expressed in cognitive ways, such as forgetting details, making errors, and failing to use good judgment. From this description it is easy to recognize the emotional, behavioral, and cognitive distortions that are the hallmark of crisis (Shubin, 1978).

Burnout can be a devastating experience for the professionals who experience it and for the clients receiving care. One of the prevailing features of burnout is decreased productivity. Burned out staff members often call in sick or simply fail to perform well when they do come to work. Dissatisfaction with the job increases. Complaining and arguing increase among staff members, and sometimes clients are pulled into the patterns of nontherapeutic communication. When one or two staff members are burned out, the responsibilities of the rest of the staff become heavier, thereby increasing the probability of burnout becoming epidemic (Parker, 1978).

In addressing the problem of burnout among nurses, two acknowledgments must be made. The first acknowledgment is that inadequate staffing is a relatively common problem for nurses. The second is that the nurses who become burned out are often those who contribute most to client care, sometimes at the expense of their own well-being. Nurses without genuine commitment to their profession are unlikely to experience burnout, because they are rarely ignited or motivated by a genuine desire to give the best possible care to their clients. In short, nurses suffering burnout are well worth salvaging and indeed may have been the most energetic workers on the staff (Chenevert, 1978; Pines and Kanner, 1982).

Burnout need not be a permanent condition, but the question is: How can it be reduced or alleviated? There are some measures that sound simplistic but can be highly beneficial. All nurses should try to develop the introspective skills to ascertain signs of burnout in themselves and in their co-workers. Forsyth and Cannady (1981) have provided excellent guidelines for assessing burnout signs and symptoms:

1. Be aware of your own emotional reactions. Recognize what you are thinking and feeling. If your reactions are negative, identify the cause or target so that you don't displace these reactions onto innocent bystanders.

2. Analyze your usual coping patterns. For example, if an unpleasant episode occurs at work, do you take it home with you? If an unpleasant episode occurs at home, do you bring it with you to work and burden yourself and others with it during the working day?

3. Develop new methods of coping if your behavioral analysis reveals questionable patterns. Persons who work hard and conscientiously need adequate rest and relaxation. Rescheduling home responsibilities may be necessary to get you off the treadmill of rushing home to take on new chores without any respite.

4. Develop the ability to say no to tasks that are exploitive. Burned out people behave aggressively, but people who are assertive enough to say no when the situation demands it are more likely to avoid getting burned out.

When a large number of staff members on a unit are burned out, a mutual support group may be the answer. Peer support can do a great deal to assuage the tension and fatigue of burnout. Specific problems can be dealt with more effectively when the entire staff is involved in a discussion. A support group for nurses who feel the effects of burnout can also be a place to share feelings and ideas, to delineate themes of interest to all, and to solve common problems. Topics of interest might include the use of assertive techniques instead of aggressive exchanges and the management of household responsibilities in single-parent or dual-career homes (Meichenbaum, 1977). One of the perennial complaints of people who are burned out is that they are unappreciated and their hard work is unrecognized. A support group might be a place where peer recognition can be given and where misunderstandings can be erased.

In organizing a support group to prevent or alleviate burnout, it is important to establish a well-defined contract and to agree upon group goals. Without such preparation the group sessions are likely to deteriorate into forums for airing complaints and reviving old disputes. Leadership should be democratic and egalitarian, but some form of leadership is essential. Group leadership might be conferred on a nurse with special knowledge of group theory and process, or it might be shared among members on a rotating basis. There are also advantages in having the group meet out-

side the borders of the actual unit or facility so that an atmosphere of collegiality and neutrality can be established (Pines and Kanner, 1982).

SUMMARY

Nobody can escape the emergence of crises at recurrent points of the life cycle, and most people are called upon at some time to intervene in crisis situations in the lives of others. The range of crisis theory includes the precipitating event, the person's response systems, and the results of responses to the precipitating event. If the responses elicited by the hazardous event are adequate and functional, the person is not propelled into the state of disorganization known as crisis. But if the person's responses to the hazardous event are inadequate and dysfunctional, a state of crisis follows.

The development of crisis theory is fairly recent, but in practice crisis intervention is as ancient as the human race. Families, friends, and communities have always sought or extended help in conditions of crisis. Whenever one distraught, confused person turns to another for help or advice, a form of crisis intervention takes place. Nurses working in acute care settings, in birthing centers, in schools, in outreach clinics, in homes, and in hospices all participate formally or informally in the problem-solving activities on which crisis intervention is based.

Sometimes it is difficult to apply strict standards to the selection of crisis clients, for in many respects this population is self-selected. The problem is compounded by the fact that many generalist nurses without advanced preparation in psychodynamics and without access to consultation services are called upon to offer crisis counseling in the context of their professional practice. It is important, then, for all nurses to have an understanding of crisis work and of the ways in which it can augment other treatment approaches.

At times crisis work is supportive and limited to the immediate event. At other times, depending on the characteristics and motivation of the client, the crisis worker may decide that it is advisable to explore issues beyond the current crisis and to consider the client's general coping patterns in addition to the behaviors necessary to resolve the current crisis. These exploratory approaches demand greater psychological strength from the client and greater psychodynamic knowledge from the clinician.

During the period of acute disequilibrium that accompanies crisis, clients experience high levels of

453

CLINICAL EXAMPLE

ANXIETY-SUPPRESSING AND
ANXIETY-PROVOKING APPROACHES
TO THE CRISIS OF AN ADOLESCENT

Noreen is a seventeen-year-old high school senior in the process of making a career choice. She is a quiet, attractive girl whose manner is shy and somewhat reserved. She has a few close girlfriends but her social experience has been limited, partly because of her protective and intrusive mother. Noreen is an average student, but music is an important part of her life. She belongs to the high school dramatic society and was chosen for an important role in the musical comedy presented by the senior class. As a result of winning the role Noreen has become convinced that she has discovered her true vocation: the stage. This conviction has become a source of controversy in her family, since for years her mother has planned for Noreen to enter college and prepare herself for a career in teaching. The girl herself wants to use the money her parents have saved for her college education to subsidize a year in New York City, where she could take singing and dancing lessons and begin looking for theatrical work. Noreen's mother is opposed to any change of plans and has insisted that she and Noreen begin to visit nearby colleges with strong teacher education departments.

During her first interview with a college administrator, Noreen began to perspire freely, tremble, and hyperventilate. Her heart beat rapidly and she gasped for air. When she fainted in the college office, an ambulance was summoned, and she was taken to the nearest hospital, with her mother accompanying her. Thirty minutes after arriving at the hospital Noreen was calm and her symptoms had subsided. She was kept under observation for several days, but a medical workup revealed no organic problem. After talking with a number of staff members and disclosing her feelings of being coerced by her mother, Noreen was discharged and referred to a crisis team that functioned as an assessment, treatment, and referral team for individuals without any previous psychiatric history.

ASSESSMENT
Noreen's anxiety attack was interpreted as a response to her mother's insistence that she become a teacher. During the intake interview Noreen was shy and withdrawn except when her musical ambitions were discussed. She described her feelings of becoming another person when she was performing on stage and said that she couldn't bear the thought of giving up her ambition to be a musical comedy star. In assessing Noreen's situation, the crisis team identified her as experiencing a transitional crisis that was aggravated by her unrealistic dreams and by her mother's excessive domination.

Nursing Diagnoses
Coping, ineffectual family: compromised

Anxiety: ranging from severe to panic

Communication, impaired verbal

Knowledge deficit

Multiaxial Psychiatric Diagnoses
Axis I   309.24 Adjustment disorder with anxious
                  mood
          V62.89 Phase of life problem
          V61.20 Parent-child problem

Axis II   None

Axis III None

Axis IV   Code 5—Severe psychosocial stressors

Axis V   Level 3—Slight impairment in social and
          occupational functioning over the last year

PLANNING
In discussing treatment approaches for Noreen, the crisis team identified deficits on the part of both Noreen and her mother. There was no doubt of the mother's commitment to Noreen, but she was unable to accept the fact that her once docile daughter was growing up and wanted more autonomy. At the same time the mother's misgivings about her daughter leaving for New York City to look for theatrical work were realistic. Because mother and daughter were angry and stubborn, communication had broken down. Each saw the other only as a source of frustration and selfishness.

The alternative approaches considered by the crisis team consisted of anxiety-suppressing crisis work or anxiety-provoking crisis work.

IMPLEMENTATION:
ANXIETY-SUPPRESSING APPROACH
It was the opinion of the crisis team that interaction between Noreen and her mother was dysfunctional in several ways. The father was a relatively passive man who left most family decisions to his wife. Noreen knew that her father was opposed to her plan to go to New York City, but she considered him less controlling than her mother. Because the crisis had many family implications, the mental health nurse who assumed responsibility for implementing treatment invited Noreen's parents to two of the eight counseling sessions that had been arranged.

During the meetings attended by all three family members, the nurse tried to facilitate communication among them. Noreen's father proved an unexpected catalyst in the interactions. He was able to tell Noreen that he did not disapprove of her desire to become a performer but that he didn't think she should go to New York City without preparation or experience in theatrical arts. Tears came to his eyes as he expressed fears for his daughter's safety if she carried out her plan. With encouragement from the nurse, he was able to ask why the family could not reach a compromise. Turning to his wife, he asked whether she would consider allowing Noreen to enter a college with a strong dance and drama department where she could acquire professional skills. When Noreen's mother realized that her husband and daughter apparently had formed an alliance, she agreed to the plan but stipulated that Noreen should earn a teaching degree as well so that she could teach dance and drama if theatrical success eluded her. Subsequent meetings were devoted to helping Noreen accept the plan that had been negotiated. The nurse supported Noreen in her wish to remove herself from her mother's control but pointed out that the separation process had already begun despite the mother's opposition.

EVALUATION: ANXIETY-SUPPRESSING APPROACH

With Noreen's consent, the entire family was present at the last meeting. This session was devoted to discussing schools to which Noreen had applied and emphasizing the benefits of preparing thoroughly before entering a highly competitive field. Noreen's mother was more or less reconciled to the compromise and even seemed a little proud of Noreen's stubbornness. She told the nurse that perhaps Noreen was more like her mother than she had realized. Noreen's father obviously enjoyed his position as the family member who had resolved the impasse. Jokingly he told his family that the next time they disagreed with each other, he would help them find a compromise without calling in an ambulance and a crisis team.

IMPLEMENTATION: ANXIETY-PROVOKING APPROACH

In adopting this approach the crisis counselor also used a family focus but directed more attention to the unwholesome interactional patterns in the family. Noreen's anxiety attack was interpreted as a means of communicating her feelings to a mother who dominated her and a father who ignored her. Until the episode of the acute anxiety attack, Noreen had been docile and obedient. However, Noreen saw her performance in the school play and the favorable attention it evoked from classmates as proof that she truly belonged on the professional stage, even though she had given no other indication of interest or talent through the years. In the crisis counselor's view, Noreen's statement that she "felt like somebody else" when she was performing indicated that she was dissatisfied with herself as she was. As Noreen described her work in the play, the crisis counselor wondered silently whether the girl's successful performance might have been due to inspired casting. Although Noreen's career goals were ridiculed by her mother, there was a lack of realism in the girl's dreams for the future. It was the opinion of the counselor that the impasse over the direction that Noreen's life should take was not the only

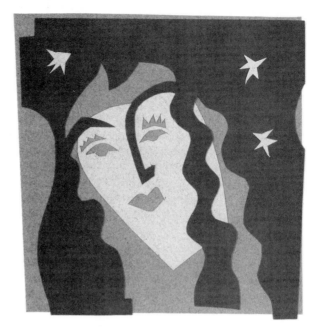

issue—that it was symptomatic of a parent-child relationship that was dysfunctional for everyone concerned.

The crisis counselor and Noreen established a contract for eight sessions, after which renegotiation for additional meetings would take place. The parents were invited to the first session, and with Noreen's collaboration the following goals were formulated:

1. Explore the possibility that Noreen's ambition for a theatrical career is an indication of an adolescent identity crisis.

2. Examine Noreen's reasons for believing she will become a successful performer without acquiring training or experience.

3. Support Noreen's right to express major input concerning her choice of a career.

4. Identify the intrusiveness of Noreen's mother and the indifference of her father, both of which increase her resistance to the legitimate concerns of her parents.

5. Suggest career counseling for Noreen to discover whether her ambitions and her aptitudes are compatible.

6. Discuss with Noreen the fact that other forms of recognition and fulfillment are available even if theatrical success eludes her.

By the end of the sessions there was no definite closure on Noreen's immediate career options, but a number of options had been explored. One option was for Noreen to apply for admission to a professional school in New York City. Another option was for her to enter a college where she could earn a teaching degree in addition to acquiring skills in drama and dance.

As a result of crisis counseling, Noreen became aware that the peer approval she had received through her work in the play was very precious to her. Until the play she had been so retiring that few people noticed her; therefore, she came to believe that the only way to obtain attention was to become a professional performer. The crisis counselor encouraged Noreen to be more assertive and outgoing if she wished to have more friends. Even though conflict continued between Noreen and her mother, it was seen as the result of Noreen's honest but inept efforts to be more autonomous. Noreen's parents were invited to the last session, at which Noreen's mother, rather than being labeled an overbearing tyrant, was accepted as an intense but worried parent who feared for the safety of her cherished daughter. The crisis counselor suggested that the choice of a vocation belonged to Noreen but that the decision-making process should not exclude the parents. In the last session the counselor spent some time reviewing the developmental tasks of adolescents and invited the parents to support Noreen in her struggle to discover who and what she was.

EVALUATION: ANXIETY-PROVOKING APPROACH

Because this approach produced heightened anxiety, it was decided that Noreen should continue seeing the crisis counselor while aptitude tests were being arranged. Noreen was referred to a social learning group made up of young people near her own age with similar interpersonal problems. She was anxious about joining the group but was encouraged by the crisis counselor, who wanted Noreen to face the future with new allies, more confidence, and better coping skills. By the time of termination Noreen and her parents had begun to talk more calmly and to listen to one another. There was no recurrence of anxiety attack. At Noreen's insistence she began visiting colleges and institutions unaccompanied by her mother, although she did discuss with her parents the advantages and disadvantages the colleges offered. Noreen's controversial plan to leave for New York City immediately after high school graduation had been put aside for the moment.

456

anxiety. Reduction of anxiety and subjective distress is the initial goal of crisis intervention, even if a decision is ultimately made to refer the client for exploratory psychotherapy. At this point the generalist nurse should indicate to the client the need for help from other practitioners qualified to offer more intensive forms of psychotherapy.

Review Questions

1. In sequential order, list the progression that leads to the disorganization and disequilibrium of crisis.

2. Crisis represents both danger and opportunity. What is meant by this statement?

3. What are the major differences between an emergency and a crisis?

4. What forms of distortion are present in a crisis? How might the nurse deal with these distortions?

5. What selection criteria are used to determine whether a client is a suitable candidate for an anxiety-provoking approach?

6. What distinctions did Baldwin use to formulate a typology of crises?

7. Give a brief example of a transitional crisis, using Baldwin's typology.

8. What crises listed by Baldwin are appropriate for intervention by a generalist nurse? Give an example of a crisis situation in which a generalist nurse might utilize the nursing process.

9. Define the term *burnout* as a professional risk for nurses.

10. Describe two possible methods of dealing with burnout experienced by nursing staff.

References

Adler, A. 1954. *Understanding Human Nature*. Greenwich, Conn.: Fawcett.

Adler, A. 1969. *The Science of Living*. New York: Doubleday.

Baldwin, B. A. 1978. A Paradigm for the Classification of Emotional Crises: Implications for Crisis Intervention. *American Journal of Orthopsychiatry*, 48:538–551.

Caplan, G. 1964. *Principles of Preventive Psychiatry*. New York: Basic Books.

Caplan, G. 1974. *Support Systems and Community Mental Health*. New York: Behavioral Science Press.

Cassel, J. 1979. Psychosocial Processes and Stress: Theoretical Formulations. In *Stress and Survival*, ed. C. E. Garfield. St. Louis: C. V. Mosby.

Chenevert, M. 1978. *Special Techniques in Assertiveness Training*. St. Louis: C. V. Mosby.

deChesnay, M. 1983. Problem Solving in Nursing. *Image*, 15(1):8–11.

Dubos, R. 1959. *Mirage of Health*. New York: Harper & Row.

Engel, G. 1964. Grief and Grieving. *American Journal of Nursing*, 64:93–96.

Fell, J. 1977. Grief Reactions in the Elderly following Death of a Spouse: The Role of Crisis Intervention and Nursing. *Journal of Gerontological Nursing*, 3(6):17–20.

Forsyth, D. M., and Cannady, J. 1981. Preventing and Alleviating Staff Burnout Through a Group. *Journal of Psychosocial Nursing and Health Services*, 19(9):35–38.

Freud, S. 1936. *Problems of Anxiety*. New York: W. W. Norton.

Garfield, C. A. ed. 1979. *Stress and Survival: The Emotional Realities of Life-Threatening Illness*. St. Louis: C. V. Mosby.

Glazer, G. 1981. The Good Patient. *Nursing and Health Care*, 2:144–146.

Haack, M., and Jones, J. W. 1983. Diagnosing Burnout Using Projective Drawings. *Journal of Psychosocial Nursing and Mental Health Services*, 21(7):8–16.

Janosik, E. H., ed. 1984. *Crisis Counseling: A Contemporary Approach*. Monterey, Calif.: Wadsworth.

Joel, L. A., and Collins, D. I. 1978. *Psychiatric Nursing: Theory and Application*. New York: McGraw-Hill.

Lindemann, E. 1944. Symptomatology and Management of Acute Grief. *American Journal of Psychiatry*, 101: 141–148.

Lindy, J. D.; Grace, M. C.; and Green, B. L. 1981. Survivors: Outreach to a Reluctant Population. *American Journal of Orthopsychiatry*, 51:468–478.

Loomis, M. E., and Wood, D. J. 1983. Cure: The Potential Outcome of Nursing Care. *Image*, 15(1):4–7.

Meichenbaum, D., 1977. A Self-Instructional Approach to Stress Management. In *Stress and Anxiety*, vol. 2, eds. C. Speilberger and I. Saranson. New York: John Wiley & Sons.

Morgan, A. J., and Moreno, J. W. 1973. *The Practice of Mental Health Nursing: A Community Approach*. Philadelphia: J. B. Lippincott.

Parad, H. J., and Resnik, H. L. P. The Practice of Crisis Intervention in Emergency Care. In *Emergency Psychiatric Care and Management of Mental Health Crises*, eds. H. L. P. Resnik, and H. L. Rubin. Bowie, Md.: Charles Slack.

Parker, R., 1978. *Emotional Common Sense*. New York: Harper & Row.

Parks, R. 1977. Parental Reactions to the Birth of a Handicapped Child. *Health and Social Work*, 2(77):52–56.

Peplau, H. E. 1952. *Interpersonal Relations in Nursing*. New York: Putnam.

Peplau, H. E. 1982. Some Reflections on the Earlier Days of Psychiatric Nursing. *Journal of Psychosocial Nursing and Mental Health Services*, 20(8):17–23.

Pines, A. M., and Kanner, A. D. 1982. Nurse Burnout: Lack of Positive Conditions and Presence of Negative Conditions as Two Independent Sources of Stress. *Journal of Psychosocial Nursing and Mental Health Services*, 20(8):30–35.

Searl, S. 1978. Stages of Parental Reaction: Mainstreaming. *The Exceptional Parent*, (April):23–27.

Shubin, S. 1978. Burnout: The Professional Hazard You Face in Nursing. *American Journal of Nursing*, 78 (1):22–27.

Sifneos, P. E. 1967. Two Different Kinds of Psychotherapy of Short Duration. *American Journal of Psychiatry*, 123:1069–1074.

Sifneos, P. E. 1972. *Short-Term Psychotherapy and Emotional Crises*. Cambridge, Mass.: Harvard University.

Sifneos, P. E. 1980. Brief Psychotherapy and Crisis Intervention. In *Comprehensive Textbook of Psychiatry*, 3rd ed., eds. H. I. Kaplan, A. M. Freedman, and B. J. Sadock. Baltimore: Williams & Wilkins.

Smith, D. W. 1979. Survivors of Serious Illness. *American Journal of Nursing*, 79:441–445.

Sullivan, H. S. 1953. *The Interpersonal Theory of Psychiatry*. New York: W. W. Norton.

Supplementary Readings

Barnhill, L. R., and Longo, D. Fixation and Regression in the Family Life Cycle. *Family Process*, 17(1978): 469–478.

Bellak, L., and Small, L. *Emergency Psychotherapy and Brief Psychotherapy*. New York: Grune & Stratton, 1978.

Borrel, L. M. Crisis Intervention: Partnership in Problem Solving. *Nursing Clinics of North America*, 9(1974):5–17.

Chamberlin, H. The Psychological Aftermath of Disaster. *Journal of Clinical Psychology*, 41(1980):238–243.

Chansky, E. R. Reducing Patient's Anxieties: Techniques for Dealing with Crises. *AORN Journal*, 40(1984): 375–377.

Finkleman, L. The Nurse Therapist: Outpatient Crisis Intervention with the Chronic Psychiatric Patient. *Journal of Psychiatric Nursing and Mental Health Services*, 15(1977):27–32.

Fitzpatrick, J. J. Stress in the Crisis Experience: Nursing Interventions. *Occupational Health Nursing*, 28(1980): 19–21.

Goldstein, D. Crisis Intervention: A Brief Therapy Model. *Nursing Clinics of North America*, 13(1978): 657–663.

Hall, J. C., and Weaver, B. R. *Nursing of Families in Crisis*. Philadelphia: J. B. Lippincott, 1974.

Hansell, N. *The Person in Distress*. New York: Human Services Press, 1976.

Harrison, D. F. Nurses and Disaster. *Journal of Psychosocial Nursing*, 19(1981):34–36.

Hatch, C., and Schert, L. Description of a Crisis-Oriented Psychiatric Home Visiting Service. *Journal of Psychiatric Nursing and Mental Health Services*, 18(1980):31–34.

Hiff, L. A. *People in Crisis: Understanding and Helping*. Menlo Park, Calif.: Addison-Wesley, 1978.

Johnson, R. *Using Crisis Intervention Wisely*. Horsham, Pa.: International Communications, 1982.

Krouse, H. J. Cancer as Crisis: The Critical Elements of Adjustment. *Nursing Research*, 31(1982):96–101.

McGee, R. K. *Crisis Intervention in the Community*. Baltimore: University Park Press, 1974.

Polk, G. C. Crisis Theory: Application and Utilization with Hemodyalysis Patients and Families. *Nephrology Nursing*, 4(1982):8–10.

Sifneos, P. E. *Short-Term Dynamic Psychotherapy: Evaluation and Technique*. New York: Plenum, 1979.

Walker, P. Community Homes as Hospital Alternatives for Youth in Crisis. *Journal of Psychiatric Nursing*, 19(1981):17–19.

Warner, C. G. Conflict Intervention for Victims of Human Violence. *Topics in Emergency Medicine*, 3 (1982):77–83.

BEHAVIOR MODIFICATION
The Scientific Method in Psychology
Classical Conditioning
Operant Conditioning
Learning Theorists

BEHAVIOR MODIFICATION TECHNIQUES
Systematic Desensitization
Aversion Techniques
Operant Techniques

BASIC GUIDELINES FOR THE USE OF
BEHAVIOR MODIFICATION

LIMITATIONS OF BEHAVIOR THERAPY

C H A P T E R

17

Behavioral Theory and Practice

Learning Objectives

After reading this chapter, the student should be able to:

1. Describe the contributions of the major behavioral therapists.

2. Integrate concepts of behavior modification into the nursing process.

3. Formulate appropriate assessment and intervention strategies for use with behavior modification.

4. Discuss the implications of providing behavior therapy for clients.

460

Overview

Regardless of philosophical orientation, the ultimate goal of all therapeutic approaches is to introduce functional change. The client has, over the course of time, developed some undesirable ways of dealing with internal and external stress. Therapy is aimed at helping the client find more desirable strategies to take their place. Unlike some other psychotherapeutic approaches, behavior modification, or behavioral therapy, does not concern itself with the causes of undesirable behaviors but rather with the behaviors themselves.

The behavioral therapist concentrates exclusively on helping clients unlearn troublesome behaviors and learn new, more adaptive ones. This chapter will help the student learn to understand the ways in which a problem may be conceptualized behaviorally and to apply techniques that may be used to change behavior. This chapter also covers behavioristic terminology and the philosophies that have contributed to modern behavioral therapy.

There is nothing more difficult to take in hand, more
perilous to conduct or more uncertain in its success than
to take the lead in a new order of things.
NICOLO MACHIAVELLI

461

How do individuals develop ineffective strategies for dealing with stress? What is necessary to change these strategies? These are questions around which all psychotherapeutic approaches have arisen. For example, Freud's psychoanalytic theory proposes that unconscious conflicts, usually of a sexual or aggressive nature, are at the core of an individual's psychological problems. Using techniques such as free association, interpretation, and analysis of the transference neurosis, the psychoanalyst can probe the client's unconscious mind to bring the conflict into conscious awareness, where the individual can begin to deal with it. Once the client is aware of unmet sexual or aggressive needs, he or she can endeavor to meet those needs in socially acceptable ways. The basic objective in psychoanalytic therapy is to help clients develop new behaviors that begin to meet their needs, rather than frustrate them.

Carl Rogers's client-centered therapy is based on the idea that it is normal for people to grow, to actualize their potential, to evolve into the fullness of their being. Unfortunately, individuals often encounter obstacles along the way and misperceive their needs and direction in life, which hinders their growth. In client-centered therapy, the therapist assists the client in discovering the obstacles to growth and removing them so that the self-actualization process may continue. The therapist does this by creating an atmosphere of total acceptance so that the client may feel free to explore any aspect of her personality without fear of rejection. This attitude of therapeutic acceptance is called *unconditional positive regard*. By trying to identify with the client during the exploration, the therapist can

help the client clarify her needs and feelings. Facilitating self-actualization thus also produces behavioral change.

Behavior modification, or *behavioral therapy*, does not concern itself with unconscious conflicts, obstacles to self-actualization, or other subjective inferential concepts. Its central concern is simply "with human behavior and learned changes in behavior" (Franks, 1969). According to this school of thought, all behavior, both appropriate and inappropriate, is *learned*. The behavior modifier, armed with principles of learning that have been observed, replicated, and validated under controlled experimental conditions, helps clients unlearn troublesome behaviors and learn new, more adaptive behaviors in their place.

This represents quite a deviation from other therapeutic approaches. The *content* of what a client has learned previously is of little or no importance to the behavioral therapist. For instance, if Mr. Jones has a fear of flying, the therapist seeks no symbolic meaning for his distress, looks for no issues of self-doubt, sexual inadequacy, or death wish in devising a treatment plan. Rather it is the *process* of learning that is central to the resolution of the problem. In Mr. Jones's case, the inappropriate behavior is considered to be an avoidance response to a stimulus. The essential questions to be answered are: What principles of learning are keeping Mr. Jones's ineffective behavior entrenched? What principles and techniques must be used to bring about the desired behavior change? Behavioral therapy is a direct attack upon symptoms because it is the symptoms that are seen as the problem.

The nice thing about behavior modification, besides the fact that it works so well, is that anyone can learn to use it, with only a moderate amount of training. Moreover, you can use behavior modification on yourself in order to promote greater self-control. If you stop to think about it, self-control—or actually, a lack of it—underlies many of the personal problems that we struggle with in everyday life. Problems such as losing weight, increasing studying, decreasing drinking or drug use, giving up smoking and diminishing anxiety can be tackled very effectively with behavior modification techniques.

WAYNE WEITEN (1983)

462

BEHAVIOR MODIFICATION

The principles of behavior modification have been derived from careful observations and have been validated by experimental data. Although scientific methods have been applied to the study of behavior since the nineteenth century, the most influential studies were done early in this century by Ivan Pavlov, the Russian physiologist, and B. F. Skinner, the American psychologist. Their two models of conditioned learning, *classical conditioning* and *operant conditioning*, respectively, form the basis upon which the modern school of behaviorism rests.

The Scientific Method in Psychology

Explanations for why humans behave the ways they do have been sought for centuries. What does it mean to be human? What is the nature of human existence? Why do individuals act the way they do? These and other questions have been asked by many of the great thinkers of history, and one aspect of modern day psychology remains firmly rooted in this philosophical tradition. Unmeasurable concepts such as the nature of the mind, consciousness, and emotions have been argued, debated, and their ramifications explored.

The other aspect of psychology is an offshoot of a much different tradition, namely, physiology. Physiology is the science concerned with the life processes, activities, and functions within the body. Objects of study in physiology include the brain, physiological responses, and *measurable* behaviors, not abstract constructs such as "consciousness" and "mind." In most scientific endeavors, objectively measurable data are the only kind of data considered relevant, and the experimental method is the only method considered acceptable for testing the validity of a hypothesis. Working from facts and observable phenomena, scientists develop theories and larger concepts, which they test by further observations or experiments. This scientific process of working from observable phenomena toward theories is called *inductive reasoning*.

In summary, the discipline of psychology encompasses both the philosophical questions that have arisen over the nature of man, mind, and consciousness and the scientific method of exploration from physiology.

The hallmarks of the *scientific method* are observation and experimentation, which is the controlled manipulation of one variable (the independent variable) in order to observe (measure) its effect on another variable (the dependent variable).

How this method varies from the more philosophical approaches to answering questions might be best demonstrated by looking at the ways in which the philosophical and scientific schools might examine the old myth that handling toads causes warts. A casual observer may be aware that toads appear to have warts. He may have heard the myth that touching toads causes warts, and, indeed he may even know someone with warts who has had some contact with toads. Based on what the observer has been told and seen, it is reasonable for him to deduce that touching toads and contracting warts are related. This deductive method is similar to that used by the philosophical school.

On the other hand, a scientist faced with such a question will try to draw his conclusions from observations and results based on the scientific method. Trying to hold all independent variables

Almost all our major problems involve human behavior, and they cannot be solved by physical and biological technology alone. What is needed is a technology of behavior, but we have been slow to develop the science from which a technology might be drawn. One difficulty is that almost all of what is called behavioral science continues to trace behavior to states of mind, feelings, traits of character, human nature and so on. Physics and biology once followed similar practices and advanced only when they discarded them . . . The environment is obviously important, but its role has remained obscure. It does not push or pull, it selects, *and this function is difficult to discover and analyze.*

B. F. SKINNER (1972)

constant except one (contact or no contact with toads), the scientist will let the examination of the dependent variable (presence or no presence of warts) speak for itself. For example, assembling a group of volunteers, the scientist will randomly assign them to one of two groups. Each subject in Group 1 (the experimental group) will be asked to hold a toad in both hands for a certain period of time. Each subject in Group 2 (the control group) will be given a bumpy rock to hold for a comparable time period. Subjects are then sent home and called back for examination of their hands in a specified period of time. If the experimental group has significantly more warts than the controls, then it is logical to induce from the data that toads and warts are related. If no difference exists, the hypothesis is at least weakened, if not totally disproven. If the controls were to have more warts than the experimental group, the scientist would induce from the data a connection between bumpy rocks and warts, even though logically this makes no sense.

Psychology as a science was officially born in 1879, when Wilhelm Wundt (1832–1920) founded the first psychology laboratory in Leipzig, Germany. Wundt attempted to systematize psychology in order to make it a bona fide science. Wundt's early work explored the functioning of the senses. His subjects were often asked to introspect and then to put their experiences and sensations into words. Although critics would argue that introspection is hardly an objective scientific measure, Wundt's contribution was his emphasis on objective and quantifiable data, which began to move psychology from pure philosophy to an emerging science. However, psychology remained a rather subjective and introspective science for a long time.

In 1913, John Watson (1887–1958) introduced *behaviorism*, a new branch of psychology. Like Wundt, Watson wanted psychology to become an objective science. He believed that observable behavior, not "consciousness" or the other vague concepts that preoccupied the philosophers, was the true domain of psychology. Watson's goal was to predict and control behavior, not to speculate about unmeasurable mental states. He moved psychology from an introspective to an objective science. Watson believed that behavior could be described in terms of observable stimuli and responses. If the behavior could not be measured or recorded, then for all intents and purposes it did not exist. A term such as "emotion" was of little scientific use unless certain measurable physiological changes were considered to be indices of that emotion.

Classical Conditioning

Even before the principles of behaviorism were widely known or accepted, data concerning how learning occurs and how behavioral change takes place were being collected in Russia. Ivan Pavlov (1849–1936) was a Russian professor of physiology originally interested in doing research on digestion and the automatic reflexes associated with it, including the salivation response. However, chance observations in the course of this research sent him on a new track of study, and he ultimately demonstrated and introduced a model of learning that has come to be known as *classical conditioning*.

It was in 1904 that Pavlov noticed that a dog being used in digestion experiments began to salivate not only when food was in its mouth but also at the very sight of food. Salivation when eating is a reflexive, unlearned response, so Pavlov called it an

Figure 17-1. Pavlov's classical conditioning paradigm.

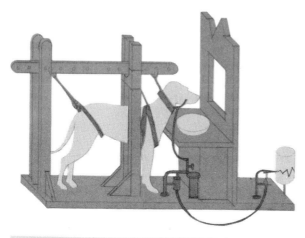

464

Before conditioning

CS (tone) → No response or irrelevant response

US (food) → UR (salivation)

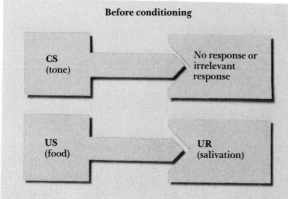

During conditioning

CS (tone)

US (food) → UR (salivation)

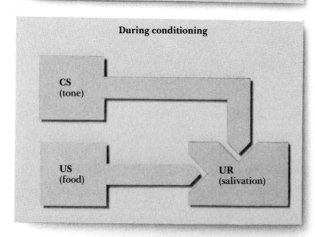

After conditioning

CS (tone) → CR (salivation)

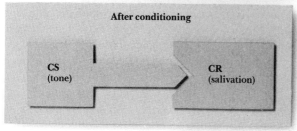

unconditioned response (UCR). But salivation at the mere sight of food was a new, learned response, which Pavlov named a *conditioned response* (CR).

Pavlov went on to explore and examine how this conditioned response might have been learned. In his experiments, the dog was securely strapped in place. A bowl into which meat powder was automatically dispensed was placed in front of the dog. The dog's salivary gland was connected to a device that measured salivary flow.

At the start of the experiment, a neutral stimulus, such as a tone from a tuning fork, was presented to the dog. The stimulus had no previous control over or association with food. Then several trials were made in which the tone was quickly followed by the presentation of food. As the dog ate, its natural salivation response was recorded.

The procedure was then changed again. This time the tone was presented, but without food. Pavlov found that the dog salivated in response to the tone, even in the absence of food. A new association had been made between a neutral stimulus (the tone) and an old response (salivation). In short, Pavlov demonstrated one way that *learning* (stimulus-response links) can take place. He showed that when a neutral stimulus is repeatedly paired with another stimulus (unconditioned stimulus, UCS) that already elicits a given response (unconditioned response, UCR), the neutral stimulus (conditioned stimulus, CS) will become connected with that response (now termed the conditioned response, CR) and become capable of eliciting the response on its own. This model of learning, called classical conditioning, is diagrammed in Figure 17-1.

Using variations of this basic experiment, Pavlov made some fundamental behavioral discoveries.

The learning theorist John B. Watson was a radical in his own time. He was the person who proclaimed that he could take a dozen healthy infants and train them to be whatever he chose—doctor, lawyer, beggar, and so on—regardless of their backgrounds or ancestry. This statement alone was sufficient to raise more than a few eyebrows. Watson also believed that the psychologists of his day were wasting their time studying subjective, "mentalistic" concepts such as sensation, volition, and emotion. On many occasions he argued that subjective, nonobservable phenonema are best left to philosophy; surely they have no place in a science *of psychology.*

DAVID R. SHAFFER (1985)

Each pairing of the CS and UCS was called a *trial*; and, generally speaking, the more trials, the stronger the association. The recorded weakening of the new CS–CR bond when the tone was no longer followed by food demonstrated a process called *extinction*. But even after the CR was extinguished, Pavlov found that, days later, a rested animal again presented only with the tone would begin to salivate. This recurrence of the CR after extinction is referred to as *spontaneous recovery*. Initially, the animal might respond to any tone, no matter what the pitch. This responding to any and all similar stimuli is called *stimulus generalization*. By hearing different pitched tones, an animal could learn, under proper training, that only one tone would be followed by food, and would learn to salivate to only that tone. This ability to distinguish between stimuli is called *stimulus discrimination*.

Operant Conditioning

Classical conditioning is helpful in explaining how an existing response (such as salivation) can come under the control of a new stimulus (such as a tone), but it tells us nothing about how new behaviors or habits are learned. For example, what unconditioned stimulus is needed to induce a rat to run a maze? Or to teach a bear to ride a motorcycle in the circus? Whereas Pavlov's paradigm occurred with a passive subject (the dog) from which an involuntary autonomic nervous system response was obtained, most actions in life involve an active organism emitting voluntary responses (without any identifiable controlling stimulus) that are followed by consequences. The process of learning brought about by a reinforcing stimulus or consequence following a response is called *operant conditioning*.

Edward R. Thorndike's (1911) *law of effect* was the starting point for B. F. Skinner's development of operant conditioning. The law of effect states that behavior is a function of its consequences. *Reinforcement* is any stimulus that increases the probability of the recurrence of a response that it follows. A *positive reinforcer* is any stimulus that, by its *presence*, increases the probability of the recurrence of a response. A *negative reinforcer* is anything that, by its *absence*, increases the probability of the recurrence of a response. Giving a child a piece of cake (positive reinforcer) for finishing dinner increases the probability of his finishing dinner the next time. If Mr. Smith stays home, his wife nags him. If he goes out, he escapes the nagging. Therefore, his "going out" behavior is strengthened by the absence of the nagging (a negative reinforcer).

Some inherently desirable stimuli are naturally reinforcing and do not have to be learned. Such *primary reinforcers* include food, water, and sex. Other stimuli are not in themselves reinforcing but have become learned reinforcers for us. Money has no natural inherent reinforcing value, but it can buy things that have reinforcing value. Therefore, money is a learned, or *secondary reinforcer*.

To help control stimulus-response contingencies, Skinner devised an experimental "box" that has come to be associated with his name. The *Skinner box* is a small animal cage with a lever or pecking disk on the inside that, when depressed by the animal, dispenses food. The Skinner box creates an easily measured dependent variable that is usually automatically recorded: the number of presses. The box is usually equipped with a small light located close to the lever or disk. Independent variables that can be manipulated by the experimenter might include the type of food (reinforcer), the time interval between pressing and the dispensing of the food, the hours of food deprivation in the animal before the trial, the type of animal, or the schedule of reinforcement (the interval or number of responses preceding reinforcement). In a typical operant conditioning experiment, the experimenter waits for the desired behavior to occur spontaneously, immediately after which the animal receives reinforcement. After this procedure is repeated many times, the frequency of the recurrence of the desired behavior will have significantly increased over its preexperiment base rate.

SHAPING An important behavioral concept demonstrated in Skinner's work is *response discrimination*, more popularly known as *shaping*. If a rat is placed in a Skinner box, some time may elapse before the rat presses the bar and is rewarded. The experimenter may choose to save some time and "shape" the rat's behavior by trying to break down the lever-pressing behavior into its component parts and reinforcing successive approximations that resemble the desired behavior. For example, if the experimenter wishes to have a rat press a lever with its left front paw only when a red light is on, he may first reward any movement that the rat makes *toward* the bar. As the rat begins to spend more time near the bar, the animal may next be rewarded if it stops *in front of* the bar. The next step might reward the rat when it accidentally hits the bar with any leg. When the rat begins to hit the bar in many different ways, it is rewarded each time. Then the experimenter may decide only to reinforce the rat for pressing the bar with its front paws. Once that response is established, the experimenter may decide to reinforce only *left paw* pushes. Finally, left paw pushes might be rewarded only *when the red signal light above the bar is lit*. A great deal of learning has taken place—complex learning that could not have occurred within the context of a classical conditioning model.

MODELS The establishment and maintenance of connections between stimuli and responses can be made in several different ways depending on how reinforcers are dispensed (Ferster and Skinner, 1957). These various methods, or models, can help one analyze a given situation and thus can have therapeutic implications. The simplest is the *reward model*, whose goal is to strengthen behavior. For the rat in the Skinner box, the lever-pressing response is followed by the presentation of a reward, food, which makes the rat more likely to press the lever in the future. The child who finishes his dinner to receive his cake is another example of the reward model.

A second model aimed at strengthening be-

BEHAVIORAL TERMINOLOGY

- *Stimulus.* An internal or external event.
- *Response.* An internal or external reaction to stimulus.
- *Unconditioned response.* A reflexive, unlearned response.
- *Conditioned response.* A learned response.
- *Conditioned stimulus.* An internal or external event that is the result of learning.
- *Extinction.* The abolition of a given behavior.
- *Spontaneous recovery.* The recurrence of a response after it has been extinguished.
- *Stimulus generalization.* The same response to similar stimuli.
- *Discrimination.* The ability to distinguish among stimuli.
- *Positive reinforcer.* A stimulus whose presence increases the probability of the recurrence of a behavior.
- *Negative reinforcer.* A stimulus who absence increases the probability of the recurrence of a behavior.
- *Primary reinforcer.* An unlearned, naturally occurring reinforcer.
- *Punishment.* An undesirable reinforcement given to suppress a behavior.

havior employs a negative reinforcer. If a rat is placed in a Skinner box where the floor is electrified, and if, when the rat presses the lever, the shock stops, then the termination of the shock is said to be a negative reinforcer. A model that uses a negative reinforcer is called an *escape model*. The husband who avoids the company of his nagging wife is another example of the escape model.

A third model of operant conditioning is the *avoidance model*, in which a response by the organism can prevent the presentation of a negative event. For example, a rat that is given 10 seconds to press a lever and prevent 30 seconds of shock will quickly learn to push that lever. A diabetic who takes insulin is also demonstrating a learned avoidance behavior.

A fourth model is *punishment*, in which the goal is not to strengthen a response but to suppress one already in existence. If a rat that seems to enjoy exercising in its running wheel is shocked every time it enters the wheel, the rat will eventually be less likely to enter it. For the behavioral therapist, the punishment paradigm is generally the last resort considered in trying to change a behavior. Aside from being unpleasant for the client, the procedure has certain drawbacks: The behavior is only suppressed, not extinguished, and often it is only suppressed in the presence of the punishing agent. Too severe a punishment can create a need for revenge on the part of the recipient. These are two important aspects of punishment of which every parent should be aware.

Learning Theorists

Although the decades of the 1920s and 1930s were characterized by extensive behavioral research, there was little direct application of behavioral techniques to clinical practice. Freud's theories of personality and psychoanalytic psychotherapy were the dominant models of the day. Then, in the 1940s, John Dollard, a sociologist, and Neil Miller, a psychologist, made the first serious attempt to integrate the work being done in the laboratory by the behaviorists with the psychoanalytic applications being used by many clinicians (Miller and Bugelski, 1948). Miller and Dollard tried to translate psychoanalytic theory into learning theory terms. Unlike the psychoanalysts who attend to internal conflicts while ignoring environmental influences, Miller and Dollard saw the need to look at influences both outside and within an organism to explain its behavior. Movement from one conceptual framework toward another may sound like a mere exercise in semantics, but, in this context, it served an important function. Freudian theory is based on concepts that are difficult to measure. Translating those concepts into operational definitions made them measurable. Familiar hypotheses could be evaluated in the light of test data, and new ideas could be explored. Psychoanalysis provided the concepts; learning theory provided the means to test them. For example, conflict could be examined and explained in terms of the strength or weakness of approach responses and avoidance responses to a given stimulus. With the vital link between learning theory and clinical practice established, behavior modification techniques began to emerge.

BEHAVIOR MODIFICATION TECHNIQUES

Arnold Lazarus (1967), a behavioral researcher and therapist, has promoted what he terms a "broad spectrum" behavioral approach to therapy. This broad spectrum is an eclectic and pragmatic approach to helping people change their behaviors with whatever means produces the desired result. Concepts such as insight, rapport, and interpreta-

tion are important in certain situations, and they should not be excluded simply because they do not fit neatly into a behavioral paradigm. But the broad spectrum behavioral therapist has access to a broad repertoire of clinical tools that includes behavioral techniques in addition to traditional techniques.

The behavioral point of view itself can be a useful tool in assessing a person's problems. Sometimes a client can overwhelm a caregiver with difficulties, and no behavior modification technique appears to be immediately appropriate or applicable. How can a therapist begin to understand the problems, let alone select a treatment technique? If the therapist thinks in terms of maladaptive learned responses, the reinforcers that are holding them in place, and the appropriate behaviors that could take the place of the inappropriate ones, then a useful framework is available to conceptualize the problem. Frequently, therapeutic strategies (behavioral or otherwise) will become apparent from such an analysis.

With the behavioral perspective in mind, it becomes possible to understand and explain three major types of behavior modification: systematic desensitization (counter-conditioning), aversion therapy, and general operant procedures.

Systematic Desensitization

In the 1950s, Joseph Wolpe devised a technique specifically for treating what may be the most common neurotic symptom: *maladaptive anxiety*, in which an inappropriate connection has been learned between a stimulus and anxiety. The therapist's task is to break that connection. One possibility is extinction; that is, helping the client face the anxiety-producing stimulus. If no terrible consequence were to follow, the anxiety response would weaken and eventually disappear. Although extinction paradigms might work on people with low to moderate levels of anxiety, a person troubled enough to seek therapy is unlikely to stay in the presence of a feared object long enough for extinction to occur.

Wolpe (1958) believed the way to treat such a conditioned fear is through *counter-conditioning*, or associating a new, antagonistic response to take the place of the anxiety response (see Figure 17-2). This new response would inhibit the anxiety response (the principle of *reciprocal inhibition*) and weaken it. Counter-conditioning has the added benefit of reducing the client's avoidance behaviors toward the feared object. It increases the likelihood of her coming into contact with the object without negative consequences and thus facilitates extinction.

Wolpe adopted Jacobson's (1938) deep muscle relaxation procedure because he believed the relaxation response is incompatible with anxiety. By having a client systematically tighten and loosen the

Figure 17-2. In counter-conditioning, a fear response to a stimulus is replaced with a relaxation response.

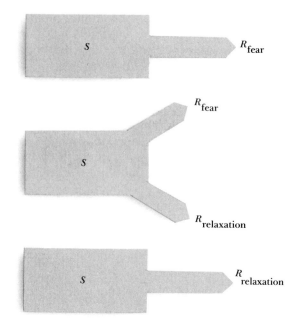

468

various muscle groups in his body, the physiological and muscular components of anxiety could be decreased. Wolpe found that after a couple of weeks of practice, a client became capable of relaxing deeply in a very short period of time. Wolpe found that other counter-conditioning responses could be used as well. For example, a young retarded woman who had difficulty learning the relaxation response was scheduled for therapy at noon and was asked to bring her favorite lunch to the session. Food was used as a primary reinforcer. The therapist had her think of anxiety-arousing situations while she was experiencing the pleasant sensations associated with eating.

In vivo desensitization is possible (using the feared object itself as the stimulus during treatment), but it can be difficult to control and is often overwhelming for the client. Therefore, Wolpe asked his clients to imagine scenes involving the feared object and to arrange these scenes from the least anxiety provoking to the most (in a *hierarchy* of anxiety). An important behavioral rationale is at work here. Attacking the most feared scene first would be impossible, but starting with a low-anxiety scene increases the chances of the strong relaxation response replacing the anxiety. Working up the ladder step by step is a form of shaping. Success at the lower levels of the hierarchy tends to generalize, making success at the higher levels more likely.

Once the client has acquired the learned relaxation response and has described the hierarchy, the desensitization procedure begins. The client is asked to relax and is given a few minutes to do so. The first item from the hierarchy is read, and the client is asked to imagine the scene and to signal the therapist when she begins to feel anxious. At that

point, the client is told to wipe the scene from her mind and to take a minute or so to get relaxed again. The same item is presented until two trials can occur (perhaps 60 seconds and 90 seconds, although timing is optional) without the client signaling that the scene is producing anxiety. At this point, the therapist moves on to the next item of the hierarchy, repeats the procedure for two successive successful trials, and then continues up the ladder until the hierarchy is completed.

The extinction paradigm for anxiety, or *implosion therapy,* is a technique by which the client is graphically talked through his hierarchy of anxiety-provoking stimuli, literally bombarded with scenes involving the feared object (Stampfl and Lewis, 1967). As the client relives the anxiety-producing scenes in his imagination, the therapist attempts to extinguish the future influence of the material over the client's behavior and feelings and to replace previous avoidance responses with more appropriate responses. Implosion presents more risk and discomfort to the client than does desensitization, especially when severe anxiety is present, but it may be quicker than systematic desensitization and a quite effective method for mild or moderate anxieties. It should not be used with clients who have a history of depression or attempted by a therapist inexperienced with the technique.

Aversion Techniques

The goal of *aversion therapy* is to suppress an undesirable response by using escape-avoidance paradigms to train the client in a new response. It is used most commonly to treat problems such as alcoholism and sexual deviance—behaviors the client finds undesirable but, at the same time, reinforcing. The alcoholic with three DWIs (driving while intoxicated) who has lost his job and family may see the destructiveness of his behavior, but the immediate gratification that accompanies alcohol is a strong reinforcer for his alcoholic behavior pattern. Likewise, the man with a shoe fetish may be appalled by it, but when the sight of six-inch spiked heels is followed by the primary reinforcement of sexual arousal, the result is a strong habit formation and maintenance.

Aversion therapy may be seen in one of two ways: as an attempt to associate an undesirable behavior pattern with unpleasant stimulation (the classical conditioning model) or as an attempt to establish the expectation of an unpleasant stimulus as a consequence of undesirable behavior (operant conditioning). Drugs, shock, and learned nausea (taught much as relaxation training is taught) are three possible ways of inducing unpleasant stimuli in conjunction with inappropriate behavior.

Overt sensitization is the use of naturally noxious stimuli (such as shock or drugs) to weaken a response. An alcoholic is given an injection of a drug that produces nausea and vomiting. After the injection, she is shown pictures of alcohol as she begins to feel sick and vomits. After she vomits and begins to feel better, the pictures are removed. This classical conditioning paradigm is forming a new association between drinking (a conditioned stimulus) and the nausea and vomiting (the conditioned response).

Disulfiram (Antabuse) is a drug that induces respiratory distress and gastrointestinal response in the person who drinks after taking it. The alcohol is followed not by the usual high but by a very punishing experience. The aim is to weaken the old stimulus-response bond. Unfortunately, most alcoholics are wise enough to stop taking the Antabuse pills a few days before they drink. If they stay on the drug, however, they experience an avoidance paradigm: the "not drinking" response is followed by the prevention of a negative experience and is therefore strengthened. Giving alcoholics a mild electrical shock when they reach for a drink is also an attempt to punish their response to alcohol and weaken it.

Covert sensitization produces an aversion response indirectly with imagery rather than directly with pain or nausea. A man with homosexual tendencies who wishes to be heterosexual in his behavior might use covert sensitization as part of his treatment (Gold and Neufeld, 1965). With training, a person can be taught to produce a mild feeling of nausea in response to undesirable behavior without the aid of chemicals. The advantage of this response is that it is directly under the client's control. The technique can be taken out of the therapy session and into the real world.

With covert sensitization the client would also be taught the relaxation response and be asked to produce a hierarchy. For example, the client could be given a set of pictures showing males in different stages of undress. He would be asked to select ten to fifteen pictures and arrange them in order from least sexually arousing to most. Once the hierarchy is set and the client has mastered the relaxation and nausea responses, the covert sensitization procedure can be begun.

In the case of the homosexual client, he first would be told to get himself relaxed. Then he would be instructed that, upon opening his eyes, he would see the first picture from his hierarchy. He would be told to signal the therapist as soon as he feels sexually attracted to the picture. At that point, the nausea response would be induced for 10 to 15 seconds in the presence of the picture. Then the picture would be withdrawn and the client would be told to take a few seconds to get relaxed again. After he completed two trials without indicating feelings of sexual attraction, the next picture would be shown, and so on, up the hierarchy. Upon conclusion of the procedure, the attraction to males should be weakened by the association of the unpleasant stimulus with the once arousing stimuli.

This procedure would be only *one part* of a total treatment program for such a client. Inquiry might reveal that the man is anxious around females. In that case, desensitization to females might also be in order. A client might also lack appropriate behaviors necessary to interact successfully with women. Failure to interact would punish him for attempting new heterosexual behaviors, and he might revert to his old homosexual patterns. Therefore, role playing and assertion training would be used to help him acquire the new behaviors necessary for success with women.

Another approach might be shaping, or breaking down complex behaviors to smaller components, with appropriate reinforcement at each step to encourage generalization and to make the next step easier. For example, a young man with a history of homosexual inclinations and experiences who wants to be heterosexual might express early in therapy that he would like to test his new inclinations upon completion of therapy by going to a prostitute. Such an encounter would put him at the top of his hierarchy of anxiety-provoking heterosexual interactions (the most anxiety-producing), where his likelihood of success would be the lowest. Instead, he should be taught the smaller steps along the way to intercourse: how to ask a woman out on a date, what to talk about, how to hold hands, and how to kiss her goodnight. Success at each of these levels would be more likely to get him to the top of his hierarchy without major setbacks.

Operant Techniques

Techniques based on principles of reinforcement include *time out* (an extinction paradigm), assertion training (a complex process involving role playing, modeling, feedback, and other social reinforcers), and token economics (a reward paradigm that often produces dramatic results in chronic psychiatric clients).

TIME OUT A good example of how inappropriate behavior is learned and how it can be analyzed behaviorally is a three-year-old's temper tantrum. Suppose Bill, a ten-year-old, has been watching television when his three-year-old brother, Erik, comes in and wants to turn the channel to watch cartoons. Dad is in the kitchen trying to prepare supper and entertain the baby. Suddenly, he hears Erik screaming and kicking. Bill runs into the kitchen and tells Dad that Erik is throwing a tantrum. He tells Bill to go back and watch his program and to ignore his brother.

Fifteen minutes later, Erik is still screaming; Bill is yelling at his brother because he can't hear his show; supper is burning; the baby has joined in the hysteria; and Dad feels a migraine on the way. Finally, out of desperation, he tells Bill to let Erik change the channel. Bill goes off to his room and closes the door; Erik is quiet now that he has gotten his way; the baby settles down; and, finally, there is peace and quiet. What has this experience taught the participants?

1. Erik has found a behavior (or behavior pattern) that works for him. The tantrum was rewarded, so he is more likely to throw a tantrum the next time he desires something.

2. Dad has learned that giving in to the tantrum is followed by a pleasant event: peace and quiet. So he is also more likely to give in when Erik acts up again.

3. Bill learned that telling Dad didn't solve his problem, so next time he may try something else, such as hitting his brother or throwing a tantrum of his own.

A better solution to the tantrum would have been to isolate Erik in another room until he remained silent for a few minutes. This isolation procedure is called "time out," meaning "time out from reinforcement" (Ferster, 1958). What is the reinforcement Erik is being denied by isolation? *Feedback*, for one. Watching Dad, brother, and the baby getting agitated during a tantrum is reinforcing because it is a sign that the behavior is working. During time out he is denied this reinforcement and also the reinforcement of interacting with other people and of moving freely.

Once begun, time out must be followed through to completion. If, after thirty minutes, Erik is still having a tantrum in isolation, and Dad gives in, he will have learned something worse than before: if he keeps a tantrum up long enough, it will eventually work. He must learn that it doesn't *ever* work. Also, the good behavior modifier (in this case, the father) should think in terms of reinforcing *competing* responses. If Erik does *not* cause a scene, this competing behavior should be reinforced with praise or a promise to have his turn watching the TV in a half hour. This kind of positive approach, in conjunction with time out, will be doubly effective.

ASSERTION TRAINING *Assertion training*, or teaching people how to stand up for their rights in ways that do not violate the rights of others, is another operant technique. Unassertive people tend to feel taken advantage of by others. They can't say no when they want to, and they tend to avoid people and potentially conflicting circumstances as a defense. Assertion training is aimed at teaching such persons the behavioral repertoire needed to successfully interact with others.

Assertion training is generally taught in two parts: relaxation training and role playing. For example, if Mary knows exactly how to say no to sex with her boyfriend but is too anxious at the time to get the words out, she may end up doing something she doesn't want to do. Relaxation training alone may be enough to help her control her anxiety (if it is mild or moderate) so that she can assert herself. If her anxiety level is high in such situations, desensitization might be a necessary adjunct to therapy.

Role playing might also be employed in Mary's case. The therapist could act as a high-pressure salesman to whom Mary is trying to say no. If role playing is conducted in a group (as is usually the case), Mary could get *feedback* (social reinforcement) from other members on her performance. She would be encouraged to practice both in the group and outside of it, but in a controlled way, saying no in low-level anxiety situations first and then working her way up to highly anxiety provoking situations with her boyfriend. This shaping procedure increases the likelihood of success, and the generalization effect and history of reinforcements will make each step easier.

TOKEN ECONOMICS *Token economics* are operant programs that have produced dramatic successes with long-term inpatient psychiatric clients (Ayllon and Azrin, 1968). *Tokens* are secondary reinforcers that are given to a client contingent on his performing certain desired behaviors. The tokens can be exchanged for food, snacks, library time, or any other reinforcers. One key to success is finding something that is reinforcing for a given client. One person might do anything for a candy bar; for another, 15 minutes alone might be highly valued. A second factor important to success is total staff cooperation. Each person interacting with the client must understand what the targeted behavior is, what reinforcers are being used, how and when they are being administered, and what the details of the treatment program are. If the goal is to get Mr. Smith to make his bed, a plan must be devised and understood by the whole staff so appropriate and timely reinforcement can be made. The first week, for example, the goal must be set low enough so that Mr. Smith will be reinforced and get a "taste" of success. Aside from leaving his bed unmade, Mr. Smith also throws his pillow around, so the contingency of reinforcement for the first week might be a token every day the morning nurse comes in and finds the pillow anywhere on the bed. After that behavior is occurring consistently, the program changes as the shaping procedure continues: the pillow must be at the head of the bed for Mr. Smith to receive the token. The next step might be to have Mr. Smith pull up the sheet and blanket, and so on. As each step becomes more demanding, manipulations can also be made with the tokens: more or less can be given at each occasion, and they can buy more or less as time goes by. Initially, every appropriate behavior should be promptly rewarded with a token that is immediately redeemable for the backup reinforcers. A variable ratio schedule (rewarding him only occasionally for making the bed) might later be introduced to encourage the long-term performance of the new behavior.

Stickers are a good reinforcer for children. Toilet training a child, for example, can be made a lot easier by thinking operantly and using shaping and reinforcing behaviors. A parent might start by giving the child a sticker for every time she asks to sit on the potty. After that behavior becomes common, a sticker might be awarded only if she urinates in the potty, and two stickers if she has a bowel movement in the potty. An additional sticker might be awarded if her pants are dry when she asks to use the potty. Then, a sticker might be awarded only every couple of times or every day she remains dry. The behavioral framework can help a parent (or therapist) attack almost any behavioral problem.

One complaint leveled against the use of stickers or other such secondary reinforcers is that they are bribes and that desirable behavior cannot and should not depend on bribes indefinitely. The behavior modifier responds with this advice: giving the sticker, candy, or token should be accompanied by social reinforcement. In the case of the child, the parent should tell her how proud he is of her. "Bribes" can help shape an appropriate behavior

into existence. Backing up such "artificial" reinforcers with social reinforcement makes them less important to the maintenance of the behavior. They can eventually be phased out, and the appropriate behavior can continue to be reinforced solely by praise or other signs of approval.

BASIC GUIDELINES FOR THE USE OF BEHAVIOR MODIFICATION

In setting up any behavioral treatment program, the behavior modifier prefers to use a *reward* paradigm whenever possible. Aversion techniques have a place only if a reward approach fails or is impractical. Using the toilet training example, the good behavior modifier thinks in terms of rewarding the correct toilet behavior, not of punishing the wetting or soiling. As mentioned earlier, punishment is not only unpleasant for the subject, it also only suppresses, *not* extinguishes, a response. Suppression may occur only in the presence of the punisher (in this case, the parent). The punisher ends up associating himself and the whole toilet training experience with unpleasantness. Equally important, the suppression of an inappropriate response does not ensure the learning of a more appropriate response to take its place.

Sometimes a combination of reward and punishment can be helpful, however. The five-year-old who continually runs into the street without looking puts his life in danger, and a mild punishment (such as withdrawal of permission to play on the sidewalk) when he does so may be in order. But it makes a great deal of behavioral (and common) sense to show him the proper way to safely cross a street and to reinforce this appropriate behavior when it occurs. Suppressing the inappropriate response while at the same time rewarding the good one is a reasonable approach in such a case.

Since most therapists prefer reward over punishment, it stands to reason that desensitization is likely to be used more frequently than implosion for treating anxiety. In the case where implosion seems to be the treatment of choice, the procedure must be understood and agreed upon by the client in advance.

When speaking of punishment, an obvious ethical question arises: What right does a therapist have to shock a person or to induce physical illness? One must remember that aversion techniques are used with people (alcoholics, sexual deviants, homosexuals) who have shown little ability to change their behaviors with conventional treatment modalities. Such clients should be told that a technique is available that might help them but that it

471

472

involves a low-level shock, a chemically induced reaction, or a self-induced discomfort response. It is important to explain the procedure, to ascertain whether the client understands what will happen to him, and to tell him that treatment can be terminated at any time he chooses. Given the strong positive reinforcement associated with the behaviors mentioned, the aversive approach may be the most appropriate means of changing them. Most behavior modifiers have no qualms about offering aversive therapy as a choice.

However, even in cases where aversive therapy is used, the therapist should employ more than just punishment, to increase the probability of success. The therapist should verbally reinforce the client throughout treatment for her hard work and motivation. New behaviors should be shaped and reinforced to replace the suppressed ones. The client should become a partner with the therapist, making suggestions, constructing hierarchies, and doing homework.

The behavior modifier should also think like a scientist. A simple observation that a client seems to be doing better after a therapeutic intervention is no real proof of the intervention's effectiveness. Although one can't expect laboratory controls in the therapist's office, some care can be taken to objectively assess a program's effectiveness. In the case of the tantrum thrower, the first step should be to clearly define the problem behavior. His parents should be sent home to get a *base rate*, that is, to describe how often in a given time period (say two weeks) the child throws a tantrum. Time out can then be explained to the parents, and, as they implement it, they should continue to keep track of tantrums. Baseline data are vital to assess the effective-

ness of the technique as time goes by. Charting progress can also be a real reinforcement to the parents, who can see actual reductions in the inappropriate behavior and are thus encouraged to continue behavior modification.

LIMITATIONS OF BEHAVIOR THERAPY

Dramatic results have been demonstrated in the shaping of behaviors with behavior modification in chronic psychotic clients confined to hospital wards. These techniques are no more a "cure" for psychosis than any other treatment approaches, but they have proven quite successful in helping to alter neurotic, anxiety-related behaviors. They are especially effective with simple phobias but less so with more complex problems, such as obsessive-compulsive disorder. They have made inroads in controlling serious behavior problems such as alcoholism and sexual deviations, with which most other treatment modalities have failed. Treatment programs based on behavioral principles have also been used successfully with problems as diverse as obesity, anorexia nervosa, stuttering, tics, enuresis and encopresis, delinquent behavior, and smoking.

The simpler the problem behavior involved, the more effective the behavioral technique is likely to be. Unfortunately, the complexities of human behavior are usually the results of years of reinforcement, multiple conditioning, and complex contingencies. Cognitive learning theorists hold that looking at stimulus-response connections is too simplistic. As Kanfer and Phillips (1970) have stated, the human capacity for language and thought provides behavioral capacities to bypass

C L I N I C A L   E X A M P L E

BEHAVIORAL THERAPY
FOR A CLIENT WITH PHOBIA

Susan Long was a twenty-eight-year-old who had recently been diagnosed with a form of anemia that demands continued follow-up with regular blood analysis. She was terrified of having blood drawn and at such times would hyperventilate and occasionally lose consciousness. She presented for therapy to help her overcome her fear of having blood drawn.

ASSESSMENT

The therapeutic interview showed an otherwise psychologically healthy woman with a clear-cut, simple phobia. She functioned well in all other areas of her life, and her phobia was of limited proportions in that only one stimulus (drawing blood) elicited the anxiety response.

Nursing Diagnoses

Anxiety

Fear

Multiaxial Psychiatric Diagnoses

Axis I   300.29 Simple phobia

Axis II   None

Axis III   Anemia

Axis IV   Code 2—Minimal psychosocial stressor: recent diagnosis of chronic illness

Axis V   Level 2—(Very good)

PLANNING

In collaboration with a behaviorally oriented clinician, plans were made to teach Susan the Jacobson relaxation technique with the following sequential hierarchy:

1. You look at your calendar and notice you have an upcoming appointment for blood work.

2. You wake up and realize your appointment is this afternoon.

3. You are getting dressed and specifically pick out a short-sleeved blouse to make blood drawing a little easier.

4. You back out of your driveway and are on the way to the hospital.

5. You park in the lot nearest the door where the lab is located.

6. Entering the hospital, you see the sign and arrow directing you to the lab.

7. You walk down the stairs and check in at the door.

8. As you wait, you see an aide carrying vials of blood from the lab.

9. Your name is called.

10. You sit down in the chair and extend your arm to the technician.

11. She tightens the rubber strap around your upper arm.

12. She wipes your arm with alcohol.

13. You see the needle.

14. You feel mild discomfort as the needle goes in.

15. The strap is loosened.

16. You feel the needle being withdrawn.

IMPLEMENTATION

Susan was seen two times a week during the desensitization stage, going through the hierarchy about three times a session. After approximately four weeks, the hierarchy was completed, and she felt confident about her ability to remain calm during blood drawing.

EVALUATION

Susan came back two weeks after completion of therapy with a smile on her face and a bandage on her arm. She had just had the necessary blood work done and indicated that although she didn't like it, her maladaptive anxiety responses (the hyperventilation, excessive sweating, and avoidance responses) were gone.

Aspects of the feared stimuli had been paired with a response incompatible with anxiety. This weakened the maladaptive stimulus-response connection enough to allow Susan to approach the feared experience and to discover that it didn't have the punishing consequences that she had feared. This would make it easier for her the next time, and each successive trial without anxiety would continue to weaken the fear and maybe even make it disappear totally.

473

simple conditioning arrangements. Researchers such as Julian Rotter (1954) have made important contributions by trying to apply learning theory to the complexities of human social behavior.

It seems that the more applied and useful a theory attempts to be, the further away it begins to move from proven laboratory principles. This is representative of the friction that has always existed between "pure" and "applied" science. The purist is like the behaviorist of old interested only in data and objectivity. The applied scientist, or therapist in this case, is faced with clients in the real world who come for help with their maladaptive behaviors. If there are no proven techniques available to help the client, the therapist must do what she thinks may be helpful and withstand the criticism of purist colleagues working in the laboratory who frown on less than perfect attempts to apply science.

The good therapist knows that there is no specific behavioral technique that will prove effective with every problem behavior with which a client may present. Therefore, the therapist may choose to restrict services to a specific kind of clientele (such as phobics). Or, the therapist may adapt Lazarus's broad spectrum behavior therapy approach, using behavioral techniques where appropriate as well as giving support and developing the therapeutic relationship. This does not mean that the therapist should stop thinking behaviorally, only that she not be so naive as to believe that she has all the answers at her fingertips. Most practitioners would agree (some grudgingly) that rapport is still an important factor in therapy, that a good history is essential (especially a history of the problem behavior), and that an assessment of the client's behavioral strengths and weaknesses is invaluable.

SUMMARY

Beginning with the efforts of Wundt and Watson in the late 1800s and early 1900s, psychology has steadily moved from a philosophical perspective to a scientific one based on observation and experimentation. Learning, or the acquisition of relatively permanent new behaviors, has become a central area in the study of psychology. The behaviorists have described the relationships between stimuli and responses and the principles that result in the acquisition, strengthening, or extinction of learned responses.

Ivan Pavlov demonstrated that if a conditioned stimulus (CS) is paired with an unconditioned stimulus (UCS), the CS will become capable of eliciting the response that was once under the control of the UCS. This model of learning has been called respondent or classical conditioning. It explains how autonomic nervous system responses become associated with different stimuli.

B. F. Skinner's operant conditioning model addresses the issue of how new behaviors are learned. According to Skinner, behavior is a function of its consequences, and reinforcement becomes the key to new stimulus-response bonds. Through his painstaking research and his emphasis on observation and experimental procedures, Skinner has amassed a wealth of data that demonstrate such concepts as extinction, generalization, spontaneous recovery, and schedules of reinforcement—concepts and principles that have applications to humans as well as to the animals used in psychological studies.

Dollard and Miller helped bridge the gap between laboratory studies and clinical practice by applying operational terms to existing clinical concepts. In the aftermath of World War II, behavior therapy techniques began to emerge.

Behavior modification represents a collection of techniques that have some basis in laboratory study. The most commonly applied techniques include desensitization, aversion therapy, time out, assertion training, and token economics. These techniques are used in the real world by therapists of diverse backgrounds with different theoretical and philosophical orientations. They share a tendency to think in terms of reinforcements and contingencies, but they also generally realize that the complexities of human behavior defy simple applications of specific behavioral techniques in every circumstance.

Review Questions

1. The SAT scores of fifty left-handed males were compared with those of fifty right-handed males to see if handedness has any relation to intelligence. Is this an experiment? If yes, what are the independent and dependent variables? If no, why not?

2. Why is the classical conditioning model of learning inadequate in explaining how a dog learns to roll over?

3. Give examples of stimulus generalization, discrimination, and spontaneous recovery.

4. Make a list of secondary reinforcers that operate daily in our lives and keep us doing the day-to-day tasks that need to be done.

5. Explain why a reward learning paradigm is generally preferred over a punishment model in helping a person modify a behavior.

6. In systematic desensitization, why does the hierarchy begin with the least anxiety-provoking scene?

474

7. Why is systematic desensitization also referred to as counter-conditioning?

8. When Mary turns up her stereo very loudly, she cannot hear her parents fighting downstairs. Why is it likely she will continue to play her music loudly? "Parents fighting" is an example of what type of reinforcement? What paradigm of learning does this situation represent?

9. The parents of a ten-year-old have been using a "time out" procedure to suppress their son's habit of slapping his younger brother whenever he becomes angry. Although the slapping has dramatically decreased, they are concerned that their son has now become more withdrawn and apparently unhappy. What have they overlooked in their program?

10. Twelve-year-old Gina barely passed last semester. Her parents want her to do better this semester. Thinking in terms of shaping, what component parts make up "getting better grades," and how might these steps be reinforced along the way?

References

Ayllon, T., and Azrin, N. H. 1968. *Token Economy: A Motivational System for Therapy and Rehabilitation*. Englewood Cliffs, N.J.: Prentice-Hall.

Ferster, C. B. 1958. Withdrawal of Positive Reinforcement as Punishment. *Science*, 126:509.

Ferster, C. B., and Skinner, B. F. 1957. *Schedules of Reinforcement*. New York: Appleton-Century-Crofts.

Franks, C. M. ed., 1969. *Behavior Therapy: Appraisal and Status*. New York: McGraw-Hill.

Gold, S., and Neufeld, I. 1965. A Learning Theory Approach to the Treatment of Homosexuality. *Behavior Research and Theory*, 2:201–204.

Hall, C. S., and Lindsey, G. 1967. *Theories of Personality*. New York: John Wiley & Sons.

Jacobson, E. 1938. *Progressive Relaxation*. Chicago: University of Chicago Press.

Kanfer, F. H., and Phillips, J. S. 1970. *Learning Foundations of Behavior Therapy*. New York: John Wiley & Sons.

Lazarus, A. A. 1967. In Support of Technical Eclecticism. *Psychological Reports*, 21:415–416.

Miller, N. E., and Bugelski, R. 1948. Minor Studies in Aggression, II: The Influence of Frustrations Imposed by the In-group on Attitudes Expressed Toward Out-groups. *Journal of Psychology*, 25:437–442.

Pavlov, I. P. 1927. *Conditioned Reflexes*. London: Oxford University Press.

Rotter, J. B. 1954. *Social Learning and Clinical Psychology*. Englewood Cliffs, N.J.: Prentice-Hall.

Shaffer, D. R. 1985. *Developmental Psychology: Theory, Research, and Application*. Monterey, Calif.: Brooks/Cole.

Skinner, B. F. 1972. *Beyond Freedom and Dignity*. New York: Random House.

Stampfl, T. G., and Lewis, D. J. 1967. Essentials of Implosive Therapy: A Learning-Theory-Based Psychodynamic Behavior Therapy. *Journal of Abnormal Psychology*, 72:496–503.

Thorndike, E. L. 1911. *Animal Intelligence*. New York: Macmillan.

Welton, W. 1983. *Psychology Applied To Modern Life*. Monterey, Calif.: Brooks/Cole.

Wolpe, J. 1958. *Psychotherapy by Reciprocal Inhibition*. Stanford, Calif.: Stanford University Press.

Supplementary Readings

Brookes, D. J. A Behavioral Approach to Psychiatric Rehabilitation. *Nursing Times*, 77(1981):367–370.

Burton, M. The Behavioral Approach to Nursing the Elderly. *Nursing Times*, 77(1981):268–272.

Cinciripini, P. M. A Behavioral Program for the Management of Anorexia and Bulimia. *Journal of Nervous and Mental Diseases*, (1983):186–189.

Clark, D. B. Behavioral Training for Parents of Mentally Retarded Children. *American Journal of Mental Deficiencies*, 87(1982):14–19.

Cole, R. J. A Coping Skills Approach to the Treatment of Adult Psychiatric Outpatients. *Canada's Mental Health*, 28(1980):5–7.

Davis, J. Treatment of a Medical Phobia Including Desensitization Administered by a Significant Other. *Journal of Psychosocial Nursing and Mental Health Services*, 20(1982):6–8.

Foa, E. B. Success and Failure in the Behavioral Treatment of Obsessive Compulsives. *Journal of Consulting Clinical Psychology*, 51(1983):287–297.

Gudjonsson, G. Behavior Modification in an Interim Secure Unit. *Nursing Times*, 79(1983):25–27.

Guydish, J. Behavioral Modification: Doing Battle in the Ethical Arena. *Journal of Behavior Therapy and Experimental Psychiatry*, 13(1982):315–320.

Hafer, R. J. Behavior Therapy for Agoraphobic Men. *Behavioral Research Therapy*, 21(1983):51–56.

Henthorn, B. S. Disengagement and Reinforcement in the Elderly. *Research in Nursing and Health*, 2(1979):1–8.

Jain, S. Operant Conditioning for Management of Non-compliant Rehabilitation Cases After Stroke. *Archives of Physical Medicine and Rehabilitation*, 63(1982):374–376.

Kazdin, A. E. *History of Behavior Modification*. Baltimore: University Park Press, 1978.

Kirk, J. W. Behavioral Treatment of Obsessive-Compulsive Patients in Routine Clinical Practice. *Behavioral Research Therapy*, 21(1983):57–62.

Klein, D. F. Treatment of Phobias: Behavior Therapy and Supportive Psychotherapy. *Archives of General Psychiatry*, 40(1983):139–145.

Knowles, R. D. Handling Depression Through Positive Reinforcement. *American Journal of Nursing*, 81(1981):1353.

Leitenberg, H. *Handbook of Behavior Modification and Behavior Therapy*. Englewood Cliffs, N.J.: Prentice-Hall, 1976.

Lindly, P. Behavioral Approaches. *Nursing* (Oxford), 1(1980):808–809

McArdle, M. Training the Mentally Handicapped at Home. *Nursing* (Oxford), 1(1980):840–844.

McArdle, M. Behavior Modification. *Nursing Mirror*, 19(1983):52–54.

McMordie, W. R. Reality Therapy: Icing on the Cake of Behavior Modification. *Journal of Contemporary Psychotherapy*, 12(1981):137–144.

Nakaniski, D. A. Behavioral Treatment of Psychogenic Vomiting Among Children. *Journal of Psychosocial Nursing and Mental Health Services*, 20(1982):17–20.

Nath, C. Effects of Individual and Group Relaxation Therapy on Blood Pressure in Essential Hypertension. *Research in Nursing and Health*, 2(1979):119–126.

Newnes, C. Short Span Time Out—A Behavioral Approach Aimed at Reducing Undesirable Behavior. *Nursing Times*, 79(1983):69–71.

Power, J. Teaching Assertive Behavior to Psychiatric Patients. *Canadian Nurse*, 78(1982):52–57.

Prehn, R. A. Applied Behavioral Analysis for Disturbed Elderly Patients. *Journal of Gerontological Nursing*, 8(1982):286–288.

Ryan, D. Skills Training and Heterosexual Social Difficulties. *Canadian Journal of Psychiatric Nursing*, 12(1982):13–15.

Smith, A. Token Economy: Does It Work? *Nursing Times*, 80(1984):64–65.

Stiorkey, C. T. Desensitization of Anxiety in Health Care. *Health and Social Work*, 7(1982):14–18.

Trower, P. The What, Who, and How of Social Skills Training. *British Journal of Hospital Medicine*, 27(1982):608–614.

Williams, M. T. Fear of Flight: Behavior Therapy Versus a Systems Approach. *Journal of Psychology*, 111(1982):193–203.

ORIGINS OF FAMILY THEORY AND THERAPY

CONCEPTUAL APPROACHES
Developmental Concepts
Systems Theory Concepts
Psychodynamic Concepts
Structural Concepts
Functional Concepts
Communication Concepts
Learning Theory Concepts

SOME PRACTICALITIES IN FAMILY
INTERVENTION

C H A P T E R

18

Family Theory and Practice

Learning Objectives

After reading this chapter, the student should be able to:

1. Differentiate the viewpoint that the dysfunction of an identified client *originates in* the family from the viewpoint that the dysfunction *is caused by* the family.

2. Describe major approaches in family theory and the significant concepts of each approach.

3. Identify and describe the following tools used in gathering and organizing family data: family mapping, family geneogram, family chronology, family sociogram.

4. Describe types of dysfunctional communication and explain the purposes they serve in family life.

5. Discuss the influence of role function and role expectations in traditional and nontraditional families.

6. Describe appropriate behaviors by nurses in an initial family meeting, in the working sessions, and in the termination sessions.

Overview

Family *theory* is based on the premise that the dysfunction of an identified client usually originates in the context of family life and may reflect problems within the family itself rather than within the client. Family *therapy* carries this premise even further and substitutes interest in the family *as* the client instead of interest in the family *of* the client. For a family therapist, the focus of attention is not the individual client but the whole interpersonal field of family interaction (Carter and McGoldrick, 1980). In their commitment to holistic, comprehensive care, all nurses should carefully consider family variables even if they may not be prepared to undertake family therapy in the strict sense of the term. Family therapy per se may be restricted to practitioners with special preparation, but family-focused care is within the scope of the generalist nurse (Mereness, 1968). A basic understanding of family theories and concepts is essential to comprehensive health care. Therefore, a number of major theories and key concepts related to family assessment and intervention are presented in this chapter.

*Greatness in the father oftimes overwhelms the son: they
stand too near one another. The shadow kills the growth.*

BEN JONSON

479

As a separate, formal treatment modality, *family therapy* is relatively new. Only in the last few decades has family therapy become a method of describing, explaining, and alleviating numerous psychological and behavioral problems (Cohen, Younger, and Sullivan, 1983). It evolved from the separate activities of a number of theorists and clinicians, including Harry Stack Sullivan (1953), who emphasized the presence of anxiety in all interpersonal situations, especially in transactions between the young child and its mother.

ORIGINS OF FAMILY THEORY AND THERAPY

During the 1950s, family theory was concerned primarily with interactional patterns in the families of schizophrenic clients, especially young persons with schizophrenia. There were a number of reasons for this interest. To begin with, these families offered an accessible laboratory for study and investigation. In addition, young clients with schizophrenia were usually at a developmental point where family factors contributing to dysfunction could be identified. Studying the families of these clients offered some possibility for primary prevention of schizophrenia in other families at risk and for promoting secondary and tertiary prevention in families already dealing with the disorder (Cohen, Younger, and Sullivan, 1983). Family theory and family therapy thus developed in tandem. Theoretical concepts were applied to clinical situations, and an innovative, significant treatment modality was born.

Although family theory and family therapy were initiated by clinicians working with psychiatric clients, many concepts derived from their work proved applicable to families without identified psychiatric disorders. Even in the absence of psychiatric illness, certain interactional patterns seem to differentiate functional from dysfunctional families (Friedman, 1981).

The early family theorists believed that the family is a social unit in which all members interact with each other, and this belief has been supported by sustained observation. The interdependent, reciprocal quality of family life has led some theorists to claim that there is a cause and effect relationship between family interactional patterns and the dysfunction of the client. Other family theorists have asserted that family interactional patterns might increase a client's dysfunction without necessarily causing it (Foley, 1974).

No less a person than Florence Nightingale is among those who have attributed psychological distress to flawed family interaction. With her mother and sister united against her determination to lead a useful life, Nightingale wrote, "The family uses people, not for what they are, nor for what they are intended to be, but for what it wants them for—its own uses. It thinks of them not as God made them but as the something which it has arranged that they shall be. If it wants someone to sit in the drawing-room, then that someone is supplied by the family, though that member may be destined for science or for education . . . This system dooms some minds to incurable infancy" (Payne, 1983, p. 163).

Not all families attempt to frustrate the ambitions of nonconforming members, and such extreme bitterness is not characteristic of all rebellious members, particularly successful ones like Nightingale. Nevertheless, many family theorists, even those who do not accept causal connections between client

Table 18-1. Forms of Family Therapy

Form of Therapy	Characteristics of Therapy
Conjoint family therapy	The family meets with one therapist or a pair of co-therapists. This is the most usual form of family therapy, especially for marital counseling or nuclear family meetings that include parents and children.
Multiple impact family therapy	The family or subgroups of the family meet with several therapists simultaneously or concurrently. In this form of family therapy the impact of treatment is increased by the teamwork of a group of therapists working with the family.
Network family therapy	A nuclear family is joined by the extended family group and by significant friends and neighbors to meet with a therapist or a pair of co-therapists. This form of therapy reduces the isolation of a small family unit and mobilizes a strong supportive network.
Multiple family therapy	A number of families meet together with one or two therapists. Families with common problems or shared interests profit from this form of therapy, in which group leadership tactics are used by the therapists.

480

dysfunction and family interaction, believe that family patterns often influence the development and the course of dysfunction in one or more members.

Family therapy is an accepted but complex treatment modality that requires graduate preparation and supervised clinical experience from those who practice it. It is a multidisciplinary approach, and practitioners are drawn from medicine, nursing, psychology, and social work. It is also an interdisciplinary modality, in that co-therapists often represent more than one health care profession. Nurses who perform family therapy should possess at least a master's degree in psychiatric mental health nursing. Even though extensive family therapy may not lie within the competence of the generalist nurse, this is not true of family assessment and planning. Nurses and other care providers who exclude family considerations from their care plan limit their effectiveness and jeopardize the welfare of clients (Mereness, 1968).

Family therapy may be offered in one of several ways, depending on the needs of the family, the availability of staff, the preferences of the therapists, and the policies of the agency where care is given. Table 18-1 indicates different forms of family therapy.

The pioneers in the field of family theory and family therapy had to develop new terminology to explain the phenomena evident in the families with whom they worked. A central issue to be resolved was simply "What constitutes a family?" There is general agreement that the family is the basic social unit of humankind, but there are numerous variations in the composition of families and in how they operate, as is demonstrated in the accompanying box.

The family is the primary or central group in the life of most individuals. The family is also the primary or central group that, when joined by other families, causes communities to be formed. Thus, few families exist in isolation, because there is a constant exchange of energy in the form of transactions between the family and the surrounding community (Howells, 1975; Langsley, 1980). A community can survive only as long as its values, customs, and norms are upheld by the majority of family units. In turn, family units can survive only as long as they manage to satisfy some needs of their individual members.

Contemporary society contains a variety of structural arrangements that differ from the traditional family comprising a married heterogeneous couple, their offspring, and some extended family members. There are a number of possible explanations for the diversity of present-day families. The soaring divorce rate, the tendency of divorced persons to remarry, the ability of unwed mothers to keep their children with them, and increased tolerance toward homosexual households are a few of the reasons for family variations in contemporary life (Fleck, 1980). Regardless of the forms that families take, the variations are usually the result of individual efforts to gratify needs within a social unit that represents a central or primary group for its members (Bohannon, 1980).

Another reason that contemporary families are so diversified is economic. For centuries, families were units of production, working together on farms or in cottage industries, but this is less true today in spite of the trend toward sharing household and parental tasks. In the marketplace it is the individual who constitutes the work unit, even in dual-

VARIATIONS IN FAMILY COMPOSITION

- *Natural or biological family.* Family into which the individual is born or is related by consanguinity.

- *Adoptive family.* Family to which an individual belongs through adoption, usually by legal means.

- *Family of origin.* Family into which an individual was born.

- *Nuclear family.* Family created by a marital or ongoing relationship between two individuals and their offspring, if any.

- *Family of procreation.* Family created by individuals entering a relationship into which children are born.

- *Extended family.* Family group that includes one or more nuclear families plus other individuals related by blood or marriage.

- *Intact family.* Family that includes two parents and their natural or adopted children living in one household.

- *Single-parent family.* Family consisting of children and one parent, either father or mother, living in one household.

- *Reconstituted family.* Family created by the remarriage of one or both parents; this family may include children of the present marriage as well as children from previous marriages of one or both spouses.

career families (McNally, 1980). Other important family tasks, such as the formal education of children, that once were accomplished within the family have been delegated to larger institutions, such as schools. It may be that emotional gratification and self-fulfillment have become the major surviving purposes of family life. The current high priority placed on emotional satisfaction helps explain variations in families that result from the pursuit of fulfillment within family settings (Bohannon, 1980).

CONCEPTUAL APPROACHES

The point has been made that family theory can ignore neither the individual nor the community (Howells, 1975), for families are the interface or connecting mechanism between the individual and the community. Family-centered nursing and fam-

481

ily-focused care are often discussed philosophically in educational programs for nurses without receiving adequate theoretical and clinical attention. What is needed in nursing is general knowledge of family dynamics, based on credible theories and concepts that can be communicated to others and applied to clinical situations. A basic understanding of various conceptual approaches to family theory is essential to assessing, planning, implementing, and evaluating the impact of family factors on individuals and communities (Krauss, 1984).

Family theory is relatively new, and many of the innovators in this area have worked independently of one another, which has led to a certain amount of conceptual confusion. This redundancy, added to the undeniable complexity of family life, makes the body of family knowledge seem formidable to beginners. One way to simplify the task of describing theories and concepts is to categorize them according to conceptual approach. Although such categorization may seem arbitrary, it does help produce a degree of order out of disorder.

Specific conceptual approaches help the practitioner recognize and describe family structure and function. Having mastered basic family theories and concepts, a nurse should be able to assess obvious strengths and weaknesses in the family, to distinguish between functional and dysfunctional interactions, and to plan appropriate interventions. Initially, a nurse may prefer to rely on a single conceptual approach, gradually drawing on others as needed. Whether used in a pure or in an eclectic manner, a conceptual approach guides the selection and organization of observable data, thereby facilitating assessment of family dynamics (Janosik and Miller, 1979).

Table 18-2. Comparison of Duvall's Family Critical Tasks and Erikson's Individual Critical Tasks

Family Stages and Critical Tasks	Individual Critical Tasks
Marital stage: Establishing a marriage	Trust versus mistrust
Childbearing stage: Adjusting to parenthood and maintaining a home	Autonomy versus shame and doubt
Preschool stage: Nurturing children	Initiative versus guilt
School-age stage: Socializing and educating children	Industry versus inferiority
Teenage stage: Balancing teenagers' freedom and responsibility	Identity versus role confusion
Launching stage: Releasing children as young adults; developing postparental interests	Intimacy versus isolation
Middle-aged stage: Reestablishing the marital dyad; maintaining links with older and younger generations	Generativity versus stagnation
Aging stage: Adjusting to retirement, aging, loneliness, and death	Ego integrity versus despair

SOURCES: Adapted from Duvall (1977) and Erikson (1963).

Some conceptual approaches are more widely used than others, but most have a unique contribution to make to family theory. In this section, a number of different conceptual approaches will be described. As each approach is presented, representative theorists will be identified and notable concepts will be explained in terms of family theory.

Developmental Concepts

The developmental approach views families from a life cycle perspective; families are seen as changing not only from day to day but also from year to year. An important contributor to family developmental theory was Evelyn Duvall (1977), who formulated an eight-stage model of the family life cycle, similar to the eight-stage model of individual development offered by Erikson (1963) (see Table 18-2). Duvall divided family development into two broad phases: expanding family life and contracting family life. The expanding period lasts from the establishment of the marital dyad until the children are grown and launched. Contraction begins when the first child leaves home and ends with the death of the surviving spouse. Figure 18-1 illustrates the family life cycle formulated by Duvall.

By contrasting the eight stages of Duvall's family life cycle with the eight stages of Erikson's individual life cycle, it is possible to recognize hazards related to the negotiation of family and individual life cycle tasks. According to Erikson, each critical or developmental task is related to the preceding ones, and there is a time of "ascendance" during which a specific task can be performed most effectively. This time of ascendance is determined by the physiological maturation of the individual, by psychological impulses, and by cultural expectations.

Sometimes it is difficult for a family to integrate the individual tasks of all its members into the developmental scheme of family life. For example, the resolution of the identity crisis requires that an adolescent begin to separate from parental influence. This separation may take place at a rate unacceptable to parents who are unwilling or unready to exchange the characteristics of a teenage family for those of a launching family. Reluctance to move into the next stage of family life may also be apparent in the behavior of a couple moving uneasily from the relatively carefree activities of a marital dyad to the responsibilities of a childbearing family. Unless this couple can be assisted and reassured as they enter early parenthood, their young children may be impeded in moving toward trust and autonomy, the first two individual tasks in Erikson's life cycle model.

Ideally, the family adjusts to the changing needs of its members so that individual critical tasks may be resolved. In families that are inflexible, the needs and aspirations of individual members may meet with resistance because the family unit fails to advance to its next developmental stage. A nurse using the developmental approach to assess families begins by identifying the appropriate life cycle stage of the family as a whole and then notes the progress being made by individual members in achieving their critical tasks. If the attainment of individual tasks has been or is being impeded, it may be possible to recognize the source of the impediment and

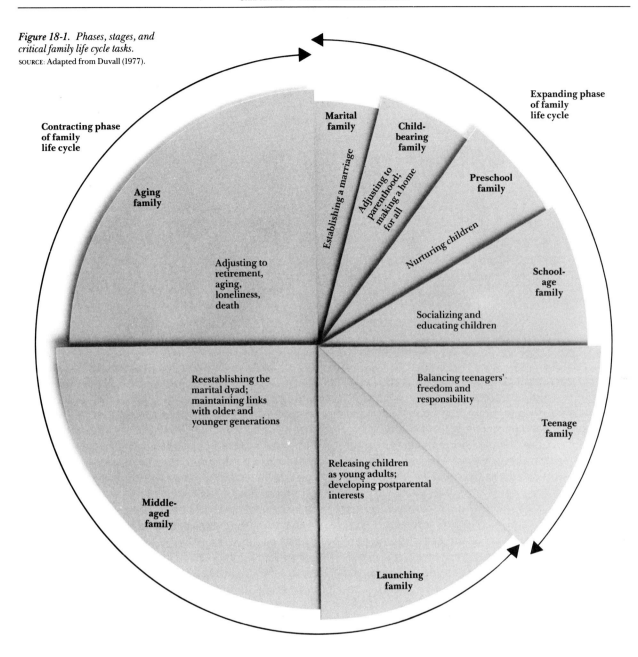

Figure 18-1. *Phases, stages, and critical family life cycle tasks.*
SOURCE: Adapted from Duvall (1977).

Contracting phase of family life cycle

Expanding phase of family life cycle

Marital family

Child-bearing family

Preschool family

School-age family

Establishing a marriage

Adjusting to parenthood; making a home for all

Nurturing children

Aging family

Adjusting to retirement, aging, loneliness, death

Socializing and educating children

Reestablishing the marital dyad; maintaining links with older and younger generations

Balancing teenagers' freedom and responsibility

Teenage family

Releasing children as young adults; developing postparental interests

Middle-aged family

Launching family

483

to assess the seriousness of the situation. Sometimes merely teaching families the importance of stage-appropriate developmental tasks is enough to reduce family resistance. At other times the nurse may decide not to intervene directly but to make a referral, if conditions are serious enough to warrant extensive family therapy. In some instances a generalist nurse may remain involved with the family and work collaboratively with the family therapist.

Systems Theory Concepts

Von Bertalanffy (1974) has described the family unit as a *system* whose components engage in mutual interactions according to rules and patterns developed over time so that the system may survive. As a system, the family is composed of separate but interdependent components separated from the external environment by *boundaries*. Boundaries are an indispensable part of family systems. They surround individual family members and groups or subsystems composed of family members, and they surround the entire family unit. Individual boundaries help family members maintain their separate identity; other boundaries determine who belongs to the family system, who is placed in family subsystems, and how and with whom various members may interact inside and outside the family unit.

Depending on the characteristics of its boundaries, a family system may be totally open, totally closed, or somewhere in between. Energy, in the

A slogan which most patients seem to find amusing and useful . . . consists of three letters: GDM. This grew out of observing again and again the reactions of parents in their own rights to the presence of their parents—that is, to the grandparents—in the household, whether for brief visits or long periods. Sometimes the grandparents do not live in the household but only exert their influence from a distance, succeeding nevertheless in playing an important part in the lives of the married couple. Perhaps sometimes the three generations really are able to make a harmonious go of it, but . . . that would be the rare experience. GDM means "generations don't mix." Usually the effect of using this slogan is to give the parents of young children some perspective on the difficulties of having the grandparents exert any appreciable influence in their lives. After all, probably it is only in human beings among all animals that the individual can grow up, pass adolescence, marry and have his or her own family without being thoroughly separated physically and psychologically from his or her own parents.

LOUIS PAUL (1963)

form of tension within the system, preserves the interdependence of the components. All families, functional or dysfunctional, contain a certain amount of tension generated by the emotional connections among members. Although excessive tension may cause strain on the system, a family without tension would cease to be a viable system.

BOUNDARIES AND HOMEOSTASIS In order to accomplish their life cycle tasks families need a degree of stability, or *homeostasis*. Homeostasis is a state of balance that maintains family stability but also permits families to change in response to internal and external conditions. Stability should not be confused with stagnation, for a capacity of families to adapt to changing circumstances is essential to their survival (Kraft and DeMaio, 1982). For example, the adaptation of families in a launching stage is unlike that of families in earlier stages. Launching-stage families must deal with separation issues; earlier stage families must deal with nurturing children and integrating them into family life.

Boundaries enable families to maintain homeostasis by regulating the amount of input or feedback into the family from external sources. Family systems whose boundaries are partially open and somewhat penetrable have the best chance of remaining functional. Such systems are capable of responding to input from their external surroundings and can discharge internal tension across their boundaries in the form of output. In closed systems there is little likelihood of discharging tension except on other family members. This behavior results in rising internal tension that increases the dysfunction of the system.

The concept of family boundaries may be used by nurses to assess and diagnose some forms of family dysfunction. Family boundaries that are too easily penetrated threaten family equilibrium by fostering a climate of instability. An example of family boundaries that are too open occurs in some upwardly mobile families who hastily discard old customs in order to imitate the behaviors of a higher socioeconomic group regardless of their relevance or appropriateness. On the other hand, family boundaries that cannot be penetrated prevent the transmission of input from outside that might improve the family's ability to cope. An example of close or impenetrable boundaries is seen in some immigrant families in which parents resist the influence of the mainstream culture and try to preserve accustomed values despite opposition from their children.

Awareness of the quality of family boundaries helps nurses understand puzzling family behaviors and the origin of certain types of conflict. Family growth can be promoted by helping families maintain protective but penetrable boundaries. Functional families can adjust to changing conditions within the system and in the outside environment. Dysfunctional families, on the other hand, tend to oppose change and growth in their members. In dysfunctional families, inflexible rules are used to maintain the status quo, regardless of the cost to individual members (Bowen, 1965; Wynne, 1978).

FEEDBACK *Feedback* is an important concept in systems theory. By means of feedback the family transmits output to the environment in the form of emotional and behavioral responses. The surrounding environment, in the form of neighborhood, church, or school, reacts by sending responses (input) to the

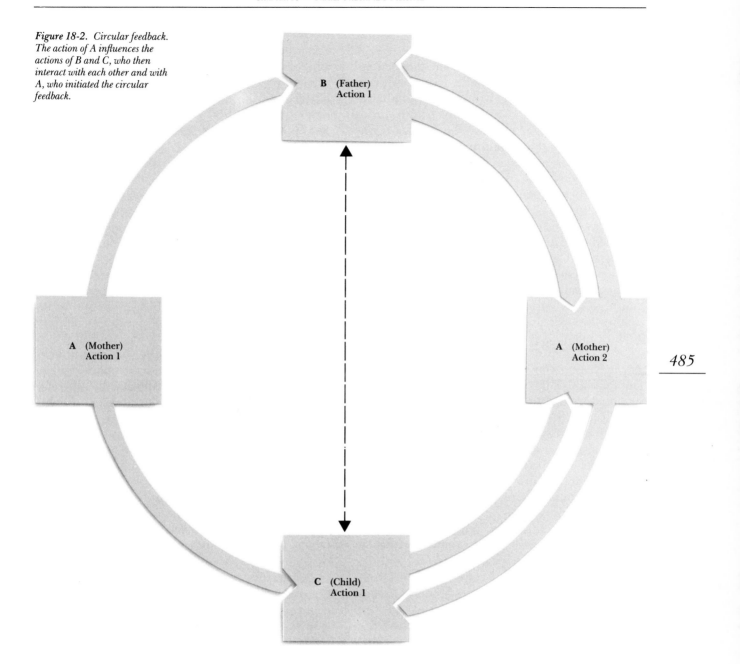

Figure 18-2. *Circular feedback. The action of A influences the actions of B and C, who then interact with each other and with A, who initiated the circular feedback.*

family. Sometimes the feedback from environmental sources is informal and takes the shape of unspoken community approval or disapproval of family actions. An illustration might be neighborhood gossip about family quarrels or criticism of a family for failing to live up to community standards in caring for their home. A more formal type of feedback might consist of complaints to the family from personnel at the children's school or a summons issued by the local police (Sedgewick, 1974, 1981).

Feedback is not a series of linear events but rather a circular process in which all elements of the system and the immediate environment surrounding the system reciprocally influence one another. In circular feedback the action of A influences the actions of B and C. Thereupon, B and C react toward each other and toward A, who instigated the circular events. Figure 18-2 illustrates circular feedback.

Feedback is a continuous process of positive and negative exchange between families and the environment they inhabit. By analyzing feedback nurses can identify the characteristics of family boundaries and, if necessary, work to increase a family's awareness of their actions and of community norms. When input from the community indicates that a family should modify its behavior, the community feedback is negative. When input from the community indicates that the family should continue its present behavior, the feedback is positive. Whether positive or negative, feedback is helpful in promoting adaptive family functioning (Powers, 1980).

An advantage of using a systems theory approach to family assessment and intervention is the avoidance of heaping blame on one or another of the family members. If the family is perceived as a system in which parents, children, extended family members, and the community influence one another reciprocally, then interactions become a shared responsibility. Systems theorists contend that alterations in one part of the family inevitably lead to alterations in other parts of the family. Health care professionals who adopt a systems approach tend to see family strengths as well as weaknesses. They try to reinforce the confidence and competence of family members, especially the parents, so that they can learn to provide an internal climate in which everyone can flourish without exploiting individuals or subgroups in the system (Collins, 1984).

Psychodynamic Concepts

The founder of the psychodynamic approach was Sigmund Freud. During his long career, Freud revised his early belief that childhood sexual trauma was the cause of neurosis and became more attentive to constitutional factors. In other words, Freud came to believe that many individuals become dysfunctional not because of externally imposed sexual trauma but because of their own instinctual drives and impulses. His preoccupation with constitutional factors caused him to overlook the contributions of parents and families in the development of psychological disturbance in their children. Although in some respects he was a skeptic who questioned the prevailing beliefs of his day, Freud seemed to accept the idea that parents love their children in benign ways and that psychological problems are largely attributable to constitutional drives (Freud, 1949; Thompson, 1957; Brown, 1967).

At first Freud believed that the frequent accounts by his patients of having been sexually assaulted in childhood were factual. Later he reported that such accounts were not substantiated, and he considered them to be fantasies representing the patients' unconscious wish fulfillment of forbidden impulses. This reversal in Freud's thinking continues to arouse controversy today. Feminists assert that the Freudian position has made it difficult for women and children to establish their credibility as victims of sexual trauma. Among other writers, Masson (1984) has suggested that Freud's failure to uphold his initial conviction reveals a lack of moral courage. It must be acknowledged that Freud's original view on this subject met with public disapproval, and Masson alleges that when Freud labeled the traumatic reports of his patients as fantasies or wishful thinking he was intellectually dishonest. There is no way to reach a definitive conclusion on this issue, but Freud continues to be held responsible for encouraging distrust by establishment figures, such as physicians and lawyers, toward self-reports by women and children of traumatic sexual experiences.

Freud made other observations regarding families that are more readily acceptable. He suggested, for example, that there exists within each family a collective psychological life that is simultaneously created and shared by the family members. The family's collective psychological life may be compared to the psychological processes of individual members, but the family psyche possesses unique dimensions of its own. Through the intrapsychic life of the family, older generations, living and dead, can transmit family values and attitudes to newer generations. Although Freud was referring primarily to the transmission of dysfunctional, neurotic behaviors, his formulations emphasized the presence of a collective psychological life in every family, functional or dysfunctional (Anthony, 1971). Certainly the idea of the transmission of family attitudes and values can be seen in families in which there is a collective, intergenerational commitment to certain occupations, such as teaching, or a collective disregard of certain goals, such as accumulating material possessions. The idea of a collective family psyche has implications for nurses working with families because it recognizes the impact of family traditions on individual members regardless of whether they adopt or challenge these traditions. In many families there is a long-standing tradition for members to choose a particular field of endeavor or to enter a family business upon reaching adulthood. The member who deviates is likely to arouse negative reactions within the family and to seek support outside.

PSEUDOMUTUALITY AND PSEUDOHOSTILITY Psychodynamic theory is concerned with the conflict between the wish of individuals to be cared for and nurtured and their opposing urge to be separate and assertive. Some families nurture their members but are unwilling to permit the formation of a separate identity. In more dysfunctional families, individual differences are not tolerated at all, and family members are expected to conform to family standards even if personal identity is sacrificed.

Wynne et al. (1958) described a form of family interaction in which any deviation from family standards was thought to threaten family survival. In this type of family interaction, a surface harmony was maintained even if it required a denial of identity and selfhood by one or more members. A family characterized by false harmony, or *pseudomutuality*, tends to be rigid, inflexible, and intolerant of change or individual differences among its members. The result is a family unit in which compliance is valued more than individuality. Family harmony may appear to be preserved, but growth is sacrificed. Pseudomutuality is maintained, but some members may be exploited in order for the family to continue just as it is.

Wynne et al. (1958) used the term *pseudohostility* to describe families that habitually engage in bickering and rancor in order to avoid intimacy or closeness. Unlike pseudomutual families, where closeness is highly regarded, pseudohostile families go to considerable lengths to avoid harmonious involvement. Even though conflict and argumentation are prominent in family interactions, the genuine conflict is seldom identified and resolved. Resolution of a conflict may pave the way for closer relationships, which is what pseudohostile families are trying to avoid. Pseudomutuality and pseudohostility are equally destructive methods for dealing with the universal human difficulty of relating to others while maintaining a separate identity (Foley, 1974).

In applying the concepts of pseudomutuality and pseudohostility to family situations, the nurse might first identify the prevailing style of family interaction. If the family displays apparent harmony but has unresolved problems, the nurse might try to analyze whose rights are being ignored in order to preserve peace. Not infrequently, the family member who is being exploited or neglected becomes the identified client, or the family "problem." For example, open marital discord can sometimes be avoided if parents unite in their behavior toward a school-aged child who is a chronic bedwetter or an adolescent who is rebellious. Even when the parents disagree on how to treat a problem child, their disagreement about the child helps them avoid dealing with marital issues.

In families where there is a great deal of quarreling and disagreement, the issue to be resolved is, what is the true nature of the conflict and what are the real goals of the contenders? Are the participants confronting each other honestly, or are other family members forced to choose sides and join the hostilities? Are genuine problems being addressed, or are peripheral issues being used to avoid dealing with more crucial matters? One example is the husband who is excessively preoccupied with his career and indifferent to the delinquent behavior of his son. This indifference incites rage in the mother, but whenever the father does attempt to talk with his son, his wife intervenes. As the pivotal member of the household, she interprets each of them to the other; this gives her the power to isolate the two. She secures the allegiance of her son by protecting

him from his father. But because her son's behavior is upsetting to her, she occasionally berates him. At the same time she avoids taking responsibility by blaming her husband for not being a more attentive father. At first glance the mother may seem justified, but further assessment shows the pseudohostility that conceals the mother's inconsistent behavior toward her son and her desire not to share her son with his father despite her protestations to the contrary (Frias and Janosik, 1980).

RUBBER FENCES In some dysfunctional families, the boundaries are neither clear nor stable but instead expand and contract in ways that are inconsistent and unpredictable. The term "rubber fences" has been used to describe such undependable, elastic boundaries. Persons living in a family with such boundaries find themselves in an emotional field in which behaviors and rules change continually. As a result, most of the members are bewildered and confused about what is acceptable or unacceptable within the family. Secrecy, inconsistency, and disorder characterize family interactions, and very little that goes on in the family can be predicted or expected (Wynne et al., 1958; Foley, 1974).

MARITAL SCHISM AND MARITAL SKEW The early family theorists were interested in tracing the etiology of various psychiatric disorders, especially schizophrenia, to questionable interactional patterns in the family. Few theorists alleged that families actually *cause* schizophrenia; rather, they suggested that maladaptive patterns of interaction are found in many families with a schizophrenic member (Lidz, 1973). One longitudinal study of patients with schizophrenia led to the conclusion that all the patients had suffered destructive experiences within the family (Lidz and Lidz, 1949).

Lidz (1958) found two specific interactional patterns to be conspicuous in the families of persons with schizophrenia. The first pattern is that of a dominant spouse whose specific ideas on what a family should be like are followed by the less dominant partner. This family is superficially compatible, but there is an underlying hostility that is not directly expressed. Lidz labeled these families as *skewed* and found the skewed family arrangement to be more common in families with a schizophrenic son. In families that Lidz labeled *schismatic* there is open dissension and acrimony. In these families it is usually a daughter who becomes the identified patient.

In skewed families the mother is usually dominant and intrusive, especially in her son's affairs. She resists her son's efforts to separate and looks to him, rather than her husband, for gratification of her needs. Because of his passivity, the father does

487

Requests for behavior change are a normal part of living together as a family. Interestingly enough, they are usually concerned with "little things." How does a wife go about getting her husband to pick up his clothes that he leaves lying about every day? This is a small thing. On the other hand, he does it every day. If one after another of these small things pile up and do not change, their accumulative effect is to produce large scale conflicts. Each small problem is added to the growing pile of unresolved problems. In many instances, the victim spends a good deal of time brooding about the various grievances, but feels powerless to change the situation. Over an extended period of time, this accumulation of "little things" can change the way we feel about each other. Finally, one day the accumulation bursts like an avalanche upon the relationship and the other person may be presented with an astonishing collection of ancient grievances . . . It is important to discuss problems as they arise.

GERALD R. PATTERSON (1975)

488

not actively intervene on his son's behalf. He either tolerates the excessively close relationship between mother and son or else adopts sibling-like behavior and competes with his son for his wife's attention. The dominance of the mother and the passivity of the father deprive the son of a positive role model with which to identify. The result is a stunting of personality development in the son, sometimes to the extent of psychiatric illness (Frias and Janosik, 1980).

In schismatic families the father generally dominates while the mother is aloof and detached. Although the mother may appear affectionate toward her daughter, her behavior is covertly antagonistic. Since the daughter finds it difficult to identify with a mother who subtly rejects her, she may turn to her father for affection. The father often cooperates in this because his marital relationship is so unrewarding. The psychoanalytic explanation for the girl's dilemma is that she has failed to resolve the Electra conflict (the female counterpart of the Oedipal conflict). The daughter cannot renounce her father and identify with her mother because she is trapped by the hostility of the parents toward each other. She cannot entirely please one parent without risking loss of the other. Regressive behaviors, in the form of truancy, delinquency, or psychiatric symptoms, may seem to be the only solution available to her (Lidz, 1958; Lidz, Fleck, and Cornelison, 1965; Wynne and Singer, 1963a, 1963b).

Parents in skewed and schismatic families have the power to scapegoat a child. Although the interactions of the parents are self-destructive, their status in the family enables them to continue to function, but their self-centered behaviors impair

their children's normal psychological growth. When a son or daughter is especially vulnerable, a process of loneliness, withdrawal, distrust, and regression may eventually lead to psychiatric illness.

Structural Concepts

Every family is organized along structural lines that reveal relationships among family members. Within the family, patterns develop governing how, when, and to whom family members relate. This patterning of relationships helps reduce frustration and inefficiency, because family members know what interactions are likely to be acceptable at a particular point in time. Of course, family structure is altered whenever family members join or leave the unit.

Family *subsystems* are divisions within the family based on age, gender, and responsibilities (Minuchin, 1974). Families begin with a marital dyad that becomes the parental subsystem when children enter the family. The children form a sibling subsystem. In large families there may be several sibling subsystems, and in many families female members form one subsystem and male members another. In general, any one family member belongs to several subsystems that help the family operate in a relatively orderly fashion.

In some families homeostasis is maintained by exploiting one of the children. Disagreements between the parents may be avoided by displacing conflict to a particular child who performs the function of family scapegoat. It is not unusual for the scapegoated child to develop psychological, physiological, or behavioral symptoms. Conflict between the parents can be avoided or detoured as the parents become preoccupied in dealing with the child,

Table 18-3. Mapping Family Structure

Organizational Structure	Symbol	Organizational Consequences
Clear boundaries	————	Differentiation and autonomy
Diffuse boundaries	....	Enmeshment and over-inclusiveness
Rigid boundaries	———	Disengagement and isolation
Detouring	——→	Displacement of conflict and problems to another family member
Subsystems	▭	Natural family subdivisions
Conflict	⊐│ │⊏	Hostility between two or more family members or subgroups

SOURCE: After Minuchin (1974).

who may actually serve the function of preserving the family unit.

Boundaries that are clearly defined uphold family and subsystem functioning. When boundaries between members are extremely rigid, family members remain separate and disengaged from one another. When boundaries between members are weak or diffuse, there is little differentiation or separation of members. In families where boundaries are diffuse the members are so close that they become enmeshed with each other. The members may enjoy a sense of belonging, but they sacrifice their individuality and autonomy (Minuchin, 1974).

Structural family therapists use a technique called family mapping to help assess characteristics of the family system. The family map can help nurses identify possible goals and can be used to demonstrate spatial and organizational relationships to family members. Table 18-3 shows the symbols most commonly used in family mapping.

The foremost exponent of structural family intervention is Salvador Minuchin (1974), who advises clinicians to enter the family system in order to restructure family relationships and alter positions in the family. To accomplish this restructuring, the therapist may (1) strengthen individual boundaries to increase separation and individuation of members who are enmeshed, (2) reinforce natural subsystems such as the parental subsystem and sibling subsystems by suggesting age-appropriate behaviors and tasks, and (3) strengthen the parental subsystem by emphasizing parental responsibilities and by challenging inappropriate alliances that weaken the parental subsystem.

In a family where the mother and father are dis-tant and disengaged from each other, the parental subsystem may have ceased to function as a dyad. The mother or father may have given a selected opposite-sex child the position in the parental subsystem that rightfully belongs to the spouse. The result may be family dysfunction in which the misplaced child is exploited and in which left-out siblings are resentful. In such an instance the structural therapist would intervene to alter distances and closeness between various members in an attempt to reestablish communication between the spouses and return the child to the subsystem with the other siblings (Nye and Bernardo, 1973).

Functional Concepts

Many functional aspects of family life have been dealt with by Murray Bowen (1971, 1974, 1976), who originally described his approach as part of systems theory but later became attentive to the emotional unity of the family. However, Bowen continued to accept the idea of the family as an operating system in which forces and counterforces are always present (Cain, 1980). Bowen's theory is directed toward the emotional functioning of families. He (1971b) delineated eight major concepts that may be applied to the assessment of family function: the nuclear family emotional system, differentiation of self, triangles, multigenerational transmission, family constellation, family projection, emotional cutoff, and societal regression.

NUCLEAR FAMILY EMOTIONAL SYSTEM   Bowen used the terms *undifferentiated ego mass* and *fusion* to describe nuclear families in which members do not see themselves as separate individuals but rather as

STRUCTURAL REALIGNMENT IN A MULTIGENERATIONAL FAMILY

Rosalie was a teenage mother who chose not to marry the father of her child. Because Rosalie wanted to finish high school, she lived at home and relinquished the care of her baby to her mother. Rosalie was a good student who was eager to return to school and to resume some of the social activities she had enjoyed before the birth of the baby. At the same time she was dismayed to find that her mother took full charge of the infant, making all decisions and indicating to Rosalie that the girl was incapable of taking proper care of the baby. Rosalie had expected that having a baby would make her more mature and independent. Instead she discovered that both she and her baby were being treated as children. The conflict between Rosalie and her mother over the baby became evident to the nurse in charge of the well baby clinic where the health of the infant was supervised. Aware of the struggle, the nurse began to deal with Rosalie's mixed feelings about motherhood and with the reluctance of the older woman to accept her proper place as grandmother and relate to Rosalie as the baby's mother.

When Rosalie brought the baby to the clinic, the nurse tried to reinforce her confidence in handling the baby. At the same time the nurse acknowledged the contribution that Rosalie's own mother was making. Because the grandmother had moved into the position of mother to her granddaughter as well as to Rosalie, positions in the family were confused. Generational boundaries were unclear because the grandmother related to the baby in a way that excluded Rosalie, who needed help in order to finish high school but resented the price her mother exacted. It became the objective of the clinic nurse to define responsibilities in the family in order to reduce conflict. In attempting this the nurse supported the contributions of the grandmother as teacher and advisor for Rosalie. The nurse also encouraged Rosalie to perform mothering tasks while seeking guidance and support from her mother. The nurse's interventions produced some structural changes in the family that are illustrated in the accompanying family maps.

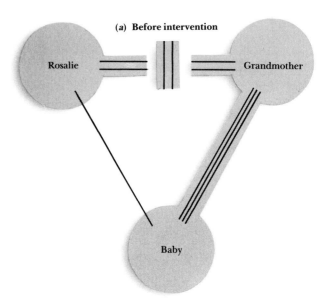

(a) Before intervention

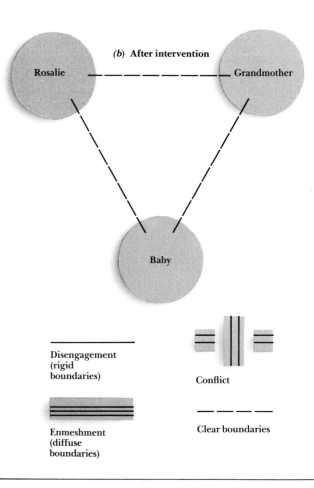

(b) After intervention

Disengagement (rigid boundaries)

Enmeshment (diffuse boundaries)

Conflict

Clear boundaries

Figure 18-3. Bowen's
differentiation of self scale.

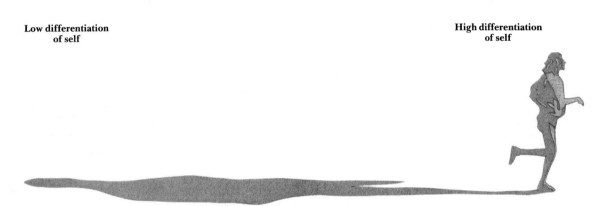

**Low differentiation
of self**

**High differentiation
of self**

Pseudoself

Automatic responses
Subjective reactions
Emotional dependence
Low self-identity
High vulnerability to stress
High incidence of illness
Prone to recurrent crisis

Solid self

Self-directed
Objective reactions
Rational
Flexible
High self-identity
Good coping skills
Lower incidence of illness

joined or fused to each other. When emotional fusion exists among family members, it is difficult for them to distinguish between thinking and feeling. As a consequence, they manage rational processes rather poorly. Irrationality then impairs their ability to handle life's problems.

DIFFERENTIATION OF SELF   Central to Bowen's theory is the importance of *self-differentiation*, which requires that individuals distance themselves from the emotional system of their family of origin. Self-differentiation does not forbid ongoing interaction between adult family members and their family of origin, but it does mean that the emotional forces of the original family do not dominate members.

In explaining the concept of differentiation of self Bowen made a distinction between "solid self" and "pseudoself." He developed a continuum called the differentiation of self scale, with the solid self at one end and the pseudoself at the other (see Figure 18-3). All individuals fall at some point on the continuum, depending on the amount of self-differentiation they have attained. One's position on the continuum is not static but may move in either direction during a lifetime.

The solid self is made up of rational, firmly held principles and attitudes that are deeply ingrained. The solid self evolves gradually and may change as an individual learns or fails to learn from life experiences. Because the solid self depends on rational thinking and is an intrinsic part of the personality, it does not succumb to pressure from external sources. The pseudoself, on the other hand, lacks intrinsic values and therefore must depend on and respond to external emotional influences. Individuals who have managed to separate only slightly from domination by the emotional system of their family of origin are likely to be located near the pseudoself end of the differentiation of self continuum. They have a propensity to react emotionally rather than cognitively and to exhibit greater degrees of emotional fusion with others. Thus, in appraising relative amounts of solid self and pseudoself in individuals, Bowen first determines whether individuals react on a feeling or a thinking level.

Use of the differentiation of self scale is helpful in assessing individuals and family units. Having made an assessment of self-differentiation (even though this is an impressionistic rather than an ex-

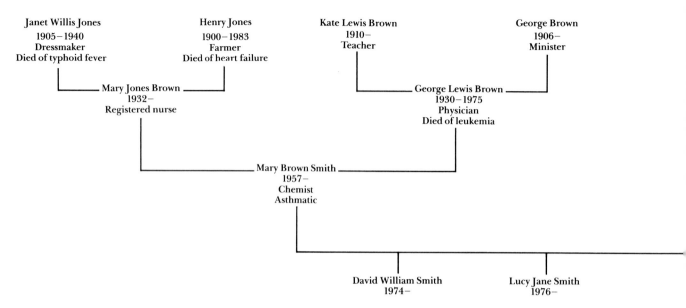

Figure 18-4. Example of a geneogram.

act measurement), the practitioner can begin to develop goals directed toward helping family members separate themselves from the emotional fusion and undifferentiation that contribute to dysfunction. However, Bowen points out that the differentiation of self scale should be used to examine family patterns over extended periods rather than to assess at a particular point in time.

It is useful to obtain a complete family history to ascertain the extent of self-differentiation in individuals and in the family. For this reason it is advisable for the family therapist to construct a *geneogram* that traces family events over several generations. Demographic data regarding family illnesses, longevity, occupations, and lifestyles all help the practitioner develop a geneogram that is informative and helpful in developing goals for clients who have failed to differentiate from the family of origin. A sample geneogram is shown in Figure 18-4.

The nuclear family emotional system and self-differentiation are complementary. Every person brings to marriage and long-term relationships remnants of behaviors and attitudes learned in the family of origin. Thus, as a matter of habit one partner may naturally assume a dominant role in the relationship while the other partner accepts a subservient role. When this kind of interaction is prolonged, the less dominant member may become unable to function autonomously. Because one partner is overassertive, the second partner is overly passive. A state of homeostasis may exist for a time, but the intrusion of stressful events may threaten the fragile balance of the relationship. Changes may necessitate a more even distribution of power and responsibility in the family, but the two partners are likely to be unable to adapt. The illness of the more dominant partner, for example, may cause family disorganization when the passive spouse is faced with new responsibilities. In marriages where both partners compete for dominance, prolonged conflict may prevail. The conflict may be expressed in open hostility between the partners, in emotional distancing of the partners, or in the projection of conflict onto one or more of the children.

FAMILY PROJECTION In *family projection*, the anxiety of one or both parents is transmitted or projected to a child. The selected child is made the focus of attention, with one parent becoming overly protective and involved. Although the child may continue to function after a fashion, his or her psychological development is endangered, because it is difficult for the child to separate and differentiate from the parent who is so close. Even when the child's psychological development is not seriously impaired, the closeness of one parent may cost the child the affection of the second parent and the acceptance of siblings who resent the special position conferred on one of their number. An inevitable consequence of the family projection process is that the selected child does not remain in the sibling subsystem but is "triangled" or drawn into the parental subsystem in order to absorb the parents' negative feelings toward each other. Family projection is used by immature parents with poor self-differentiation in order to avoid dealing with actual issues. Bowen believes that children on whom parental anxiety and conflict are projected may be unable to move in the direction of establishing a solid self (Cain, 1980).

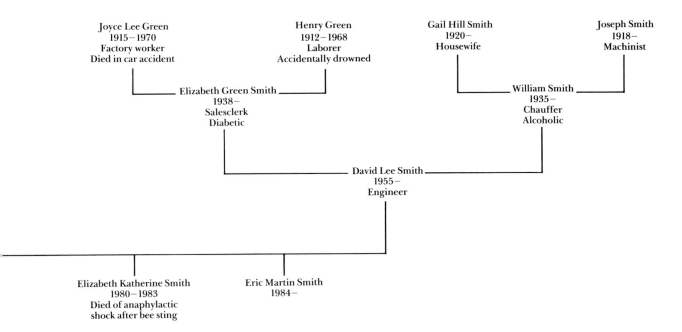

Joyce Lee Green
1915–1970
Factory worker
Died in car accident

Henry Green
1912–1968
Laborer
Accidentally drowned

Gail Hill Smith
1920–
Housewife

Joseph Smith
1918–
Machinist

Elizabeth Green Smith
1938–
Salesclerk
Diabetic

William Smith
1935–
Chauffer
Alcoholic

David Lee Smith
1955–
Engineer

Elizabeth Katherine Smith
1980–1983
Died of anaphylactic
shock after bee sting

Eric Martin Smith
1984–

EMOTIONAL CUTOFF Bowen (1976) used the concept of *emotional cutoff* to describe the detachment from one's family of origin that individuals must try to accomplish. When deep attachment to the family of origin continues even after the individual has established a new family of procreation, conditions of pseudoselfhood continue. This pattern of prolonged attachment and emotional dependency on the family of origin can become a source of contention between marital partners and can threaten the existence of the family of procreation. Bowen does not advise individuals to abandon their families of origin but rather to develop a solid sense of self that allows them to be autonomous in their thoughts and actions without feeling anxious and disloyal.

TRIANGLES According to Bowen, the triangle is the basic "molecule" of the family (Bowen, 1971b). Whenever the relationship between two people in a family becomes difficult, one person will pull in, or "triangle," a third party in order to relieve tension. A wife who sees her husband as detached or uncaring may turn to a son in order to fulfill her unmet needs. This exploits the son in many ways but reduces the anxiety of the mother and permits the father to continue his behavior. Often the father in such a situation is content with the status quo. Sometimes, however, the father resents his isolated position and moves toward the son, thereby becoming his wife's rival for the son's affection.

Triangulation is not confined to family members. The married man who takes a mistress has constructed a classic triangle, and the man who devotes most of his energy to his job creates a different kind of triangle. So has the woman who turns to alcohol to relieve marital boredom. In one case the apex of the triangle is the husband's job; in another case the apex of the triangle is the wife's alcoholism.

The solution to the dysfunctional family triangle is *detriangulation*. Bowen suggests that this be done by showing clients the difference between responding (acting in a manner that meets their own needs) and reacting (acting in a manner that meets the needs of others). For Bowen, reacting means being manipulated by others, whereas responding means being free to recognize the perspectives of other people but not to be ruled by this alone (Foley, 1974).

MULTIGENERATIONAL TRANSMISSION The concept of *multigenerational transmission* was anticipated by Freud in his description of the collective emotional life of families as allowing certain values to be perpetuated across generations (Anthony, 1971). As postulated by Bowen, movement toward one extreme or the other on the differentiation of self continuum can occur from one generation to the next. Progression or regression in one generation has an effect on succeeding generations, which also have the ability to reverse direction. After several generations of decreasing self-differentiation in families, mental disorders may become apparent in offspring made vulnerable by dysfunctional family patterns such as triangling or projection.

FAMILY CONSTELLATION The effects of sibling rank and order in the family were recognized by Toman (1976), who suggested that sibling positions, gender differences, and family configurations influence the personality characteristics and social

SOCIETAL REGRESSION DURING
THE GREAT DEPRESSION

The unemployed had been put to work on certain road jobs, to be built by the towns with a certain amount of state aid. The towns had no money, and state money would not be available until sometime in December. The result was that some of the men had as much as $300 due in back pay! In some towns the school teachers were actually on relief. Some of them hadn't received any money since last January. And before that their pay had been cut down to practically nothing. In one town they were going to close the schools, but the teachers, having no place to go and no way to earn a living, said they preferred to keep on

working—for food orders. Their offer was accepted . . .

Largely because it was handled by public officials, inexperienced and unsympathetic in their attitude, the relief administration in some places was awful. Weekly food orders were written out by men who apparently hadn't the slightest idea of the food needs of a family. Nor its other needs. It had never occurred to some of them that people need soap, for instance. One food order . . . contained, in fact, practically nothing except starch, a little fat, and a little molasses.

SOURCE: Richard Lowitt and Maureen Beasley, eds., *One Third of A Nation* (Chicago: University of Chicago, 1981), p. 39.

494

tendencies of offspring. Toman listed eight significant positions in addition to being an only child or one of twins:

Oldest brother of brother(s).

Youngest brother of brother(s).

Oldest brother of sister(s).

Youngest brother of sister(s).

Oldest sister of sister(s).

Youngest sister of sister(s).

Oldest sister of brother(s).

Youngest sister of brother(s).

Each of these positions is thought to be accompanied by certain behavioral and personality qualities.

The concept of sibling position does offer clues to the understanding of certain predispositions. One assumption is that children who are oldest siblings tend to feel responsible and to be somewhat directive, whereas those who are youngest siblings are apt to feel dependent and to accept direction. This concept is a broad generalization, however, and does not take into account relevant family events, past and present. As part of a tentative or provisional appraisal, the concept may be helpful, but careful validation is needed to recognize discrepancies and exceptions. Toman's work on family constellations and sibling positions may be used in assessing families, and his concepts have been incorporated into Bowen's formulations.

In constructing a family geneogram it is useful to ask what sibling position the spouses held in their respective families of origin, what responsibilities

and privileges were attached to various sibling positions, and what emotional reactions were aroused in them and in their siblings by these responsibilities and privileges. The wife who grew up as the oldest girl in a family with five younger boys is apt to have a different perception of family life than her husband who was the baby brother of five doting older sisters. Helping the partners to resolve discrepancies in their early experiences of family life is possible only after identifying the discrepancies. Utilizing the concept of sibling position can be an effective way of introducing this issue.

SOCIETAL REGRESSION Bowen suggested that society itself is an emotional system resembling the family. Just as families must struggle to deal with rationality versus emotionality, so society must work to avoid regressive, dysfunctional behavior. Under stressful conditions such as illness or loss, families become dysfunctional. Under stressful conditions such as crop failure, economic fluctuation, and environmental pollution, society becomes dysfunctional. The consequence is that legislative and administrative decisions are made on an emotional rather than a rational basis, so that problems are worsened rather than solved.

The concept of societal regression is important because all families are affected by conditions of the society in which they exist. Poverty, bureaucracy, and occupational and industrial obsolescence are only a few of the negative aspects of society that operate to transform functional families into dysfunctional ones. As advocates for families and as care providers for families, nurses should be informed about social and political developments in communities where they practice and should make

. . . today a great deal of misunderstanding has arisen in childrearing. In the belief that children go through phases (which they do) many parents adopt an attitude of Spartan endurance for the term of "the phase" in the expectation that spontaneous growth or evolution will take place at its conclusion. While it is true that each phase has its own characteristics, the progress through successive phases of development is largely influenced by the child's environment.

SELMA H. FRAIBERG (1959)

informed judgments about the logic and rationality of legislative and administrative actions.

Communication Concepts

Several theorists have devoted themselves to the application of communication concepts to family work. Communication theorists rarely conceptualize personality except in terms of communication and interaction. Their central purpose is to improve the ways in which families communicate, nonverbally as well as verbally. *How* messages are sent and received is just as important to communication theorists as the content of the messages that are transmitted.

DOUBLE BINDS A classic paper titled "Toward a Theory of Schizophrenia" proved to be of considerable importance in family theory and family therapy (Bateson et al., 1956). In this paper, Gregory Bateson and his colleagues made a distinction between situations in which it is possible to choose one course of action over another and situations in which options seem to be offered but no choice is available. The term they coined for these latter situations is *double bind*.

In a double bind transaction, a primary command or message is given followed by a secondary command or message that contradicts the first. The recipient of the message is in essence told, "Do not take this action or you will suffer consequences," followed by "Do take this action, for if you do not you will suffer consequences." For double bind messages to create the greatest harm to the recipient, the practice must occur repeatedly and the recipient must be unable to escape the situation.

Although the double bind concept grew out of observations of families with a schizophrenic mem-

ber, this phenomenon is also evident in many families that might appear to be quite functional; it is only after study of family interactional patterns that the double binding of one or more members is revealed. Because of their immaturity and dependency, children are often the target of double bind messages, although it may also be one of the spouses who is victimized in this fashion.

The secondary message in the double bind is often communicated nonverbally. For example, a mother might ask her young son to come to her for a kiss and then proceed to ward off his attention because his face or hands are dirty. Another example is provided by parents who consider themselves permissive, assuring their children that they are free to choose any occupation they wish, and who then show disappointment when a preference is expressed.

What do people do when they are constantly subjected to double binds? First they suspect that something mysterious is happening to them that they could figure out if they just tried hard enough. But the more they ruminate about their situation, the more confused they become. Some of them adopt the attitude that since nothing makes sense, why bother trying to understand anything. Others react by becoming rigid and literal in their thoughts and actions as they try to obey every command given them, no matter how paradoxical the commands become. Still others give up so completely that they withdraw from interpersonal involvement, thus avoiding confusion and entrapment (Watzlawick, Beaven, and Jackson, 1967).

The concept of the double bind has proven quite useful in family therapy (Wynne, 1978). Because double bind transactions are often beyond the

The child will be slapped and scolded if he tries to break the bars of his crib, bangs his head, throws his bottles around, spills his milk, throws his toys on the floor, etc. If, on the other hand, he is quiet, can be left alone in his room for long periods, doesn't get in anyone's way, doesn't "bug" anyone, he will be ignored. Thus the child learns that his parents will give him strokes (i.e. recognition) for being bad and forget that he exists if he is good. And now he is in a quandary. If he is recognized, he hurts; but if he does nothing to deserve a spanking or scolding, and that is the only way he can attract his parents' attention, he is lonely—and loneliness is infinitely more painful.

ROBERT GOULDING (1972)

496

awareness of family members, senders and receivers alike, caregivers are in a position to identify contradictory messages and to offer feedback to correct the confusion. Recognizing double binds and helping families clarify messages are activities within the scope of nurses who have had sufficient opportunity to observe and assess family communication patterns (Smoyak, 1975).

COMMUNICATION AND COGNITION   Jackson and Lederer (1967) consider communication to be the means by which homeostatic balance is maintained in families. They have noted that families operate within certain limits. That is, even though families interact and communicate in dynamic ways, their transactions are governed by certain norms and patterns. Theirs is a cognitive approach to the analysis of communication patterns.

One notable family characteristic they identified is *equifinality*, which refers to the idea that the same assessment of a family will be made regardless of when the assessment is made. Take, for example, a marriage in which the wife is at first a reckless spendthrift and the husband is a frugal planner. Over time, the behavior of each partner changes so that the partners' attitudes toward spending become reversed. After decades together, the husband and wife have exchanged positions, but family homeostasis has been maintained because the marriage continues to consist of a spendthrift and a saver. The frugality of one partner perpetuates the extravagance of the other, regardless of the identity of either partner. Equifinality thus reveals the reciprocal nature of family transactions. In other marriages the passivity of one partner makes possible and reinforces the dominance of the other.

One therapy technique advocated by Jackson (1968) is *relabeling*. This strategy consists of taking behavior that is considered negative by the family and emphasizing its positive aspects. For example, in a family with a school nonachiever whose parents are angry and impatient, the therapist might interpret the child's behavior as a self-sacrificing effort to distract the attention of parents from their disillusionment with each other. In another context, a violent argument between husband and wife might be interpreted as a dysfunctional attempt to get closer to each other.

COMMUNICATION AND POWER   Jay Haley (1971) has focused on power tactics between family members. In most human relationships, power is a troublesome issue, regardless of whether it is equally or unequally shared. Haley has referred to unequal relationships between individuals as being *complementary* and to equal relationships as being *symmetrical*. In complementary relationships the participants tend to assume superior versus inferior positions; in symmetrical relationships competition for dominance often develops.

Haley has also categorized communication into two levels. Content, or *what* is said, constitutes one level. Process, or *how* things are said, constitutes another level. Tone of voice, body language, inflection, and tempo are all aspects of the communication process that deserve attention.

Haley considers family therapists to be referees in the power struggle between family members. In his view, dysfunction is not the fault of any one family member but rather a property of the whole unit. Therapy, according to Haley (1971, 1973, 1976) is a process in which the therapist assumes

---

FAMILY CHRONOLOGY

1950–1973 Richard Grant was born and raised in California. He has two older sisters. His father is a practicing lawyer and his mother manages a dress shop.

1955–1973 Rosemary Cooper was born and raised in Cleveland, Ohio. After high school she attended a business college, where she earned an associate degree. Her father died the year Rosemary found her first job. Rosemary is an only child.

1973–1975 Richard graduated from college and began working for an insurance company. He attended a sales conference in Cleveland, where Rosemary was working as a secretary. The couple met when Rosemary was assigned to help Richard finish a report.

1975–1977 Rosemary and Richard corresponded and saw each other as much as possible. They were married in June 1977 and moved to California.

1978 Rosemary's mother had a stroke and she returned to Cleveland to look after her mother. The stay lasted eight months and although he visited occasionally Richard became increasingly unhappy with the separation.

1979 Rosemary became pregnant and agreed to return to California if her mother could come live with her. Twin boys were born in November 1979. The first year after the birth was hectic but the couple managed well by sharing parenting tasks.

1981 Richard left the insurance company to go into business for himself. The move was financially successful, but Richard was absent from home much of the time.

1982–1983 Rosemary and her mother, who still lived with the couple, formed a coalition that excluded Richard. Rosemary often felt torn between her mother and her husband, who did not get along well with each other. She felt lonely at times, was impatient with her sons, and resented Richard's absences from home. Richard was proud of the way he had provided for his family, was devoted to his sons, was resentful of his mother-in-law's presence, and worried about Rosemary, who did not seem like the bright, confident young woman he had married.

1984 At Richard's insistence, the couple went to a marriage counselor to try, in Richard's words, to "revitalize the marriage."

control of family interactions by guiding, teaching, and interpreting in a benevolent but directive fashion. The therapist should also educate or enlighten the family about its internal struggles.

COMMUNICATION AND EMOTION Like Haley, Virginia Satir (1967) has assessed communication and interaction in families. But unlike Haley, she has not been interested in power struggles; rather, she has focused on the way family members feel about one another. Satir's approach brings an empathy to family work that is absent from the work of many other communication theorists. This empathetic quality makes her interventions very compatible with the nursing process.

It is Satir's contention that the husband and wife are the architects of the family and that the causes of dysfunction lie in their relationship. Assessment therefore begins with the marital dyad. Satir's assumption is that at one point in their lives the partners both thought their mutual needs would be met through their relationship. Therefore, it is important to take a family history or chronology dealing with how the partners met, what their expectations of marriage were, and what memories they have of their early years together. Gathering a family chronology has two benefits: it traces the divergent memories and expectations of the partners, and diverts the partners from current feeling of hostility as they recall happier times (Satir, Stachwiak, and Taschman, 1977). A sample chronology is provided in the accompanying box.

SELF-ESTEEM A basic tenet of Satir's approach is that low self-esteem is the fundamental problem in dysfunctional marriages, not sexuality. In rela-

Table 18-4. Types of Dysfunctional Communication

Type	Purpose
Blaming	Family members are fearful of being blamed and therefore attribute responsibility for error or failure to others.
Placating	Family members adopt a pretense of being inadequate but well meaning in order to preserve peace at any price.
Generalizing	Family members make global statements using terms like *always* and *never* instead of dealing with specific issues or problems.
Computing	Family members emphasize cognitive and literal transactions, ignoring emotional issues in order to appear in control and fully reasonable.
Distracting	Family members introduce irrelevant details into problematic issues in order to avoid functional problem solving.

SOURCE: Adopted from Satir (1967).

498

tionships where the self-esteem of one of the partners is threatened, rising levels of anxiety and aggressiveness appear in their transactions. Children are often brought into the world as a way of increasing the self-esteem of the parents. This may become a heavy burden for the child who cannot live up to unrealistic parental expectations.

In order to acquire adequate self-esteem, children need physical care, continuity of relationships, parental consistency, and reassurance that they are valued for themselves rather than for their accomplishments. If these qualities were markedly deficient in the family of origin, they are likely to be deficient in the family of procreation as well.

Three ideas are basic to Satir's approach to family assessment and intervention:

1. Everyone wants to survive, to grow, and to be close to other significant people. All behavior, however bizarre it may seem, is directed toward these ends.

2. Behavior that appears to be "sick" or "crazy" is usually an effort to transmit distress signals to others.

3. Thoughts and emotions are closely connected; to understand thinking one must get in touch with what oneself and others are feeling.

COMMUNICATION PATTERNS One result of failure to maintain the self-esteem of family members, particularly between the partners, is that unclear, ambiguous communication patterns develop (Satir, 1967). According to Satir, family members should be able to express their needs and feelings openly but with regard for the needs and feelings of other members. She has identified several dysfunctional ways in which families communicate. These are described in Table 18-4.

In order to assess family communication patterns, Satir uses a *sociogram*—a technique for noting the frequency and direction of messages sent between family members. After a family meeting has ended, the health professional can diagram the spatial positions of family members, who spoke to whom and how often, and who failed to speak to other family members. An example of a communication sociogram is shown in Figure 18-5. This tool can be used for evaluation as well as assessment purposes. If a sociogram is developed soon after every family session, it is possible to note changes in communication patterns that occurred as family intervention proceeded.

Although sociograms are helpful in permitting the professional to recall communication direction and frequency more accurately, they have some deficiencies. Unless the sessions are videotaped and later analyzed or there is a skilled observer taking notes, total accuracy is impossible. As an impressionistic measurement, however, the sociogram has definite advantages.

Sociograms can also be used as reminders of the qualitative differences in family communication. The following qualitative aspects of family communication should be part of the assessment process:

1. How are messages transmitted in the family? Directly? Indirectly?

2. How are disagreements dealt with in the family? By avoidance? By confrontation? By negotiation?

Figure 18-5. A sample sociogram. Each arrow represents communication from one person to another. The daughter, for example, communicated four times more frequently to the son than the son to the daughter.

499

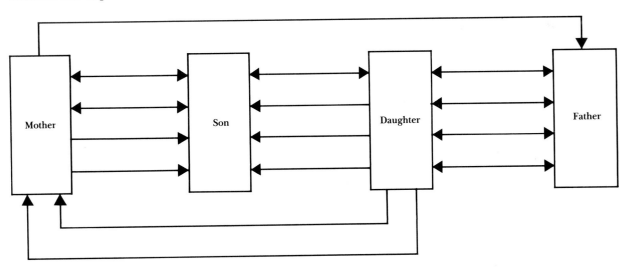

3. What subjects are not discussed by the family?

4. What issues absorb the attention of the family?

Communication theorists believe that communication can be a major assessment, implementation, and evaluation tool in working with individuals and families—a belief that has particular applicability for nurses. Any message, verbal or nonverbal, that occurs in the presence of another person reveals something about the nature of their relationship. Only the more sophisticated professionals need decide whether power, emotion, or cognition is the most significant influence in family communication. The generalist nurse can be effective merely by using and understanding basic principles of communication theory and by learning to observe carefully and listen actively to the multiple levels on which communication takes place.

Learning Theory Concepts

Social learning is an ongoing process in which people teach others how to behave. The teaching is accomplished through reward and punishment methods that have the power to perpetuate or alleviate dysfunctional behavior (O'Neill, 1980). Although strict behaviorists such as B. F. Skinner believe that behavior can be reduced to simple stimulus-response patterns (Carpenter, 1974), most learning theorists are more apt to recognize the impact of intervening influences.

Human beings have the capacity to interpret events in an individualistic manner. This means that the same event will be perceived differently by different people, because people who share the same physical environment inhabit an internal symbolic environment that is entirely their own (Mead, 1933; Speigel, 1971). Human beings also have the capacity to analyze their own actions and to understand the reactions of other people. This means that people can predict the behavior of others at least some of the time and can modify their own behavior based on these predictions. To understand how this operates one has only to compare the behavior of schoolchildren when an experienced, organized teacher is present and the behavior of the same children when an unfamiliar, insecure substitute teacher enters their classroom.

In attempting to promote change in families, the nurse enacts a social learning role not simply by teaching appropriate behaviors but by modeling them. Instead of telling the family how to interact, the nurse can demonstrate desirable ways of interacting with one another. In family meetings the nurse should not become the ally of any single coalition or subsystem but should recognize the existence of all subsystems and coalitions. The nurse may agree or disagree with family members, indicating by these actions that it is acceptable to express one's opinions. Without relying on verbal directives, the nurse models a more functional way of interacting.

As has been noted by various family theorists, a great deal of human behavior is learned in the family of origin and transferred to the family of procreation. If conditions in the more recently established family are such that the old behaviors are rewarded, there is no doubt that they will continue. If in the family of origin an action taken in response to certain stimuli has been rewarded, similar stimuli will tend to produce the same behavior. For example, a young woman who becomes accustomed to functioning in a managerial role in her family of origin and who has enjoyed a reputation for competence will try to perform the same role in her family of procreation, especially if she receives positive rewards from her husband and children. If, however, her executive functions are resented by her new family, she will undoubtedly be disappointed. Disappointment over not being rewarded may lead her to modify her managerial tendencies, but this is likely to happen only if family members are able to express their feelings and she is willing to listen. If she does not receive expected rewards, she may react with anger and disapproval. Such feelings may lead to avoidance of appropriate role enactment or to retaliation against family members who have not provided the expected rewards. If she is aggressive enough, she will retain the executive role in the family, but other members will experience mounting tension in the form of unexpressed resentment.

In this example, the young woman became accustomed to enacting a role that was rewarded in her family of origin. In other words, she learned to behave in a way that was appreciated and therefore reinforced in that family. The most powerful reinforcers in family life are social. For most people a smile, an expression of approval, an embrace, or a touch is enormously effective in promoting social learning. Single episodes of reinforcement are unlikely to have sustained impact, but repeated reinforcement can have profound effects on human expectations and behavior (Patterson, 1975; Bandura, 1977).

Roles are an important aspect of family theory. Roles can be analyzed in terms of status or position (structure) and performance or enactment (function). In families roles may be assigned or ascribed to certain individuals by reason of the position they hold in the family. The husband/father role is assigned to the person who completes the marital dyad and sires the children. A number of functions are expected from the person who fills this role. Not too many years ago, it was a common expectation that the husband/father would be the primary breadwinner and that major family decisions would be his to make. In present-day families the husband/father may or may not be present in the home. When he is physically absent, many role functions formerly assigned to him are discharged by the mother, perhaps with the help of older children. When role functions are performed by family members not usually associated with enactment of that particular role, this is called *achieved* rather than *assigned* role performance (Parsons, 1951; Lambert and Lambert, 1984).

Variations in the structure of contemporary families have lessened emphasis on assigned roles in favor of achieved roles. This pattern may be necessary, but it often introduces new problems. One danger is that a single parent trying to fill two roles may become overwhelmed by responsibility (Franklin and Hibbs, 1980). Another danger is that immature family members may be pushed into achieved roles for which they are not ready, and resolution of critical life cycle tasks may not be handled as well as they might be. Maturation, readiness, aptitude, and experience are factors that affect adequate role performance. These considerations are sometimes overlooked in single-parent families, dual-career families, and families where the partners are not in agreement concerning role expectations. Men who have grown up in traditional families of origin where tasks were assigned on the basis of gender differentiation may cling to familiar patterns in households where both partners hold jobs outside the home (Janosik, 1984).

Table 18-5 summarizes the learning approach along with the several other approaches to family theory that have been discussed in this chapter.

Table 18-5. Approaches to Family Theory

Conceptual Approach	Representative Theorists	Concepts	Nursing Process Actions
Developmental theory	Erikson Duvall	Individual life cycle tasks Family life cycle tasks	1. Identify stage-specific individual tasks. 2. Identify stage-specific family tasks. 3. Recognize impediments to resolution of individual and family tasks. 4. Help families identify and reduce impediments to individual and family task resolution.
General systems theory	Von Bertalanffy	Interdependence Boundaries Feedback	1. Emphasize interdependence of all members to avoid placing blame on any one member. 2. Help families acknowledge circular effects of their actions on all members. 3. Promote boundary maintenance that protects the family from excessive input from external sources. 4. Promote boundary maintenance that allows the family adequate input from external sources. 5. Encourage families to recognize the reciprocal effects of their actions on all members.
Psychodynamic theory	Freud Wynne Lidz	Collective family psyche Pseudomutuality Pseudohostility Rubber fences Marital schism and skew	1. Identify significant family attitudes and values. 2. Differentiate genuine harmony from surface harmony (pseudomutuality). 3. Differentiate conflict around authentic issues from conflict used to avoid authentic issues (pseudohostility). 4. Help families establish consistent, functional family boundaries. 5. Discourage excessive closeness between a parent and a selected child. 6. Strengthen the relationship between the partners.

Structural theory	Minuchin	Boundaries
		  Clear
		  Rigid
		  Diffuse
		Subsystems
		  Parental
		  Sibling
		Scapegoating
		Family mapping
			1. Use a family map to show emotional closeness and distance between members and family organizational structure.
			2. Identify boundary characteristics.
			3. Promote clear, functional boundaries between members.
			4. Help the family realize that the symptoms of the identified client may be keeping the family together.
			5. Encourage family members to reduce their preoccupation with the symptoms of the identified client.
			6. Restructure family positions so that parents form a parental dyad and children form a sibling subsystem.

Functional theory	Bowen
	Toman
		Family emotional systems
		Differentiation of self
		  Pseudoself
		  Solid self
		Geneograms
		Family projection
		Emotional cutoff
		Multigenerational transmission
		Family constellation
		  Sibling position
		Societal regression
			1. Promote separation and individuation of members in nuclear families.
			2. Encourage rational rather than irrational thoughts and behaviors.
			3. Attempt to modify inappropriate family triangles.
			4. Help families avoid placing any child in a special position in relation to a parent.
			5. Assess family direction across generations toward or away from developing a solid self (rational) or pseudoself (irrational).
			6. Teach families the effects of age, gender, and rank order on the behavior and development of adults and children.

(continued)

501

Table 18-5. *Continued*

Conceptual Approach	Representative Theorists	Concepts	Nursing Process Actions
Functional theory			7. Encourage encounters with family of origin that foster autonomy and differentiation of adult members. 8. Help families cope with stressful environmental conditions such as unemployment, poverty, overcrowding, and environmental pollution. 9. Formulate a geneogram showing marriages, births, deaths, and other events across generations.

Communication theory	Bateson
	Jackson and Lederer
	Haley
	Satir
		Double binds
		Equifinality
		Symmetrical relationships
		Complementary relationships
		Dysfunctional communication
		  Blaming
		  Placating
		  Generalizing
		  Distracting
		  Computing
		Self-esteem
		Family chronology
		Family sociogram
			1. Reinforce self-esteem of all members.
			2. Use relabeling techniques to interpret behaviors in a positive way.
			3. Analyze communication in terms of cognition (thinking), power (control), and emotion (feeling).
			4. Encourage specific, clear messages.
			5. Help families identify behaviors that reinforce or complement each other (dominant wife/passive husband).
			6. Help families identify behaviors that are symmetrical or parallel (spouses compete for nurture/spouses compete for dominance).
			7. Formulate a family chronology or history of events.
			8. Develop family sociograms showing the frequency and direction of communication between members.

Learning theory	Skinner Mead Parsons	Stimulus-response Interactional symbolism Role expectations Role performance Rewards	1. Use operant behavioral concepts to modify behavior. 2. Identify and apply intervening variables to reinforce or reduce socially learned behavior. 3. Help families recognize how inappropriate role expectations and role performance increase family dysfunction. 4. Teach families appropriate ways of rewarding desirable behaviors.

SOME PRACTICALITIES IN FAMILY INTERVENTION

This chapter has presented an overview of major approaches to assessing and assisting families. Some of the concepts are quite sophisticated, but many are relatively simple and can be used safely by generalist nurses. Assessment of family needs is within the scope of every nurse, but it is essential for generalist nurses to consult with colleagues prepared on the graduate level before offering family intervention. If consultation and supervision are available, an experienced generalist nurse may undertake family intervention around a specific problem. Otherwise a referral for family intervention is more appropriate.

Family theory is a fairly new field, and systematic and clinical investigation continues at a rapid rate. Nevertheless, there are some established guidelines to help nurses as they begin to enter this complex field.

THE INITIAL INTERVIEW Families who seek professional help have already made a difficult decision. They are anxious, they are confused, and they are afraid of what may be revealed in family sessions. A good rule is for the nurse to discover first what the family's perception of the problem is. This should be one of the goals of an initial family meeting.

The initial interview is primarily a time for getting acquainted with the family members who are present, for observing their interactions with one another, and for trying to reduce the levels of anxiety that are present. It is important to know who initiated the referral. Was a recommendation made by another professional or by a relative or neighbor, or was the contact initiated by a family member?

If the family behaves as if there is an identified patient who is the family problem, this is important to know.

The nurse should tell the family the purpose of the meeting and disclose enough identifying information to decrease the family's fears of the nurse as a powerful, intrusive stranger. It may even be appropriate for the professional to share some personal feelings regarding the family meeting. While trying to establish a calm, unhurried atmosphere, the nurse should also bring up contractual matters, such as how often they will meet and how long the sessions will last. If the family can tolerate exploration at the initial meeting, the nurse might ask what the members would like to accomplish as a result of the sessions. Usually some but not all the family members will respond to this request.

ORGANIZING DATA A great deal goes on at family meetings, and a number of tools have been suggested to organize data in a coherent way. The family map suggested by Minuchin, the geneogram adapted by Bowen, and the family chronology and sociogram devised by Satir are all useful mechanisms for data organization, especially in the early sessions.

When family members give inaccurate information, their distortion may not be deliberate but rather may indicate feelings of embarrassment or anxiety. Distortion can be reduced considerably if the nurse carefully avoids indications of shock or disapproval as information is given. Emotionally charged words should be avoided. Instead of asking what the family problem is, the nurse should simply ask, "What has been happening in the family to bring you here?" It is permissible and even desirable to refer to what was discussed at the previous meeting. Very often the most important data are not revealed until the very end of a session. Referring back to such unresolved issues is an excellent way to provide continuity from session to session and to demonstrate to the family that what they say is important.

WORKING PHASE As families begin to trust their therapist, they move into the working phase of the therapy. Even then, hazards persist, and many families find the prospect of change so difficult that they drop out of treatment. For families who continue to meet, it is necessary to continue to word questions carefully. Interpretations of statements and challenges of actions should be done in the form of suggestions or reflective comments. Examples of this strategy are: "How have things changed in the family since we've been meeting?" "You both may be right, but there is another way of looking at what happened." "I wonder whether you were really as hurt as you say you were. Is it possible that you were hurt and angry, too?"

TERMINATION SESSIONS Sometimes the family terminates the meetings prematurely and without the concurrence of the therapist. Even the most adept therapist cannot change the family. The therapist can only offer the family an opportunity to change; it is the family that decides whether or not to grasp the opportunity. A wide gulf may exist between what the family is willing to change and what the therapist would like to see changed. When there is discrepancy between the therapist's and the family's

CLINICAL EXAMPLE

███████████████████████

*FAMILY INTERVENTION FOR
A SCHOOL PHOBIC CHILD*

████████████████

Joshua is a bright, engaging six-year-old in the first grade. Shortly after the school year began, Joshua's father lost his job as a salesman and his mother accepted employment as a secretary. Previously, this had been a traditional family in which Joshua's father had been the family provider and his mother, the homemaker. Joshua is an only child, and he and his mother are very involved with each other.

The financial problems and role reversal created difficulties between the parents. At night, Joshua would go to sleep with the sound of parental quarreling in his ears and would awaken to the same noise. Sometimes he believed that his parents never slept but spent the entire night yelling at each other. Within a short time, he became reluctant to go to school. Although Joshua's father was available to care for the child during the day, Joshua began to cling to his mother, begging her not to go to work. After trying to reason with Joshua, his father would storm angrily from the house. By this time Joshua was hysterical, crying, retching, and out of control. His mother would then have to give up her plans to go to the office in order to stay home with the child. She missed so many days that her job was endangered. This increased the quarrels between the parents, which in turn aggravated Joshua's fears of leaving his mother. In desperation, Joshua's mother arranged a joint interview with the school nurse, the school psychologist, and Joshua's teacher.

ASSESSMENT

After interviewing Joshua, the nurse and psychologist arrived at the following nursing and psychiatric diagnoses for Joshua and his family:

Nursing Diagnoses
Anxiety: Moderate

Coping, ineffective individual

Coping, ineffective family: compromised

Family process, alteration in: roles

Fear

Multiaxial Psychiatric Diagnosis
Joshua:
Axis I   309.21   Separation anxiety disorder

Family:
Axis I   V61.10   Marital problem
          V61.20   Parent-child problem

Axis IV   Code 5—Severe

Axis V   Level 3—Good

A number of different theoretical approaches could be taken to assessing the situation of Joshua and his parents.

Developmental Approach
According to Erikson's psychosocial model, Joshua is at the stage of resolving the conflict between initiative and guilt. When his family life was untroubled, he was able to demonstrate initiative and growing competence as he entered school. He is aware that he has contributed to the problems between his parents, feels guilty about this, but does not know what to do to improve the situation. His solution is to cling to his mother, believing that if he goes to school, she might not return to him. The family is at the school-age stage of its expanding period. It is a traditional family whose major developmental tasks are threatened by economic reverses caused by the father's joblessness and the role reversal of the parents.

Psychodynamic Approach
Psychodynamic theory explains Joshua's situation in terms of the need to resolve the Oedipal conflict: giving up close attachment to his mother in order to identify with his father. This task is impeded by problems between his parents. Joshua feels frightened and anxious because of changes in the home. His behavior has regressed to early levels in order to obtain the gratification that he needs from his mother. In this family the collective expectation of all the members was that roles would continue to be performed in accustomed ways. When circumstances made this impossible, the parents resorted to regressive behaviors as well. This has perpetuated and aggravated Joshua's anxiety.

General Systems Approach
Every family member acts and reacts in ways that affect all other members. Boundaries protect families from excessive input from the surrounding environment but can be penetrated by outside influences and events. An example of external input in Joshua's case is the joblessness of his father and the need for his mother to become the primary wage earner. Disagreement between the parents has increased Joshua's feelings of stress and has led to somatic complaints that allow him to stay home from school to make sure that he will not be abandoned by his mother. Staying home from school has solved Joshua's immediate problem temporarily but has added to the rising levels of tension within the family system.

Structural Approach

Joshua's fear of going to school is not only an effort to avoid losing his mother but also an attempt to reconcile his parents. Some of his behavior is motivated by a wish to keep his parents together even though the result of his actions is to keep his mother home and to drive his father from the house. The absence of his father is more acceptable than the absence of his mother, since his father's absence has been the usual pattern. Over the years Joshua's mother had been overly involved with Joshua (enmeshed) and underinvolved with his father (disengaged). This structural pattern became inoperative when more cooperation between the parents was required. Family subsystems were not functional because Joshua had become an intruder into the marital subsystem. This structural alignment was not disruptive to the family until it became necessary for the parents to behave in a different way toward each other and for Joshua to move toward the family position that is appropriate for his age, a position equidistant from both mother and father.

Functional Approach

Conflict between the parents has been generated by their emotional reaction to changed patterns in the family. In their respective families of origin, both parents had been accustomed to sex role differentiation. When their roles became reversed, Joshua's mother and father responded emotionally rather than rationally. Joshua's position as an only child had contributed to the fusion between him and his mother. Separating from her to begin school would have been difficult in any case, but it was aggravated by the fact that Joshua is part of a family triangle and the marital dyad is not a functioning unit. Joshua's father and mother have blamed each other for the conflict. This conflict has been projected onto Joshua and absorbed by him. His mother and father have not been able to separate emotionally from their traditional-minded families of origin in order to accept the joblessness of the father and the economic contributions of the mother in a rational rather than irrational manner.

Communication Approach

Loss of his job has resulted in lowered self-esteem for Joshua's father. When Joshua's mother went to work, she did not see this as an accomplishment but as an indication that she had made an unwise choice when she married and that she could no longer enact the role of a "good" mother. When her husband had been the primary provider, she gave him the respect that she believed was due him. When he lost his job, she made no effort to provide emotional support. Her major concern was the welfare of her son and the threats to her own self-image. Joshua's father has been so preoccupied with his feelings of inadequacy that he has not acknowledged the contributions his wife is making to keep the family solvent. As a result, endless blaming, tirades, and reproaches have characterized family communication. Instead of viewing the dilemma as a family problem in which everyone has a responsibility to cope, each parent

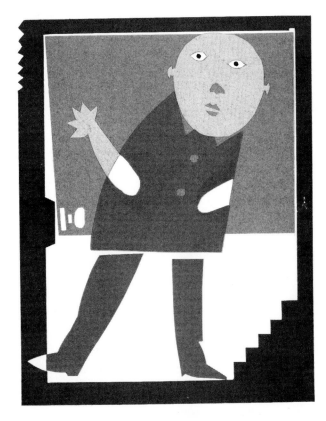

has thought only of his or her own deprivation. Joshua, in particular, has been the victim of double bind messages. He has been told by both parents that he should attend school. Yet he also knows that his mother resents working and wants to stay at home. Verbally Joshua is given one message; behaviorally his mother sends another message. Joshua's phobic behavior toward going to school is his way of dealing with the entrapment of such double bind messages.

Learning Approach

The fear of leaving his mother to begin first grade would probably have been present to some extent in Joshua even if family problems had been minimal. As circumstances have grown worse, discounted fears have emerged and have taken on the proportions of a school phobia. The phobic behavior is a learned response reinforced by parental reactions, especially the willingness of Joshua's mother to stay home with him. Even though his father is available to look after him, Joshua prefers the companionship of his mother. Joshua also knows that once his mother decides not to go to work, she is usually in good humor. It is acceptable for him to recover quickly as soon as this decision is made. With his angry father out of the house, Joshua and his mother can spend a pleasant day together.

PLANNING

Regardless of the approach chosen or the combination of approaches used by the nurse, the following questions facilitate planning:

505

1. What does the family identify as the major problem?

2. What are the developmental tasks of the family as a unit?

3. What are the developmental tasks of the individual members?

4. What changes occurred in the family shortly before the present problem emerged?

5. What reactions, other than the emergence of the major problem, followed recent changes in the family?

6. What is the composition of the family? What are the tasks or responsibilities expected of family members?

7. How are disagreements usually resolved in the family?

8. What has been done thus far to deal with the major problem identified by the family?

IMPLEMENTATION

Family therapists who are committed to one or two conceptual approaches often base their interventions on the approach being used. For a generalist nurse or a nurse therapist using an eclectic approach, the following interventions are useful with many families:

1. Ask the partners to describe their early relationship with each other, including how they met and what each found attractive in the other.

2. Ask the partners to describe and contrast their present relationship.

3. Ask the partners and other family members to explain what they think is happening in the family.

4. Promote functional communication by asking each member to speak only for himself or herself.

5. Comment on nonspecific statements that include words such as "always" and "never."

6. Encourage members to be less sure that they are always right. Suggest that they begin sentences with "I think" or "It seems to me." This will arouse less resentment in others.

7. Assure the family that change is difficult but can be an opportunity to grow.

8. Support the self-esteem of every family member.

9. Restructure the family by helping the partners move closer and by strengthening subsystems in which the children belong.

10. Help members see the identified problem as a family, not an individual, problem. This will encourage everyone to become involved in finding a solution.

EVALUATION

Outcome evaluation is possible only if goals are clear, attainable, and accepted by the family. In dealing with

Joshua's school phobia, the school nurse, psychologist, and teacher limited themselves to fairly simple goals. Long-range marital issues were not directly addressed. This would not have been in keeping with school policy, nor did the marital problems seem severe enough to warrant referral for additional help. Goals were based on the consensus of the family and the school personnel that the family problems were largely situational. The goals included:

1. Mother will go to her job every day unless herself is ill.

2. Joshua will attend school every day unless seen by a physician. If Joshua feels upset or ill in the morning, father will bring him to school as soon as Joshua recovers. Lateness will be excused by his teacher, but not absence.

3. Father will have responsibility for Joshua on school days and will not leave the house whenever Joshua complains of being too upset to go to school.

4. Father will take more time to look for another job while Joshua is at school and his wife is working.

5. Father will verbally recognize the help he receives from his wife and son as he looks for another job.

6. The parents will discuss day-to-day events without accusing each other or yelling so that Joshua can't sleep.

7. Two evenings a week will be devoted to inexpensive activities in which all members can participate, such as making popcorn or watching television.

8. One evening a week will be spent doing something Joshua and his father can do together, such as playing ball or making a model airplane.

The formulation of specific behavioral goals helped the parents modify their actions. Joshua was no longer able to manipulate his parents into letting him avoid school; this alone helped eliminate a source of contention between the parents. Although no direct attention was given to the relationship between the parents, the suggested behaviors helped bring them closer, increased Joshua's involvement with his father, and encouraged disengagement from his mother.

The support of school personnel was crucial, especially for Joshua's mother, who was apprehensive that her son might feel unloved and neglected. There was some restructuring of the family as Joshua and his father found common interests. As Joshua's father grew less critical of the way his mother treated Joshua, their relationship improved. Because the mother was accustomed to family patterns in which male members formed an alliance, she did not object to Joshua's new identification with his father. Eventually Joshua's father found suitable employment and his mother was able to resume her role as a full-time homemaker. She found that Joshua's new relationship with his father gave her time to pursue interests of her own, all within the context of traditional values to which this family was committed.

507

views on what should be altered, some agreement must be reached.

During the earlier family meetings, specific goals must be formulated so that the family has a sense of direction and a sense of achievement if the goals are reached. Without specific goals being negotiated, neither the family nor the therapist has standards by which to evaluate progress.

SUMMARY

Family theory and family therapy are based on the premise that dysfunction originates in the family rather than in the client. There is disagreement as to whether the family causes dysfunction or perpetuates it. Family therapy is a treatment modality that has developed within the last few decades and is widely used, but it demands special preparation from practitioners. However, a number of family concepts are available that may be used to advantage by generalist nurses adopting a family-focused approach to health care.

Because many of the early family theorists and therapists worked independently of one another, there is considerable overlap in their conceptual approaches. Some approaches are more compatible with nursing process than others, but most of them have some unique contribution to make. Seven conceptual approaches were described in this chapter: developmental theory, general systems theory, psychodynamic theory, structural theory, functional theory, communication theory, and learning theory.

Although early family theorists worked mostly with families that had a schizophrenic member, many of the dysfunctional patterns found in these families are present in families without any identified psychiatric disorder. Among the notable concepts from psychiatric theory that have contributed to the understanding of dysfunctional family dynamics are the double bind, rubber fences, pseudohostility, pseudomutuality, equifinality, and schismatic and skewed families.

The communication theorists offer concepts that are especially compatible with nursing process, since effective communication is a skill well within the scope of the generalist nurse. Communication theorists disagree to some extent in their focus. Jackson and Lederer have emphasized communication and cognition, Haley has emphasized communication and power, and Satir has emphasized communication and emotion. It is not necessary for nurses to choose among these three emphases. However, the empathetic qualities of Satir's approach make it very compatible with nursing process and nursing interventions.

A number of methods have been devised to help professionals working with families collect and organize data. Minuchin developed the technique of family mapping to show the structural characteristics of family organization. General systems theorists emphasized the influence of circular feedback and the interdependence of the family as an operating system. Bowen, a theorist who viewed the family as an emotional system, proposed eight concepts that support his insistence on personal autonomy and emotional separation from the family of origin.

Learning theory augments the contributions of other conceptual approaches to family work. Changing role expectations and structural variations in present-day families help explain some causes of conflict in families. Assessment of role expectations and structural organization can help nurses understand reasons for conflict when people raised in traditional families of origin find themselves in nontraditional families of procreation.

Family therapy requires advanced preparation from its practitioners, but family interventions are within the scope of generalist nurses who have a basic knowledge of family theory. Attrition rates are high in family therapy, but the nurse who can sustain a climate of nonjudgmental acceptance is more apt to forestall premature termination. Even the most experienced family therapist cannot alter family interactional patterns unless the family is willing to change. When there is disagreement between the family and the therapist regarding goals, accommodation is necessary to resolve areas of dispute. Without specific goals being set, neither the family nor the therapist has a sense of direction or standards by which to evaluate progress.

508

Review Questions

1. How might individual and family life cycle tasks be used as a basis for assessment?

2. Describe what is meant by the interdependence of family members, using systems theory terminology.

3. Explain the difference between pseudomutuality and pseudohostility in families.

4. Using a diagram, illustrate clear boundaries, rigid boundaries, and diffuse boundaries in a family. What are the effects of these diverse boundaries on family members?

5. What is a family subsystem? What function do subsystems perform in a family?

6. What are the major differences between pseudoself and solid self? Which is considered more functional?

7. Explain the concept of triangling. Give an example of a family triangle.

8. What is a double bind? How does it affect family members?

9. Identify three types of dysfunctional communication in families and describe situations in which they may be used.

10. Contrast assigned and achieved roles in terms of role expectations and role performance.

References

Anthony, J. R. 1971. An Introduction to Family Group Therapy. In *Comprehensive Group Psychotherapy*, eds.

H. I. Kaplan and B. J. Sadock. Baltimore: Williams & Wilkins.

Bandura, A. 1977. *Social Learning Theory*. Englewood Cliffs, N.J.: Prentice-Hall.

Bateson, G.; Jackson, D. D.; Haley, J.; and Weakland, J. H. 1956. Toward a Theory of Schizophrenia. *Behavioral Science*, 1:251–264.

Bohannon, P. 1980. Marriage and Divorce. In *Comprehensive Textbook of Psychiatry*, 3rd ed., eds. H. I. Kaplan, A. M. Freedman, and B. J. Sadock. Baltimore: Williams & Wilkins.

Bowen, M. 1965. Family Psychotherapy with Schizophrenia in the Hospital and in Private Practice. In *Intensive Family Therapy*, eds. I. Boszormenyi-Nagy and J. Framo. New York: Harper & Row.

Bowen, M. 1971a. Family and Family Group Psychotherapy. In *Comprehensive Group Psychotherapy*, eds. H. I. Kaplan and B. J. Sadock. Baltimore: Williams & Wilkins.

Bowen, M. 1971b. The Use of Family Theory in Clinical Practice. In *Changing Families*, ed. J. Haley. New York: Grune & Stratton.

Bowen, M. 1974. Toward the Differentiation of Self in One's Family of Origin. In *Georgetown Family Symposia: A Collection of Selected Papers*, eds. F. Andres and J. Loria. Washington, D. C.: Georgetown University, 1974.

Bowen, M. 1976. Theory in the Practice of Psychotherapy. In *Family Therapy*, ed. P. Guerin. New York: Gardner.

Brown, J. A. C. 1967. *Freud and the Post-Freudians*. Baltimore: Pelican Books.

Cain A. 1980. Assessment of Family Structure. In *Family-Focused Care*, eds. J. R. Miller and E. H. Janosik. New York: McGraw-Hill.

Carpenter, F. 1974. *The Skinner Primer: Beyond Freedom and Dignity*. New York: Free Press.

Carter, E. A., and McGoldrick, M., eds. 1980. *The Family Life Cycle*. New York: Gardner.

Cohen, M. W.; Younger, R.; and Sullivan, J. M. 1983. Treating the Family of Chronically Emotionally Impaired Adults. *The Family Therapist*, 4(1):2–12.

Collins, G., 1984. A Dean of Pediatricians Looks at Today's Family. *The New York Times*, May 28.

Duvall, E. M. 1977. *Marriage and Family Development*, 5th ed. Philadelphia: J. B. Lippincott. 1977.

Erikson, E. H. 1963. *Childhood and Society*. New York: W. W. Norton.

Fleck, S. 1980. The Family and Psychiatry. In *Comprehensive Textbook of Psychiatry*, 3rd ed., eds. H. I. Kaplan, A. M. Freedman, and B. J. Sadock. Baltimore: Williams & Wilkins.

Foley, V. D. 1974. *An Introduction to Family Therapy*. New York: Grune & Stratton.

Fraiberg, S. H. 1959. *The Magic Years*. New York: Scribner's.

Franklin, R. L., and Hibbs, B. 1980. Child Custody in Transition. *Journal of Marital and Family Therapy*, 6:285–292.

Freud, S. 1949. *Outline of Psychoanalysis*. New York: W. W. Norton.

Frias, C., and Janosik, E. H. 1980. Mental Illness in the Family. In *Family-Focused Care*, eds. J. R. Miller and E. H. Janosik. New York: McGraw-Hill.

Friedman, M. M. 1981. *Family Nursing: Theory and Assessment*. New York: Appleton-Century-Crofts.

Goulding, R. 1972. New Directions in Transactional Analyses: Creating an Environment for Redecision and Change. In *Progress in Group and Family Therapy*, eds. C. J. Sager and H. S. Kaplan. New York: Brunner/Mazel.

Haley, J. 1971. *Changing Families*. New York: Grune & Stratton.

Haley, J. 1973. *Uncommon Therapy: Psychiatric Techniques of M. H. Erickson*. New York: W. W. Norton.

Haley, J. 1976. *Problem Solving Therapy*. San Francisco: Jossey-Bass.

Howells, J. G. 1975. *Principles of Family Psychiatry*. New York: Brunner/Mazel.

Jackson, D. D. 1968. *Communication, Marriage, and Family*. Palo Alto, Calif.: Science and Behavior Books.

Jackson, D. D., and Lederer, W. 1967. *The Mirages of Marriage*. New York: W. W. Norton.

Janosik, E. H. 1984. Adults in Crisis. In *Crisis Counseling: A Contemporary Approach*, ed. E. H. Janosik. Monterey, Calif.: Wadsworth Health Sciences.

Janosik, E. H., and Miller, J. R. 1979. Theories of Family Development. In *Family Health Care*, eds. O. Hymovich and M. Bernard. New York: McGraw-Hill.

Kraft, S. P., and DeMaio, T. J. 1982. An Ecological Intervention with Adolescents in Low Income Families. *American Journal of Orthopsychiatry*, 52(1):131–140.

Krauss, J. B. 1984. *Nursing in the Community*. New York: John Wiley & Sons.

Lambert, V. A., and Lambert, C. E. 1984. Role Theory and the Concept of Powerlessness. *Journal of Psychosocial Nursing*, 11(9):11–14.

Langsley, D. L. 1980. Community Psychiatry. In *Comprehensive Textbook of Psychiatry*, 3rd ed., eds. H. I. Kaplan, A. M. Freedman, and B. J. Sadock. Baltimore: Williams & Wilkins.

Lidz, R. W., and Lidz, T. 1949. The Family Environment of Schizophrenic Patients. *American Journal of Psychiatry*, 106:332–345.

Lidz, R. W.; Fleck, S.; and Cornelison, A. 1965. *Schizophrenia and the Family*. New York: International Universities Press.

Lidz, T. 1958. Intrafamilial Environment of Schizophrenic Patients: Marital Schism and Skew. *American Journal of Psychiatry*, 114:241–248.

Lidz, T. 1973. *The Origin and Treatment of Schizophrenic Disorders*. New York: Basic Books.

Masson, J. M. 1984. *The Assault on Truth: Freud's Suppression of the Seduction Theory*. New York: Farrar, Straus, and Giroux.

McNally, S. 1980. Historical Perspectives on the Family. In *Family-Focused Care*, eds. J. R. Miller and E. H. Janosik. New York: McGraw-Hill.

Mead, G. H. 1933. *Mind, Self, and Society*. Chicago: University of Chicago Press.

Mereness, D. A. 1968. Family Therapy: An Evolving Role for the Psychiatric Nurse. *Perspectives in Psychiatric Care*, 6:256–259.

Minuchin, S. 1974. *Families and Family Therapy*. Cambridge, Mass.: Harvard University Press.

Nye, I. F., and Bernardo, F. 1970. *The Family: Its Structure and Interaction*. New York: Macmillan.

O'Neill, S. M. 1980. Behavioral Intervention of Family Feedback Processes. In *Family-Focused Care*, eds. J. R. Miller and E. H. Janosik. New York: McGraw-Hill.

Parsons, T. 1951. *The Social System*. New York: Free Press.

Patterson, G. R. 1975. *Families: Applications of Social Learning to Family Life*. Champaign, Ill.: Research Press.

Paul, L., ed. 1963. *Psychoanalytic Clinical Interpretation*. New York: Free Press.

Payne, K., ed. 1983. *Between Ourselves: Letters of Mothers and Daughters*. New York: Houghton Mifflin.

Powers, P. 1980. *Creating Environments for Troubled Children*. Chapel Hill: University of North Carolina.

Satir, V. 1967. *Conjoint Family Therapy: A Guide to Theory and Technique*. Palo Alto, Calif.: Science and Behavior Books.

Satir, V.; Stachwiak, J.; and Taschman, H. 1977. *Helping Families to Change*. New York: Jason Aronson.

Sedgewick, R. 1974. The Family as a System: A Network of Relationships. *Journal of Psychiatric Nursing and Mental Health Services*, 12(2):17–20.

Sedgewick, R. 1981. *Family Mental Health: Theory and Practice*. St. Louis: C. V. Mosby.

Smoyak, S., ed. 1975. *The Psychiatric Nurse as a Family Therapist*. New York: John Wiley & Sons.

Speigel, J. 1971. *Transactions: Interplay Between Individual, Family, and Society*. New York: Science House.

Sullivan, H. S. 1953. *The Interpersonal Theory of Psychiatry*. New York: W. W. Norton.

Thompson, C. 1957. *Psychoanalysis: Evolution and Development*. New York: Grove Press.

Toman, W. 1976. *Family Constellation*. New York: Springer.

Von Bertalanffy, L. 1974. General Systems Theory in Psychiatry. In *American Handbook of Psychiatry*. New York: Basic Books.

Watzlawick, P.; Beaven, J.; and Jackson, D. P. 1967. *Pragmatics of Human Communication*. New York: W. W. Norton.

Wynne, L. 1978. *Beyond the Double Bind*. New York: Brunner/Mazel.

Wynne, L., and Singer, M. 1963a. Thought Disorder and Family Relations of Schizophrenics—A Research Strategy. *Archives of General Psychiatry*, 9:191–198.

Wynne, L., and Singer, M. 1963b. Classification of Forms of Thinking. *Archives of General Psychiatry*, 9:199–206.

Wynne, L.; Rykoff, I.; Day, J.; and Hirsch, S. I. 1958. Pseudomutuality in Family Relations of Schizophrenics. *Psychiatry*, 21:205–220.

Supplementary Readings

Ackerman, N. W. *The Psychodynamics of Family Life*. New York: Basic Books, 1958.

Beavers, W. *Psychotherapy and Growth: A Family Systems Perspective*. New York: Brunner/Mazel, 1976.

Berman, E. M., and Lief, H. I. Marital Therapy from a Psychiatric Perspective: An Overview. *American Journal of Psychiatry*, 6(1975):583–592.

Bowers, J. Family-Focused Care in the Psychiatric Inpatient Setting. *Image*, 15(1983):26–31.

Clements, I., and Buchanon, D. *Family Therapy: A Nursing Perspective*. New York: John Wiley & Sons, 1982.

Dunn, G. When the Family Must Change Too. *Nursing Mirror*, 155(1982):28–29.

Feldman, L. B. Psychiatric Symptoms of Maritally Distressed Wives and Their Husbands. *International Journal of Social Psychology*, 29(1983):140–145.

Greenbaum, H. On the Nature of Marriage and Marriage Therapy. *Journal of the American Academy of Psychoanalysis*, 11(1983):283–289.

Johnson-Soderberg, S. Theory and Practice of Scapegoating. *Perspectives in Psychiatric Care*, 15(1977):154–159.

Jones, S., and Dimond, M. Family Theory and Family Therapy Models: A Comparative Review with Implications for Nursing Practice. *Journal of Psychiatric Nursing and Mental Health Services*, 20(1982):12–19.

Kressel, K., and Deutsch, M. Divorce Therapy: An In-Depth Survey of Therapists' Views. *Family Process*, 16(1977):413.

Laing, R. D. *The Politics of the Family*. New York: Vintage Books, 1972.

Miller, S., and Winstead-Fry, P. *Family Systems Theory and Nursing Practice*. Reston, Va.: Reston Publishing, 1982.

Rosenfield, A. H. Closing the Revolving Door Through Family Therapy. *Hospital and Community Psychiatry*, 33(1982):893–894.

Sedgewick, R. *Family Mental Health: Theory and Practice*. St. Louis: C. V. Mosby, 1981.

Shynner, A. C. *Systems of Family and Marital Therapy*. New York: Brunner/Mazel, 1976.

Sluzki, C. E., and Ronson, D. C. *Double Bind: The Foundation of the Communicational Approach to the Family*. New York: Grune & Stratton, 1976.

Weltner, J. S. One to Three Session Therapy with Children and Families. *Family Process*, 21(1982):281–289.

CATEGORIES OF GROUPS

HISTORICAL INFLUENCES ON GROUP TREATMENT

PSYCHODYNAMIC ISSUES

ORGANIZING THE GROUP
Assessing Needs and Resources
Planning the Group
Implementing the Plan
Evaluating Group Progress

STAGES OF GROUP DEVELOPMENT
Initial Stage
Middle Stage
Final Stage

LEADERSHIP IN GROUPS
Leadership Styles
Coleadership

MEMBERSHIP ROLES IN GROUPS

CURATIVE FACTORS IN GROUPS

GROUP RESEARCH ISSUES

C H A P T E R

19

Group Theory and Practice

Learning Objectives

After reading this chapter, the student should be able to:

1. Trace the historical development of group methods as a therapeutic modality.

2. Differentiate between primary, secondary, and reference groups.

3. Present guidelines for organizing, leading, and observing groups.

4. Classify group development according to the stages and dominant issues characteristic of each stage.

5. Identify the primary and secondary tasks of groups and relate them to leadership styles and functions.

512

Overview

Nurses often work with groups, whether for the purposes of psychotherapy (group therapy) or for the purposes of accomplishing interpersonal, cognitive, or behavioral change (therapeutic groups). This chapter examines the theoretical basis for group therapy and therapeutic groups and details methods of organizing a group, the stages of group development, issues in group leadership and membership, the curative factors in groups, and methods of research in group practice.

Men grind and grind in the mill of a truism and nothing
comes out but what was put in. But the moment they desert
tradition for spontaneous thought, then poetry, wit, hope,
virtue, learning, and anecdote all flock to their aid.

RALPH WALDO EMERSON

513

Group therapy and therapeutic groups have become very important in the health care system, especially in the field of mental health. One reason for the increased utilization of group methods is that the geographic and social mobility of individuals and families in the modern world has often resulted in the unavailability of extended support systems. Human beings are social animals with a desire to interact with and be understood by others. This deep social human need can be met or partially met by interaction within a structured group.

In this chapter a distinction is made between group therapy and therapeutic groups. *Group therapy*, or group psychotherapy as it is sometimes called, is a treatment modality in which selected clients with psychiatric disorders are treated in groups led by a qualified therapist for the purpose of alleviating intrapsychic distress or modifying personality traits. *Therapeutic groups*, on the other hand, include formal and informal groups of individuals in which interpersonal, cognitive, or behavioral change, rather than a deeper psychological alteration, is the objective (Sadock, 1980).

Nurses have been involved in working with groups of clients for many decades, especially with families. Although only nurses with advanced preparation are qualified to act as group therapists, the numerous ways in which nurses are called on to interact with groups of clients necessitate an understanding of the basic principles of group theory and practice for all nurses (Armstrong and Rouslin, 1963).

Group interaction is a proven method of promoting adaptive change, whether cognitive, emotional, or behavioral. Groups offer health care providers an efficient method of transmitting didactic information to clients and families. Group dynamics can help modify members' behavior, and groups can provide a safe environment in which clients can share emotional experiences. Even though intrapsychic change is not a goal of therapeutic groups, many of these groups provide a setting in which members can learn and practice new ways of interacting.

A number of factors have enhanced the opportunities available to nurses wishing to engage in group work (Lancaster, 1982). The sense of isolation felt by many persons in contemporary life is one factor. Another factor is the soaring cost of health care and the quest for cost-efficient treatment modalities. Equally important is the current emphasis on community rather than institutional treatment, the trend toward distributive rather than episodic care, and the commitment to the three levels of prevention (primary, secondary, and tertiary) introduced by Caplan (1964, 1970). Even though generalist nurses rarely function as group psychotherapists, they lead groups that address the three prevention levels. Examples of therapeutic groups directed at various levels of prevention are shown in Table 19-1. The examples include groups with a professional leader, self-help groups without a professional leader, and groups where leadership is shared among members on a rotating basis.

CATEGORIES OF GROUPS

Most individuals belong to groups either by birth, by circumstance, or by choice. A group is characterized by boundaries that determine who belongs to the group and who does not. More interaction

Table 19-1. Therapeutic Groups at Three Levels of Prevention

Level	Goal	Leadership	Example
Primary prevention	Reduce incidence of illness or dys-function	Designated leader(s)	Childbirth education, premarital counseling
Secondary prevention	Decrease prevalence of illness or dys-function	Designated leader(s) or shared leadership	Alcoholics Anonymous, Parents Anonymous, hypertensive groups, weight reduction groups, stop smoking groups
Tertiary prevention	Diminish impairment due to illness or dysfunction	Designated leader(s) or shared leadership	Vocational rehabilitation groups, cardiac rehabilitation groups, re-socialization groups

goes on within the boundaries of a group than across its boundaries at a particular time. A collection of individuals waiting for a bus may start to interact as a group if they begin talking about their common problems related to riding buses. Only persons waiting at that place at that time are part of the group, and more interaction goes on among persons within the waiting group than with persons outside the group.

The groups to which people belong may be divided into three major categories: primary groups, secondary groups, and reference groups. Probably the most influential group in the life of an individual is the *primary group*, or the family. This is the group that shapes one's identity, influences one's values, and provides emotional support in return for allegiance (Miller and Janosik, 1980). *Secondary groups* are limited in time and purpose. They exert less influence on their members than the primary group, but they may incite intense loyalty and generate extensive interaction for a while. Some secondary groups, such as a committee charged with a specific task, have a very brief life. Others, such as a board of directors that meets intermittently for many years, develop a quasi-permanent status.

Reference groups are formal or informal groups that influence the attitudes, values, and behaviors of those who consider themselves members. Membership in a reference group implies that the individual has identified with the group, so aspects of selfhood are evaluated according to the standards of the reference group (Marram, 1978). Some reference groups are those based on occupation, race, national origin, or religion. Membership in a reference group may be constructive or destructive, depending on the values perpetuated by the group and the stigma or pride that accompanies membership. A reference group for one person may be only a secondary group for another. For example, for some alumni, graduation means the end of their association with their college. For others, their association continues to influence them throughout their lives. The phrase "Harvard man" conjures up vivid images that indicate the extent to which some institutions can become reference groups.

HISTORICAL INFLUENCES ON GROUP TREATMENT

Joseph Pratt, a Boston internist, is considered the founder of group treatment. Pratt organized group meetings for his patients suffering from tuberculosis in 1905, a time when tuberculosis patients were isolated from their families for many months and ostracized by the community. Pratt lectured groups of twenty to thirty patients once or twice a week about the course, treatment, and prognosis of their disease. Patients who had progressed satisfactorily were invited to tell the group about the success of their treatment. In this atmosphere of hope and encouragement, very ill patients could identify with those who were recovering, much as alcoholics do today in meetings of Alcoholics Anonymous (Scott, 1976). Difficult patients who resisted the therapeutic regimen were seen individually by a nurse called a "friendly advisor."

The first to employ group methods with mentally ill clients was L. Cody Marsh, a psychiatrist and clergyman. Like Pratt, Marsh called his meetings classes and referred to patients as students. Lectures were given on a range of mental disorders as stu-

[Without organization a group] is excessively emotional, impulsive,
violent, fickle, inconsistent, irresolute, and extreme in action,
displaying only the coarser emotions and the less refined sentiments;
extremely suggestible, careless in deliberation, hasty in judgment,
incapable of any but the simpler and imperfect forms of reasoning;
easily swayed and led, lacking in self-consciousness, devoid of
self-respect and of sense of responsibility, and apt to be carried away by
the consciousness of its own force, so that it tends to produce all the
manifestations we have learned to expect of any irresponsible and
absolute power. Hence its behavior is like that of an unruly child or
an untutored savage in a strange situation, rather than like that
of its average member; and in the worst cases it is like that of
a wild beast, rather than like that of human beings.

W. McDougall (1920)

515

dents took notes. Attendance was taken, homework was assigned, and examinations were given. Students who did poorly were assigned a tutor or were required to repeat the course. Marsh was one of the first mental health professionals to realize the importance of the transactions between patients and the staff of a psychiatric facility. He included physicians, nurses, social workers, and aides in discussion groups with patients. In effect, he was one of the first persons to consider a psychiatric facility a therapeutic community (Sadock, 1980).

Another pioneer in the introduction of group treatment methods was Trignant Burrow. In 1927 Burrow, an American psychiatrist, applied the term "group analysis" to meetings in which persons with psychiatric disorders were encouraged to share their thoughts and feelings with each other. Burrow emphasized the role of the participant-observer—that is, the individual who observes while being observed. He insisted that most emotional experiences are universal and that sharing emotions with others in a group reduces feelings of loneliness and isolation. Burrow did not think of group members as sick people being treated by a healthy leader; rather, he thought of all those present as participants in a shared experience.

Samuel Slavson (1964, 1974), an engineer, conceived of the idea of play therapy by watching the behaviors of children at play. He initiated a form of play therapy in which groups of children were encouraged to act out conflicts spontaneously under the supervision of a permissive therapist. Slavson's approach allowed children to discharge aggressive impulses in a secure environment. Using toys as props the children improvised spontaneous domestic dramas that revealed their feelings about significant people in their lives. The premise was that the children would become aware of their feelings, would realize that others had similar feelings, and would learn that there were appropriate and inappropriate ways to express feelings. According to Slavson, similar group techniques may be used to teach withdrawn, fearful, and even psychotic children new ways of behaving.

The fact that Slavson was an engineer and not a physician helped open the field of group work to nonmedical practitioners. The American Group Therapy Association, which Slavson helped establish in 1948, remains an interdisciplinary group concerned with sharing information and maintaining professional standards and qualifications among the practitioners of group work. A minimum of master's level preparation in an appropriate discipline has been endorsed by the AGTA for persons undertaking group therapy leadership.

Psychodrama, a variation of group treatment, was introduced into the United States in 1925, although it had been used in Europe more than ten years earlier. Jacob Moreno, a psychiatrist, introduced psychodrama as a therapeutic tool. He used a method of role playing called "the theater of spontaneous man," in which patients acted out problem situations for the purpose of gaining insight into their own problems. In psychodrama the therapist (the "director") encourages a client (the "protagonist") to enact extemporaneously a problem or conflict drawn from her own experience. Other members of the group (the "alter egos") make suggestions concerning the drama being portrayed and frequently connect their own feelings and experiences to the events unfolding before them (Coleman, Butcher, and Carson, 1984).

Figure 19-1. Two ways of looking at groups.

Group as family

Leaders as parents

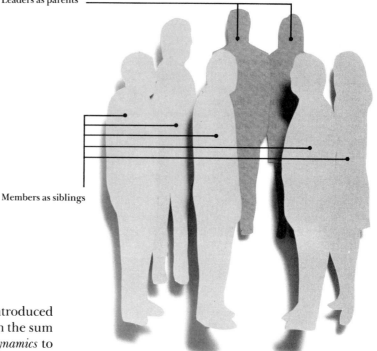

Members as siblings

Kurt Lewin, a social psychologist, introduced the idea that a group consists of more than the sum of its parts. He coined the phrase *group dynamics* to describe forces, counter-forces, and changes within a group. He used the phrase *group pressure* to describe influences exerted by the group on its members, which he believed could alter behavior. It was Lewin's contention that each member wields influence in a group and that groups function as interdependent units even though they are composed of separate individuals (Lewin, 1957; Anthony, 1971).

Group work advanced during World War II, when the number of psychiatrists was inadequate to deal with emotional trauma suffered by Allied soldiers. American and European psychiatrists working at a military center in Northfield, England discarded army rules and regulations in order to adopt innovative group treatment methods. One innovation was the *community network*, which consisted as much as possible of friends and family members who had significant relationships with the client at the onset of the breakdown. The experiments in group treatment at Northfield were forerunners of today's therapeutic communities and milieu therapy.

After World War II, many disciplines became interested in group therapy and practice. Programs in sociology, psychology, education, psychiatry, nursing, and social work added courses in group methodology to their curriculum. Wellesley College was the first institution to introduce group theory in a nursing program in 1952. In order to ease the entry of Wellesley College freshmen into the nursing role the group experiences of students were explored. As masters' programs in psychiatric nursing proliferated, sensitivity training was introduced to enhance the self-awareness of students. By means of groups, students learned to analyze their own feelings and reactions in the context of group dynamics (Racy, 1969; Adams, 1971).

Industry and government soon realized the importance of understanding how groups operate and provided financial support for the application and study of group theory. In 1947, the National Training Laboratory for Applied Behavioral Science was established. The purpose was to acquaint corporate and industrial executives with the effects of group dynamics on human relationships. The National Training Laboratory used training groups, or *T-groups*, to increase the members' ability to handle difficult interpersonal situations and to transfer this ability to the work place.

During the prosperous years after World War II, there was intense popular interest in achieving self-actualization and personal fulfillment. In this period, lower level needs, as outlined by Maslow (1968), were easily met, and popular yearning grew for "peak experiences" to overcome the tedium and boredom of everyday life. Although Maslow did not equate self-actualization with peak experiences, the ideas seemed to merge in the public mind. This contributed to enormous interest in groups whose goal was a vaguely defined but emotionally exciting experience. The demand for self-actualization was the impetus for the *encounter groups* of the 1960s and 1970s. Many diverse groups, led by both qualified and unqualified leaders, fell into the broad classification of encounter groups; most sought to fulfill

Group as social microcosm

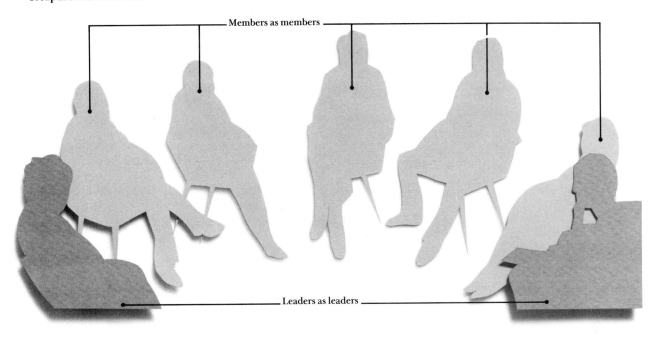

Members as members

Leaders as leaders

people's need to be loved and to belong. Encounter groups were based on the belief that the open expression of feelings is an end in itself (Sayre, 1979). For a time the encounter group movement was regarded as a cureall for emotional alienation, but systematic studies eventually questioned its worth. One study of encounter groups suggested that while the groups did provide opportunity for self-expression, they produced few lasting positive changes in members and negative effects in some (Lieberman et al., 1973).

PSYCHODYNAMIC ISSUES

Nurses do not often lead psychoanalytically oriented groups that attempt to promote personality change, but they do utilize a number of concepts contributed by psychoanalytic theorists, sometimes without being aware of the source. Since various psychoanalytic concepts are likely to surface in therapeutic groups as well as psychotherapy groups, a brief discussion of psychodynamic issues is included in this section.

There are two general ways of examining a group experience (see Figure 19-1). To psychoanalytic theorists, a group is a replication of the early family experience, and members bring to the group residual feelings and behaviors from their family of origin. Although this perception of the members is seldom conscious, they react to the leaders as if they were surrogate parents and to the other members as if they were siblings. The corrective reenactment of

experiences that first occurred within the original primary group is thought to modify emotional conflicts and dysfunctional defenses developed in early life (Maluccio, 1981).

The other view of group dynamics is less psychoanalytic. In this perspective, the group is seen as a microcosm of society. Interactions between members are thought to reduce feelings of alienation, to clarify communication, and to teach alternative ways of acting and reacting. Regardless of whether the group is perceived as a family or as society in miniature, a number of psychodynamic phenonema are likely to become evident, including transference, countertransference, resistance, acting out, and insight (Lego, 1978).

Transference is an unconscious distortion in which individuals transfer to others the wishes and fears associated with significant persons in early life. For example, a group member who was "daddy's little girl" in the original family configuration may continue to enact that role, especially with a male group leader. If the underlying dynamics of the behavior are recognized by the leader and by other members, the urge to behave like "daddy's little girl" may be replaced by more mature actions. The leader and the group thus have the potential to correct transference (Freud, 1957; Gibbard, 1974).

Countertransference is an unconscious distortion in which the group leader transfers to one or more members wishes and fears associated by the leader with people in his early life. A group leader who becomes enraged by the actions of a member may be responding to his internal distortion rather than to

Some think that nature having established paternal authority, the most natural government was that of a single person. But the example of paternal authority proves nothing. For if the power of a father relates to a single government, that of brothers after the death of a father, and that of cousins after the decease of brothers, refer to a government of many . . . Better is it to say that the government most conformable to nature is that which best agrees with the humor and disposition of the people in whose favor it is established.

FRANCIS WILLIAM COKER (1946)

518

the reality of group events. Like other mortals, group leaders may not always be aware of the underlying causes of their reactions and may engage in denial, rationalization, or other defensive maneuvers. But if the leader is aware of countertransference, it can more easily be controlled. The leader is a powerful person in the eyes of group members, and only a mature group will be able to deal directly with countertransference issues. This is one reason why supervision, observation, and consultation are important for all group leaders but are crucial for psychotherapy groups whose members are likely to be very vulnerable.

Resistance is unwillingness on the part of members to relinquish distortions or to turn their attention to accomplishing the purpose for which the group was formed. Resistance may be individual or collective, open or hidden, conscious or unconscious. Some indications of resistance are inattention, flippancy, superficiality, anger, tardiness, or absences. Like transference and countertransference, resistance can be a complex issue. It may be directed toward the leader or toward group members in ways that are not immediately identified but that sooner or later become apparent.

Acting out is often confused with simple acting up, although the latter is usually a sign of resistance. Acting out is deeper and more profound, for it means that a member is expressing internal conflicts through symbols or actions instead of openly. An example of acting out is the behavior of a member who is very frightened that confidentiality will be broken and therefore avoids personal disclosure. The unresolved conflict may center on issues of trust versus mistrust (Erikson, 1963). Acting out behavior is usually unconscious and in therapy groups

should be confronted by the leader or other members who notice it. If the behavior is confronted or interpreted, the acting out member may reject the meaning but later may come to accept its accuracy, and thus take a step toward insight.

Insight is the conscious connection ultimately made between one's behavior and one's underlying motives. Acquiring insight is often a slow process of which intellectual understanding is only the beginning. Gaining insight into the meaning of one's acting out behavior is a long process that requires a state of readiness and a willingness to work through the connections between behavior and motives. Without emotional as well as intellectual readiness, genuine commitment to change will not be made. This is one of the reasons that group psychotherapy devoted to the goal of promoting intrapsychic change is of long duration (Robinson, 1983).

ORGANIZING THE GROUP

There are some instances when prospective members become aware of their own needs and can organize a group that meets their requirements. Alcoholics Anonymous, an international movement with a proven record of success in helping members maintain sobriety, is a prominent example. More often, however, prospective members lack the resources or are ignorant of the possibilities of using a group approach to health care. Therefore, it is usually a nurse or other health care professional who must identify a target population from which to recruit members and begin to assess their needs (Marvin, 1982). Nurses who determine that the needs of certain clients may be met through group

REQUIREMENTS FOR GROUP ORGANIZATION

According to Freud (1957), there are five basic requirements for group organization:

- First there must be continuity of existence in the group: The same individuals must exist for some time or the same fixed positions must exist even though occupied by successive individuals.

- Individual members should have a definite idea of the nature, functions, capacities, and composition of the group in order to develop emotional relationships to the group as a whole.

- The group should be brought into some interaction, perhaps in the form of rivalry, with other groups similar in some respects but differing from it in many respects.

- The group should possess traditions, customs, habits especially those that determine the relation of its members to one another.

- The group should have a definite structure, expressed in the specialization and differentiation of the functions of its members.

methods can turn to the nursing process for direction.

Assessing Needs and Resources

The process of organizing a group should begin by asking whether the prospective leaders are equipped by temperament and preparation to act as leaders. The answer to this question depends to a large extent on the kind of group that is being considered. Nurses are accustomed to working on health teams, teaching families, and interacting with groups of clients in hospital and community settings. Basic nursing programs emphasize self-awareness and usually provide students with some knowledge of group dynamics, but it is important for generalist nurses to realize their limitations. If the proposed group involves psychotherapy, the prospective leaders should meet the standards of the American Nurses' Association, which state that psychotherapy groups should be led by nurses with graduate preparation at least at the master's level. The availability of qualified supervision, the group composition, and the group objectives should also be considered when deciding whether a nurse can lead a group safely and effectively.

Before deciding that a group is needed, the status of the target population should be reviewed in relation to existing resources and services. It is important to decide whether the needs of the target population are already being met by existing services. If so, there is no need to organize a new group. For example, a community health nurse concerned with the problem of child abuse might attempt to discover what groups are available for parents who are potential abusers. If programs such as Parents Anonymous are already active in the community, the nurse might refer troubled parents to this support group. If no appropriate group is found, the nurse might, with the approval of the employing agency, take steps to organize a support group or activate a chapter of Parents Anonymous. The degree of support of the sponsoring agency can be a significant factor in a group's success (Loomis, 1979).

Planning the Group

Experienced group leaders stress the importance of advance planning in ensuring successful outcomes. Before interviewing prospective members, the leader or leaders should decide what the selection standards will be. Group objectives must be clearly stated and conveyed to the members so that the understanding of leaders and members coincides. The formulation of specific goals also reassures members about what they may expect and later permits an adequate evaluation of group outcomes.

Authorities on group work disagree on whether homogeneous groups are consistently superior to heterogeneous groups. Some feel a degree of homogeneity may be beneficial in helping members relate to one another, but others claim that heterogeneity in a group helps members learn from one another (Yalom, 1975). Some groups benefit from homogeneity of problems and interests among members—groups of substance abusers, for example. But in virtually all groups a certain amount of heterogeneity is inescapable. Individual differences in defenses, coping mechanisms, and interactional styles persist in all groups.

It is impossible to predict with total accuracy whether a particular individual will do well in a group because the success or failure of the experience may depend less on the characteristics of the client than on the characteristics of the group itself. Each group, whether it is considered group therapy or a therapeutic group, will develop its own constellation of relationships, behaviors, and values based to a large extent upon the composition of the membership and the orientation of the leader.

In selecting and preparing prospective group members, Marvin (1982) recommended that the following questions be considered:

What specific needs does this client have?

Can her needs be met effectively through a group experience?

Will the client tolerate the anxiety engendered by a group experience?

What previous experience has the client had with primary, secondary, and reference groups?

Is there evidence of willingness to participate in the group?

Is the client motivated to work on achieving group goals?

Group cohesion—the sense of belonging in the group—constitutes a powerful factor in maintaining a viable group. Group cohesion can be promoted by choosing members on the "Noah's Ark" principle, which states that the isolation felt by any group member will be decreased by the presence of another member with similar characteristics who can serve as his compeer or companion. Age, gender, occupation, and interests are among the characteristics that may be used in matching group members. Examples of unfortunate group selection would include a solitary male or female member, a middle-aged member among a group of adolescents, or a young, vigorous member among a group of elderly, infirm retirees.

During the process of selecting and preparing members for the group experience, a group contract or agreement should be discussed. The group contract should be clearly stated and agreed to by the leader(s) and members. Provisions of the contract, once accepted, should be carefully followed as originally outlined. If it becomes necessary to alter provisions of the group contract, the decision should be made jointly by the members and leader(s).

Negotiating the group contract requires collaboration and open communication between leaders and prospective members. Provisions of the contract should also be shared with members of the sponsoring agency. Sharing general information about group goals and the contract can be done

without betraying confidentiality, and it encourages support from the sponsoring agency. When prospective members are interviewed, they should be asked whether they understand and accept the group contract. In some cases the leader may devise a written contract that is cosigned by members and leaders. If used, the written contract should note the time and place of the meetings, the agreed-upon goals for the group, and the commitments and expectations shared by members and leaders. Although it is not mandatory and not always appropriate, a written contract reduces any discrepancy between what members would like the group to be and what the leader has promised.

The length and frequency of group sessions may vary according to the time frame and the goals of the group. A psychotherapy group might meet twice a week for an hour or once a week for an hour and a half. A teaching group for hypertensive or for diabetic clients might meet for only 45 minutes at weekly or biweekly intervals. A group for recovering cardiac clients and their spouses might meet daily for 30 minutes over a period of several months. In all cases, the surroundings in which the group meets should be as comfortable as possible, and sessions should convene at the same place and at the times designated during the preparatory period.

Group size depends on the composition of the group and the nature of the group goals. There is little agreement on the optimal size for a group, but there is consensus on the optimal range of group size. The generally accepted range for small groups is from five to fifteen members. Groups with fewer than five or more than ten members are unlikely to generate maximum therapeutic exchange. Groups of more than ten members tend to form subgroups; groups of less than five members are inclined to be inhibited in their participation. Therefore, groups with five to ten members fall within the ideal range, although these are not hardfast rules but merely guidelines. A nurse contemplating group work with an elderly population might limit the group to three or four members if reality orientation is the objective. If the proposed group is designed to promote reminiscing or life review for elderly members, the leader might be advised to increase the number of members. One shortcoming in the field of group research is the lack of systematic investigation needed to correlate successful outcomes with group size (Burnside, 1984).

Another issue to be decided is whether a group is to be closed or open to new members. There are arguments supporting both decisions. Closed groups tend to become more cohesive, but groups that admit new members at specified times benefit from the orienting activities extended by senior members toward new arrivals. Another decision that must be made is whether to allow members to leave the group if they feel they have made sufficient progress or to insist that termination be collectively experienced by all members. These are decisions that should be made during the preparatory phase of organizing the group.

Early in the group sessions the question will arise as to whether group members should meet outside the scheduled sessions, and this is an issue that leaders should consider even before the sessions begin. There is no denying the fact that outside meetings between two or three members may fragment the group and impede group progress. Nevertheless, there will be times when group members have an affinity for other members and therefore arrange meetings that do not include the entire group. One solution is to acknowledge the possibility that such meetings will take place but insist that they not be kept secret from the rest of the group. This suggestion may not satisfy purists who believe with some justification that group interaction should be confined to meetings at which all members are present. Since it is almost impossible for the leader to enforce prohibitions against meeting outside the scheduled sessions, the suggested compromise may be the answer.

Implementing the Plan

Once assessment and planning have been completed, implementation of the group can proceed. Yalom (1975) suggested that private screening interviews consisting of two or three meetings be arranged to select and prepare each member. Questions directed to prospective members should be based on the objectives of the group. If mastering cognitive knowledge, changing behavior, learning new skills, or promoting insight is a major goal, the interviewees should be appraised for their potential capacity to achieve this goal.

In these preparatory meetings the leader should be prepared for questions and challenges from the interviewees. The prospect of a group experience is apt to evoke some anxiety, and candidates are entitled to have their questions answered at this time. Interviewees often ask the leaders about their qualifications and previous group experiences. Essentially what is being asked is whether the leader can guarantee that the group will be a safe place for the members. Questions about the leader should be answered truthfully and without resentment. Before requesting a prospective member to make an immediate decision about joining the group, time should be allowed for mutual consideration.

Evaluating Group Progress

Evaluating the progress of the whole group and of individual members allows leaders to determine the effectiveness of their interventions and of the group experience. In evaluating group progress, the stated goals are a good standard of measurement, especially if the goals have been expressed behaviorally and if adequate records have been kept. Judging the extent to which group goals have been met helps evaluate group outcomes, but this is not always easy to do. Members' subjective impressions of the progress they have made are of questionable reliability and validity, but these factors can be increased if pretests and posttests are used. These questionnaires are more helpful if the items are ranked so that quantitative comparisons are possible. Figure 19-2 illustrates what is meant by ranking questionnaire items. Ongoing observation of group development in terms of movement from dependence to interdependence is another subjective way of evaluating the effectiveness of the group. Later in this chapter, group development is described in terms of observable behaviors that emerge at various stages of the group life cycle.

Evaluation of group progress is facilitated by using a log or journal to record changes noted in the group by the leader or by observers. Some results of the group experience are indisputable, even though external variables may intrude. Losing 10 pounds, getting a job, maintaining normal blood sugar readings, or reducing blood pressure readings provides tangible evidence that in all likelihood the group experience has proved to be successful for that member.

Evaluation of group progress can be a difficult task. This is one reason for using a coleadership model in which two leaders can compare observations, engage in validation, and correct false impressions. Any systematic method of observing and recording group data will make evaluation an easier task. One-way mirrors and electronic taping, either audio or audiovisual, can be helpful. All observation and recording methods must be disclosed to prospective members during contract negotiations, and written consent must be obtained in advance from every member. Observers or supervisors are valuable, for they can review group proceedings while events are recent and give immediate feedback to the leader in a postsession.

In the absence of electronic taping or live supervision, a log or journal of the sessions may be substituted. This record should be made as soon as possible after a session has concluded and should identify group themes, describe interventions, and note the impact of interventions on individual members and on whole-group interaction. Although less objective

521

Figure 19-2. Sample items showing quantitative rank order. These items deal with self-reported distress of a client. Items are given a numerical value of one to four, with one indicating the lowest index of distress and four representing the highest index. By means of rank order it is possible to compare individuals or groups of individuals.

Name _____ Age _____ Sex _____ Date _____	1. Never or rarely	2. Some of the time	3. Much of the time	4. Most or all of the time
I feel down-hearted, blue, and sad				
I find it hard to make decisions				
I have crying spells or feel like crying				
I have trouble sleeping through the night				
I get tired for no reason				

522

than other methods, the log enables the leader to review group events, recall sequential actions, analyze interactions, and clarify relationships within the group.

STAGES OF GROUP DEVELOPMENT

Group development refers to the changes that occur in the life cycle of a group, from a tentative beginning into a productive phase, and eventually to the end. Some groups enjoy a full and vigorous life span; some do not survive infancy; still others reach maturity without ever achieving their potential. Most groups go through stages in which conflict arises around various issues that are characteristic of the developmental stage of the group. Accepting the idea that groups go through stages of development helps leaders and observers interpret various tumultuous group events as constructive rather than destructive.

There is some danger in taking the stages of group development too literally. Groups resemble individuals in that they are prone to periods of progression and regression. Realizing that groups do not always progress steadily and without interruption helps eliminate disappointment or surprise when "settled" issues are revived in the group and must be dealt with again. It is also important to recognize that few groups move as a single unit through developmental stages. Some members may be more willing than others to confront the group task. Usually a group does not become productive until a majority of members indicate readiness. Although group development has been described in

many ways, one of the simplest and most useful divisions of group development is into an initial stage, a middle or working stage, and a final stage.

Initial Stage

In the early stage of group development, the dominant issues are dependency and authority. The leader is assumed to possess great power and may be perceived by members as a parental figure. Feelings of rivalry may exist in the group, with members wishing to be the favorite of the leader but fearing exclusion by other members if the wish is realized. All members hope for a safe and secure place in the group but may be afraid of giving up too much individuality in order to be accepted. In this early period politeness and conformity are used by the members to control anxiety. Because silence often heightens anxiety, there is a tendency on the part of leaders and members to avoid silences at any cost. Controversy and differences also generate anxiety, so the members search for similarities and common interests among themselves.

After most of the members have managed to become part of the group without sacrificing too much of their individuality, a struggle against the leader may follow. Now the members begin to assert themselves and to challenge the authority of the leader. In this period of competition some members are more active than others. The movement of group members from attitudes of dependency to struggles for power is an indication that the group is beginning to mature. Rather than resenting the growing strength and autonomy of the group, the leader should tolerate and even encourage questions and criticisms that represent challenges to au-

---

> ### VARIATIONS IN GROUP LEADERSHIP ROLE ENACTMENT
>
> ■ *Leaderless Groups:* Most experienced member functions as leader; leadership is shared; leadership resides in commitment to a creed or goal.
>
> ■ *Leaderless Sessions:* Alternate meetings are conducted without the presence of a designated leader.
>
> ■ *Leader as a Background Figure:* Leader functions mostly behind the scenes in that his or her influence is felt but presence is subtle and unobtrusive.
>
> ■ *Leader as a Foreground Figure:* Leader is dominant presence in the group: directs, stimulates, extends, interprets.
>
> SOURCE: Adapted from H. I. Kaplan and B. J. Sadock, eds., *Comprehensive Group Psychotherapy* (Baltimore: Williams & Wilkins, 1975), p. 112.

thority and renunciation of dependency by the members (Mills, 1967).

The challenge to the leader by the group requires a rational and careful response. For example, a head nurse whose staff meetings are disrupted by criticisms about work assignments or complaints about time schedules may decide not to consider the validity of the objections that are raised and choose instead either to ignore or dismiss the opinions of staff members. The head nurse could then continue the usual practice of making unilateral decisions about staffing, thereby retaining full control in this matter. On the other hand, the head nurse might decide to rotate responsibility for assignments and schedules among the nurses working on the unit. By sharing power with the group, the head nurse would foster self-direction and independence among the nursing staff. As they experienced leadership responsibility, staff members would realize how many factors intrude when assignments are made. The result in most cases would be growing maturity of the staff members and greater respect for the designated leader.

Another example of therapeutic response when leadership is challenged might occur in a psychiatric day treatment center where clients habitually deface bulletin boards with graffiti. Instead of invoking punitive measures, the nurse administrator might arrange to set aside one bulletin board for the clients. At a community meeting they could be told that one bulletin board is theirs on which to write whatever they choose. This concession would make the problem of defacing informational bulletin boards no longer the focus of prolonged discussion at community meetings.

The initial stage of group development may be divided into a dependency phase and a power phase. The first phase represents the willingness of individual members to become part of the group; the second represents the reluctance of individual members to merge fully with the group. In group terminology the first part of the initial stage deals with dependency and inclusion; the second part deals with power and authority (Schutz, 1966).

Middle Stage

By the end of the initial stage of group development, problems of dependency and power should be resolved for the most part. At this stage cohesion has developed among the members and the group should be ready to undertake productive work. Some tension and anxiety may be present, because members must now confront the task for which the group was organized, even though they may hesitate to do so.

A group in the working stage has accumulated a shared history. Group norms have evolved, and members have formulated standards that define which behaviors are acceptable and which are unacceptable. There is a marked difference between group rules and group norms. *Group rules* can be established by the leader or agreed upon by the leader and the members even before the group begins to meet. *Group norms* cannot be imposed but rather emerge gradually as the group begins to move toward interdependence and task performance. One example of the difference between rules and norms is the fact that the leader may enforce a rule that no member who is more than 5

*Conflict cannot be eliminated from human groups, whether we
consider dyads, small groups, macrogroups, or such megagroups as
nations and blocs of nations. If conflict is denied or suppressed,
invariably it will manifest itself in oblique, corrosive, often ugly ways.
Although our immediate association with conflict is
negative—destruction, bitterness, war, violence—a moment of
reflection brings to mind positive associations; conflict brings drama,
excitement, change, and development to human life and
societies . . . Conflict is inevitable in the course of the group's
development; its absence, in fact, suggests some impairment of the
developmental sequence. Furthermore, conflict can be harnessed
in the service of the group; the group members can, in a variety
of ways, profit from conflict, provided its intensity does not
exceed their tolerance and provided that proper group
norms have been established.*

IRVIN D. YALOM (1975)

524

minutes late will be admitted to a session. This is an explicit rule that is part of the group contract and that has been in effect since the first meeting. Because of the rule all of the members are punctual. Gradually a group norm develops that the members consistently arrive 15 minutes early to have coffee together. Group rules are generally enforced for everyone, but norms may not be applied uniformly. For instance, a member who works irregular hours might not be expected to be part of the premeeting socializing (a norm) but is expected not to be late for the session (a rule). Norms are usually unwritten and may not even be verbalized; rules are usually verbalized and are more explicit and well defined than norms.

The working stage is usually a satisfying time for the members. Each of them has moved toward achieving a position in the group that feels comfortable. Problems will inevitably arise that require decisions and solutions. Anxiety and resistance to the task may be evident from time to time, but the general direction of the group is progressive. The leader may be less active than in the initial stage but continues to intervene to help resolve problems, to protect the exploitation of weaker members by stronger ones, and to monitor the anxiety level of the group so that no member is overwhelmed (Whitaker, 1976).

Final Stage

As in every therapeutic interaction, the process of termination begins with the first meeting. It may already have been discussed during preparatory interviews with group members in terms of how long the group will meet. In open-ended groups, members may terminate individually; in closed-end groups, the group terminates as a unit. Premature termination occurs when a member drops out or when a group disbands without completing its primary task. Even though termination has been mentioned during negotiation proceedings and alluded to during meetings, it usually seems to come as a surprise to members. The element of unexpectedness that surrounds termination is a form of denial, especially if the group has become meaningful to members.

Often it is the more successful groups that have the most difficulty with termination, and this is true of leaders as well as members. It is helpful to divide termination into two phases: disengagement and actual dissolution. The period of disengagement, which precedes dissolution, is a time when members begin to recognize the fact that the group will end soon. Problems of dependency and authority may reappear. Members may display anger, perhaps because anger is a less painful emotion than grief (Sampson and Marthas, 1977; Rubin, 1981). Avoiding discussion of termination is dysfunctional, and members should be encouraged to talk about the history and meaning of the group. Appropriate leadership tactics during termination include reminiscing, review of group themes, and discussion of group outcomes. It is also useful if leaders and members can identify authentic feelings of sadness at the end of the group experience. Termination is an important part of the group life cycle and should neither be denied, avoided, or ignored.

There is danger that group leaders and observers who use a chronological, stage-specific model will note only conspicuous clusters of behavior and ignore subtle changes in the group. However, dividing group development into stages helps in the

Table 19-2. Stages of Group Development

Stage	Schutzian Conflict Issues	Eriksonian Tasks	Tuckmanian Sequence
Initial	Dependency Authority	Trust vs. mistrust Autonomy vs. shame and doubt Initiative vs. guilt	Storming Forming
Middle	Intimacy Cooperation Productivity	Industry vs. inferiority Identity vs. role confusion Intimacy vs. isolation Generativity vs. stagnation	Norming Performing
Final	Disengagement Dissolution	Ego integrity vs. despair	Mourning

assessment of group progress. The work of a number of group theorists has dealt with stage-specific behaviors. Schutz (1966) conceptualized group conflicts likely to appear at various stages; Tuckman (1965) formulated a well-known sequence of group behaviors that has the advantage of being recalled easily. The sequential nature of group development is even more obvious when the psychosocial framework of Erikson (1963) is superimposed. Table 19-2 synthesizes the concepts of these three theorists and applies them to developmental group stages.

LEADERSHIP IN GROUPS

Freud (1957) described leaderless groups as mobs capable of violent, excessive behavior. Freud compared groups with a leader to families in which the members behaved like siblings bound to the leader and to each other by ambivalent feelings of identification that were sometimes loving and sometimes hostile (Mills, 1967).

Marram (1978) differentiated leadership functions from leadership interventions. *Leadership functions* are essential responsibilities that the leader does not delegate or share with members. Leadership functions include providing a safe environment within the group, fostering autonomy and maturation of the group, and meeting the needs of members in a growth-enhancing manner. *Leadership interventions* refer to specific acts or behaviors that facilitate progress toward the group task, and these may be delegated or shared among group members.

Groups have primary and secondary tasks. The primary task is the purpose for which the group was formed. The secondary task is group maintenance so that the group survives long enough for the primary task to be accomplished (Rioch, 1975). The existence of a primary and secondary group task means that group leaders always have two functions: to meet the emotional needs of the members so that the group is preserved and to mobilize abilities and resources within the group so that the primary task can be completed. If a group has only one leader, she must perform both socioemotional functions and task or instrumental functions. When there are two leaders these functions can be divided between them.

In psychoanalytic terminology, the socioemotional leader is commonly thought of as the group nurturer or "mother," while the task leader is thought of as the group "father." Needless to say, leadership functions should not be allocated merely on the basis of gender. If a group is composed of passive, ineffectual female members it may be wise to assign a female coleader the role of task or instrumental leader. Conversely, if a spouses' group contains male members who consider nurturing and caring to be signs of weakness, it may be advisable to assign a male coleader the responsibility for meeting the socioemotional needs of the group. The most important consideration is that the primary task (achieving the purpose of the group) cannot be met if the secondary task (maintaining and preserving the group) is neglected or left to chance.

In order to fulfill leadership functions an individual must possess a working knowledge of content and process. *Content* is the substantive, explicit, factual material that is brought up in a group, in other words, *what* is said or done in a group meeting.

Table 19-3. Theme, Content, and Process Analysis in Group Sessions

Group Theme	Content Analysis	Process Analysis
Cardiac clients in an outpatient health teaching group during their rehabilitation program	Protracted discussion and indecision about time, place, and agenda for future meetings	Covert ambivalence about being in the group, resistance to accepting a changing lifestyle, and a need to be in control
Diabetic clients in a health teaching group that emphasizes dietary control and general measures of coping with a chronic illness	Complaints about spouses, relatives, and physicians who don't have diabetes and therefore don't understand what it's like to live with so many prohibitions	Covert dissatisfaction with the leader, partial denial of the severity of the illness, anger about being ill, and skepticism about the value of the group
Recent nurse graduates in a staff orientation program preparing them for their first professional position	Discussion of their residences, how near or far they live from work, commuting problems, car accidents, driver's licenses	Covert fear of giving up student status, of enacting the professional role, and of making errors
Pregnant teenagers in a childbirth education class dealing with labor and delivery, as well as care of the newborn	Ridicule directed to the leaders' emphasis on nutrition, coupled with refusal to give up favorite junk food for a balanced diet	Covert expression of unmet needs for nurturance, reluctance to give up adolescent attitudes and accept responsibility in the new role soon to be thrust upon them

SOURCE: Adapted from Boyer (1982).

Group process is less easily observed; it includes covert, subtle, implicit forces present in the group. Process deals with *how* and *why* interactions develop in the group. Questions that help a leader understand group process are: How do the members relate to each other? How do the members and the leader interact? Why do group interactions take the form they do?

The importance of analyzing both content and process cannot be overstated, for the two are equally significant. Analyzing group content permits the leader to uncover recurrent themes and patterns in the group. Analyzing content also helps the leader understand process and to make assumptions on which to base interventions. By observing and analyzing group process a leader is better able to understand and meet the needs of group members. Monitoring group process requires attention to both nonverbal and verbal messages, as well as sensitivity to subtle behaviors that indicate the needs of the group. In most group meetings one or more themes dominate or recur, and they can be identified. A leader who analyzes a group session by identifying the dominant themes can then explore the substantive content of the theme in order to recognize the process factors that were present in the session. Table 19-3 shows how identifying a group theme can be a prelude to understanding group process.

Yalom (1975) called the strategy of linking content and process *process illumination*. Egan (1982) used the term *alternative frames of reference*, while Sampson and Marthas (1977) called such interventions *processing the here and now*. Regardless of the terminology used, group leaders should examine content and process of interactions as they occur and reexamine them later. This enables the leader to extrapolate themes or patterns noted in a session and to base future interventions on prevailing group modes of interaction.

Leadership Styles

The style of leadership is determined primarily by the needs of the group, the composition of the group, and the goals that are to be achieved. The preferences and personal characteristics of the leader also influence the style of leadership. One of the first issues to be determined by a leader is whether to choose an authoritarian, democratic, or laissez-faire style of leadership. An *autocratic* leader is clearly in charge of group proceedings, guiding and directing the members and holding them to the group task. A *democratic* leader remains responsible for the well-being of group members during the sessions and may remind members of the group task but shares leadership functions with them by permitting considerable autonomy. The *laissez-faire* leader may monitor group proceedings but offers little guidance, allowing the group members to shape the group sessions without interventions or reminders from the leader. Even though the first consideration should be the needs of the group, the personal biases of the leader have a way of intruding. If, for example, a leader believes that most people do not enjoy working and need to be harnessed to the task, that leader will likely be more authoritarian. On the other hand, if the leader believes that most people are willing to work and are capable of self-direction, that leader is likely to be democratic and to engage in collaborative efforts (Sampson and Marthas, 1977).

These three leadership styles have been studied

Table 19-4. Comparison of Characteristics of Three Leadership Styles

Democratic	Autocratic	Laissez-faire
Member-oriented	Leader-oriented	Diffuse orientation
Problem-solving approach	Persuasive approach	Style drifts and changes
Member-defined goals	Leader-defined goals	Few clear goals
Facilitates participation	Limits participation	Unclear participation
Group evaluates process and progress by means of extensive feedback and extensive activity	Limited feedback	Little evaluation of process; minimal feedback; decreased effectiveness
Leader influences group and may share leadership functions with members	Leadership retained by one or two designated persons	Leadership neither centralized nor distributed
Complex approach	Direct approach	Confused approach
Diversity encouraged	Limited tolerance of diversity	Diversity neither encouraged nor discouraged

SOURCE: Adapted from White and Lippitt (1953), Shaw (1976), Sampson and Marthas (1977), and Lego (1978).

Table 19-5. Comparison of the Results of Three Leadership Styles

527

Democratic	Autocratic	Laissez-faire
Increased member participation	Decreased participation	Decreased cooperation
Increased member enthusiasm, cohesiveness, morale	Decreased morale, cohesiveness	Decreased morale, emotional satisfaction, cohesiveness
Increased member commitment	Decreased innovation	Increased scapegoating
Increased productivity, but less than autocratic	Highest productivity level	Decreased productivity
Increased initiative	Consistent surveillance required Increased dependency	Decreased learning of leadership skills
Leadership skills learned by members	Decreased individuality	Decreased quality of work
Self-corrective feedback maximizes member's potential	Conversations restricted and related to task	Increased requests for information
	Increased uniformity	
	Repressed aggression leads to scapegoating, resentment, passive-aggressive, acting out behaviors	

SOURCE: Adapted from White and Lippitt (1953), Shaw (1976), Sampson and Marthas (1977), and Lego (1978).

using dependent variables of group productivity and morale (White and Lippitt, 1953). Autocratic or authoritarian leadership seems to result in greater productivity but lower morale compared to democratic leadership. Hostility, scapegoating, and aggression have been found to be significantly greater in groups with an autocratic leader. Democratic leadership has been found to result in less productivity, but groups with such leadership are more cohesive, self-directed, and better able to mobilize group resources on their own. Laissez-faire leadership has been found to be the least effective in terms of productivity and morale.

Table 19-4 compares the characteristics of the three leadership styles. Table 19-5 compares the results of the three styles.

Flexibility on the part of the leader is necessary, and the choice of leadership style should be determined by the situation. For many groups a direct, authoritative approach is advisable. This is very true of groups where the members are acutely anxious,

adolescent, elderly and confused, or even marginally out of touch with reality. Other situations that require authoritarian leadership include:

1. When the group is on the verge of dissolving prematurely and an immediate decision must be made if the group is to remain viable. In a scout troop where attendance has become erratic, the leader may issue an ultimatum that members who miss more than three meetings are barred from attending the midsummer camping jamboree.

2. When the task is very structured, and few, if any, alternative approaches are available. A class of nursing students practicing a technical procedure may be limited to step-by-step actions that are needed to ensure safe practice. In this instance the instructor (leader) would not allow deviation or improvisation, regardless of group pressure to accept alternative behaviors.

Table 19-6. Styles of Leadership and Types of Groups

Leadership Style	Type of Group
High in caring	Support
High in executive function	Task
High in caring and executive function	Socialization
High in meaning attribution and executive function	Behavior change
High in emotional stimulation and meaning attribution	Sensitivity group
Moderate in emotional stimulation, moderate in executive function, high in caring, high in meaning attribution	Psychotherapy

SOURCE: Adapted from Janosik and Phipps (1982).

528

3. When members desire and expect a strong, central leader and are unwilling or unable to accept a share of leadership. A group of pregnant teenagers preparing in childbirth education classes for labor or delivery is likely to respond to a kind but knowledgeable leader who accepts and does not delegate leadership functions to members.

Situations in which democratic leadership is more suitable include:

1. When there are several alternatives in the way the task may be accomplished. In health team meetings where client care is being planned, discussion should be free and open. The suggestions of each team member should receive consideration.

2. When the members are capable of and can benefit from increased self-direction and responsibility. A group of recovering alcoholics engaged in planning a Christmas party may well derive benefit from being permitted to take charge of the arrangements with minimal supervision from the leader.

3. When there is a need to alter attitudes and opinions as well as promote behavioral change. High school students who are studying the adverse consequences of drug abuse are more likely to believe an instructor who listens to their views and does not reject or totally discount their opinions.

A classic study of leadership style in encounter groups showed that some leadership styles corre-

lated with persistent, severe psychological dysfunction of some members (Yalom and Lieberman, 1972). Intrusive, aggressive confrontation of members by an authoritarian but charismatic leader seemed to produce the highest incidence of psychic trauma among vulnerable members. It appeared that leaders with these characteristics sought immediate change in members and therefore exerted great pressure on the group. In the study, four basic styles based on the prevailing behavioral characteristics of the leaders were identified:

Emotional stimulation and confrontation.

Caring, support, and nurture.

Meaning attribution and explanation.

Executive and managerial activities.

The group leaders who brought about the most positive results were those who provided high amounts of caring and explaining combined with only moderate amounts of managerial activities and emotional stimulation or confrontation (Lieberman et al., 1973). Loomis (1979) suggested that the four leadership styles cited in this study could be used to designate leadership styles for specific kinds of groups. Table 19-6 presents various types of groups that might respond well to a particular style of leadership.

A group leader is often the target of ambivalent feelings on the part of members. In the early stages of group development the leader is thought to possess enormous power. The leader is assumed to be wise and kind but is also considered a taskmaster.

CHARACTERISTICS OF SELF-HELP GROUPS

■ The members share a common interest, problem, situation, or experience.

■ The groups are largely self-governing, self-regulating, and self-supporting.

■ The groups cooperate with professionals but rely primarily on fellowship among members.

■ The groups conform to a particular organizational code for conducting meetings, accepting members, integrating new members, and accomplishing the group task.

■ The groups frequently emphasize

commitment and responsibility to other members expressed through visitation and phone services that are available to all without charge.

■ The groups disregard or blur strict distinctions between consumers, professionals, and boards of directors, combining and exchanging functions in order to serve the membership at large.

■ There are a wide variety of self-help groups in the United States; the number appears to be growing and they greatly augment professional and community resources.

SOURCE: Adapted from Burnside (1984).

This contradictory perception of the leader creates problems for groups that want the leader to be human but also larger than life. Dependent members, in particular, exaggerate the leader's abilities and minimize their own. Other members may also wish to receive care and attention from the leader but resent the wish. These members become assertive or even aggressive toward the leader, dealing with their conflict by becoming counterdependent (Dick, Lesseer, and Whiteside, 1980).

Three specific techniques have been suggested for dealing with the excessive expectations and ambivalence of members toward the leader. The recommended techniques are (1) turning to the group for validation in order to correct biases, (2) engaging in careful self-disclosure in order to make the leader known or transparent to the group, and (3) using status denial in order to reduce the belief of members that the leader is all-knowing and infallible. A leader using status denial or self-disclosure should recognize the developmental stage of the group. Timing is important; a mature group can tolerate more self-disclosure and status denial by a leader than an immature group can. Inexperienced leaders occasionally engage in self-disclosure in response to their own needs rather than to the group's needs. When engaging in self-disclosure or status denial, the leader must not exploit the group as a vehicle for personal catharsis. On the contrary, the leader should be mindful of his or her role, remaining enough apart from the group to observe, reflect, and analyze so that corrective experiences in the group can be generalized to everyday life by the members (Yalom, 1975).

Coleadership

There are advantages and disadvantages to adopting a coleadership model. Data collection regarding content and process is facilitated by the observations, validation, and feedback that occur between coleaders. Mutual support may lower leader anxiety and increase the reserves of leader energy. Group continuity is assured should one of the leaders become ill or go on vacation. The fact that every group requires two leadership functions—socioemotional responsibility and task responsibility—produces a natural distribution of leader functions when this model is used.

A number of disadvantages have been cited for coleadership (Davis and Lohr, 1971; Dick, Lesseer, and Whiteside, 1980). Coleadership is an arrangement that necessitates respect, compatibility, and trust between the leaders. If rivalry exists between the leaders, a power struggle that inhibits group development may develop. Before organizing the group, coleaders must discuss relevant issues and reach agreement. A protocol must be developed that distributes leadership responsibilities and determines procedural matters. If one leader has more experience than the other, a choice must be made as to whether an egalitarian relationship will exist between them during group sessions or whether one will be the senior and the other a junior partner. Similarly, the prospective leaders must decide whether one will be responsible for socioemotional issues and the other for task issues, or whether these two essential functions will be shared or rotated. As much attention should be devoted to the matching of coleaders and the resolution of co-

To win our deepest respect the individual must both find himself and lose himself. This is not so contradictory as it sounds. We respect the man who places himself at the service of values which transcend his own individuality—the values of his profession, his people, his heritage, and above all, the religious and moral values which nourished the idea of individual fulfillment in the first place. But this "gift of himself" only wins our admiration if the giver has achieved a mature individuality and if the act of giving does not involve an irreparable crippling of that individuality.

JOHN W. GARDNER (1962)

530

leadership issues as to the selection and preparation of group members.

MEMBERSHIP ROLES IN GROUPS

Role enactment refers to the behavioral patterns that are exhibited by individual group members during the life span of the group. Role enactment is usually the result of the personal characteristics and emotional needs of the individual combined with the complex relationships that develop in the group. Role enactment is expressed behaviorally in the form of sustained verbal and nonverbal communication patterns. Usually role enactment is explicit and durable enough to permit leaders and observers to identify the roles that various members assume.

Regardless of its purpose, a group tends to adhere to a constellation of roles that evolve gradually over successive meetings. The role enactment of some members may promote group development, whereas the role enactment of other members may impair group development. Every role enacted in a group produces shared expectations that make group events predictable and understandable. Thus, the member who assumes a certain role in the group may find that the group will not permit that member to relinquish his role. Enacting a certain role in the group may give a member an identity, but it also burdens him with fulfilling the inflexible expectations that others have formed.

One of the obligations of the leader is to unlock fixed or inflexible role enactment that is detrimental to any member or to the group as a whole (Bogdanoff and Elbaum, 1978). This may be done by

leader interventions based on meaning attribution (explaining) and supportive nurture (caring). For example, a single group member may become the target of hostile, negative remarks by other members. The leader might intervene by giving the member some positive recognition. Pointing out similarities between the member under attack and other members with more status is an indirect but effective intervention that protects one member without blaming others.

Group roles have been classified along the following lines (Marram, 1978):

1. Task roles that are essentially administrative and goal oriented.
2. Maintenance roles that enhance group participation and interaction.
3. Egocentric roles that express individual emotional needs.

Egocentric roles are not directed toward maintenance or task accomplishment but are enacted to fulfill personal needs and express inner conflicts. Members who enact egocentric roles often act against the best interests of the group, and their behaviors may become problematic for the group leader (Phipps, 1982). The accompanying box presents a comparison based on role enactment classified as task, maintenance, or egocentric.

A number of roles commonly enacted in groups deserve explanatory comments and basic definitions. *Role differentiation* is the patterned behaviors of group members that can be distinguished and identified. *Role specialization* is the result of the adherence of individual members to persistent and

GROUP ROLE SPECIALIZATION

Task Roles

Initiator—Defines problem, proposes solution, mobilizes group toward problem solving.

Elaborator—Illustrates ideas, predicts, and plans.

Information and opinion seeker—Requests data, opinions, ideas related to problem.

Information and opinion giver—Brings own experiences, opinions, and suggestions regarding group goals and values.

Coordinator—Clarifies ideas, offers suggestions to demonstrate relationships between them, harmonizes activities of members.

Evaluator—Measures group decisions and achievements against group standards and goals.

Energizer—Stimulates group to perform at a higher level.

Orienter—Summarizes discussion, raises questions regarding group's direction.

Liaison—Performs bridging function between group and external authorities, communicates group needs and concerns.

Maintenance Roles

Encourager—Accepts ideas with understanding, approval, and praise.

Diplomat—Mediates group conflicts and relieves tension, is sensitive and tactful.

Process observer—Reflects observation of group process back to group.

Communication facilitator—Uses skillful communication to enhance consensual

validation, encourages other members to participate.

Follower—Passive member, frequently an audience in decision-making situations.

Egocentric Roles

Aggressor—Expresses behavior that reduces others' status and contributions, attacks the group or its task.

Seducer—Engages in openness and self-disclosure that promotes group intimacy but, if premature, may inhibit group progress and increase the anxiety of some members.

Blocker—Uses resistive, negative behavior, returns to issues that have been rejected or discarded previously.

Playboy—Is aloof, displays lack of concern and involvement through "horseplay" or other irrelevant behavior.

Monopolizer—Assumes responsibility for maintaining communication; dominates group, creating group hostility.

Recognition seeker—Attempts to gain admiration and attention by boasting of accomplishments, dressing flamboyantly, arriving late.

Scapegoat—Experiences criticism and/or rejection in the group by doing or saying what other members may wish to do or say but dare not.

Deviant—Reinforces group standards by opposing rules and norms, thereby demonstrating what is and is not acceptable to the group.

Silent member—Remains silent for a variety of reasons such as anxiety, fear of self-disclosure, or desire for attention, but often participates nonverbally.

SOURCE: Compiled from Benne and Sheats (1948), Bales (1953), and Kreigh and Perko (1979).

consistent patterns of behavior. Among the commonly encountered role specialists is the member who becomes the group seducer. No sexual connotations are attached to this label, for the group seducer is merely the member who is least afraid of interpersonal closeness and therefore weakens group defenses against intimacy. At times the seducer can be a very effective group member, but if attempts to become close are made too early in the

life of the group, other members may become frightened by premature intimacy. The counterpart of the seducer is the aggressor. This role is enacted by a member who fears intimacy and self-disclosure and therefore resorts to distancing maneuvers of one kind or another. Humor, superficiality, or anger may characterize the behavior of the aggressor who feels safe only at a distance.

Many groups need a scapegoat, and the mem-

Everyone involved, the newcomer and the others whom he joins, have new experiences with each other. The members of a group tend to influence the newcomer more strongly and determine to a greater extent than he does just what his place should be in the group. This is even more true the longer the group has been in existence and the more frequently and regularly the group members have met . . . If the newcomer wants to change his role or position, he meets with resistance from the group. They may force him not to deviate from the direction of development they have chosen for him, whatever his own inclinations may be.

WALTER TOMAN (1976)

532

ber enacting this role often performs a constructive function, even though appearances may belie this fact. The scapegoat may begin by being a seducer or an aggressor, but as time passes he begins to express feelings that other members would like to express but dare not. When group members hear the scapegoat say what they have been refusing to express, they deny their own feelings by attacking the scapegoat. At times it may be necessary for a leader to assume the role of the scapegoat deliberately in order to protect a candid member from group hostility and to demonstrate that negative opinions are not forbidden. As groups mature and settle down to the task, they have less need of a scapegoat. At this point, the scapegoat, in turn, may find it less necessary to express negative or opposing views (Hare, 1976).

The group deviant is a member who performs a constructive function in the group, even though she appears to be disruptive. The positive function performed by the group deviant is to define, reinforce, and strengthen group norms by separating acceptable from unacceptable behaviors. In a vague way the group majority seems to recognize the value of the deviant, for the group exerts considerable effort trying to convince the deviant to accept group norms. The deviant therefore receives considerable attention from other members and often is persuaded to comply. Occasionally the deviant may drop out of the group rather than accept group standards, and at times the group majority may eventually expel a deviant who fails to conform to a satisfactory extent.

Another member whose behavior may seem disruptive is the group monopolizer. This is usually a garrulous member who demands that all attention

be paid to his personal needs. He may also operate as an unofficial group leader, dispensing advice and information to other members. The motivation of the monopolizer may vary, and it is important for the leader to assess whether the monopolizing behavior stems from anxiety, self-centeredness, fear of closeness, fear of inadequacy, or rebellion against authority. If possible, the leader should not intervene directly to silence the monopolizer, for this may be interpreted by other members as an indication that the leader does not welcome participation. A better tactic is to label monopolizing behavior so that it appears to be constructive. The leader might comment to the group that the monopolizer is doing all the work for other members while they remain aloof, safe, and silent. Such an intervention conveys to other members that their participation is invited but does not display to the group the stark power of the leader (Gibbard, 1974; Kernberg, 1978).

Another member with whom leaders have difficulty is the silent, nonparticipating individual. As in the case of the monopolizer, the motivation of the silent member may vary. Silence may be an attention-getting ploy, or it may indicate anxiety, fear of self-disclosure, or difficulty in verbalizing. The leader might begin by speculating on the meaning of the silence and soliciting the help of the group in identifying the underlying feelings of the silent member. It must be remembered that many nonverbal members are actively participating and getting something out of the interaction of other members. While the leader may comment on the behavior of the silent member, allowances should be made for individual differences. It is necessary to accept the fact that all members may not be equally ready to speak and that excluding a silent member prohibits any possibility of verbalization in a later session.

In addition to the roles enacted by single members, role pairing often appears in a group. Two members may enact the paired roles of lovers who are lost in mutual admiration of each other and therefore are joined in their resistance to change. Another common pairing is that of enemies; this emerges when two members oppose each other regardless of the issue involved or the cost to themselves or the group. These are members whose decisions are not determined by logic or reason but are controlled by a need to frustrate the opposing member who is enacting the role of enemy. Group performance may be enhanced by paired members who work well together as collaborators but refuse to become more than a task-oriented team. Their avoidance of intimacy is detrimental only if socioemotional satisfaction is essential to achieving the group task. The pairing most effective is that of members who consider themselves comrades. Such pairing encourages members to work, fight, love, and respect each other in the interests of the group and for the benefit of all members (Bion, 1959; Dunphy, 1974).

CURATIVE FACTORS IN GROUPS

Yalom (1975) described group curative factors as interpersonal experiences or transactions that propel individual members and the group toward productivity, competence, and a sense of well-being. Certain curative factors have been identified as present in groups to varying degrees. The curative factors

---

GROUP CURATIVE FACTORS

■ *Guidance*. Experiences in the group that include suggestions and advice on the modification of destructive social attitudes and behaviors.

■ *Altruism*. Actions that demonstrate mutual caring and concern among members.

■ *Cohesion*. Shared belief that the group is meaningful to members and that members are meaningful to the group.

■ *Catharsis*. Therapeutic ventilation and expression of feelings, both positive and negative, within the group.

■ *Identification*. Adoption of functional behaviors and problem-solving techniques patterned after those of the leader or other group members.

■ *Family reenactment*. Reliving early family experiences in a conscious, corrective manner.

■ *Interpersonal learning: input*. Activities related to having events or experiences explained, described, or interpreted by others.

■ *Interpersonal learning: output*. Activities related to explaining, describing, or interpreting events and experiences to others.

■ *Universality*. Recognition that one's problems, fears, and emotions are not unique.

■ *Insight*. Understanding the causes and sources of conflicted attitudes and behaviors.

■ *Instillation of hope*. Growing belief that one's problems can be solved.

■ *Existentialism*. Accepting the need for self-direction and self-determination, in order to improve the quality of existence.

---

identified by Yalom are listed in the accompanying box.

Curative factors that are process oriented include guidance, altruism, cohesion, catharsis, identification, universality, insight, instillation of hope, and existentialism. Each operates in ways that promote growth from immature to mature group behaviors. The curative factors that are almost entirely content based are interpersonal learning: input and output. If the information is relevant to group needs or to the group task, the members enjoy reduced anxiety as their cognitive understanding increases. One example of the effect of these curative factors is the reduced tension in a class-

---

JUDGMENTAL VERSUS NONJUDGMENTAL NURSING BEHAVIORS

■ *Moral Judgments:* Forms of blaming that have no place in nursing theory or practice.

■ *Speculative Judgments:* Untested choices that may contribute to nursing theory but prove risky in nursing practice until validated.

■ *Pragmatic Judgments:* Decisions based on practicality and on recollection of what measures proved effective in the past.

■ *Professional Judgments:* Optimal judgments that integrate tested theoretical formulations, situational factors, and clinical and ethical considerations with nursing process and role.

SOURCE: Adapted from Mary Ellen Doona, *Travelbee's Intervention in Psychiatric Nursing*, 2nd ed. (Philadelphia: Davis, 1979).

534

room situation when the group is able to master the material presented by the instructor. Yet even these two curative factors have some process elements, in that exchanging information within a group leads to a realization of common interests or universality, which in turn leads to group cohesion.

Group leaders often use verbal and nonverbal language to encourage the emergence of various curative factors. This may be done by modeling clear, direct communication or by commenting on interactions between members in which certain curative factors were present. For instance, one member might reveal difficulties being experienced in a personal relationship. The leader might refer to a similar problem previously revealed by another member and solicit help from that member. Such an intervention would promote the process factors of universality and group cohesion. If one member was observed giving support or encouragement to another member, recognition of this by the leader would reinforce the curative factor of altruism and promote imitative behavior from other members. Curative factors are helpful even when members do not call attention to their presence but are usually more beneficial if attention is directed to them because cognitive and emotional understanding of what is happening in the group strengthens the positive reactions in the members (Boyer, 1982).

GROUP RESEARCH ISSUES

Group research, like other aspects of group work, can be extraordinarily complex, especially if undertaken in a clinical setting. General guidelines were offered by Loomis (1979), who listed the following sources of group data:

Individual group members.

Group leaders or coleaders.

The group as a whole.

Significant persons in the lives of members.

Group observers and supervisors.

Relying on these sources of data does not guarantee reliability or validity, because reports from any of these sources may be highly subjective. Some nurse leaders compare data by using pretests and posttests. However, even carefully designed instruments may not accurately reflect group dynamics or group outcomes. Members and leaders alike may overestimate or underestimate the outcomes of the group experience. Reports of changes observed by significant others may be equally unreliable.

Even though group research can be formidable, nurses are beginning to look beyond customary clinical approaches and to subject their work to more rigorous examination. Nurses starting to organize a group project can easily incorporate a research tool that will elevate their work from the level of intuition to the realm of theory building.

An essential decision is to decide what aspect of group work can be included in the research process. Will the research be focused on leadership versus membership behaviors? Will process or content be studied? Will group productivity or emotional satisfaction be compared?

Having determined the scope of the study, the nurse must begin to formulate clear, concise hypotheses based upon the defined goals set for the

---

BALES' INTERACTION PROCESS ANALYSIS

Social-Emotional Behavior
A. Positive reactions
   1. Shows solidarity: jokes, raises others' status, gives help.
   2. Shows tension release: laughs, shows satisfaction.
   3. Shows agreement: passive acceptance, understands, complies.
B. Negative reactions
   4. Shows disagreement: passive rejection, formality, withholds help.
   5. Shows tension: asks for help, withdraws from field.
   6. Shows antagonism: deflates others' status, defends or asserts self.

Task Behavior
A. Problem-solving
   7. Gives suggestions: direction, implying autonomy for others.
   8. Gives opinion: evaluation, analysis, expresses feelings, wishes.
   9. Gives information: orientation, repeats, clarifies, confirms.
B. Questioning
   10. Asks for information: orientation, repetition, confirmation.
   11. Asks for opinion: evaluation, analysis, expression of feelings.
   12. Asks for suggestions: direction, possible ways of acting.

SOURCE: Adapted from Bales (1953).

---

group. An illustration of a goal-related hypothesis is "Elderly members of a daily reminiscing group will demonstrate lower depression levels as measured by a valid and reliable self-evaluation scale." To prove or disprove the hypothesis pretesting and posttesting are necessary so that comparisons may be made.

As in any research study, the protection of human subjects is of great importance and agency policies must be strictly followed. How well these requirements have been fulfilled may be determined by asking the following questions (Maher, 1978; Zastowny and deFrank, 1982):

■ Have specific goals been determined and clearly defined?

■ Is there an explicit hypothesis based on the goals?

■ Is the hypothesis compatible with the goals of the group, the composition of the group, and the leadership style that has been selected?

■ Will the addition of systematic data collection impair group progress and affect group outcomes?

■ Is the group membership adequately protected from intrusiveness or invasiveness resulting from data collection?

■ Is the sponsoring agency in agreement with data collection procedures?

■ Have proper procedures been followed to secure permission for data collection from the members, from the sponsoring agency, and from the appropriate human subjects research committee, if one exists?

There are a number of ways for a nurse to proceed once the working hypothesis has been determined (Liddle, 1982). It is possible to compare phenonema in different groups or to examine contrasting leadership styles. A number of interesting tools are available to nurses beginning to try their research skills. Among the tools are the Bales Interaction Process Analysis (Bales, 1953; Hare, 1976), which categorizes group behaviors and can be used to measure leader and member behaviors (see the accompanying box). The Bales interaction scoring method conceptualizes the group as an ordered system and helps the scorer attend to each transaction as it occurs. Some deficiencies of the scoring method have been cited by Mills (1967) as follows:

1. Substantive aspects of interaction are not recorded either in detail or thematically.

2. The intent, purpose, or aim of the actors is not recorded.

3. The affective content of actors is not recorded.

4. Cognitive experiences that stimulate or are stimulated by the interactions are not recorded.

Another provocative tool is the questionnaire based on Yalom's (1975) curative factors, which can be used to compare leader and member opinions of what is helpful within a single group, or leader and member opinions across groups. A number of authorities in the field of group research have urged that leader and member responses to group experiences be compared in order to formulate optimum treatment combinations for various group populations (Zastowny and deFrank, 1982).

The physical environment in which a group meets can affect group content, process development, and outcomes (Hare, 1976). Ecology is the study of the relationship of human beings to the environment they inhabit. The Ward Atmosphere Scale has been developed to measure ecological variables and the Group Atmosphere Scale is available to assess the perceptions members have of the psychosocial climate within the group (Silbergeld, Manderscheid, and Koenig, 1977). Although designed for psychotherapy groups, these and similar tools may be used with many types of therapeutic groups.

Another way of making systematic observations is to assign a specific task for the group to accomplish. Such a procedure enhances group comparisons because the task on which different groups work is standardized. Analyzing the actions used by the group to complete the task can be employed to identify intragroup behavior and to note intergroup differences. Bales' Interaction Process Analysis is concerned mostly with verbal exchanges in the group, but it is also possible to study spatial differences as an assigned task if confronted. Noting the manner in which group members position themselves so as to preserve, increase, or decrease distances from one another can provide additional data on the nature of group interactions (Shaw, 1976). Group research is not a simple matter, but it is possible for a generalist nurse to incorporate a measurement tool when planning a group project with clients.

SUMMARY

Group work may be divided into therapy groups and therapeutic groups. The first category includes groups that deal with intrapsychic problems, while the latter includes groups concerned with interpersonal, cognitive, or behavioral change. Nurses have been working with groups and families for many years, but only nurses who possess advanced degrees are considered qualified by the American Nurses' Association to function as group psychotherapists.

Joseph Pratt, a Boston internist, is credited with being the founder of group work as a treatment modality. Samuel Slavson, an engineer, used play therapy as a method of dealing with the problems of children. Slavson was instrumental in founding the American Group Therapy Association, an interdisciplinary organization that opened group work to disciplines other than medicine. The use of psychodrama was introduced by Jacob Moreno, who used spontaneous dramatization of life experiences as a way of dealing with the life problems of

C L I N I C A L   E X A M P L E

ANTICIPATORY PROBLEM SOLVING IN A SHORT-TERM THERAPY GROUP

ASSESSMENT

One of the most discouraging obstacles for group leaders is lack of involvement on the part of the members, which leads to sporadic attendance, low morale and cohesion, and occasionally the dissolution of the group. The problem was avoided in this instance because of several measures adopted by two co-therapists, a female psychiatric nurse and a male psychologist, in order to facilitate a successful group experience in a partial hospitalization unit.

The group studied consisted of eight clients, four males and four females, all attending a metropolitan day hospital facility and identified as psychiatrically disabled. Their ages ranged from seventeen to forty years; five of them were between the ages of nineteen and thirty. The group met for fifteen sessions over a period of eight weeks. Clients considered appropriate for group therapy were selected for a short-term group chiefly on the basis of the length of their expected stay in the day hospital. Those likely to remain for more than three months in the treatment facility were generally invited to join another group that offered long-term, open-ended therapy.

The two co-therapists sought to foster group cohesion and commitment by introducing certain innovations. The previous short-term group in the day hospital had terminated prematurely, largely because of the inability of one co-therapist to sustain the group during the three-week illness of the other co-therapist. Although the staff had tried to deal therapeutically with these developments, some of the clients in the day hospital expressed negative views concerning the usefulness of group therapy and a disinclination to engage in any future sessions. It was for these reasons that the new group therapists chose to allow several weeks to elapse between the expiration of one group and the start of theirs.

PLANNING

Nine clients were approached and interviewed by the therapists; eight were ultimately invited to join the group. The one client who did not become a member withdrew from day hospital during the selection process for unrelated reasons. Each candidate met two, three, or even four times with the therapists. Usually three or four interviews were undertaken when a client was undecided or was inclined to establish his own conditions for membership. All but one client came to take an active role in the interviews; one client asked the therapists what their

qualifications were, and another threatened that he might "take over" the group if he didn't like the way the therapists were working.

During this time, the therapists stressed that this short-term group would be extremely rigorous in its pursuit of its goals and that only serious, committed members were being sought. The primary goal was to increase the social skills and decrease social anxiety of the members. The therapists stated that they and the members would share the responsibility for making the group experience a meaningful one. Therefore, potential members were urged to make a firm commitment to the group, should they decide to join. At no time did the therapists allow any client to assume that he would automatically be accepted as a group member, so that the choosing eventually became a mutual process in which the client's decision to accept membership became as significant as the therapists' decision to offer it. At the initial interview each candidate was given a copy of the following group contract:

Short-Term Group Contract

1. There will be no forcing of people into this group. However, we ask a verbal commitment to attend regularly. We are interested in prospective members who have problems in relating to people.

2. We shall try to face our life problems honestly and to share them.

3. We expect therapists and members to work hard during the sessions.

4. We promise confidentiality.

5. Group contract:
   a. to meet twice a week for one hour on Tuesdays and Thursdays.
   b. to attend all fifteen sessions, as far as possible.
   c. to deal in the group with whatever happens in the group.

IMPLEMENTATION

A few days before the first session, a short questionnaire was given to each member asking how much he or she expected to benefit from the short-term group. Members were asked to complete the questionnaire and return it to therapists at the first session. They were also told that they would be asked to fill out an evaluation of the group at the conclusion of the sessions. At this time each member was given a short letter welcoming him into the group and listing the names of all group members. Rather significantly, all members returned the first questionnaire promptly, and one member insisted on reading his aloud to the group at the first meeting so that everyone would know what his expectations were.

Expectations Questionnaire

How much do you expect your group experience to help you? Please circle one of the numbers below.

1. Not at all
2. A little
3. An average amount
4. A considerable amount
5. A very great amount

In your own words, what are your goals of participating in this group? What do you hope to gain from the group experience?

During the preliminary interviews and at the group sessions, the therapists tried to encourage full participation of the members without censure or undue control. Both therapists were democratic rather than authoritarian, intervening primarily to lead all members into involvement. The therapists consciously tried to avoid setting themselves above the group and presented themselves as flexible and accepting figures. Although they did not admit illness or pathology in their own personalities, they stressed the universality of emotions and the prevalence of certain behavior patterns. They interpreted rarely, believing that interpretations in a short-term group should come from the members. When making interpretations, the therapists were tentative rather than didactic, except when discussing their own feelings. As group members became more active, the therapists became less so. In a few situations when the group behaved harshly toward a member, the therapists tried to give the beleaguered member a measure of support without denying the accuracy of the group's assumptions or its freedom to deal with any member or action.

Each session lasted one hour and was held twice weekly. Every session was followed by a critique lasting 30 minutes that was attended by a designated staff observer and by other interested staff members, who attended as their schedules permitted. The members also were informed of the presence and identity of the staff member who functioned as an observer during the sessions behind a one-way mirror. They also realized that post-group meetings followed their sessions. In the first meeting, each member was assigned an alphabetical letter by the observers that was not known to the leaders.

EVALUATION

At the next-to-the-last session, group members were asked to complete the following evaluation form and return it unsigned (except for the alphabetical letter) in a sealed envelope at the final meeting.

Evaluation Questionnaire

How much has your group experience helped you? Please circle one of the numbers below.

1. Not at all
2. A little
3. An average amount
4. A considerable amount
5. A very great amount

In your own words tell what you have gained from this group experience. How many sessions did you attend?

The emphasis on commitment and the early development of group cohesion may have induced the risk taking, which several members were willing to assume. Most members seemed to remember keenly the lengthy selection process and some of the considerations of the interviews. Often they would remind one another that this was a group pledged to hard work and to solving relationship problems. There seemed agreement that whatever troubled one member was the concern of all, and that any topic, however intimate, was allowable. When it became apparent that the therapists would suggest, but not control, the group began to exercise its own control and to make its own judgments. Explicit language was used throughout the sessions, not for shock value, but to communicate, in tacit awareness that within the group honesty was safe and that all present understood and spoke the same language.

Although subjective, the comments on their group experience in the members' own words were poignant to read and showed the prevailing desire to be part of a successful group experience. Some brief excerpts:

> I have been able to talk about things I never thought I could. I feel freer and more open . . . the group helped me accept myself.

> I wanted a friendship with D. but I didn't get it. I had to keep things going though. I've solved all my problems. The therapists weren't bossy. They acted equal. I helped them do this.

> More awareness, more self-confidence, less fear of risk and what people can do to hurt me.

> I felt a certain moral support from the group which helped to give me the strength to continue to do better.

> It helped me be more sociable.

> This group has helped me to be (a) better person so that I can speak more freely with other people and get better adjusted to the public life outside the hospital.

If a positive group experience is rewarding for the group members, it is equally rewarding for the therapist. For the therapist there is the joy derived from carrying an arduous task to a successful conclusion. Perhaps the

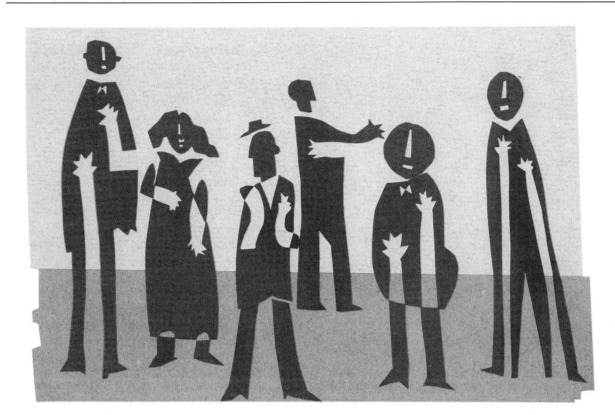

chief value of the measures used in this short-term group can be found in the fact that they extended to members the sense of accomplishment usually reserved for therapists. The gains made by members as a result of group therapy are often more evident to the trained observer than to the member himself, who is less conscious of the progress already made than of the distance he still must go. The simple comparison of pregroup expectations with postgroup evaluations afforded group members a sense of improvement they might not otherwise have admitted (see Table 19-7).

Group cohesion was evidenced by the concern expressed almost from the first meeting whenever members were absent and by the overt annoyance at unwarranted absence or lateness. At the end of each session, the members displayed a noticeable reluctance to leave.

Table 19-7. Comparison of Pregroup and Postgroup Ratings

Members	Pretest Expectations	Posttest Evaluation	Number of Sessions Attended
A	2	4	13
B	3	3	12
C	1	*	8
D	3	4	11
E	2	4	15
F	2	*	5
G	1	*	5
H	1	4	13

*Questionnaire not returned.

Several proposals were made to extend the number of sessions or to meet outside the treatment facility merely "to talk." As the last session approached, sadness was expressed and finally anger, especially toward the male therapist, who was not a full-time member of the day hospital staff.

The prolonged selection process and the cohesion that developed early in the life of the group seemed to reduce the resistance that often emerges. Absenteeism for the entire group was at the satisfactory figure of 28 percent and would have been lower except that two members left the day hospital to take advantage of Christmas employment opportunities. Another member simultaneously terminated her connection with the day hospital and with the short-term group. One member attended all meetings; two members attended all but two sessions and had valid reasons for missing these. No client reported receiving less from the short-term group than had been expected and half of them reported receiving more.

No two groups are identical, yet there are characteristics common to all groups. Some of these are constructive, but many are not. Certainly, the means used here to encourage motivation and commitment would not be suitable for every group of clients. For some therapists the lengthy interviewing would be tedious and the techniques used would seem mechanical and simplistic. Should the suggested practices cause discomfort to the leader, there is no better reason for avoiding them. If, however, a therapist can use them easily and naturally, they may prove worth a trial. At least in this limited sample, they allowed group members and group therapists to share a sense of accomplishment.

the actors and the audience. The Northfield experiment during World War II was another important development that expanded the clinical application of group methods.

A number of psychoanalytic concepts are evident in groups even though the group may be devoted to here-and-now events. According to psychoanalytic theory, the group represents a corrective reenactment of the original family experience. A less psychoanalytic view is that the group is a social microcosm.

In organizing a group, nurses are advised to follow the nursing process, devoting sufficient attention to assessing the needs of a target population, planning group objectives and negotiating a group contract, implementing the design, and evaluating the impact of the group experience.

Assessing and evaluating the effectiveness of the group experience is facilitated by dividing group development into three stages: the initial stage, the middle stage, and the final stage. Each stage is likely to be dominated by clusters of behaviors, some of which may appear to be disruptive to group progress and troublesome to the leader.

Group leadership involves two major functions: maintaining the group and accomplishing the purpose for which the group was formed. In addition, the leader should analyze group content and group process in order to base interventions on the needs of the group. Several leadership styles are available, each of which has certain advantages and disadvantages. Choice of a leadership style is dependent on the needs of members and the goals of the group.

There are a number of egocentric roles that may be enacted by group members. Some of these may seem to impede group progress but in fact may not. Among the egocentric roles are those of group seducer, aggressor, scapegoat, and deviant. Group leaders should analyze the reasons members enact these roles and formulate interventions accordingly.

A number of curative factors are present in groups to varying degrees. Knowledge of the curative factors enables the leader to recognize some of the forces that are operative in the group. In addition, identification of the curative factors present in groups may become the basis of systematic investigation by generalist nurses and others who wish to incorporate research in their clinical practice.

Review Questions

1. What characteristics make a reference group different from a secondary group?

2. What was the significance of the Northfield experiment on the expansion of group work?

3. Explain what is meant by the "Noah's Ark Principle."

4. List the dominant issues that are likely to emerge in the first stage of group development.

5. In helping members deal with termination of the group, what interventions might prove facilitative?

6. Describe the characteristics of different leadership styles and their probable effect on the group.

7. Differentiate group content from group process. Why is it important to include both when analyzing group development?

8. What are the advantages of using coleadership?

9. Define the term "role specialization" and give examples of task role enactment, maintenance role enactment, and egocentric role enactment in groups.

10. What is meant by the term *group curative factors*?

References

Adams, J. 1971. Student Evaluations of an Interactional Group Experience. *Journal of Psychiatric Nursing and Mental Health Services*, 9(4):28–36.

Anderson, S. A., and Russell, C. J. 1982. Utilizing Process and Content in Designing Paradoxical Interventions. *American Journal of Family Therapy*, 10:48–60.

Anthony, E. J. 1971. The History of Group Psychotherapy. In *Comprehensive Group Psychotherapy*, eds. H. I. Kaplan and B. J. Sadock. Baltimore: Williams & Wilkins.

Armstrong, J., and Rouslin, J. 1963. *Group Psychotherapy in Nursing Practice*. New York: Macmillan.

Bales, R. F. 1953. *Interaction Process Analysis: A Method for the Study of Small Groups*. Cambridge, Mass: Addison-Wesley.

Benne, K. D., and Sheats, P. 1948. Functional Roles of Group Members. *Journal of Social Issues*, 4(2):41–49.

Bion, W. R. 1959. *Experiences in Groups*. New York: Basic Books.

Bogdanoff, M. A., and Elbaum, P. L. 1978. Role Lock: Dealing with Monopolizers, Mistrusters, Isolates, Helpful Hannahs and Other Assorted Characters in Group Psychotherapy. *International Journal of Group Psychotherapy*, 28(2):247–262.

Boyer, V. B. 1982. Process and Content: Distinctions and Implications. In *Life Cycle Group Work in Nursing*, eds. E. H. Janosik and L. B. Phipps. Monterey, Calif.: Wadsworth Health Sciences.

Burnside, I. 1984. *Working with the Elderly*. Monterey, Calif.: Wadsworth Health Sciences.

Caplan, G. 1964. *Principles of Basic Psychiatry*. New York: Basic Books.

Caplan, G. 1970. *Theory and Practice of Mental Health Consultation*. New York: Basic Books.

Coker, F. W. 1946. *Readings in Political Philosophy*. New York: Macmillan.

Coleman, J. C.; Butcher, J. N.; and Carson, R. C. 1984. *Abnormal Psychology in Modern Life*, 7th ed. Glenview, Ill.: Scott, Foresman.

Davis, F. B., and Lohr, N. E. 1971. Special Problems with the Use of Cotherapists. *International Journal of Group Psychotherapy*, 21(2):143–158.

Dick, B.; Lesseer, K.; and Whiteside, J. 1980. A Developmental Framework for Cotherapy. *International Journal of Group Psychotherapy*, 30(3):273–285.

Dunphy, D. C. 1974. Phases, Roles, and Myths in Self Analytic Groups. In *Analysis of Groups*, eds. G. B. Gibbard, J. J. Hartman, and R. D. Mann. San Francisco: Jossey-Bass.

Egan, G. 1982. *The Skilled Helper*, 2nd ed. Monterey, Calif.: Brooks/Cole.

Erikson, E. H. 1963. *Childhood and Society*. New York: W. W. Norton.

Freud, S. 1957. Group Psychology and the Analysis of the Ego. In *Standard Edition of Complete Psychological Works of Sigmund Freud*, Vol. 18. London: Hogarth Press.

Gardner, J. W. 1962. *Excellence*. New York: Harper & Row.

Gardner, K. 1979. Small Groups and Their Therapeutic Force. *Principles and Practice of Psychiatric Nursing*, eds. G. Stuart and J. Sundean. St. Louis: C. V. Mosby.

Gibbard, G. S. 1974. Individuation, Fusion, and Role Specialization. In *Analysis of Groups*, eds. G. S. Gibbard, J. J. Hartman, and R. D. Mann. San Francisco: Jossey-Bass.

Hare, A. P. 1976. *Handbook of Small Group Research*, 2nd ed. New York: Free Press.

Janosik, E. H., and Phipps, L. B., eds. 1982. *Life Cycle Group Work in Nursing*. Monterey, Calif.: Wadsworth Health Sciences.

Kernberg, O. F. 1978. Leadership and Organizational Functioning: Organizational Regression. *International Journal of Group Psychotherapy*, 28(1):3–25.

Kreigh, H. Z., and Perko, J. E. 1979. *Psychiatric and Mental Health Nursing: A Commitment to Care and Concern*. Reston, Va.: Reston.

Lancaster, J. 1982. Communication as a Tool for Change. In *The Nurse as Change Agent*, eds. J. Lancaster and W. Lancaster. St. Louis: C. V. Mosby.

Lego, S. 1978. Group Dynamic Theory and Application. In *Comprehensive Psychiatric Nursing*, eds. J. Haber, et al. New York: McGraw-Hill.

Lewin, K. 1957. *Field Theory in the Social Sciences*. New York: Harper & Row.

Liddle, H. A. 1982. On the Problems of Eclecticism. *Family Process*, 21:243–250.

Lieberman, M. A.; Yalom, I. D.; and Miles, M. B. 1973. Encounter Groups: The Leader Makes the Difference. *Psychology Today*, 6(10):69–76.

Loomis, M. K. 1979. *Group Process for Nurses*. St. Louis: C. V. Mosby.

Maher, B. A. 1978. A Reader's, Writer's and Reviewer's Guide to Assessing Research Reports in Clinical Psychology. *Journal of Consulting and Clinical Psychology*, 46:643–647.

Maluccio, A. N. 1981. A Task Based Approach to Family Treatment. In *Understanding the Family*, eds. C. Gelty and W. Humphrey. New York: Appleton-Century-Crofts.

Marram, G. W. 1978. *The Group Approach in Nursing Practice*. St. Louis: C. V. Mosby.

Marvin, L. K. 1982. Group Organization: Selection Criteria, Member Preparation, Contractual Issues. In *Life Cycle Group Work in Nursing*, eds. E. H. Janosik and L. B. Phipps. Monterey, Calif: Wadsworth Health Sciences.

Maslow, A. 1968. *Toward a Psychology of Being*. New York: Van Nostrand.

McDougall, W. 1920. *The Group Mind*. Cambridge, England: University Press.

Miller, J. R., and Janosik, E. H. 1980. Evaluation of Family Process. In *Family-Focused Care*, eds. E. H. Janosik and J. R. Miller. New York: McGraw-Hill.

Mills, T. M. 1967. *The Sociology of Small Groups*. Englewood Cliffs, N.J.: Prentice-Hall.

Ofshe, R. J., ed. 1973. *Interpersonal Behaviors in Small Groups*. Englewood Cliffs, N.J.: Prentice-Hall.

Phipps, L. B. 1982. Membership Role Enactment. In *Life Cycle Group Work in Nursing*, eds. E. H. Janosik and L. B. Phipps. Monterey, Calif.: Wadsworth.

Racy, J. 1969. How a Group Grows. *American Journal of Nursing*, 69(11):2396–2400.

Rioch, M. J. 1975. Group Relations: Rationale and Technique. In *Group Relations Reader*, eds. A. D. Colman, and W. H. Bexton. Sausalito, Calif.

Robinson, L. 1983. *Psychiatric Nursing as a Human Experience*. Philadelphia: W. B. Saunders.

Rubin, S. 1981. A Two Track Model of Bereavement: Theory and Application in Research. *American Journal of Orthopsychiatry*, 51(1):101–109.

Sadock, B. J. 1980. Group Psychotherapy, Combined Individual and Group Psychotherapy, and Psychodrama. In *Comprehensive Textbook of Psychiatry*, 3rd ed., eds. H. I. Kaplan, A. M. Freedman, and B. J. Sadock. Baltimore: Williams & Wilkins.

Sampson, E., and Marthas, M. 1977. *Group Process for the Health Professions*. New York: John Wiley & Sons.

Sayre, J. 1979. Alternative Healing Therapies. In *Psychiatric Nursing*, eds. H. S. Wilson and C. R. Kneisl. Menlo Park, Calif.: Addison-Wesley.

Schutz, W. C. 1966. *FIRO: A Three-Dimensional Theory of Interpersonal Behavior*. New York: Holt, Rinehart, and Winston.

Scott, E. M. 1976. The Alcoholic Group: Formation and Beginnings. *Group Process*, 7:95–116.

Shaw, M. E. 1976. *Group Dynamics: The Psychology of Small Group Behavior*. New York: McGraw-Hill.

Slavson, S. R. 1964. *A Textbook In Analytic Group Psychotherapy*. New York: International Universities Press.

Slavson, S. R. 1974. *Child-Centered Guidance of Parents*. New York: International Universities Press.

Silbergeld, S.; Manderscheid, R. W.; and Koenig, G. R. 1977. The Psychosocial Environment in Group Therapy Evaluation. *International Journal of Group Psychotherapy*, 27:153–163.

Toman, W. 1976. *Family Constellation*, 3rd ed. New York: Springer.

Tuckman, B. W. 1965. Developmental Sequence in Small Groups. *Psychological Bulletin*, 63:384–389.

Whitaker, D. S. 1976. A Group-Centered Approach. *Group Process*, 7:37–57.

White, R., and Lippitt, R. 1953. Leader Behavior and Member Reaction in Three Social Climates. In *Group Dynamics, Research, and Theory*, eds. D. Cartwright and A. Zandeu. Evanston, Ill.: Row Patterson.

Yalom, I. D. 1975. *Theory and Practice of Group Psychotherapy*. New York: Basic Books.

541

Yalom, I. D., and Lieberman, M. A. 1972. A Study of Encounter Group Casualties. In *Progress in Group and Family Therapy*, eds. C. J. Sagaw and H. I. Kaplan. New York: Brunner/Mazel.

Zastowny, J. R., and deFrank, R. J. 1982. Empirical Investigation: Research Strategy. In *Life Cycle Group Work in Nursing*, eds. E. H. Janosik and L. B. Phipps. Monterey, Calif.: Wadsworth Health Sciences.

Supplementary Readings

Brabender, V. A Study of Curative Factors in Short-Term Group Psychotherapy. *Hospital and Community Psychiatry*, 34(1983):643–644.

Clark, C. C. *The Nurse as Group Leader*. New York: Springer, 1977.

Durkin, H. E. Change in Group Psychotherapy: Therapy and Practice—A Systems Perspective. *International Journal of Group Psychotherapy*, 32(1982):431–439.

Fielding, J. M. Verbal Participation and Group Therapy Outcome. *British Journal of Psychiatry*, 142(1983): 524–528.

Gorden, V. C. Themes and Cohesiveness Observed in Depressed Women's Support Group. *Issues in Mental Health Nursing*, 4(1982):115–125.

Johnson, D. R. Principles of Group Treatment in a Nursing Home. *Journal of Long Term Care Administration*, 10(1982):19–24.

Jordan, F. T. Group Process in Action: A Detoxification Unit for Alcoholics. *Free Association*, 10(1983):7–10.

Kansas, N. Homogeneous Group Therapy for Acutely Psychotic Schizophrenic Inpatients. *Hospital and Community Psychiatry*, 34(1983):257–259.

Kibel, H. D. A Schema for Understanding Resistance in Groups. *Group Process*, 7(1977):221–236.

Levinger, L. A Values Clarification Group with Adolescents. *Social Work and Health Care*, 8(1982):95–98.

Matteson, M. A. Group Reminiscing Therapy with Elderly Clients. *Issues in Mental Health Nursing*, 4(1982): 177–189.

Ruffin, J. E. Racism as Countertransference in Psychotherapy Groups. *Perspectives in Psychiatric Care*, 11 (1973):173–178.

Schwartzberg, S. L. A Comparison of Three Treatment Group Formats for Facilitating Social Interaction. *Occupational Therapy in Mental Health*, 2(1982):1–16.

Sewall, K. S. Peer Group Reality Therapy for the Pregnant Adolescent. *American Journal of Maternal Child Nursing*, 8(1983):67–69.

Toker, E. The Scapegoat as an Essential Group Phenomenon. *International Journal of Group Psychotherapy*, 22(1972):320–332.

Weiner, M. F. Termination of Group Psychotherapy. *Group Process*, 5(1973):85–93.

Williams, K. Use of Small Group with Chronically Ill Children. *Journal of School Health*, 53(1983):205–207.

Yalom, I. D. Problems of Neophyte Group Therapists. *International Journal of Social Psychology*, 15(1966):52–59.

THE DIMENSIONS OF COMMUNITY
Community as Group
Community as Place
Community as Culture

EPIDEMIOLOGICAL CONCEPTS
Host, Agent, and Environment
Epidemiological Terminology
Risk Factors

COMMUNITY HEALTH CARE DELIVERY

THE IMPACT OF DEINSTITUTIONALIZATION

*THE ROLE OF THE COMMUNITY MENTAL
HEALTH NURSE*

COMMUNITY PROGRAM EVALUATION

C   H   A   P   T   E   R

20

Community Theory and Practice

Learning Objectives

After reading this chapter, the student should be able to:

1. Describe the concept of community as place, group, and culture.

2. Define epidemiological terms related to community health.

3. Differentiate biological, psychological, and environmental risk factors.

4. Analyze the impact of the deinstitutionalization process on clients and on communities.

5. Describe various aspects of the role of the community mental health nurse.

6. Identify variables important to the evaluation of community health programs.

Overview

What constitutes a healthy or unhealthy community in regard to mental health? Are the indicators of mental health or mental illness the same for communities as for individuals and families? Since individuals and families have the right and responsibility to participate in their own health care, who has responsibility for the health of a community, especially in regard to issues as vast and imprecise as those concerning mental health?

These questions arouse lively discussion among health professionals and lay persons alike, most of whom realize that the planning and management of collective health issues require collaborative efforts from health care workers and health care consumers. In collaborative efforts to

deal with community health issues, health professionals are perceived as experts and resource persons. Therefore, they need extensive knowledge concerning the community that is being served. Knowledge of health issues that once existed in the community, that presently exist in the community, or that are likely to exist in the future is essential to realistic planning and the best use of community resources. This is true of community health in general and of community mental health in particular. In this chapter, *community* is defined along several dimensions, and such important aspects of community care as epidemiology, deinstitutionalization, and program evaluation are discussed.

*Good laws lead to the making of better ones; bad ones
bring about worse. As soon as anyone says of the affairs
of the state, "What does it matter to me?" the state may
be given up for lost.*
JEAN-JACQUES ROUSSEAU

545

THE DIMENSIONS OF COMMUNITY

In order to discuss community mental health, it is necessary first to determine what is meant by the word *community*. The American Heritage Dictionary defines community as "a group of people living together in the same locality and under the same government; the district or locality in which they live; a social group or class having common interests." Thus, the term community may be applied to a variety of settings, interests, and groups.

Community can mean different things to different people. Communities may be geographic areas, such as neighborhoods, contained within spatial limits. Communities may consist of individuals drawn together for special reasons. Students may be part of a school community for only a few years, while teachers may be part of the school community for their entire working lives. The school community demonstrates that community membership not only has different time frames for various members but also imposes different role expectations for members who serve in different capacities: Any school community expects one set of behaviors from students and another set from teachers (Stuart, 1981).

Common experiences or shared cultures may lead to the formation of a community. Religious orders are communities created around shared missions and values. Membership in a particular ethnic group with a common history establishes another kind of community. Belonging to the black community in the United States does not depend on geography but is based on shared experiences, historical and contemporary. Thus, a community may

not always be the place where one lives but may be a collective way of life or state of mind.

There are also communities within larger communities. One area may contain several subdivisions or enclaves existing within the larger community of neighborhood. Essential to the meaning of community is the idea that individuals and families are not solitary but exist in relation to other individuals and families. Because community is an ambiguous term, it is crucial that one understand clearly what is meant when the word is used (Greenblatt, 1980).

When it comes to community mental health, the term *community* also has a specific political meaning. Recall from Chapter 1 that enabling legislation dealing with mental health centers defined a community as a *catchment area* delineated by geographic boundaries that cut across established neighborhoods and social class differences. Homogeneity was not an important consideration in setting up catchment areas. More important considerations included the range of the catchment population in terms of size, income, and social class. Heterogeneity within a catchment area was thought to be more desirable than homogeneity. Thus, although community mental health nurses work within a specific geographic area, they come into contact with, and must be knowledgeable about, communities that vary along the dimensions of group, place, and culture.

Community as Group
Any ethnic or racial group with shared values and a common culture may be regarded as a community regardless of whether they reside close to one another. Hispanics living anywhere in a city are apt to consider themselves part of the Spanish Amer-

Plato and Aristotle believed that the best social order was the one that experienced the fewest changes; there was no room in their world for the concept of continued change and growth. Growth, after all, did not signal greater value and order in the world but the exact opposite. If history represented the continued chipping away of the original perfect state, and the using up of the original fixed bounty, then the ideal state was the one that slowed down the process of decay as much as possible. The Greeks associated greater change and growth with greater decay and chaos. Their goal, then, was to hand down to the next generation a world as much preserved from "change" as possible. The Christian world view provided a unified and all-encompassing picture of history. There was no room for the individual in this grand theological synthesis. It was duties and obligations, not freedom and rights, that cemented and unified the historical frame of medieval life . . . society was viewed as an organic whole, a kind of divinely inspired moral organism in which each person had a part to play.

JEREMY RIFKIN (1981)

546

ican community when certain issues such as education or employment are involved.

The community mental health nurse must be sensitive to the customs and habits of clients being served and to changes, obvious and subtle, that take place in community groups. Just as individuals and families change over time, so do the communities they form. What happens outside the community may have profound effects within the community. Sometimes change is so extreme that the quality of community life is altered beyond recognition.

Such was the case with Chinese who immigrated to California between 1850 and 1870. They were seeking relief from conditions of drought, military defeat, and burdensome taxation by the Manchu government in their homeland. Their original intent was to earn a living, provide for their families in China, and eventually return home. When such a large number of immigrants enter a community, the change affects both the newcomers and the established residents. In California, the treatment given the immigrants by other residents was harsh enough to prevent them from achieving their goals. The Chinese immigrants accepted jobs scorned by others and were willing to work under very adverse conditions. As a result of their willingness to work long hours for little pay, anger and prejudice against them mounted. American workers, organized in the Workingman's Party, advocated punitive measures against the Chinese. Discrimination included taxes, physical abuse, and even the murder of Chinese workers. Ultimately legislation was adopted that excluded future Chinese immigration (Orque, 1983). The response of the Chinese immigrants was to retreat from their persecutors and to establish homogeneous neighborhoods known as "Chinatowns" within larger localities. In their homogeneous neighborhoods the Chinese felt safer, survival networks evolved, and language and cultural heritage flourished.

Residual discriminatory attitudes toward the Chinese and toward other racial and ethnic groups persist today. One Chinese American noted that regardless of where a Chinese American lives, barriers are likely to be encountered and the individual is likely to experience inner conflict between acquired American values of individualism, freedom, and egalitarianism and Chinese values of filial piety, order, and authoritarianism. Traditional customs upholding family loyalty rather than individual expressiveness then become a cause of intergenerational struggle and intrapsychic turmoil, leading at times to mental health problems (Orque, 1983). Conflict between traditional values and those of the dominant culture occurs in many transplanted groups and is by no means limited to Chinese Americans.

Another example of community as group is provided by Irish Americans. The potato famine in Ireland, which lasted from 1847 to 1850, led thousands of Irish men and women to immigrate to the United States. Although many of these immigrants had been agricultural workers, they landed in American cities and stayed there, eventually becoming urban rather than rural workers. The Catholicism of the Irish immigrants was distrusted by the Protestant majority in the United States. Irish immigrants continued to draw strength from their religious beliefs, and the church responded by establishing parishes, where a church building and parochial school were conveniently located. These Irish neighborhoods resembled little villages, in

Table 20-1. Population Groups in the United States

Group	Population
White	188,340,790
Black	26,488,218
Hispanic	14,605,883
American Indian	1,418,195
Asian	3,500,636
Other	6,756,986

which the people knew each other and formed a strong social network (Janosik, 1980).

Many other racial and ethnic groups have managed to find protection and affirmation of their group identity within similar segregated neighborhoods, whether these neighborhoods have been established forcibly or voluntarily. Some observers believe that the United States is not a melting pot but a pressure cooker and that the pressure is sometimes contained by the survival of neighborhoods known as "Chinatown" or "Little Italy" or "The Barrio." This belief should not be construed as a defense of ghettos but as one explanation of why segregated enclaves continue to exist. Of course, external discrimination remains a significant factor in the perpetuation of segregated neighborhoods and may even be the primary reason. Another explanation for the survival of segregated neighborhoods is that the residents feel comfortable among people whose customs and traditions are familiar and reassuring.

The history of the United States indicates that immigrants have enriched and strengthened the nation. At the same time every wave of immigration has brought assimilation problems to the newcomers and to established residents. For the health care professional, awareness of the diversity of the national population is a first step toward meeting the needs of individuals and communities. A breakdown of national population groups, as determined in the 1980 census, is shown in Table 20-1.

The 1980 census revealed that the percentage of white residents in the United States diminished in the decade from 1970 to 1980. The extent of change is not fully known, partly because the 1980 census included self-reported data not obtained in 1970.

The 1980 census data on ethnic and racial groups were based on self-identification by respondents, who selected the race or group to which they believed they belonged. In previous decades the census taker was involved in the designation of race and ethnicity.

Immigration records for those persons who entered the United States legally since 1970 show that most of them were of non-European origin. Changes in immigration law that became effective in 1968 lifted the quotas limiting the entry of Asians and others who were not like the white Americans who constituted the majority of the population. Illegal aliens, who were unlikely to appear in the 1980 census, constitute another segment of the population. No one knows their actual number, but few are thought to be of European descent. Arguments continue between persons who oppose the reimposition of immigration quotas and residents of regions like Florida and California who fear the effects of a large influx of refugees on the labor force and on state social services (Herbers, 1981).

Community as Place

In the United States the management of community affairs is largely accomplished at the local level, although there may be input in the form of regulation or financial subsidy from state and federal agencies. The mental health nurse viewing community as a place must consider a number of variables, beginning with geographic location and physical environment. Among other important considerations are the geographic and environmental factors listed in Table 20-2. These factors contribute to community assessment because of their impact on the physical and mental health of the resi-

Table 20-2. Variables in Assessing Community as Place

Variables	Assessment Data
Size	What are the boundaries of the community? What is the total population? What is the population density (how many people per square mile or acre)?
Climate	Is the community located in a tropical, temperate, or arctic zone? Are there seasonal changes in climate? If seasonal changes occur, are there two seasons (dry and rainy) or four seasons?
Basic characteristics	Is the community rural, suburban, urban, or a mixture? Is the community homogeneous or comprised of several racial or ethnic groups?
Natural resources	Is the water supply adequate and safe? Is the community in mountainous area, in a valley, or in an area that encompasses mountains and valleys? What vegetation, if any, grows in or near the community?
Hazards	Are natural hazards present, such as rivers that flood or dry areas where widespread fires occur? Are hazards present in the form of air, soil, or water pollution?
Housing	Is adequate housing available at reasonable prices for families of various sizes and income levels?
Transportation	Is adequate and appropriate transportation available for workers living in the community? Is more than one means of transportation available?
Recreational facilities	Is there diversity in the types of recreational activities available? Is there diversity in the cost of recreational activities available?

dents and on the quality of life in the community. In turn, the quality of life experienced by residents has considerable influence on the promotion and maintenance of mental health. Population density, housing, and environmental hazards, whether natural or of human origin, are factors that profoundly affect the lives of community residents.

Community as Culture

Culture may be described as the total of socially determined characteristics handed down from one generation to the next. The United States is a pluralistic society made up of many different groups, each with a different historical past, each with different traditions and priorities. Although some of them are concentrated in particular neighborhoods, many families prefer to live in heterogeneous communities even though their cultural heritage may not conform to their neighbors'.

At the beginning of the twentieth century the disappearance of cultural and ethnic diversity was predicted as newcomers tried to become "Americanized." More astute observers argued to the contrary, and for some years there has been resurgent interest in searching for one's cultural roots. Indeed, cultural inheritance has become a positive force and a statement of individual and collective worth. Minority status and cultural values seem to require less apology than in the past. In the present climate of cultural and ethnic assertiveness, it is not enough for nurses to be open-minded and accepting of people who are different. They must also be aware of historical, anthropological, and sociological factors that affect cultural attitudes toward health and illness.

The concept of community as culture is so complex that a subspeciality has developed called *transcultural nursing*. Transcultural nursing was developed by nurse anthropologists such as Madeline Leininger (1970, 1978). Anthropologists and sociologists, some of whom are nurse scientists, have a great deal to offer community nurses. Although anthropologists are well known for their studies of primitive societies, they are beginning to look carefully at the subcultures that compose the population of the United States.

Leininger studied the health beliefs of a Spanish-speaking community living in an urban center in the western part of the United States. The group consisted of 550 people living in a circumscribed area that was popularly known as the "Spanish community." Within a twenty-two-year period, this group had moved from a rural setting to a semirural setting and finally to an urban setting. Leininger found that the group members retained many of

> ### CONDITIONS CHANGING HEALTH-RELATED BEHAVIORS IN A SPANISH-SPEAKING COMMUNITY
>
> ■ Ineffective results obtained from traditional folk remedies already tried.
>
> ■ Extreme or critical illness or injury where there was possible death of a family member.
>
> ■ Curiosity among community members who were more willing to conform to norms of the dominant culture.
>
> ■ Pressure from official sources to attend clinics and utilize health services. Compliance seemed to be motivated by fear rather than cultural change.
>
> SOURCE: Adapted from Leininger (1978).

their customary attitudes toward health, illness, and treatment. It became apparent that the world of modern medicine was alien to the group culture, and only under threatening conditions were modern methods accepted. Conditions under which professional help was sought are listed in the accompanying box.

NURSING AND CULTURE   Professional caregivers are often unaware of the extent to which their particular cultural orientation influences the way they present themselves to clients and families. An important fact to remember is that each of us interprets our experience in an individualistic way but that we continue to be influenced by the culture in which we were socialized when young. Nurses must therefore be sensitive to the effects of their own cultural biases as well as those of clients. In addition to sensitivity, nurses dealing with cultural or ethnic groups different from their own need to know about how members of the particular culture eat, sleep, and interact with others in order to communicate effectively with clients from that culture (Taylor, 1973). Nurses can also benefit from:

■ Knowledge of the historical experience, recent and long term, of ethnic groups composing the community.

■ Demographic data that include family size, socioeconomic status, and future expectations characteristic of diverse ethnic groups.

■ Recognition of folk beliefs and cultural attitudes toward health and illness, including

sick role behaviors, use of folk healers, and folk remedies.

■ Awareness of the nature of problems encountered by ethnic group members when they enter the health care system. Problems include fear and distrust of new methods, language barriers, and discrimination by caregivers.

This information is important to the nurse's understanding of why cultural differences prevail and how they affect behavior.

Holistic nursing demands attention to the habits, expectations, and prohibitions found within various subcultures. Folk beliefs concerning health and illness may not be substantiated by scientific research, but many of them have been tried and tested across generations. Leininger (1978) found that in extreme circumstances the Spanish Americans in her study became willing to try modern methods. As nurses become more knowledgeable about and more attentive to cultural differences, it is possible that clients from such subcultures will seek professional help before conditions become extreme. The successful nurse is the one who respects cultural values, however unusual they appear, and who can provide care that is compatible with the cultural beliefs and lifestyle of clients.

SOCIAL CLASS VARIABLES Social class differences can have marked effects on attitudes toward health and illness. Admittedly, there is some danger in con-

As the nurse uses a comparative analysis approach, she avoids labeling all people with the same values and beliefs. She learns to assess differences in order to provide therapeutic nursing care. The dynamic comparative approach of identifying contrasts in values and behaviors and their origins provides the basis for variations in nursing care goals, plans, and services. The use of unicultural norms in nursing is still far too prevalent in which nurses tend to believe and act as if all human beings are alike or need to be treated alike in order to avoid favoritism or "special considerations." Treating people alike limits the opportunity for culture-specific care based upon the specific values of people, and may lead to the "cult of efficiency," in which all nursing activities are performed quickly and in a similar way for everyone.
MADELEINE LEININGER (1978)

550

signing clients to a specific socioeconomic category, since there are many variations within each category. Many individuals and families are inconsistent, in that they may seem to belong in one socioeconomic category on the basis of some characteristics and to another category on the basis of other characteristics. For example, a couple who belonged to the middle-class socioeconomic level most of their lives may in later life have the financial resources of a lower socioeconomic level but continue to adhere to middle-class values.

It is often hard to determine the social class of an individual, family, or group because numerous indicators may be used to classify social class, including income, occupation, and education. In addition, where a family happens to live may influence designation of social class. Depending on the cost of living, a family in one city might exist at a lower-class level while another family with the same income in another city might be considered middle class. In many instances it is the individual's or family's perception of its social class that proves to be the determining factor, since this is the class with which they identify and whose values they adopt (Otto, 1977).

In working with children, the educational background of the parents is an important variable. If there is a wide discrepancy between the educational levels of the parents, it is especially useful to work with the parent who has the most contact with the children. However, both parents should be part of a care plan if there is disagreement between them on how the children should be handled.

Differences exist between classes in regard to parent-child interactions. Zegiob and Foreband (1975) found that middle-class mothers were less directive with their children and engaged in more verbal exchanges than did lower-class mothers. Mothers in both upper and middle classes behaved similarly toward their children when involved in similar situations. When exerting control over their children, mothers at all levels employed directive, prohibitive, restraining behaviors. When the mothers took on the role of experts, all engaged in teaching, explaining, and demonstrating behaviors. Little differences were observed between lower- and middle-class mothers in showing interest, affection, and friendship toward their children. Differences between the mothers seemed to be differences of degree rather than differences in the type of maternal behavior.

Difficulties may arise when parents are moving from one class to another. Values and expectations of different socioeconomic classes may create confusion and dissension in the family. Families that are upwardly or downwardly mobile may suffer loneliness and confusion along the way. Nurses working with such families may serve as resource persons as the family decides which values and behaviors should continue and which should be discarded in view of their transition from one socioeconomic class to another (Hawkins, Weisberg, and Ray, 1977; Miller and Janosik, 1980).

EPIDEMIOLOGICAL CONCEPTS

Epidemiology is the study of disease occurrence in human populations. Epidemiologists are concerned with disease patterns in particular populations, such as those living in a particular place or those representing a particular age, gender, or ethnic group.

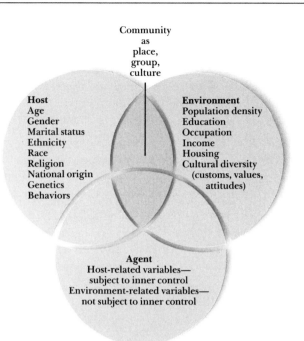

Community
as
place,
group,
culture

Host
Age
Gender
Marital status
Ethnicity
Race
Religion
National origin
Genetics
Behaviors

Environment
Population density
Education
Occupation
Income
Housing
Cultural diversity
(customs, values,
attitudes)

Agent
Host-related variables—
subject to inner control
Environment-related variables—
not subject to inner control

*Figure 20-1. Trifactorial
epidemiological balance.*

551

Initially epidemiologists were concerned primarily with communicable diseases, but their interests have expanded to include other phenomena, such as congenital, degenerative, and chronic health problems in various populations. Investigators who analyze patterns of births in the United States have learned, for example, that the number of babies born with some physical or mental defect has doubled over the last twenty-five years. Identification of this alarming trend will give direction to a search for the causes (Lyons, 1983). Reliable epidemiological studies show that a positive association exists between physical and psychiatric disorders and that the strength of the association varies among different populations. Again, the epidemiological findings help researchers and funding sources establish priorities to guide future investigations into suspected biochemical, psychodynamic, or sociocultural factors (Lipowski, 1975).

Host, Agent, and Environment

Three concepts are important in understanding epidemiological approaches to health and illness: host, agent, and environment. These concepts emerged with the development of epidemiology as a scientific endeavor. During the nineteenth century, environmental factors such as poor sanitation and filth were acknowledged as contributing to the development of illnesses. The growing field of bacteriology substantiated these beliefs and directed attention to finding the actual causative *agents*. In the twentieth century, immunology, or the study of the resistance or vulnerability of certain individuals and groups to various disorders, led to investigation of *host* factors or characteristics influential in the occurrence, nonoccurrence, or prognosis of an ill-

ness. At present the term "host" may refer to an individual, a family, a community, or any segment of the population. Investigation of agent factors and host factors led naturally to interest in environmental factors that might explain variations in the interactions between agent and host. The modern epidemiologist examines the balance between host factors and agent factors within a changing environment. Figure 20-1 shows the trifactorial balance that concerns the epidemiologist.

Environmental factors are instrumental in maintaining a balance between host and agent factors. When there is a shift in the environment that produces imbalance in favor of the host, both the *incidence* (number of new cases) and the *prevalence* (total number of cases at a given point in time) of the illness decrease. When the environment shifts in favor of agent factors, there is increased susceptibility of the host to the illness; consequently both incidence and prevalence are likely to increase. Examining relationships between host, agent, and environment not only expands knowledge of causative agents but also permits manipulation of host, agent, and environment variables to reduce the incidence and prevalence of a disorder.

If community is conceptualized as a place, an epidemiologist might begin by examining environmental factors of the area inhabited by the population being studied, then move to agent factors and to host factors. If an outbreak of encephalitis developed in a region during summer months, for example, the epidemiologist would realize the connection between the illness and a certain type of mosquito and would begin investigating the presence of environmental factors such as swamps or stagnant waters where mosquitos breed. If com-

> ## COMMON EPIDEMIOLOGICAL TERMS
>
> - *Rate.* A quantitative measure used to describe phenomena in a group or to compare similar phenomena in different groups. Comparing suicide rates of Afro-Americans and of Asian Americans is an example of using a rate for comparisons.
>
> - *Incidence.* A quantitative measure used to describe the number of new cases of a disorder or phenomenon in a group. The daily incidence of assaults in an American city, for example, is a matter of great concern to individuals, families, and communities.
>
> - *Prevalence.* A quantitative measure used to describe the total known number of cases of a disorder or phenomenon in a group at a particular point in time. In discussing prevalence, the time frame, whether a year or a decade, should be clearly stated.
>
> - *Mean rate.* A quantitative measure used to describe the average rate of occurrence of phenomena in a group.

munity is conceptualized as a group, an epidemiologist might be concerned about high levels of alcoholism among recruits in an army base. Here investigation might well begin by looking at the characteristics of the recruits; demographic data such as age, marital status, and education would be important, in addition to data as to whether the recruits were draftees or volunteers. Agent factors might include discovering whether the recruits had any control over where they were sent and how severe the training conditions were. Environmental factors would include food, housing, and recreational outlets available to the recruits.

Community conceptualized as culture might be the perspective from which to begin an epidemiological investigation of hypertension. Here the investigation might begin by identifying stressors characteristic of a particular culture, followed by identification of host characteristics, followed by a study of environmental conditions such as isolation, overcrowding, or time pressures that influence host and agent factors.

Epidemiological Terminology

Epidemiology is largely a quantitative science that applies statistical tools to data about populations and patterns of illness. A major concern of epidemiologists is to "find and enumerate appropriate denominators (variables) in a useful and meaningful way" (Friedman, 1974, p. 8). Epidemiologists can often use relevant data to obtain probabilities regarding frequency, risks, and prognoses for particular disorders in a population.

Community mental health nurses need to understand basic epidemiological terminology in order to evaluate research in the field and to describe characteristics of a population in knowledgeable terminology. Some of the most commonly used terms are defined in the accompanying box. These terms can be used to demonstrate a number of different phenomena. For example, Bourne (1973) investigated suicides among Chinese Americans in San Francisco in the years between 1958 and 1968 and arrived at the following quantitative measures:

- The mean suicide rate for subjects in the sample population was 27.9, compared to a mean suicide rate for the national population of 10.0.

- The highest suicide rate for all subjects in the sample population was for those between fifty-five and sixty-five years of age.

- The suicide rates for female subjects in the sample increased significantly from 1964 to 1968.

- A significant number of suicide victims in the sample population (67 percent) were foreign born.

Risk Factors

Bourne's findings indicate the presence of certain *risk factors* associated with suicide in the sample

SOCIETAL REGRESSION IN ACTION

Some social observers fear that divorced women and their children constitute a huge deprived class. Reportedly, this group has suffered a decline of 73 percent in their living standards after divorce while the men involved saw their own living standards raised 42 percent.

Revised divorce laws that were passed in California in 1970 and adopted in some form by every state except Illinois and South Dakota were intended to erase marital misconduct as grounds for divorce, and to base financial awards on need and resources rather than moral considerations. The child support system now addresses only property and tangible assets, overlooking education, career status, career prospects, pension plans, and so on, which generally favor men. In addition, the child support system enforces its awards ineffectively. While 90 percent of custodial parents are women, 60 to 80 percent of all fathers, regardless of income, fail to adhere to support orders. In many divorce settlements an assumption is made that women—even those who have not held a job for many years, or must care for young children—can become economically self-sufficient within two or three years.

SOURCE: Adapted from Lenore J. Weitzman, *The Divorce Revolution* (New York: Free Press, 1985).

population. One risk factor was age and another was having been foreign born. Risk factors are important not only to epidemiologists but to all health care providers, regardless of discipline. Risk factors are interrelated and may be biological, psychosocial, or environmental. Risk factors may also be differentiated according to the place, group, or culture being discussed. When identified, risk factors can assist in planning for populations most likely to suffer illness or injury. This is rarely a simple matter, for in clinical practice the interrelationships among biological, psychosocial, and environmental factors may be difficult to distinguish.

Among risk factors of biological origin are genetic traits that make certain individuals, families, and groups susceptible to particular disorders. (The influence of genetics in the development of various disorders was traced in Chapter 10.) Techniques have been developed that enable scientists to understand the genetic code that transmits human traits. Prenatal screening can already detect genetic errors and predict whether the fetus is likely to suffer specific ailments or defects, a few of which can even be treated in utero. Future discoveries may lead to diagnosing disorders before they develop, thus giving primary prevention a whole new direction (McAuliffe and McAuliffe, 1983).

Psychosocial risks include developmental or situational events occurring at a point in the life cycle when individuals are especially vulnerable. Adolescents, for instance, have a high suicide rate, and jobless workers are prone to depression, illness, and marital conflict. A sociological study at Johns Hopkins University reported that a community that experiences a 1 percent increase in the unemployment rate can expect to have 5 percent more suicides, 3 to 4 percent more hospitalizations for mental illness, 4 to 6 percent more homicides, 6 to 7 percent more admissions to prisons, and a 2 percent increase in the overall death rate (Bird, 1982).

Some population groups are at greater risk than others because they are more likely to live under unfavorable environmental conditions. Disparity between income and employment opportunities for black Americans and white Americans has not changed greatly since the 1960s. In 1959, 66 percent of blacks under age eighteen lived in households at or below poverty level as defined by the federal government. By 1981 this proportion had declined to 45 percent. Among young whites, 21 percent lived at or below poverty levels in 1959; by 1981 this proportion had declined to 15 percent. Thus, despite gains, young blacks remained three times more likely to live in poverty than their white counterparts. The result is that many black children continue to be affected by living in impoverished environments characterized by high population density and poor housing (Herbers, 1983). These statistics underline the interrelated risk factors encountered by the black community across the United States. The same data point to psychosocial stress when individual and family hopes are unfulfilled.

Sometimes environmental factors are not restricted to one group or segment of the community but endanger all inhabitants. Flood, earthquake, and nuclear contamination are not discriminatory in their choice of victims, yet even here characteristics of the host operate to safeguard some residents and endanger others. Whenever a nuclear reactor accident happens, for example, vigorous efforts are made to remove young children and pregnant women from the vicinity as quickly as possible because of their excessive vulnerability to radiation.

Mental health nurses are aware of the unity of mind-body interactions and realize that mental distress is not confined to persons with identified psychiatric diagnoses but is so widespread that identifying risk factors for emotional problems can be extremely complex. Coleman and Patrick (1978) found that 15.7 percent of the clients visiting a general health center over a two-year period exhibited emotional problems. Of these, 72 percent were treated only by a primary health care nurse and were not seen by a mental health professional. From this it may be inferred that awareness of interrelated risk factors should be part of every nurse's clinical knowledge.

COMMUNITY HEALTH CARE DELIVERY

In the United States health care delivery is implemented by persons, agencies, and organizations working in one of three sectors: the private sector, the voluntary sector, and the public sector. As the terms imply, the *private sector* is maintained largely by private funding and the *public sector* by public funding. *Voluntary* organizations are supported by their own fund-raising drives or share in the resources obtained by community fund raising. Some voluntary organizations are not wholly health related but have an interest in or support health causes to some extent. Other voluntary organizations limit themselves to specific health problems, such as cancer or heart disease, in order to concentrate their resources. One example is the American Cancer Society; another is Compeer, a group with a single mission: to provide lonely psychiatric clients with suitable volunteers who befriend the client and reduce interpersonal isolation.

In the public sector, health care delivery is carried out at federal, state, and local levels. The federal government regulates some medical services, personnel, and facilities, in addition to providing financial support. Direct service from the federal government is available to American Indians, veterans, military personnel, merchant seamen, and, in a limited way, migrant workers. The involvement of the federal government is coordinated through state agencies and is carried out by local agencies.

States have the responsibility for inspecting public areas such as state parks, for licensing professionals, for licensing hospitals and other health care facilities, and for controlling the spread of communicable disease. The states maintain institutions for the care of the mentally ill and the physically disabled who cannot be cared for elsewhere. At the local level, the official health department is charged

with providing direct care in homes, clinics, and other facilities. The nursing staff of a health department delivers many of the direct services offered by the department and cooperates with official agencies such as Child Protection Units and with voluntary agencies such as shelters for battered women.

Client advocacy has been accepted as a necessary part of the nursing role. In order to be effective advocates at the local level, nurses are becoming more involved with community planning and community organization. The best way for nurses to prepare for an influential role in the community is, as always, to start with a knowledge base. It is useful to identify the components of the community as a social system, to identify relationships among the components, and to explore popular opinion, especially on controversial issues.

Usually a nurse will have little difficulty learning what problems the community considers important. It may be more difficult to discover how and where decisions are made regarding community health issues. Often decisions are not made by the officially designated health agency or its board of directors. It is not cynical, but only realistic, to say that decisions announced by designated persons may have originated elsewhere. Knowing as much as possible about how the social system of a community operates and where power is vested can be invaluable to nurses trying to meet consumer needs.

Nurses practicing in the community have the opportunity to judge the value of various health programs and to observe deficiencies. When major change seems to be needed, nurses should observe how the health care system is influenced by individuals and groups in the community. What value do the majority of community residents place on physical and mental health needs? What mandate has been given to elected officials concerning the scope and cost of health care services in the community?

Relationships between health care delivery and other aspects of the community social system are constantly changing. The needs and expectations of health care consumers also change. A majority of people now believe that health care is less a privilege than a right but the costs of health care are burdensome for many communities. Advanced technology and scientific developments have made life-saving measures possible, and this has fostered governmental interest in the policies and actions of health care agencies. The increased longevity of Americans has introduced new problems, both economic and ethical. With medical costs escalating, there is greater emphasis on primary prevention and on holistic health care than on medical care alone. This increased emphasis means that the nursing role is broadened and that nurses must be aware of the many forces that have an impact on the health care system.

THE IMPACT OF DEINSTITUTIONALIZATION

When state asylums or mental institutions were originally founded, they were perceived by society as humane refuges for persons who could not manage on their own. More recently, society has become disenchanted with such institutions. Basuk and Gerson (1978) wrote that "the reform movement, having seen its original objectives apparently accomplished, had ceased to be a significant influence. By early in this century the network of state mental hospitals, once the proud tribute to an era of reform, had largely turned into a bureaucratic morass within which patients were interned, often neglected, and sometimes abused" (p. 47).

Disenchantment with the system of state mental institutions coincided with the emergence of the community mental health movement. The result was *deinstitutionalization*, or the discharge of large numbers of hospitalized psychiatric clients into the community. Consequently, over the past twenty-five-years mental hospital populations have dropped significantly; whereas 559,000 persons were in institutions in 1955, only 150,000 were in 1978.

Deinstitutionalization is a dramatic example of the impact that one health care trend can have on communities. When the community mental health movement undertook the task of returning large numbers of psychiatric clients to the community, the results were mixed. Many persons who had supported deinstitutionalization in principle became opposed to it in fact when it became evident that discharged psychiatric clients might become their neighbors. Deinstitutionalization aroused fears among established residents, particularly when they were not informed or reassured about the presence of discharged psychiatric clients in their midst. Some people interpreted deinstitutionalization as a legitimate wish by society to free individuals from confinement and restraint; others saw it as neglect and abandonment of chronic psychiatric clients (Coleman, Butcher, and Carson, 1984).

In theory, deinstitutionalization seemed workable. It was believed that the staffs of the newly organized community mental health centers would be equal to the task of providing adequate follow-up care and that government costs would be less than were needed to support state mental institutions. But despite the best efforts of many well-intentioned professionals and lay persons, unexpected problems arose. According to one source, "The needs of chronic patients had no place in the original federal mandate for the community

mental health center" (Pepper and Ryglewiecz, 1982, p. 389).

Lamb (1979) observed that problems arose because there were so many different kinds of chronic mental health patients and they varied so greatly in the extent to which they could be rehabilitated. Many persons discharged to the community found it difficult, if not impossible, to adjust to community living. Apparently, community mental health centers were better equipped to help clients during acute episodes of psychological impairment than to deal with chronic impairment.

One critic of deinstitutionalization used the example of a young male client who had been admitted to psychiatric hospitals or wards thirty-one times in eleven years (Smith, 1981). Between hospital admissions, the client was arrested more than a dozen times. He was assaulted, beaten, and raped. He made numerous suicide attempts by jumping off bridges, slashing his wrists, and taking drug overdoses. The revolving door through which this client and others move is a consequence of current methods of dealing with the mentally ill. These methods include limited hospitalization and permissive forms of confinement in which clients are relatively free to wander about in the community. According to Smith (1981), the policy of trying to care for mental patients in the community has not meant better or more humane care but only recurrent worry and frustration for clients, their families, and the community. Others have pointed out that perhaps deinstitutionalization and return to the community were oversold and that benefits were lost because of the inability of the mental health care system to adjust to sudden changes in the delivery of mental health services (Bachrach, 1980; Estroff, 1981; Larson, 1983).

Pepper and Ryglewiecz (1982) have expressed concern regarding another population, referred to as the "uninstitutionalized." They describe them as persons who in the past might have been institutionalized for lengthy periods but who now spend just enough time in an institution to be stabilized and are then returned to the same stressful community conditions that they left.

Some community mental health programs are working satisfactorily. In Madison, Wisconsin an integrated program has been developed to stabilize chronic mental patients in the community and to improve their quality of life. Hospital admissions are discouraged through crisis intervention, extensive community support services, work programs, and independent living arrangements. This program was developed by the director of a community mental health center who realized that patients living in the community were becoming disoriented and were being rehospitalized repeatedly.

> ### PRINCIPLES FOR SUCCESSFUL DEINSTITUTIONALIZATION PROGRAMS
>
> 1. Identify target chronic patients.
>
> 2. Integrate treatment and social services through broad-based planning.
>
> 3. Offer a full range of services so that community care is not inferior to institutional care.
>
> 4. Provide services, including social casework and crisis intervention, on a 24-hour basis.
>
> 5. Take cultural and ethnic group attitudes into consideration.
>
> 6. Prepare staff members so that they recognize stresses and problems encountered by patients in the community.
>
> 7. Maintain a liaison with psychiatric inpatient facilities so that readmission is facilitated when needed.
>
> 8. Continue internal evaluation and review processes in order to monitor program effectiveness.

Introduction of the program followed a three-year systematic investigation of patients in both community and hospitalized settings. One group of patients consisted of sixty-five persons seeking admittance to a state psychiatric institution for the sixth time. Instead of being admitted, they were treated in the community for twelve months and were followed every four months for two years. A control group of sixty-five patients similar in age, sex, and illness were hospitalized in the state facility until well enough for discharge. Concerted efforts were used to make mental health services available to the patients treated in the community. A contingent of hospital staff members were placed in a house in the community, where they worked in shifts so that someone was always available to the patients. The staff accepted the task of doing whatever seemed necessary to keep the patients in the community. That included negotiating with landlords, going shopping with patients in stores near their homes, and teaching them to cook and to take care of their personal needs. At the same time, neighbors and shopkeepers were educated about the actions and behaviors in which the patients sometimes engaged. It was explained to them that dressing and acting differently from the majority is permitted in a free society as long as laws are not broken and no one is victimized.

The results of this experiment were significant. Of the sixty-five patients in the control group, fifty-eight were rehospitalized within one year. Of the sixty-five patients in the sample population, only twelve were rehospitalized in the same period. These results led to modification of the mental health care system in Madison. In that city all public funding for mental health is given to community-based programs, which then pay state institutions whenever any of their patients needs hospitalization (Smith, 1983).

Deinstitutionalization is a major issue in New York City. Concern over the large numbers of homeless people is growing, and this population constitutes an enormous drain on municipal resources. State hospitals that once housed 93,000 housed only 21,000 in 1982. Mental patients are returning to the community with only the most severe aspects of their illness under control (Westermeyer, 1982). Such people need a slow, gradual introduction to the activities of daily living and a step-by-step return to independence, living for a time in facilities where food, clothing, and medications are supervised before moving back with their families or finding housing of their own. Yet most patients are not provided with this intermediate stage.

In spite of the obvious problems, some investigators support the concept and practice of deinstitutionalization. Braun et al. (1981) concluded that selected patients receiving care in a community in controlled, experimental programs do no worse than, and in some instances demonstrate outcomes superior to, hospitalized patients. Nevertheless, reliable data concerning the outcomes of deinstitu-

INTANGIBLE ASPECTS OF DEINSTITUTIONALIZATION

Deinstitutionalization and the community mental health movement have achieved mixed results, depending on the demands made of the community for aftercare and the cost of meeting the demands. One result of deinstitutionalization is seldom mentioned, and that is the opening up of large mental hospitals so that clients and staff are not enshrouded in medieval darkness. Having become aware of patterns of chronicity and dependency, nurses and other staff members are using corrective rather than custodial approaches. Remotivation, resocialization, reality orientation, and recreational groups have introduced a new social interest on the part of clients and greater expectation on the part of staff members that improvement is possible after all.

tionalization are hard to come by, partly because the target population is transient and elusive.

Bachrach (1980) has identified a number of principles common to successful programs developed to return chronic mental patients to the community; these principles are listed in the box on page 556. Braun et al. have pointed out that deinstitutionalization is unlikely to be successful if continuity of care is not available through community mechanisms.

THE ROLE OF THE COMMUNITY MENTAL HEALTH NURSE

During the deinstitutionalization era of the community mental health movement, leaders of the nursing profession disagreed about who should care for the mentally ill in the community. Because this role was one with autonomy and independence, Mereness (1963) argued that nurses with graduate level preparation in psychiatric nursing were the most appropriate providers of care for mentally ill persons in the community. Another viewpoint was expressed by Wolff (1964), who said that the needs were so great and the supply of adequately prepared psychiatric nurses so limited that community health nurses already skilled in providing family and community care were qualified to serve mentally ill persons living in the community. As more nurses completed graduate work in mental health and community health, the problem of supply and demand became less pressing, and collaboration between mental health nurses and community health nurses proved to be the answer.

Today, a community mental health nurse may be employed by a state or local psychiatric hospital or by a community mental health center. A community mental health nurse who works with individuals, families, or groups as a primary therapist or a co-therapist should have a master's degree. Other nurses who work under closer supervision may use the title of community mental health nurse but lack advanced preparation. In any case, the community mental health nurse works with clients having a range of psychological problems and is concerned with clients' stress levels, adaptation, and coping abilities. According to Sheehy (1976), helping individuals and families anticipate the course of events is a preventive measure that is quite effective. Consumer participation is actively encouraged in developing policies and in evaluating the services provided by the community mental health nurse and related personnel.

The role of community mental health nurse is one that carries considerable independence, even though the nurse has support resources in the person of other professionals who are available as consultants. In addition, the community mental health nurse often functions as a consultant to others, professional and paraprofessional. She may, for example, act as client advocate in a supervised residence where client needs are not being met adequately, or she may become a consultant and guide for families who must place an aged relative in a long-term care facility. A community mental health nurse may function as a counselor for individuals or groups or may be a liaison between clients and community agencies. Krauss (1984) has described community health nursing roles in the context of five models of

Table 20-3. Nursing Models of Care and Community Role Functions

Model of Mental Health Care	Community Nursing Role Functions
Service models of care (found in community mental health centers where emphasis is on assessment, treatment, education, and consultations)	Engaging in case finding Making appropriate referrals Identifying and educating high-risk groups Providing consultation to caregivers and consumers Monitoring medication for clients living in the community Assessing adjustment of clients to life in the community Assessing family coping and adjustment to clients living at home or elsewhere in the community
Living models of care (found in rehabilitation settings such as vocational programs, alternative living placements, or socially oriented drop-in centers)	Serving as consultant for rehabilitation programs or working directly with clients to provide health service and health teaching Providing supportive intervention to families: natural, adoptive, foster, and extended
Learning models of care (found in schools or community settings where emphasis is on problem solving and social learning)	Offering cognitive, didactic instruction to community groups
Working models of care (may be found in occupational settings ranging from sheltered workshops to free enterprise corporations; preemployment counseling is part of the working model, as is on-the-job health coverage and protection)	Serving as *ad hoc* counselor and employee advocate for groups of workers employed by a company or corporation Providing on-site health coverage for workers in the free market and in sheltered workshops
Family models of care (include systematic observation and surveillance in order to identify dysfunctional behaviors in families and to promote healthy family interaction)	Monitoring family interactions Leading or providing consultation to family groups Referring dysfunctional families to appropriate sources for help

558

mental health care. These models and roles are summarized in Table 20-3.

In whatever capacity a nurse functions, assessment of the status of clients, families, and groups is ongoing. Assessment should include biological, psychological, and sociological factors, and the nurse must be cognizant of all three in order to recognize changes in health status. In community mental health, nurses frequently find no clear separation between assessing, planning, implementing, and evaluating activities (Morgan and Moreno, 1973). The holistic goal of the community mental health nurse is to assist individuals to live in the community, to anticipate and manage stress, and to learn to cope with the anxieties and frustrations of everyday life.

COMMUNITY PROGRAM EVALUATION

Most nurses have learned to define specific goals to be met by clients and families with whom they are working. Evaluation of community goals and program outcomes is more complicated but is essential to determining the success or failure of a program. *Progress* evaluation analyzes the degree to which program implementation has reached or approached stated goals. For example, a community concerned with the prevalence of teenage pregnancies in the local high school and the frequency of teenage mothers dropping out of school might con-

sider offering a program in which the following goals are outlined:

- Pregnant teenagers enrolled in the school will receive prenatal care.

- Prenatal care will include preparation for labor and delivery in addition to instruction on child development and child care.

- After delivery, babies will be admitted to a day care facility with services that permit the teenage mothers to return to school.

- Counseling will be provided by school personnel during pregnancy, after delivery, and upon the mothers' return to school.

- Teenage mothers in the program will acquire marketable job skills.

- The rate of school dropout among the teenage mothers will decrease.

- The incidence of second teenage pregnancies among the mothers will decrease.

With these goals defined, a program could be planned and inaugurated to achieve the goals, which are clearly stated and measurable. By comparing data collected before the program and at regular intervals during the program, it would be possible to ascertain what progress is being made toward goal achievement.

A program such as this would be both costly and controversial. Thus, evaluation of the program should include *efficiency* measures to determine whether program progress and outcomes are justifying the expenditure of time, money, and resources. It would be possible to ascertain the immediate effects of the program in terms of how many teenage mothers remain in school and obtain job skills. However, it would take somewhat longer to discover how many mothers in the program avoid a second teenage pregnancy and even longer to learn how many of them enter the labor force as stable workers. Only if it could be shown statistically that teenagers in the program finish school, do not become pregnant again within two years, and find jobs rather than join welfare lists would the program be justified in terms of efficiency or cost effectiveness. Another long-term way of evaluating program cost effectiveness would be to compare the health of babies born to teenage mothers in the sample and the health of babies born to mothers in a control population with similar characteristics, even though the health of the babies is not a primary consideration.

Subjective changes resulting from the program, such as increasing the self-esteem of the young mothers and improving the quality of life for them and their babies, are rarely part of community program evaluation. These outcomes are important, of course, but community programs are concerned with target populations and with social change rather than with individual change, important as the latter may be (Shore, 1981).

Community programs are often continued in the absence of solid evidence that they are helping the target population and contributing to the well-being of the community as a whole (Monro, 1983). In fact, traditional evaluation has often depended

on subjective responses rather than on concrete evidence. If the deinstitutionalization process were to be evaluated, for example, the results would depend on the attitudes of the respondent. In order to avoid subjectivity, evaluation of community programs should incorporate the following questions:

1. What stated goals have been achieved, and to what extent?

2. How effective has the program been in terms of cost effectiveness; that is, do the results justify the expenditures?

3. What impact has the program had on the target population and on the community as a whole?

SUMMARY

Because the concept of community is subject to different interpretations, it is essential to know exactly what is meant when the term is used. Community may be conceptualized as a group, a place, or a culture. Assessing community needs is not an easy task, but deciding how the term is being used in a specific instance helps organize the many variables included in a comprehensive community assessment.

Community always involves relationships between people; therefore, concepts drawn from epidemiology are helpful in examining factors related to health and illness in various populations. Epidemiologists employ the concepts of agent (causes), host (population), and environment (surroundings) to explain the presence or absence of ill-

CLINICAL EXAMPLE

A COMMUNITY-ORIENTED APPROACH
IN A NURSING FACILITY FOR THE ELDERLY

A nursing home for the elderly is a community in more than one sense of the word. For elderly persons residing in a nursing home, the daily routine represents a collective lifestyle based on the customs and traditions of the facility. The implications of being placed in a nursing home are painful for family members and for the elderly person. Placement is a statement that the elderly person is no longer considered fully competent. When an elderly person enters a nursing home, personal preferences must be left behind, privacy is invaded, and personal freedom is greatly limited.

A particular nursing home was owned and operated by a corporation that wanted a fair return on its investment but also wished to provide good care. In order to raise the standards of care, a nurse gerontologist was hired. Some budgetary restrictions were placed on the gerontologist, but otherwise she was given a free hand. In accepting the position, the gerontologist made it clear to the owners that certain needs of staff members should be taken into account if the needs of the elderly residents were to be met satisfactorily.

The nurse gerontologist did not immediately make changes but spent a number of weeks studying records and observing the daily routine of the nursing home.

Her assessment of the facility, of staff members, and of the residents was comprehensive and detailed.

ASSESSMENT
The Facility

The three-story building was located within city limits but was surrounded by several acres of lawn, shrubbery, and woods. Parking for visitors was adequate. On the first floor was an entrance lobby and two large day rooms that were used for meetings of administrative staff and for occupational therapy. The first floor also had a dining room that was spacious and bright but that provided few amenities. Windows were curtainless, table covers were dark brown vinyl, and eating utensils were plastic.

The nursing home had a capacity of 100 residents. Some of the rooms were private and had one occupant; other rooms were shared by two occupants. Each room had its own toilet and bath.

The second floor had a room that opened onto an open deck or porch with a low, ornamental railing. The room adjoining the deck was called the solarium. Although residents had access to the solarium, the doors to the deck were locked. Because the railing was low, staff members were afraid to allow residents to use the deck even in the best of weather.

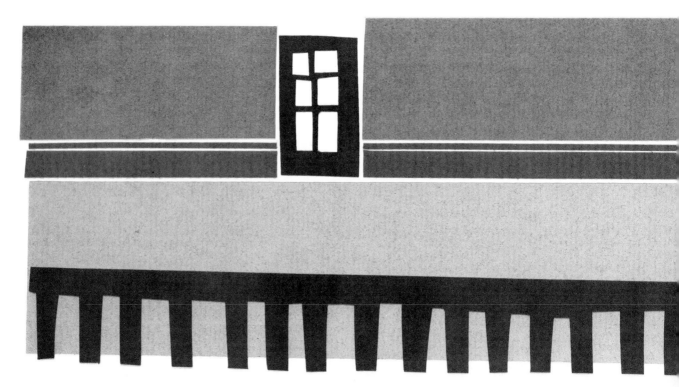

The Staff

The nursing home complied with legal standards that required a ratio of registered nurses to be employed on all three shifts. Most of the needs of the residents were met by health aides with varying amounts of preparation. The health aides, dietary staff, and other paraprofessionals were paid minimum wage rates, with very few exceptions.

Turnover rate among employees was very high, even for registered nurses who were paid more than other employees. Registered nurses were employed in supervisory capacities and did little bedside nursing. Except for giving medication and talking occasionally with family members, record keeping occupied most of their time.

The Residents

The gerontologist realized that the elderly, as a group, are subject to distress related to acute and chronic illnesses, loss of loved ones, decreased physical strength, social isolation, financial reverses, and low self-esteem.

The nurse gerontologist noted that the needs of the elderly clients were being met to some extent but were not being fully met in the nursing home. Among the needs she identified were:

Care and attention based on individual needs.

Respect from care providers.

Comfortable sleeping quarters with some privacy.

Nutritious, balanced, attractive meals.

Single-purpose day rooms for occupational activities/diversional activities, reading or letter writing, and conversation or TV watching.

Regular, consistent medical care, including foot care, eye care, and dental care.

Maintenance of normal motion and activity to the fullest possible extent.

PLANNING

Some obvious changes could be made in the facility without incurring great expense. One of the two large day rooms, used infrequently for administrative meetings, could be divided in two, creating a room that could be used by small groups of residents for reading, playing cards, or writing letters. The dining room could be brightened by adding bright table coverings and bouquets of artificial flowers. Replacing plastic eating utensils with stainless steel ones would enable the residents to cut their own meat instead of asking an aide for help.

The gerontologist strongly recommended that a protective railing be installed around the deck so that residents could sit outside in good weather. One or two aides could be assigned to remain in the deck area while it was being occupied by the residents.

Many of the practices that had developed in the nursing home were objectionable to the nurse gerontologist. Some of the problems were attributable to underpaid staff aides who had little or no understanding of the special needs of the elderly. An obvious deficiency was the fact that staff members showed impatience with the slow movements of elderly residents. In helping clients get dressed, staff members did not take the time to fasten garments properly or comb hair attractively. The result was that the residents looked clean but unkempt, except when family members assumed some of the grooming tasks. Another problem was that residents who were not ambulatory were rarely taken from their rooms,

561

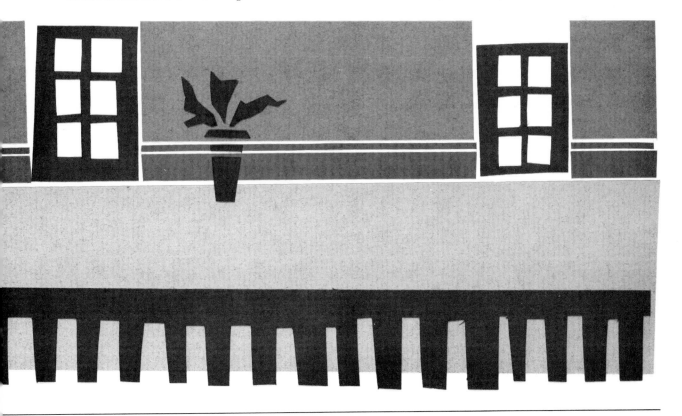

even though their beds were modern, on wheels, and easily moved.

Perhaps the most disconcerting feature of the nursing home routine was the excessive use of restraints. Residents who were even slightly confused were restrained in bed or, if they were ambulatory, in a chair. The reason given was fear of the staff that confused residents might fall or wander into neighboring rooms. Even in the early weeks of observation and assessment, the gerontologist could see the deterioration of restrained residents, who received little sensory input, whose limbs stiffened from lack of use, and who became incontinent because the staff was inattentive to their requests to be taken to the bathroom.

The gerontologist saw no evidence of mistreatment of the residents, but there were signs of thoughtlessness. In general, the routine followed in the nursing home seemed to encourage regression in the residents and indifference in staff members.

IMPLEMENTATION

562

In presenting recommendations to administrative staff, the gerontologist shared her observations concerning the facility, the staff, and the residents. The following recommendations were presented, voted upon, and implemented by the corporation:

The Facility

Purchase new table covers and eating utensils for the dining room. Decorate the room for various holidays.

Divide the day room area into three rather than two rooms.

Provide a safety railing for the deck; assign staff members to supervise the area; transport bedridden residents to the deck in good weather.

Construct safety railings in all corridors to facilitate movement of ambulatory residents.

Place large signs with the occupant's name on the doors of bedrooms.

The Staff

Offer an intensive inservice and orientation program for staff members to help them understand the needs of the elderly.

Arrange regular meetings between administrators and all staff members in order to share ideas and information.

Establish a career ladder within the facility so that staff performing well or staff with seniority can be recognized. Recognition could be in the form of merit increases, commendations, and job titles that indicate higher status.

Develop routine assignments for each shift so that every staff member is aware of specific responsibilities to the residents.

Adopt a system of team nursing so that the residents are given care each day by the same person or group of persons.

The Residents

Residents should be addressed by their proper surnames and titles, such as Mr., Mrs., or Miss, except in unusual circumstances.

Current visiting hours (1 to 3 P.M. and 7 to 8 P.M.) restrict family visits. Therefore, new visiting hours should be arranged, lasting from 10 A.M. to 8 P.M.

Family members should be permitted to join residents for meals by paying a nominal sum.

Registered nurses working in supervisory roles should make rounds three times in each eight-hour shift to check the appearance, general condition, and comfort level of each resident.

An ombudsman or "troubleshooter" should be available to clients and families, functioning as a liaison between care providers and care consumers.

Confused residents who are ambulatory should be restrained as little as possible. When restraints are considered necessary, the resident will be restrained for no more than 30 minutes without being freed from restraints in order to eat, walk, or go to the bathroom with the help of a staff member.

A system of 15-minute rounds should be established and staff members should be assigned to make rounds for an hour at a time. When a second staff member takes over the assignment, an accounting of the whereabouts of all residents should be given by the person previously assigned rounds. This method of professional watchfulness would eliminate much of the need for physical restraints.

EVALUATION

The recommendations of the gerontologist required some additional expenditure of funds but were within the allocation that had been agreed to by the corporation. In objective measures, the following outcomes were attributed to the recommendations of the nurse gerontologist:

- Decreased staff turnover due to greater involvement and recognition.
- Greater satisfaction expressed by family members.
- Measurable improvement in the mobility of residents.
- Reduced self-care deficits in residents.
- Enhanced reputation of the nursing home in the area.
- Greater willingness of family and physicians to use the facility for placement purposes.
- Fewer indices of depression, regression, and apathy of residents.

563

ness. Initially, epidemiologists were concerned with communicable disease, but their interests have expanded to include congenital health problems, degenerative health problems, and chronic health problems. Quantitative measures developed by statisticians and others enable health professionals to describe and compare health-related phenonema within a particular group or between groups.

The Community Mental Health Center legislation passed by Congress in 1963 supported mental health centers in all fifty states and was an enabling force in the deinstitutionalization process that returned thousands of mental patients to the community. This process represented a shift in the locus of care for the mentally ill from long-term hospitalization to flexible, community-based care. Deinstitutionalization was implemented in the hope of achieving the following goals:

■ To save clients from the debilitating effects of lengthy, restrictive periods of hospitalization.

■ To return the client to home and community life as soon as possible after hospitalization.

■ To maintain the client in the community for as long as possible thereafter.

Deinstitutionalization remains a controversial issue with its share of supporters and critics. Many communities have found their municipal resources drained by large numbers of discharged mental patients living with little supervision or follow-up care. On the other hand, experimental programs that are based on proven principles have shown that deinstitutionalization can work in practice as well as in theory. Until now, little systematic research has been directed to the study of deinstitutionalization, and evaluations are largely subjective (Altman, 1984).

The evaluation of community programs is relatively complex but is essential. In evaluating these programs, progress toward achieving the stated goals should be measured. The efficiency or cost effectiveness of the program should be evaluated to determine whether the outcomes justify expenditures of time, money, and resources. The impact of the program on the target population and on the community at large should be included in the evaluation process.

Review Questions

1. Identify major differences between conceptualizations of community as group, place, and culture.

2. In assessing communities, what positive and negative aspects of homogeneous communities should be considered?

3. Define the following epidemiological terms: agent, host, environment.

4. Briefly describe the relationship between agent, host, and environment in the incidence of illness in a community.

5. Give an example of a biological risk factor and explain its significance.

6. Give an example of an environmental risk factor and explain its significance.

7. What sectors are involved in the delivery of community health care?

8. Identify three causes for the failure of deinstitutionalization in some communities.

9. What considerations are important in transferring clients from institutional to community care?

10. In what ways does community program evaluation differ from evaluation of health care provided to individuals and families?

References

Altman, L. E. 1984. New Focus on World Health. *The New York Times*, January 17.

Bachrach, L. L. 1980. Overview, Model Programs for Chronic Patients. *American Journal of Psychiatry*, 132:1023–1031.

Basuk, E. L., and Gerson, S. 1978. Deinstitutionalization and Mental Health Services. *Scientific American*, 238(2):46–53.

Bird, C. 1982. Joblessness Scars Deeper than Simple Totals Tell. *The Plain Dealer*, Cleveland, Ohio, April 10.

Bourne, P. 1973. Suicide Among Chinese in San Francisco. *American Journal of Public Health*, 63:744–750.

Braun, P.; Kochansky, G.; Shapiro, R.; Greenberg, S.; Gudeman, J. E.; Johnson, S.; and Shore, M. 1981. Overview: Deinstitutionalization of Psychiatric Patients: Critical Review of Outcome Studies. *American Journal of Psychiatry*, 138:736–749.

Coleman, J., and Patrick, J. L. 1978. Psychiatry and General Health. *American Journal of Public Health*, 68:451–457.

Coleman, J. C.; Butcher, J. N.; and Carson, R. C. 1984. *Abnormal Psychology and Modern Life*. Glenview, Ill.: Scott, Foresman.

Estroff, S. 1981. *Making It Crazy*. Berkeley: University of California Press.

Fleck, S. 1980. The Family and Psychiatry. In *Comprehensive Textbook of Psychiatry*, 3rd ed., eds. H. I. Kaplan, A. M. Freedman, and B. J. Sadock. Baltimore: Williams & Wilkins.

Friedman, G. D. 1974. *Primer of Epidemiology*. New York: McGraw-Hill.

Greenblatt, H. R. 1980. Psychopolitics. In *Comprehensive Textbook of Psychiatry*, 3rd ed., eds. H. I. Kaplan, A. M. Freedman, and B. J. Sadock. Baltimore: Williams & Wilkins.

Hawkins, J.; Weisberg, C.; and Ray, I. D. 1977. Marital Communication Style and Social Class. *Journal of Marriage and the Family*, 39:479–490.

Herbers, J. 1981. The New Population Mix. *The New York Times*, September 6.

Herbers, J. 1983. Income Gaps Between Races as Wide as in 1960. *The New York Times*, July 18.

Janosik, E. H. 1980. Variations in Ethnic Families. In *Family-Focused Care*, eds. J. R. Miller and E. H. Janosik. New York: McGraw-Hill.

Krauss, J. B. 1984. *Nursing in the Community*. New York: John Wiley & Sons.

Lamb, H. R. 1979. Roots of Neglect in the Long Term Mentally Ill. *Psychiatry*, 42:201–207.

Larson, R. 1983. The Deinstitutionalized Environment: A Case for Better Planning. *ORB*, 3(May):126–130.

Leininger, M. 1970. *Nursing and Anthropology: Two Worlds to Blend*. New York: John Wiley & Sons.

Leininger, M. 1978. *Transcultural Nursing: Concepts, Theories, Practices*. New York: John Wiley & Sons.

Lipowski, Z. J. 1975. Psychiatry of Somatic Diseases: Epidemiology, Pathogenesis, Classification. *Comprehensive Psychiatry*, 16(2):105–123.

Lyons, R. D. 1983. Physical and Mental Disabilities in Newborns Double in 25 Years. *The New York Times*, July 18.

McAuliffe, K., and McAuliffe, S. 1983. Keeping Up with the Genetic Revolution. *The New York Times Magazine*, November 6:40–44+.

Mereness, D. 1963. The Potential Significant Role of the Nurse in Community Mental Health Services. *Perspectives in Psychiatric Care*, 1(34):18–22.

Miller, J. R., and Janosik, E. H. 1980. Social Class Influences on Family Structure and Function. In *Family-Focused Care*, eds. J. R. Miller and E. H. Janosik. New York: McGraw-Hill.

Monro, B. H. 1983. A Useful Model for Program Evaluation. *Journal of Nursing Administration*, (March):23.

Morgan, A. J., and Moreno, J. W. 1973. *The Practice of Mental Health Nursing: A Community Approach*. Philadelphia: J. B. Lippincott.

Orque, M. S., ed. 1983. *Ethnic Nursing Care: A Multicultural Approach*. St. Louis: C. V. Mosby.

Otto, L. B. 1977. Class and Status in Family Research. *Journal of Marriage and the Family*, 39:479–490.

Pepper, B., and Ryglewicz, H. 1982. Testimony for the Neglected: The Mentally Ill in the Post-deinstitutionalized Age. *American Journal of Orthopsychiatry*, 52:388–392.

Poussaint, A. F. 1980. Interracial Relations and Prejudice. In *Comprehensive Textbook of Psychiatry*, 3rd ed., eds. H. I. Kaplan, A. M. Freedman, and B. J. Sadock. Baltimore: Williams & Wilkins.

Rifkin, J. 1981. *Entropy: A New World View*. New York: Bantam.

Sheehy, G. 1976. *Passages: Predictable Crises of Adult Life*. New York: Dutton.

Shore, M. F. 1981. Marking Time in the Land of Plenty: Reflections on Mental Health in the United States. *American Journal of Orthopsychiatry*, 51:391–402.

Smith, S. 1981. Arrests, Suicide Tries, and a Frustrated Family. *Times Union*, Rochester, N.Y., April 28.

Smith, S. 1983. How an Idea Works in Wisconsin. *Times Union*, Rochester, N.Y., November 7.

Stuart, G. W. 1981. Role Strain and Depression: A Causal Inquiry. *Journal of Psychosocial Nursing and Mental Health Services*, 19(12):20–28.

Swanson, A. R., and Hurley, P. M. 1983. Family Systems: Values and Value Conflicts. *Journal of Psychosocial Nursing and Mental Health Services*, 21(7):24–30.

Taylor, C. 1973. The Nurse and Cultural Barriers. In *Family Health Care*, eds. D. P. Hymovich and M. U. Barnard. New York: McGraw-Hill.

Weitzman, L. J. 1985. *The Divorce Revolution*. New York: Free Press.

Westermeyer, J. 1982. Bag Ladies in Isolated Cultures, Too. *Behavior Today*, 13(21):1–2.

Wolff, I. 1964. The Psychiatric Nurse in Community Health: A Rebuttal. *Perspectives in Psychiatric Care*, 2(11):10.

Zegiob, L. E., and Foreband, R. 1975. Maternal Interaction Behavior as a Function of Race, Socioeconomic Status, and Sex of the Child. *Child Development*, 46(2):564–568.

Supplementary Readings

Archer, S. E.; Kelly, C. D.; and Besch, S. A. *Implementing Change in Communities: A Collaborative Process*. St. Louis: C. V. Mosby, 1984.

Bachrach, L. L. Psychiatric Services in Rural Areas: A Sociological Overview. *Hospital and Community Psychiatry*, 34(1983):215–226.

Biegel, A. Community Mental Health Centers: A Look Ahead. *Hospital and Community Psychiatry*, 33(1982): 741–745.

Carter, J. H. Treating Black Patients: The Risks of Ignoring Critical Social Issues. *Hospital and Community Psychiatry*, 32(1981):279–280.

Clemen, S. A.; Ergsti, D. G.; and McGuire, S. L. *Comprehensive Family and Community Health Nursing*. New York: McGraw-Hill, 1981.

Dawe, A. M. A Case for Community Psychiatric Nurses. *Journal of Advanced Nursing*, 5(1980):485–490.

Dawe, A. M. Community Psychiatric Nurses: Value for Money. *Nursing Mirror*, 29(1981):36–37.

Elliott-Cannon, C. Do the Mentally Handicapped Need Specialist Community Nursing Care? *Nursing Times*, 77(1981):77–80.

Ellison, E. S. Social Networks and the Mental Health Care System: Implications for Psychiatric Nursing Practice. *Journal of Psychosocial Nursing and Mental Health Services*, 21(1983):18–24.

Felton, G. Research and the Nurse in Community Mental Health. *Michigan Nurse*, 55(1982):7–12.

Fitzgerald, A. Maintaining the Elderly Mentally Frail in the Community. *Nursing* (Oxford), (1981):1097–1098.

Flasherud, J. H. Community Mental Health Nursing: Its Unique Role in the Delivery of Services to Ethnic Minorities. *Perspectives in Psychiatric Care*, 20(1982): 37–43.

Hagebak, J. E. Serving the Mental Health Needs of the Elderly. *Community Mental Health Journal*, 16(1980): 263–275.

Hall, V. The Community Mental Health Nurse: A New Professional Role. *Journal of Advanced Nursing*, 7(1982):3–10.

Krauss, J. The Chronic Psychiatric Patient in the Community—A Model for Care. *Nursing Outlook*, 28(1980): 308–314.

Lanoil, J. The Chronic Mentally Ill in the Community—Case Management. *Journal of Psychosocial Rehabilitation*, 4(1980):1–6.

McLaughlin, J. S. Toward a Theoretical Model for Community Health Programs. *Advances in Nursing Science*, 5(1982):7–28.

Miller, J. C. Theoretical Basis for the Practice of Community Mental Health Nursing. *Issues in Mental Health Nursing*, 3(1981):319–339.

Paykel, E. S. Community Psychiatric Nursing for Neurotic Patients. *British Journal of Psychiatry*, 140(1982): 573–581.

Reingold, C. D. Community Nursing Care for the Mentally Retarded. *Curatonis*, 3(1980):14–19.

Roberts, S. J. Oppressed Group Behavior. *Advances in Nursing Science*, 5(1983):21–30.

Slavinsky, A. T. Two Approaches to the Management of Long Term Psychiatric Outpatients in the Community. *Nursing Research*, 31(1982):284–289.

Spence, G. G. Factors Affecting the Performance of a Prescribed Community Psychiatric Role for Nurses. *Canadian Mental Health*, 29(1981):36–39.

Stanfield, I. Weeding Out the Victims: Detecting Mental Illness in Its Early Stages. *Community Outlook*, (1984): 238–240.

Stanhope, M., and Lancaster, J. *Community Health Nursing: Process and Practice for Promoting Health*. St. Louis: C. V. Mosby, 1984.

Sullivan, G. Community Care: A Day in the Life of a Community Psychiatric Nurse. *Nursing Mirror*, 154 (1982):37.

Thomson, R. Community Nursing with Mentally Handicapped Adults. *Nursing Times*, 76(1980):2007–2010.

Williams, R. A Community Nursing Service for Mentally Handicapped Children. *Nursing Times*, 76(1980): 2011–2012.

Wilson, H. S. Usual Hospital Treatment in the United States Community Mental Health System: A Dispatching Process. *International Journal of Nursing Studies*, 20(1983):75–82.

REALITY THERAPY

RATIONAL EMOTIVE THERAPY

IMPLOSIVE THERAPY

PRIMAL THERAPY

*MILIEU THERAPY AND THE THERAPEUTIC
COMMUNITY*

CLIENT-CENTERED THERAPY

RELATIONSHIP THERAPY AS NURSING PROCESS
Assessment in Relationship Therapy (The Introductory Phase)
Planning in Relationship Therapy (The Testing Phase)
Intervention in Relationship Therapy (The Working Phase)
Evaluation in Relationship Therapy (The Termination Phase)

C　　H　　A　　P　　T　　E　　R

21

Eclectic Theory and Practice

Learning Objectives

After reading this chapter, the student should be able to:

1. Describe various therapeutic modalities used in delivering health care to clients with maladaptive alterations.

2. Discuss the implications and usefulness of various therapeutic approaches and their relevance for psychiatric nurses.

3. Compare the strengths and limitations of specific therapeutic modalities.

4. Formulate a viable, integrated clinical approach based on the therapeutic relationship between nurse and clients.

Overview

Eclectic psychotherapy involves the selection and application of traditional methods augmented by current approaches to specific clinical situations. The eclectic approach matches the most suitable clinical methods to the needs of specific clients and takes into consideration indications and contra-indications in determining what is appropriate for individual clients. This chapter presents various psychotherapeutic approaches that may be used alone or in combination, depending on the needs of individual clients, in the context of the nursing process.

The philosophies of one age have become the absurdities of the next, and the foolishness of yesterday has become the wisdom of tomorrow.

SIR WILLIAM OSLER

569

Countless new types of therapeutic approaches for emotional problems have emerged in the United States and Europe since the 1950s and 1960s. Usually, new therapies are associated with a single therapist who is identified as the founder and who often claims to obtain spectacular cure rates. Torrey (1972) wrote that the effectiveness of new approaches may be due to the fact that the founder transmits to clients an utmost faith in the new methods and this certainty increases their expectations of being helped.

It is difficult to determine absolutely the effectiveness of specific therapies for several reasons. For one thing, therapists are seldom purists and they usually employ more than one type of therapy at a time. Typically, physiological, psychosocial, and group milieu therapies are used in combination in the hope of achieving optimum results. No school of psychology has the complete answer to all problems accompanying emotional disorders, and no single method of treatment is universally applicable and successful. Furthermore, there is a wide range of competence among mental health practitioners, and methods employed for evaluation of the success or effectiveness of therapy are often inadequate. Because it is impossible to control for differences in therapists and the effects of combinations of various therapeutic approaches, it is often difficult to identify which factors produce which effects.

The choice of a therapy seems to be influenced by various cultural, philosophical, and religious values. In addition, therapeutic goals may reflect the basic values held by the therapist. Also, a client's choice of therapist tends to reflect the client's beliefs about the causes of his or her psychological discomfort. If a client believes psychic pain is caused by traumatic childhood experiences, that client is likely to choose a therapist whose beliefs are compatible. Compatibility of beliefs and the client's perception of the adequacy of a therapist's credentials and preparation may also contribute to the client's expectations of being helped.

The value placed by society on the ability to think rationally, to be responsible and independent, and to work and be productive is reflected in the therapeutic approaches used in the United States today. Since there is no consensus in psychotherapy, an eclectic approach broadens the resources available to caregivers as they adapt various forms and aspects of psychotherapy to specific situations. The therapies discussed in this chapter are summarized in Table 21-1.

REALITY THERAPY

Reality therapy reflects many of the current values in our culture. William Glasser (1965), the founder of reality therapy, emphasizes the importance of *responsibility*, which he defines as the ability to fulfill one's needs in a way that does not deprive others of the ability to fulfill their own needs. Glasser believes that people do not act irresponsibly because they are ill; rather, they are ill because they act irresponsibly. It follows from this premise that responsible persons behave in functional ways that enhance their sense of self-worth.

According to Glasser, two basic psychological needs of most people are the need to love and be loved and the need to be valued by oneself and others. Difficulties arise when an individual is unable to meet these basic human needs. He adds that

Table 21-1. Comparison of Various Approaches to Therapy

Therapeutic Approach	Basic Premise
Reality therapy	People should engage in responsible behavior in order to enhance their sense of self-worth.
Rational emotive therapy	People tend to engage in irrational, immature thinking that is essentially dysfunctional. This form of thinking should be replaced with logical thought patterns.
Implosive therapy	A process called *flooding* is used to reduce anxiety precipitated by a dreaded object or situation. Flooding involves repeated intense exposure to feared objects and situations under controlled conditions.
Primal therapy	People who experience unmet needs and conditional acceptance by parents and significant others develop unhealthy defenses that must be discarded if people are to become aware of their true selves. Regression is sought in order to help clients abandon maladaptive defense patterns.
Milieu therapy	A therapeutic environment is provided that involves staff members and clients in planning and decision making. Unity, group cohesiveness, participation, and mutuality are emphasized.
Client-centered therapy	Therapy is a journey of self-discovery embarked on by the client, with the therapist functioning as guide and companion.
Relationship therapy	Clients are encouraged to express feelings and needs within a therapeutic relationship with the nurse or other caregivers. Clarification, validation, affirmation, and reinforcement are offered in an accepting relationship that utilizes communication constructively.

in order to feel worthwhile, one must maintain a socially acceptable standard of behavior. Adherence to society's standards, values, and views of right and wrong help individuals maintain their sense of self-worth. Rejecting important social values results in societal disapproval or rejection and leads to a sense of being unloved, unappreciated, and devalued.

In reality therapy, responsibility for one's actions is equated with mental health, and irresponsibility is equated with various manifestations of mental illness. In order to be effective, the reality therapist must promote responsibility and self-determination. Although the reality therapist should be warm, sensitive, caring, and emotionally involved, she must also be willing to allow the client to experience the consequences of any irresponsible behavior. Hostility is never encouraged, and acting out impulsively or irresponsibly is believed to compound problems. This approach helps motivate clients to try out new, more responsible patterns of behavior that are therefore more likely to produce rewarding consequences.

Another premise of reality therapy is that frustration or unhappiness does not justify irresponsible behavior. The reality therapist does not accept or excuse irresponsible behavior or allow the client to blame parents or other people, past circumstances, or the present situation for his actions. The therapist should focus on the present and on ethical values and morality as critical issues. The past should be regarded as history that cannot be changed. Parents or significant other persons are neither censured nor blamed, no matter how irresponsibly they may seem to have acted in the past. Because the past cannot be changed, the client should be encouraged to find ways to live responsibly with or without the influence of significant others.

Avoiding responsibility may help the client feel better temporarily, but ultimately it causes him to cling to dysfunctional behaviors and to become disillusioned with treatment. In reality therapy it is thought that merely listening to a recital of a client's problems provides a measure of comfort, but the client eventually discovers that talking about problems does nothing to alleviate them. The reality therapist focuses on *what* the patient is doing, not *why*.

At the same time, the therapist focuses on the client's strengths and on the areas in which he behaves responsibly. The reality therapist explores the client's range of interests by discussing many different topics, including politics, marriage, sex, religion, sports, and hobbies, always focusing on values, standards, and responsibility as underlying issues. In this way, the client is reminded that he is a part of the world and his confidence in his ability to cope with the world is reinforced.

In their unsuccessful effort to fulfill their needs, no matter what behavior they choose, all patients . . . deny the reality of the world around them. Some break the law, denying the rules of society; some claim their neighbors are plotting against them, denying the improbability of such behavior. Some are afraid of crowded places, close quarters, airplanes, or elevators, yet they freely admit the irrationality of their fears. Millions drink to blot out the inadequacy they feel . . . and far too many people choose suicide rather than . . . solve their problems by more responsible behavior. Whether it is a partial denial or the total blotting out of all reality of the chronic back ward patient in the state hospital, the denial of some or all of reality is common to all patients. Therapy will be successful when they are able to give up denying the world and recognize that reality not only exists but that they must fulfill their needs within its framework.

WILLIAM GLASSER (1965)

571

The function of the therapist is to become involved with the client and to encourage acceptance of reality, as painful or problematic as it may be. The therapist then helps the client deal with reality and learn better ways of meeting needs through more adaptive patterns of behavior. Reality therapy emphasizes the therapist's role as an educator and as a role model of responsibility.

Reality therapy can be the basis of interventions with clients on a daily basis. The nurse's attitude of genuine concern and involvement permits gentle encouragement of the client to be more responsible. A client who believes that she is being pursued by foreign agents can be reminded that the nurse has no reason to believe this is so, but the nurse also acknowledges it must be frightening to harbor this belief.

A nurse may support the client experiencing the discomfort of chronic mental illness yet find ways to foster more appropriate interactions with others. For example, the nurse may have to suggest to a client who hears internal voices that it is unwise to respond to them in public places such as the checkout counter in a grocery store. The nurse denies the reality of the voices but acknowledges the reality of the client's experience with the voices. At the same time the nurse reinforces the necessity of behavioral controls. Reality therapy focuses on the client's daily activities as they relate to social standards regarding what is acceptable or unacceptable. The client is taught alternative patterns of behavior and alternative ways of relating to others. Reality therapy encourages involvement that will contribute to a greater sense of self-worth and to an increased ability to give and receive love, so that ultimately the client feels more valued and more fulfilled.

RATIONAL EMOTIVE THERAPY

Albert Ellis, a clinical psychologist, formulated *rational emotive therapy* (RET) in 1955 after he found psychoanalysis to be ineffective with many clients. According to Ellis, no matter how much insight a person may gain into his early childhood experiences and their connection with his current emotional state, he can seldom overcome his present distress solely by gaining insight. On those rare occasions when presenting symptoms are eradicated, new disturbing traits tend to surface.

Ellis maintains that virtually all serious emotional dysfunction results from magical, superstitious, immature thinking and asserts that if disturbing thoughts are rigorously disputed and principles of logical thinking are emphasized, the disordered thought processes can be eliminated. The unwarranted dogmatic, irrational, and unexamined beliefs are not thought to be related to reality and therefore are expected to dissolve if they are carefully and logically attacked.

The philosophical basis for RET can be traced back to the early Greek philosophers, one of whom, Epictetus, wrote during the first century that men are less disturbed by things than by the view that they take of them (Ellis, 1973b). Centuries later Shakespeare supported this belief with his statement that "There is nothing either good or bad but thinking makes it so." Ellis was influenced by the work of Alfred Adler, a modern theorist and psychotherapist who was convinced that a person's behavior springs from his ideas and that his attitudes toward life determine his relationship to the outside world (Ellis, 1973a). Thus, Ellis notes that

Figure 21-1. Theoretical premises of rational emotive therapy.

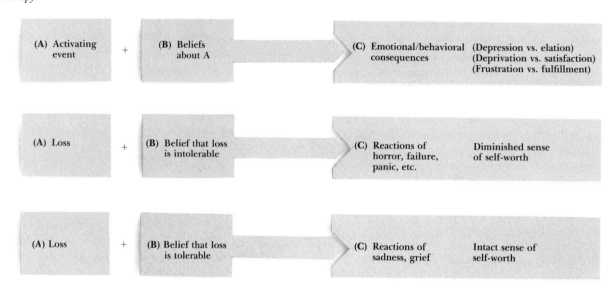

572

life experiences themselves do not make an individual a success or a failure; rather, the individual's *view* of his experiences and the meaning he attributes to them determine his destiny.

The theoretical premises of RET may be described as the ABC's. "A" stands for *activating event*. Some event occurs and the individual reacts. "B" represents the individual's *beliefs* about "A." "C" represents emotional and behavioral *consequences*. According to RET, traumatic occurrences at point "A" do not automatically cause depression or strong feelings of deprivation at point "C." Rather, one's beliefs about the event at point "B" result in the feelings of depression and sense of deprivation, or consequences, at point "C." This is illustrated in Figure 21-1.

For example, if the traumatic occurrence is the loss of a love relationship, and an individual believes that the loss of this relationship is intolerable, not just unfortunate, then the consequences might include feelings of horror, worthlessness, panic, and profound depression. If, on the other hand, the loss of the relationship is viewed as unfortunate (but not intolerable), then the consequences would tend to be sadness (but not profound depression) and regret (but not panic). The sense of being a worthwhile individual would remain intact.

Once an individual accepts that external events influence her feelings but do not cause them, her control over her own emotions is significantly increased and she is less likely to give in to profound depression, hostility, panic, and self-belittling thoughts and feelings. When an individual accepts the fact that not an event but her perception of an event gives rise to her feelings, she has taken a step toward controlling her feelings.

The therapist then searches for irrational perceptions, statements, and conclusions that distort reality and make situations seem worse than they actually are. Detrimental perceptions of events are termed *masturbatory ideologies* (Ellis and Grieger, 1977). An example of a masturbatory ideology is the feeling that "I must excel and win approval for my performance or else I am a mediocre person." Major supporting ideas for this notion are:

1. I must have sincere love and approval almost all the time from all the people I find significant.

2. I must prove myself thoroughly competent, adequate, and achieving, or at least have real competence or talent at something important.

3. My emotional misery comes almost completely from external pressures that I have little ability to change or control. Unless these pressures change, I cannot help making myself feel anxious, depressed, belittled, or hostile.

4. If events occur that put me in real danger or that threaten my life, I have to react by making myself exceptionally preoccupied with and upset by them.

5. My past life has influenced me immensely and remains all-important. If something once strongly affected me, it has to keep determining my feelings and behavior today. My early childhood gullibility and conditionability still remain, and I cannot surmount them and think for myself.

6. I must have a high degree of order or certainty in the universe around me to enable me to feel comfortable and to perform adequately.

Except for those affiliated with teaching units and low-cost clinics, psychoanalysts are not even interested in brief psychotherapy. The community and its mental health problems are remote to the psychoanalyst. Most of his patients have already been screened by the referring doctors, who, well aware of the cost of psychoanalysis in time and money, send those patients who can afford both. Of these patients, only those poorly motivated or those with insufficient ego strengths are refused. Since the rest meet the psychoanalyst's requirements, modification of treatment is unnecessary. If not all the patient's conflicts are examined, if the transference neurosis is not resolved, the analyst does not feel he has permanently helped the patient . . . The psychoanalyst scorns brief psychotherapy as a stopgap measure.
KARL KAY LEWIN, (1970)

573

7. I desperately need others to rely and depend on. Because I shall always remain so weak, I also need some supernatural power on which to rely, especially in times of crisis.

8. I must understand the nature or meaning of the universe in order to live happily in it.

9. I can only rate myself as good or worthy if I perform well, do worthwhile things, and have people generally approve of me.

10. If I make myself depressed, anxious, ashamed, angry, or disturbed in response to people and events, I perform incompetently and shamefully. I amount to a thoroughly weak, rotten person if I react in such ways.

11. Beliefs held by respected authorities or by my society must be correct and I have no right to question them in theory or action; if I do, people have a right to condemn and punish me, and I cannot bear their disapproval.

Another masturbatory ideology is the belief that "Others must treat me with consideration, in exactly the way I want them to treat me. If they fail in this, they should be severely blamed, damned, and punished for their unkindness to me." Major supporting ideas for this notion include:

1. People must treat others in a fair and just manner; if they act unfairly or unethically, they amount to rotten people and deserve severe punishment. The universe will almost certainly see that they get this kind of retribution.

2. If others behave incompetently or stupidly, they are idiots and ought to feel ashamed of themselves.

3. If people have the ability to do well but actually choose to shirk and avoid their responsibilities, they are worthless and should feel ashamed of themselves. People must achieve their full potential for happy and worthwhile living or else they have little or no value as humans.

A third masturbatory ideology states that "Conditions in which I live must be arranged so that I get whatever I want comfortably, quickly, and easily and I receive nothing that I don't want." Major supporting ideas for this notion include:

1. Things must go the way I would like them to go, because I need what I want. Life is awful, terrible, and horrible when I do not get what I prefer.

2. When fearsome people or things exist in my world, I must continually preoccupy myself with and upset myself about them; in that way I will have the power to control or change them.

3. I find it easier to avoid facing many of life's difficulties and responsibilities than to undertake self-discipline. I need immediate comfort and cannot go through present pain to achieve future gain.

4. People should act better than they usually do. If they don't act well and do create needless hassles for me, I view it as awful, and I can't stand the problems that they create.

5. Once handicaps exist in my life, either because of my hereditary tendencies or the influences of my past or present environment, I can do practically nothing to change them. I must

continue to suffer endlessly because of these handicaps. Therefore, life hardly seems worth continuing.

6. If changing some obnoxious or handicapping element in myself or my life proves hard, that difficulty ought not exist. I find it too hard to do anything about it; I might as well make no effort, or very little effort, to change it.

7. Justice, fairness, equality, and democracy must prevail. When they don't, I can't stand it and life seems too unbearable to continue.

8. I must find correct and practically perfect solutions to my problems and others' problems. If I don't, catastrophe will result.

9. People and external events cause practically all my unhappiness, and I have to remain a helpless victim of anxiety, depression, feelings of inadequacy, and hostility unless these conditions and people change and allow me to stop feeling disturbed.

10. I find it completely unfair and horrible to think about the possibility of my dying and no longer having any existence.

11. As long as I remain alive, my life has to have some unusual or special meaning or purpose. If I cannot create this meaning or purpose for myself, the universe must give it to me.

12. I can't stand the discomfort of feeling anxious, depressed, guilty, ashamed, or otherwise emotionally upset. If I really went crazy and wound up in a mental institution, I never could stand that horror and might well have to kill myself.

13. When things have gone badly for me for a long period and no guaranty exists that they will change or that anyone will take over my life and make things better for me, I can't bear the thought of living any longer and have to seriously consider killing myself.

This is an incomplete but representative list of irrational, self-defeating, and dysfunctional beliefs that, according to Ellis, release individuals from responsibility for changing unrewarding ways of thinking and acting.

RET proposes that the tendency to think, emote, and behave in irrational ways has an innate, biological basis as well as an acquired one. Because of the genetic or biological nature of this characteristic, a vulnerable individual is naturally inclined toward self-defeating or self-destructive tendencies and has difficulty modifying them. As a result, a sense of personal worthlessness prevails, and social relationships or productive goals are impeded.

Ellis believes that many individuals are indoctrinated with erroneous perceptions of their own lack of worth learned when they were young and that these erroneous perceptions continue in adult life (Ellis, 1973a).

Ellis alleges that humans tend to misinterpret themselves, frequently mistaking desires for love, approval, success, and pleasure as basic needs. According to Ellis, humans are not simply products of social or environmental learning. Instead, because they are human, they experience complex family-centered transactions that all too often endorse and perpetuate maladaptive behaviors. When erroneous ideas originating in the past intrude on adult interactions, individuals behave in ways that cause them to be labeled deviant, disturbed, or mentally ill.

Basic to RET is the belief that individuals are born with a potential to be rational as well as irrational in their thinking. Other inherent potentials include predispositions toward creativity, language, self-preservation, organization, self-actualization, sexuality, love, and belonging. Paradoxically, individuals also have opposing tendencies toward self-destruction, hedonism, irresponsibility, procrastination, hatred, callousness, superstition, intolerance, perfectionism, and grandiosity. Also, most individuals tend to repeat their mistakes and frequently fail to anticipate future consequences of their current behavior.

The RET approach is cognitive, directive, and discipline oriented. The RET therapist does not believe that involvement or warmth between the client and the therapist is necessary to achieve personality change. The RET therapist does believe that rapport and unconditional acceptance of the client are desirable. While the therapist may criticize dysfunctional behavior, the client is seen as a fallible but forgivable human being. The therapist refuses to disparage the client even when the client disparages himself. The therapist accepts the client without necessarily extending great warmth or showing high regard for the client's behavior.

Implementation of rational emotive therapy requires debating, challenging, disputing, and debunking each of the client's irrational beliefs. The therapy helps clients differentiate between what they want and what they actually need. The goal of the rational emotive therapist is to help clients gain control over irrational beliefs and modify their overreactive emotions and behaviors. This approach allows a more objective, realistic assessment of events, beliefs, and responses, which helps the individual let go of previously incapacitating behavioral consequences. According to Ellis, real and lasting changes can occur through habituation, or repetition and practice, in a conscious, action-oriented effort.

RET is a useful therapeutic tool that, with preliminary preparation, can be implemented by psychiatric nurses for use with specific client populations. In general, the attitude of the nurse should be one of acceptance of the client as a fallible human being. The client herself should not be criticized, but maladaptive behaviors may be examined in light of the activating event (A), beliefs about the event (B), and the emotional/behavioral consequences (C). This approach can be implemented in an individual or group setting.

The masturbatory ideologies to be avoided can be printed on posters and placed in group or individual therapy rooms as continual reminders of the human tendency to overreact to certain life events. A variety of impersonal therapeutic aids may also be used, such as films, didactic discussions, activity-oriented homework assignments, and approaches that are not essentially empathetic or sympathetic. A combination of behavior therapies such as desensitization, assertiveness training, and operant conditioning may be employed to help the client make a compelling cognitive change.

Persons susceptible to disorders with strong psychological components, such as peptic ulcer, coronary artery disease, hypertension, and migraine headaches, may find this form of therapy especially helpful in reducing excessive reactivity to life stresses and keeping such stresses in perspective.

IMPLOSIVE THERAPY

As explained in Chapter 17, *implosive therapy* is based on the general behavioral principle that a person can overcome maladaptive anxiety elicited by situations or objects by approaching the feared situation while in a psychophysiological state that inhibits anxiety. Implosive therapy is used specifically for persons disabled by phobias and anxiety. The patient is desensitized to anxiety-producing stimuli by intense exposure to fear-producing situations, either through imagination or through actual exposure to the fear-producing situation. This process of repeated intense exposure is called *flooding*. An important difference between flooding and traditional behavior modification procedures is that exposure to feared objects or situations is repeatedly intensified in flooding. Relaxation training and medication are sometimes used to facilitate implosive techniques and shorten the process.

Flooding means that the client confronts the anxiety-producing object or situation at full intensity for prolonged periods of time. This results in the client's being allowed to experience anxiety rather than being protected from overwhelming discomfort. For example, a client who fears heights might be brought to the top of a tall building and required to remain there long enough for excessive anxiety to dissipate. Anxiety tends to diminish to lower levels within the first 25 minutes of the initial intense exposure. Subsequent sessions would be held, preferably within an interval of a few days. In the second session the anxiety level would be lowered more quickly. With repeated exposure to the feared situation, less effort would be required for the client to reach a state of calmness. The flooding process would be repeated until little or no anxiety was experienced. To prevent a return of previous levels of anxiety, additional sessions would be held, with longer periods of time elapsing between each session, until the client was able to remain calm and be aware of a sense of mastery. The entire treatment of flooding usually requires from five to twenty sessions, depending on the severity and durability of the problem.

One disadvantage to using flooding techniques is the extent of discomfort produced in the client. Therefore, the flooding approach is suitable only for carefully selected clients. Persons who have a history of cardiac problems or hypertension would certainly not be candidates for this form of therapy. Clients who are susceptible to extremely generalized rather than focused anxiety are inappropriate for this form of therapy. For such clients a psychotic reaction in which contact with reality is lost might be triggered by the induction of overwhelming anxiety. Thus the vulnerability, actual or potential, of any client may preclude the adoption of this form of therapy.

An alternative form of implosive therapy that avoids flooding a client with anxiety is *graded exposure*, which is similar to flooding except that the feared object or situation is introduced gradually.

Imagery is an approach that can be used to help clients cope with fear-inducing measures such as chemotherapy or other painful treatments. When faced with unpleasant experiences, the client is encouraged to detach emotionally from what is happening and to focus on another, more pleasant memory. This approach encourages the client to achieve greater control over emotional and physiological fear responses. Imagery is based on the theory that people are able to modify, through processes of self-monitoring and self-reinforcement, physiological activity or processes of consciousness (Tart and Fadiman, 1975). By means of imagery (for example, visualizing heartbeats or the pressure with which blood moves through veins and arteries) clients can voluntarily control some autonomic functions that previously had been thought beyond voluntary control. A principle underlying the effectiveness of imagery is the psychophysiological principle proposed by Green, Green, and Holmes

575

A VARIANT FORM OF EXISTENTIAL THERAPY

Logotherapy, developed by Victor Frankl (1963), is a humanistic type of therapy that emphasizes the importance of finding meaning in one's existence. Suffering is regarded as an inescapable fact of life to be met bravely. It is the meaning of our lives that sustains us; love and endeavor are the most valuable human behaviors. Frankl introduced two therapeutic procedures. One is *dereflection,* or the refocusing of the individual's attention from the self to others. The other procedure is called *paradoxical intention.* A paradox is an apparent contradiction: here the individual is encouraged to engage in problematic activities that are distressing. When the distressing activity is consciously brought about, the individual must take some responsibility for its occurrence. Feelings of being in control rather than being controlled remove feelings of helplessness, thereby reducing distress and anxiety.

576

(1980), which states that each change in physiological conditions is accompanied by commensurate changes in cognition and emotions, conscious or unconscious. Conversely, every change in the mental-emotional state is accompanied by commensurate changes in the psyiological state of the individual, conscious or unconscious.

Human beings have a biological but not conscious awareness of their physical state down to the level of a single cell. In essence, this means that physiological activity of a single cell induces a reactive response in other cells. It is possible to control the direction and flow of nerve impulses throughout their body and to monitor physiological functioning to some extent. Because the mind is capable of controlling some of the physical activity of cells, it follows that some diseases may even originate in mental processes. Health is affected by stresses largely because the mind confronts situations that are perceived as threatening and that cannot be coped with effectively (Brown, 1980).

The belief that physical and psychological processes are interdependent can help clients deal with painful and feared procedures and can assist them in contributing to their own recovery by monitoring their own cognitive and emotional responses.

Imagery and visualization approaches have proved successful in a variety of health problems thought to have strong psychological components, such as migraine headaches, hypertension, peptic ulcers, and asthma. It must be acknowledged that considerable systematic research in the form of controlled studies must be undertaken to validate and evaluate the effectiveness of imagery and visualization techniques.

PRIMAL THERAPY

Primal therapy, originated by Arthur Janov (1970), is based on the idea that infants are born without symptoms of neurosis or psychosis but that when needs for food, tenderness, and acceptance are unmet, difficulties arise. Unmet needs create pain, and the pain continues until the infant separates his needs from his painful feelings and suppresses or disconnects himself from his feelings in an effort to avoid feeling pain. In time, suppressed needs contribute to a continuous state of tension, which, in later life, can be acted out in a variety of behaviors ranging from disrupted sleeping patterns to sociopathic disorders.

The neuroses, or anxiety disorders, are seen as dysfunctional feeling responses that are symbolic substitutes for the original unmet needs. Experiences in which basic needs go unmet may not necessarily be sudden, overwhelming, traumatic events. Instead, they may be subtle and occur insidiously over a period of time. Janov's examples include being forced to say "please" and "thank you," not being allowed to complain or cry when unhappy, being left with an insensitive babysitter too often, or being asked to recite poetry, perform, catch a ball, or solve abstract problems before one is able. Whatever the demands, the child learns that to be loved or to receive approval, she must comply with whatever she is asked to do. The feeling that love is conditional and is withheld unless parental expectations are met produces intolerable feelings of hopelessness and distress. The child's attempt to please the parents is called *the struggle.* This endless

THE PHENOMENON OF PRIMAL THERAPY

Arthur Janov, the originator of primal therapy, reported that his therapeutic approach grew out of an experience in a psychotherapy group of which he was the leader. Upon being asked to call out for "Mommy" and "Daddy," a group member became increasingly agitated; his body trembled and his movements became convulsive. Finally the member uttered a piercing scream, followed by subjective feelings of clarity and understanding. Janov began using similar techniques with other clients and noted that the sequence of agitation and an anguished scream was followed by greater capacity for insight. By using variations of his methods with large numbers of people, Janov formulated a theory to explain the impact of the approach known as primal therapy. The detractors of this approach consider it to be a cathartic emotional experience rather than a rational, proven form of psychotherapy.

struggle prevents the child from feeling hopeless but rather makes her strive ever harder to meet self-imposed standards of high performance. These activities are undertaken in an effort to be loved. Eventually, the behaviors become automatic or unconscious, and the person believes them to be a part of her real self. Although the struggle begins with trying to please the parents it is later generalized to trying to please everyone. The wish to please controls and motivates the person's activities from then on. The real self, as defined by Janov, is the person one is before discovering that such a person is not acceptable to one's parents. A person is born real, but the authentic self is lost in the struggle to please.

The injuries resulting from the accumulation of unmet needs are stored in what Janov calls the *primal pool*. Because substitutes for unconditional love are never fully satisfying, the resulting frustration is acted out through a variety of behaviors that may be symbolic of the pain. Such behaviors may take the form of overachievement, obesity, substance abuse, anxiety, or phobias, depending on the personality traits of the individual.

The primal therapist believes that the real self is disconnected and, along with the original feelings of pain, is encased in a protective shell. When the defense behaviors of the struggle are not present, as during a vacation, the individual may feel strange or unreal. In some vulnerable individuals the absence of the struggle may lead to psychiatric disability.

Janov's "shell" differs from the Freudian defense system. A strong defense system, according to Freudian theory, helps maintain a functional, integrated personality. In contrast, Janov believes that the person who is well-defended is likely to be dys-functional or "unreal." According to Janov, the healthy, well-integrated person is the one without defenses. In troubled persons the real self is rejected in favor of the unreal self. At the same time most persons continue to wish to be real. This conflict, according to Janov, results in disruption of the endocrine system, causing strain on other organ systems. Thus, the troubled individual does not function smoothly or normally on physiological and psychological levels.

The troubled individual can be freed from his or her unreal self by reexperiencing the original *primal pain* through primal therapy, which is described as a systematic assault on the unreal self. Janov believes that feeling the original agony of unmet needs eventually results in discovery of the real or true self. Experiencing primal pain is severe enough to cause the individual to react by expressing *primal screams*; the unmet needs of the individual will be fulfilled, paradoxically, when the defenses are removed and the pain is felt. The unreal self is destroyed and the real self can emerge.

The therapeutic approach involves reliving key early events, or *primal scenes*. The client feels the distress of primal hopelessness once again. By reliving the agony and feeling the pain completely, the individual can give up the unreal hope of being loved for what she is. When the unrealistic hope of unconditional love is given up, the individual can then give up the struggle to please, which has caused so much anguish.

Because defenses against pain are viewed as unhealthy, the goal of therapy is for the client to relinquish defenses that prevent recalling and experiencing the pain of early hurts. In primal therapy, the client is isolated in a hotel room for 24 hours before the first session. Customary activities, such as reading, smoking, watching television, and making phone calls, which may provide outlets for release of tension, are prohibited. Some individuals who are especially well defended might be asked to remain awake all night. Sleeplessness is thought to break down the defenses, partly because dreaming, a usual outlet for tension, is prevented. With his defenses weakened and his pain threshold lowered by isolation, the client is brought closer to a primal experience.

During the first three weeks of primal treatment, the therapist works intensively with the client. Later, the client usually becomes a part of a primal group that emphasizes reliving painful early scenes. The primal group ordinarily meets for a period of six to nine months.

Treatment usually takes place in a soundproof office where clients lie supine in a defenseless position. Some patients may complain of tight feelings in the throat and chest or may begin to gag and retch in early sessions. As the clients are encouraged to name the pain they feel, they may writhe and thrash about. The therapist continues to encourage the clients to let their feelings out; often a client screams with utterances of "Daddy, be nice!" or "Mommy, hurt!" or just "Hate!" or "Help!" A client may clutch his abdomen and fall to the floor convulsing. The scream is described as a liberating event, orgasmic in nature and involuntary. It represents a reenactment of experiences from the past.

Primal screaming may take place by the third day of therapy, sometimes it may not take place for weeks. When it does occur, it is believed that barriers between thought and feelings are broken. The person becomes open to feelings and may have spontaneous primal experiences outside therapy sessions. This is considered an indication that the client is on the way to health. Many more primal experiences may occur over a period of months, each one diminishing the unreal self and expanding the real self, until the client is free of distress.

The goal of the therapist is to evoke pain in order to produce a functioning, feeling person. As the primal process continues, the client may regress into childhood or infancy, speaking with a lisp or using infantile manners as the primal scenes are relived. Some clients have been reported to relive the traumatic birth experience itself.

Being cured means that an individual is able to feel, without outside help, whatever feelings are present. Defenses are relinquished and therefore not available to hide feelings or to cause acting-out behaviors. Total happiness is not the goal of primal therapy, and clients who are cured will have moments of pain. Because they are able to feel what is

happening in the here and now, events may upset the postprimal client, but neurotic behavior induced by tensions does not return, and the results are said to be lasting. The struggle is no longer necessary, so life is made easier and the client is able to enjoy life without artificial aids such as chemicals.

Advocates of primal therapy allege that other forms of therapy that treat only symptoms ignore the totality of the psychophysical self and actually continue fragmenting the self. Tension, they believe, continues and disturbs the client's emotional and physical well-being. Primal therapy is thought to provide a unifying experience that makes the individual whole again.

Primal therapy advocates claim to have discovered the definitive cure for mental disorders and state that it cannot be integrated with other therapeutic approaches. Janov (1972) wrote that all other forms of therapy are obsolete and invalid and that primal therapy is the only valid approach to treating neurotic and psychotic clients. Primal therapy is therefore rarely used in an eclectic way.

MILIEU THERAPY AND THE THERAPEUTIC COMMUNITY

In *milieu therapy* the maintenance of an atmosphere that encourages recovery or optimal functioning is stressed. Early forms of milieu therapy included a form of moral therapy, which advocated "compassionate and understanding treatment of innocent sufferers" (Almond, 1974, p. 33). Moral therapy emphasized discussion of difficulties and the daily pursuit of purposeful activities. Between 1900 and 1930, Herman Simon, a German psychiatrist, developed the system of active hospital treatment known as *milieutherapie* or *aktivere behandlung*, meaning "more active therapy." Simon believed that clients responded to the expectations of those around them. Clients were carefully assessed for psychopathology and for strengths, especially past or recent work successes. They were then placed in work situations consistent with their abilities and social functioning levels. As clients demonstrated success at one level, they were encouraged to undertake higher level tasks.

During the 1920s milieu therapy was widely used in Germany, but the establishment of the Third Reich interfered with the growth of this modality. Nevertheless, using the hospital as a therapeutic environment was undertaken during the 1930s in other countries, including the United States. The Menninger brothers in Topeka, Kansas introduced milieu therapy in their in-patient treatment settings, where individualized regimens were devised for each client. Every client received individual psychotherapy, and specific approaches were prescribed for individual clients (Almond, 1974).

Milieu therapy is defined by Cummings and Cummings (1962) as "the scientific manipulation of the environment aimed at producing changes in the personality of the patient" (p. 5). Nurses and other caretakers are not supervisors of work but are co-workers and participants with clients. Designated tasks take into account the ability of the individual. Since overexpectations may be harmful, initial expectations of performance should be modest, and work should be broken down into simple steps. Milieu therapy uses the entire environment, physical and social, therapeutically, and no psychiatric limitation is considered a complete barrier to graded activity (Almond, 1974).

Milieu therapy provides for a more rational, flexible, and democratic decision-making process among those persons affected by the consequences of the decisions. This approach represents a major change from the authoritarian administration of traditional institutions. It is thought that clients who have a voice in making rules are more likely to conform to them, so client government is an important part of milieu therapy. It allows clients to develop constitutional by-laws, hold regular meetings, and elect officers to leadership positions that are recognized by clients and hospital administrators alike. Ward meetings are attended by clients, staff, and the unit administrator, but by no one higher in the administrative hierarchy. Clients are permitted to vote on issues and to make suggestions and recommendations to hospital authorities based on the consensus of the client population rather than on any one person's opinion. Clients can organize, assign, and carry out unit duties and can urge changes in unit rules. They can organize and carry out social activities or related projects, such as editing a hospital newsletter. Committees can be formed by clients for the betterment or beautification of the treatment facility. But above all, the client government is responsible for making and enforcing most of the unit rules and regulations.

The concept of the *therapeutic community* is similar to that of milieu therapy. Both emphasize the importance of using all aspects of the clients' hospital experience in a therapeutic manner. The major difference, according to Almond (1974), is that milieu therapy adheres more closely to the medical model; the psychiatrist heads the treatment team and instructs unit staff about the approach to be used with each client. The therapeutic community is less likely to be organized along hierarchical lines, and planning and implementation of the therapeutic regimen are usually delegated to members of an interdisciplinary team.

Like milieu therapy, the therapeutic community stresses group treatment, group activities, and joint decision making by both clients and staff. Community meetings, client government meetings, activities programs, job training, planning meetings, social and recreational groups, psychodrama, and family group meetings are all part of the therapeutic community. Democratic processes and egalitarianism are greatly emphasized.

Maxwell Jones was a pioneer in the development of the therapeutic community at Belmont Hospital in England in the 1950s. Jones described an industrial rehabilitation unit and the meetings and activities considered important to structuring a client's day. Unity, cohesiveness, and the social culture of the therapeutic community were emphasized, with clients and staff participating in the decisions dealing with everyday problems of living. The focus was on the present and on friendliness and informal sociability rather than on the causes of problems or dissension. All clients and staff were considered part of the therapeutic community. Symbols of rank such as white coats or uniforms were conspicuously absent (Jansen, 1980).

Any therapeutic community should promote a sense of belonging, of shared membership, and of responsibility toward others in the community. Behavioral expectations should be made clear, as is shown in the box on page 580.

According to Jansen (1980), in therapeutic communities there is a transmission of healing, which can be shared by members and experienced even by newcomers. A therapeutic community provides a communal experience that fosters open communication and promotes intrapsychic and interpersonal adjustment to the maximum potential of each individual.

The therapeutic aspect of the community environment serves as an adjunct to individual therapy, medication, and group and activities therapy. Social therapies, behavior therapy, individual psychotherapies, or eclectic approaches may also be incorporated to meet individual needs of clients.

The introduction and expansion of milieu therapy has had a profound effect on psychiatric nursing. Prior to its introduction, nurses were delegated the responsibility of managing a safe, secure psychiatric unit. With the advent of milieu therapy, the role of the nurse changed from custodial to therapeutic and rehabilitative. Instead of taking charge *of* clients, nurses could now focus on involvement in goal-directed activities *with* clients.

The nurse in the therapeutic community plays an active part in making the decisions affecting the community. The nurse's comments, opinions, and suggestions about medication choices and dosages and about client discharge and placement receive serious consideration. Because the nurse is in close

579

<table>
<tr><td>

BEHAVIORS EXPECTED FROM MEMBERS OF A THERAPEUTIC COMMUNITY

1. Clients are expected to try to control their own behaviors.

2. Clients are encouraged to engage in social interactions.

3. Clients are urged to speak out in community and group meetings.

4. Clients are encouraged to talk about their problems with staff, among themselves, and with significant others.

5. Clients are expected to attend meetings, activities, and therapy sessions.

6. Clients are expected to care about others and to value community interests.

7. Clients are urged to trust the staff and client members of the therapeutic community.

8. Clients are expected to show concern for others in the community.

</td></tr>
</table>

580

touch with and has extensive data on clients, the opinions and observations of the nurse are greatly respected by others on the mental health team.

One responsibility of the nurse in a therapeutic community is to help clients express feelings and conflicts appropriately and to help them find healthier ways of relating to others. The focus is on helping clients to function at their optimum capacity and thus avoid further regression. Limits on client behavior are set whenever necessary to help the client maintain control. The nurse may also use permissive approaches when appropriate and endeavor to provide protection and support when necessary.

Since a substantial portion of the nurse's energies are directed toward various group activities within the therapeutic community, the nurse must be knowledgeable about group dynamics and skilled in group process. A basic assumption in the therapeutic community is that clients have strength and potential, and therefore should be actively involved in developing the treatment plan. This concept of client participation is consistent with the basic assumptions of the nursing process.

The concept of the therapeutic community is applicable to inpatient units and to community residences or partial care programs, regardless of setting. Torrey (1972) reported the experience of a Nigerian psychiatrist who was educated in England and returned to develop in his native country a hospital village system in which the clients live in four villages surrounding a central hospital. Results reported thus far indicate a higher discharge rate and lower rate of relapse in these partially hospitalized clients, at lower costs for treatment than would occur with total hospitalization.

In Denver, Colorado, the Community Support Systems Program offers additional evidence that a therapeutic community can be effectively implemented outside a hospital. Approximately 350 lower functioning clients residing in surrounding boarding homes come daily to an old but spacious building. Each day begins with a community meeting attended and cooperatively led by staff and clients. The schedule for the day is listed on a blackboard and read aloud by a client. Various clients volunteer for the activities required to ensure smooth operation of the facility. Some clients agree to work in the kitchen preparing food for "Cafe Broadway," where lunches are served at cost. Other clients offer to serve as waiters. Those who work at the cafe receive free lunches and may keep any tips. Others volunteer to staff the resource desk for hourly periods in order to provide assistance for clients or visitors who come to the facility. Still other clients volunteer to share their special talents in performances of an in-house drama company. The performances help raise funds for the center as well as provide amusement for clients.

Some supervision is provided by staff. Clients are seen by a psychiatrist who supervises their medications. A nurse practitioner assesses clients for physical problems that may require treatment, and all staff members observe the clients for medication side effects as well as for the therapeutic effects.

An interdisciplinary health team coordinates

Prior to therapy the person is prone to ask himself, often unwittingly, "What do others think I should do in this situation? What would my parents or my culture want me to do? What do I think ought to be done?" He is thus continually acting in terms of the form which should be imposed on his behavior. This does not mean that he acts in accord with the expectations of others. He may . . . act so as to contradict the expectations of others. He is nevertheless acting in terms of the expectations . . . of others. During the process of therapy the individual comes to ask himself, in regard to the ever-widening areas of his life space, "How do I experience this? What does it mean to me?" . . . He comes to act on a basis of what may be termed realism—a realistic balancing of the satisfactions and dissatisfactions which any action will bring to himself.

CARL R. ROGERS (1961)

581

treatment activities and provides a supportive environment that addresses the clients' needs for medical care, psychotherapy, financial management, skill development, socialization, stress management, job counseling, and adequate housing. This program is a good example of a therapeutic community that helps clients raise their functioning level by participating in a structured treatment environment with an interpersonal and vocational focus.

CLIENT-CENTERED THERAPY

Originated by Carl Rogers in the 1940s, *client-centered therapy* is concerned with developing the client's potential. It focuses on present rather than past experiences. The therapist offers a caring, listening presence. The therapist's knowledge and technical skills are not emphasized. Instead, three attitudes are considered necessary to effect a change in the client: (1) empathy, or understanding, (2) genuineness, or congruence, and (3) nonpossessive caring. An individual's growth is thought to be enhanced by a caring, nonjudgmental, empathetic relationship with a helping individual. The therapist endeavors to understand the client's experience, and to monitor his or her feelings.

The therapist's unconditional regard for the client's individuality facilitates the process of self-actualization as the client discovers appropriate directions to take. The client-centered therapist does not give advice or direction but rather functions as a companion and guide for the client's journey of self-discovery.

Any techniques that place the therapist in control rather than the client, such as formal psychological testing, manipulation, or the use of specialized language, are avoided. Control or criticism by the therapist is thought to undermine the client's confidence in his ability to discover and mobilize his own resources. Other therapeutic techniques that place the therapist in the role of expert and reduce the client's reliance on personal resources, such as rational emotive therapy or primal therapy, are also avoided. The Rogerian model of therapy emphasizes trust in the client's rational, orderly progress toward growth and fosters constructive behaviors that are conducive to self-fulfillment.

A major goal of client-centered therapy is to facilitate self-discovery and the abandonment of masks, disguises, or facades. Rather than trying to be what others think they should be, clients are helped to reveal themselves, to accept themselves, and to value themselves for what they are. As a result of therapy, clients gradually allow themselves to be more open to experiences and more aware of their inner feelings and attitudes. Clients are also helped to replace their stereotyped views of events with more realistic perceptions that are more flexible and more tolerant of ambiguity. Clients learn to trust their own perceptions of themselves more, and to look less to others as models for behaviors, choices, values, and standards to live by. They learn to accept free choice and to judge their lives by whether they are living in a satisfying and expressive way (Rogers, 1960).

Torrey (1972) cited historical psychiatric evidence supporting the effectiveness of empathy, genuineness, and warm regard. At the peak of the humanitarian movement in mental hospitals during the early to mid-1800s, when therapists made an effort to demonstrate interest and kindness toward their clients as human beings, more clients improved. For example, between 1833 and 1846 at Worcester State Hospital in Massachusetts, 70 percent of the clients shown interest and kindness while hospitalized were reported much improved or cured within one year of admission and were discharged. This impressive improvement and discharge rate compares favorably with that of state hospitals today. In addition, this rate of improvement occurred before psychotropic medications or electroconvulsive therapy were available. The explanation offered was that the humanitarian movement encouraged use of caregiver attitudes considered therapeutic: warmth, genuineness, and empathy.

The Rogerian approach has a wide range of usefulness in nursing, counseling, social work, and education. It is effective with many types of clients, ranging from relatively functional to chronically dysfunctional. It is especially applicable to individuals living in stressful situations in which they feel insecure, inferior, or trapped. When used by caregivers, this approach helps reduce feelings of loneliness, isolation, and alienation. Nurses can actively transmit positive regard to the client by reflecting or rephrasing the client's words and by communicating acceptance. This allows the client to become aware of any self-image distortions. The nurse should avoid interpreting, explaining, or changing the client. Consistent use of a client-centered approach can be effective in establishing a positive relationship, which in turn can be beneficial in enhancing the client's sense of self. With Rogers' approach, therapy becomes a journey into self-understanding in which the nurse is a trusted companion rather than a leader.

RELATIONSHIP THERAPY AS NURSING PROCESS

Relationship therapy combines the therapeutic nurse-client relationship and nursing process in a therapeutic plan whose purpose is to facilitate the development of more adaptive responses in the client. The therapeutic relationship differs from a social or friendly relationship in that both nurse and client enter into the relationship for the purpose of helping the client and the relationship is time limited and goal oriented. Although the nurse is warm, genuinely caring, and accepting of the client, the relationship must remain professional in order for it to be therapeutic. A social relationship develops spontaneously in response to mutual needs; a therapeutic relationship is planned in order to meet the needs of the clients. A social relationship has no time limits expressed or implied, and verbal ex-

changes are limited by society's norms. In a therapeutic relationship, the client is encouraged to express feelings and thoughts that might not be acceptable in social settings, although an ultimate goal might be to help the client develop socially acceptable expressions of feelings and thoughts.

Communication is the basic tool of relationship therapy and of the nursing process. It is a complex, dynamic process through which people send and receive verbal and nonverbal messages in order to understand and be understood by others, respond to the environment, and transmit ideas to one another (Lippincott, 1982). Communication in a therapeutic relationship is monitored by the nurse, who consciously develops and employs communication skills. Superficial, social conversation is limited and communication is directed toward assessment of client needs, identification of goals, and implementation of therapeutic nursing interventions.

Communication skills facilitate the nursing process and the therapeutic relationship. By active listening, the nurse communicates respect for the client. Eye contact and occasional nods or comments indicate that the client has been heard and understood. Broad opening statements and open-ended questions encourage verbalization of relevant information. General leads, such as "Go on . . ." or "And . . ." indicate the nurse's wish for the client to continue. Restating what the client has just said encourages clarification. Validation of perceptions reduces the chance of misunderstanding or misperception by either the nurse or the client. Opportunity should be provided for the client to validate or dispute the nurse's observations. Since communication is a two-way process, feedback from the nurse is also important. Feedback provides the client with information regarding the effect the client's behaviors may have on the interviewer. Focusing and selective reflecting encourage communication of specific information. As relationship therapy progresses, the nurse guides communication in order to help the client remain on important issues or themes the nurse has identified.

Silences during an interaction can be valuable in providing opportunities for both the client and the nurse to reflect upon what has been said. However, some silences indicate anger or resistance on the part of the client. Some silences can become awkward and provoke anxiety, especially if the nurse or client believes that interactions must be filled with conversation. However, a silence may also indicate resolution of one topic and readiness to bring up other issues.

Reassurance is sometimes used inappropriately to reduce the nurse's anxiety, in which case it may cause a breakdown in communication. On the other hand, sincere reassurance can contribute to a sense of security or provide positive reinforcement, affirmation, or validation of the client's thoughts, feelings, and behaviors.

Throughout a therapeutic interaction, it is important for the nurse to maintain an awareness of his or her own feelings in order to serve the client's best interests. Communication of the nurse's own values or judgments in the form of lectures or "pep talks" is countertherapeutic because such messages belittle the significance of the client's own values and experiences. Judgmental attitudes can block communication and increase anxiety in the client. A nurse may convey stereotyping or prejudice by means of subtle innuendo and phrasing. Clients are often aware of negative attitudes in the nurse even though these attitudes have not been directly communicated. Psychiatric clients are often acutely sensitive to others and soon recognize when a nurse is not wholly accepting. Since negative responses do nothing to promote an effective helping relationship, it is the nurse's responsibility to engage in sufficient introspection so as to develop an awareness of negative personal feelings and to discuss them with an experienced staff person. Once recognized, these problem feelings can be dealt with and their influence diminished.

Offering advice is also counterproductive for most clients. It indicates that the nurse believes the client's decision-making abilities are inadequate, and it places the client in a dependent position and weakens the client's confidence and self-esteem. The client's interests are better served by an approach that encourages clients to make their own decisions once they have had the opportunity to explore their options. In this way, the client's problem-solving abilities are emphasized. Because the client is encouraged to choose a course of action, the responsibility for decisions remains with the client.

Therapeutic use of the nurse's own personality is an integral part of relationship therapy. Qualities that have been identified as helpful include those described by Carl Rogers: empathy, genuineness, and warm regard. These promote therapeutic interaction and contribute to the attainment of mutually agreed-upon goals.

Showing empathy rather than sympathy is in accord with the general principle that the nurse should refrain from doing for clients what they are able to do for themselves. In offering empathy, the nurse feels *with* the client not *for* the client. Sympathy tends to make the nurse assume excessive responsibility for providing relief and reduces the client's potential for growth.

Genuineness implies sincerity and open, authentic communication. Throughout relationship therapy, the nurse strives to understand the client's feelings, remain professionally involved, and be-come aware of her own feelings that might threaten the therapeutic quality of her relationship with the client.

Involvement, another therapeutic quality, entails caring for another and standing by that person through difficult situations, while doing something with and for that person. The nurse should be involved with clients as a caring human being, but at the same time, her involvement must be shaped by the professional role. Clients who have difficulty relating to others can benefit from a human relationship that models skills in communication and interpersonal transactions. Involvement, however, is different from identification; objectivity is retained even though the client is perceived as a unique individual. Nurses must be able to respond first to the needs of the client, not to their own needs for control or approval.

Both the nursing process and the therapeutic relationship are collaborative processes directed toward the development of adaptive coping mechanisms and behavioral change in the client. The therapeutic relationship can be separated into four sequential phases: (1) the introductory or orientation phase, (2) the testing phase, (3) the working phase, and (4) the termination phase. These parallel the four steps of the nursing process: assessment, planning, implementation, and evaluation.

Assessment in Relationship Therapy (The Introductory Phase)

During the first phase of the therapeutic relationship, the *introductory* or *orientation phase*, the nurse and client become acquainted and reach an agreement on the time, place, and initial goals of their interactions. Together they discover relevant information that helps identify needs, formulate nursing diagnoses, and establish initial goals. During this initial phase, rapport is established between nurse and client. Unless the client begins to develop trust in the nurse, the prospect of a successful outcome is diminished. They discuss expected length of time needed to meet defined goals, the nature of their relationship, and their respective responsibilities.

During the first phase of the therapeutic relationship, the client's behaviors are assessed and her strengths and vulnerabilities are identified. Maladaptive patterns of behavior (those that compound rather than relieve the client's problems) are the focus of interventions. The client's strengths and functional behaviors can serve as the basis for developing alternatives to maladaptive behavior patterns.

In assessing a client, the nurse must first recognize those behaviors that are self-defeating, ineffective, or inappropriate. Second, the nurse might assess those factors that preceded or seemed to precipitate the problem behavior. She should attempt to identify reinforcing events that encourage the continuation of the problem behavior. One goal is to prevent, if possible, the recurrence of those events that reinforce negative behaviors and to replace them with events that reinforce more constructive cognitive, affective, and behavioral responses. This should be done with the client's consent.

The nurse should also suggest that the client undergo physical assessment to rule out any physiological basis for maladaptive behaviors. Thyrotoxicosis, brain or adrenal tumors, and withdrawal from drugs or alcohol are only a few of the disorders that can mimic conditions of psychiatric disorganization.

Assessment for side effects of psychiatric medications should continue throughout the nurse-client relationship. The psychiatric nurse must also remember that clients may become ill with any disorder that affects the general population. Certain physical conditions may prohibit the use of specific medications designed to relieve psychiatric symptoms. Mental and physical health are interrelated, each one affecting the other. Thus, assessment of client needs must be done on a comprehensive and continuing basis.

Sources of data for assessing maladaptive responses are numerous. The primary source is the client, but the family or other significant persons in the client's life may also contribute information that can be utilized in the plan of care. Here again the client must assent.

Planning in Relationship Therapy (The Testing Phase)

Arriving at a treatment plan is the second step in the nursing process. At this point, the nurse should encourage the client's participation in recognizing and assessing his own maladaptive responses. The origin, perpetuation, and consequences of the client's self-defeating behaviors should be cooperatively determined, and the client should continue to be involved in the problem-solving process.

Goals should be collaboratively developed, mutually agreed upon, and stated in behavioral terms and in clear language that can be understood by the client. Vague abstractions are not useful in describing goals because clients are often unable to understand abstract, ambiguous concepts.

Goals may be differentiated into long-term and short-term ones. Long-term goals are those that resolve the problems that led the client to become involved in relationship therapy. Short-term goals are the intermediate steps required to meet the long-term goals. Discharge, or outcome, goals that will

lead to the termination of therapy should be identified at the beginning of the relationship. This can be done by evaluating progress, anticipating the client's future needs, and identifying specific behaviors needed for more independent living. The entire nursing process should be aimed at encouraging the highest level of adaptation possible within the limits of the client's capabilities.

As the relationship evolves into the second phase, the nurse should expect considerable testing of the relationship. The client who lacks self-esteem and who cannot conceive of another's genuine concern for her may try to prove that the nurse is not trustworthy. Appointments may be missed if the client feels especially vulnerable or fearful. The client may be late for an appointment and then covertly try to determine whether the agreement to set aside a specific period of time for the client was sincere. It is important at this critical time for the nurse to demonstrate her trustworthiness by not turning to other activities when a client fails to keep an appointment. The nurse should simply wait for the client. If the client appears for the meeting, the nurse can remind her of the agreed-upon starting time in order to encourage punctuality. Even when a client is late, the interaction should be terminated according to the initial time frame. In this way limits are reinforced. Most clients feel more secure when given clear limits. The nurse demonstrates acceptance of the client but at the same time sets limits on unacceptable behaviors. Consistency is an essential aspect of relationship therapy and should extend to other matters, as well.

During early phases of the relationship, the client is usually allowed considerable freedom in introducing topics to discuss. Typically, the client will begin by revealing factual information on an intellectual level. Good interviewing skills are helpful in eliciting information about the client's emotional level. This helps the nurse to assess the client's needs and establish nursing diagnoses. The nurse should promise confidentiality but must not agree to withhold information from others on the health team.

Achievement of goals can lead to a sense of accomplishment in the client. Therefore, care should be taken to avoid establishing goals incompatible with the client's abilities, values, or level of functioning. It is preferable initially to set goals the nurse and client are reasonably certain of being able to fulfill. The nurse may then use positive, low-key reinforcement to increase the client's confidence and self-esteem. Higher-level goals are usually introduced after lower-level goals have been met. Unrealistic goals only frustrate the nurse, discourage the client, and compound the client's feelings of inferiority and worthlessness.

Intervention in Relationship Therapy (The Working Phase)

Implementing relevant nursing actions, the third step in the nursing process, parallels the third phase of the therapeutic relationship, the working phase. It is during this phase that the client verbalizes her feelings more readily and the nurse can suggest adaptive behaviors to take the place of maladaptive or problematic responses. This is usually the longest and most productive of the four phases of the therapeutic relationship. By this time, the nursing care plan has undergone considerable change. The care plan has been evaluated in terms of goal outcomes, and additional information concerning the client has led to modifications of the chosen therapeutic approaches.

During the working phase, the tendency is toward more open expression of feelings. Self-defeating or maladaptive responses expressed by the client may be analyzed cooperatively by the client and nurse. Therapeutic approaches are formulated by the nurse or the mental health team. The selection of suitable approaches is made on the basis of an ongoing assessment of the client and an evaluation of the client's progress.

During the working phase, the nurse should anticipate plateaus where little progress is observed. These may take the form of resistance to therapy manifested by the rejection of or hostility toward the nurse, avoidance behaviors, or denial of issues related to the client's maladaptive responses. The nurse can respond by facilitating the client's expression of feelings and identifying possible issues that appear to threaten the effectiveness of the relationship therapy. However, the client, not the nurse, must take responsibility for controlling undesirable or maladaptive responses. The nurse can only provide opportunities for trying out alternative behaviors and help the client work through the anxiety that change often brings. Throughout the therapeutic relationship, the client's gains should be given positive reinforcement by the nurse.

It is not necessary to cling to a narrow approach in relationship therapy. For example, clients who express aggression in inappropriate or maladaptive ways may need a therapeutic milieu that provides security both for them and for the intended objects of their aggression. Group meetings in the milieu setting provide the opportunity for the clients and staff to discuss their reactions and feelings about others' excessively aggressive behaviors. In meetings, disputes resulting from inappropriate expression of aggression can be confronted and resolved, and agreement can be reached on the consequences of aggressive acts. In a therapeutic community the client can be exposed to peer pressure and to role modeling in learning how to deal with aggressive impulses.

Another approach to dealing with the client who expresses aggression in maladaptive ways might draw from reality therapy. The nurse could emphasize to the client that it is possible to satisfy one's needs without acting irresponsibly toward others. He could emphasize the client's needs to love, to be loved, and to feel worthwhile. The client could be told that in order to fulfill these needs he must maintain satisfactory standards of behavior. The client would not be allowed to project blame for her aggressiveness on early childhood experiences or a traumatic event. Reality therapy thus would attempt to foster in the aggressive client a sense of responsibility for her behavior.

A nurse using rational emotive therapy with an aggressive client would point out the error of believing that *desires* for love, approval, or success are *needs*. The nurse would criticize dysfunctional aggressive responses, yet accept the client as a fallible human being. The ABC's of RET would be applied to aggressive acts. The event that activated the aggressive act would be identified, and the client would be asked to share her beliefs about the activating event. It would be emphasized that the activating event alone did not result in the aggressive act but that the client's *beliefs* about the activating event resulted in her aggressive responses. As the client learned to accept that an activating event may influence responses but not truly cause them, she could attain greater control over her emotions and behaviors. The client would be encouraged to realize that it is not necessary to yield to feelings of anger, hostility, or depression. The client would then be helped to detect her irrational beliefs that distort reality and make situations seem worse than they actually are. Irrational beliefs might cause a sense of worthlessness, or difficulty with interpersonal relationships or self-actualization. Each of the irrational beliefs would be debated and disputed. The client would be encouraged to differentiate between her needs and desires and to modify her ineffectual responses by controlling and managing them. The goal of rational emotive therapy would be the development of a more objective, realistic assessment of events, beliefs, and responses.

Should acts of aggression be thought to result from a fear-producing situation, the technique of implosive therapy might be utilized. In implosive therapy, the client would be encouraged to see the relationship between the fear stimulus, his feelings, and the act of aggression that follows. If desensitization is the chosen route, relaxation training could be begun with the client. Sessions with the therapist may be supplemented with tape-recorded proce-

586

dures that would enable the client to practice self-relaxation on his own.

As relaxation techniques were mastered, an escalating list of anxiety- or fear-producing situations would be prepared and rank ordered, with the least fearsome situation placed in a graded sequence with more fearsome situations. Then the relaxation skills would be used while the client is exposed to the prepared fear scenes. The client, while in a deeply relaxed state, would be encouraged to imagine vividly the least fearsome situation. When he can do so with minimal anxiety, he would progress to the next situation, until, after several sessions, he could imagine the most fearsome situation and experience only minimal anxiety. The client would then be ready to encounter fear-producing situations in real life. The expectation or goal would be that the client would be able to tolerate the actual life situations without experiencing the anxiety or fear that previously precipitated aggressive feelings and actions. Implosive therapy would have the additional advantage of helping the client gain insight into the events and feelings that led to his aggression.

Evaluation in Relationship Therapy (The Termination Phase)

Evaluation, the fourth step in the nursing process, determines the degree to which goals have been met. Evaluation data may also be used to revise goals and intervention strategies as needed. All responses to interventions should be assessed according to the stated goals. Should the interventions be evaluated as having successfully met the identified goals, then termination of the therapy is undertaken.

Termination, the fourth phase of the therapeutic relationship, is often the most poorly planned and executed of all the phases of the relationship. Ideally, the nurse and the client will mutually determine the date of the last interaction, having reviewed the list of goals and determined whether they have been successfully completed. Typically during this phase, the client may regress to an earlier communication style and exhibit resistance to planning for the future. This is often due to the client's reluctance to end the therapeutic relationship. Reactions of clients to termination vary greatly, depending on circumstances of previous terminations, the type of treatment approach used, and the length and strength of the relationship. The longer the relationship, the longer the time required for termination. The more meaningful the relationship is to the client, the more likely he is to show grief, anger, or a mixture of both. During the termination phase, the nurse should encourage the client to explore and evaluate the course of the relationship therapy and to express his feelings regarding termination. Accomplishments should be reviewed cooperatively. Sometimes a client will have made great progress but will deny having profited from the therapeutic relationship. Other clients will claim progress that may not be apparent to the nurse. Such issues should be examined by the nurse and the client.

Grief reactions to the impending loss of the therapeutic relationship should be anticipated. Feelings of sadness and hostility may be expressed, and earlier maladaptive responses may threaten to return. Denial of termination may be revealed by a lack of emotional response that actually represents a profound reaction to the expected loss. Both nurse and client can be expected to react to impending

C L I N I C A L   E X A M P L E

███████████████████████

*ECLECTICISM IN
RELATIONSHIP THERAPY*

██████████████████

Daphne was an eighteen-year-old girl who was hospitalized as the result of a violent outburst during which she attempted to injure her mother and grandmother, with whom she lived, by attacking them with a meat cleaver. Daphne's father had deserted her mother when the girl was a baby and his present whereabouts were unknown. Daphne had been restrained forcibly by the police and hospitalized involuntarily. Shortly after hospitalization, Daphne was quiet but unresponsive to overtures from the staff or other clients on the unit. She spent most of her time sitting in the day room chain-smoking cigarettes, most of which she begged from other clients. When asked, she could give no reason for her behavior toward her mother and grandmother except to say that they were always "bugging" her. Her only visitor was her twenty-year-old boyfriend, who came every day to see her.

When Daphne's boyfriend visited, the couple were very affectionate toward one another. It was obvious that their embraces and kisses were upsetting to other clients. A nurse mentioned this to Daphne and suggested the couple modify their demonstrations of affection or at least meet in a less conspicuous corner of the day room. Daphne responded that the other clients were just jealous of her. When her boyfriend next visited, their behavior was even less inhibited than before. Another client objected to their lovemaking and accused Daphne of being a "slut." This evoked a verbal tirade from Daphne that caused her boyfriend to say goodbye hurriedly and leave the unit. As soon as he was gone, Daphne picked up a glass ashtray, broke it in half and went after the client who had criticized Daphne's actions with her boyfriend. Before staff members could bring the situation under control, the other client suffered severe lacerations and several staff members were bruised. By shielding themselves with a mattress from one of the beds, some staff members were able to wrest the broken ashtray from Daphne and place her in seclusion. She pounded the walls, swore, and sobbed bitterly before falling asleep. While secluded, Daphne was visited regularly by staff members as required by hospital regulations. The house physician was called to evaluate Daphne and her adversary. Daphne was released from seclusion the next morning and was allowed to go to the dining hall, provided she remained in control of herself. She complied and joined the other clients for breakfast, although many of them avoided her. The injured client was able to come to the dining room and was the focus of solicitude from the other clients.

ASSESSMENT

The incident involving Daphne was discussed at the health team meeting the next morning. The history taken shortly after Daphne was admitted to the hospital had shown that the girl had been pregnant a few months earlier and had had an abortion at her mother's and grandmother's insistence. Daphne's boyfriend had been the father and had not opposed the wishes of her female relatives regarding the abortion. Interviews with the girl's mother and grandmother had persuaded staff members that the older women, especially the mother, were intrusive yet rejecting toward Daphne. Her mother showed excessive interest in her daughter's social and sexual life, boasting that "I know more about Daphne than she knows about herself." Although the mother said she was sorry that Daphne had to have an abortion, she also showed satisfaction that Daphne had finally discovered what "life is all about."

It was the consensus of the staff that Daphne had been victimized by her mother, who was sometimes overinvolved with the girl and sometimes quite indifferent. Because her mother's attitude toward her was ambivalent and inconsistent, Daphne had not learned to develop self-control or to verbalize her emotional reactions. She eagerly sought affection from men because her mother had been so withholding of love and approval. The following diagnoses were made:

Nursing Diagnoses

Violence, potential for

Coping, ineffective family

Multiaxial Psychiatric Diagnoses

Axis I   312.34   Intermittent explosive disorder

Axis II   301.50   Histrionic personality disorder

Axis III None

Axis IV   Code 4—Moderate

Axis V   Level 5—Poor

PLANNING

A treatment plan was developed based on Daphne's needs. The plan drew from a number of different therapeutic approaches.

Reality Therapy Goals

Daphne will begin to modify tendencies to blame others for her problems.

Daphne will begin to develop internal sources of control.

587

Rational Emotive Goals

Daphne will utilize a cognitive review of events in order to establish connections between her thoughts, motives, and actions.

Implosive Therapy Goals

Daphne will use relaxation techniques and imagery to distance herself from anxiety-provoking situations in order to increase her self-control.

Milieu Therapy Goals

Daphne will attend client government meetings regularly, initially as an observer, if she prefers, but later as a participant, as her comfort increases.

Daphne will follow a schedule of occupational therapy activities and group meetings agreed upon by her and by the staff.

Relationship Therapy Goals

Daphne will begin to trust others as a result of consistent staff behaviors.

Daphne will begin to express negative feelings verbally instead of behaviorally.

IMPLEMENTATION

In order to foster trust, Daphne was assigned a mature female nurse who functioned as a companion, mentor, and guide. The primary nurse led Daphne through the following stages:

Initial Stage. In this stage efforts were devoted to increasing Daphne's trust in staff members, particularly her primary nurse. Rules were made clear and were enforced firmly but not punitively. Daphne became dependent on her primary nurse for direction and explanation; this dependency was permitted temporarily in the belief that Daphne needed time to develop the trust necessary for her to move toward autonomous functioning and internal control. Appropriate behaviors were acknowledged and rewarded; inappropriate behaviors were also acknowledged, but the patient herself was never made to feel unworthy or "bad."

Working Stage. During this stage Daphne became an active participant in therapy groups, member government, and occupational therapy activities. She remained dependent on her primary nurse and often became angry and belligerent when her primary nurse had a day off. Various methods were used to oppose these regressive tendencies. Anticipatory guidance was used to explain to Daphne the work schedule of her primary nurse. The nurse assigned to care for Daphne in the absence of the primary nurse was introduced to her, and she accompanied the primary nurse in activities involving Daphne. None of these methods was effective; other staff members found themselves dreading the absences of the primary nurse. Daphne's primary nurse brought up the issue with Daphne, and a search for a solution began. A strategy gradually evolved of leaving Daphne some object or article that she and the primary nurse had shared.

This transitional object could be compared to a security blanket or teddy bear carried by a small child who needs reassurance that the world is stable and predictable and that valued persons who are absent will return. The transitional objects were carefully selected and were always approved by Daphne. Sometimes the object was a book or picture that Daphne and the nurse had discussed together. It might be a small bouquet brought by the nurse or a note pad on which Daphne could write down some thoughts she wanted to share with the nurse on her return. The transitional objects were trivial in themselves, but they represented a powerful connection to the rational world that Daphne was learning to live in.

During the latter part of the working stage, Daphne was encouraged to move from dependency to greater autonomy. Other staff members became more active in her treatment. Her boyfriend was encouraged to visit; family meetings were held to help Daphne's mother deal more constructively with her daughter and to tolerate the probability of separation.

Termination Phase. During this period Daphne was given time to mourn the imminent loss of the primary nurse, who had become in effect her "good mother." There was no sudden separation, and it was agreed that occasional communication between Daphne and the primary nurse would be beneficial, provided they were integrated into the follow-up plan for care. Because of the long-standing problems between Daphne and her mother, and because separation was an appropriate life-cycle task for someone approaching the age of twenty, plans were made for Daphne to enter a halfway house rather than return home. There she would have the advantage of some staff supervision, peer support, and the opportunity to test the new coping methods she had learned. A mature female outpatient therapist was found to continue the consistent, accepting relationship established with the primary nurse while Daphne was hospitalized.

EVALUATION

The outcome evaluation of Daphne's progress was facilitated by the previous establishment of specific goals. Evaluation was subjective, but there was agreement between Daphne and the staff members who worked with her that, in the two months of hospitalization, Daphne had discarded her extreme tendency to blame others for her problems, even though it was true that her mother had often provoked Daphne's violent outbursts. Daphne gradually became able to verbalize her negative feelings rather than act on them, although her mother continued to provoke aggressive reactions from her. Daphne used relaxation techniques to monitor her internal reactions to such episodes with her mother and others. As a result of her increased ability to relax and to trust, she was able to make friends more easily and to keep the friends she made. This development also reduced her vulnerability to her mother. Relationship therapy, supplemented by other treatment modalities, was very therapeutic for a young woman who had never before encountered a wholesome, constructive, accepting relationship with another human being.

589

termination with a degree of grief. The ability of the nurse to recognize and discuss his own thoughts and feelings can serve as a role model for the client. Successful termination of a therapeutic relationship is the result of a well-planned and carefully executed process orchestrated by the nurse and experienced by both parties.

SUMMARY

There is much to be learned about the causes of psychiatric disorders and the effectiveness of different forms of treatment. No school of psychology has the complete answer to all emotional disorders, and no single method of treatment is universally applicable and successful. Combinations of available therapeutic modalities in an eclectic approach are most likely to result in successful outcomes in the clinical situations encountered by nurses.

Reality therapy is based on the assumption that people need to love and be loved and that in order to fulfill these needs people must maintain satisfactory standards of behavior. Clients are taught appropriate patterns of behavior that will increase their acceptance by others and therefore result in an enhanced sense of their own worth.

Rational emotive therapy is based on the belief that virtually all serious emotional illnesses result from magical, superstitious, invalid thinking and that if the disturbing thoughts are regularly and rigorously disputed and principles of logical thinking are emphasized, the disordered thought processes can be eliminated.

Implosive therapy is based on the principle that a person can overcome maladaptive anxiety elicited by situations or objects by approaching the feared situation while in a psychophysiological state that inhibits anxiety.

Primal therapy is based on the idea that unmet childhood needs for food, tenderness, or acceptance result in a primal pain that later causes an individual to encase his real self in a protective shell. Primal therapy is a systematic assault on the protective shell. It is believed that feeling the original agony of unmet needs eventually results in discovery of the real self and, therefore, mental health. Primal therapy advocates claim that this approach cannot be integrated with other therapeutic approaches.

Milieu therapy is the maintenance of an atmosphere that encourages recovery or optimal functioning. It is based on group treatment, activities geared to the abilities of individual clients, and joint decision making by both clients and staff.

Client-centered therapy is based on the belief that an individual's growth is enhanced by a caring, nonjudgmental, empathetic relationship with a helping individual. A major goal of this type of therapy is to facilitate the abandonment of facades and to help the client learn to accept and value herself for what she is.

Theoretical concepts of the therapeutic relationship and the nursing process are strikingly similar and virtually inseparable in actual practice. Yet the simultaneous application of these therapeutic tools would not be effective without the use of facilitative skills of communication, acute awareness of one's own feelings and attitudes, and authentic personal qualities of warmth, acceptance, and genuine concern.

Review Questions

1. What is the meaning of the term "eclectic" as it relates to the application of psychotherapeutic approaches?

2. List some of the cultural and religious values in the United States that might affect the choice of a particular form of psychotherapy.

3. How are these cultural and religious values reflected by the various eclectic approaches, including relationship therapy?

4. Which of the eclectic therapeutic approaches would you feel comfortable using with a particular client? Support your choice with rationale based on chapter content.

5. How can the various eclectic therapies be applied by nurses? Give examples from your own experience.

6. Which of the eclectic therapeutic approaches are applicable in a multidiscipline treatment milieu? Which are not, and why?

7. Give examples of conditions listed in DSM-III that might respond to each of the therapeutic approaches discussed in this chapter. Identify those from DSM-III that would preclude use of these therapeutic approaches. Explain your reasons.

8. How could the nurse benefit a client in a general nursing situation other than a psychiatric setting with:
   a. the various eclectic therapeutic approaches discussed in this chapter?
   b. relationship therapy?

9. Which of the eclectic approaches lend themselves to group involvement? Which do not?

10. Which of the eclectic approaches are applicable to stresses of everyday living encountered by the general population? Give examples of how these therapeutic approaches can be implemented to counteract stress.

590

References

Almond, R. 1974. *The Healing Community*. New York: Jason Aronson.

Brown, E. 1980. *Supermind: The Ultimate Energy*. New York: Harper & Row.

Cummings, J., and Cummings, E. 1962. *Ego and Milieu*. Chicago: Aldine.

Ellis, A. 1973a. Rational Emotive Therapy. In *Current Psychotherapies*, ed. R. Corsini. Itasca, Ill.: F. E. Peacock.

Ellis, A. 1973b. Rational Emotive Therapy. In *Direct Psychotherapy*, ed. R. M. Jurjevich. Coral Gables: University of Miami Press.

Ellis, A., and Grieger, R., eds. 1977. *Handbook of Rational-Emotive Therapy*. New York: Springer.

Frankl, V. 1963. *Man's Search for Meaning*. Boston: Beacon Press.

Glasser, W. 1965. *Realtiy Therapy*. New York: Harper & Row.

Glasser, W., and Zunin, L. M. 1973. Reality Therapy. In *Current Psychotherapies*, ed. R. Corsini. Itasca, Ill.: F. E. Peacock.

Green, K. W.; Green, W. B.; and Holmes, D. W. 1980. Speech Reading Abilities of Young Deaf Children. *American Annals of the Deaf*, 25:906–908.

Janov, A. 1970. *Primal Scream*. New York: Putnam's.

Janov, A. 1972. *The Primal Revolution: Toward a Real World*. New York: Simon & Schuster.

Jansen, E. 1980. *The Therapeutic Community*. London: Croon Helm.

Lewin, K. K. 1970. *Brief Encounters*. St. Louis: Green.

Lippincott Manual of Nursing Practice. 1982. Philadelphia: J. B. Lippincott.

Rogers, C. R. 1960. *On Becoming a Person*. Boston: Houghton Mifflin.

Tart, C., and Fadiman, J. 1975. The Case of the Yellow Wheatfield: A Dream Style Exploration of a Broadcast Telepathic Dream. *Psychoanalytic Review*, 61:607–618.

Torrey, E. 1972. *The Mind Game*. New York: Emerson Hall Publishers.

Supplementary Readings

Ascroft, B. Token Power: Token Rewards Are Backed Up with Praise and Social Approval. *Nursing* (Oxford), (1980):832–834.

Bernard, M. E., and Joyce, M. R. *Rational-Emotive Therapy with Children and Adolescents: Theory, Preventive Methods, and Treatment Strategies*. New York: John Wiley & Sons, 1984.

Berne, E. *What Do You Say After You Say Hello?* New York: Grove Press, 1972.

Chapmen, S. Cash on Delivery—A Token Economy Scheme in Which Patients Were Rewarded for Good Behavior. *Nursing Mirror*, 156(1983):38–41.

Ellis, A., and Harper, R. *A Guide to Rational Living in an Irrational World*. Englewood Cliffs, N. J.: Prentice-Hall, 1971.

Fagan, J., and Shepard, I. *Gestalt Therapy Now*. New York: Harper & Row, 1971.

Frances, G. The Therapeutic Use of Pets. *Nursing Outlook*, 29(1981):6–9.

Harris, T. *I'm OK, You're OK*. New York: Harper & Row, 1967.

Janov, A. *The Anatomy of Mental Illness: The Scientific Basis of Primal Therapy*. New York: Putnam's, 1971.

Jones, M. *The Therapeutic Community*. New York: Basic Books, 1953.

Kamjug, T. A New Approach to Token Economy. *Nursing Times*, 79(1983):31–32.

Kleen, S. Token Economy for Developing Independent Living Skills in Geriatric Patients. *Psychosocial Rehabilitation Journal*, 4(1980):1–11.

Landgarten, H. B. *Clinical Art Therapy*. New York: Brunner/Mazel, 1980.

Lehman, A. F. First Admission Psychiatric Ward Milieu Treatment Process and Outcome. *Archives of General Psychiatry*, 39(1982):1293–1298.

MacPhail, D. Brief Therapy. *Nursing Mirror*, 157 (1983):38–42.

Menos, N. The Value of the Psychosocial Approach in the Treatment of Long-Term Hospitalized Patients. *Hospital and Community Psychiatry*, 34(1983):456–458.

Merchant, M., and Saxley, P. Reality Orientation: A New Way Forward. *Nursing Times*, 77(1981):1442–1445.

Mitchell, S. F. Use of Ward Support by Psychiatric Patients in the Community. *British Journal of Psychiatry*, 142(1983):9–15.

Paul, G. L., and Lentz, R. J. *Psychosocial Treatment of Chronic Mental Patients*. Cambridge, Mass.: Harvard University Press, 1977.

Roberts, C. M. RET: Rational/Emotive Therapy—A Cognitive Behavior Treatment System. *Perspectives in Psychiatric Care*, 20(1982):134–138.

Van Patten, T. V. Milieu Therapy: Contraindications? *Archives of General Psychiatry*, 29(1973):640–643.

Wadeson, H. *Art Psychotherapy*. New York: John Wiley & Sons, 1981.

Wexler, D. A., and Rue, L. N. *Innovations in Client-Centered Theory*. New York: John Wiley & Sons, 1974.

Yablanszky, L. *Psychodrama: Resolving Emotional Problems Through Role Playing*. New York: Basic Books, 1980.

591

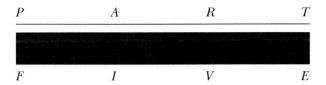
ISSUES IN PSYCHIATRIC MENTAL HEALTH NURSING

HEALTH CARE TEAM STRUCTURE

MODELS OF NURSING CARE DELIVERY
Team Nursing in Mental Health Settings
Primary Nursing in Mental Health Settings

CONSULTATION AND LIAISON WORK
Types of Mental Health Consultation
Implementation of Consultation and Liaison Work
Implications of Consultation and Liaison Work

THE REFERRAL PROCESS IN PSYCHIATRIC NURSING
Sequence of Referrals
Themes of Referrals

COLLABORATION AND COORDINATION IN HEALTH
CARE DELIVERY

C H A P T E R

22

Case Management and Collaboration

Learning Objectives

After studying this chapter, the student should be able to:

1. Contrast the nurse's role as leader with the nurse's role as member of the health team.

2. Compare and contrast the functions of nurses as case managers in team and in primary nursing.

3. Describe the process of consultation and its implications.

4. Discuss collaboration among nurses, and between nurses and other health professionals, as a way of increasing overall effectiveness of case management.

5. Describe the implications of the referral process.

596

Overview

The delivery and management of nursing care in mental health settings has experienced several changes throughout this century. Different models of nursing care delivery have been implemented at various times. Currently, the primary care model is popular because of its value in comprehensive care planning and its accountability.

Along with these changes, the delivery of health care in general has become multidisciplinary and has expanded to include several types of client services. The role of the psychiatric nurse in

the health care setting has been expanded to include liaison and consultation work, both in the mental health arena and in the psychiatric and medical-surgical settings.

This chapter describes types of nursing care delivery models and the structure of the health care team, with emphasis on the necessity of collaboration and coordination for health care. The expanded role of the psychiatric nurse in the consultation and liaison process and the use of referral systems are also discussed.

*Mind is the great lever of all things; human thought is the
process by which human ends are ultimately answered.*
DANIEL WEBSTER

HEALTH CARE TEAM STRUCTURE

Three types of teams are commonly used in health care settings. A *unidisciplinary* team is composed of members of the same discipline, as exemplified by team nursing. A *multidisciplinary* team is composed of members of different disciplines who each provide discipline-specific services to the same client, but with no formal arrangement for interaction between the members; no one is required to give up power, authority, or territory. An *interdisciplinary* team is made up of members from different disciplines all involved in a formal team arrangement, which facilitates opportunities for educational interchange and delivery of service. Challela (1979) described an interdisciplinary health team as one in which responsibility for assessment, decision making, delivery of services, and evaluation is shared among the health professionals on the team.

Most mental health care settings utilize an interdisciplinary team approach, the most complex of the three types. Interdisciplinary teams have been used by mental health professionals since the late 1940s (Sienkilewski, 1983). The early interdisciplinary teams were composed of a psychiatrist, a psychologist, a psychiatric social worker, and a psychiatric nurse (Robinson, 1950). In recent times additional team members have been added, such as an activities therapist, an occupational therapist, and a dietitian.

Philosophy and organizational structure are the major determinants of which team member will head the interdisciplinary health care team. In 1951 Mereness reflected the norm of the times in describing the psychiatrist as "best equipped" to be the team leader "because of his superior professional equipment and his maturity of judgment." Status and professional identity are not the only factors to be considered in choosing the interdisciplinary team leader. Different disciplines have different areas of expertise, and matching these areas with the problems of the client should receive consideration.

The role of the leader is to help team members resolve disagreements and conflicts related to planning and providing care. The leader's role also is to foster effectiveness of the team as a mechanism of achieving optimal client care (Crawshaw and Key, 1961). Regardless of which team member assumes the official leadership role, each discipline retains specific responsibilities to the client based on his or her particular education and clinical expertise.

The role of the nurse as an interdisciplinary team member differs from the role of the nurse as a person charged with responsibility for total client care. As an effective team member, the nurse is guided by the need to understand and respect the contributions and expertise of others on the team (Mereness, 1951). Identifying with the team as a whole minimizes the problems of hierarchy, status, and communication (Crawshaw and Key, 1961). Benfer (1980) emphasized that each team member should display communication skills along with maturity, trust, professional confidence, and problem-solving ability. Each team member collects relevant information that is then combined with information obtained by other team members in order to form a data base that assures development of a comprehensive care plan.

Challela (1979) raised four issues that the nurse must acknowledge and deal with as a member of an interdisciplinary team: (1) defining the nursing role to achieve role identity, (2) recognizing the need for overlap between disciplines, (3) knowing what other disciplines can do, and (4) developing influence and sharing in the power distribution. Other issues for consideration include communication problems among team members (Benfer, 1980) and personal characteristics of team members as a potential barrier to effective functioning of the team (Given and Simmons, 1977).

It is usually within an interdisciplinary context that nursing care is delivered. However, the way in which care is given can vary from setting to setting, depending on the model of nursing care delivery being utilized.

MODELS OF NURSING CARE DELIVERY

Historically, four major models of nursing care delivery have been identified and utilized: the case method, functional nursing, team nursing, and primary nursing. The *case method* was the earliest type used by nurses. In this model, one nurse planned and administered total care for one client for the entire time the nurse was on duty. The case method is still used in acute care settings, such as intensive care units, that demand continuity of care and that involve complex nursing care. However, private duty nursing in the home, hospital, or other care facility such as a nursing home is rarely used in our present-day system of health care delivery (Langford, 1981).

Functional nursing evolved from the industrial concepts of division of labor that were popular from the 1920s through the 1940s. The result was a fragmentation of nursing care, and the client had no identified nurse to provide care for the whole person. Some aspects of functional nursing, such as assigning a medication nurse to pass all medications on one unit for each shift, are still used in some nursing care settings, but otherwise this model is rarely used.

Team nursing began in the post–World War II years, when hospitals were flooded with technical health care workers, such as nurse's aides and vocational nurses, and there was a lack of registered nurses. Team nursing is based on a hierarchical structure, with the most prepared caregiver, the registered nurse, placed in the role of team leader. In this model team members are assigned groups of clients and tasks according to their ability and to the acuteness of client needs, while the team leader is responsible for guiding and supervising all aspects of nursing care provided to that particular client group. Clients are assigned to one nursing team for

the duration of their hospital stay, and the same team members are responsible for their care. A major disadvantage of team nursing is that the supervisory functions of the team leader detract from the time spent delivering care; consequently, the person best prepared to provide direct care, the nurse team leader, is least available to do so.

The most recently developed model of nursing care delivery is *primary nursing*, in which one nurse is assigned a client for the duration of the client's hospitalization. This model is similar to the case method in this one-to-one aspect, but rather than being responsible for only an 8-hour shift, in primary nursing the nurse's responsibility extends for 24 hours a day, every day, throughout the client's hospitalization. The primary nurse assesses the total client needs and collaborates with the client and other health care providers in developing a comprehensive care plan. A secondary nurse (also called an associate nurse) is assigned to the client when the primary nurse is not on duty. However, the primary nurse retains responsibility and may even be called at home during off-duty hours to make a decision regarding the client's nursing care. The requirements of autonomy, authority, and accountability that characterize primary nursing are thus ensured (Marram, Shlegel, and Bevis, 1974). In this model, head nurses and supervisors function as nursing care consultants and do not interfere with the primary nurse's responsibilities (Miller and Janosik, 1978).

The functions of nurses as case managers in team nursing and in primary nursing merit discussion. *Case management* refers to the nurse's responsibility for delivery of comprehensive nursing care to more than one client. Benfer (1980) outlined six basic case management functions of the psychiatric nurse:

1. Collecting data and making a nursing assessment.
2. Implementing planned interventions.
3. Meeting client needs through environmental change.
4. Meeting client needs through health teaching.
5. Coordinating client activities to maximize therapeutic effects.
6. Predicting and altering maladaptive behaviors.

The next two sections describe how these functions are performed in both team and primary nursing.

Team Nursing in Mental Health Settings

The first and most basic nursing function is obtaining a client history and making a nursing assessment. For the assessment to be adequate, inclusion of family issues is essential. A comprehensive assessment culminates in conceptualization of an appropriate nursing diagnosis and development of a care plan that can be implemented, documented, and evaluated. In team nursing the team leader is responsible for seeing that all clients are the focus of ongoing nursing assessment and planning. If the team includes paraprofessional mental health aides, the team leader will delegate the responsibility for assessment and planning to other nurses on the team or will personally assume these tasks. When the health team approach is used, nurses may be writing nursing diagnoses and developing care plans on clients for whom they are not primary caregivers.

The second basic function is implementing planned interventions, evaluating effects, and documenting client responses to the interventions used. In team nursing individual nurses carry out this function on their assigned shift only and do not maintain this responsibility 24 hours a day as primary nurses do. Consistency in implementing the care plan depends on how clearly specific nursing approaches are described in the care plan and are understood by all team members. Evaluation of outcomes depends greatly on the quality of documentation in the client's nursing record. Continuity of care and consistency among health team members are necessary for successful outcomes in team nursing. Since the case manager in team nursing may not have responsibility for providing direct client care on a continuing basis, outcomes may be unclear unless documentation of interventions and clients' responses are provided for all team members.

The third basic function is determining how the needs of the client can be met within the surrounding milieu. This requires maintenance of a therapeutic environment in which clients are helped to achieve adaptive interpersonal coping skills by means of structured and unstructured group and individual transactions. An aspect of this function includes the impact of significant events in the milieu, such as seclusion of an assaultive client. As an effective case manager, the team nurse will explore the client's response to the seclusion and devise strategies for encouraging ventilation of feelings. In team nursing the case manager is responsible for planning strategies that help the client cope with the experience of seclusion.

The fourth function is client teaching, including such topics as communication skills, stress management, and the rationale for the use of psychotropic medications. Client education should not be delegated to one discipline alone but should be done by all caregivers involved with the client's plan of care. Nurses are frequently in the ideal position to act as coordinators of the client's education.

The fifth function is coordination of client activities. The nursing team conference is a useful means for evaluating the client's behavior in the milieu. Interdisciplinary conferences provide data regarding the patient's behavior in off-unit activities. The team leader integrates data obtained from all caregivers into the care plan and arranges conferences to discuss needed revisions.

The sixth function is prediction and prevention of maladaptive client behavior. This function is particularly important when the client has a history of suicidal or homicidal behavior. The team nurse will need to be cognizant of such impulses and alert for patterns of behavior that indicate beginning loss of control. Knowledge of risk factors predictive of suicidal and homicidal behavior is necessary in order for the team nurse to identify early warning signs and to share observations with other team members.

For all six nursing functions, there is sharing of responsibility and delegation of tasks among nursing team members. The team leader is expected to be able to guide and supervise the team members in executing all these functions for every client assigned to the team. Ciske's (1974) observation that shared responsibility and accountability often results in *no* responsibility or accountability is a caution worthy of consideration. The team leader is ultimately responsible for ensuring that the needs of all clients are met to the utmost possible extent.

Primary Nursing in Mental Health Settings

Primary nursing in mental health settings also entails Benfer's six functions. Since the first function is obtaining a client history and making a nursing assessment, the primary nurse initiates an admission history, including a family assessment, and writes the initial nursing diagnosis. The primary nurse makes ongoing nursing assessments during each nurse-client interaction and revises the nursing diagnoses if indicated. The primary nurse is accountable for the development and documentation of a care plan designed to meet the client's needs over a 24-hour time frame. The primary nurse develops this plan collaboratively with the client.

The second function is implementing planned interventions, assessing the effects of interventions, and documenting patient behavior. The primary nurse implements the care plan when on duty and maintains communication with the secondary nurse to assure continuity of care when off duty. The primary nurse documents the specific interventions

*Each profession uses conceptual frameworks for practice that are
consistent with its mandates and concerns. If psychosocial problems are
the focus of concern, then logically the model of the client should promote
the collection of psychosocial information; if disease is the phenomenon of
interest, then attention is directed toward pathophysiological or
psychopathological manifestation. The focusing of attention leads to the
naming and classification of conditions the profession can address . . .
Essentially the same cognitive processes are applied by each profession but
the focus for their application differs. The information collected, the
concepts used to interpret information, and the problems addressed vary.
Generally these differences are reflected in professional care.*

M. GORDON (1982)

600

used and describes the client's behavioral response. During off-duty hours, the primary nurse is available by telephone to discuss questions about implementation of the plan with secondary nursing staff. Specific aspects of nursing implementation may be delegated to the secondary nurse.

The third function is determining how to meet the needs of the client within the milieu. The primary nurse needs to analyze the environment and its potential supports and stressors in terms of the client's specific needs. This analysis includes examination of the milieu during all three shifts. For example, if a client goal is to increase skill in initiating conversation in groups, the primary nurse may assign the client the task of initiating at least one topic during each evening community meeting. If the primary nurse works days, he or she may have the secondary nurse on evening duty follow up with the client after the community meeting to provide him with feedback.

Regarding the fourth function, the primary nurse is responsible for assessing the client's learning needs and for developing a comprehensive teaching plan to meet these needs from admission until discharge. This includes teaching the client and the family adaptive coping mechanisms to facilitate the client's reentry to family and community. The primary nurse needs to monitor and evaluate the client's responses to the teaching interventions and should revise approaches as needed.

The fifth function, coordinating client activities, is enhanced by use of interdisciplinary conferences. The primary nurse may function as leader of such conferences or may develop a collegial relationship with the psychiatrist to present client data

and recommendations for care from their respective viewpoints. Coordination includes designing strategies to involve the family in the client's care. The interdisciplinary conference is an appropriate time to identify the collaborative functions of the various disciplines in carrying out this important aspect of care. For example, the primary nurse, the psychiatrist, and the social worker may all decide to participate jointly in one or more family meetings. To ensure comprehensive and ongoing coordination of care, the primary nurse may plan a home visit before or after discharge.

Primary nursing facilitates implementation of the sixth function of the psychiatric nurse, the prediction of behavior and prevention of problems. Because the primary nurse is familiar with the client's past behavior and because the client's history includes documentation of known precipitants of the current hospitalization, the primary nurse is in a position to watch for early signs of potential problems. Included in the data are identification of the client's usual coping mechanisms, both adaptive and maladaptive, in response to stressors. With this data base, the primary nurse is able to identify and describe high-risk situations that the client may encounter during hospitalization and to collaborate with interdisciplinary team members to develop contingency plans to be implemented as needed. Again, the 24-hour availability of the primary nurse to consult with secondary nurses about potential behavioral problems lessens the risk of clients engaging in behavior destructive to themselves or others.

Table 22-1 summarizes the similarities and differences between nursing functions within the two delivery systems, team nursing and primary nursing.

Table 22-1. Nursing Functions in Team and Primary Nursing

Function	Team Nursing	Primary Nursing
Benfer's basic functions		
1. Collecting data and making assessments	Assigned team nurse is responsible for 8-hour shift assessment Team leader is responsible if team member not qualified	Nurse is responsible for admission history and for ongoing assessment.
2. Implementing planned interventions	Team member or team leader initiates individual written care plan Team member or team leader implements plan Team leader is responsible for 8-hour shift Team nurse is responsible for documentation of client behavior and nursing interventions	Nurse is responsible for written nursing care plan to cover client needs on 24-hour basis; client is involved in planning Nurse may implement plan or delegate Nurse is available to guide decisions regarding nursing care on a 24-hour basis Nurse is responsible for documentation of client behavior and nursing interventions
3. Meeting clients' needs in the environment	Team maximizes use of therapeutic milieu Each team member is responsible for 8-hour shift	Nurse analyses therapeutic benefits available in total milieu and communicates this to other nurses Nurse is responsible for 24-hour care plan
4. Client teaching	Team member or team leader assesses learning needs and develops, implements, and evaluates teaching plans	Nurse is responsible for assessment of learning needs and for developing, implementing, and revising teaching plans
5. Coordinating client activities	Each member is responsible for 8-hour shift Team members participate in nursing team conference; team leader leads nursing team conference Team member or team leader collaborates with other disciplines to provide family-focused nursing care	Nurse considers client needs over 24-hour time frame, every day Nurse participates in and leads client-centered nursing conference Nurse collaborates with other disciplines to provide family-focused care
6. Predicting and preventing maladaptive behaviors	Members identify and document adaptive and maladaptive behavioral responses to stressors observed during 8-hour shift	Nurse documents client's usual adaptive and maladaptive responses to stressors, identifies high-risk situations client may encounter during any twenty-four hour period, and collaborates with team members to develop contingency plan
Quality of care functions		
1. Accountability	Team leader is accountable for team members' nursing care	Nurse is accountable for all aspects of nursing care
2. Continuity of care	Not consistent; team stable but leaders may vary	Continuity is built into delivery system; same primary or secondary nurse is assigned to client throughout hospital stay
3. Communication lines	Vertical, hierarchical	Triangular, collaborative

CONSULTATION AND LIAISON WORK

According to Caplan (1970), *consultation* is a process of interaction between two professionals: the *consultant*, who is a specialist, and the *consultee*, who seeks the consultant's help in regard to a current work problem. The consultee accepts the fact that the work problem falls within the consultant's area of specialized competence and solicits assistance. In Caplan's model, the consultant accepts no direct responsibility for implementing remedial action for the client, and professional responsibility for the client remains with the consultee. The consultee is free to accept or reject all or part of the consultant's advice. In addition to helping the consultee with the work problem, the consultant endeavors to add to the consultee's knowledge and to decrease areas of misunderstanding so that in the future the consultee will be able to cope independently with similar problems.

According to Lipowski (1974), *liaison* involves a linking of groups for the purpose of effective collaboration. The groups are usually a liaison team (consisting of one or more psychiatrists, a psychologist, a psychiatric nurse, and a psychiatric social worker) and a health care team on a general hospital unit. The teaching of mental health concepts and care to the medical and surgical staff on general hospital units is an accepted component of liaison work

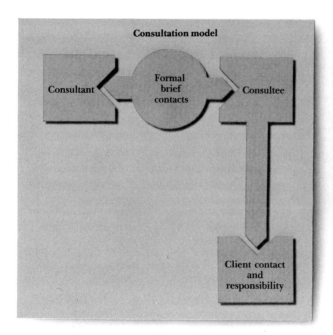

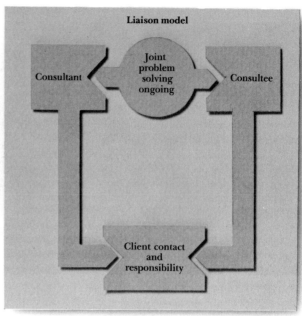

(Kimball, 1979; Pasnau, 1982). A major goal of liaison work is to enhance the quality of psychological care provided to the medically ill (Strain and Grossman, 1975).

Consultation and liaison in nursing have developed in parallel with consultation and liaison in psychiatry. Consultation in nursing was first reported in the literature by Johnson (1963), who described a cross-service consultation program developed at Duke University in response to nursing requests for assistance on complex client care problems. The nursing consultants were experienced head nurses, nursing supervisors, and instructors and included a psychiatric nurse who had primary responsibility on a psychiatric unit but could be called to consult on medical/surgical units. The expectation was that the consultants would not work directly with clients; their focus was to assist the nursing staff (consultees) to solve problems and to become sensitive to the psychological needs of clients and the influence these needs played in the client's response to altered health states (Nelson and Schilke, 1976). As the consultant role evolved, the model of an ongoing relationship between the consultant and the consultee became established, and this model was eventually labeled *psychiatric liaison nursing*.

Davis (1983) has compared consultation and liaison nursing models on three parameters: type of contact, determination of concerns, and responsibility for the care of clients (see Figure 22-1). In the consultation model, contact between consultant and consultee is episodic, sporadic, formal, and initiated by the consultee. The consultant has brief contacts with the consultee, provides suggestions, and leaves the setting. In the liaison model, contact is ongoing,

is informal, and may be initiated by either consultee or consultant. The liaison nurse becomes part of the health team and attends staff rounds and conferences. Whereas the consultee determines the focus for consultation work, in the liaison model the consultant may raise issues related to the care of clients or identify clients who need intervention. Finally, in the consultation model responsibility for the care of clients remains largely with the consultee, whereas in the liaison model the consultant may collaborate with the consultee throughout the process and therefore share responsibility to some extent.

Nursing literature has documented the growth of consultation/liaison nursing since Johnson's early paper in 1963. Psychiatric nurses have written descriptive accounts of their experience as collaborative members of a psychiatric consultation/liaison team on general hospital units (Barton and Kelso, 1971; Burch and Meredith, 1974; Moreau, Kahn, and Lai, 1974; Stickey, Moir, and Gardner, 1981; Tringali, 1982), in emergency departments and ambulatory settings (Issacharoff et al., 1970; Severin and Becker, 1974), and in nursing homes (Covert, 1979). From such accounts, one can appreciate the gradual evolution of the consultation/liaison nursing role over the past twenty years. Liaison nursing is now widely accepted as a subspecialty of psychiatric mental health nursing (Davis, 1983).

Types of Mental Health Consultation

Caplan (1970) described four types of consultation: client-centered case consultation, consultee-centered case consultation, program-centered administrative consultation, and consultee-centered administrative consultation.

Client-centered case consultation, also called direct

Figure 22-1. Comparison between the consultation and liaison nursing models.

THE GOALS OF CONSULTATION

Lewis and Levy (1982) have identified the goals of case consultation in psychiatric nursing as follows:

1. Demonstrating and teaching mental health concepts and their application to clinical nursing practice.
2. Effecting appropriate psychiatric and nursing interventions.
3. Supporting nurses to continue to provide high-quality nursing care.
4. Promoting and developing the professional and personal self-esteem of the nurse.
5. Encouraging tolerance among the nursing staff for situations that preclude immediate or effective intervention or resolution.

consultation, focuses on the client's immediate problem. The primary goal is to communicate to the consultee how the client can be helped. A secondary goal is to enhance the nurse's ability to apply the same concepts to similar problems in the future. *Consultee-centered case consultation*, also called indirect consultation, focuses on trying to understand the nature of the nurse's (consultee's) difficulty in working with a client, and the goal is to improve the consultee's functioning.

Program-centered administrative consultation focuses on development of a program for nursing staff. An example of this type of consultation is teaching assertiveness skills to a group of nurses as a way of improving interdisciplinary communication. The program could be run as a series of hour-long workshops or as a day-long conference. *Consultee-centered administrative consultation* focuses on helping nurses with administrative or organizational structure, such as consulting to a group of head nurses who will be guiding their staff in changing from team to primary nursing.

Implementation of Consultation and Liaison Work

Lewis and Levy (1982) have delineated five basic steps in the consultation process as applied to psychiatric liaison nurses: (1) request consultation, (2) define the problem, (3) diagnose the consultation issues, (4) make recommendations, and (5) develop the interventions and evaluate. These steps are the same whether the setting is a general hospital unit or a community setting such as a school or visiting nurse service.

Lewis and Levy describe the process of consultation as egalitarian, while Caplan (1970) sees the relationship between consultant and consultee as

coordinate, meaning there is no inherent hierarchial authority, which tends to decrease tension throughout the process. Freedom to accept or reject the consultant's suggestions increases the consultee's willingness to consider and to adopt any ideas that seem useful. As part of the overall consultation process, the nurse consultant should develop a contract with the consultee, regardless of setting or context. A contract clarifies mutual expectations and may be verbal or written.

In the first step of the consultation process, the consultant is invited by the consultee to participate in problem solving. Such a request may be made by a nurse, a physician, or another health care provider. One of the next tasks is to set up communication with the nursing staff before and after the actual consultation. Initial communications begin with the head nurse and other involved nursing personnel. Communication is necessary to establishing and maintaining a viable relationship with the nursing staff, an essential element in the consultation process. Face-to-face contact with key individuals early in the process serves to introduce the liaison nurse (the consultant) and to define the scope of consultation. The nurse consultant can instill hope in the consultee group during the initial phase of contact by explaining the consultant's role. In one study, visibility was found to be more important than availability in terms of the utilization of psychiatric nurse consultants (Zahaurek and Morrison, 1974). However, development of a trusting relationship between the consultant and the consultee is strengthened by both availability and visibility.

Another early task is building channels of communication between the nurse consultant, the nursing staff, and other involved health care providers. Identification of a staff member who will serve as a gatekeeper, transmitting messages between staff and consultant and among staff members, is an essential aspect of building a communication network (Caplan, 1970). Larkin and Crowdes (1976) described this gatekeeper as an individual who controls the consultant's access to the workers and the workers' access to the consultant. The consultant needs to develop a trusting relationship with the person acting as a gatekeeper and must ensure that the gatekeeper is a person who has ready access to significant staff and to the authority system (Fife, 1983).

The second step of the consultation process is to define the problem. Although a consultation request often indicates a concern for some aspect of client care, such as management issues or staff attitudes and feelings, the actual problem may be covert. Application of Caplan's concept of theme interference is helpful in understanding such covert problems. Caplan described *theme interference* as loss of objectivity by the consultee because of unresolved present or past problems that are unconsciously displaced onto the work situation. Such unresolved problems block the nurse's ability to use knowledge and skills effectively. For example, if the nurse consultee believes that all alcoholics are hopeless and resistant to help, he or she is less likely to refer a client to an alcoholism treatment program or AA. Referrals are more likely if the caregiver believes that alcoholics can be helped even though they may have relapses. To reduce theme interference, Caplan (1970) suggests initially accepting the consultee's care plan and later helping the consultee reexamine the data to allow the consultee to see that some favorable outcomes are possible, thus encouraging a more objective approach. For instance, the consultant may use an analogy such as "I worked with a man like your client last year, and with the aid of an AA member who visited after discharge the client became willing to join AA." This type of intervention will cast doubt in the consultee's mind about the "doomed to failure" viewpoint that operates to the disadvantage of the client.

During this period of defining the problem, the consultant must keep in mind that the focus of the consultation is always the care of the client, not the personal dynamics or problems of the consultee. The role of the consultant is not to provide therapy to the consultee but to address client needs. During this phase, the consultant may need to collaborate with other disciplines. For example if psychotropic medication is indicated, the nurse consultant will

work with the psychiatrist or encourage nursing staff to do so (Lewis and Levy, 1982).

The third step in the consultation process is diagnosing the total consultation. Stanton and Schwartz (1954) found that on a psychiatric unit patients frequently act out conflicts originating among the professional staff, and Bursten (1963) noted that this phenomenon also occurred on general hospital units. Such findings provide a rationale for the nurse consultant to engage in diagnosing the total scope of consultation problems.

Many consultation requests that are stated in terms of client behavioral problems are symptomatic of more complex processes involving patients, nurses, physicians, and the social system of the unit (Bursten, 1963). Because distrust, misunderstanding, and lack of meaningful communication between staff and clients interfere with optimal care and with the therapeutic functioning of the hospital unit, it is important to assess staff and client interactions (Lipowski, 1974; Pasnau, 1975).

Assessment of the client and the system as one integral unit has been described as a "comprehensive consultation" by Barton and Kelso (1971). Comprehensive consultation is accomplished by assessing: (1) the consultation request, (2) the unit nurse and physician, (3) the client's chart, (4) the family and unit culture, (5) the client's medical illness, and (6) client interviews. These assessments facilitate identification and understanding of the overt and covert consultation problems and in clarifying expectations of the consultee. From this assessment the consultant can also decide whether direct or indirect consultation will be more beneficial and what types of intervention are indicated.

The fourth step involves interventions and recommendations based on the comprehensive consultation. At first, suggestions need to be as simple and as nonintrusive as possible; they may be increased in complexity if necessary. Suggestions must also be practical and realistic in terms of the limits of the clinical setting; otherwise they will be inappropriate to the setting or unacceptable to the consultee. If the consultee perceives the suggestions as increasing the work load rather than relieving stress, the suggestions will be ignored or attempted in a half-hearted manner. The consultant needs to avoid use of excessive psychiatric jargon in making suggestions and to refrain from statements that might be taken as criticisms.

Client behavior that results in a consultation request is often behavior that consultees believe is beyond the range of their clinical skills or that has not responded to interventions already tried. Usually the identified behavior is actually or potentially disruptive to unit functioning or to client care. The introduction of an expert such as a nurse consultant who can help manage problem behavior has been shown to reduce tension on a unit. A nurse consultant who is willing to accept ongoing involvement with a clinical problem may serve to change the consultee's attitudes, which in turn may lead to more therapeutic interactions with clients. During this phase of the consultation process, the nurse consultant observes and evaluates both client and consultee responses to interventions and makes recommendations as indicated while retaining a focus on client needs.

The fifth and final step is follow-up and reassessment. The nurse consultant needs to encourage feedback from the consultee and other significant caregivers in order to evaluate the situation. The consultant will want to find out whether suggested interventions have been tried, and if so, what the results were. The consultant will also want the consultee to consider whether interventions suggested in a particular case can be generalized to similar cases in the future. As part of follow-up procedures, the nurse consultant may look for documentation in the progress notes and care plans to evaluate consistent implementation of suggestions among all the nursing shift rotations. Poor communication among members of different shifts may indicate lack of acceptance of or resistance to the consultant's suggestions.

Another aspect of follow-up is evaluation of the teaching of mental health principles to consultees, since this is one of the goals of consultation. The consultee may have implemented the consultant's recommendations and the client may have improved, yet the learning needs of the consultee may not have been met. To illustrate, if a consultant repeatedly receives requests for consultation on terminally ill patients even when staff members usually implement recommendations with good results, the consultant might surmise that the staff's learning needs related to issues of death and dying should be addressed through consultation or education for the staff.

This final step in the consultation process provides data to the consultant about what has been learned about the client, the consultee, the setting, and the recommendations made. These data are useful in stimulating the consultant's professional growth and expertise. It is important that the consultant remain visible for a time after the consultation, so that the consultee does not feel prematurely abandoned. Support can be provided by means of a phone call if a personal follow-up visit is not possible. Requests for future consultation will depend on the consultant maintaining communication with the consultee.

The question of accountability of the nurse consultant has relevance for the consultation process in a clinical setting. Nursing literature emphasizes that the nurse consultant in a general hospital should be based in the department of nursing (Garant, 1977; Lewis and Levy, 1982). The power and influence derived from this base are an important support when problems arise as part of providing psychiatric liaison nursing service. In some hospitals the nurse consultant may participate as a team member of the department of psychiatric liaison but maintains alliance and accountability to nursing.

Since psychiatric nurses began, some twenty years ago, to provide consultation to nurses on medical and surgical units in a general hospital, practitioners have recognized the need for development of a theoretical framework around which to organize their clinical work. Such a framework is still evolving, but most nursing literature currently emphasizes synthesis and application of theoretical models from nursing, psychiatry, systems theory, crisis theory, adult learning theory, and group process (Hendler, Wise, and Lucas, 1979; Lewis and Levy, 1982).

Implications of Consultation and Liaison Work

Nursing literature on consultation contains many descriptions, mostly anecdotal, of the outcomes of consultation work. The most common outcome has been an increased awareness by staff nurses of the psychological needs of patients hospitalized on general medical/surgical hospital units. One study of a program of mental health nursing consultation in a general hospital found that at the end of three years more collaboration was occurring among nurses, physicians, and ancillary staff in achieving care goals and in increasing the satisfaction and well-being of clients and families (Hedlund, 1978). Among the identified benefits were more effective counseling practices by nurses, increased respect for psychosocial aspects of patient care, and enhanced staff interest in developing competency in this area. Nurses also demonstrated greater recognition of counseling and teaching as important functions.

There are many descriptions in the literature of specific and creative interventions developed by nurse consultants to improve the ability and willingness of nurses to provide psychological care to clients on general hospital units. In developing a consultation program, Langman-Dorwart (1979) focused on Caplan's four categories of work problems: lack of knowledge, lack of skills, lack of self-confidence, and lack of professional objectivity. In addressing these problems, Langman-Dorwart used an assertiveness training program that empha-

Whatever the type of consultation, the effect of the consultant's intervention is mediated by the relationship between the consultee and himself. This must be a relationship of mutual trust and respect, so that what each expresses has importance and significance for the other. The consultee must be open to the cognitive and affective influence of the consultant, but at the same time he must feel sufficiently independent to accept only those aspects of the consultant's ideas about the case that fit in with his own needs and with his subjective impressions of the realities of his current professional situation.

GERALD CAPLAN (1970)

606

sized role-play of situations encountered by nursing staff. For example, nurses on a unit had felt powerless with physicians and behaved either nonassertively or aggressively in their interactions with physicians. After the nurses were taught assertive communication skills, they became more self-confident and adopted alternative ways to negotiate problematic work issues with physicians.

Another useful program developed by consultants has been an inservice model to help staff nurses cope with grief (Baker and Lynn, 1979). It is commonly believed that confronting the death of a client is the most devastating problem nurses must face. Nurses experience feelings of helplessness, despair, and anger when dealing with the anticipated or actual death of a client; they need a way to ventilate these feelings so as to develop an understanding of their emotional responses and to build a supportive network among themselves. Baker and Lynn found that nurses who participated in the inservice program on death and grieving scored lower for depression on Zuckerman's multiple affect adjective checklist than did a control group of nurses not participating in the inservice program.

Another example of application of liaison psychiatric nursing principles was a pilot project designed to improve undergraduate nursing students' ability to integrate principles of psychiatric mental health nursing in clinical areas outside the psychiatric setting (Jansson, 1979). Using Caplan's consultee-centered approach, senior students functioned as nursing consultants to junior students. This was a collaborative situation in which the junior students retained responsibility for direct client care. Jansson found that consultees' skill in coping with "difficult"

patients improved, leading to better nurse-client relationships and client care.

An essential aspect of the nurse consultant role is education. The examples of inservice programs on assertiveness and grief illustrate two models of educational strategies. Other opportunities for teaching arise during interdisciplinary health team conferences, nursing staff conferences, Kardex-rounds, walk rounds, and formal workshops. Informal teaching also occurs by means of modeling interviewing skills during unplanned staff contacts on the unit (Weinstein, Chapman, and Stallings, 1979; Tringali, 1982; Fife, 1983). As the nurse consultant helps nursing staff develop a therapeutic environment on general hospital units, the quality of client care will generally improve. Consultation often leads to increased awareness of the stress and anxiety experienced by clients as a result of hospitalization and illness (Isaacharoff et al., 1970).

Psychiatric nurse consultants have advocated the use of support groups to prevent staff burnout and to minimize stress in nursing staff (Lewis and Levy, 1982; Tringali, 1982). Nurses in special care settings, such as renal dialysis units, intensive care units, and burn units, are at risk for burnout because of the constant high level of stress in such environments. Because psychiatric nurses have greater understanding than psychiatrists of the demands and conflicts experienced by staff nurses working on such units, the psychiatric nurse consultant is well qualified for this type of consultative work (Barton and Kelso, 1971).

There is impressive evidence for the belief that nurse-to-nurse consultation has advantages over consultation from outside experts, such as psychol-

Mental health consultation is a method which has emerged from clinical practice but also has roots in organizational theory and consultation. The experience and research derived from clinical practice has gradually led from a narrow physiological and psychological perspective on individual patients toward a social-systems approach focused on organizational dynamics and influences. The method combines elements of both, making it possible for a mental health professional to work within an organization toward mental health objectives.

ARNOLD R. BEISSER AND ROSE GREEN (1972)

607

ogists or psychiatrists (Stickey, Moir, and Gardner, 1981; Fife, 1983). The nurse consultant possesses first-hand understanding of the personal and professional stressors that nurses experience. This knowledge enhances the nurse consultant's ability to identify consultee strengths as well as needs. In addition, a trusting relationship may more easily be achieved in a nurse-to-nurse consultation because both view client care from a holistic perspective. It has been found when psychiatric nurse consultants establish credibility with staff and have the support of the nursing administrator, their effectiveness in planning and coordinating improved client care is impressive (Barbiasz et al., 1982).

THE REFERRAL PROCESS
IN PSYCHIATRIC NURSING

Hospitalization and illness evoke a variety of emotional responses in clients. Thus, any person receiving care in a general hospital is a potential referral for psychiatric mental health consultation (Marcus, 1976). The psychiatric nurse consultant in a general hospital functions in a variety of ways. For example, the consultant may function as a member of a psychiatric liaison consultation team or as part of a crisis team that offers help on demand (Hart, 1982). Consultation may also be offered through a service-based system, such as being assigned to a burn unit or a renal dialysis unit.

Because the expertise of psychiatrists and psychiatric nurses differs, one might expect that there would be a difference in the type of clients re-

ferred to these different professional groups, and this proves true. A study by Stickey and Hall (1981) found that requests for nursing consultations were indeed different than requests for psychiatric consultations. The most common requests for nurse consultant interventions were for clients who were withdrawn and depressed. Nurses were found to be more likely to be called in with cases involving death and dying or when family or staff support was in question. Intervention with nursing staff was primarily in the form of support when they felt angry, were experiencing a loss, or were in disagreement over a client's care. Requests for psychiatric nurses to consult with nursing staff on orthopedic units often focused on dependency secondary to patient disability. On burn units nursing staff frequently needed nurse consultants to help them cope with their feelings about the pain they inflicted on patients while delivering care. Pain in general is a major concern to nursing staff (Stickey, Moir, and Gardner, 1981).

Psychiatrists were requested to see clients in critical care units three and a half times more often than psychiatric nurses, and they were also called more often for clients with organic mental disorders and for clients who needed evaluation for psychotropic medication. However, psychiatric nurses were called to consult with staff regarding nursing management of patients on psychotropic medications. Nurse consultants were also called more often than psychiatrists to intervene with manipulative patients, which testifies to the psychiatric nurse's expertise in milieu management. Other "difficult" patients typically referred for psychiatric nursing consultation were those who used excessive denial

Figure 22-2. Sample consultation request form.

Request for Consultation

Date: _____ To: _____

Client's name _____

Location _____

Identified problem: _____

_____

_____

_____

Assistance required/expected outcomes: _____

_____

_____

_____

Preferred date and time of initial consultation:

_____

Requested by: _____

Name: _____

Department: _____

608

or who were uncooperative, hostile, anxious, agitated, or self-destructive (Goldstein, 1978).

Sequence of Referrals

Who initiates referrals to psychiatric nurse consultants? Any member of the nursing staff may initiate such a referral, as may members of any other discipline. However, nurses are sometimes reluctant to seek nursing consultation and may instead call psychiatrists or psychologists to consult on a nursing problem. Polk (1980) offers two explanations for this paradox. One explanation is related to the socialization of women, which encourages them to depend on men for authority. Since nurses are primarily female and psychiatrists are primarily male, nurses who are socialized in this manner are more inclined to request a psychiatric consultation than a nursing consultation. The other explanation comes from the way nurses are socialized into the profession itself. Nurses are frequently made to believe that they should know everything about nursing, and so they consider it an inadequacy to have to ask another nurse for guidance.

In setting up a referral system, three administrative steps are needed. First is the development of a *referral protocol* (Burch and Meredith, 1974). This includes formalizing such things as who may make the request, what channels of communication should be used, who contacts the consultant, when the consultant is available, and how soon to expect the consultant to respond. An important aspect of the referral protocol is to ensure that the head nurse sanctions the consultant's entry onto the hospital unit. The head nurse is the most powerful person on the unit, and her support is necessary if the con-

sultant is to be successful. On units with primary nursing, the primary nurse may initiate the nurse consultant request, but the primary nurse collaborates with the head nurse in making the referral (Hart, 1982). The referral protocol should include development of a written referral form that includes reasons for the request and a definition of the problem (Hart, 1982). Such a form (see Figure 22-2) helps organize data for the consultant and helps the consultee think through the purpose and goals for the consultation request.

The second step is publicizing the nurse consultation service to all involved hospital units in the general hospital, and the third step is to devise a system to assure feedback to the consultee. A written report, documentation in the client's chart, a phone call to the staff, or a conference to evaluate the interventions—all are different ways this feedback can be provided (Burch and Meredith, 1974).

Research on psychiatric nursing consultation is extremely sparse. Wolff (1978) did study factors that contributed to decisions by surgical nurses to request psychiatric nursing consultation. Wolff found that a variety of factors were involved and that those patients who were referred manifested more psychopathology and evoked more negative responses in the nurse than did clients who were not referred for consultation. Wolff also found that

There is no such thing as nonbehavior or, to put it even more simply: one cannot not behave. Now, if it is accepted that all behavior in an interactional situation has message value, i.e., is communicaiton, it follows that no matter how one may try, one cannot not communicate. Activity or inactivity, words or silence, all have message value: they influence others and these others, in turn, cannot not respond to these communications and are thus themselves communicating.

PAUL WATZLAWICK, JANET BEAVIN, AND DON JACKSON (1967)

609

nurses' observations of clients, not their own subjective reactions, were the most significant factors underlying referral. Behaviors most commonly observed in the referred clients were depression, tension, anger, withdrawal, suicidal tendencies, manipulation, dependence, and need for family support. The most significant factor leading to request for consultation was depression in the client. Because depression is a common emotional response to hospitalization and to illness, this finding is not unexpected.

Themes of Referrals

From this discussion of the referral process, two main themes emerge, one involving nursing education and the other involving nursing research. Basic content in undergraduate nursing programs includes some content on the consultation process, on the role of the psychiatric nursing consultant, and on types of appropriate referrals. More research is necessary to identify the types of clients and the staff issues that might benefit from expanded nursing consultation services. Other research is needed to determine which interventions are most effective in specific consultation situations and how referrals to nurse consultants can be evaluated.

The occasional need arises for a psychiatric nurse consultant to refer a medical client for psychotherapy. Although crisis intervention is an accepted aspect of consultation/liaison work, if long-term therapy is indicated, the consultant may not be able to assume this responsibility because of policy or time constraints. Additionally, if a client has a complex medical illness and also requires psychotropic medication, a psychiatric referral may

be appropriate. Such complexities do not rule out a psychiatric nurse providing psychotherapy for the client if the nurse has adequate preparation and is allowed to offer such services by the employer. In such cases the medical and psychiatric aspects of care must be carefully coordinated.

The psychiatric nurse consultant can play an important role in preparing a medical client for a psychiatric referral. The consultant may do so directly by working with the client or indirectly by working with the client's primary nurse or team leader. Clients invariably have fears about psychotherapy and believe it denotes they are crazy or incurable. A nurse can play a major role in fostering acceptance of psychotherapy regardless of who provides such therapy.

On a psychiatric inpatient unit, the discharge plan often calls for referrals to support networks, such as a day treatment program, a medication clinic, or a halfway house. To preserve confidentiality, the nurse must obtain the client's permission to make such referrals. Most hospitals use a standardized release of information form for referral purposes. When referrals are made between different departments within the same hospital, a written release may not be required; however, the client's verbal agreement for the nurse to initiate such a referral is indicated and should be documented.

When making referrals to another service or agency, the referring nurse must be assured that this agency provides services to meet the client's needs, that it is accessible to the client, that the care providers are competent and qualified, and that payment for service can be made by third-party coverage, private funds, or other means. It is helpful to provide more than one choice of agency or care provider wherever possible, in order to increase the client's sense of control over his or her life (Litwack, Litwack, and Ballou, 1980). It is also necessary to be direct in explaining to the client the reason for the referral, such as saying, "You have told me you have no friends and you stated that one goal of hospitalization was to strengthen your social supports, so I am recommending we make a referral to the volunteer companion service." Litwack, Litwack, and Ballou (1980) noted that it is important to counsel the client about the limitations as well as the advantages of the service or agency to which the client is referred.

COLLABORATION AND COORDINATION IN HEALTH CARE DELIVERY

Collaboration refers to the process whereby health care providers share feelings, ideas, and information within a noncompetitive atmosphere focused on the general goal of providing optimal client care (Lewis and Levy, 1982). Collaboration involves sharing responsibilities for the client. It occurs between two colleagues, each of whom is expected to carry out role-appropriate behaviors (Caplan, 1970). Nurses collaborate with one another and with clients as well as with other professionals. The purpose of collaboration is to utilize various skills of the mental health team members to provide the most effective and comprehensive client care (Wilson and Kneisl, 1983).

Nurses may collaborate with each other on a one-to-one basis or within team conferences, whether unidisciplinary or interdisciplinary. For ex-

ample, the psychiatric nurse consultant may assess a female client for abnormal grief after a mastectomy while the primary nurse evaluates the client's performance of arm muscle strengthening exercises. The nurse colleagues would then meet to discuss client needs and goals and then plan intervention strategies.

An example of collaboration between a psychiatric nurse and another health care provider would be a psychiatric nurse and a dietitian working with an anorectic depressed client who has lost 20 pounds in six months. While the dietitian and client meet to determine food likes and dislikes and to develop a specific meal plan for one week, the psychiatric nurse simultaneously sets up a plan with the client for progressing from eating one meal a day to eating three meals a day in the dining room in the presence of others.

The psychiatric nurse on a primary nursing unit may refer a client with a history of poor medication compliance to a community health nurse for follow-up after discharge. The two nurses would then collaborate in the development of an approach to ensure medication compliance. The psychiatric nurse might review therapeutic and possible side effects of the medication with the client and the family prior to discharge, and the community health nurse would monitor compliance through weekly medication counts at home with the client after discharge.

Coordination is the organizing activity necessary to assure delivery of comprehensive health care. The psychiatric nurse, whether the primary nurse or team leader, generally assumes the coordinating role during the client's hospitalization. Coordination frequently involves seeing that the client's basic

CLINICAL EXAMPLE

PSYCHIATRIC CONSULTATION IN THE CONTEXT OF PHYSICAL DISABILITY AND COGNITIVE DEFICITS

Mrs. Brown, age eighty-two, is widowed and the mother of one daughter. She was living in her own apartment until she was hospitalized for bowel cancer and a colostomy was performed. Subsequently, she was an inpatient on the surgical unit of the local general hospital.

ASSESSMENT

During her hospitalization it became apparent that Mrs. Brown had moderately severe cognitive impairments. As a result she was diagnosed as having primary degenerative dementia. Every day she talked about wanting to return home to her apartment. She insisted she would be fine and that she did not need any help. She had been shown how to irrigate her colostomy but was unable to remember the steps in the procedure and could not handle the equipment. However, she said she was sure that once she got home she would have no trouble irrigating her colostomy.

Mrs. Brown's daughter approached her mother's primary nurse, saying that she knew her mother could not manage at home alone but she couldn't face up to telling her mother this. The daughter had always looked to her mother for advice and guidance, and she said that she fell apart even thinking of confronting her mother with the fact that she couldn't return home alone. Mrs. Brown has been a widow for twenty years and has been fiercely independent, always making her own decisions and taking care of herself.

In addition to coping with discharge plans for her mother, the daughter was shocked at the diagnosis of dementia. She couldn't understand how it seemed to show up so suddenly. She stated that she had not noticed any change in her mother's functioning except that she had decreased her usual outings with friends and had been asking the daughter to shop for her the past few months. The daughter was decreasing the frequency and length of her hospital visits because she didn't know how to respond to Mrs. Brown's pleas to go home.

While hospitalized Mrs. Brown showed a great deal of agitation, calling out for her daughter and ringing the call bell frequently. She was not sleeping well at night and was found wandering in the hall disoriented as to time and place. After talking with Mrs. Brown's daughter, her primary nurse decided that a request for a psychiatric nursing consultation would be helpful to plan interventions in response to Mrs. Brown's changed behavior and to develop a discharge plan for the client with the daughter's involvement. The primary nurse reviewed the referral with the head nurse who agreed this was a good idea, and the primary nurse filled out the formal referral form.

Based on the history and the clinical presentation, the following diagnoses were made:

Nursing Diagnoses

Coping, ineffective family

Family processes, alteration in

Knowledge deficit

Self-care deficit

Sleep pattern disturbance

Multiaxial Psychiatric Diagnoses

Axis I 290.00 Uncomplicated primary degenerative dementia, senile onset

Axis II None

Axis III Cancer of colon

Axis IV Code 5—Hospitalization, serious illness

Axis V Level 2—Very good

PLANNING

After receiving the consultation request, the psychiatric nurse consultant went to the surgical unit. Initially she arranged a meeting with the primary nurse and then reviewed the client's chart. She met again with the primary nurse and together they discussed interventions to decrease Mrs. Brown's agitation and improve her orientation. The nursing consultant then met with the head nurse and the primary nurse and suggested that an interdisciplinary team conference with the surgeon and social worker would be beneficial to develop a comprehensive care plan for the client's discharge. This strategy was agreed upon, the primary nurse contacted the other involved team members, and the conference was held the next day.

The primary nurse opened the meeting and the psychiatric nurse consultant encouraged the members to focus on identifying their unique contributions to the client's care. The surgeon stated that Mrs. Brown would not require further treatment for her cancer and he would see her in surgery ambulatory clinic for routine

611

follow-up visits. The team then developed a list of disposition options, including nursing home placement, home care with 24-hour aides in Mrs. Brown's own apartment, and moving in with her daughter, with aides during the day and community health nurse visits every week to monitor overall health and colostomy irrigation and function. The psychiatric nurse consultant and the social worker arranged to meet together with the daughter to discuss these options and to be supportive figures to her. In addition, the consultant counseled the daughter about dementia and its usual course.

IMPLEMENTATION

The psychiatric nurse consultant met with the head nurse to suggest a series of four weekly inservice meetings to focus on the care of clients with dementia and their families. Information on support services available in the community for the daughter, such as the group for Alzheimer's clients' family members, and an adult day care program was presented to the staff, along with specific teaching about dementia and communication techniques used to decrease client anxiety and to convey empathy to the client.

EVALUATION

As a result of these interventions, the following outcomes were achieved after one week: Mrs. Brown's agitation and calling out decreased, her sleep improved, and her daughter was able to make the decision to place her in a nursing home. The consultant then met with the daughter and the primary nurse for short visits every afternoon for one week to help her work through her grief about the loss of her once intact, independent mother.

As a result of this consultation, the primary nurse felt more confident to plan future interventions to cope with Mrs. Brown's cognitive impairment and was more aware of how the daughter's feelings had affected her. The nursing staff felt better prepared to cope with clients like Mrs. Brown in the future, and they acquired increased awareness of the psychological impact of dementia on the client and the family.

612

daily needs, such as food and safety, are not only met but are delivered in an individualized and timely fashion. If, for example, the client's favorite dish of lasagna is served cold because it was late arriving on the unit, the nurse will need to call the dietary department to ensure that future meal delivery will be on time. Coordination of higher-level needs, such as self-esteem and creativity, may be implemented by developing an activity schedule that allows extra time in music and art if these are meaningful to the client. In this case, the primary nurse would need to meet with the activities therapist and plan for coverage of the client's extra time in art and music.

Coordination of the planning for psychiatric follow-up care is a critical task for the psychiatric nurse. The nurse must ensure that the client has an appointment with the outpatient therapist, has the therapist's phone number, and knows how to get to the psychiatric clinic or office. Providing the client with a list of emergency phone numbers before discharge is also a coordination task. The local crisis intervention hotline and the psychiatric emergency department should be on such a list, along with the client's medical care provider and any other relevant support services, such as a transportation service. The coordination of activities related to discharge planning is a responsibility assumed by the psychiatric nurse because he or she is knowledgeable of the client's needs and the services available to support the client in the community. Knowledge of community health care systems will aid the nurse in delivering optimal health care to the client and will facilitate the client's effective interaction with the system.

SUMMARY

This chapter has examined the role and functions of psychiatric nurses as members of health care teams within the two delivery systems of team nursing and primary nursing. The process of consultation as currently practiced by psychiatric nurses emphasizes consultee-centered and client-centered types of consultation within the general hospital. These are exemplified by the psychiatric nurse's consultant/liaison role. Referral and collaboration among nurses and between nurses and other health professionals should follow sequential steps. The process of nursing consultation is facilitated by a formal written referral, by the visibility and accessibility of the nurse consultant, and by careful documentation and record keeping. Ongoing use of consultation makes nurses more sensitive to the psychosocial needs of clients and promotes effective coordination of care and collaboration between nurses and between nurses and other care providers.

Review Questions

1. Compare and contrast a unidisciplinary team, a multidisciplinary team, and an interdisciplinary team.

2. Discuss the components of the consultation process.

3. Describe the four models of nursing care delivery and the advantages and disadvantages of each.

4. Outline the functions of a nursing team in a mental health setting.

5. Describe the role of a primary nurse in a mental health setting.

6. Compare and contrast the consultant and liaison models in nursing.

7. Discuss the advantages and disadvantages of being a psychiatric nurse consultant on a unit with team nursing as compared with a unit with primary nursing.

8. What other health care providers might be part of the health care team if Mrs. Brown in the clinical example were transferred to an inpatient psychiatric unit?

9. Review the steps of the referral process as exemplified in the clinical example.

10. Using the clinical example, discuss the collaborative aspects of the primary nurse's role.

References

Baker, B., and Lynn, M. 1979. Psychiatric Nursing Consultation: The Use of an Inservice Model to Assist Nurses in the Grief Process. *Journal of Psychiatric Nursing*, 17(5):15–19.

Barbiasz, J., et al. 1982. Establishing the Psychiatric Liaison Nurse Role: Collaboration with the Nursing Administrator. *Journal of Nursing Administration*, 12(2):14–18.

Barton, D., and Kelso, M. S. 1971. The Nurse as a Psychiatric Consultation Team Member. *Psychiatry in Medicine*, 2(2):108–115.

Beisser, A. R., and Green, R. 1972. *Mental Health Consultation and Education*. Palo Alto, Calif.: National Press Books.

Benfer, B. A. 1980. Defining the Role and Function of the Psychiatric Nurse as a Member of the Team. *PPC*, 18(4):166–177.

Burch, J. W., and Meredith, J. L. 1974. Help with Problem Patients: Nurses as the Core of a Psychiatric Team. *American Journal of Nursing*, 74:2037–2038.

Bursten, B. 1963. The Psychiatric Consultant and the Nurse. *Nursing Forum*, 2(4):6–23.

Caplan, G. 1970. *The Theory and Practice of Mental Health Consultation*. New York: Basic Books.

Challela, M. 1979. The Interdisciplinary Team: A Role Definition for Nursing. *Image*, 11(1):9–15.

Ciske, K. L. 1974. Primary Nursing: An Organization That Promotes Professional Practice. *Journal of Nursing Administration*, 4(1):28–31.

Covert, A. B. 1979. Community Mental Health Nursing: The Role of the Consultant in the Nursing Home. *Journal of Psychiatric Nursing*, 17(7):15–19.

Crawshaw, R., and Key, W. 1961. Psychiatric Teams: A Selective Review of the Literature. *Archives of General Psychiatry*, 5:397–405.

Davis, D. S. 1983. Psychiatric Mental Health Nursing Consultation in the General Hospital: Liaison Nursing. In *Handbook of Psychiatric Mental Health Nursing*, eds. C. Adams and A. Macione. New York: John Wiley & Sons.

Deloughery, G. W.; Gebbie, K. M.; and Neuman, B. M. 1971. *Consultation and Community Organization in Community Mental Health Nursing*. Baltimore: Williams & Wilkins.

Fife, B. 1983. The Challenge of the Medical Setting for the Clinical Specialist in Psychiatric Nursing. *Journal of Psychiatric Nursing*, 21(1):8–13.

Garant, C. A. 1977. The Psychiatric Liaison Nurse— An Interpretation of the Role. *Supervisor Nurse*, 8(4):75–78.

Given, B., and Simmons, S. 1977. The Interdisciplinary Health Care Team: Fact or Fiction? *Nursing Forum*, 16(2):165–184.

Goldstein, S. 1978. The Psychiatric Clinical Specialist in the General Hospital. *Journal of Nursing Administration*, 9(3):34–37.

Gordon, M. 1982. *Nursing Diagnosis: Process and Application*. St. Louis: McGraw-Hill.

Hart, C. A. 1982. Psychiatric Mental Health Nursing Consultation: A Two-Model System in a General Hospital. *Issues in Mental Health Nursing*, 4(2):127–147.

Hedlund, N. L. 1978. Mental Health Nursing Consultation in the General Hospital. *Patient Counseling and Health Education*, 1(2):85–88.

Hendler, N.; Wise, T. N.; and Lucas, M. J. 1979. The Expanded Role of the Psychiatric Liaison Nurse. *Psychiatric Quarterly*, 51(2):135–143.

Isaacharoff, A., et al. 1970. Psychiatric Nurses as Consultants in a General Hospital. *Hospital Community Psychiatry*, 21(11):361–367.

Jansson, D. P. 1979. Student Consultation: A Liaison Psychiatric Experience for Nursing Students. *Perspectives in Psychiatric Care*, 17(2):77–94.

Johnson, B. S. 1963. Psychiatric Nursing Consultation in a General Hospital. *Nursing Outlook*, 11:728–729.

Kimball, C. P. 1979. Liaison Psychiatry: Approaches and Ways of Thinking About Behavior. *Psychiatric Clinics of North America*, 2(2):201–210.

Langford, T. L. 1981. *Managing and Being Managed: Preparation for Professional Nursing Practice*. Englewood Cliffs, N.J.: Prentice-Hall.

Langman-Dorwart, N. 1979. A Model for Mental Health Consultation to the General Hospital. *Journal of Psychiatric Nursing*, 17(3):29–33.

Larkin, M., and Crowdes, N. E. 1976. Nurse Consultation: The Instilling of Hope. *Supervisor Nurse*, 7(11):54–58.

Lewis, A., and Levy, J. S. 1982. *Psychiatric Liaison Nursing*. Reston, Va.: Reston Publishing.

Lipowski, Z. J. 1974. Consultation—Liaison Psychiatry: An Overview. *American Journal of Psychiatry*, 131:623–630.

Litwack, L.; Litwack, J. M.; and Ballou, M. B. 1980. *Health Counseling*. New York: Appleton-Century-Crofts.

Marcus, J. 1976. Nursing Consultation: A Clinical Specialty. *Journal of Psychiatric Nursing*, 14(11):29–31.

Marram, G. D.; Schlegel, M. W.; and Bevis, E. O. 1974. *Primary Nursing: A Model for Individualized Care*. St. Louis: C. V. Mosby.

Mereness, D. 1951. Preparation of the Nurse for the Psychiatric Team. *American Journal of Nursing*, 51(5):320–322.

613

Miller, J. R., and Janosik, E. H. 1978. The Hospital Nurse. *Exceptional Parent*, October: 43–50.

Moreau, D.; Kahn, P.; and Lal, S. 1974. Role of a Nurse on a Psychiatric Consultation Service. *Canadian Psychiatric Association Journal*, 19:453–456.

Nelson, J. K. N., and Schilke, D. A. 1976. The Evolution of Psychiatric Liaison Nursing. *Perspectives of Psychiatric Nursing*, 14(21):60–65.

Pasnau, R., ed. 1975. *Consultation-Liaison Psychiatry*. New York: Grune & Stratton.

Pasnau, R. 1982. Consultation-Liaison Psychiatry at the Crossroads: In Search of a Definition for the 1980s. *Hospital and Community Psychiatry*, 33:989–1005.

Polk, G. C. 1980. The Socialization and Utilization of Nurse Consultants. *Journal of Psychiatric Nursing*, 18(2):33–36.

Robinson, A. 1950. Changing of the Guard. *American Journal of Nursing*, 50(3):152–154.

Severin, N. K., and Becker, R. E. 1974. Nurses as Psychiatric Consultants in a General Hospital Emergency Room. *Community Mental Health Journal*, 10(3):261–267.

Sienkilewski, K. 1983. Evolution of Inpatient Psychiatric Nursing. In *Principles and Practice of Psychiatric Nursing*, 2nd ed., eds. G. Stuart and S. Sundeen. St. Louis: C. V. Mosby.

Stanton, A. H., and Schwartz, M. S. 1954. *The Mental Hospital: A Study of Institutional Participation in Psychiatric Illness and Treatment*. New York: Basic Books.

Stickey, S., and Hall, R. 1981. The Role of the Nurse on a Consultation Liaison Team. *Psychosomatics*, 22(3):224–235.

Stickey, S.; Moir, G.; and Gardner, E. 1981. Psychiatric Nurse Consultation: Who Calls and Why? *Journal of Psychiatric Nursing*, 19(10):22–26.

Strain, J., and Grossman, S. 1975. *Psychological Care of the Medically Ill*. New York: Appleton-Century-Crofts.

Tringali, R. 1982. The Role of the Psychiatric Nurse Consultant on a Burn Unit. *Issues in Mental Health Nursing*, 4:17–24.

Watzlawick, P.; Beavin, J.; and Jackson, D. 1967. *Pragmatics of Human Communication*. New York: W. W. Norton.

Weinstein, L. J.; Chapman, M. M.; and Stallings, M. A. 1979. *Perspectives in Psychiatric Nursing*, 17(2):66–71.

Wilson, H. S., and Kneisl, C. R. 1983. *Psychiatric Nursing*, 2nd ed. Menlo Park, Calif.: Addison-Wesley.

Wolff, P. 1978. Psychiatric Nursing Consultation: A Study of the Referral Process. *Journal of Psychiatric Nursing*, 16(5):42–47.

Zahaurek, R., and Morrison, K. 1974. Help with Problem Patients: Mental Health Nurses as Consultants to Staff Nurses. *American Journal of Nursing*, 74:2034–2036.

Supplementary Readings

Bergman, A. S. Psychiatric and Social Work Collaboration in a Pediatric Chronic Illness Hospital. *Social Work and Health Care*, 7(1981):45–55.

Green, B. Primary Nursing in Psychiatry. *Nursing Times*, 79(1983):24–28.

Groves, J. Management of the Borderline Patient on a Medical or Surgical Ward. *International Journal of Psychiatry in Medicine*, 25(1969):1365–1370.

Hegyvary, S. *The Change to Primary Nursing: A Cross-Cultural View of Professional Nursing*. St. Louis: C. V. Mosby, 1982.

Kurtz, L. F. Case Management in Mental Health. *Health and Social Work*, 9(1984):201–211.

Marram, G., and Flynn, K. *Cost Effectiveness of Primary and Team Nursing*. Rockville, Md.: Aspen, 1976.

Martin, M. The Role of the Psychiatric Consultant in Psychosomatic Medicine. *Psychosomatics*, 16(1975):7–11.

Pati, B. Nursing Consultation: A Collaborative Process. *Journal of Nursing Administration*, 10(1980):33–37.

Robinson, L. *Liaison Nursing: Psychological Approach to Patient Care*. Philadelphia: F. A. Davis, 1976.

Slickney, S. K. The Role of the Nurse on a Consultation Liaison Team. *Psychosomatics*, 22(1981):224.

Slokoloff, S. Psychiatric Nurse Consultant. *Canadian Nurse*, 79(1982):42–45.

Stickey, S. K. Psychiatric Nurse Consultation: Who Calls and Why. *Journal of Psychosocial Nursing*, 19(1981):22–26.

Talley, S. Psychiatric Consultation and Collaboration: The Availability of Mental Health Services to Primary Care Clients. *Nurse Practitioner*, 8(1983):55–58.

Termini, M. The Consultation Process. *Issues in Mental Health Nursing*, 3(1981):77–78.

Von Schilling, K. The Consultant Role in Multidisciplinary Team Development. *International Nursing Review*, 29(1982):73–75.

NURSING AND ETHICS
The Rights of Mental Health Clients
Institutional Responsibilities Regarding Client Rights
The Right to Refuse Treatment
Restrictive Treatment
Involuntary Commitment
Nursing Implications of Clients' Rights

PROFESSIONAL ACCOUNTABILITY AND LIABILITY
Standards of Practice
Peer Review
Professional Liability

ADVOCACY
The Nurse as Client Advocate
Cautions Relative to the Advocacy Role

THE MENTAL HEALTH NURSE AS CHANGE AGENT

C   H   A   P   T   E   R

23

Advocacy, Legality, and Ethical Values

Learning Objectives

After studying this chapter, the student should be able to:

1. Discuss the interplay of values, ethics, rights, and the law in the practice of mental health nursing.

2. Outline the rights of clients guaranteed by the U.S. Constitution and the Patients' Bill of Rights.

3. Describe the implications of standards of practice and peer review for professional accountability and liability.

4. Present the pros and cons of the nurse as client advocate.

5. Describe the role of the psychiatric mental health nurse as change agent.

Overview

This chapter examines the interplay of ethical values, clients' rights, and legal issues in the practice of mental health nursing. It explores the unique rights of psychiatric clients and their importance to professional nursing practice. Finally, it examines the role enactment of the mental health nurse as client advocate and change agent in promoting a social and professional climate that respects the rights and needs of clients with mental health problems.

Truth crushed to earth shall rise again
The eternal years of God are hers.
But error, wounded, writhes in pain,
And dies among its worshippers.
WILLIAM CULLEN BRYANT

Figure 23-1. The inter-relationship of values, ethics, human rights, and the law.

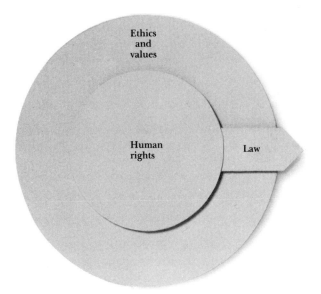

Values, ethics, human rights, and the law are inextricably intertwined. *Values* represent the ideals, customs, and institutions for which individuals have enormous regard. Values that address human relationships at the level of society are called ethics. *Ethics* are guiding principles that define what individuals should do in relation to one another on the basis of general values held by most members of the society. These principles, in their abstract form, are considered essential to the maintenance and promotion of a moral and just society. In effect, the principles delineate the societal member's right to individuality, freedom, and self-determination in behavior and decision making. The legal system defines in a formal and less abstract way what members of society may or may not do according to prescribed doctrine or law. Law is created within society to make explicit the rights of the members according to an ethical value system; the law, then, serves society in protecting the individual's autonomy and rights through formal judgments and actions (see Figure 23-1).

NURSING AND ETHICS

Nursing has special obligations to society in regard to ethics, human rights, values, and the law. Members of the nursing profession are charged with a responsibility for performing the functions of the professional in a way consistent with the ethics and guiding principles of the society, as well as consistent with accepted formal standards of practice and conduct set for and by the profession.

The same law that protects the rights of all members of society is applicable to the professional practice of nursing. This law demands that professionals practice their discipline in such a manner that the rights of the client are never unreasonably compromised. Should professional practitioners violate the ethical code and the standards of professional practice derived from that code, they are accountable to the larger society under the law.

Individual practitioners of a profession therefore reflect the ethical values of their society and their profession in their philosophy of professional practice and their basis for decision making. Internal consistency among the various levels of values—social, legal, professional, and individual—enhances the development of a discipline. When individual or professional values are not congruent with prevailing social values, one result is a potential

618

for creating change in the society (Chinn and Jacobs, 1983). Another result is the potential for creating change within the profession.

The nursing profession upholds the larger society's ethical values for the protection of basic human rights. This is evident in the Code for Nurses (American Nurses' Association, 1976), which identifies the general duties, powers, and obligations of members of the profession regarding clients' rights (see the accompanying box). This code guides the nurse in the performance of professional duties in such a way that the rights of the client are explicitly valued and protected.

In addition to seeing that the practice of nursing is aligned with society's ethics, the ethical code provides direction, self-regulation, and self-evaluation for the members of the profession. "The Code and the Interpretive Statements together provide a framework for the nurse to make ethical decisions and discharge responsibilities to the public, to other members of the health team, and to the profession" (American Nurses' Association, 1976, p. 1).

The Rights of Mental Health Clients

Webster's defines *right* as "that which is due to anyone by just claim." The Constitution of the United States sets forth specific rights for all individuals in accordance with the ethical values held by the larger society; these rights are protected by civil laws and are accepted and assumed as expected outcomes. While the protection of civil rights for all is generally assumed, much attention has recently been given to the protection and enforcement of the rights of individuals seeking or requiring health care. A number of professional policy-making or-

---

ANA CODE FOR NURSES

1. The nurse provides services with respect for human dignity and the uniqueness of the client unrestricted by considerations of social or economic status, personal attributes, or the nature of health problems.

2. The nurse safeguards the client's right to privacy by judiciously protecting information of a confidential nature.

3. The nurse acts to safeguard the client and the public when health care and safety are affected by the incompetent, unethical, or illegal practice of any person.

4. The nurse assumes responsibility and accountability for individual nursing judgments and actions.

5. The nurse maintains competence in nursing.

6. The nurse exercises informed judgment and uses individual competence and qualifications as criteria in seeking consultations, accepting responsibilities, and delegating nursing activities to others.

7. The nurse participates in activities that contribute to the ongoing development of the profession's body of knowledge.

8. The nurse participates in the profession's efforts to implement and improve standards of nursing.

9. The nurse participates in the profession's efforts to establish and maintain conditions of employment conducive to high-quality nursing care.

10. The nurse participates in the profession's effort to protect the public from misinformation and misrepresentation and to maintain the integrity of nursing.

11. The nurse collaborates with members of the health profession and other citizens in promoting community and national efforts to meet the health needs of the public.

SOURCE: Used with permission of American Nurses' Association.

A PATIENT'S BILL OF RIGHTS

1. The patient has the right to considerate and respectful care.

2. The patient has the right to obtain from his physician complete current information concerning his diagnosis, treatment, and prognosis in terms the patient can be reasonably expected to understand. When it is not medically advisable to give such information to the patient, the information should be made available to an appropriate person in his behalf. He has the right to know, by name, the physician responsible for coordinating his care.

3. The patient has the right to receive from his physician information necessary to give informed consent prior to the start of any procedure and/or treatment. Except in emergencies, such information for informed consent should include but not necessarily be limited to the specific procedure and/or treatment, the medically significant risks involved, and the probable duration of incapacitation. Where medically significant alternatives for care or treatment exist, or when the patient requests information concerning medical alternatives, the patient has the right to such information. The patient also has the right to know the name of the person responsible for the procedures and/or treatment.

4. The patient has the right to refuse treatment to the extent permitted by law and to be informed of the medical consequences of his action.

5. The patient has the right to every consideration of his privacy concerning his own medical care program. Case discussion, consultation, examination, and treatment are confidential and should be conducted discreetly. Those not directly involved in his care must have the permission of the patient to be present.

6. The patient has the right to expect that all communications and records pertaining to his care should be treated as confidential.

7. The patient has the right to expect that within its capacity a hospital must make reasonable response to the request of a patient for services. The hospital must provide evaluation, service, and/or referral as indicated by the urgency of the case. When medically permissible, a patient may be transferred to another facility only after he has received complete information and explanation concerning the needs for and alternatives to such a transfer. The institution to which the patient is to be transferred must have accepted the patient for transfer.

8. The patient has the right to obtain information as to any relationship of his hospital to other health care and educational institutions insofar as his care is concerned. The patient has the right to obtain information as to the existence of any professional relationships among individuals, by name, who are treating him.

9. The patient has the right to be advised if the hospital proposes to engage in or perform human experimentation affecting his care or treatment. The patient has the right to refuse to participate in such research projects.

10. The patient has the right to expect reasonable continuity of care. He has the right to know in advance what appointment times and physicians are available and where. The patient has the right to expect that the hospital will provide a mechanism whereby he is informed by his physician or a delegate of the physician of the patient's continuing health care requirements following discharge.

11. The patient has the right to examine and receive an explanation of his bill regardless of source of payment.

12. The patient has the right to know what hospital rules and regulations apply to his conduct as a patient.

619

ganizations, associations, and accrediting groups have taken the issue of patients' rights beyond mere assumption and have devoted special policy statements or publications to this important issue (American Hospital Association, 1980; Joint Commission on Accreditation of Hospitals, 1983). A Patient's Bill of Rights devised by the American Hospital Association is reproduced in the accompanying box.

Psychiatric illness presents particular threats and challenges to the assumptions that underlie client rights. Psychiatric clients are often stereotyped in a manner that is a direct affront to individuality and uniqueness. The psychiatric client is commonly considered to be incompetent and therefore incapable of exercising autonomy in behavior and decision making. The right to legal counsel, the right to refuse medicine that may be prescribed to control behavior, and the right to oppose involuntary hospitalization are a few of the civil rights threatened in care of the psychiatric client.

In caring for the mental health client, the health professional is often faced with the fact that acknowledging a client's civil rights may mean the withdrawal of a treatment, which ultimately will have an impact on the client's well-being. Conversely, to medicate or restrain a client in order to promote ultimate health and well-being can be interpreted as an infraction of the client's rights. The distinctions between what is ethical, what is legal, and what is needed to safeguard the psychiatric client's rights are not always apparent.

Institutional Responsibilities Regarding Client Rights

The institution or agency and health care providers share the responsibility of explaining to individuals their rights as clients in that facility. It is expected that the clients' rights will be explained to them in a manner that they understand. In the explanations of rights, it is necessary to inform clients of the facility's rules or regulations that have an impact on their conduct and behavior. Clients should be assured of their right to impartial access to treatment and should receive care that respects their personal dignity. Providers should make it clear to clients and families that an individualized treatment plan will be instituted and mutual planning will establish the therapeutic goals.

Clients and their families must be informed about the care and treatment being given. Clients should be told about who is responsible for their care, the professional status of caregivers, and their role in the health care team of the treatment facility. If there is a change in the professional team responsible for the client, or if a transfer to another facility or ward is necessary, this must be explained to the client in understandable terms. Informing clients about the personnel ultimately responsible for their care may seem to be simplistic and elementary, but in large teaching facilities it may not be clear to clients just who is responsible for various aspects of their care.

Health professionals should pay attention to clients' preferences for and reactions to their treat-

ment. Information concerning the benefits, side effects, and risks of treatment should be explained. Alternate treatment options should also be made clear and presented in such a manner that clients can make an informed choice for themselves and their families.

With the increasing involvement of clients in institutional and individual research, special emphasis must be given to the rights of clients as research subjects. All clients must be informed and must give written consent for participation in research projects. What is more, such consent should be obtained without coercion, unfair inducements, or persuasion on the part of the health care provider (Watson, 1982). Written consent is also required for the use of audiovisual equipment in the treatment process, for the performance of surgical procedures, for invasive diagnostic procedures, for electroconvulsive therapy, and for the use of any unusual medication. If the client is unable to give consent or is incompetent, the next of kin or legal guardian must give consent prior to implementing the procedure or treatment.

The Right to Refuse Treatment

A major issue in clients' rights is the right to refuse treatment. This right is implied and supported by certain amendments to the Constitution of the United States, including the First Amendment, which protects the freedoms of speech, thought, and expression; the Eighth Amendment, which grants the right to freedom from cruel and unusual punishment; and the Fifth and Fourteenth Amendments, which grant due process of law and equal protection for all.

The Patient's Bill of Rights states that the client has the right to refuse treatment to the extent permitted by law. The "extent permitted by law," however, may vary from state to state. This necessitates being familiar with the mental health laws in the state in which one practices. Statements on clients' rights clearly mandate that health care providers explain to the client what steps the facility will take when refusal of treatment occurs (Joint Commission on Accreditation of Hospitals, 1983). These steps may include involuntary commitment and other legal alternatives, such as a competency hearing or discharge of the client.

In psychiatric settings refusal of treatment primarily concerns the administration of psychotropic medication. Advocates of refusal of treatment point out that psychotropic medication alters thought process and controls behavior rather than cures the illness (Davis, 1978). Those who are concerned with the ethical implications of psychotropic medication argue that the individuality and autonomy of the client are compromised when drugs are given to make behavior conform with what is considered "normal" (Curtin, 1979a).

Some limits have been placed on the psychiatric client relative to the right to refuse treatment. In emergency situations where there is substantial evidence to predict or support the possibility that clients may harm themselves or others, it is admissible to temporarily medicate forcibly (Regan, 1981a; Arkin, 1983). For inpatients who are involuntary admissions and deemed incompetent, the right to refuse treatment requires intervention from the client's legal guardian or the legal system. Here again it is important to know the laws of the particular county or state and to be familiar with the facility's policy.

The right to refuse ongoing treatment that necessitates residence in an institution has aroused much attention (Bandman, 1978). *O'Connor* v. *Donaldson* established that it is unconstitutional to hold persons involuntarily in an institution primarily for custodial reasons (Carroll, 1980). Involuntary commitment is a denial of the individual's autonomy and is a direct challenge to the ethical values of our society. If a person's independence is being denied by involuntary commitment, it is crucial that full efforts be directed toward providing therapeutic treatment and not merely custodial care.

Restrictive Treatment
Another area of controversy has been the concept of least restrictive treatment. Carroll (1980) pointed out that "the more intrusive or restrictive a technique, the more the person's autonomy is diminished" (p. 288). While this may be true, most clinicians would agree that restrictions, at times, do provide necessary controls. The use of physical restraints (the most restrictive form of treatment) may be necessary if less restrictive measures have proven ineffective in providing safety for the client and others (Miller, 1982).

With hospitalization, the least restrictive treatment alternatives must be followed. In trying to maintain the least restrictive treatment alternative, it is imperative not to allow the client to become dangerous to himself or to others. While respecting individual rights is important, it is also necessary to respect and assure the safety of everyone concerned. It is unreasonable to think that seclusion or restraints should never be employed. It is equally unreasonable to use seclusion or restraint procedures when other alternatives are available.

Health professionals must make a judgment as to when a restrictive measure is warranted. When a client unexpectedly becomes disturbed and violent, it is the responsibility of the facility and the staff to ensure the safety of the client and others. The nurse should be knowledgeable concerning the policy and procedure of placing a client in seclusion or restraints. In most facilities a nurse may make an independent judgment but must immediately obtain a retroactive physician's order for the restrictive procedure.

It is equally important to know when a client must be released from seclusion or restraint. Most states and most facilities have strict limits on the time that seclusion and restraint measures can be used, even with a written medical order. If the client's behavior no longer warrants seclusion or restraints, he or she should be released immediately. To maintain a person in seclusion or restraints without adequate behavioral justification is subjecting the client to treatment that is a violation of the right to mutually agreed treatment.

Involuntary Commitment
In most states there are specific criteria for involuntary commitment. In general, the criteria are centered on the person's posing a clear danger to himself or others (Roth, 1980; Tancredi, 1980). With involuntary commitment, the treating facility has a legal responsibility for the client's care and well-being. The length of time a commitment is effective varies from state to state, as do the application procedures for commitment.

Many states specify a detention period in which the family or hospital can begin necessary legal proceedings for commitment. When the initial detention period has lapsed and there are no pending legal plans for involuntary commitment, the individual is free to leave the treating facility. Detention after the expiration of the legal time frame is considered false imprisonment (Cazalas, 1978).

Once an individual is legally committed to a health care facility, does she still have the right to refuse treatment? The answer is yes, the person who is an involuntary admission does maintain the right to refuse treatment (Regan, 1981b). This concept may be difficult to comprehend, as the criteria for involuntary commitment clearly specify that the person must pose a clear danger to self or others. However, the person who has been committed has not lost his or her civil rights. Those rights may only be lost if the person is judged incompetent (Tancredi, 1980; Arkin, 1983). A hearing for incompetency is separate from a commitment hearing.

To be judged *incompetent* means that the person has difficulty in comprehending the full impact of binding legal transactions and that questionable thinking contributes to impaired judgment. Thus, individuals who are judged incompetent cannot marry, divorce, enter into any contractual agree-

621

In recent decades, and in American society especially, social research has shifted its attention from the contrasts between sacred ideals and secular practices to the discrepancies between public ideologies and privileged deliberations and decisions. Such study can be intellectually rewarding and socially valuable, although neither result is inevitable. And there is clearly a place in such work for protective procedures, in investigation as well as in publication. But that place is often misconceived, as scientific rather than political and moral. It is also often misrepresented, as protecting informants' personal rights more than researchers' professional interests. As a result, much social research has become misanthropic, making scholars themselves distrust and discourage the very sort of empathy which gives all men a personal sense of human identity.

RICHARD COLVARD (1967)

622

ments, or vote. Their license to operate a motor vehicle is also revoked. Persons who are ruled incompetent have no power to consent to or refuse treatment.

Nursing Implications of Clients' Rights

The issue of clients' rights has many implications for nursing. One major implication is that nursing personnel must be knowledgeable about the rights of clients and must be aware of their facility's policies and of procedures concerning client rights. They should also be aware of the mental health laws in their state.

In the administration of medication, the nurse must realize that both inpatients and outpatients have the right to refuse medication (Appelbaum and Gutheil, 1980). To forcibly administer medication may result in the client filing suit for assault and battery. The Supreme Court of Colorado has ruled that an involuntary client has the right to refuse treatment when alert, oriented, and aware of the illness and of what treatment is proposed (Regan, 1980). If a client refuses medication, the nurse may try to elicit reasons for the refusal and encourage the client to voice concerns. The nurse may try to persuade the client but should not try to coerce him into taking the medication.

Nursing staff must also learn what constitutes the least restrictive treatment alternatives. They must know what interventions or measures should be taken before more restrictive treatment is instituted. Using the least restrictive form of treatment implies that the client's treatment plan should be individualized and that placement of treatment (as inpatient or outpatient) should be appropriate and responsive to the degree of illness. That is, if the client can be treated on an outpatient basis, then outpatient care is preferable to hospitalization.

The nurse should also be aware of society's ethical values as they apply to the mental health client. Every effort should be made to acknowledge and respect the client's individuality and to promote the client's autonomy to the fullest extent possible. The client should be viewed as an active, not passive, participant in the planning and implementation of care. The nurse must be vigilant concerning the form of care rendered by nursing personnel and by other professionals as well.

There are those who would argue that the practice of mental health nursing provides nurses with insurmountable ethical problems. From the ethical viewpoint, certain measures are contrary to what nurses might prefer if they were free to follow their own values only. The use of behavior-controlling drugs, environmental and mechanical restraints, and other prescribed therapeutic approaches, for example, is sometimes a direct attack on the nurse's belief in the client's right to individuality and autonomy (Curtin, 1979a). Nevertheless, nurses must fulfill professional standards of practice that are directed toward helping the client progress to an improved health state.

There are inevitable circumstances in the practice of mental health nursing that necessitate the use of measures that infringe on the client's individuality and autonomy in decision making. The nurse must be clear in the knowledge of state laws and of the ethical rights of the client before implementing these measures. Once they are implemented, every precaution should be taken to see that any restrictive or controlling measures are withdrawn as soon as the safety and well-being of the client will permit.

CLINICAL VIGNETTE

REFUSAL OF TREATMENT

*B*ill Shaeffer, a hospitalized patient, complains that his medication is making him dizzy and that he therefore does not want to continue with the treatment. Bill has a history of severe hypertension and has been diagnosed as having a bipolar disorder, depressed type. On admission his blood pressure was 182/108. He is extremely suspicious of the staff and fears they will harm him.

Although Bill had willingly taken his hypertensive and antidepressant medication for two days, he now refuses all medications and is becoming more withdrawn. Among the relevant questions to be addressed are:

1. Is Bill a candidate for involuntary admission? Yes. With a history of an affective disorder and untreated, uncontrolled hypertension, he is a danger to himself. His judgment at present is impaired.

2. Can Bill be forcibly medicated for his hypertension and not his antidepressant medication? No. Until he is committed for treatment to an appropriate facility or is legally ruled incompetent, he may not be forcibly medicated. If he becomes violent and poses a serious threat to himself or others, he may be medicated; once he has been medicated, the nurse or physician should contact the legal system for guidance.

3. What measures should the nurse take concerning Bill's medication? Until Bill is committed to the facility or is judged incompetent, nursing measures are somewhat limited. The nurse may encourage Bill to verbalize his reasons for refusing the medication but may not coerce him into taking the medications. The nursing staff should monitor his blood pressure and physical activity frequently, record the results, and inform the physician.

623

To the extent that the nurse is attentive to professional responsibilities outlined in the Code for Nurses, as well as to the basic rights of her patients, the ethical values of society and the mental health client's well-being will be safeguarded.

PROFESSIONAL ACCOUNTABILITY AND LIABILITY

Nurses function within an enormously complex system involving a delicate balance between protection of clients' rights and implementation of health care directed at improving the clients' well-being. The responsibility of the professional nurse within this complex system is to maintain the standards of nursing practice. To the extent that the standards of care are violated, nurses can be held accountable and liable for negligence. This section of the chapter deals with nursing accountability and liability for actions that are committed or omitted in care of the psychiatric client.

Standards of Practice

Nursing as a professional discipline has structured its practice principles so that it may (1) judge the competency of its members, (2) evaluate the quality of the services rendered to clients, and (3) safeguard client rights (American Nurses' Association, 1973). This structuring is partially represented in the development of nursing practice standards. *Standards of practice* are authoritative statements or approved concepts that provide guidance to the profession and its members in the actual delivery of care. Both generic and specific standards for each major division of nursing practice have been developed by the American Nurses' Association.

The Standards of Psychiatric and Mental Health Nursing Practice were developed in 1973. These standards provide guidance and direction in the delivery of care as well as in defining professional roles and expectations for mental health nurses (see Appendix C). Each standard is written with a supporting rationale statement and a list of assessment factors. The assessment factors identify nursing behaviors that, if employed, assure achievement of the standard.

For example, Standard III is "The problem-solving approach is utilized in developing nursing care plans" (p. 3). The rationale states that a nursing diagnosis that encompasses the individual and the environment and the interaction between the two is utilized in the development of a plan of care. This standard gives direction to the specific aspects that must be addressed in the daily delivery of care. The assessment factors specify that attention should be given to the individual, to response to the environment, and to behavioral patterns. These specific elements must not only be observed, but an assessment must be drawn. The statement implies that the assessment process is ongoing. The assessment factors further state that input should be obtained from others who know the patient and that the

The confluence of the health rights movement, consumerism, and the escalating cost of health care have turned the delivery, organization, financing, and control of health care into a highly politicized issue. As a result, pressure has increased for the more rigorous application of principles of internal accountability, and there is growing evidence that self-regulation, as currently practiced, must eventually give way to a more pluralistic system of accountability which includes both the consumer and the body politic. Within this broader context, utilization and peer review offer not only systematic approaches toward achieving professional accountability, but also mechanisms for involving service providers in establishing parameters to determine both the effective utilization of services and the quality of care provided.

GARY TISCHLER AND BORIS ASTRACHAN (1982)

624

plans of nursing care are shared with other caregivers. These plans of care are used as guides for each client-nurse interaction and are periodically reviewed and revised. Utilization of the assessment factors facilitates the successful attainment of the mental health standard, thereby improving the quality of care. Failure to utilize the assessment factors places the nurse in a vulnerable position that ultimately could lead to a negligence or malpractice suit.

Standardization of nursing care eliminates reliance on individual values and standards, thereby improving the quality of care and consistently defining clear expectations of the professional nurse. Standards of practice facilitate the definition and delineation of standards of care. *Standards of care* have been defined as acts committed or omitted that an ordinary prudent person would have committed or omitted. Standards of care are a measure of what ought to be done in a given situation by a nurse carrying out professional duties and responsibilities. An individual nurse may be judged by peers who compare the nurse's actions with those described by the standard of care. Knowledge of the standards of care is the basis for providing quality care as well as for ensuring against a lawsuit for malpractice.

Peer Review

"Peer review is the process by which nursing care delivered by a group of nurses or an individual nurse is evaluated by individuals of the same rank or standing according to established standards of practice" (Dunkley, 1973, p. 17). The process of *peer review* uses the standards of nursing practice as guidelines for evaluating the quantity and quality of nursing care.

The assessment factors within the standards of practice provide a mechanism for objective evaluation of the level of achievement for each standard. They also help develop criteria that may be used in the peer review process. The stages in the peer review process, as defined by Gold et al. (1973), are: (1) establishment of criteria by consensus, (2) self-evaluation utilizing the established criteria, and (3) group review. The first element in the process, the establishment of criteria, should be derived from the standards of nursing practice. This process forces one to identify specific nursing behaviors, which then must be accepted or ratified by other nurses. The ratification process provides the opportunity for a critical review of the criteria and an opportunity to share with others the expected and appropriate nurse behaviors. Self-evaluation provides for not only a self-assessment but a working knowledge of the criteria and an opportunity to identify those areas that require improvement. This step emphasizes personal accountability for one's actions and continued professional growth. Feedback from peers is obtained through group review. Usually one or two peers are asked to observe clinical performance and to review clinical documentation. The implementation of this step may vary, but the principle of peers providing feedback is the essence of peer review. Feedback promotes collaboration and validation and facilitates the structuring of personal growth and goal setting.

The advantages of peer review are many. The degree of peer collaboration and the analysis of the care rendered does much to enhance personal growth and to improve the quality of nursing care rendered. Peer review is a self-regulatory mechanism that should be used as a continual evaluation

*Autonomy has not been imposed on nurses. The nurse probably could
have remained safely within the protective shadow of medicine if such
behavior had not been contrary to the very nature of nursing. From the
beginning of modern nursing, the profession has struggled to gain
stature, and to provide the means for continuing intellectual growth that
would ensure the right and obligation of nurses to share in the expansion
of health services. Today, the professional nurse demands the right to
think and act responsibly and, in doing so, must and
does stand ready to be held accountable.*

I. MURCHISON, T. NICHOLS, AND R. HANSON (1978)

625

tool for professional nurses in any setting. It provides an impetus for individual professional growth and accountability and is a mechanism for evaluating and enhancing the quality of nursing care.

Peplau (1980) pointed out that "peer review is more essential in psychiatric nursing practice than in general practice because of the ambiguity of the field" (p. 132). Perhaps the most important aspects of peer review are the disclosure and assessment of clinical data from nurse-client relationships in a supervising review process in which nurse colleagues openly check each other's work. In such review it becomes possible to know whether a nurse is practicing in a way that fosters professional growth, clinical judgment, and personal control. By means of peer review it is possible to note whether the nurse is using theory in considering a range of nurse actions and in foreseeing the probable consequences of actions taken.

Professional Liability

The nurse is held responsible for her nursing judgments and actions and is responsible for the safety and well-being of designated clients receiving care. There are three important legal concepts that every nurse should be familiar with: malpractice, negligence, and liability. *Malpractice* is defined as "professional misconduct, an improper discharge of professional duties, or a failure to meet the standard of care by a professional which results in harm to another." *Negligence* is defined as "carelessness, failure to act as an ordinary prudent person, or action contrary to the conduct of a reasonable person." *Liability* is "an obligation one has incurred or might incur through any act or failure to act" (Cazalas, 1978, p. 258).

Although nurses are intellectually aware that a malpractice claim may arise in the course of their practice, most cannot imagine such an event happening to them personally. Many nurses believe that they are protected by their employer's insurance policy. While it is true that the employer may be liable for the actions of its employees (doctrine of respondent superior) and must therefore pay for damages incurred, there is no guaranty that the employer will not file a later claim against the negligent individual to recover damages paid. This practice, called *subrogating the claim*, is quite common.

In order for nurses to protect their professional careers, they should have professional liability insurance. Most people have insurance on possessions they consider valuable, such as jewelry, home, and automobile, but fail to consider their professional career as a valued possession. Professional liability insurance does not absolve accountability for actions; it simply means that the damages awarded in a liability suit are paid by the insurance company and not by the individual nurse. Most individuals would have difficulty paying for the awarded damages and legal fees. Malpractice insurance provides some protection if a suit is brought against an individual practitioner. The payment of damage awards is outlined in the individual policy. In general, liability insurance will pay for the attorney fees and for bond, if the latter is required during an appeal (Creighton, 1974).

Professional liability insurance policies usually consist of five parts: (1) the insurance agreement, (2) defense and settlement, (3) period of coverage, (4) amount payable, and (5) conditions (Cazalas, 1978). The insurance agreement is basically that the insurer will pay all sums of money up to the policy

CLINICAL VIGNETTE

PROFESSIONAL LIABILITY

John Noth sought admission to a hospital's emergency room where he was well known. Mr. Noth had been discharged the previous day from one of the hospital's psychiatric units. He was seen by Mrs. Warren, one of the registered nurses, for an initial assessment. Mr. Noth stated that he wanted to kill himself. Mrs. Warren noted that both the client's arms had superficial scratches, which he said he put there with a piece of broken glass. Mrs. Warren documented that Mr. Noth was agitated, had rambling, slurred speech, became loud, and cursed frequently during the initial assessment process.

When Mrs. Warren completed her interview, she asked the client to wait for the physician in the emergency room receiving area. Mr. Noth left the examining room and went to the receiving area. The nurse then paged for the psychiatrist on duty to report to emergency. Left unattended in the receiving area, Mr. Noth walked out of the hospital onto a busy street and was hit by an automobile; he died at the scene.

1. At which point did Mrs. Warren fail to use good judgment? When she left Mr. Noth and did not arrange to have him observed by anyone in her absence.

2. Was Mrs. Warren negligent? Yes, because the client stated he wanted to kill himself. She noted this in the medical record but took no precaution to observe or have someone observe the client. With the client's presenting complaints and his behavior during the interview process, the nurse was negligent and her actions were not those of a "reasonable" person.

limit for the insured in cases in which he or she becomes legally liable. The defense and settlement section states that the insurer will defend the insured in any case brought against him or her as a consequence of his or her nursing services. The insurance company also has the power to obtain a settlement prior to the case going to trial.

The insurance contract covers a specified period of coverage. Policy coverage can be either "occurrence" or "claims made." *Occurrence* covers the insured for lawsuits that stem from any incidents that occur during the time of the policy coverage. For example, if a person was insured during an incident in 1980 but the malpractice suit was not filed until 1983 when the person was no longer insured, the person would still be covered since the incident occurred during the time when the policy was active. With *claims made* coverage, the person is insured for any claim that is filed during the policy time frame. If a lapse in coverage occurs, the person is not covered for any events that happen during the lapse in coverage. In this situation the nurse should check on the statute of limitations for client claims for his or her respective state (Trandel-Korenchuk and Trandel-Korenchuk, 1980).

The amount payable to the injured party will be no more than the maximum coverage stated in the policy. If the awarded damages are more than the policy's maximum coverage, the individual must pay the difference.

In the conditions section of the insurance policy, the responsibility of the insured to notify the insurance company is spelled out. If there is any indication that a suit may be filed or that an actual injury has occurred, it is the responsibility of the insured to notify the insurance company. There is usually a clause concerning the cooperation of the insured in working with the insurance company. Also included is a clause concerning changes in the policy and cancellation of the policy.

Nurses must realize that they are accountable for their actions at all times. If nurses are provided with liability coverage by their employing agency, they must realize that the coverage is only for the time they are at work. There is no coverage for nonwork hours in which individuals may be volunteering their time to community activities or when a neighbor may seek their help. Individual professional liability insurance provides a broader coverage.

Although there is no foolproof way of avoiding the chance of being sued, adherence to nursing standards of practice is one way to decrease the likelihood. No one is totally immune, but knowledge of the facility's policies and procedures and the use of sound nursing judgment will help protect the nurse from litigation and assure clients of the highest quality nursing care.

ADVOCACY

Despite general efforts on the part of health professionals and the legal system to safeguard the rights of clients, several issues specific to mental health clients have yet to be addressed. Clients with histories of psychiatric illness have begun to bring violations of their rights by care providers and insti-

Public access to medical records is increasing in a dramatic way. . . .
Documentation of patient care is the principal way in which
governmental agencies approach the cost-cutting solutions to escalating
hospital costs. . . . Private, nongovernmental third party payors are
responding to sky-high hospital costs by probing into patients' charts to
determine what the record reveals as to the quantity and quality of patient
care. All of this authorized invasion of the once-privileged precincts of
medical records means that such charts must now be clean as hounds'
teeth in terms of accurate documentation. No room for conspiracy, no
room for cover ups, no "professional lies," no justification for the old
adage, "What the public doesn't know won't hurt 'em."
WILLIAM A. REGAN (1983)

627

tutional policies to the attention of legislators, attorneys, and the general public. One of their main grievances is that they are not given the legal representation they require. Prior to a commitment hearing, legal counsel is appointed without the client's consent or knowledge. Such appointed attorneys are often poorly prepared because of lack of time to confer with the client, lack of competence in mental health law, and limited commitment to the client's interests.

Similarly, psychiatrists are called in on short notice to evaluate clients whom they have not previously seen. Their assessment is often made on the basis of a short interview. Yet their judgments and subsequent recommendations are seldom questioned or challenged. Because the appointed lawyer lacks mental health law expertise, his or her only recourse is usually to defer to the psychiatrist. Thus, the client's welfare is placed in the hands of one individual, whose competency in assessing the client may be limited or compromised.

As a result of these and other problems, concerned citizens, health professionals, and even institutions have begun to participate in the client advocacy movement. Concerned individuals and organizations have joined forces to see that care providers, the legal system, and clients themselves join in safeguarding the rights of mental health clients. Many hospitals and health care agencies philosophically or financially support the existence of formal client advocacy systems. People functioning within these formal systems are charged with: (1) informing clients of their rights, (2) advocating and protecting those clients whose rights have been violated, and (3) fostering a public perception of mental health clients that accepts their capacity to

challenge the status quo of the health care system and to defend their civil rights.

The Nurse as Client Advocate

"Client advocacy" and "nurse as advocate" are certainly not new terms in nursing. The need for someone to act on the behalf of clients, as well as the feasibility of the nurse's assumption of this role, has emerged as a significant issue in psychiatric nursing. There is no general agreement, however, as to what exactly the advocate's role should be or even as to whether the nurse should act as the client's advocate.

The definition of *client advocacy* within nursing ranges from a broad philosophical interpretation to a more narrow, concrete definition with legal and political implications. Curtin (1979b), for example, defined advocacy as the very essence of nursing. She viewed it as the foundation upon which the nurse and client determine the form of their relationship—child-parent, client-counselor, friend-friend, colleague-colleague, and so on. She suggested that the ideal of advocacy is based on the commonality of the rights and needs of both client and nurse.

Mauksch (1980) emphasized that the true advocate appreciates the holism of the individual and the uniqueness of each individual's needs. If one is truly a client advocate, one will respect the total integrity of the client—mind, body, and spirit—and will put the needs expressed by the client above the needs of care providers, institutions, significant others, and oneself. While client needs may not always be rational in the eyes of others, they are real to the client and should receive the utmost patience and tact. This position is clearly derived from society's

There are three things which a nurse ought to possess to fulfill her professional duties, to respect the rights of others and to be the sort of nurse she herself would require. The first is character, the second professional knowledge, and the third sufficient professional skill. With these three qualifications the nurse can give due service. Without any one of them, she cannot be just to others as a nurse, not give to them the sort of service she herself would expect.

A. FAGOTHY (1963)

628

basic ethical values of protection of individuality and autonomy.

Some nurses have viewed client advocacy more concretely, as a way of defining the structure of the relationship that exists between the client and the nurse. Brower (1983) defined advocacy as a political process that directs its activities toward redistributing the power and resources to the individual or group that has a demonstrated need. Thollaug (1980) similarly defined advocacy as a type of reform movement that seeks to structure the client-nurse relationship strictly according to the expressed interests of the client. Both Brower and Thollaug have argued that forces other than client interests currently determine the power distribution in provider-client encounters. Financial reimbursement for providers, the bureaucracy behind today's health care delivery, and the medical dominance of health care all contribute to provider-centered priorities as opposed to client-centered priorities. This situation automatically predisposes the client to physical, emotional, and financial vulnerability. Advocacy as a defined role is an effective way to offer the client protection from such vulnerability.

In strictest legal terms, advocacy is "the act of defending or pleading the case of another." This definition represents the traditional role of the legal defense counselor—the practice of law within the defense of individual legal rights (Durel, 1981). Kohnke (1980) has offered a parallel definition for nursing as the act of informing and supporting a client, who can then make the best possible decisions. Two actions of the advocate are implied here: (1) informing the client of exactly what his rights are and supplying the client with information sufficient

to make an informed decision, and (2) supporting the client once a decision has been made.

While nursing viewpoints on advocacy vary, all embody the tenets and philosophy undergirding many conceptual frameworks of nursing practice. These frameworks have traditionally emphasized the concept of advocacy without specifically describing it. Holism of the individual, the promulgation of client-centered interaction, and protection of the client's autonomy in determining her health state and in choosing measures to restore, maintain, or advance that health state—all are elements of advocacy that have been described and supported by various conceptual views on nursing practice (Nightingale, 1860; Hall, 1966; Levine, 1971; Cox, 1982).

Thus, in principle, the concept of advocacy has long been an integral part of the practice of nursing. As the principles of client advocacy become more visible, they are increasingly subject to intra- and extra-professional scrutiny and to legal interpretation. As a consequence, issues and controversies related to the nurse's assumption of the formal client advocate role have emerged and broadened.

THE PROS AND CONS OF THE NURSE AS CLIENT ADVOCATE Although most nurses agree in principle that the nurse should be the client's advocate, they are divided as to whether the nurse should assume a formal advocate role with clients. Those who would champion the formalized advocate role argue that the nursing profession is particularly well suited to assume this role. First, nurses spend more time with clients than do any other providers and thus are afforded more potential opportunities to learn about the clients as individuals, noting their

CLINICAL VIGNETTE

THE NURSE AS ADVOCATE

A number of clients in a mental hygiene day clinic were concerned that their group sessions had become less effective because of the simultaneous participation by several nursing students. While the clients welcomed the students' participation in general, they felt that the introduction of more than one student per session significantly altered the context and character of the group process. The nurse/group leader asked permission from group members to serve as spokesperson to the faculty member in charge of the students. The nurse promised to express their concerns exactly as they were presented and to report the results of the discussion with the faculty member at the next group session.

In this example, the nurse was taking a direct advocacy action in that she was serving as the group representative to express concerns on a matter that had implications for institutional policy and practice. If the nurse had arranged a meeting to allow direct confrontation between the faculty person and the clients themselves, it would have been an act of indirect advocacy.

concerns, strengths, and limitations. Second, nurses have traditionally emphasized client teaching as a primary professional function. In the teaching role, nurses provide clients with knowledge sufficient to enable them to make informed decisions about their health care. This, of course, is a primary function of the advocate (Kohnke, 1980; Thollaug, 1980).

An additional argument for nurses' assumption of the advocate role comes from their position as employees of a specific agency or institution. Internal advocates, as opposed to advocates outside the institution, have a number of advantages. They have greater access to information about the client and are more familiar with the inner workings of the institution or agency. At the same time, they may be seen as a lesser threat to administrators than external advocates would (Willetts, 1980).

A final point that provides support for the nurse as advocate is economic. Nursing services within agencies and institutions are, for the most part, not directly reimbursable. Decisions that clients make regarding their health status do not serve as financial incentives for the nurse. Unlike the physician or the attorney, therefore, the nurse in the advocate role is more likely to be client-centered rather than provider-centered (Thollaug, 1980). Decisions are more likely to be made for the benefit of the client rather than to enhance any benefits for the provider.

The same arguments presented as supportive of the nurse as client advocate have been suggested by others to be the very reasons why nurses should *not* assume the advocate role. For example, the fact that the nurse is with the client more than other providers are is thought to set up a dependent relationship that negates the intent of the advocacy role. If the client has to depend on the nurse for basic care, it would seem that clients would come to rely on the nurse for extensive decision making. Because the role of advocate is enacted in order to enable the individual to make independent decisions, potential for conflict between the nurse and client is increased and the risk of invading a client's rights is exacerbated when nurses assume advocacy roles (Castledine, 1981).

A second argument against the nurse as advocate is based on educational background. Most nurses have an inadequate knowledge base to support the formalized role of conservator or legal advisor. Although increasing numbers of nurses are preparing themselves for joint nursing-legal careers, they remain in the minority. General nursing education simply has not prepared nurses to enact a formalized advocate role that assumes legal expertise.

A third factor that makes the nurse an undesirable client advocate is that clients would have no choice of who would act as their advocate. If the advocacy role is to be assumed by the nurse charged with the client's primary nursing care—independent of client input—the client's rights have already been violated.

The final argument against the nurse as advocate comes from the constraints placed on the nurse by the institution or authority who employs him or her (Castledine, 1981). Very often the major functions of advocacy are antagonistic to the institution. The advocate often acts as "informer" and is labeled a troublemaker or insubordinate if he or she supports the client in a decision that is contrary to the thinking of other health care providers or the institution.

CHARACTERISTICS AND RESPONSIBILITIES OF THE MENTAL HEALTH CLIENT ADVOCATE Despite controversies over the nurse's general assumption of the advocate role, advocacy as a psychiatric nursing function has been clearly described. The psychiatric nurse's advocacy role is not only to defend client rights but to monitor the safety of services rendered to mental health clients. Durel (1981) sees the advocacy role for mental health nurses as a logical blending of professional, legal, and ethical responsibilities. For example, the mental health nurse should monitor whether:

1. Clients' medications are being reduced in order to determine lowest maintenance dosages.

2. Treatment plans are periodically evaluated for their contribution to the patient's well-being.

3. Alternatives to hospitalization are being offered to clients and their families.

4. Safeguards are being provided for those clients who may be unable to communicate effectively.

5. Clients are routinely informed of the potential side effects of psychotropic drugs.

6. Diagnostic labels are used as therapeutic tools rather than applied for bureaucratic or administrative reasons.

Durel has proposed that the mental health nurse as client advocate assumes two types of functions: direct and indirect. *Direct* advocacy includes those actions taken by the nurse to speak as the client's representative to those who have control over the client's treatment. *Indirect* advocacy refers to those nursing actions that place the client in a favorable position to speak for himself to those having the power to satisfy his needs or interests.

In keeping with the basic philosophical tenets of nursing practice, indirect advocacy or a combination of direct and indirect advocacy is often preferred to direct advocacy. Direct advocacy is reserved for those situations that (1) reflect institutional practices or policy, (2) cannot be addressed by the client because of emotional or cognitive limitations, (3) would be ineffectively addressed by the client because of lack of social power, or (4) would potentially elicit negative interpersonal responses from those holding power, resulting in loss of self-esteem for the client (Durel, 1981).

Cautions Relative to the Advocacy Role

Caution must be exercised by the mental health nurse in executing the advocacy role. Advocacy acts can be in direct conflict with the traditional image of nursing as a discipline that offers professional ex-

pertise. Professional education and experience tend to reinforce the image of "experts" who know what is best for the client and who are paid to make clinically relevant decisions. The tendency, then, is to make decisions *for* the psychiatric client as opposed to supporting the client in making his or her own decisions. Making choices for the client not only violates his or her rights but also places the nurse in the position of being blamed if the choice turns out to have been a poor one (Kohnke, 1980).

Another caution concerning advocacy is the potential for conflict of values between the mental health nurse and the client. To faithfully represent the rights and interests of clients without interjecting a personal set of values is difficult, at best. Mauksch (1980) pointed out that at times "fending for" can easily lead to "control of." The mental health nurse must continually ask whether actions taken as advocate represent the interests of the client or actually reflect his or her own personal biases and perspectives on the issue.

Clearly, there will be times when clients make decisions that are in direct opposition to the values of the nurse. If possible, however, it is the client's values that should prevail. When compromise is essential to protect the client's health and well-being, the compromise that is most acceptable to the client should be the one enacted.

THE MENTAL HEALTH NURSE AS CHANGE AGENT

The mental health nurse is in a position to create a climate that supports the rights and needs of psychiatric clients and to institute progressive change. Although nurses have been most comfortable in activities that are directly client centered, they are beginning to move into activities that reflect broader social and political influences. Advocacy includes not only addressing the rights and needs of individual clients but engaging in activities at the local, community, state, and national levels as well.

The effective advocate must develop expert communication skills. Through the written and spoken word, the mental health nurse can amass support for psychiatric clients' rights and bring pressure to bear on influential governmental and community agencies (Brower, 1982). Media publicity can be a tool for nurse advocates, because newspapers, television, and news magazines reach large audiences and have the potential to generate support on significant issues.

Mental health nurse advocates can influence legislative bodies through such activities as public relations work and door-to-door visiting to disseminate information on specific mental health issues. Sending letters to community, state, and national legislators, appearing at public hearings, and even participating in litigation proceedings can be part of the advocacy role (Brower, 1982). Being familiar with the legislative process, obtaining copies of bill drafts for review, and making presentations at state and federal hearings are additional ways mental health nurses can function as effective change agents.

Mental health nurse advocates should actively seek membership on community committees or councils that recommend or formulate policy. Local health systems agencies and state health care coordinating councils are powerful policy change groups; local and state mental health boards are further channels for making advocacy issues known. Some communities have developed ombudsman systems that serve as an advocacy mechanism; mental health nurses should acquaint themselves with the leadership of these groups and strive to obtain membership or influence. In these ways the nurse can work formally or informally as a community organizer for the mental health client's rights and needs.

SUMMARY

The practice of mental health nursing involves an interplay of ethical values, clients' rights, and legal issues. Nurses have obligations to society, to their profession, to their clients, and to themselves. Achieving the proper balance among these obligations necessitates a knowledge of clients' rights, of the responsibilities of institutions, of the use of restrictive treatments, and of the implications for nursing in these areas.

Because the care of mentally ill clients can be overwhelmingly complex, nurses need to be aware of their professional accountability and liability when working with these clients. The Standards of Psychiatric and Mental Health Nursing Practice and the peer review process are necessary for establishing guidelines and promoting excellence in care of mentally ill clients.

The complexity of the health care system dictates the need for advocates for clients, especially those who are mentally ill. While there are conflicting views about the amount of involvement that nurses should have in client advocacy, most nurses find themselves in a position of helping clients in obtaining the best care available. It is imperative that nurses be aware of the various roles that they may perform in this capacity. Perhaps the most powerful and influential of these roles is that of change agent, promoting change in the larger arena

of health care, thereby ultimately benefiting the individual client.

Review Questions

1. What is the purpose of the ANA Code for Nurses?

2. What are the major responsibilities of an institution or agency in delineating clients' rights?

3. Under what circumstances would detention of a client be considered false imprisonment?

4. How or when is the use of restraints considered a violation of the client's rights?

5. Under what conditions might a nurse be sued for administering the correct medication to a client?

6. What is the purpose of the standards of practice?

7. What are the three components of the peer review process?

8. What is the difference between malpractice and negligence?

9. List three arguments for nurses to *not* assume the client advocate role.

10. Identify four ways in which mental health nurses can serve as change agents to formulate mental health policies and address mental health issues.

631

References

American Hospital Association. 1975. *A Patient's Bill of Rights.* Chicago: American Hospital Association.

American Nurses' Association. 1973. *Standards of Psychiatric Mental Health Nursing Practice.* Kansas City, Mo.: American Nurses' Association.

American Nurses' Association. 1976. *Code for Nurses with Interpretive Statements.* Kansas City, Mo.: American Nurses' Association.

Appelbaum, P., and Gutheil, T. 1980. Drug Refusal: A Study of Psychiatric Inpatients. *American Journal of Psychiatry,* 137:340–345.

Arkin, H. 1983. Forcible Administration of Antipsychotic Medication. *Journal of American Medical Association,* 249:2784–2785.

Bandman, B. 1978. Some Remarks on the Mentally Disabled Patient's Right to Receive and Refuse Treatment. *Issues in Mental Health Nursing,* Winter: 46–50.

Brower, H. 1982. Advocacy: What Is It? *Journal of Gerontological Nursing,* 8:141–143.

Carroll, M. A. 1980. The Right to Treatment and Involuntary Commitment. *The Journal of Medicine and Philosophy,* 5:278–290.

Castledine, G. 1981. The Nurse as the Patient's Advocate: Pros and Cons. *Nursing Mirror,* 153:38–40.

Cazalas, M. W. 1978. *Nursing and The Law,* 3rd ed. Rockville, Md.: Aspen Systems.

Chinn, P., and Jacobs, M. 1983. *Theory and Nursing: A Systematic Approach.* St. Louis: C. V. Mosby.

Colvard, R. 1967. Interaction and Identification in Reporting Field Research: A Critical Reconsideration of Protective Procedures. In *Ethics, Politics, and Social Research*, ed. G. Sjoberg. Cambridge, Mass.: Schenkman.

Cox, C. 1982. An Interaction Model of Client Health Behavior: Theoretical Prescription for Nursing. *Advances in Nursing Science*, 5:46–57.

Creighton, H. 1974. *Law Every Nurse Should Know*. Philadelphia: W. B. Saunders.

Curtin, L. 1979a. Clarity and Freedom: Ethical Issues in Mental Health. *Issues in Mental Health Nursing*, 2:102–108.

Curtin, L. 1979b. The Nurse as Advocate: A Philosophical Foundation for Nursing. *Advances in Nursing Science*, 1:1–10.

Davis, J. 1978. The Ethics of Behavior Control: The Nurse as Double Agent. *Issues in Mental Health Nursing*, Winter: 2–16.

Dunkley, P. 1973. Accountability: The Implications. *South Carolina Nursing*, 21:7–21.

Durel, S. 1981. Advocacy: A Function of the Community Mental Health Nurse. *Virginia Nurse*, 49:33–36.

Fagothy, A. 1963. *Right and Reason*. St. Louis: C. V. Mosby.

Gold, H.; Jackson, M.; and Sachs, B. 1973. Peer Review: A Working Experiment. *Nursing Outlook*, 21:634–636.

Hall, L. 1966. Another View of Nursing Care and Quality. In *Community of Patient Care: The Role of Nursing*, eds. K. Staub and K. Parker. Washington, D.C.: Catholic University Press.

Joint Commission on Accreditation of Hospitals. 1983. *Consolidated Standards Manual/83 for Child, Adolescent, and Adult Psychiatric, Alcoholism and Drug Abuse Facilities*. Chicago: Joint Commission on Accreditation of Hospitals.

Kohnke, M. 1980. The Nurse as Advocate. *American Journal of Nursing*, 80:2038–2040.

Levine, M. 1971. Holistic Nursing. In *The Nursing Clinics of North America*, eds. L. Germain and G. Alfano. Philadelphia: W. B. Saunders.

Mauksch, I. 1980. Advocacy or Control: Which Do We Offer the Elderly? *Geriatric Nursing*, 1:278.

Michels, R. 1981. The Right to Refuse Treatment: Ethical Issues. *Hospital and Community Psychiatry*, 32:251–255.

Miller, R. D. 1982. The Least Restrictive Alternative: Hidden Meanings and Agendas. *Community Mental Health Journal*, 18:46–55.

Murchison, I.; Nichols, T.; and Hanson, R. 1978. *Legal Accountability in the Nursing Process*. St. Louis: C. V. Mosby.

Nightingale, F. 1860. *Notes on Nursing*. New York: Appleton.

Peplau, H. 1980. The Psychiatric Nurse Accountable? To Whom? For What? *Perspectives in Psychiatric Care*, 18: 128–134.

Regan, W. 1980. Force-Medicating the Mental Patient: Assault. *The Regan Report on Nursing Law*, 20(11).

Regan, W. 1981a. Mental Patients and Forced Medication. *The Regan Report on Nursing Law*, 21(10).

Regan, W. 1981b. N.J.: No Forced Meds for Mental Patients. *The Regan Report on Nursing Law*, 22(6).

Regan, W. 1983. *The Regan Report on Nursing Law*, 24(7):1.

Roth, L. H. 1980. Mental Health Commitment: The State of the Debate. *Hospital and Community Psychiatry*, 31:385–395.

Tancredi, L. R. 1980. The Rights of Mental Patients: Weighing the Interests. *Journal of Health, Politics, Policy and Law*, 5:199–204.

Thollaug, S. 1980. The Nurse as Patient Advocate. *Imprint*, 27:37+.

Tischler, G., and Astrachan, B. 1982. *Quality Assurance in Mental Health: Peer and Utilization Review*. Rockville, Md.: National Institute of Mental Health.

Trandel-Korenchuk, D., and Trandel-Korenchuk, K. 1980. Current Legal Issues Facing Nursing Practice. *Nursing Administration Quarterly*, 5(1):37–45.

Watson, A. 1982. Informed Consent of Special Subjects. *Nursing Research*, 31:43–47.

Willetts, R. 1980. Advocacy and the Mentally Ill. *Social Work*, 25:372–377.

Supplementary Readings

Appelbaum, P. S. Refusing Treatment: The Uncertainty Continues. *Hospital and Community Psychiatry*, 34(1983): 11–12.

Barry, A. The Importance of Mental Health Advocacy. *Psychosocial Rehabilitation Journal*, 6(1983):35–41.

Bellamy, C. Political Advocacy for the Chronic Mental Disabled. *Psychosocial Rehabilitation Journal*, 4(1980): 7–11.

Berg, W. E. Working with Physically Handicapped Patients: Advocacy in a Nursing Home. *Health and Social Work*, 6(1981):26–32.

Bullough, B. *The Law and the Expanding Nursing Role*. New York: Appleton-Century-Crofts, 1980.

Curtin, L. Should We Feed Baby Doe? *Nursing Management*, 15(1984):22–28.

Cushing, M. Wronged Rights in Nursing Homes. *American Journal of Nursing*, 84(1984):1213–1218.

Davidhizar, R. Can the Client with Chronic Schizophrenia Consent to Nursing Research? *Journal of Advanced Nursing*, 9(1984):381–390.

Donnelly, G. F. *The Nursing System: Issues, Ethics and Politics*. New York: John Wiley & Sons, 1980.

Fasano, M. A. The Long-Term Care Ombudsman. *Journal of Gerontological Nursing*, 6(1980):717–720.

Jameton, A. *Nursing Practice: The Ethical Issues*. Englewood Cliffs, N.J.: Prentice-Hall, 1984.

Jolly, H. Have Parents the Right to See Their Children's Medical Reports? *Archives of Disease in Childhood*, 59(1984):601–602.

Laben, J. K., and MacLean, C. P. *Legal Issues and Guidelines for Nurses Who Care for the Mentally Ill*. Thorofare, N.J.: Charles Slack, 1983.

Slack, A. Killing and Allowing to Die in Medical Practice. *Journal of Medical Ethics*, 10(1984):82–87.

Taub, S. Psychiatric Malpractice in the 1980s: Some Areas of Concern. *Law, Medicine and Health Care*, 11(1983): 97–103.

Thompson, I. E., and Thompson, H. O. *Ethics in Nursing*. New York: Macmillan, 1981.

632

NURSING AND THE DRGs
Historical Perspectives
The Yale Study
Implications for Nursing

NURSING AND QUALITY ASSURANCE
Components of Quality Assurance
Establishing a Quality Assurance Program

NURSING RESEARCH
Historical Perspectives
The Research Process
The Importance of Writing

C   H   A   P   T   E   R

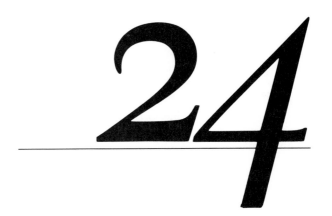

Trends and Research in Nursing

Learning Objectives

After studying this chapter, the student should be able to:

1. Trace the development of the prospective payment system for health care and describe its implications for nursing.

2. Discuss the implementation and utilization of a quality assurance program in nursing.

3. Discuss clinical opportunities for nursing research.

4. Compare and contrast experimental, quasi-experimental, and survey designs for research.

5. Describe the direction of nursing research in mental health.

634

Overview

Health care delivery in the United States has become problematic and controversial. Costs are spiraling and access to care is unequally distributed. Changes are being demanded on a national basis, and the nursing profession is now in a position to influence these changes and to advance its standing as a profession while offering greater benefits to health consumers. There are many avenues open to nurses to accomplish these tasks. This chapter describes several areas that must receive attention if nurses are to establish the relevance and the credibility of the profession. One such area is the institution of prospective payment for health care based on Diagnostic Related Groups (DRGs), which will have a decided influence on health care delivery. In addition, nursing must continually and thoroughly evaluate its own functioning through appropriate and comprehensive quality assurance programs. The basis for quality assurance programs and for self-evaluation within nursing must be careful and thorough development and use of clinical and laboratory research by nurses, so as to advance the body of knowledge that is nursing theory and practice.

He who ascends to mountain tops shall find
The loftiest peaks most wrapt in clouds and snow.
LORD BYRON

635

NURSING AND THE DRGS

On April 20, 1983, President Ronald Reagan signed into law H.R. 1900 (P.L. 98-21), the Social Security Amendments of 1983. This legislation established a *prospective payment system* that allows for pretreatment diagnosis billing categories. This legislation will permanently alter the nature of health care delivery and is hoped to help resolve the long-standing problem of rising health care costs.

Historical Perspectives

The trend toward uncontrolled cost expansion for health care can be traced back to the 1940s. In 1946, the Hill-Burton program provided for postwar replenishment of hospital facilities. The institution of Medicare and Medicaid in the 1960s encouraged utilization of hospital facilities. Third-party payers, such as Blue Cross and Blue Shield, provided few incentives for cost containment. Everyone in the health care system became aware that the patient would not be paying for the majority of the expenses incurred.

In the 1960s and 1970s hospital costs continued to rise at a higher rate than general inflation. In the 1980s hospital costs have increased 12.6 percent while general inflation has dropped to 3.9 percent. There have been no effective limits on costs that are reimbursed, since hospitals are guaranteed payment without having to worry about cost containment. Payments are made retroactively, after the client has received the care. The more a hospital spends, the more money it receives from third-party payers. The sky is the limit, and hospitals have taken full advantage of this opportunity for profit making (Shaffer, 1983).

The 1970s saw some attempts at cost containment, with efforts focused on regulating the cost per day of hospital stay. However, these methods still encouraged longer lengths of stay in hospitals. The time was at hand for reform of the system rather than attempts at regulation.

The Yale Study

The concept of *Diagnostic Related Groups* (DRGs) was developed at Yale University in the late 1960s and early 1970s (Shaffer, 1984a, 1984b). The primary purpose was to define types of cases that could be expected to receive similar amounts of services from the hospital. The length of stay (LOS) was used as a measure of hospital services.

DRGs were an attempt to define the "product" of the health care industry, which had not been done previously. The Yale group defined this product as a set of services, or "outputs," received by clients, such as hours of nursing care, medications, and laboratory tests. The "inputs," or costs, of these services are labor (including salaries), materials, and equipment. The box on page 636 provides definitions of terms that are necessary for understanding the DRG system.

The hospital output is conceptualized as hospital products that can be as extensive as the number of clients. The particular product is defined as the diagnosis. Some "products" or diagnoses require more resources than others and are more complex and expensive. The proportions of the various types of cases treated by a hospital is called its "case mix."

Currently there are 467 DRG categories into

DRG TERMINOLOGY

■ *Diagnostic Related Groups (DRGs)*. A client classification scheme in which client types are defined by the client's diagnosis, procedures, age, sex, and discharge status. Each DRG ordinarily requires approximately equal resource consumption measured by length of stay and cost.

■ *Case mix*. Proportion of various types of cases (diagnoses) in a particular hospital.

■ *Prospective payment system (PPS)*. Payment rates set in advance and considered fixed for a certain period of time.

■ *Trim points*. Range of usual length of stay for a particular DRG.

■ *Outliers*. Client cases falling outside the range of the trim points.

636

which each case can be classified, based on the primary diagnosis responsible for the hospitalizations, the treatment procedure, the discharge status, and the client's age and sex. DRGs rely on discharge abstracts, and assignment to a DRG is dependent on the documentation of the physician. The performance of surgery usually categorizes a client into a more complex DRG.

With DRGs, payment for inpatient costs is based on a fixed amount, determined in advance for each case, depending on the diagnostic group. This payment is considered payment in full. If the treatment costs the hospital less than the DRG allotment, the hospital keeps the extra as profit. If the treatment costs more than the specified rate, the hospital must absorb the loss. Because hospitals vary in their expertise in different categories, some DRGs will make money and some will lose money for specific hospitals.

The DRG system is expected to provide incentives for efficiency and to decrease demand for inpatient hospital services. Although the length of stay is not as accurate an indicator as actual costs, it is being used because of its practical availability at a time when cost cutting is required on a near-emergency basis (Plomann and Shaffer, 1983).

Implications for Nursing

All nurses should be educated about the prospective payment system. Traditionally, nurses have performed their duties with very little thought about the cost of their care. It will be difficult for some nurses to become cost conscious and think of their services with a dollar value.

The first task of nursing under the system of DRGs will be to define essential nursing services under reduced financial conditions. Monies will become less available, and nurses will be faced with justifying the necessity of nursing care to top management. Within hospitals, the nursing service is the largest portion of the hospital's budget. As a result, nursing will be vulnerable to cost-containment policies. As the DRG method of reimbursement is implemented, nurses will be called upon to operate more efficiently while still providing quality client care. Nurses will need good negotiation skills to ensure that resources are obtained for nursing. Up until this time, specific costs of nursing services have never been clearly identified. There will be a growing need to document the cost of nursing care. Nursing services are currently included in overhead costs, but there is evidence that nursing departments will be required to justify costs according to the client's acuity, which must correlate with the client's DRG.

At present, research is being conducted to develop an appropriate patient classification system. The most notable of these is the RIM (relative intensity measures) methodology. RIMs are cost-allocation statistics that specifically relate a client's consumption of nursing resources to the client's medical condition. Nursing resources are minutes of nursing care that a client reserves. Relative intensity increases as more nursing resources are used; as the RIMs increase, so does the cost. While RIMs are still in the experimental stage, the method provides a better measure of nursing care than does the per diem method.

Without a workable and meaningful client classification system, the control of staffing and budget

We cannot predict with any certainty what the future of health care will be. We cannot assume either a medical holocaust or a health nirvana. We can, however, assume that America's future will depend on better use of resources, and that fuller use of the nation's human resources will be related to the health of those resources. If nurses are to play a positive role in shaping the future, then nursing must be in the forefront of policymaking.

JIM BINDER (1983)

637

could easily be removed from nursing's control. Without appropriate data, decisions may be made by others about nursing practice that could have far-reaching, detrimental consequences (Hamilton, 1983). Nurses should be members of hospital budget committees, as their understanding of clients' needs mandates that nursing be involved in the planning of the distribution of hospital resources.

Nurses must begin to focus more intensively on the discharge planning process. Because the prospective payment system rewards efficiency, efforts will be made to discharge the client as soon as possible. Effective discharge planning can be an effective means of monitoring quality client care. Discharge planning will be improved by a system which dictates that length of stay is understood at the time of admission. Nurses must become responsible for educating the client and the family at the time of admission about the length of stay and discharge.

Decentralization should be considered by nursing departments. A decentralized structure will diminish the demands made on nursing administration and allow more time for focusing on hospital-wide policy issues. Decentralization moves decision-making authority down the organization and involves staff nurses in making decisions about client care, which often results in greater productivity, more commitment, and better morale.

Nurse managers need to develop skills in all management areas. They need to learn staffing and scheduling skills, with special attention to client acuity; they need to learn cost control and budget preparation; and they need to use the full potential of their staff and develop unit and individual objec-

tives. First-time nurse managers are the key figures in facing the challenges of the prospective payment system.

Nurses need to become acquainted with the use of computer information systems. Nurses gather and generate large amounts of data that need to be utilized accurately and appropriately. Statistics are needed to prepare meaningful reports to top management.

Finally, nursing services must take steps to control nursing staff involvement in nonnursing functions. Under DRGs, nursing services will lose money when providing services other than direct client care. Nonnursing duties should be delegated to appropriate staff.

Hospitals are the primary employers of nurses. Unless nurses can begin to quantify their contribution to client care, autonomy for nursing will not become a reality. If nurses can demonstrate that hospitals can provide quality client care within budget restrictions, nursing will become the key ally for hospital management, and nursing will acquire an increasingly greater responsibility for coordinating client care.

NURSING AND QUALITY ASSURANCE

Because of their continuous contact with clients on a 24-hour basis, nurses should be the leaders in quality assurance. Changes caused by the implementation of DRGs must be monitored to assure that the quality of care is not reduced. It is hoped that clients who really need care will receive it and that ones who do not need care, will not. The nursing department can emphasize its commitment to quality

*As an evaluative endeavor, quality assurance encompasses both
obtaining measurements based on predetermined criteria for the purpose
of decision making and acting on that information by introducing
change directed toward the improvement of patient care. Quality
assurance is more than assessment, more than a review. It adds the
actions component of attempting to "make care better." Making
care better may mean making nursing care more effective,
economical and efficient.*

U. E. WESTFALL (1980)

638

client care by implementing and utilizing a strong quality assurance program.

Quality assurance programs began to develop in the early 1970s as a result of government requirements for evaluating client care in facilities that used Medicare and Medicaid funds. The programs of Professional Standards Review Organizations (PSROs) and Utilization Review required hospitals to show appropriate use of resources. The Joint Commission on Accreditation of Hospitals (JCAH) also established a requirement that a minimum number of chart audits be done to show evidence of quality of care provided. Currently, there is no requirement that a specific number of audits be done; each facility determines its own type of quality assurance activity. In order to receive accreditation by JCAH, hospitals must simply have a program that is designed to solve client care problems (Larsen, 1983).

Components of Quality Assurance

Quality assurance is a systematic inquiry designed to evaluate client care and to identify, study, and correct deficiencies in the client care process. Quality assurance activities are usually aimed at solving immediate problems, and they rely on use of descriptive data. The primary purpose is to change and improve nursing practice. Quality assurance should not be rigid; there is no right or wrong way to utilize the concept. It can be used to solve everyday problems, to provide data to promote change in procedure and policy, to provide feedback, and to develop a basis for decision making.

Frequently, quality assurance activities focus on two areas: (1) problem solving (such as performance of nonnursing duties), and (2) monitoring the achievement of a standard (such as following protocols for isolation techniques). When quality assurance studies are done, some aspect of client care is assessed, a written record is kept of the results, and some action is taken to either maintain the appropriate care or correct the deficiencies.

The American Nurses' Association (1982) has proposed a conceptual model of quality assurance that provides an overall philosophy and framework. There are five steps in this model:

1. Designing the study.
2. Establishing the criteria.
3. Gathering the data.
4. Interpreting the data.
5. Taking action.

According to this framework, the process can be entered at any step. If nurses know that a problem exists and have already discovered a possible solution, emphasis should be placed on step 5. After taking action, it may be appropriate to start at step 1 to evaluate the effectiveness of the action. If a study is repeated, the effort goes into the data collecting, interpretation, and action (steps 3, 4, and 5). In other cases, all steps may require a great deal of time and commitment, especially if the problem is great and the topic difficult to define. By using this five-step process, nurses can become more familiar with the techniques and can apply the procedure quickly and accurately to a variety of problems.

Establishing a Quality Assurance Program

Before evaluation of nursing care can occur, a systematic quality assurance program should be de-

. . . a quality assurance program is intrinsically related to the nature of practice at a particular point in time. To the extent that current images of care are based upon limited knowledge, or even misconceptions, a quality assurance program may be used to reify improper practice. Review practices, criteria, and standards should, therefore, be regularly reevaluated and updated. In the 18th century, adequate psychiatric practice would have involved bleeding and purging patients, spinning patients rapidly in revolving chairs, and alternating hot and cold baths; in later times, patients were subject to extraction of teeth to remove assumed foci of infections. In the 1950s good care generally implied lengthy hospitalization. As knowledge accumulates and practice changes, so too must standards and criteria.

GARY TISCHLER AND BORIS ASTRACHAN (1982)

veloped within the institution. The quality assurance activities of nursing services should be directed and coordinated by nursing personnel with communication and participation in the hospital quality assurance activities as well. Nursing quality assurance programs are usually designed and implemented by a quality assurance committee. This group often develops standards of care, suggests topics for review, organizes the program, sets deadlines, and serves as a resource for nurses in conducting reviews and in analyzing data.

Nursing evaluation and review activities are frequently called *audits*. There are three types of audits: concurrent, retrospective, and prospective. A *concurrent audit* is a method of evaluating ongoing activities and may involve an assessment of one particular aspect of care. For example, nurses may wish to assess the care of clients placed in leather restraints to determine whether proper attention is given to hygiene needs of the client, whether restraints are removed at intervals to administer skin care, whether the emotional needs of the client are attended to, and whether documentation is done at appropriate intervals. This type of audit can provide immediate feedback to nurses to improve any deficiencies that may be identified.

In a *retrospective audit*, activities of nurses are reviewed after the care has been given. For example, a review of records of clients who have been discharged may be evaluated to assess compliance with predetermined standards, such as whether a nurse conducted an initial assessment of the client within a certain period of time. The Joint Committee on Accreditation of Hospitals requires that there be evidence of a professional nurse having assessed, planned, implemented, and evaluated a client's

care. Goals should be established for each client, and there should be evidence that the client or the family has been given instruction in the use of medication and other appropriate aspects of care. These criteria should be incorporated in a retrospective chart audit.

In a *prospective audit*, criteria are set in advance and the study is conducted over a designated period of time. For example, nurses may wish to evaluate the implementation of a teaching program for clients who will receive certain tests. For a three-month period, all clients who receive radiological tests would be interviewed after the test to determine whether patient teaching has taken place, whether it has been effective, and whether it has been helpful to the client.

Once a problem or topic has been identified and the appropriate type of audit has been chosen, criteria are developed for the study. Criteria include what is to be measured, how the data will be collected, and, in some instances, what level of compliance is expected. For instance, in an audit of records, documentation of client education may be expected to be present in 95 percent of the records.

The proposed audit is usually reviewed by the quality assurance committee before it is undertaken. When the study has been approved, data may be collected by nurses on a particular unit, by quality assurance committee members, or by personnel designated by the committee. After the data are collected and analyzed, the appropriate nursing personnel are informed of the results. If problems are identified, a plan of corrective action is formulated and a follow-up method is devised. As part of the plan, a reaudit may be scheduled after suggested corrective action has been taken.

EXAMPLE OF A PROBLEM-FOCUSED PROSPECTIVE AUDIT: OFF-TOUR ADMISSIONS

Nursing personnel who worked a hospital's evening and night shifts voiced their concerns that an increasing number of clients were being admitted to the units on the off tours, when there was less staff available. Since the admission process demanded considerable nursing time to properly assess the clients and devote considerable attention to helping the clients adjust to the new environment, the staff on these tours of duty did not feel they were able to meet clients' needs adequately. In addition, the staff members felt that clients admitted during the evening and night shifts were usually in greater distress and were potentially more volatile than those admitted during the day. In order to obtain objective data about the extent of the problem, an audit was conducted for a three-month period.

Purpose

The purpose of the audit was to obtain descriptive data related to off-tour admissions in order to determine changes that might be indicated in staffing distributions.

Objectives

1. To determine the percentage of off-tour admissions as compared to admissions during the day shift.
2. To document the diagnosis, presenting complaints, and presenting behaviors of clients who were admitted during the off tours.
3. To determine the incidence of acting-out behavior on the off tours as compared with the amount that occurred on the day shift.

Procedure and Criteria

Over a three-month period, data were collected by the nurses on each unit using a data collection sheet with the following criteria:

1. Date.

2. Total number of admissions on day shift, evening shift, night shift.
3. Time of admissions.
4. Diagnoses of clients arriving on off tours.
5. Presenting behavior of clients arriving on off tours.
6. Number of incidents of acting-out behavior on each shift that required the use of seclusion or a call for additional help to subdue the client.

Results

1. Of the 1,623 admissions to the psychiatric units during the three-month period, 650 admissions (40 percent) occurred on either the evening or night shift.
2. The most common diagnoses of these 650 clients were alcoholism and schizophrenia.
3. Four hundred of these clients presented with potential acting-out behavior, as determined by the presence of high anxiety level, tremors, and verbalization of reluctance to be in the hospital.
4. During the time period, 47 instances occurred that required the use of seclusion or a call for additional help. Of these, 35 occurred during the evening or night shift.

Conclusions and Recommendations

Since 40 percent of the admissions to the psychiatric units occurred on the off tours and many of the clients presented with potential acting-out behavior, a change in staffing patterns was recommended. Although the nursing department did not receive additional staff, the new distribution of available staff reflected concern for client care as well as for the safety of personnel on the off tours. Instead of a concentration of nurses on the day shift, the staff was redistributed to allow for increased numbers on the tours.

Table 24-1. Comparison of Nursing Research and Quality Assurance

Dimension	Research	Quality Assurance
Focus	Answering questions; contributing knowledge	Solving immediate problems
Audience	General, beyond study population	Local, usually within institution
Study methods	Exploratory, descriptive, experimental	Usually descriptive only
Analysis	Usually uses some form of statistical testing	Usually summarizes raw data
Applicability	May not provide immediate change; may contribute to theory	Used primarily to change practice

Components of a quality assurance program are usually planned on a yearly basis. A comprehensive one-year schedule might include the following:

1. Monthly record reviews on each nursing unit.

2. Assessment of adherence to protocol for administration of medications.

3. Review of medication errors on each unit.

4. A study of client accidents and falls.

5. An ongoing assessment of client satisfaction with care received.

6. Compliance with JCAH standards.

7. Safety inspections of nursing units.

8. Use of restraints and seclusion.

9. Review of nursing referrals to community agencies.

10. Three or four problem-focused reviews.

Quality assurance activities may also include nursing research activities, but the goals of these programs are frequently different. Larsen (1983) compared nursing research and quality assurance in five dimensions, as shown in Table 24-1.

NURSING RESEARCH

Nursing research is a systematic, detailed attempt to discover or confirm facts that relate to a problem in the field of nursing. The goal of nursing research is the provision of scientific knowledge in nursing. Research with the ultimate goal of application of sci-entific knowledge to improve nursing practice is referred to as *clinical research in nursing* (Abdellah, 1970). Research by nurses is just beginning to come into its own. Ever-increasing numbers of nurses are being prepared for doing and are doing research. Findings from this research are having an impact on clinical practice, nursing education, nursing administration, and the relationships between nursing and other disciplines in providing health care to all segments of the population. Yet many nurses, particularly staff nurses who are "where the action is" in clinical practice, regard nursing research as something to be avoided. This unwillingness to engage in research is due to many factors: lack of knowledge about conducting research, other demands on available time, fear of attempting something new, and lack of realization concerning the value of nursing research.

Nurses prepared at the masters or Ph.D. level are schooled in sophisticated methods of research, and these nursing scholars are important to the advancement of nursing science through research. But clinical nursing research also needs to be conducted by nurses who are experiencing the everyday problems of delivering nursing care. These are the nurses who can help bridge the gap between theory and practice and who can contribute knowledge based on hands-on experience. The nurses in clinical practice are in a position to know what does and doesn't work and to share these experiences with others.

The student should keep in mind that research does not have to be complicated and sophisticated to be important. Many times the basic premise and methodology of a study are relatively simple. An ex-

Nursing, like other occupations seeking to establish themselves as a profession, is experiencing concerns for the development of a service orientation, the continual growth of a scientific base from which members practice, and the evolution of a fairly distinct body of knowledge that separates nursing from other professions. The increasing awareness by nurses of research as an integral part of professional nursing behavior is accelerating rapidly in several areas. Nurses recognize a need to extend the base of nursing knowledge as part of professional responsibility and are endorsing scientific investigations as a way to broaden the body of knowledge.

DENISE POLIT AND BERNADETTE HUNGLER (1978)

642

ample of such a simple project would be evaluating the effects of a patient teaching program by comparing client knowledge and compliance before and after the instruction.

The problems in delivering good-quality nursing care are painfully evident to all nurses. These problems should be the basis of nursing research. One way to discover the basis for a study is to ask "Isn't there a better way to do . . . ?" The process of discovering, implementing, and evaluating such "better ways" is nursing research.

Historical Perspectives

The first clinical nursing research was done by Florence Nightingale during the Crimean War. Her investigations and use of statistics revealed the deplorable conditions in military and civilian hospitals and brought about widespread reforms (Stewart, 1962).

The three schools of nursing that were established in the United States in 1873—Bellevue in New York, Massachusetts General in Boston, and the Connecticut School in New Haven—adhered to the principles of accurate recording and data collection set forth by Nightingale. Unfortunately, later schools did not follow these guidelines. From 1900 to 1930, schools of nursing were established at a rapid rate as hospitals discovered that the easiest and cheapest way to obtain nurses was to have their own school. The bulk of the work was done by students, as most graduates went into private duty. Physicians, the public, and nurses themselves began to think of the practicing nurse as one who followed the directions of physicians and other authority figures. These conditions did not promote the

growth of nursing research (Gortner and Nahm, 1977).

Practice-related research began again in the 1920s and 1930s, when the need for systematic evaluation of nursing procedures was recognized. Descriptions of nursing care plans and case studies predominated in the literature and reflected a gradual change in emphasis from focusing on case studies as teaching tools to case studies as a method for improving patient care.

During the 1940s and 1950s, as a result of the shortage of nurses that was demonstrated during World War II, research turned to studies of nursing resources (kinds, numbers, and uses of nurses) and of the organization and delivery of nursing services. Studies about the nurse outnumbered studies about nursing practice ten to one.

In 1952 the journal *Nursing Research* was established. It provided an avenue for nurses to publish and share their findings with one another. Concern for improvement of nursing services was particularly acute in psychiatric and maternal-child health nursing at this time. These fields received major research thrusts from federal grant and training programs. Federal funds supported the development of graduate programs in these two areas of nursing, and the Russell Sage Foundation provided grants for studies related to the functioning of psychiatric nurses. Typical of these studies were those by Schwartz and Shackley (1956), which focused on the role of the nurse with the psychiatric patient, and by Stanton and Schwartz (1954), which studied the social context of psychiatric institutions.

The 1960s witnessed an increase in studies related to specific groups of clients, such as dying

---

RESEARCH PRIORITIES FOR THE FUTURE

Several gaps in the existing body of knowledge have been identified in the literature. Nursing has not yet reached the stage where one study builds upon another. Replication and follow-up studies are rarely done. A scientific body of knowledge that is uniquely nursing has yet to be defined to provide a basis against which nursing practice can be measured. Without these criteria, nursing practice is one of trial and error rather than one of solid scientific foundation.

The American Nurses' Association Commission on Nursing Research (1976) has enumerated several research priorities relating to the area of nursing practice and to the profession of nursing (Tornyay, 1977). Areas of nursing practice included:

1. Studies to reduce complications of hospitalization and surgery.
2. Studies to improve the outlook for high-risk parents and infants.
3. Studies to improve health care of the elderly.
4. Studies of life-threatening situations, anxiety, pain, and stress.
5. Studies of adaptation to chronic illness and the development of self-care and group-care systems.
6. Studies to facilitate the successful utilization of new technology.
7. Studies of interventions to promote health.

8. Studies to facilitate application of new knowledge to client care.
9. Studies to define and delineate healthy states.
10. Studies of addictive and adherence behaviors.
11. Studies of undernutrition and overnutrition.
12. Studies to evaluate outcomes and effectiveness to consumers and providers of different patterns of delivery of nursing services.

Topics pertaining to the profession of nursing included:

1. Studies of manpower for nursing education, practice, and research.
2. Studies of quality assurance and of criterion measures for practice and education.
3. Studies of cost effectiveness of nurse utilization and preparation in relation to acute, long-term, and extended care and community health.
4. Studies in the history and philosophy of nursing.
5. Studies of nursing curriculum.
6. Studies of the organization of the nursing profession.

---

clients and cardiac clients, and to the areas of geriatrics, ambulatory care, and pediatrics. In 1970, the emphasis turned to the topic of assuring quality nursing practice, with a search for direct cause-effect relationships between the process of nursing care and client outcomes. Practice-related research is gaining momentum because of the interest in increasing the knowledge base for nursing (Gortner and Nahm, 1977).

Within psychiatric nursing specifically, the focus of nursing research has changed. Prior to World War II, the emphasis was on the individual as the unit of study. In the 1950s, the conceptualization of illness turned from a "within the person" approach to a "within the relationship" framework,

and studies about the nurse-patient relationship came into being. The following decade brought a pattern of collaborative work between social scientists and nurses and some "within the social system" studies. There was a trend toward the investigation of psychosocial variables related to physical illness states. The interdisciplinary approach to research had begun. Nursing needs to continue to study what is within its boundaries and to study collaboratively with other disciplines what is within the larger boundaries of health care (Sills, 1977).

The Research Process

A research study can range from the simple to the highly complex in its design, management, and

RESEARCH TERMINOLOGY

■ *Design*. A plan for the research that specifies what, who, how, and when.

■ *Hypothesis*. The researcher's statement concerning the relationship between the elements being studied; what the researcher expects to find. *Example*: Clients who are given a course of instruction in the use of their medications will have greater compliance in taking the medication than those clients who have not had instruction.

■ *Instrument or tool*. The device used for collecting the data, such as a questionnaire.

■ *Operational definition*. Communicating exactly what the researcher means by a certain concept used in the research.

■ *Reliability*. Consistency of the measurement tool; its ability to perform in a similar manner each time it is used. *Example*: A blood pressure cuff that registers 140/80 is expected to register this same value every time the blood pressure is taken and the client's pressure remains at that level.

■ *Validity*. Measuring what is claimed to be measured. *Example*: Does an instrument designed to measure attitudes toward alcoholism really measure those attitudes, or does it measure something else, such as responding in the expected, usually accepted manner?

■ *Variable*. An entity that can take on several values; usually the focus of the study. *Example*: Age is a variable that can range from birth to any number of years.

■ *Independent variable*. The variable that is manipulated or changed in the study. *Example*: A teaching program is given or not given to groups of clients.

■ *Dependent variables*. Variables to be explained. Values of the dependent variable are the result of the manipulation of the independent variable.

■ *Experimental research*. Research in which the researcher makes a change or an intervention and observes the results.

■ *Nonexperimental relationship*. Research in which the researcher observes a phenomenon without making an intervention.

■ *Population*. The universe available for study. *Example*: All cardiac clients in the United States.

■ *Sample*. A representative group of the population. *Example*: All cardiac clients at one hospital treated during a certain time period.

■ *Random sampling*. Sampling in which every subject has an equal chance of being assigned to any group.

■ *Experimental group*. Group that receives the experimental intervention.

■ *Control group*. Group that does not receive the experimental intervention.

■ *Descriptive statistics*. Statistics that describe and summarize data, such as means and frequency distributions.

■ *Inferential statistics*. Statistics that infer a relationship among variables.

644

analysis. However, certain elements are incorporated in any study. The following section is designed to give the student a basic introduction to the process of research (Polit and Hungler, 1978). For further study, the student is referred to the supplementary readings at the end of this chapter.

In order to understand the research process, the student needs a basic understanding of some terms that are frequently used when discussing research. A brief glossary of research terms is provided in the accompanying box.

The research process involves several sequential steps: defining the problem, reviewing the literature, defining the variables, formulating the hypotheses, designing the study, collecting the data, analyzing the data, interpreting the results, and communicating the findings.

DEFINING THE PROBLEM Getting started on a research project and defining the problem is frequently the most difficult aspect of doing research. Many nurses may wonder what there is to be studied, while others may have a variety of ideas and have difficulty choosing among them. The problem statement may arise from a difficult situation encountered in practice or from the nurse's particular area of interest. For example, a nurse may be interested in remotivation therapy for groups of

Examination of one's work can be a painful experience especially since nurses are taught, like doctors, that they are infallible, if not omnipotent. Perhaps part of the reason many nurses are uneasy with the thought of research is that to question what is not being done amounts to criticism. Yet nurses are constantly modifying their own practice in the light of new information, whether based on continued experiences or on more formally gathered knowledge. Research simply helps the modification process along, and if carefully constructed, makes appropriate use of clinical experience in designing and conducting studies that have maximum potential for improving practice. In fact, the closer the relationship between nursing practice and nursing research, the better the research and the better the practice.

DONNA DIERS (1979)

clients. Her experience has indicated that clients who receive remotivation therapy are able to socialize better with other clients on the unit. The nurse would like to determine whether her observations can be demonstrated to have merit by researching the effect of the therapy on socialization. The research question or problem may become: Does remotivation therapy make a difference in socialization of clients?

Other factors that must be considered when designing the research question are: Is the problem of significance to nursing? Are there facilities available to conduct this research? Is there access to enough subjects? Is the cooperation of others needed, and will it be available?

Once the problem is defined, the problem is stated as the purpose of the study. Using the example of remotivation therapy, the purpose would be stated as:

The purpose of this study is to examine the differences in the amount of time clients spend socializing with other clients and staff before and after receiving ten sessions of remotivation therapy.

REVIEWING THE LITERATURE A review of the literature is necessary as a beginning step in the research process. The researcher needs to be familiar with studies that have already been done in the area that has been chosen for study. The review of the literature can provide (1) a justification for doing the study, (2) a baseline upon which to build the study, (3) a comparison of a variety of views and opinions on the subject, and (4) suggestions for the methodology for performing the study. A comprehensive review of the literature should not be limited to nursing literature alone but should encompass

other related fields, such as sociology, psychology, law, economics, or medicine, depending on the subject of the research.

The research should also be linked to a basic theoretical framework. Without a theoretical underpinning to guide it, the research is unlikely to be useful in explaining the phenomenon being studied. The theory need not be complicated or inhibitive for the student. For example, the theoretical framework for the remotivation study might be Sullivan's or Peplau's theories of interpersonal relations, which emphasize the need for interpersonal experiences for the development of self-concept. Or behavioral theory could be used: The researcher might see the positive experiences in group sessions as reinforcers that promote the continued social behavior after the group sessions are finished.

DEFINING THE VARIABLES The next step in the process is to define the variables in a way that they can be measured. In the remotivation study, the independent variable to be manipulated is the remotivation sessions. The purpose, objectives, and content of these sessions should be clearly defined and described. The dependent variable is the socialization scores of the clients after they have experienced ten remotivation sessions.

FORMULATING THE HYPOTHESES The hypotheses are statements of the relationship between the variables. A hypothesis is the researcher's interpretation of the outcome of the research. Hypotheses are developed before the study to give the study a direction and to facilitate the interpretation of the data. The hypotheses may be directional or nondirectional; that is, they may or may not specify a direction of the relationship of the variables. In the remotivational study, a directional hypothesis would be most appropriate, since the nurse's first interest in the topic was generated by the observation that remotivation sessions increased the socialization of clients. The hypotheses might be stated: There will be a positive relationship between attendance at ten remotivation therapy sessions and the socialization scores of the clients.

DESIGNING THE STUDY The research design is the overall plan to obtain answers to the research question. Research can be either *experimental* (in which the researcher makes an intervention with participants and then observes the results) or *nonexperimental* (in which data are collected without making any changes or interventions).

Experimental Designs A true experimental design must have three elements: (1) the researcher must make some kind of intervention with some of the subjects, (2) there must be some control over the research situation, usually provided by the use of a control group, and (3) the subjects must be assigned to either experimental or control groups on a random basis. An experimental design is often considered to be the ideal form of research because direct cause and effect can be hypothesized from it. Unfortunately, much research that is needed in nursing cannot be conducted in this manner. Many times the variables that nurses need to study cannot be manipulated or experimentally controlled. There are also many ethical considerations in this type of research. For example, depriving some clients of treatment or giving controversial treatments to clients could create ethical dilemmas.

In a true experimental design, an experimental and a control group are used. Both are initially assessed, an intervention is made with the experimental group, and then both groups are reassessed. Any changes observed in the experimental group are attributed to the intervention if no change occurs in the control group over the same time.

Quasi-experimental Designs A quasi-experimental design resembles the experimental design except that one or more of the three essential elements is lacking. Sometimes there is no suitable control group available; at other times, randomization is not possible. However, quasi-experimental designs do involve an intervention.

If, in the remotivation study the clients are given a socialization score before the ten sessions and again after the sessions but no control group is used, the study would be quasi-experimental. Without a control group, any changes in the socialization

scores may be due to a variety of factors besides the remotivation session—changes in personnel, institution of another program during the same period of time, growth in general comfort level because of increased familiarity with the surroundings, and so on. The use of a control group would help eliminate these alternative explanations.

Survey Designs Survey research is designed to assess an existing situation within a group of people. Surveys are frequently conducted in all aspects of life. During an election year, surveys are continually made of samples from the population to assess the popularity of various candidates. Mail surveys are commonly used to determine buying preferences of consumers.

Surveys are the most common method of descriptive research. Surveys are often needed to aid in defining a research question or in delineating the pertinent variables. In many instances, it is necessary to find out what *is* before the researcher can decide what needs to be. Various methods can be used for survey designs, including face-to-face interviews, questionnaires, and telephone interviews. Information obtained by surveys is usually relatively superficial, since surveys lack the ability to probe deeply into behavior and feelings. However, this type of research is especially needed in nursing today. Nursing is at a stage where descriptive studies are necessary to define phenomena before progress can be made in experimental research on these phenomena. The practice of nursing is not well understood. Descriptive studies are needed to understand and explain functions and forms of nursing care in meeting the needs of society and in helping individuals regain or maintain health.

COLLECTING THE DATA Data can be collected in a variety of ways, depending on the design of the research. Some frequently used methods include:

1. Physiological measurements, such as changes in blood pressure, sweat gland activity, eye blinks.

2. Observational measurements, such as observing behaviors, activities, communication, the environment.

3. Interviews and questionnaires.

4. Scales and psychological measures, such as Rorschach tests and the Minnesota Multiphasic Personality Inventory.

In the remotivation study, observation measures would be used to compile a socialization score for each client. For a two-week period prior to the sessions, the number of times that a client approached another client or staff member and the length of time of the contact would be noted. The same observations would be made for a two-week period following the sessions. In order to collect the data, the researcher would need the cooperation of a nurse on each shift. The same observations might be made again two months later to assess sustaining effects.

ANALYZING THE DATA The data collected in a study need to be analyzed to provide meaning to the study. For descriptive studies, statistics such as means and frequency distributions are used. These statistics describe the results; they do not make any inferences about the relationships between variables. Experimental or quasi-experimental studies frequently make use of inferential statistics, which do make inferences about the relationships between the variables. Inferential statistics provide the means for drawing a conclusion about the population studied based on the results obtained from the sample.

Several statistical tests are available to determine whether the scores obtained by one group are statistically different from scores obtained by another group. Statistical significance means that the differences in scores are probably not due to chance. There will always be some differences in scores, but whether the difference is great enough to be significant can be determined by the statistical tests. In the remotivation study, the scores obtained prior to and after the remotivation sessions could be tested for significance using the T-test and Dependent Samples.

The beginning researcher should not be overwhelmed by lack of knowledge about statistics. In most institutions, there are people available who can help with the statistical analysis and interpretation if this is needed. In many instances, basic computation of averages and frequencies will be sufficient.

INTERPRETING THE RESULTS After the data are collected and analyzed, it is the task of the researcher to make some sense of the results and to draw conclusions based on the findings. If the findings fit the hypothesis, the explanation is easier. But alternative explanations should also be listed. If the hypothesis is not supported, the researcher must develop some possible explanations, such as that measurement was poor or that the sample was too small. Suggestions for future research should be made.

COMMUNICATING THE FINDINGS In preparing the report of the research, the writer should be as clear and objective as possible, realizing that the reader will not be familiar with the research. Reports will vary in style and length, but the basic format outlined in this chapter should be followed. Many researchers hesitate to report negative findings, perhaps because most journals do not report studies with negative findings. However, in many instances negative findings are as important as positive ones in guiding others for future research. The importance of writing and sharing research findings and ideas with other nurses cannot be overemphasized. Yet many nurses, after laboriously planning and researching, are hesitant to write up their findings. Their reasons are many and varied, but nurse researchers may be assisted in their writing efforts by keeping the following thoughts in mind.

The Importance of Writing

Not too many years ago, thoughtful nurses working in clinical settings were ready and willing to share their experiences by publishing case studies that were highly personal. These early contributions to nursing literature were important, even though they lacked the sophistication provided by a strong theoretical foundation or competence in research techniques. Most of the early articles followed a familiar theme, in which physicians insisted, patients resisted, and nurses persisted until a successful denouement was achieved.

As nursing became more complex, hierarchical ranking became prevalent within the profession. The eventual result was that capable but lower-status nurses who practiced solely in clinical facilities were silenced by their feelings of inferiority. Because they lacked impressive academic credentials, nurses who were working with clients became less willing to compete with colleagues who had advanced degrees but who were more removed from hands-on client care. This hierarchical ranking can be compared to that of the army, in which only generals are encouraged to describe the battles while the silent footsoldiers listen, sometimes in awe and sometimes in disbelief. The paradox in this arrangement is that soldiers who have served in the front lines may have as much or more to tell than some of the generals. Unfortunately, nurses directly engaged in delivering care to clients are all too often like the silent soldiers.

This analogy is by no means a denigration of the leadership skills of highly educated nurses attempting to develop a body of theoretical knowledge crucial to our profession. What it does mean is that the work of identifying and testing hypotheses in structured settings is essential but is of little value unless it is validated by nurses practicing in a clinical context. The task of applying theoretical constructs under clinical conditions is one that is well within the scope of the professional nurse with no

647

CLINICAL EXAMPLE

CONTINGENCY CONTRACTING FOR WEIGHT LOSS IN AN OUTPATIENT PSYCHIATRIC SETTING

Obesity, or an excess of body weight, has been called the main public health problem in the United States and has received extensive attention from the public at large as well as from the scientific community. Efforts have been made to define, measure, and determine the etiology of this problem and to discover safe, effective means of dealing with it.

Nurses are in a unique position to assist in the treatment of obesity. Not only do they have the ability and skill to assess the individual's psychosocial needs, but they also possess the nutritional knowledge essential to any successful weight reduction program. Their direct and continued client contact allows for an in-depth relationship, creating a more trusting environment in which to implement and evaluate a program.

Obesity, like many chronic conditions, is difficult to control. The reasons for resistance of the obese individual to treatment and the recidivism rate following weight loss still remain quite vague (Wineman, 1980). However, a plausible explanation is noncompliance with the prescribed treatment or a failure of the persons to assume an active role in their own treatment (Stalones, Johnson, and Christ, 1972; Epstein and Martin, 1977; Steckel and Swain, 1977).

One approach that has been used to deal with this problem is the use of behavioral techniques. Although it should not be assumed that a behavior modification technique is a complete answer (Jordan and Levitz, 1975), several studies attest to the effectiveness of this approach. Some researchers believe that the implementation of positive reinforcement principles is potentially useable to modify outpatient behaviors in their natural life setting (Mann, 1972; Steckel, 1980). On this premise, there are several behavior modification techniques that have applied to obesity, including contingency contracting and self-monitoring for new behaviors.

The contingency contract is an explicit statement of specified behaviors linked to a terminal goal, whose occurrence would produce specific consequences (Mann, 1972). Although multidimensional, contingency contracts have identifiable components, such as increased attention from a therapist; clients' involvement in goal setting and active participation in decision making regarding their therapeutic regimen; incentives for goal achievement; and assistance in applying general information regarding a topic to the clients' own environment or social circumstances (Steckel and Swain, 1977). These components aid in the treatment of obesity because they utilize the principles of self-management so vital in successful weight reduction programs.

Self-monitoring is a technique in which the individual records verbally or in written form specific behaviors to be modified. For example, an individual may contract to slow down his eating time by chewing his food twenty times before swallowing. He therefore monitors the number of times he chews his food and must report his compliance or noncompliance to the researcher.

PURPOSE

The purpose of this study was to determine the effectiveness of a program of contingency contracting for behavior change in order to facilitate weight loss in an overweight outpatient population. Following is the report of a study on application of contingency contracting and self-monitoring in a weight loss program.

METHODOLOGY

Sample

The study took place in an outpatient clinic for psychiatric clients. Participation in this study was strictly voluntary. All male clients over the age of twenty were invited to join a weight control group to be conducted weekly for twenty weeks. Criteria were an expressed desire to lose at least 5-10 pounds and being at least 10 percent overweight using the Metropolitan Life Insurance Company's weight/height charts as guidelines.

Design

The research design was quasi-experimental. In this study each client served as his own control. His weight loss or gain during the first ten-week period, in which the group-oriented client education approach was used, was compared to the loss or gain during the second ten-week period, in which contingency contracting was used. The group-oriented client education consisted of weekly meetings of the weight control group where clients weighed in, had a 10- to 15-minute session of ambulating outdoors or performing basic stretching exercises, and engaged in a 15- to 20-minute discussion/education session. The education consisted of information on basic nutrition, caloric values of food, and suggested modifications of behavior.

Procedures

The study was conducted in two stages. During Stage I, all clients participated in the group with the client education focus. Following these ten weeks, the researcher met with each participant and obtained an eating habit record and a profile of the client's weight history. Self-monitoring was explained to the participants and instruction was given on contingency contracting, reinforcers, goal setting, and the mechanics of keeping a diary.

To facilitate the learning process, trial contracts were written with each participant. This enabled them to set a goal of weight to be lost, help identify problem behavior, and decide on meaningful reinforcers to be used during Stage II.

Stage II consisted of a ten-week period during which all participating clients contracted for some form of new behavior, such as increasing activity by taking the stairs instead of the elevator. The researcher assisted the clients in choosing the behaviors to be monitored by evaluating their individual personality and weight history pattern. Terminal and intermediate goals were set and revised as needed. Clients who were able to read and write without assistance contracted for compliance in the written diary recording. Some participants also contracted for verbal reporting to the researcher of self-monitored behaviors, such as eating smaller portions or eating one less dessert each day. The contracts were individually designed and modified regarding the behaviors chosen to be self-monitored as well as the reinforcers used. Each contract used in the study was written, signed, and dated by both the researcher and the participants each week.

Reinforcers used included fruit, extra ceramic or other craft projects, special occupational therapy privileges, and calorie-counting books. The participants were required to comply 100 percent with their contract in order to receive their chosen reinforcement.

The dependent variable, the client's weight, was measured and recorded on a flowsheet by the researcher and placed on a graph by the participants on a weekly basis. In addition, each participant submitted his written diary at the beginning of each group meeting for the researcher to review, and the diary was returned at the end of the session. The subjects also met with the researcher for approximately 5 minutes during group time to give a verbal report of their self-monitored behavior compliance. The researcher recorded all data relating to the contracts and compliance on a flowsheet, which summarized the subjects' weekly compliance and activities. Data were analyzed using T-tests for dependent samples to determine whether any significant difference existed between amount of weight gained or lost during Stage I and Stage II.

RESULTS

Eighteen persons chose to participate in the study, and sixteen completed the twenty-week program. Thirteen of the sixteen subjects had gained weight during the control period while three had lost weight. In the research study, two participants gained weight, twelve lost weight, and two remained unchanged. Thus, more participants lost weight under the experimental conditions. The T-test for dependent samples was significant at the .10 level of probability.

DISCUSSION

Before the study was undertaken, the researcher believed that all participants would progress to a point of keeping daily dietary diaries, including calorie counting. By gradually increasing their responsibility for daily recording—first contracting to record three out of seven days, then four out of seven days, and so on—the researcher assumed the subjects could handle the task. In fact, very few individuals were able to progress to this point. Although the exact reasons are not known, one can speculate that the participants' psychiatric disabilities caused a greater impairment than originally thought. They may have either forgotten to complete the diary, felt too much pressure or stress to record all meals, or lacked the confidence to complete the task and the terms of the contract. Clients easily became discouraged when they did not comply with the contract and therefore chose to contract for less diary keeping. Some individuals expressed concern over their writing abilities, which could have been a source of embarrassment and lowered self-esteem. Alleviation of this stress might be accomplished in future studies by developing a diary flowsheet, which would decrease the amount of writing necessary to complete the task.

Interestingly, participants were eager to contract for modification of other problem behaviors, such as eating too quickly, eating too many sweets, or low activity levels. These other self-monitored behaviors were reported verbally rather than in diary form.

When asked for feedback, participants gave these replies: "It made me feel better to accomplish my goals. My self-image improved." "I felt more determined and watched what I ate." "I became more conscious of my nutrition by writing down what I ate." "I felt more in control." "It made me more aware. I didn't realize I ate so much, like when I had nine slices of bread in one day." "Writing the contract and knowing I would get something by following it really helped me stay motivated."

Several individuals became more aware of their eating habits through their attempts to use the diary, however limited that was, and they did lose weight.

LIMITATIONS

There are several areas that should be considered when evaluating the effectiveness of the study. As mentioned in the discussion, the degree of impairment second to psychiatric illness must be more closely evaluated when designing contracts for such clients. Since the subjects in this study all carried a psychiatric diagnosis, a thorough review of their medications and possible side effects should have been conducted. It is a known fact that psychotropic medications and many antidepressant drugs can cause weight gain.

Many of the individuals in this study had expressed a concern about the lack of control they had in deciding on meals served to them. Because of group living situations or uncooperative families, it is possible that those individuals who lost little or no weight during the experimental conditions had a less active role in meal planning than those who lost more weight.

Because of the lack of funding, reinforcement tools were very limited. If the reinforcement had been more desirable to obtain, such as money, a greater change in eating habits and weight loss might have resulted.

academic pretentions beyond the possession of a baccalaureate degree.

Many of the most important scientific discoveries have stemmed from accidental occurrences that were noted by acute observers. This means that the clinically oriented nurse is in a favorable position to evaluate responses to conceptual innovations presented by nurse theorists, to consider viable modifications, and to disseminate this information by writing and publishing. An eavesdropper listening to a group of nurses talking about their clinical practice would find the perceptiveness and analytic thinking of the nurses remarkable. Humor, independence, compassion, judgment, and intellectual vigor are likely to characterize the attitudes of such nurses in their professional practice. Yet most lack the confidence to put in writing the opinions and ideas they verbalize so easily.

There is no denying that writing is hard work. It is one of the loneliest jobs in the world, for it is a solitary undertaking and there is no audience to give immediate applause. In order to confront the challenge of an empty page, one must first be convinced that one has something important to say. Many nurses in clinical settings must resolve the crisis of confidence that makes them believe they lack the tools for scholarly writing. They do themselves and the profession a great disservice in this regard.

The schism in nursing that is most detrimental may be the gulf between abstract nursing theory and clinical application. Only by bridging this gulf and by hearing what clinical nurses are doing and thinking can nursing theory be refined and the uniqueness of the nursing process be truly understood. The major tool of clinical scholarship is not research methodology but critical thinking.

The message being transmitted here is an invitation for nurses to exchange their burden of inferiority for the impetus of mastery. Nurses, except for a notable few, tend to underestimate their abilities and contributions. It is possible in any clinical setting to observe phenomena, to use deductive and inductive reasoning in order to accept or question established theory, and to consider new ways of thinking and acting. These behaviors are displayed every day in nursing; the challenge is to make them known to others. Intellectual vigor in the form of inquiry and evaluation exists in nursing to an extent far greater than is commonly acknowledged. Nursing and nursing theory will be enhanced if more nurses become motivated to express their ideas on paper and thus move into the ranks of published authors whose opinions and reactions carry weight within and beyond the borders of the profession.

Every nurse, regardless of predilection or position on the career ladder, has access to information that is interesting and publishable. One does not need extensive academic credentials in order to have knowledge worth sharing. For all nurses interested in personal growth and professional enrichment, the question should not be "Why write?" but rather "Why not write?" This is particularly true of nurses who have not retreated to the groves of academe but who remain closely involved with individual clients and their families.

SUMMARY

The profession of nursing has experienced a variety of changes since its beginnings in the times of Florence Nightingale. Although relatively autonomous a century ago, nursing became subservient to the medical profession throughout the years and has recently begun to make efforts to reverse this process. For nurses to retain control over nursing practice, they must take advantage of the many avenues available to them. Opportunities exist for nurses to become influential in determining the distribution of available resources for health care through the prospective payment system of care (DRGs). Quality assurance activities are necessary to identify problems with client care and to evaluate the quality of care given by nurses.

The area of clinical research has received little emphasis from nurses over the years, but in recent times more nurses are being prepared for and are conducting research. The importance of the nurses who are engaged in clinical practice doing research cannot be overemphasized. It is in the everyday, reality-based world that the gap between theory and practice can be closed. Of equal importance is the necessity for nurses to write and publish in order to share their knowledge and experiences and to build a solid foundation for the practice of nursing.

Review Questions

1. Trace the development of expanded health care services and explain some reasons for the increased cost of these health services.

2. Explain the basis for the prospective payment system of DRGs.

3. Discuss ways in which nursing can be influential under the new DRG system.

4. What are some dangers to nursing that may be realized under the DRG system?

5. Explain the components of a comprehensive quality assurance program.

6. Explain the importance of clinical nursing research.

7. Discuss reasons why nurses are hesitant to do research.

8. Using one of the priorities for nursing research, outline a brief study, including the steps in the research process.

9. Explain the difference between experimental and nonexperimental research.

References

Abdellah, F. G. 1970. Overview of Nursing Research 1955–1968, Part I. *Nursing Research*, 19:6–17.

Aldridge, M. 1982. Nursing: An Emergency Power in Health. *The Arizona Nurse*, 2:11.

American Nurses' Association. 1982. Professional Nurses Role in Quality Assurance. In *Nursing Quality Assurance Management/Training System*. Kansas City, Mo.: American Nurses' Association and Sutherland Learning Associates.

American Nurses' Association Commission on Nursing Research. 1976. Priorities. *Nursing Research*, 25:357.

Binder, J. 1983. Toward a Policy Perspective for Nursing. *Nursing Economics*, 1(July-August):47.

Diers, D. *Research in Nursing Practice*. Philadelphia: J. B. Lippincott, 1979.

Epstein, L. H., and Martin, J. E. 1977. Compliance and Side Effects of Weight Regulation Groups. *Behavior Modification*, 1:551–557.

Gortner, S. R., and Nahm, N. 1977. An Overview of Nursing Research in the United States. *Nursing Research*, 26:10–33.

Hamilton, J. M. 1984. Nursing and DRG's: Proactive Responses to Prospective Reimbursement. *Nursing and Health Care*, 3:155–159.

Jordan, H. A., and Levitz, L. S. 1975. A Behavioral Approach to the Problem of Obesity. *Obesity/Bariatric Medicine*, 4:58–69.

Larsen, E. 1983. Combining Nursing Quality Assurance and Research Programs. *Journal of Nursing Administration*, 13:32–35.

Mann, R. A. 1972. The Behavior-Therapeutic Use of Contingency Contracting to Control an Adult Behavior; Weight Control. *Journal of Applied Behavior Analysis*, 5:99–109.

Plomann, M. P., and Shaffer, F. A. 1983. DRG's as One of Nine Approaches to Case Mix in Transition. *Nursing and Health Care*, 10:438–443.

Polit, D. F., and Hungler, B. P. 1978. *Nursing Research: Principles and Methods*. Philadelphia: J. B. Lippincott.

Schwartz, M. S., and Shackley, E. L. 1956. *The Nurse and the Mental Patient: A Study in Interpersonal Relations*. New York: Russell Sage Foundation.

Shaffer, F. A. 1983. DRG's: History and Overview. *Nursing and Health Care*, 9:388–396.

Shaffer, F. A. 1984a. A Nursing Perspective of the DRG World, Part I. *Nursing and Health Care*, 1:48–51.

Shaffer, F. A. 1984b. Nursing: Gearing up for DRG's, Part II: Management Strategies. *Nursing and Health Care*, 2:93–99.

Sills, G. M. 1977. Research in the Field of Psychiatric Nursing, 1952–1977. *Nursing Research*, 26:201–207.

Stalones, P. M.; Johnson, W. G.; and Christ, M. 1978. Behavior Modification for Obesity: The Evaluation of Exercise, Contingency Management and Program Adherence. *Journal of Consulting and Clinical Psychology*, 46:463–469.

Stanton, A. H., and Schwartz, M. A. 1954. *The Mental Hospital: A Study of Institutional Participation in Psychiatric Illness and Treatment*. New York: Basse Books.

Steckel, S. B. 1980. Contracting with Patient-Selected Reinforcers. *American Journal of Nursing*, 80:1596–1599.

Steckel, S. B., and Swain, M. A. 1977. Contracting with Patients to Improve Compliance. *Journal of the American Hospital Association*, 51:81–84.

Stewart, I. M. 1962. Remarks on Research in Nursing. *Nursing Research*, 2:5–6.

Tischler, G. and Astrachan, B. 1982. *Quality Assurance in Mental Health: Peer and Utilization Review*. Rockville, Md.: National Institute of Mental Health.

Tornyay, R. 1977. Nursing Research—The Road Ahead. *Nursing Research*, 26:404–407.

Westfall, U. E. 1980. Nursing Diagnosis: Its Use in Quality Assurance. *Topics in Clinical Nursing*, January:80.

Wineman, N. M. 1980. Obesity: Focus of Control, Body Image, Weight Loss and Age-at-Onset. *Nursing Research*, 29:231–237.

Supplementary Readings

Abdellah, F. G. Overview of Nursing Research 1955–1968, parts II and III. *Nursing Research*, 19(1970):151–162, 239–251.

Abdellah, F. G., and Levine E. *Better Patient Care Through Nursing Research*. New York: Macmillan, 1978.

Ackerman, W. B., and Lohnes, P. R. *Research Methods for Nurses*. New York: McGraw-Hill, 1981.

Beck, C. T. The Conceptualization of Power. *Advances in Nursing Science*, 4(1982):1–17.

Bullough, B., and Bullough V. *Nursing Issues and Nursing Strategies for the Eighties*. New York: Springer, 1980.

Bush, C. T. *Nursing Research*. Reston, Va.: Reston Publishing, 1985.

Davis, M. Promoting Nursing Research in the Clinical Setting. *Journal of Nursing Administration*, 11(1981):22–26.

DeChesnay, M. Cross-Cultural Research: Advantages and Disadvantages. *International Nursing Review*, 30 (1983): 21–23.

Downs, F. *A Sourcebook of Nursing Research*. Philadelphia: F. A. Davis, 1983.

Duespohl, T. A. *Nursing in Transition*. Rockville, Md.: Aspen, 1982.

Edwardson, S. R., and Anderson, D. I. Hospital Nurses' Valuation of Quality Assurance. *Journal of Nursing Administration*, 13(1983): 33–39.

Ellis, J. R., and Hartley, C. L. *Nursing in Today's World: Challenges, Issues and Trends*, 3rd ed. Philadelphia: J. B. Lippincott, 1984.

Fuller, E. O. Preparing an Abstract of a Nursing Study. *Nursing Research*, 32(1983):316–317.

Gilliss, C. L. The Family as a Unit of Analysis: Strategies for the Nurse Researcher. *Advances in Nursing Science*, 5(1983):50–59.

Hardy, L. K. Nursing Models and Research—A Restricting View. *Journal of Advanced Nursing*, 7(1982): 447–451.

Jacox, A. J., and Prescott, P. Determining a Study's Relevance for Clinical Practice. *American Journal of Nursing*, 78(1978):1882–1889.

Johnson, M. Some Aspects of the Relation Between Theory and Research in Nursing. *Journal of Advanced Nursing*, 8(1983):21–28.

Kaluzny, A. S. Quality Assurance as a Management Innovation: A Research Perspective. *Health Services Research*, 17(1982):253–268.

Karch, A. M. *Concurrent Nursing Audit: Quality Assurance in Action.* Thorofare, N.J.: Charles Slack, 1980.

Knapp, R. G. *Basic Statistics for Nurses*, 2nd ed. New York: John Wiley & Sons, 1985.

Krueger, J., and Nelson, A. *Nursing Research: Development, Collaboration and Utilization.* Rockville, Md.: Aspen, 1979.

Leininger, M. Power—Use It or Lose It. *National League for Nursing*, Publication #52–1675, (1977):6–18.

Leininger, M. Creativity and Challenges for Nurse Researchers in this Economic Recession. *Journal of Nursing Administration*, 13(1983):21–22.

Lelean, S. R. The Implementation of Research Findings into Nursing Practice. *International Journal of Nursing Studies*, 19(1982):223–230.

Lindeman, C. A., and Schantz, D. The Research Question. *Journal of Nursing Administration*, 12(1982):6–10.

Miller, M., and Flynn, B. *Current Perspectives in Nursing: Social Issues and Trends.* St. Louis: C. V. Mosby, 1977.

Muff, J. *Socialization, Sexism, and Stereotyping: Women's Issues in Nursing.* St. Louis: C. V. Mosby, 1982.

Numerof, R. Conflicts and Power in the Nurse Role. *Health Services Manager*, 6(1978):7–8.

Phaneuf, M. *The Nursing Audit: Self-Regulation in Nursing Practice*, 2nd ed. New York: Appleton-Century-Crofts, 1976.

Phippen, M. L. Power: What Nursing School Never Taught. *AORN Journal*, 33(1981):650–656.

Schantz, D., and Lindeman, C. The Research Design. *Journal of Nursing Administration*, 12(1982):35–38.

Schroeder, P. S., and Mailbusch, R. M. *Nursing Quality Assurance: A Unit-Based Approach.* Rockville, Md.: Aspen, 1984.

Smeltzer, C. H. Organizing the Search for Excellence: Nursing Can Use a Quality Assurance Program. *Nursing Management*, 14(1983):19–21.

Stevens, K. R. *Power and Influence: A Sourcebook for Nurses.* New York: John Wiley & Sons, 1983.

Tinkle, M. B. Toward a New View of Science: Implications for Nursing Research. *Advances in Nursing Science*, 5(1983):27–36.

652

NURSING DIAGNOSES ACCORDING TO PATTERNS OF ALTERATION

ALTERED PATTERNS OF HEALTH PERCEPTION AND MANAGEMENT

Noncompliance (Specify)
Explanatory note: Noncompliance is considered present when the client makes an informed decision not to follow all or part of a therapeutic regimen.

Comfort, Alteration in: Pain
Explanatory note: The presence of pain may be indicated by subjective verbal complaints and/or observable nonverbal signs such as facial expression, body movement or lack of movement, autonomic responses, and social behaviors.

Communication, Impaired Verbal
Explanatory note: Impaired communication may be attributable to developmental or cultural language deficits, cognitive impairment, emotional distress, or physical problems.

ALTERED NUTRITIONAL AND METABOLIC PATTERNS

Skin Integrity, Impairment of: Potential
Explanatory note: The potential impairment of skin integrity may be due to environmental or physiological factors for which primary prevention measures may be indicated.

Skin Integrity, Impairment of: Actual
Explanatory note: Actual impairment of skin integrity may be due to environmental or physiological factors for which secondary or tertiary prevention measures may be indicated.

Nutrition, Alterations in: Less Than Body Requirements
Explanatory note: Altered nutritional patterns result in deficient food intake, absorption, or metabolism.

Nutrition, Alterations in: More Than Body Requirements
Explanatory note: Altered nutritional patterns result in the ingestion of excessive food due to dysfunctional eating habits.

Nutrition, Alterations in: Potential for More Than Body Requirements
Explanatory note: Altered nutritional patterns result in the possibility or potential for ingesting excessive food requirements due to familial, social, cultural, or emotional influences.

Fluid Volume Deficit: Potential
Explanatory note: This refers to the potential for excessive loss of body fluids by various routes.

Fluid Volume Deficit, Actual (1) and (2)
Explanatory note: This refers to fluid volume imbalance due to (1) deficits of regulatory mechanisms or (2) active loss of body fluids.

ALTERED PATTERNS OF ELIMINATION

Urinary Elimination, Alteration in Patterns
Explanatory note: This includes any alteration of urinary elimination patterns such as frequency, incontinence, retention, hesitation, urgency, dysuria, or nocturia due to various causes.

Bowel Elimination, Alteration in: Constipation
Explanatory note: This includes alterations in bowel elimination patterns that result in decreased bowel activity, infrequent evacuation, subjective feelings of distention.

Bowel Elimination, Alteration in: Diarrhea
Explanatory note: This includes alterations in bowel elimination patterns that result in increased bowel activity, frequent evacuation, loose stools, and subjective feelings of urgency.

Bowel Elimination, Alteration in: Incontinence
Explanatory note: This refers to the involuntary evacuation of stool.

ALTERED PATTERNS OF ACTIVITY AND EXERCISE

Home Maintenance Management, Impaired
Explanatory note: This refers to the inability of an individual to maintain for himself or herself a safe, wholesome environment.

653

Mobility, Impaired Physical
Explanatory note: This is the inability to maintain a satisfactory range of motion for various physiological and/or psychological reasons.

Self-Care Deficit: Feeding, Bathing/Hygiene, Dressing/Grooming, Toileting
Explanatory note: This refers to the inability to maintain patterns of self-care without assistance for various reasons.

Sleep Pattern Disturbance
Explanatory note: This is the disruption of sleep patterns to an extent that causes distress to the individual or interferes with routines of living.

Diversionary Activity, Deficit
Explanatory note: This refers to the disruption of leisure time interests and activities.

ALTERED PATTERNS OF
EXCHANGE AND PERFUSION

Tissue Perfusion, Alteration in: Cerebral, Cardiopulmonary, Renal, Gastrointestinal, Peripheral
Explanatory note: This refers to interruption of venous or arterial flow due to exchange problems.

Breathing Pattern, Ineffective
Explanatory note: This refers to impaired respiratory patterns of function due to physiological or psychological causes.

Cardiac Output, Alteration in: Decreased
Explanatory note: This includes any altered pattern that results in decreased cardiac output such as arrythmias, blood pressure changes, rales, and dyspnea, among others.

Airway Clearance, Ineffective
Explanatory note: This refers to changes in patterns of respiration commonly attributed to infection, obstruction, or secretion that prevent adequate clearance.

Gas Exchange, Impaired
Explanatory note: Altered patterns of gas exchange result in deficient ventilation and perfusion.

ALTERED PATTERNS OF
COGNITION AND PERCEPTION

Knowledge Deficit
Explanatory note: This refers to lack of information, misinterpretation of information, disinterest, and poor recall of pertinent information.

Sensory-Perceptual Alterations: Visual, Auditory, Kinesthetic, Gustatory, Tactile, Olfactory Perception
Explanatory note: This refers to altered patterns of sensory perception due to environmental factors, physiological factors, or psychological factors.

Thought Processes, Alteration in
Explanatory note: Altered interpretation of external environmental conditions due to thought processes not oriented to reality.

ALTERED PATTERNS OF
SELF-PERCEPTION AND SELF-CONCEPT

Fear
Explanatory note: This is a subjective feeling of dread that can be attributed to identifiable causes.

Anxiety
Explanatory note: This is a subjective feeling of dread that frequently cannot be attributed to identifiable causes. There are four levels of anxiety: mild, moderate, severe, and panic.

Self-concept, Disturbance in: Body Image, Self-esteem, Role Performance, Personal Identity
Explanatory note: Disturbances in self-concept manifest themselves through alterations in the way an individual perceives his or her body image, self-esteem, role performance, and/or sense of personal identity.

ALTERED FAMILY PATTERNS

Parenting, Alterations in: Actual or Potential
Explanatory note: This is the inability of responsible person or persons to maintain a safe, wholesome environment for the growth and development of others.

Coping, Ineffective Family: Compromised
Explanatory note: This is the inability, complete or partial, of a family member or support person to provide sufficient comfort and assistance for persons needing help in meeting health needs.

Coping, Ineffective Family: Disabling
Explanatory note: This is the inability of a family member or significant support person to meet his or her health needs, or to perform tasks essential to the health needs of other family member(s).

Coping, Family: Potential for Growth
Explanatory note: The family demonstrates readiness and willingness to meet the health needs of its members.

ALTERED ROLE RELATIONSHIP PATTERNS

Grieving, Anticipatory
Explanatory note: This refers to a range of emotional reactions expressed verbally and nonverbally, precipitated by the imminent loss of a significant person or object.

Grieving, Dysfunctional

Explanatory note: This refers to altered patterns of daily life involving behavioral, somatic, and emotional responses to the actual or perceived loss of a significant person or object.

Sexual Dysfunction

Explanatory note: This refers to altered biopsychosocial patterns of sexuality attributable to various causes and influences.

ALTERED VALUE AND BELIEF PATTERNS

Spiritual Distress

Explanatory note: This refers to distress of the human spirit for reasons that go beyond biopsychosocial causes and represent disintegration or transgression against the individual's innate nature.

ALTERED PATTERNS OF RESPONSIBLE/PRECAUTIONARY BEHAVIOR

Injury, Potential For

Explanatory note: This is an interactive situation in which conditions of the environment and characteristics of the individual result in the potential for injury to the individual.

Trauma, Potential For

Explanatory note: This refers to accentuated possibilities of risk to the individual in the form of tissue injury or trauma.

Poisoning, Potential For

Explanatory note: This refers to accentuated possibilities of risk to the individual in the form of exposure to or ingestion of substances in amounts large enough to cause poisoning.

Suffocation, Potential For

Explanatory note: This refers to accentuated possibilities of risk to the individual of accidental suffocation.

Violence, Potential For (Self-directed or Directed at Others)

Explanatory note: This refers to accentuated possibilities of violent, aggressive behavior expressed toward others or of violent self-destructive acts committed against oneself.

ALTERED REACTIVE PATTERNS TO TRAUMA

655

Rape Trauma Syndrome

Explanatory note: This refers to the disorganization that follows forced sexual penetration without the consent of the victim. The period of disorganization may be prolonged and reorganization may be a lengthy process.

███████████████████

DSM-III CLASSIFICATION:
AXES I AND II CATEGORIES AND CODES

███████████████████

The long dashes indicate the need for a fifth-digit subtype or other qualifying term.

DISORDERS USUALLY FIRST EVIDENT IN INFANCY, CHILDHOOD, OR ADOLESCENCE

Mental Retardation
(Code in fifth digit: 1 = with other behavioral symptoms [requiring attention or treatment and that are not part of another disorder], 0 = without other behavioral symptoms)
- 317.0(x) Mild mental retardation, _____
- 318.0(x) Moderate mental retardation, _____
- 318.1(x) Severe mental retardation, _____
- 318.2(x) Profound mental retardation, _____
- 319.0(x) Unspecified mental retardation, _____

Attention Deficit Disorder
- 314.01 With hyperactivity
- 314.00 Without hyperactivity
- 314.80 Residual type

Conduct Disorder
- 312.00 Undersocialized, aggressive
- 312.10 Undersocialized, nonaggressive
- 312.23 Socialized, aggressive
- 312.21 Socialized, nonaggressive
- 312.90 Atypical

Anxiety Disorders of Childhood or Adolescence
- 309.21 Separation anxiety disorder
- 313.21 Avoidant disorder of childhood or adolescence
- 313.00 Overanxious disorder

Other Disorders of Infancy, Childhood, or Adolescence
- 313.89 Reactive attachment disorder of infancy
- 313.22 Schizoid disorder of childhood or adolescence
- 313.23 Elective mutism
- 313.81 Oppositional disorder
- 313.82 Identity disorder

Eating Disorders
- 307.10 Anorexia nervosa
- 307.51 Bulimia
- 307.52 Pica

- 307.53 Rumination disorder of infancy
- 307.50 Atypical eating disorder

Stereotyped Movement Disorders
- 307.21 Transient tic disorder
- 307.22 Chronic motor tic disorder
- 307.23 Tourette's disorder
- 307.20 Atypical tic disorder
- 307.30 Atypical stereotyped movement disorder

Other Disorders with Physical Manifestations
- 307.00 Stuttering
- 307.60 Functional enuresis
- 307.70 Functional encopresis
- 307.46 Sleepwalking disorder
- 307.46 Sleep terror disorder (307.49)

Pervasive Developmental Disorders
Code in fifth digit: 0 = full syndrome present, 1 = residual state.
- 299.0x Infantile autism, _____
- 299.9x Childhood onset pervasive developmental disorder, _____
- 299.8x Atypical, _____

Specific developmental disorders (These are coded on Axis II):

- 315.00 Developmental reading disorder
- 315.10 Developmental arithmetic disorder
- 315.31 Developmental language disorder
- 315.39 Developmental articulation disorder
- 315.50 Mixed specific developmental disorder
- 315.90 Atypical specific developmental disorder

ORGANIC MENTAL DISORDERS
Section 1. Organic mental disorders whose etiology or pathophysiological process is listed below

Dementias Arising in the Senium and Presenium

Primary degenerative dementia, senile onset,
- 290.30 With delirium
- 290.20 With delusions
- 290.21 With depression
- 290.00 Uncomplicated

Code in fifth digit: 1 = with delirium, 2 = with delusions, 3 = with depression, 0 = uncomplicated.

290.1x Primary degenerative dementia, presenile onset, _____

290.4x Multi-infarct dementia, _____

Substance-induced

Alcohol

303.00 Intoxication

291.40 Idiosyncratic intoxication

291.80 Withdrawal

291.00 Withdrawal delirium

291.30 Hallucinosis

291.10 Amnestic disorder

Code severity of dementia in fifth digit: 1 = mild, 2 = moderate, 3 = severe, 0 = unspecified.

291.2x Dementia associated with alcoholism, _____

Barbiturate or similarly acting sedative or hypnotic

305.40 Intoxication (327.00)

292.00 Withdrawal (327.01)

292.00 Withdrawal delirium (327.02)

292.83 Amnestic disorder (327.04)

Opioid

305.50 Intoxication (327.10)

292.00 Withdrawal (327.11)

Cocaine

305.60 Intoxication (327.20)

Amphetamine or similarly acting sympathomimetic

305.70 Intoxication (327.30)

292.81 Delirium (327.32)

292.11 Delusional disorder (327.35)

292.00 Withdrawal (327.31)

Phencyclidine (PCP) or similarly acting arylcyclohexylamine

305.90 Intoxication (327.40)

292.81 Delirium (327.42)

292.90 Mixed organic mental disorder (327.49)

Hallucinogen

305.30 Hallucinosis (327.56)

292.11 Delusional disorder (327.55)

292.84 Affective disorder (327.57)

Cannabis

305.20 Intoxication (327.60)

292.11 Delusional disorder (327.65)

Tobacco

292.00 Withdrawal (327.71)

Caffeine

305.90 Intoxication (327.80)

Other or unspecified substance

305.90 Intoxication (327.90)

292.00 Withdrawal (327.91)

292.81 Delirium (327.92)

292.82 Dementia (327.93)

292.83 Amnestic disorder (327.94)

292.11 Delusional disorder (327.95)

292.12 Hallucinosis (327.96)

292.84 Affective disorder (327.97)

292.89 Personality disorder (327.98)

292.90 Atypical or mixed organic mental disorder (327.99)

Section 2. Organic brain syndromes whose etiology or pathophysiological process is either noted as an additional diagnosis from outside the mental disorders section or is unknown

293.00 Delirium

294.10 Dementia

294.00 Amnestic syndrome

293.81 Organic delusional syndrome

293.82 Organic hallucinosis

293.83 Organic affective syndrome

310.10 Organic personality syndrome

294.80 Atypical or mixed organic brain syndrome

SUBSTANCE USE DISORDERS

Code in fifth digit: 1 = continuous, 2 = episodic, 3 = in remission, 0 = unspecified.

305.0x Alcohol abuse, _____

303.9x Alcohol dependence (Alcoholism), _____

305.4x Barbiturate or similarly acting sedative or hypnotic abuse, _____

304.1x Barbiturate or similarly acting sedative or hypnotic dependence, _____

305.5x Opioid abuse, _____

304.0x Opioid dependence, _____

305.6x Cocaine abuse, _____

305.7x Amphetamine or similarly acting sympathomimetic abuse, _____

304.4x Amphetamine or similarly acting sympathomimetic dependence, _____

305.9x Phencyclidine (PCP) or similarly acting arylcyclohexylamine abuse, _____ (328.4x)

305.3x Hallucinogen abuse, _____

305.2x Cannabis abuse, _____

304.3x Cannabis dependence, _____

305.1x Tobacco dependence, _____

305.9x Other, mixed or unspecified substance abuse, _____

304.6x Other specified substance dependence, _____

304.9x Unspecified substance dependence, _____

304.7x Dependence on combination of opioid and other nonalcoholic substance, _____

304.8x Dependence on combination of substances, excluding opioids and alcohol, _____

657

SCHIZOPHRENIC DISORDERS

Code in fifth digit: 1 = subchronic, 2 = chronic,
3 = subchronic with acute exacerbation, 4 = chronic
with acute exacerbation, 5 = in remission,
0 = unspecified.

Schizophrenia
    295.1x Disorganized, _____
    295.2x Catatonic, _____
    295.3x Paranoid, _____
    295.9x Undifferentiated, _____
    295.6x Residual, _____

PARANOID DISORDERS
    297.10 Paranoia
    297.30 Shared paranoid disorder
    298.30 Acute paranoid disorder
    297.90 Atypical paranoid disorder

PSYCHOTIC DISORDERS NOT ELSEWHERE CLASSIFIED
    295.40 Schizophreniform disorder
    298.80 Brief reactive psychosis
    295.70 Schizoaffective disorder
    298.90 Atypical psychosis

AFFECTIVE DISORDERS

Code major depressive episode in fifth digit: 6 = in
remission, 4 = with psychotic features (the unofficial
non-ICD-9-CM fifth digit 7 may be used instead to
indicate that the psychotic features are mood-
incongruent), 3 = with melancholia, 2 = without
melancholia, 0 = unspecified.

    Code manic or mixed episode in fifth digit: 6 = in
remission, 4 = with psychotic features (the unofficial
non-ICD-9-CM fifth digit 7 may be used instead to
indicate that the psychotic features are mood-
incongruent), 2 = without psychotic features,
0 = unspecified.

Bipolar disorder,
    296.6x Mixed, _____
    296.4x Manic, _____
    296.5x Depressed, _____

Major depression,
    296.2x Single episode, _____
    296.3x Recurrent, _____

Other Specific Affective Disorders
    301.13 Cyclothymic disorder
    300.40 Dysthymic disorder (or depressive
            neurosis)

Atypical Affective Disorders
    296.70 Atypical bipolar disorder
    296.82 Atypical depression

ANXIETY DISORDERS

Phobic disorders (or phobic neuroses)
    300.21 Agoraphobia with panic attacks
    300.22 Agoraphobia without panic attacks
    300.23 Social phobia
    300.29 Simple phobia

Anxiety states (or anxiety neuroses)
    300.01 Panic disorder
    300.02 Generalized anxiety disorder
    300.30 Obsessive-compulsive disorder (or
            obsessive-compulsive neurosis)

Posttraumatic stress disorder
    308.30 Acute
    309.81 Chronic or delayed

    300.00 Atypical anxiety disorder

SOMATOFORM DISORDERS
    300.81 Somatization disorder
    300.11 Conversion disorder (or hysterical
            neurosis, conversion type)
    307.80 Psychogenic pain disorder
    300.70 Hypochondriasis (or hypochondriacal
            neurosis)
    300.70 Atypical somatoform disorder (300.71)

DISSOCIATIVE DISORDERS (OR HYSTERICAL NEUROSES, DISSOCIATIVE TYPE)
    300.12 Psychogenic amnesia
    300.13 Psychogenic fugue
    300.14 Multiple personality
    300.60 Depersonalization disorder (or
            depersonalization neurosis)
    300.15 Atypical dissociative disorder

PSYCHOSEXUAL DISORDERS

Gender Identity Disorders
Indicate sexual history in the fifth digit of
transsexualism code: 1 = asexual, 2 = homosexual,
3 = heterosexual, 0 = unspecified.

    302.5x Transsexualism, _____
    302.60 Gender identity disorder of childhood
    302.85 Atypical gender identity disorder

Paraphilias
    302.81 Fetishism
    302.30 Transvestism
    302.10 Zoophilia
    302.20 Pedophilia
    302.40 Exhibitionism
    302.82 Voyeurism
    302.83 Sexual masochism
    302.84 Sexual sadism
    302.90 Atypical paraphilia

Psychosexual Dysfunctions
- 302.71 Inhibited sexual desire
- 302.72 Inhibited sexual excitement
- 302.73 Inhibited female orgasm
- 302.74 Inhibited male orgasm
- 302.75 Premature ejaculation
- 302.76 Functional dyspareunia
- 306.51 Functional vaginismus
- 302.70 Atypical psychosexual dysfunction

Other psychosexual disorders
- 302.00 Ego-dystonic homosexuality
- 302.89 Psychosexual disorder not elsewhere classified

FACTITIOUS DISORDERS
- 300.16 Factitious disorder with psychological symptoms
- 301.51 Chronic factitious disorder with physical symptoms
- 300.19 Atypical factitious disorder with physical symptoms

DISORDERS OF IMPULSE CONTROL NOT ELSEWHERE CLASSIFIED
- 312.31 Pathological gambling
- 312.32 Kleptomania
- 312.33 Pyromania
- 312.34 Intermittent explosive disorder
- 312.35 Isolated explosive disorder
- 312.39 Atypical impulse control disorder

ADJUSTMENT DISORDER
- 309.00 With depressed mood
- 309.24 With anxious mood
- 309.28 With mixed emotional features
- 309.30 With disturbance of conduct
- 309.40 With mixed disturbance of emotions and conduct
- 309.23 With work (or academic) inhibition
- 309.83 With withdrawal
- 309.90 With atypical features

PSYCHOLOGICAL FACTORS AFFECTING PHYSICAL CONDITION
Specify physical condition on Axis III.
- 316.00 Psychological factors affecting physical condition

PERSONALITY DISORDERS
(These are coded on Axis II):
- 301.00 Paranoid
- 301.20 Schizoid
- 301.22 Schizotypal
- 301.50 Histrionic
- 301.81 Narcissistic
- 301.70 Antisocial
- 301.83 Borderline
- 301.82 Avoidant
- 301.60 Dependent
- 301.40 Compulsive
- 301.84 Passive-aggressive
- 301.89 Atypical, mixed, or other personality disorder

V CODES FOR CONDITIONS NOT ATTRIBUTABLE TO A MENTAL DISORDER THAT ARE A FOCUS OF ATTENTION OR TREATMENT
- V65.20 Malingering
- V62.89 Borderline intellectual functioning (V62.88)
- V71.01 Adult antisocial behavior
- V71.02 Childhood or adolescent antisocial behavior
- V62.30 Academic problem
- V62.20 Occupational problem
- V62.82 Uncomplicated bereavement
- V15.81 Noncompliance with medical treatment
- V62.89 Phase of life problem or other life circumstance problem
- V61.10 Marital problem
- V61.20 Parent-child problem
- V61.80 Other specified family circumstances
- V62.81 Other interpersonal problem

ADDITIONAL CODES
- 300.90 Unspecified mental disorder (nonpsychotic)
- V71.09 No diagnosis or condition on Axis I
- 799.90 Diagnosis or condition deferred on Axis I

V71.09 No diagnosis on Axis II
799.90 Diagnosis deferred on Axis II

659

A P P E N D I X C

███████████████████████

STANDARDS OF PSYCHIATRIC AND MENTAL HEALTH NURSING PRACTICE

███████████████████████

The Standards of Psychiatric and Mental Health Nursing Practice were developed in 1973 and revised in 1982 by the Division on Psychiatric and Mental Health Nursing Practice of the American Nurses' Association. Only the basic standards are reprinted here; in their entirety the standards are accompanied by specific rationales and measurement criteria. The rationales explain the basic premise on which each standard is based. The criteria suggest various mechanisms that may be employed to judge adherence to or attainment of a particular standard.

The Standards of Psychiatric and Mental Health Nursing are written in broad terms and are intended to guide practitioners regardless of the setting or the population being served. In the standards a distinction is made between generalist nurses and specialist nurses. All standards apply to generalists and specialists alike, except for Standard V-F and Standard X. The first of these deals with psychotherapy and the second with community health systems; both of these standards are addressed to clinical specialists in psychiatric and mental health nursing.

The Standards of Psychiatric and Mental Health Nursing are organized according to the dimensions of nursing process and include data collection (assessment), diagnosis, planning, implementation, and evaluation. The first standard deals with theory and makes a strong case for scholarly and knowledgeable utilization of theoretical concepts as the foundation of all professional nursing practice, whether the practitioner is a generalist or a specialist in psychiatric and mental health nursing.

Most of the eleven standards are concerned with professional practice, but an important few are concerned with aspects of professional performance beyond offering clinical care. The performance standards focus on peer review as an evaluation tool, acceptance of lifelong learning as a professional obligation, and collaboration with other health care disciplines. The importance of nursing research is addressed in the final standard of professional performance. In effect, the Standards of Psychiatric and Mental Health Nursing Practice support and guide the enactment of expanded roles for nurses within the framework of professional accountability, lifelong growth, and commitment to excellence in client care.

Reprinted by permission of the American Nurses' Association, Kansas City, Missouri.

PROFESSIONAL PRACTICE STANDARDS

Standard I: Theory
The nurse applies appropriate theory that is scientifically sound as a basis for decisions regarding nursing practice.

Standard II: Data Collection
The nurse continuously collects data that are comprehensive, accurate, and systematic.

Standard III: Diagnosis
The nurse utilizes nursing diagnoses and standard classification of mental disorders to express conclusions supported by recorded assessment data and current scientific premises.

Standard IV: Planning
The nurse develops a nursing care plan with specific goals and interventions delineating nursing actions unique to each client's needs.

Standard V: Intervention
The nurse intervenes as guided by the nursing care plan to implement nursing actions that promote, maintain, or restore physical and mental health, prevent illness, and effect rehabilitation.

Standard V-A: Psychotherapeutic Interventions
The nurse (generalist) uses psychotherapeutic interventions to assist clients to regain or improve their previous coping abilities and to prevent further disability.

Standard V-B: Health Teaching
The nurse assists clients, families, and groups to achieve satisfying and productive patterns of living through health teaching.

Standard V-C: Self-care Activities
The nurse uses activities of daily living in a goal-directed way to foster adequate self-care and physical and mental well-being of clients.

Standard V-D: Somatic Therapies
The nurse uses knowledge of somatic therapies and applies related clinical skills in working with clients.

Standard V-E: Therapeutic Environment
The nurse provides, structures, and maintains a therapeutic environment in collaboration with the client and other health care providers.

Standard V-F: Psychotherapy
The nurse (specialist) utilizes advanced clinical expertise in individual, group, and family psychotherapy, child psychotherapy, and other treatment modalities to function as a psychotherapist and recognizes professional accountability for nursing practice.

Standard VI: Evaluation
The nurse evaluates client responses to nursing actions in order to revise the data base, nursing diagnoses, and nursing care plan.

PROFESSIONAL PERFORMANCE STANDARDS

Standard VII: Peer Review
The nurse participates in peer review and other means of evaluation to assure quality of nursing care provided for clients.

Standard VIII: Continuing Education
The nurse assumes responsibility for continuing education and professional development and contributes to the professional growth of others.

Standard IX: Interdisciplinary Collaboration
The nurse collaborates with interdisciplinary teams in assessing, planning, implementing, and evaluating programs and other mental health activities.

Standard X: Utilization of Community Health Systems
The nurse (specialist) participates with other members of the community in assessing, planning, implementing, and evaluating mental health services and community systems that include the promotion of the broad continuum of primary, secondary, and tertiary prevention of mental illness.

Standard XI: Research
The nurse contributes to nursing and the mental health field through innovations in theory and practice and participation in research.

ETHICAL CODE FOR NURSES

1. The nurse provides services with respect for human dignity and the uniqueness of the client unrestricted by considerations of social or economic status, personal attributes, or the nature of health problems.

2. The nurse safeguards the client's right to privacy by judiciously protecting information of a confidential nature.

3. The nurse acts to safeguard the client and the public when health care and safety are affected by the incompetent, unethical, or illegal practice of any person.

4. The nurse assumes responsibility and accountability for individual nursing judgments and actions.

5. The nurse maintains competence in nursing.

6. The nurse exercises informed judgment and uses individual competence and qualifications as criteria in seeking consultation, accepting responsibilities, and delegating nursing activities to others.

7. The nurse participates in activities that contribute to the ongoing development of the profession's body of knowledge.

8. The nurse participates in the profession's efforts to establish and maintain conditions of employment conducive to high-quality nursing care.

9. The nurse participates in the profession's efforts to implement and improve standards of nursing.

10. The nurse participates in the profession's effort to protect the public from misinformation and misrepresentation and to maintain the integrity of nursing.

11. The nurse collaborates with members of the health professions and other citizens in promoting community and national efforts to meet the health needs of the public.

Reprinted by permission of the American Nurses' Association, 1976.

████████████

MENTAL HEALTH PATIENTS'
LIBERATION PROJECT

████████████

This is a voluntary organization designed to help hospitalized psychiatric patients and discharged patients who suffer job discrimination or educational discrimination or mistreatment at the hands of any agency or personnel, professional or otherwise. Persons in need of assistance or interested parties are encouraged to communicate with MPLP based in New York City.

1. You are a human being and are entitled to be treated as such with as much decency and respect as is accorded to any other human being.

2. You are an American citizen and are entitled to every right established by the Declaration of Independence and guaranteed by the Constitution of the United States of America.

3. You have the right to the integrity of your own mind and the integrity of your own body.

4. Treatment and medication can be administered only with your consent and, in the event you give your consent, you have the right to demand to know all relevant information regarding said treatment and/or medication.

5. You have the right to have access to your own legal and medical counsel.

6. You have the right to refuse to work in a mental hospital and/or to choose what work you shall do and you have the right to receive the minimum wage for such work as is set by the state labor laws.

7. You have the right to decent medical attention when you feel you need it just as any other human being has that right.

8. You have the right to uncensored communication by phone, letter, and in person with whomever you wish and at any time you wish.

9. You have the right not to be treated like a criminal; not to be locked up against your will; not to be committed involuntarily; not to be fingerprinted or "mugged" (photographed).

10. You have the right to decent living conditions. You're paying for it and the taxpayers are paying for it.

11. You have the right to retain your own personal property. No one has the right to confiscate what is legally yours, no matter what reason is given. That is commonly known as theft.

12. You have the right to bring grievance against those who have mistreated you and the right to counsel and a court hearing. You are entitled to protection by the law against retaliation.

13. You have the right to refuse to be a guinea pig for experimental drugs and treatments and to refuse to be used as learning material for students. You have the right to demand reimbursement if you are so used.

14. You have the right not to have your character questioned or defamed.

15. You have the right to request an alternative to legal commitment or incarceration in a mental hospital.

LEGISLATION PROTECTING MENTAL PATIENTS

Laws vary from state to state. The Massachusetts Civil Rights Law for the protection of hospitalized mental patients is an example of enlightened legislation. The following guarantees are exerpted from the law (M.G.L. ch. 23).

- No person shall be deprived of the right to manage his affairs, to contract, to hold professional, occupational or vehicle operator's licenses, to make a will, to marry, to hold or convey property, or to vote in local, state, or federal elections solely by reason of his admission or commitment to facility except where there has been an adjudication that such person is incompetent, or when a conservator or guardian has been appointed for such person. In the event of the conservatorship of a patient, a patient's civil rights may be limited only to the extent of the conservator's adjudicated responsibility.

- Under Law . . . notice shall be given to the patient and his nearest living relative that a recommendation has been made that there be an adjudication of the competency of such patient. The facility shall take reasonable means to apprise persons having dealings with such patient that such recommendation has been made or that said adjudication of competency of such patient is pending.

- A mentally ill person (receiving care as an inpatient): Shall be provided with stationery and postage in reasonable amounts. Shall have the right to have his letters forwarded unopened to the governor, the (mental health) commissioner, his personal physician, attorney, clergyman, any court, any public elected official, member of his immediate family; the superintendent (of the treating facility) may open or restrict the forwarding of any other letters written by such person when in that person's best interest. Shall have the right to be visited at all reasonable times by his personal physician, his attorney, and his clergyman. Shall have the right to be visited by other persons unless the superintendent determines that a visit by such other persons would not be in the best interests of the mentally ill person. The superintendent shall include a statement of the reasons for any denial of visiting rights. Shall have the right to wear his own clothes, to keep and use his own personal possessions including toilet articles, to keep and be allowed to spend a reasonable sum of money for canteen expenses and small purchases, to have access to individual storage space for private use, to have reasonable access to public telephones to make and receive confidential calls, to refuse shock treatment, and to refuse lobotomy. A denial of any of these rights for good cause by the superintendent or designee shall be entered in the treatment record of such person.

- Any patient involuntarily committed to any facility who believes or has reason to believe he should no longer be retained may make written application to Superior Court for a judicial determination of the necessity of continued commitment.

STATEMENT OF THE RIGHTS
OF MENTAL HEALTH PATIENTS

Many mental health facilities distribute statements similar to the following to patients receiving treatment and to their families.

Your rights to be treated with dignity and respect will be safeguarded while you are a patient.

PERSONAL RIGHTS
You have the right to wear your own clothes.
You have the right to keep your own money.
You have the right to have personal belongings.
You have the right to vote in all elections.
You have the right to hold licenses (driver's, professional).

HEALTH CARE RIGHTS
You have the right to be informed of:
  what is wrong with you;
  what treatments are possible;
  what are the risks of those treatments.
You have the right to refuse treatment.

COMMUNICATION RIGHTS
You have the right to use the telephone.
You have the right to mail letters.
You have the right to write to public officials.

VISITATION RIGHTS
You have the right to visit with family and friends.
You have the right to be visited by your clergy.
You have the right to see your own physician.

LEGAL RIGHTS
You have the right to be notified of commitment procedures.
You have the right to consult your own attorney.
You have the right to make contracts.
You have the right to own property.

665

████████████████

PSYCHOLOGICAL TESTS: PURPOSES AND
AGE RANGE OF SUBJECTS

████████████████████

Test	Type	Assesses	Age of Patient
Bayley Scales of Infant Development	Infant development	Cognitive functioning and motor development	1–30 months
Bender Visual-Motor Gestalt Test	Projective visual-motor development	Personality conflicts Ego function and structure Organic brain damage	5 to adult
Benton Visual Retention Test	Objective performance	Organic brain damage	Adult
Catell Infant Intelligence Scale	Infant development	General motor and cognitive development	1–18 months
Draw-A-Person, Draw-A-Family-House-Tree-Person	Projective	Personality conflicts Self-image (DAP) Family perception (DAF) Ego functions Intellectual functioning (DAP) Visual-motor coordination	2 to adult
Frostig (Marianne) Developmental Test of Visual Perception	Visual perception	Eye-motor coordination Figure ground perception Constancy of shape Position in space Spatial relationships	4–8 years
Gesell Developmental Schedules	Preschool development	Cognitive, motor, language, and social development	1–60 months
Illinois Test of Psycholinguistic Ability (ITPA)	Language ability	Auditory-vocal, visual motor channels of language receptive, organizational, and expressive components	2–10 years
Minnesota Multiphasic Personality Inventory (MMPI)	Paper and pencil personality inventory	Personality structure Diagnostic classification	Adolescent to adult
Otis Quick Scoring Mental Abilities Test	Intelligence	Intellectual functioning	5 to adult
Rorschach	Projective	Personality conflicts Ego function and structure Defensive structure Thought processes Affective integration	3 to adult
Stanford-Binet	Intelligence	Intellectual functioning	2 to adult
Thematic Apperception Test (TAT) Michigan Picture Stories	Projective	Personality conflicts Defensive structure	Adult—TAT Adolescent—Mich.

APPENDIX I

███████████████████████

HEALTH-RELATED ORGANIZATIONS

American Nurses' Association
2420 Pershing Road
Kansas City, Missouri 64108

American Psychiatric Association
1700 18th Street N.W.
Washington, D.C. 20009

Council of Advanced Psychiatric Mental Health
Nursing Practitioners
American Nurses' Association
2420 Pershing Road
Kansas City, Missouri 64108

National Association for Mental Health
1800 North Kent Street
Arlington, Virginia 22209

National Institute of Mental Health
56 Fishers Lane
Rockville, Maryland 20852

National League for Nursing
10 Columbus Circle
New York, New York 10019

Nursing Archive, Mugar Library
Boston University
771 Commonwealth Avenue
Boston, Massachusetts 02215

U.S. Department of Health and Social Services
200 Independence Avenue S.W.
Washington, D.C. 20201

U.S. Department of Education
400 Maryland Avenue S.W.
Washington, D.C. 20202

APPENDIX J

███████████████████████████

CONTROLLED DRUGS
███████████████████████████

The drugs that come under jurisdiction of the Controlled Substances Act are divided into five schedules. They are as follows.

SCHEDULE I SUBSTANCES
The drugs in this schedule are those that have no accepted medical use in the United States and have a high abuse potential. Some examples are heroin, marijuana, LSD, peyote, mescaline, psilocybin, tetrahydrocannabinols, ketobemidone, levomoramide, racemoramide, benzylmorphine, dihydromorphine, morphine methylsulfonate, nicocodeine, nicomorphine, and others.

SCHEDULE II SUBSTANCES
The drugs in this schedule have a high abuse potential with severe psychic or physical dependence liability. Schedule II controlled substances consist of certain narcotic, stimulant, and depressant drugs. Some examples of Schedule II narcotic controlled substances are: opium, morphine, codeine, hydromorphone (Dilaudid), methadone (Dolophine), pantopon, meperdine (Demerol), cocaine, oxycodone (Percodan), anileridine (Leritine), and oxymorphone (Numorphan). Also in Schedule II are amphetamine (Benzedrine, Dexedrine), methamphetamine (Desoxyn), phenmetrazine (Preludin), methylphenidate (Ritalin), amobarbital, pentobarbital, secobarbital, methaqualone, etorphine hydrochloride, diphenoxylate, and phencyclidine.

SOURCE: Controlled Substance Act of 1970 as interpreted by United States Department of Justice.

SCHEDULE III SUBSTANCES
The drugs in this schedule have an abuse potential less than those in Schedules I and II, and include compounds containing limited quantities of certain narcotic drugs, and non-narcotic drugs such as: derivatives of barbituric acid except those that are listed in another schedule, glutethimide (Doriden), methyprylon (Noludar), chlorhexadol, sulfondiethylmethane, sulfonmethane, nalorphine, benzphetamine, chlorphentermine, clortermine, mazindol, phendimetrazine, and paregoric. Any suppository dosage form containing amobarbital, secobarbital, or pentobarbital is in this schedule.

SCHEDULE IV SUBSTANCES
The drugs in this schedule have an abuse potential less than those listed in Schedule III and include such drugs as: barbital, phenobarbital, methylphenobarbital, chloralbetaine (Beta Chlor), chloral hydrate, ethchlorvynol (Placidyl), ethinamate (Valmid), meprobamate (Equanil, Miltown), paraldehyde, methohexital, fenfluramine, diethylpropion, phentermine, chlordiazepoxide (Librium), diazepam (Valium), oxazepam (Serax), clorazepate (Tranxene), flurazepam (Dalmane), clonazepam (Clonopin), prazepam (Verstran), lorazepam (Ativan), mebutamate, and dextropropoxyphene (Darvon).

SCHEDULE V SUBSTANCES
The drugs in this schedule have an abuse potential less than those listed in Schedule IV and consist primarily of preparations containing limited quantities of certain narcotic drugs generally for antitussive and antidiarrheal purposes.

A P P E N D I X   K

███████████████

COMPENDIUM OF COMMON DRUGS IN PSYCHIATRIC NURSING

███████████████████████

ANALGESIC NARCOTIC MEDICATION
███████████████████

All narcotic analgesics, whether natural or synthetic, are related to opium, which has been used for many centuries. In fact, the term *opiate* or *opioid* is often used as a more accurate and descriptive title for this important group of drugs.

Morphine was the first opium alkaloid to be isolated, and by the latter half of the nineteenth century pure alkaloids of opium were widely used in medical practice. Although over twenty alkaloids have been isolated from crude opium, only a few are used clinically. A number of semisynthetic opiates, produced by simple modification of the morphine molecule, and true synthetic opiates are also available.

Of the opiate analgesics, morphine is the standard to which all other opiates are compared. The semisynthetic and synthetic narcotics were developed as part of the search for a potent morphinelike analgesic without the addictive and other side effects of the opiates.

Morphine and related drugs are effective against all types and sources of pain, including deep visceral pain.

There is some difference of opinion as to whether morphine actually alters the physiologic sensation of pain or whether it only increases the ability to tolerate painful sensations—that is, raises the pain threshold.

The major effects of morphine on the central nervous system are related to the drug's depressant effects. In addition to analgesia, other manifestations are drowsiness, mental clouding, and sometimes an exaggerated sense of well-being. Although the analgesic effect occurs first, it may not be followed by sleep even though drowsiness, lethargy, and apathy are induced. Morphine has a depressant effect on the respiratory center in the medulla, causing a decrease in rate and depth of respirations. In morphine poisoning, death is caused by complete respiratory failure. Other effects on the central nervous system include pupillary constriction, depression of the cough center, and stimulation of the emetic zone in the medulla, which may cause nausea and vomiting.

The effects of morphine on the gastrointestinal tract include increased smooth muscle tone in the sphincters, which causes a delay in stomach emptying, and decreased peristalsis. The defecation reflex is depressed, and constipation may result from continued morphine use. Glandular secretions are also diminished, slowing down digestive process. Urinary bladder tone is affected, and this may cause difficulty in voiding. Urinary output may also be decreased.

In therapeutic doses, morphine has no significant effects on blood pressure or heart rate and rhythm. However, the small blood vessels in the head, neck, and chest may dilate, causing a flushed appearance and diaphoresis, even when small dosages are given.

Opiate tolerance varies with individuals and with usage patterns. The more frequently the drug is used, the more frequently the dose must be increased to produce the desired effects. Tolerance develops to the drug's euphoric, respiratory, analgesic, and sedative effects, but not to the gastrointestinal or pupillary effects; hence, an addict will still exhibit contracted pupils and constipation. When a narcotic analgesic is used continually, tolerance may develop in as little as two weeks. Moreover, if a client is addicted to one opiate, he or she will be just as tolerant to another, so that changing the prescription from one narcotic to another will not delay or prevent addiction.

NATURAL OPIUM ALKALOIDS
█████████████████████

Generic Name   Morphine sulfate, morphine hydrochloride
Trade Name   MS
Classification   Narcotic analgesic

Action   Depresses cerebral cortex; causes sleep; depresses respiratory center and cough center; causes blood vessel dilatation in face, head, and neck (causes pruritus and sweating); stimulates contraction of ureters, bladder, and other smooth muscles; decreases GI secretions and motility, increases biliary tract pressure; releases ADH and histamine; promotes contraction of bronchial musculature; may cause nausea and vomiting through stimulation of emetic center in medulla.

Indications for Drug   Relief of severe pain, anxiety; preanesthetic agent; relief of pain and dyspnea in myocardial infarction.

Contraindications Urethral stricture, head injuries, craniotomy, acute alcoholism, bronchial asthma, prostatic hypertrophy, convulsive disorders, undiagnosed abdominal disorders, pancreatitis, ulcerative colitis, hypersensitivity to opiates. Use with caution in clients with reduced blood volume or those with reduced respiratory reserve; in the presence of hepatic or renal insufficiency; toxic psychosis; arrhythmias; in the elderly or very young children.

Forms of Drug Tablets and capsules containing 10, 15, or 30 mg; oral solution containing 10 mg/5 ml or 20 mg/5 ml; 1-ml ampules containing 2, 8, 10, or 15 mg/ml; 20-mg vials containing 15 mg/ml; prefilled cartridges containing 2, 8, 10, or 15 mg/ml. Store in light-resistant containers.

Administration of Drug Adults: Oral: 5 to 30 mg every 3 to 4 hours; oral forms are seldom used because GI absorption is not reliable. Intramuscular, subcutaneous: 5 to 15 mg every 3 to 4 hours; 10 mg/70 kg for initial dose. Intravenous: 2.5 to 15 mg in 4 to 5 ml of sterile water. Children: 0.1 to 0.2 mg/kg per dose subc; single dose not to exceed 15 mg.

1. For IV route, administer slowly over a 4- to 5-minute period.
2. Assess pupillary size and vital signs, particularly respirations, before each dose. Withhold medication if respirations are below 12 per minute and notify physician.
3. Do not mix with other medications, since morphine is incompatible with many drugs.

Absorption From GI tract, nasal mucosa, lungs, and vascular system. Peak action occurs in: 20 minutes (IV), 60 to 90 minutes (subc, IM). Duration of action is 3 to 7 hours. Crosses placenta and small amounts appear in breast milk.
Distribution Concentrated in the kidneys, lungs, liver, spleen, and skeletal muscles.
Metabolism In the liver.
Excretion Mostly in urine by glomerular filtration. Also in feces via biliary tract (about 7% to 10%).

Side Effects Slow and shallow respirations, coma, pinpoint pupils, cyanosis, hypothermia, weak pulse, hypotension, nausea, vomiting, dizziness, mental clouding, constipation, cough center depression, urinary retention, dysuria, biliary colic, bradycardia, allergic dermatologic reactions. Coma, severe respiratory depression, pulmonary edema, hypothermia, and cardiac arrest occur with acute intoxication.

Interactive Effects Effects are exaggerated and/or prolonged by tricyclic antidepressants, antianxiety agents, phenothiazines, MAO inhibitors, alcohol, general anesthetics, barbiturates, and other sedatives and hypnotics. Morphine can potentiate the effects of other CNS depressants and skeletal muscle relaxants. Narcotic antagonists block the effects of morphine.

Nursing Considerations
1. Assessment and planning
   a. The most effective analgesia is achieved before client's pain becomes intense. Evaluate client's need for medication carefully and be aware that smaller doses are effective in controlling continuous dull pain.
   b. Morphine has a high abuse potential. Clients, except for those who are terminally ill, should be transferred to a less potent analgesic as soon as possible.
   c. Oxygen and narcotic antagonists should be readily available.
2. Assessment and implementation
   a. Instruct client not to ambulate without assistance after receiving drug. Postural hypotension, dizziness, and syncope are common side effects.
   b. Movement and ambulation often enhance the emetic effect of morphine. Client should be instructed to remain supine following administration until effects are ascertained.
   c. Elderly clients may become restless because of paradoxical CNS stimulation.
   d. Bedrails should be instituted for all clients during first few days of morphine therapy and maintained until effects are ascertained.
   e. Intake and output should be monitored and client assessed for urinary retention.
   f. Assess client frequently for abdominal distention, decreased peristalsis, and constipation.
3. Assessment and evaluation
   a. Clients with acute myocardial infarction may experience temporary hypotension after administration.
   b. Possible false-positive results of serum amylase, lipase, and urine glucose with Benedict's solution. May cause decreased urinary vanilmandelic acid excretion and elevated serum glutamic-oxaloacetic transaminase.

Generic Names Codeine, codeine phosphate, codeine sulfate
Classification Narcotic analgesic and antitussive agent

See morphine for contraindications and side effects.

Action Similar actions to morphine, but one-tenth the analgesic activity. Less side effects than morphine (gastrointestinal, pupillary, respiratory). Depresses cough center. Addictive, but tolerance develops much more slowly than with morphine. (See morphine.)

Indications for Drug Relief of mild to moderate pain; suppression of cough. Used in patients sensitive to morphine.

Forms of Drug   Tablets containing 15, 30, or 60 mg; vials containing 15, 30, or 60 mg/ml; elixir and syrup for coughs (combination preparation); prefilled cartridges containing 15, 30, or 60 mg/ml.

Administration of Drug   Adults: 15 to 60 mg po or subc every 3 to 4 hours; Children—3 mg/kg daily.

Interactive Effects   Aspirin and codeine have a synergistic effect. (See morphine.)

Nursing Considerations   Large doses may stimulate nerve center causing restlessness. (See morphine for further details.)

WHOLE OPIUM DRUGS

Generic Name   Opium tincture
Trade Name   Laudanum
Classification   Narcotic (antiperistaltic)

See morphine for contraindications and side effects.

Action   Similar actions to morphine, but contains only 1% morphine (10 mg/ml). Major effect is gastrointestinal (decreases propulsive peristalsis).

Indications for Drug   Diarrhea.

Forms of Drug   Liquid alcoholic solution (combination preparation).

Administration of Drug   0.3 to 1.5 ml po qid.

Nursing Considerations   (See morphine.) Dilute drug in about 50 ml of water before administering. When diarrhea is controlled, drug should be discontinued, since it has addictive potential.

Generic Name   Camphorated opium tincture
Trade Name   Paregoric
Classification   Narcotic (antiperistaltic)

See morphine for contraindications, side effects, and drug interactions. See morphine and opium tincture for nursing considerations.

Action   Opium with camphor, benzoic acid, and anise oil. Similar actions to morphine, but contains 0.25 mg morphine per millileter. Major effect is to decrease peristalsis. (See morphine.)

Indications for Drug   Diarrhea.

Forms of Drug   Liquid in light-resistant bottle containing 0.25 mg/ml.

Administration of Drug   4 to 8 ml po qid.

SEMISYNTHETIC OPIATES

Generic Name   Diacetylmorphine
Trade Name   Heroin
Classification   Narcotic

Action   Similar actions to morphine, but produces greater euphoria. Highly addictive. (See morphine.)

Indications for Drug   None—illegal.

Generic Name   Apomorphine hydrochloride
Classification   Narcotic (emetic)

See morphine for drug interactions and nursing considerations.

Action   Produced by treating morphine with acids. Has reduced analgesic potency. Stimulates emetic center in medulla causing vomiting.

Indications for Drug   Oral ingestion of poisons.

Contraindications   Corrosive poison ingestion, shock, CNS depression for any reason.

Forms of Drug   Powder; hypodermic tablets containing 6 mg. Packaged in airtight, light-resistant containers. Must be dissolved in sterile water and sterilized before use. Once dissolved, solution deteriorates rapidly. Discolored solutions should be discarded.

Administration of Drug   Acts within 10 to 15 minutes. If first dose does not produce emesis, subsequent doses will be ineffective. Do not repeat dosage. Adults: 5 mg subc; Children: 0.1 mg/kg subc.

Generic Name Hydrocodone bitartrate
Trade Names Dicodid, Mercodinone (an ingredient of Hycodan)
Classification Narcotic analgesic (antitussive)

See morphine for contraindications and side effects. See morphine and codeine for drug interactions.

Action Similar actions to morphine and codeine, but with greater antitussive activity. (See morphine and codeine.)

Indications for Drug Primarily for cough.

Contraindications Not to be used in patients with glaucoma. (See morphine.)

Forms of Drug Tablets containing 5 mg; syrup containing 5 mg/ml.

Administration of Drug Adults: 5 to 15 mg po every 4 hours; always taken after meals. Children: under 2 years: 1.25 mg po every 4 hours; Ages 2 to 12 years: 2.5 to 5 mg po every 4 hours.

Nursing Considerations (See morphine and codeine.)
1. Addictive liability is greater than for codeine.
2. Warn clients not to operate machinery if drowsiness occurs.

Generic Name Hydromorphone hydrochloride
Trade Names Dilaudid, Hymorphan
Classification Narcotic analgesic

See morphine for contraindications and side effects.

Action Similar actions to morphine, but five times more effective for pain relief. Less hypnotic effect than morphine. (See morphine.)

Indications for Drug Relief of moderate to severe pain.

Forms of Drug Tablets containing 1, 2, 3, or 4 mg; ampules containing 1, 2, 3, or 4 mg/ml; vials of 10 or 20 ml containing 2 mg/ml; suppositories containing 3 mg.

Administration of Drug 1 to 4 mg po, IM, subc, or IV every 4 to 6 hours, whenever necessary; Rectal suppository: 3 mg.

Nursing Considerations (See morphine.)
1. For IV route, administer slowly over a 3- to 5-minute period.
2. Less tendency than morphine to produce nausea, vomiting, and constipation.

Generic Name Methyldihydromorphinone
Trade Name Metopon
Classification Narcotic analgesic

See morphine for contraindications and side effects.

Action Similar actions to morphine, but more potent. Effective with oral administration. Side effects are rare. (See morphine.)

Indications for Drug Relief of pain.

Forms of Drug Tablets containing 3 mg.

Administration of Drug 3 mg po every 3 hours, whenever necessary.

Nursing Considerations Less addictive liability than morphine. (See morphine.)

Generic Name Oxycodone hydrochloride
Trade Name (An ingredient of Percodan)
Classification Narcotic analgesic

See morphine for contraindications and side effects. See morphine and codeine for drug interactions. See codeine for indications for drug.

Action Similar actions to morphine and codeine. Effective with oral administration. (See morphine and codeine.)

Contraindications Not to be used in pregnancy or children under 6 years.

Forms of Drug Tablets (combination preparation).

Administration of Drug Adults: 3 to 20 mg po every 6 hours, whenever necessary. Children: Ages 6 to 12 years: 0.5 mg po every 6 hours, whenever necessary; Over 12 years: 1 mg po every 6 hours, whenever necessary.

Nursing Considerations Addictive liability is greater than for codeine. (See morphine and codeine for further details.)

Generic Name Oxymorphone hydrochloride
Trade Name Numorphan
Classification Narcotic analgesic

See morphine for action and side effects.

Indications for Drug Relief of severe pain.

Forms of Drug Powder for injection containing 0.5 mg/ml; suppositories containing 2.5 mg. Store in refrigerator.

Administration of Drug 0.75 to 1.5 mg IM or subc every 4 to 6 hours; Rectal suppository: 2 to 5 mg every 4 to 6 hours.

Nursing Considerations (See morphine.)
1. Less tendency than morphine to produce GI symptoms and respiratory depression.
2. Peak action occurs in 10 to 20 minutes when administered parenterally.

Generic Name Pantopium
Trade Name Pantopon
Classification Narcotic analgesic

See morphine for contraindications and side effects. See morphine and codeine for drug interactions and nursing considerations.

Action Similar actions to morphine and codeine. Purified opium alkaloids containing about 50% morphine. (See morphine and codeine.)

Indications for Drug Relief of pain in patients hypersensitive to morphine.

Forms of Drug Ampules containing 20 mg/ml.

Administration of Drug 5 to 20 mg IM or subc.

SYNTHETIC OPIATES

Generic Names Meperidine hydrochloride, pethidine hydrochloride
Trade Names Demerol, Dolantin, Dolosal
Classification Narcotic analgesic

See morphine for contraindications and side effects.

Action Similar actions to morphine, but one-tenth the analgesic activity. Less hypnotic, antitussive, and pupillary effects than morphine. Less likely to cause nausea, vomiting, or respiratory depression. (See morphine.)

Indications for Drug Relief of moderate or intermittent pain; preanesthetic agent; obstetric analgesic.

Forms of Drug Tablets containing 50 or 100 mg; syrup containing 50 mg/5 ml; ampules of 0.5, 1, 1.5, or 2 ml; vials of 30 ml containing 50 mg/ml.

Administration of Drug Adults: 50 to 100 mg po or IM every 3 to 4 hours, whenever necessary; Children: 6 mg/kg po or IM daily. Intravenous: 25 mg.

1. For IV route, administer very slowly over a 3- to 5-minute period.
2. Demerol solution is not compatible with barbiturate solution; do not mix together.
3. Dilute syrup in water.

Interactive Effects Amphetamines enhance analgesic effect. (See morphine.)

Nursing Considerations
1. Constipation and urinary retention are unlikely with Demerol.
2. Addictive liability is less than for morphine.

Generic Name Alphaprodine hydrochloride
Trade Name Nisentil
Classification Narcotic analgesic

See morphine for contraindications and side effects.

Action Similar actions to morphine. Analgesic activity is between that of meperidine and morphine, but acts more quickly, and over a shorter duration (2 hours). (See morphine.)

Indications for Drug Relief of moderate to severe pain; preanesthetic agent for minor surgery and diagnostic procedures; obstetric analgesic (early labor).

673

Forms of Drug 1-ml ampules containing 40 or 60 mg/ml; 10-ml vials containing 40 or 60 mg/ml.

Administration of Drug Subcutaneous: 20 to 60 mg every 2 hours; Maximum dosage: 240 mg daily. Intravenous: 20 to 30 mg every 3 to 6 hours.

Nursing Considerations Less danger of respiratory depression than with morphine. (See morphine.)

Generic Name Anileridine, anileridine phosphate
Trade Name Leritine
Classification Narcotic analgesic

See morphine for contraindications and nursing considerations. See morphine and meperidine hydrochloride for drug interactions. See meperidine hydrochloride for indications for drug.

Action Similar actions to meperidine, but three times the analgesic activity. Unlike meperidine, anileridine seldom causes constipation.

Forms of Drug Ampules and vials containing 25 mg/ml, tablets containing 25 mg.

Administration of Drug 25 to 50 mg po, IM, or subc every 3 to 4 hours; not to exceed 200 mg daily. Intravenous: 5 to 10 mg every 3 to 4 hours.

Generic Name Diphenoxylate hydrochloride with atropine sulfate
Trade Names Colonil, Lomotil
Classification Narcotic (antidiarrhetic)

See morphine for contraindications and side effects. See morphine and meperidine hydrochloride for drug interactions.

Action Similar actions to meperidine. Strong constipating effect.

Indications for Drug Diarrhea.

Contraindications Not to be used for children under 2 years. (See morphine.)

Forms of Drug Tablets and liquid (5 ml) containing 2.5 mg diphenoxylate with 0.025 mg atropine sulfate.

Administration of Drug Adults: 20 mg po daily in divided doses; Children: 0.3 to 0.4 mg/kg po daily in divided doses.

Nursing Considerations (See morphine.)
1. Exempt from restrictions of federal narcotic law.
2. May cause slight sedation with therapeutic doses. In doses over 40 mg/day, client can be expected to exhibit side effects like those of morphine.
3. For children 2 to 12 years, use liquid preparation only.

Generic Name Fentanyl citrate
Trade Name Sublimaze
Classification Narcotic analgesic

See morphine for contraindications, side effects, drug interactions, and nursing considerations.

Action Similar actions to morphine. Analgesic activity is equivalent to 10 mg morphine or 75 mg meperidine. Respiratory depression may last longer than analgesic effect.

Indications for Drug Primarily as preanesthetic agent or anesthetic supplement.

Forms of Drug Ampules of 2 or 5 ml containing 0.05 mg/ml.

Administration of Drug Intramuscular, intravenous: 0.025 to 0.1 mg.

Generic Name Levorphanol tartrate
Trade Names Levo-Dromoran, Methorphinan
Classification Narcotic analgesic

See morphine for contraindications, side effects, drug interactions, and nursing considerations.

Action Similar actions to morphine, but more potent. (See morphine.)

Indications for Drug Relief of severe pain; preanesthetic agent.

Forms of Drug Tablets containing 2 mg; 1-ml ampules containing 2 mg/ml; 10-ml vials containing 2 mg/ml.

Administration of Drug Oral: 2 to 3 mg every 3 to 4 hours; Subcutaneous: 1 to 3 mg every 3 to 4 hours.

674

Generic Name   Methadone hydrochloride
Trade Names   Adanon, Amidone, Dolophine, Methadon, Miadone, Polamidon
Classification   Narcotic analgesic

See morphine for contraindications, side effects, and drug interactions.

Action   Similar actions to morphine, but longer duration of action (up to 72 hours). (See morphine.)

Indications for Drug   Relief of pain; treatment of narcotic withdrawal symptoms, heroin users; antitussive.

Forms of Drug   Tablets containing 5 or 10 mg; ampules containing 10 mg/ml; vials containing 10 mg/ml; elixir or syrup containing 0.34 to 1 mg/ml.

Administration of Drug
- *Relief of pain:* 2.5 to 10 mg po or IM every 3 to 4 hours.
- *Treatment of narcotic withdrawal symptoms:* 15 to 20 mg po or IM every 3 to 4 hours.
- *Cough:* 1.5 to 2 mg po.

Nursing Considerations   Withdrawal from methadone addiction is more prolonged than for other opiates, but symptoms are less severe. (See morphine.)

Generic Name   Phenazocine
Trade Names   Prinadol, Xenagol
Classification   Narcotic analgesic

See morphine for contraindications, side effects, and drug interactions.

Action   Similar actions to morphine, but causes less sedation. Effective in smaller doses than morphine. (See morphine.)

Indications for Drug   Relief of severe pain; preanesthetic agent; obstetric analgesic.

Forms of Drug   10-ml vials containing 2 mg/ml; 1-ml vials containing 2 mg/ml.

Administration of Drug   Intramuscular: 1 to 3 mg every 4 to 6 hours; Intravenous: 0.5 to 1 mg every 4 to 6 hours.

Nursing Considerations   (See morphine.)
1. Greater danger of respiratory depression than with morphine.
2. Do not mix with other medications, since phenazocine is incompatible with many drugs.

Generic Name   Piminodine
Trade Name   Alvodine
Classification   Narcotic analgesic

See morphine for contraindications, side effects, and nursing considerations. See morphine and meperidine hydrochloride for drug interactions.

Action   Similar actions to meperidine, but with slightly shorter duration of action. Less likely to cause constipation.

Indications for Drug   Relief of moderate to severe pain.

Forms of Drug   Tablets containing 25 mg; vials containing 50 mg/ml. Store in light-resistant containers.

Administration of Drug   Oral: 25 to 50 mg every 4 to 6 hours; Intramuscular, subcutaneous: 10 to 20 mg every 4 to 6 hours.

SYNTHETIC OPIATES WITH LOW POTENCY AND LOW ADDICTIVE LIABILITY

Generic Name   Propoxyphene hydrochloride
Trade Names   Darvon, Dolene, Progesic
Classification   Analgesic (mild narcotic)

See codeine for contraindications and side effects.

Action   Similar actions to codeine, but only half as potent. With aspirin, is as effective as codeine and aspirin. Has no antitussive effect.

Indications for Drug   Relief of mild to moderate pain in chronic or recurring diseases.

Contraindications   Hypersensitivity; not to be used for children.

Forms of Drug   Capsules containing 32 or 65 mg.

Administration of Drug   65 mg po q4h.

675

Interactive Effects   Has synergistic effect with aspirin. Has additive effect with alcohol, tranquilizers, and other CNS depressants.

Nursing Considerations
1. Exempt from restrictions of federal narcotic law.
2. Has very slight addictive liability, but can produce psychic and physical dependence.
3. Client should not drive or operate machinery until effect of drug is evaluated.
4. Drowsiness usually occurs only with very large doses (300 mg or more).
5. Client should not consume alcohol or any other sedatives or hypnotics while taking propoxyphene.

Generic Name   Ethoheptazine citrate
Trade Name   Zactane
Classification   Analgesic (mild narcotic)

See morphine for contraindications and side effects. See morphine and meperidine hydrochloride for drug interactions.

Action   Acts on CNS to produce analgesia. Has no antitussive, sedative, or respiratory effects. Structurally related to meperidine.

Indications for Drug   Relief of mild to moderate musculoskeletal pain. Not effective for headaches.

Contraindications   Not used in first trimester of pregnancy. Itching, dizziness, GI distress.

Forms of Drug   Tablets containing 75 mg.

Administration of Drug   75 to 150 mg po qid.

Nursing Considerations   (See morphine.)
1. Exempt from restrictions of federal narcotic law.
2. Drug is nonaddictive and rarely causes side effects, except with prolonged use.

Generic Name   Pentazocine hydrochloride
Trade Name   Talwin
Classification   Analgesic (mild narcotic)

See morphine for side effects and drug interactions.

Action   GI and CNS effects similar to morphine and codeine. Is a weak narcotic antagonist and has no antitussive effect. High doses cause elevation in blood pressure and heart rate.

Indications for Drug   Relief of moderate pain.

Contraindications   Not to be used for children under 12 years. Safety in pregnancy has not been established.

Forms of Drug   Tablets containing 50 mg.

Administration of Drug   Oral: 50 to 100 mg q4h; Intramuscular, subcutaneous, intravenous: 30 to 60 mg q4h. Total dosage should not exceed 600 mg daily.

Nursing Considerations   (See morphine.)
1. Exempt from restrictions of federal narcotic law.
2. Do not mix with barbiturates as the drugs are incompatible in solution.
3. May cause dependence in clients with a history of drug abuse.
4. Clients should not operate machinery while taking drug.
5. In respiratory depression produced by pentazocine, narcotic antagonists are not effective. Artificial respiration and respiratory stimulants are preferred methods of treatment.

NARCOTIC ANTAGONISTS

Generic Name   Nalorphine hydrochloride
Trade Names   Lethidrone, Nalline Hydrochloride
Classification   Narcotic antagonist

Action   Displaces other narcotics from cellular receptor sites. An effective antagonist against depressant effects of all narcotics. Causes abrupt withdrawal symptoms in narcotic addicts. Is not effective against other CNS depressants, barbiturates, or alcohol. May cause respiratory depression when given alone.

Indications for Drug   Acute narcotic toxicity with respiratory depression; diagnosing narcotic addiction; prevention of respiratory depression in newborns after narcotic given to mother.

Contraindications   CNS depression from sources other than narcotics. Not to be used for the treatment of addiction.

Forms of Drug   Adults: Ampules of 1, 2, or 10 ml containing 5 mg/ml; Children: 1-ml ampules containing 0.2 mg/ml. Store in light-resistant containers.

Administration of Drug   Adults: 2 to 10 mg IM, subc, or IV as needed; Newborns: 0.1 to 0.2 mg IM or IV as needed.

Absorption From tissues after subc injection.
Metabolism Detoxified in liver.
Excretion In urine.

Interactive Effects Can aggravate the effects of barbiturates and other hypnotics on the respiratory system.

Nursing Considerations
1. Exempt from restrictions of federal narcotic law.
2. Respiratory rate and volume and blood pressure should increase within 2 minutes after IV administration in clients with severe narcotic depression. Additional doses may be required to prevent recurrence of respiratory depression.
3. Large doses cause drowsiness, sweating, dysphoria, nausea, and vomiting.
4. When used on narcotic-free clients, effect is similar to that of a small dose of morphine.

Generic Name Levallorphan tartrate
Trade Name Lorfan
Classification Narcotic antagonist

See nalorphine hydrochloride for indications for drug, contraindications, side effects, drug interactions, and nursing considerations.

Action Similar actions to nalorphine, but ten times more potent. (See nalorphine hydrochloride.)

Forms of Drug Adults: 10-ml vials containing 1 mg/ml; 1-ml ampules containing 1 mg/ml. Children: Vials containing 0.05 mg/ml. Store in light-resistant containers.

Administration of Drug 0.5 to 1 mg IM, subc, or IV as needed.

Generic Name Naloxone hydrochloride
Trade Name Narcan
Classification Narcotic antagonist

See nalorphine hydrochloride for indications for drug, contraindications, side effects, and nursing considerations.

Action Similar actions to nalorphine, but 10 to 30 times more potent. When given alone, does not cause morphinelike effects and does not aggravate respiratory depression of barbiturates and hypnotics. (See nalorphine hydrochloride.)

Forms of Drug 2-ml ampules containing 0.4 mg/ml; 10-ml vials containing 0.4 mg/ml.

Administration of Drug Adults: 0.2 to 1 mg IM, subc, or IV as needed; Children: 0.01 mg/kg IM, subc, or IV as needed.

ANTIDEPRESSANT MEDICATIONS

Three major classifications of antidepressant medications are (1) tricyclic antidepressants, (2) monoamine oxidase (MAO) inhibitors, and (3) lithium carbonate.

Antidepressant medication is used to alleviate the discomfort of clients with moderate to severe signs of depressed mood and affect and to treat clients experiencing a depressed cycle of manic-depressive illness.

TRICYCLIC ANTIDEPRESSANTS

677

Generic Name Amitriptyline hydrochloride
Trade Names Amitid, Amitril, Elavil, Endep, SK-Amitriptyline
Classification Tricyclic antidepressant

Action Amitriptyline is closely related to the phenothiazines and produces an antidepressant effect without the side effects of MAO inhibitors. Although the exact mechanism of action is unknown, amitriptyline is believed to interfere with the reuptake of brain amines by nerves. It depresses the effects of epinephrine and serotonin; it is a mild CNS depressant. Amitriptyline is an effective mood elevator and promotes mental acuity and an increased level of physical activity. Its sedative effects help counteract insomnia that may accompany any depression.

Indications for Drug Treatment of depressive disorders and anxiety neuroses.

Contraindications Acute phase of myocardial infarction, severe renal or hepatic deficiency, concomitant use of MAO inhibitors, glaucoma.

Forms of Drug Tablets containing 10, 25, or 50 mg; vials containing 10 mg/ml.

Administration of Drug   Adults: 75 mg po or IM daily, usually in divided doses; can be increased gradually to a maximum dosage of 150 mg/day. Geriatrics and teenagers: 10 mg po tid and 20 mg hs.

Absorption   Readily absorbed from GI tract. Peak action occurs in 3 to 4 hours. Half-life is 2 days.
Distribution   Widely distributed in body tissues and plasma proteins.
Metabolism   In the liver.
Excretion   In urine.

Side Effects   Dry mouth, constipation, orthostatic hypotension; allergic reactions; CNS symptoms (extrapyramidal signs, anxiety, agitation, disorientation, hallucinations, ataxia, tremors, seizures); cardiovascular symptoms (arrhythmias, congestive heart failure, stroke); GI symptoms (gastric upset); endocrine and hematologic changes; altered blood sugar, blood dyscrasias, altered hepatic function.

Interactive Effects   Enhances the effects of other CNS depressants, catecholamines, adrenergics, anticholinergics, thyroid hormones, disulfiram, anticoagulants, vasodilators, and central-acting skeletal muscle relaxants. Antagonizes the effects of antihypertensives, anticonvulsants, phenylbutazone, and cholinergics. Tricyclic effects are potentiated by phenothiazines, methylphenidate, amphetamines, furazolidone, acetazolamide, MAO inhibitors, and urinary alkalizers. Tricyclic effects are inhibited by urinary acidifiers and barbiturates.

Nursing Considerations
1. Assessment and planning
   a. Drug should be discontinued at least 48 hours prior to surgery.
   b. Baseline vital signs, particularly blood pressure, should be determined prior to institution of therapy.
2. Assessment and implementation
   a. Entire daily dose may be prescribed at bedtime, since drug is long acting and has sedative effects.
   b. Monitor blood pressure frequently during initial phase of therapy.
   c. Inform client that the full therapeutic effect may occur 1 to 3 weeks after initiation of therapy.
   d. Instruct client that drug must be taken as prescribed, not merely when needed for depression.
   e. Instruct client to be alert for development of orthostatic hypotension; the elderly are particularly susceptible.
   f. Caution clients to avoid prolonged exposure to sunlight.
   g. Warn client not to drive or use heavy machinery while taking drug, since drowsiness is a frequent side effect.
   h. Instruct client that alcohol will potentiate drug effects, possibly producing extreme drowsiness and ataxia.
   i. Advise client to ingest sufficient fluids, rinse the mouth frequently, and chew gum to relieve the unpleasantness of dry mouth.
3. Assessment and evaluation
   a. Assess suicide risk carefully, since all depressed clients are potentially suicidal.
   b. Observe for slowing of normal elimination processes, since urinary retention and constipation are common side effects.

Generic Name   Desipramine hydrochloride
Trade Names   Norpramin, Pertofrane
Classification   Tricyclic antidepressant

See amitriptyline hydrochloride for indications for drug, contraindications, drug interactions, and nursing considerations.

Action   It has been theorized that desipramine is the active metabolite of imipramine and so is at least as therapeutic as imipramine. Desipramine may no longer be as effective after a few weeks, which is the amount of time needed for behavioral changes when other tricyclic antidepressants are administered. (See amitriptyline hydrochloride.)

Forms of Drug   Tablets containing 25, 50, 75, 100, or 150 mg; capsules containing 25 or 50 mg.

Administration of Drug   Adults: 25 to 50 mg po daily in divided doses; then increase gradually to a maximum dosage of 200 mg/day until desired effect; Maintenance dosage: 50 to 100 mg po daily.

Side Effects   May cause hyperthermia or a bad taste in the mouth. (See amitriptyline hydrochloride.)

Generic Name   Doxepin hydrochloride
Trade Names   Adapin, Sinequan
Classification   Tricyclic antidepressant

See amitriptyline hydrochloride for contraindications, side effects, drug interactions, and nursing considerations.

Action   Similar to amitriptyline. (See amitriptyline hydrochloride.)

Indications for Drug   Treatment of depression in psychoneurotic patients.

Forms of Drug   Capsules containing 10, 25, or 50 mg.

Administration of Drug   Adults: 75 mg po daily in divided doses; Maximum dosage: 150 to 300 mg/day.

Generic Name   Imipramine hydrochloride
Trade Name   Tofranil
Classification   Tricyclic antidepressant

See amitriptyline hydrochloride for indications for drug, contraindications, side effects, and drug interactions.

Action   Similar to amitriptyline. (See amitriptyline hydrochloride.)

Forms of Drug   Tablets containing 10, 25, or 50 mg; vials containing 12.5 mg/ml.

Administration of Drug   Adults: Outpatients: 75 mg po or IM daily in divided doses. Hospitalized clients: 100 to 150 mg po or IM daily; can be gradually increased to a maximum dosage of 300 mg/day in divided doses until desired effect; Maintenance dosage: 50 to 150 po or IM daily. Geriatrics and teenagers: Initially, 30–40 mg daily, not to exceed 100 mg daily.

Nursing Considerations   (See amitriptyline hydrochloride.)

1. Improvement in behavior may be observed as early as 3 days after onset of therapy.
2. Full therapeutic effect may not be apparent for 1 or 2 weeks.

Generic Name   Nortriptyline
Trade Name   Aventyl
Classification   Tricyclic antidepressant

See amitriptyline hydrochloride for indications for drug, contraindications, side effects, and drug interactions.

Action   Similar to amitriptyline. (See amitriptyline hydrochloride.)

Forms of Drug   Capsules containing 10 or 25 mg; concentrate containing 10 mg/5 ml.

Administration of Drug   Adults: Initial dosage: 20 to 40 mg po daily in divided doses for the first week; Maintenance dosage: 30 to 75 mg po daily; Maximum dosage: 100 mg/day. Geriatrics: 30 to 50 mg po daily.

Nursing Considerations   (See amitriptyline hydrochloride.)

Generic Name   Protriptyline hydrochloride
Trade Name   Vivactil
Classification   Tricyclic antidepressant

See amitriptyline hydrochloride for indications for drug, contraindications, drug interactions, and nursing considerations.

Action   Similar to amitriptyline. (See amitriptyline hydrochloride.)

Forms of Drug   Tablets containing 5 or 10 mg.

Administration of Drug   Adults: Initial dosage: 30 to 60 mg po daily in divided doses; Maintenance dosage: 15 to 40 mg po daily.

Side Effects   Causes more cardiovascular side effects than other tricyclic antidepressants, but produces less sedation. (See amitriptyline hydrochloride.)

MONOAMINE OXIDASE INHIBITORS

Generic Name   Isocarboxazid
Trade Name   Marplan
Classification   Antidepressant (MAO inhibitor)

Action   MAO inhibitors interfere with the enzyme monoamine oxidase, which metabolizes norepinephrine. The direct clinical result is a buildup of norepinephrine in the tissues, with all the attendant complications. These drugs affect blood pressure and hepatic function.

Indications for Drug   Endogenous depression, manic-depressive psychosis, severe reactive depression. Usually administered only after a trial with tricyclic antidepressants has proven ineffective.

Contraindications   Children under 16 years, congestive heart failure, hepatic dysfunction, phenochromocytoma, hyperthyroidism, cardiovascular disease, the elderly, debilitated clients.

Forms of Drug   Tablets containing 10 mg.

Administration of Drug   Adults: 30 mg po daily in a single dose or in divided doses; Maintenance dosage: 10 to 20 mg po daily.

Absorption   Readily absorbed from GI tract.
Metabolism   Rapidly metabolized in the liver.
Excretion   In urine.

Side Effects   Orthostatic hypotension, dizziness, insomnia, GI upsets, headache, arrhythmias, tremors, hypomania, euphoria, confusion, memory loss, ataxia, hallucinations, convulsions, dry mouth, blurred vision, dysuria, impotence, palpitations, edema, weight gain, blood dyscrasias, jaundice, photosensitivity reactions, sodium retention, hypoglycemia, glaucoma, anorexia.

Interactive Effects   Potentiates the effects of sympathomimetics, anticholinergics, antihistamines, antiparkinsonian drugs, and antihypertensives. Increases the toxic effects of barbiturates, phenothiazines, and CNS depressants. Increases the hypoglycemic effects of hypoglycemic drugs and the muscle-relaxing effect of succinylcholine. Interferes with the effect of antiepileptics. Foods containing tyramine (cheese, sour cream, yogurt, beer, wine, yeast, herring, chicken livers, aged meats, tenderizers, licorice, caffeine, chocolate) increase the risk of hypertensive crisis. Reserpine or guanethidine administered IV or IM can cause severe hypertension.

Nursing Considerations
1. Assessment and planning
   a. Drug should be discontinued at least 3 weeks prior to surgery.
   b. Baseline blood and hepatic function tests and blood pressure determinations should be done prior to institution of therapy.
2. Assessment and intervention
   a. Give with meals to reduce GI distress.
   b. Observe client carefully for toxic reactions, which can occur within hours of the first few doses.
   c. Blood pressure should be monitored between doses during initial phase of therapy.
   d. Instruct client to take no other drugs, including OTC preparations, concurrently and for 3 weeks following cessation of therapy.
   e. Instruct client to avoid tyramine-rich foods.
   f. Advise client to change positions slowly to avoid postural hypotension.
   g. Instruct client to report promptly any symptoms suggestive of hypertensive crisis (headache palpitations).
   h. Client should report any rapid or unusual weight gain or other unusual symptoms.

3. Assessment and evaluation
   a. Observe client for color blindness, which indicates eye damage.
   b. Assess lethality of client's suicidal statements, since client's mood improves with continued therapy.
   c. Since drug is long acting and may have a cumulative effect, behavioral changes may not be apparent for 1 to 4 weeks.

Generic Name   Phenelzine sulfate
Trade Name   Nardil
Classification   Antidepressant (MAO inhibitors)

See isocarboxazid for indications for drug, contraindications, and drug interactions.

Action   Similar to isocarboxazid. (See isocarboxazid.)

Forms of Drug   Tablets containing 15 mg.

Administration of Drug   Adults: Initial dosage: 45 mg po daily in divided doses; then gradually increase to a maximum dosage of 75 mg/day, if necessary, until desired effect; Maintenance dosage: 15 mg po every other day.

Side Effects   Similar to isocarboxazid, but less likely to precipitate a hypertensive crisis. (See isocarboxazid.)

Nursing Considerations   Therapeutic effect can occur after 1 to 2 weeks. (See isocarboxazid for further details.)

Generic Name   Tranylcypromine sulfate
Trade Name   Parnate
Classification   Antidepressant (MAO inhibitor)

See isocarboxazid for contraindications, drug interactions, and nursing considerations.

Action   Similar to isocarboxazid, but stimulant effect is stronger. (See isocarboxazid.)

Indications for Drug   Intractable depression. Should only be administered when other safer medications have been tried.

Forms of Drug   Tablets containing 10 mg.

Administration of Drug Adults: Initial dosage: 20 mg po daily in divided doses for 2 to 3 weeks; then gradually increase to a maximum dosage of 30 mg/day until desired effect; Maintenance dosage: 10 to 20 mg po daily.

Side Effects As the peak effect of this drug occurs much sooner than that produced by the other MAO inhibitors, there is a greater chance of precipitating a hypertensive crisis.

OTHER ANTIDEPRESSANTS

Generic Name Lithium carbonate
Trade Names Eskalith, Lithane, Lithonate, Lithotabs
Classification Antidepressant

Action Precise mechanism is unknown, but seems to act similarly to the sodium ion and enhances the excretion of sodium and potassium. Decreases circulating thyroid hormones, may block renal response to ADH, decreases glucose tolerance, and increases circulating growth hormone levels.

Indications for Drug Some controversy abounds concerning the value of lithium in treating manic-depressive illness. It has been found to be extremely effective in controlling acute manic and hypomanic behaviors, such as hyperactivity, poor judgment, flight of ideas, and aggressiveness. May be used in conjunction with phenothiazines.

Contraindications Cardiovascular or renal impairment, dehydration, clients taking diuretics, clients with sodium depletion, pregnancy, lactation, schizophrenia, organic brain disease. Safe use in children (under 12 years) has not been established.

Forms of Drug Tablets and capsules containing 300 or 600 mg.

Administration of Drug Adults: 300 to 600 mg po tid until desired effect; Maintenance dosage: 300 mg po tid.

Absorption Rapidly absorbed from GI tract. Peak action occurs in 2 to 4 hours. Half-life is 24 hours. Crosses the blood-brain barrier slowly. Crosses placenta and appears in breast milk.
Distribution Widely distributed in body water with high concentrations in the kidneys and saliva. Some drug is concentrated in bone, muscles, and liver.
Excretion About 75% in urine within 24 hours; alkalization of the urine enhances excretion.

Side Effects Dry mouth, metallic taste, thyroid enlargement, glycosuria, hyperglycemia, weight gain, edema. Lithium poisoning: nausea, diarrhea, diabeteslike symptoms, tremors. More serious symptoms include blurred vision and slurred speech. Dermatologic manifestations may also occur. In acute toxicity, convulsions, shock, coma, and death can occur. (See amitriptyline hydrochloride.)

Interactive Effects Acetazolamide, aminophylline, sodium bicarbonate, and sodium chloride enhance the renal excretion of lithium, thereby decreasing its effect. Phenothiazines may enhance hyperglycemic effects. Iodine-containing agents and tricyclic antidepressants may enhance hypothyroid effects. Thiazide diuretics, haloperidol, and methyldopa may increase lithium toxicity. Lithium may decrease the effects of amphetamines.

Nursing Considerations
1. Assessment and planning
   a. Since there is no antidote available for lithium poisoning, every effort must be made to prevent it.
2. Assessment and implementation
   a. Careful monitoring is required because there is a narrow margin between therapeutic and toxic dosages. Blood lithium levels should be determined before each morning dose during the initial treatment period and then weekly; therapeutic serum drug levels: 0.6 to 1.5 mEq/l.
   b. Give with meals or immediately after to minimize GI upset.
   c. Emphasize the importance of performing serum lithium determinations as scheduled (monthly).
   d. Stress the need to maintain adequate sodium and fluid intake and to avoid the use of diuretics.
   e. Advise client not to drive or operate machinery, since drowsiness is common.
   f. Lithium intoxication begins to develop when serum levels reach 1.5 mEq/l; if such levels occur, therapy should be discontinued for 1 day and then resumed at a lower dosage.
3. Assessment and evaluation
   a. Therapeutic response is usually evident within 10 days. If no response occurs within 2 weeks, drug should be discontinued.
   b. Client should be weighed daily. Report evidence of fluid retention.
   c. Assess client regularly for symptoms of hypothyroidism and/or thyroid enlargement.

681

ANTIANXIETY MEDICATIONS

Two major classes of antianxiety medications are benzodiazepines and propanediols. Sometimes called minor tranquilizers, antianxiety agents effectively reduce mild to moderate anxiety and the accompanying neurotic symptoms without interfering with the individual's ability to function at an adequate level.

Antianxiety agents have been especially useful in treating people with high anxiety levels or withdrawal from alcohol intoxication. The use of these drugs is said to enhance the individual's ability to participate effectively in psychotherapy.

BENZODIAZEPINES

Generic Name Diazepam
Trade Name Valium
Classification Antianxiety agent

Action Unlike the barbiturates used as antianxiety agents, diazepam produces only minor circulatory and respiratory depression, while preserving mental acuity even when administered in large dosages. Most of the brain is not depressed, but electrical impulses in the limbic system are inhibited. Diazepam is an effective skeletal muscle relaxant and a powerful anticonvulsant, but its mode of action is not clearly understood. Benzodiazepines depress the polysynaptic reflexes of the spinal cord, which reduces skeletal muscle tension, thereby inhibiting those afferent proprioceptive impulses that might aggravate existing anxiety. Benzodiazepines also inhibit stimulation of the amygdala and the hippocampus structures of the brain, which influence behavior. These drugs therefore have a mild sedative effect but do not alter the level of consciousness or the ability to perform psychomotor tasks.

Indications for Drug Anxiety states of organic or functional origin, such as anxiety due to angina pectoris, asthma, premenstrual tension, or menopause; insomnia; preoperative sedation; relaxation of tension due to arthritis and low-back pain; status epilepticus; withdrawal from alcohol intoxication.

Contraindications Severe psychoses, glaucoma, shock, children under 6 months.

Forms of Drug Tablets containing 2, 5, or 10 mg; vials of 2 to 10 ml containing 5 mg/ml.

Administration of Drug Adults: 4 to 40 mg po, IM, or IV daily in divided doses; Elderly patients require a lower dosage; Children: Over 6 months: 1 to 2.5 mg po tid.

1. IM injection must be deep into gluteal muscle.
2. Do not mix drug with other solutions. Do not add to IV fluids.
3. IV injection should not exceed 5 mg/min. Give into a large vein and avoid extravasation.

Absorption Readily absorbed from GI tract or the bloodstream. Onset of action is: 30 to 60 minutes (po); 15 to 30 minutes (IM). Peak blood levels occur in 2 hours. Half-life is 20 to 50 hours. Crosses placenta and appears in breast milk.
Metabolism Metabolized slowly in the liver; can still be found in the blood 7 days after discontinuation of therapy.
Excretion In urine, with a small amount in stool.

Side Effects Drowsiness, lethargy, ataxia, confusion, headache, syncope, vertigo, depression, stupor, excitement, dry mouth, constipation, urinary retention, blurred vision, hypotension, weight gain, cardiovascular collapse, blood dyscrasias, hypersensitivity reactions, endocrine abnormalities.

Interactive Effects Enhances the depressant effects of alcohol, barbiturates, antihistamines, phenothiazines, and narcotics. Potentiates the effects of phenytoin and skeletal muscle relaxants. Antagonizes the effects of levodopa. Smoking may inhibit the effects of benzodiazepines.

Nursing Considerations
1. Assessment and planning
   a. Since the effect of diazepam is accumulative, therapeutic results may not be apparent for 5 to 10 days after initiation of therapy.
2. Assessment and implementation
   a. Since diazepam is long acting, 1 dose per day is usually sufficient. The dose should be given at bedtime to promote sleep and relieve anxiety throughout the following day.
   b. Observe client for excessive drowsiness or ataxia.
   c. Provide bedrails and assistance with ambulation.
   d. Observe client for signs of developing physiologic or psychologic dependence. As dosage and duration of therapy increase, the risk of dependence increases.
   e. Observe geriatric clients carefully, since they are more likely to develop side effects.
   f. Advise client not to drink alcohol or take any other CNS depressant.
   g. Instruct client not to drive or operate dangerous machinery.
   h. Instruct client to change position slowly to prevent postural hypotension.
   i. Instruct client not to discontinue drug without medical supervision.

3. Assessment and evaluation
   a. Observe client for signs of drug dependence.
   b. Arrange for periodic blood and liver function tests if drug is given on a long-term basis.

Generic Names   Chlordiazepoxide, chlordiazepoxide hydrochloride
Trade Names   Libritabs, Librium
Classification   Antianxiety agent

See diazepam for contraindications, drug interactions, and nursing considerations.

Action   (See diazepam.)

Indications for Drug   Management of delirium tremens; treatment of anxiety associated with psychosomatic conditions.

Contraindications   Use with caution in addiction-prone clients.

Forms of Drug   Tablets and capsules containing 5, 10, or 25 mg; ampules containing 100 mg of dry powder.

Administration of Drug   Adults: 15 to 40 mg po, IM, or IV daily in divided doses; can be gradually increased to a maximum dosage of 300 mg/day. Geriatrics: 10 to 20 mg po, IM, or IV daily. Children: Over 6 years: 0.5 mg/kg po, IM, or IV daily.

Generic Name   Clorazepate dipotassium
Trade Name   Tranxene
Classification   Antianxiety agent

See diazepam for action, indications for drug, contraindications, and drug interactions.

Forms of Drug   Capsules containing 3.75, 7.5, or 15 mg.

Administration of Drug   Adults: 15 to 60 mg po daily in divided doses; Geriatrics: 7.5 to 15 mg po daily; Children: Over 6 years: 7.5 to 60 mg po daily in divided doses.

Generic Name   Oxazepam
Trade Name   Serax
Classification   Antianxiety agent

See diazepam for action, indications for drug, contraindications, and drug interactions.

Forms of Drug   Tablets containing 15 mg; capsules containing 10, 15, or 30 mg.

Administration of Drug   Adults: 30 to 120 mg po daily in divided doses.

Nursing Considerations   Monitor elderly clients carefully for the development of hypotension. (See diazepam.)

PROPANEDIOLS

Generic Name   Meprobamate
Trade Names   Equanil, Miltown
Classification   Antianxiety agent

See diazepam for contraindications and drug interactions.

Action   Similar to diazepam in that it reduces anxiety. Meprobamate is a skeletal muscle relaxant and an anticonvulsant. Its action is believed to be similar to phenobarbital.

Indications for Drug   Insomnia, simple nervous tension, petit mal epilepsy.

Forms of Drug   Tablets and capsules containing 200 or 400 mg; oral suspension containing 40 mg/ml; vials containing 80 mg/5 ml.

Administration of Drug   Adults: 400 mg po or IM daily in divided doses. Children: Over 6 years: 100 to 200 mg po or IM daily in divided doses; Maximum dosage: 2.4 g/day.

Nursing Considerations   (See diazepam.)
   1. Skin rash responds to antihistamines.
   2. Drug dependence may develop.

683

ANTICONVULSANT MEDICATIONS

Seizure disorders are so complex that there is no specific medication to control this range of disorders. Frequently, a seizure can only be treated symptomatically. Most anticonvulsant agents act by causing CNS inhibition, increasing the seizure threshold, and/or preventing the transmission of seizure-causing impulses.

Seizures may be classified broadly as grand mal, petit mal, and psychomotor, but the distinctions are not always clear. Seizures that originate in one part of the brain are termed *focal* and are localized in specific muscles or groups of muscles. *Psychomotor* seizures are usually localized. Both focal and psychomotor seizures are considered partial seizures. Generalized seizures are the result of bilateral, symmetrical brain disturbances. These seizures may take the form of grand mal or petit mal convulsions. Persons with more than one kind of seizure are said to have a mixed seizure disorder.

Each type of seizure disorder responds to different classes of anticonvulsant medication. Barbiturates, analogs of barbiturates, and hydantoin derivatives are helpful for grand mal seizures, focal seizures, and some generalized convulsive disorders. Valproic acid, succinimides, and oxazolidione derivatives are effective for petit mal seizures. Psychomotor seizures are usually controlled by hydantoin derivatives, phenobarbital, and primidone. Mixed seizure disturbances frequently require a combination of more than one anticonvulsant agent.

Anticonvulsant agents are administered daily to control the frequency and severity of the seizure episodes. The goal is to maintain a serum level high enough to prevent seizures yet low enough to avoid drug toxicity. For a number of anticonvulsant agents the range between therapeutic and toxic serum levels is quite narrow.

HYDANTOIN DERIVATIVES

Generic Names   Phenytoin; phenytoin sodium
Trade Names   Dihycon, Dilantin, Diphentoin, Ekko; Dilantin Sodium
Classification   Anticonvulsant

Action   Although chemically related to the barbiturates, phenytoin has little or no sedative effect, but is very effective in controlling grand mal seizures. Phenytoin inhibits the spread of seizure activity in the motor cortex. The exact mechanism of action is unknown, but phenytoin is thought to promote the loss of sodium from neurons and thereby tends to stabilize the

threshold against hyperexcitability. The maximal activity of the brain stem centers responsible for the tonic phase of grand mal seizures is reduced. Because phenytoin decreases myocardial contractility and ventricular automaticity it has been used to treat ectopic arrhythmias.

Indications for Drug   Status epilepticus (often in combination with other anticonvulsants); grand mal seizures (generalized tonic-clonic seizures); psychomotor seizures (temporal lobe); prevention and control of seizures induced by neurosurgery or head trauma. Has been used to treat Reye's syndrome, arrhythmias, and certain types of migraine headache.

Contraindications   Hypersensitivity to hydantoin derivatives, sinus bradycardia, S-A block, second and third degree heart block, Adams-Stokes syndrome. Use with caution in clients with hypotension, severe myocardial insufficiency, acute heart failure, impaired hepatic or renal function, diabetes (since plasma glucose levels may be altered), and the elderly. Not intended for use in seizure due to hyperglycemia or other types of easily identified and corrected seizure activity. Not effective for petit mal (absence) seizures, but has been used in combination with other anticonvulsant drugs. Safe use during pregnancy has not been established; may cause birth defects.

Forms of Drug   Capsules containing 100 or 300 mg; 300-mg capsules are reserved for noncompliant clients who are willing to take 300 mg daily, but not to take 100 mg tid. Suspension (Dilantin-125) containing 125 mg/5 ml; pediatric suspension (Dilantin-30) containing 30 mg/5 ml. Chewable tablets (Infatabs) containing 50 mg; yield higher serum drug levels than capsules; switch dosage form with caution. 2-ml ampules of ready-mixed solution containing 50 mg/ml; 2-ml prefilled syringes of ready-mixed solution containing 50 mg/ml; 5-ml ampules of ready-mixed solution containing 50 mg/ml. Capsules containing 100 mg phenytoin and 16 mg phenobarbital; capsules containing 100 mg phenytoin and 32 mg phenobarbital.

Administration of Drug   Highly individualized to provide maximum benefit and maintain therapeutic serum drug levels. Adults: Initial dosage: 100 mg po tid; then increase to 200 mg po tid after 7 to 10 days. Children: Initial dosage: 5 mg/kg/day in 2 or 3 divided doses; then increase as necessary after 7 to 10 days; Usual dosage range: 4 to 8 mg/kg/day; Maximum dosage: 300 mg/day.

Absorption Slowly absorbed from GI tract; absorption may vary with the drug dosage, form, and manufacturer. Slow and erratic absorption from IM sites due to drug precipitation; IM injections are avoided. Onset of action is 3 to 5 minutes after IV administration. Peak plasma levels occur in 3 to 12 hours. Therapeutic plasma concentration is 10 to 20 mcg/ml; steady-state therapeutic levels may take 7 to 10 days of therapy. Half-life is 22 hours (ranges from 7 to 42 hours), but varies greatly due to hepatic metabolism. About 70% to 95% bound to plasma proteins, but may be displaced or cause displacement of other drugs from protein-binding sites. Crosses placenta; risk of birth defects is often outweighed by risk of convulsion. Enters breast milk; lactating mothers should bottle-feed their babies. Crosses blood-brain barrier.

Metabolism By saturable liver enzyme system; hypermetabolizers may have low serum drug levels. Excessive serum drug levels may be induced by hepatic disorders, congenital enzyme deficiencies, or drug interactions.

Excretion Inactive metabolites enter bile, are reabsorbed, and then excreted by the kidneys, primarily by tubular excretion. About 5% excreted as unchanged drug. Severe renal impairment may cause retention of drugs or metabolites.

Side Effects Toxicity can occur with IV drug administration or ingestion of an overdose. The most common symptoms include hypotension that progresses to cardiovascular collapse; life-threatening arrhythmias, including ventricular fibrillation and depressed A-V conduction; and CNS depression that may induce ataxia, drowsiness, and nystagmus. Vertigo, circumoral tingling, and nausea have occurred. Death may result from respiratory depression or apnea. Supportive treatment is given since there is no antidote. Dialysis is of some value. Gingival hyperplasia, nausea, and vomiting are common. Gum overgrowth is irreversible and occurs most frequently in children. Although the gum condition may be annoying, the drug is usually continued. Meticulous oral hygiene may prevent further gum overgrowth. Neonatal hemorrhage can be prevented or minimized if the pregnant woman receives prophylactic vitamin K_1 for 1 month prior to and during delivery. The neonate should also receive vitamin K_1 if necessary. Hepatic dysfunction may occur, particularly in the elderly and clients who are critically ill. Toxic hepatitis has been reported. Allergic skin reactions can occur, particularly exfoliative dermatitis. Purpuric or bullous dermatitis, lupus erythematosus, and Stevens-Johnson syndrome have occurred. The drug should be discontinued promptly. Blood dyscrasias, including agranulocytosis, thrombocytopenia, and leukopenia have occurred and usually respond to folic

acid supplements. Lymphadenopathy, pseudolymphoma, lymphoma, and Hodgkin's disease have been reported. Osteomalacia has been reported and may be due to phenytoin's interference with vitamin D metabolism. CNS disturbances, including dizziness, insomnia, transient nervousness, twitching, and headache, have occurred. Chorea, dystonia, tremor, and asterixis have been reported, but rarely. Pain may occur at injection sites.

Interactive Effects There are numerous drug interactions reported for phenytoin, primarily because of the drug's high plasma protein binding and its method of metabolism and excretion. Clients should be monitored carefully for phenytoin toxicity. Drugs that may displace phenytoin from its protein-binding sites include salicylates, sulfonamides, phenothiazines, phenylbutazone, and phenyramidol. Drugs that inhibit the metabolism of phenytoin by the liver include oral anticoagulants, oral contraceptives, aminosalicylic acid, chloramphenicol, disulfiram (antabuse), and isoniazid. Phenytoin decreases the body's supply of folic acid and the two substances are antagonistic. Supplemental use of folic acid may decrease the anticonvulsant action of phenytoin. Phenytoin and other anticonvulsants interact with barbiturates. Concurrent therapy has an additive CNS depressant effect. Barbiturates tend to alter the hepatic metabolism and excretion of phenytoin. Tricyclic antidepressants may induce seizure activity if administered in high dosages. The ingestion of alcohol increases the hepatic metabolism of phenytoin and may induce seizure activity. Phenytoin and lidocaine have additive cardiac depressant effects; however, phenytoin may decrease the action of lidocaine through enzyme induction.

Nursing Considerations
1. Assessment and planning
   a. Obtain comprehensive history: Seizures; precipitating factors; cardiac, renal, and liver status.
   b. Obtain baseline data on vital signs, cardiac status, nepatic (blood urea nitrogen), and renal (creatinine) function.
2. Assessment and implementation
   a. Store drug at room temperature away from moisture. Discard all parenteral solutions that are cloudy or have a precipitate. If a faint yellow color occurs, the solution can be used (does not affect potency).
   b. Administer oral preparations with 4 fl oz or more of water.
   c. Avoid administering oral preparations with other drugs or food. If GI irritation occurs, phenytoin can be given 30 minutes before meals or 60 minutes after meals. Shake suspension vigorously before measuring dosage.

d. When administering IM:
- Inject deep into large muscle mass with good circulation.
- Rotate injection sites.
- Check previous injection sites for irritation.
- Switch to oral drug administration if drug is needed for more than 1 week after neurosurgery; decrease oral dose by 50% for 7 days, since IM drug sites will still be releasing drug. *Note:* IM method of administration is no longer recommended for this drug.

e. When administering IV:
- Do not dilute in IV solution, such as 5% D/W, as precipitation may occur. A precipitate will form immediately in dextrose solutions. Microcrystallization occurs within 20 to 120 minutes in normal saline solutions.
- Inject IV bolus directly into IV line or use Y port closest to IV site.
- Never mix with other drugs.
- Flush IV line with 1 to 5 ml of normal saline solution.
- Administer at the rate of 25 mg/min. Do not exceed 50 mg/min. when administering IV. A syringe pump is recommended.
- Constantly monitor the client for signs of toxicity when administering drug. EKG monitoring is highly recommended. Discontinue drug if hypotension occurs, PR intervals become prolonged (greater than 0.2), or if QRS complex widens (greater than 0.1).
- Make sure oxygen and vasopressors are immediately available.

f. Emphasize the importance of maintaining dosage schedule to maintain serum drug levels, thereby avoiding loss of seizure control. Warn client to avoid taking drug dosages too close together since toxicity may occur; there is a fine margin between lack of seizure control and drug toxicity.

g. Urge client to eat a well-balanced diet regularly. Some foods rich in folic acid, calcium, and vitamin D should be eaten daily. Consult dietitian and physician, as needed. A vitamin supplement may be indicated.

h. Caution client that adequate hydration is essential, but excessive intake of fluids should be avoided. A state of slight dehydration has been associated with a decrease in the frequency of seizures.

i. Instruct client to avoid activities requiring constant attention (driving a car) until seizure disorder is well controlled (seizure free for 1 year or longer). Some states require epileptics to have a physician's certificate before a driver's license can be issued.

j. Caution client to avoid changing dosage form or drug manufacturer, since lack of seizure control or toxicity may occur.

k. Caution client against using OTC drugs and home remedies, since drug interactions may occur.

l. Advise client to seek medical assistance for the treatment of common ailments.

m. Instruct client to avoid ingesting alcohol, as seizures may occur.

n. Periodic assessment of gums is recommended. Encourage frequent brushing of teeth (after meals), flossing daily, and regular checkups.

o. Advise client to carry identification indicating seizure disorder and anticonvulsant being used.

p. Reassure client that discoloration of urine may occur.

3. Assessment and evaluation
a. Maintain a flowchart showing the type, duration, and time (date) of convulsion.
b. Serum drug levels should be obtained every 3 to 6 months for clients on prolonged drug therapy.
c. Assess client for toxicity periodically (daily) when oral and IM preparations are administered. Constant monitoring is required with IV drug administration.
d. Serum glucose levels should be obtained daily for diabetic clients when drug is first initiated. Insulin adjustment may be necessary.
e. Complete blood cell counts should be done yearly or twice a year for clients on prolonged drug therapy. Megaloblastic anemia and other blood dyscrasias may occur. Folic acid deficiency may also occur. Folic acid supplements of 0.1 to 0.5 mg/day are usually adequate, but watch the client for loss of seizure control.
f. Duration of therapy is variable. If client is seizure free for 3 to 5 years, the physician may taper the dosage gradually over 3 to 6 months and then discontinue the drug. Abrupt withdrawal of drug may cause seizures.

Generic Name Ethotoin
Trade Name Peganone
Classification Anticonvulsant

See phenytoin for contraindications and drug interactions.

Action Similar to phenytoin, but less effective. The drug is said to be less toxic than phenytoin and lacks its arrhythmic activity. (See phenytoin.)

Indications for Drug Grand mal, psychomotor, and jacksonian seizures.

Contraindications   Hepatic impairment, hematologic disorders, hypersensitivity to hydantoin derivatives.

Forms of Drug   Scored tablets containing 250 or 500 mg.

Administration of Drug   Adults: Initial dosage: 250 mg po qid after meals; then increase slowly every 3 to 7 days until desired effect; Maintenance dosage: 2 to 3 g daily. Children: Initial dosage: 250 mg po bid; then increase, if necessary, to tid or qid; Maintenance dosage: 500 to 1000 mg daily.

Absorption   Half-life is 3 to 9 hours. Therapeutic serum drug levels: 15 to 50 mg/l.
Metabolism   In the liver.
Excretion   In bile, urine, and some in saliva.

Side Effects   Lymphadenopathy and systemic lupus erythematosus may occur. Ataxia and gum hypertrophy occur, but rarely.

Nursing Considerations   GI disturbances are decreased if drug is given after meals. (See phenytoin.)

Generic Name   Mephenytoin
Trade Name   Mesantoin
Classification   Anticonvulsant

See phenytoin for contraindications.

Action   Hydantoin homolog of the barbiturate mephobarbital with characteristics similar to barbiturates and phenytoin.

Indications for Drug   Refractory seizure disorders only, since drug causes severe untoward reactions: grand mal, focal, jacksonian, psychomotor.

Forms of Drug   Scored tablets containing 100 mg.

Administration of Drug   Adults: Initial dosage: 50 to 100 mg po daily; then increase by 50 to 100 mg every 7 to 10 days until desired effect; Maintenance dosage: 200 to 600 mg po daily; Maximum dosage: 200 mg po tid. Children: Initial dosage: 50 to 100 mg po daily; then increase by 50 mg every 7 to 10 days until desired effect; Maintenance dosage: 100 to 400 mg po daily in divided doses.

Absorption   Onset of action is about 30 minutes and duration of action is 24 to 48 hours. Therapeutic serum drug levels: 5 to 20 mcg/ml.
Metabolism   In the liver.
Excretion   By the kidneys.

Side Effects   May cause severe blood dyscrasias, including neutropenia, leukopenia, and agranulocytosis. May cause severe hypersensitivity reactions, including exfoliative dermatitis.

Interactive Effects   Additive effects may occur if taken with other CNS depressants or alcohol. (See phenytoin.)

Nursing Considerations   It is recommended that complete blood cell counts (white blood cell and differential) be done initially, then every 2 weeks until desired effect is achieved, then monthly for 1 year. If neutrophils drop below 1600/mm^3, the drug should be discontinued. Notify physician of abnormalities. (See phenytoin.)

BARBITURATES AND DERIVATIVES

Generic Name   Phenobarbital
Trade Names   Eskabarb, Luminal, SK-Phenobarbital
Classification   Anticonvulsant

687

Action   CNS depressant that increases the threshold of the motor cortex to stimuli.

Indications for Drug   Grand mal and focal seizures; other forms of epilepsy.

Contraindications   Use with caution in the elderly, young children, debilitated clients, diabetics, clients with hyperthyroidism, and clients with multiple allergies.

Forms of Drug   Elixir containing 20 mg/5 ml; tablets containing 15, 30, or 120 mg; capsules (prolonged action) containing 65 or 100 mg.

Administration of Drug   Adults: 100 to 200 mg po daily administered once hs or given in 2(q12h) or 3(q8h) divided doses; Children: 4 to 6 mg/kg po daily in 2 divided doses (q12h).

Absorption   Duration of action is 6 to 10 hours. Half-life is 2 to 5 days. Therapeutic serum drug levels: 10 to 25 mcg/ml; Maximum: 40 mcg/ml; full therapeutic effect occurs in 2 to 3 weeks. About 50% bound to plasma proteins.

Side Effects   Prolonged use may cause folic acid deficiency and osteomalacia. Abrupt withdrawal may precipitate seizures.

Interactive Effects   There are numerous drug interactions reported for phenobarbital and other barbiturates, primarily because of the drug's high plasma protein binding and its method of metabolism and excretion. Client should be monitored carefully for drug toxicity. Barbiturates interact with phenytoin and other anticonvulsants. Concurrent therapy has an additive CNS depressant effect. Barbiturates tend to alter the hepatic metabolism and excretion of phenytoin. An increase in CNS depression occurs with concurrent use of alcohol, narcotics, other sedatives, antihistamines, phenothiazines, disulfiram, MAO inhibitors, procarbazine, and methotrimeprazine. Sulfonamides increase the effect of barbiturates by inhibiting protein binding. By interfering with absorption and increasing liver enzyme activity, barbiturates can decrease the effects of oral anticoagulants, corticosteroids, digitalis glycosides, estrogens, oral contraceptives, griseofulvin, lidocaine, carbamazepine, and methyldopa.

688

Generic Name   Phenobarbital sodium
Trade Name   Luminal Sodium
Classification   Anticonvulsant

See phenobarbital for contraindications and drug interactions.

Indications for Drug   Status epilepticus; febrile convulsions in children.

Forms of Drug   Injectable solutions containing 30, 50, 65, or 130 mg/ml.

Administration of Drug   Adults: 90 to 120 mg IV bolus; then 30 to 60 mg IV every 15 minutes, as needed; Maximum dosage: 500 mg. Children: 5 to 10 mg/kg IV bolus; then repeat every 15 minutes, as needed; Maximum dosage: 20 mg/kg.

Absorption   Therapeutic serum drug levels: 10 to 40 mcg/ml.

Side Effects   Symptoms of toxicity include confusion, vomiting, nystagmus, coughing, hiccups, and coma. Extravasation causes pain and necrosis.

Nursing Considerations
1. When administering IV bolus, do not exceed 60 mg/min.
2. Several drug incompatibilities can occur; flush IV line with 1 to 3 ml of normal saline before and after drug administration.

Generic Name   Amobarbital sodium
Trade Name   Amytal Sodium
Classification   Anticonvulsant

See phenobarbital for drug interaction.

Action   Intermediate-acting barbiturate with sedative and hypnotic effects.

Indications for Drug   Seizures due to eclampsia, meningitis, tetanus, chorea, procaine reactions, poisoning (strychnine), and picrotoxin; status epilepticus.

Contraindications   Porphyria, hypersensitivity to barbiturates, severe respiratory disorder, hepatic impairment. CNS depression, including apnea, may occur in newborns if the drug was used during labor.

Forms of Drug   Ampules containing 125, 250, or 500 mg of powder for reconstitution.

Administration of Drug   Adults and children over 6 years: 65 to 500 mg slow IV bolus, repeat if necessary; Maximum dosage: 1000 mg. Children under 6 years: 3 to 5 mg/kg slow IV bolus; sometimes given IM.

1. Reconstitute powder with sterile water for injection only.
2. Prepare a 10% or more dilute solution:
   a. 125-mg ampule—add 1.25 ml or more of diluent
   b. 250-mg ampule—add 2.5 ml or more of diluent
   c. 500-mg ampule—add 5 ml or more of diluent
3. Rotate ampule to dissolve powder; do not shake.
4. Do not use solution if there is a precipitate.
5. Inject IV bolus slowly; do not exceed 1 ml/min.
6. Monitor blood pressure, pulse, and respiration continuously. Observe for toxicity (apnea, hypotension, sluggish or absent reflexes, coma).
7. Check IV site frequently for irritation; embolism has been reported.
8. Drug deterioration occurs rapidly; discard unused portion.

Absorption   Onset of action is 5 minutes and duration of action is 3 to 6 hours after IV administration.
Metabolism   In the liver.
Excretion   By the kidneys.

Generic Name Mephobarbital
Trade Names Mebaral, Menta-Bal, Mephoral
Classification Anticonvulsant

See phenobarbital for nursing considerations.

Action Mephobarbital is a long-acting barbiturate with anticonvulsant properties similar to phenobarbital. Larger dosages of mephobarbital are required to produce the same effect as phenobarbital. Sedation occurs but the drug is considered a weak hypnotic. Sedative effect is reported to be less than phenobarbital.

Indications for Drug Grand mal and petit mal (absence) seizures.

Contraindications Porphyria, hypersensitivity to barbiturates.

Forms of Drug Tablets containing 32, 50, 100, or 200 mg.

Administration of Drug Low initial dosage, then increased every 4 to 5 days. Adults: 400 to 600 mg po daily in divided doses; Children: Over 5 years: 32 to 40 mg tid or qid (6 to 12 mg/kg/day); Under 5 years: 16 to 32 mg tid or qid.

Absorption About 50% absorbed from GI tract. Onset of action is 30 to 60 minutes and duration of action is 10 to 16 hours. Half-life is unknown.
Metabolism About 85% metabolized in the liver to phenobarbital in 24 hours.

Side Effects Prolonged use may cause folic acid deficiency and osteomalacia. Abrupt cessation of drug may precipitate seizures or result in withdrawal symptoms (tremor, insomnia, confusion, weakness).

Generic Name Metharbital
Trade Name Gemonil
Classification Anticonvulsant

See phenobarbital for contraindications and drug interactions.

Action A long-acting barbiturate with anticonvulsant properties that has less toxic and fewer sedative effects then phenobarbital.

Indications for Drug Grand mal, petit mal (absence), and mixed seizure disorders.

Contraindications Porphyria, hypersensitivity to barbiturates.

Forms of Drug Scored tablets containing 100 mg.

Administration of Drug Adults: Initial dosage: 100 mg po daily, bid, or tid; Maintenance dosage: 300 to 600 mg daily in divided doses; Maximum dosage: 800 mg/day. Children: Initial dosage: 50 mg po daily, bid, or tid; Maintenance dosage: 5 to 15 mg/kg/day in divided doses. Divided doses should be given 98h or q12h over 24-hour period.

Absorption Onset of action is 2 to 4 hours and duration of action is 6 to 12 hours.
Metabolism Demethylated in the liver to barbital.
Excretion In urine.

ANALOG OF PHENOBARBITAL

Generic Name Primidone
Trade Names Mysoline, Primidone, Sertan
Classification Anticonvulsant

Action Synthetic analog of phenobarbital whose mechanism of anticonvulsant action is unknown; but primidone is known to increase the seizure threshold and alter the seizure patterns in experimental animals. The drug potentiates the action of phenobarbital and may be used concurrently with other anticonvulsants, particularly for refractory seizure disorders. The sedative effects that occur in almost one-quarter of the clients during the early weeks of drug therapy are attributed to the metabolite phenobarbital. The drug is considered to have a relatively low toxicity.

Indications for Drug Grand mal, psychomotor, and focal seizures. May control refractory grand mal seizures. May be used alone or concurrently with other anticonvulsants.

Contraindications Hypersensitivity to phenobarbital, porphyria (group of disorders that alter the metabolism of porphyrin and result in excessive production and urinary excretion of porphyrin). Abrupt withdrawal may precipitate status epilepticus or other seizure disorders. Safe use during pregnancy has not been established; may cause birth defects. Neonatal hemorrhage due to a coagulation defect resembling vitamin K deficiency has occurred.

689

Forms of Drug Scored tablets containing 50 or 250 mg; suspension containing 250 mg/ml.

Administration of Drug Dosage varies according to the individual and severity of seizure disorder. Adults and children over 8 years: Initial dosage: 100 to 125 mg po hs for 3 days; then 100 to 125 mg po bid for 3 days; then 100 to 125 mg po tid for 3 days; Maintenance dosage: 250 mg po tid; Maximum dosage: 2000 mg/day. Children under 8 years: Initial dosage: 50 mg po hs for 3 days; then 50 mg po bid for 3 days; then 100 mg po bid for 3 days; Maintenance dosage: 125 to 250 mg tid; Usual maintenance dosage: 10 to 25 mg/kg/day in divided doses.

Baseline complete blood cell count and SMA-12 should be obtained.

Absorption About 75% absorbed from GI tract. Peak levels occur in about 4 hours. Therapeutic serum drug levels: 5 to 12 mcg/ml. Half-life varies widely (3 to 24 hours) and largely depends on rate of metabolism. There is little or no binding to plasma proteins. Crosses placenta and substantial quantities enter breast milk; lactating mothers should bottle-feed their babies.
Metabolism Slowly in the liver to two active metabolites, phenobarbital and phenylethylmalonamide.
Excretion By the kidneys as unchanged drug (about 20%), active metabolites, and inactive metabolites.

Side Effects Ataxia, vertigo, and drowsiness are common during the first few weeks of drug therapy, but tend to subside with continued treatment. If the symptoms persist, dosage reduction is usually effective. GI disturbances, including anorexia, nausea, and vomiting, occur occasionally. Other reactions: fatigue, hyperirritability, emotional disturbances, sexual impotence, diplopia, nystagmus, moribilliform rash. Megaloblastic anemia has occurred, but rarely; the anemia responds to supplements of folic acid without discontinuation of the drug. Neonatal hemorrhage can be prevented or minimized if the pregnant woman receives prophylactic vitamin K_1 for 1 month prior to and during delivery.

Interactive Effects Potentiates the action of phenobarbital. Lower dosages of phenobarbital can be used when drugs are administered concurrently. Phenytoin stimulates the metabolism of primidone to phenobarbital. Toxic effects of phenobarbital may occur. The anticonvulsant effect of primidone may be reduced by folic acid supplements.

Nursing Considerations
1. Assessment and planning
   a. Porphyria should be ruled out before instituting drug therapy.
   b. When primidone is added to client's anticonvulsant therapy, the dosage of primidone is gradually increased while the dosage of the other anticonvulsant is gradually decreased until the desired balance is achieved.
2. Assessment and implementation
   a. Administer on an empty stomach with 4 fl oz or more of water.
   b. GI disturbances may be prevented by administering drug 1 hour after meals.
   c. The client's need for the drug should be stressed. Emphasize the importance of adherence to dosage schedule to maintain serum drug levels, thereby avoiding drug toxicity or loss of seizure control.
   d. Advise client against abrupt withdrawal of drug.
   e. Instruct client to avoid activities requiring constant attention (driving a car) during the first few weeks of drug therapy, since sedative effects occur. Physician should be consulted before resuming these activities.
   f. Stress the importance of periodic laboratory and medical checkups to avoid serious untoward reactions.
   g. Advise client to carry identification indicating seizure disorder and anticonvulsant being used.
3. Assessment and evaluation
   a. Serum drug levels should be monitored frequently when drug is first initiated or the dosage adjusted. Serum phenobarbital levels (therapeutic levels: 15 to 40 mcg/ml) may also be ordered. Steady-state therapeutic drug levels and therapeutic effectiveness usually take several weeks of therapy.
   b. Sedative effects may occur during the first 2 weeks or more of therapy. Sedative effects tend to subside as treatment is continued.
   c. Anorexia and sedative effects may cause the client to eat inadequately. Encourage client to eat a well-balanced diet and to eat foods rich in folic acid regularly.
   d. Assess client daily for toxicity and other untoward reactions.
   e. Complete blood cell counts and SMA-12 should be done periodically (every 3 to 6 months). If anemia occurs, folic acid supplements may be ordered.
   f. Observe client for lack of seizure control.
   g. Duration of therapy is variable. Dosage may be gradually reduced if the client remains seizure free for 1 to 3 years.
   h. Abrupt withdrawal of drug may cause seizures.

SUCCINIMIDE DERIVATIVES

Generic Name   Ethosuximide
Trade Name   Zarontin
Classification   Anticonvulsant

Action   Ethosuximide is considered the most effective succinimide for the control of petit mal (absence) seizures. Although it is less effective than trimethadione, it is often preferred because it causes fewer serious untoward reactions. The exact mechanism of action is unknown, but the drug is thought to act by causing depression of the motor cortex and elevation of the CNS threshold to stimuli. The drug decreases the paroxysmal spike and brain wave activity associated with absence seizures. The drug is ineffective against grand mal seizures and may even increase the frequency of such seizures in clients with mixed seizure disorders.

Indications for Drug   Control of petit mal (absence) epilepsy.

Contraindications   Hypersensitivity to succinimides. Use with caution in clients with hepatic or renal impairment, since ethosuximide is capable of producing morphologic and functional changes in these organs. Lupus erythematosus and fatal blood dyscrasias have been associated with ethosuximide; periodic blood counts are recommended. Safe use in pregnancy and lactation has not been established; birth defects may occur. Impairment of mental and physical abilities required for the performance of potentially hazardous tasks may occur. When used alone, ethosuximide may increase the frequency of grand mal seizures in clients with mixed seizure disorders. Abrupt withdrawal of drug may precipitate absence seizures.

Forms of Drug   Capsules containing 250 mg; raspberry-flavored syrup containing 250 mg/5 ml.

Administration of Drug   Highly individualized. Do not exceed 1500 mg daily unless close medical supervision is available. Adults and children over 6 years: Initial dosage: 500 mg po daily; then increase by 250 mg daily every 4 to 7 days until desired effect. Children 3 to 6 years: Initial dosage: 250 mg po daily; then increase, if necessary, after 4 to 7 days; Optimal dosage: 20 mg/kg/day. If excessive dosages are required, the drug can be combined with other anticonvulsants.

Absorption   Readily absorbed from GI tract. May cause GI disturbances. Therapeutic serum drug levels: 40 to 100 mcg/ml. Steady-state plasma concentration occurs within 1 week. Half-life varies widely (24 to 60 hours). There is little or no binding to plasma proteins. Crosses placenta and enters breast milk; lactating mothers should bottle-feed their babies. Crosses blood-brain barrier.
Distribution   Widely distributed in body tissues.
Metabolism   In the liver to inactive metabolites. Rate of metabolism in liver is variable; drug-induced hepatic impairment may occur.
Excretion   By the kidneys as unchanged drug (about 10%) and as metabolites. Excretion may be delayed in the elderly and in clients with renal impairment.

Side Effects   GI disturbances are common. Anorexia, vague GI upset, nausea, vomiting, cramps, diarrhea, and epigastric and abdominal pain may occur. Blood dyscrasias, including leukopenia, agranulocytosis, pancytopenia, aplastic anemia, and eosinophilia, may occur, but rarely. CNS disturbances, including ataxia, drowsiness, headache, dizziness, euphoria, hiccups, irritability, lethargy, and fatigue, may occur; these symptoms may be dose related. Psychologic disturbances, including night terrors, inability to concentrate, and aggressiveness, have occurred, particularly in clients with preexisting psychological abnormalities. Paranoid psychosis, increased libido, depression, and suicidal tendencies have been reported, but rarely. Skin reactions, including urticaria, Stevens-Johnson syndrome, systemic lupus erythematosus, and pruritic erythematosus rashes, occur, but rarely. Other reactions: myopia, vaginal bleeding, swelling of the tongue, gum hypertrophy, hirsutism. May cause a positive Coombs' test.

Interactive Effects   Concurrent ingestion of amphetamines may decrease GI absorption. Drugs that induce or retard liver enzyme systems may alter the metabolism of ethosuximide.

Nursing Considerations
1. Assessment and planning
    a. Baseline data on hepatic (blood urea nitrogen) and renal (creatinine) function should be obtained.
    b. Obtain history of the hepatic and renal disorders.
2. Assessment and implementation
    a. The client's need for the drug should be stressed.
    b. Emphasize the importance of adherence to dosage schedule to maintain therapeutic serum drug levels, thereby avoiding loss of seizure control.
    c. Advise client against abrupt withdrawal of drug.

691

d. Instruct client to avoid activities requiring constant attention (driving a car) until seizure disorder is completely controlled (seizure free).

e. Advise client to carry identification indicating seizure disorder and anticonvulsant being used.

f. Teach client and family members untoward reactions and to report symptoms to health professionals immediately.

g. Stress the importance of regular laboratory and medical checkups.

3. Assessment and evaluation

a. Elderly clients and clients with hepatic or renal impairment are susceptible to rapid toxicity.

b. Serum drug levels should be monitored frequently when drug is first initiated or dosage adjusted.

c. Maintain a seizure disorder flowchart.

d. Assess client daily for toxicity, hypersensitivity, and other untoward reactions.

e. Complete blood cell count, blood urea nitrogen, serum creatinine levels, and urinalysis should be obtained periodically.

f. Duration of therapy is variable. If the client is seizure free for 1 to 3 years, the physician may taper the dosage gradually.

g. Abrupt withdrawal of drug may cause seizures.

Generic Name Methsuximide
Trade Name Celontin
Classification Anticonvulsant

See ethosuximide for action, contraindications, and drug interactions.

Indications for Drug Refractory petit mal (absence) and psychomotor seizures. May be administered in combination with other anticonvulsants.

Forms of Drug Capsules containing 150 or 300 mg.

Administration of Drug Adults and children: 300 mg po daily the first week; dosage may be increased at weekly intervals by 300 mg; Maximum dosage: 1200 mg daily in divided doses.

Absorption Peak levels occur in 1 to 3 hours. Therapeutic serum drug levels: 40 to 100 mcg/ml. Half-life is 2 to 4 hours.
Metabolism Rapidly in the liver.
Excretion By the kidneys.

Side Effects Nearly one-third of all clients develop untoward reactions, particularly GI disturbances, blood dyscrasias, and CNS disturbances. Behavioral changes may progress to psychosis. (See ethosuximide.)

Nursing Considerations (See ethosuximide.)

1. Complete blood cell count should be done frequently (every 1 to 3 months); hepatic function tests and urinalysis should be done periodically (every 3 to 6 months).

2. Causes harmless pinkish brown color change in urine.

3. Abrupt withdrawal may precipitate seizure activity.

Generic Name Phensuximide
Trade Name Milontin
Classification Anticonvulsant

See ethosuximide for contraindications and drug interactions.

Action Less effective in controlling seizure activity than any other succinimide derivatives, but causes fewer severe untoward reactions. (See ethosuximide.)

Indications for Drug Petit mal (absence) seizures. May be administered in combination with other anticonvulsants.

Forms of Drug Capsules containing 50 mg.

Administration of Drug Adults and children: 500 to 1000 mg po bid or tid; Maximum dosage: 3 g/day.

Absorption Peak levels occur in 1 to 4 hours. Therapeutic serum drug levels: 40 to 80 mcg/ml. Half-life is about 4 hours.
Metabolism Rapidly metabolized in the liver.
Excretion By the kidneys.

Side Effects Nausea and other GI distress. (See ethosuximide.)

Nursing Considerations (See ethosuximide.)

1. Complete blood cell count should be done every 3 months and hepatic function tests and urinalysis should be done every 3 to 6 months.

2. Causes harmless pinkish brown color change in urine.

3. Abrupt withdrawal may precipitate seizure activity.

OXAZOLIDINEDIONE DERIVATIVES

Generic Name Paramethadione
Trade Name Paradione
Classification Anticonvulsant

Action Ineffective against grand mal seizures but may be used in conjunction with other anticonvulsants for mixed seizures.

Indications for Drug Petit mal (absence) refractory seizure disorders only, since drug causes severe toxic and other untoward reactions.

Contraindications Use with caution in clients with retinal or optic nerve disorders. Use with caution in clients of childbearing age, since birth defects may occur. An appropriate contraceptive should be used.

Forms of Drug Capsules containing 150 or 300 mg. Bottles of oral solution with a calibrated dropper containing 300 mg/ml (also contains 65% alcohol).

Administration of Drug Adults: Initial dosage: 300 mg po tid; then increase by 300 mg every 7 to 10 days until desired effect; Maintenance dosage: 300 to 600 mg po tid or qid. Children: Initial dosage: 300 mg po bid; then increase every 7 to 10 days until desired effect; Maintenance dosage: Infants: 150 mg po bid; Ages 2 to 6 years: 150 mg po tid or qid; Over 6 years: 300 mg po tid. Administer with 4 oz. or more of water.

Absorption Therapeutic serum drug levels: 6 to 71 mcg/ml.

Side Effects May cause severe nephrosis and blood dyscrasias, including aplastic anemia and agranulocytosis. Photophobia may occur; clients should be warned to wear screening sunglasses. Hypersensitivity reactions to FD&C No. 5 yellow, including bronchial asthma, may occur with 300-mg capsules.

Interactive Effects No significant known interactions.

Nursing Considerations Routine complete blood cell count and urinalysis should be done weekly, then monthly for a year, then periodically.

Generic Name Trimethadione
Trade Name Tridione
Classification Anticonvulsant

See paramethadione for contraindications.

Action Ineffective against grand mal seizures, but may be used in conjunction with other anticonvulsants for mixed seizures.

Indications for Drug Petit mal (absence) refractory seizure disorders only, since drug causes severe toxic and other untoward reactions.

Forms of Drug Capsules containing 300 mg; chewable tablets containing 150 mg; oral solution containing 40 mg/ml.

Administration of Drug Adults: Initial dosage: 300 mg po tid; then increase by 300 mg every 7 to 10 days until desired effect; Maintenance dosage: 300 to 600 mg po tid or qid. Children: 20 to 50 mg/kg po daily in divided doses every 6 to 8 hours. Administer with 4 oz or more of water.

Absorption Therapeutic serum drug levels: 20 to 40 mcg/ml.

Side Effects Exfoliative dermatitis and other severe rashes may occur. (See paramethadione.)

Nursing Considerations (See phenytoin.)
1. Routine complete blood cell count and urinalysis should be done weekly, then monthly for a year, then periodically.
2. If neutrophil count drops below 2500/mm^3, drug should be discontinued.

BENZODIAZEPINE DERIVATIVES

Generic Name Clonazepam
Trade Name Clonopin
Classification Anticonvulsant

See phenytoin for nursing considerations.

Action CNS depressant that also decreases the frequency, amplitude, duration, and spread of discharge in minor seizures. Suppresses the spike and brain wave discharge in petit mal (absence) seizures.

693

Indications for Drug Lennox-Gastuat syndrome (type of petit mal), akinetic and myoclonic petit mal (absence) seizures that do not respond to succinimides.

Contraindications Hypersensitivity to benzodiazepines, hepatic impairment, acute or narrow-angle glaucoma. Safe use during pregnancy and lactation has not been established; may cause birth defects. Safe use in children has not been established. Abrupt withdrawal may cause status epilepticus or result in withdrawal symptoms, including convulsions, tremor, abdominal and muscle cramps, vomiting, and sweating. May increase the frequency of tonic-clonic (grand mal) seizure activity in clients with mixed seizure disorder. Use with caution in clients with impaired renal function, the elderly, debilitated clients, and clients with respiratory disorders (since drug causes respiratory depression and excessive salivation).

Forms of Drug Scored tablets containing 0.5, 1, or 2 mg.

Administration of Drug Adults: Initial dosage: 0.5 mg po tid; then increase by 0.5 mg every 3 days until desired effect; Maximum dosage: 20 mg/day. Infants and children: Initial dosage: 0.01 to 0.03 mg/kg/day bid or tid in divided doses; then increase by 0.25 to 0.5 mg every 3 days until desired effect; Maintenance dosage: 0.1 to 0.2 mg/kg/day.

Absorption Peak levels occur in 1 to 2 hours. Therapeutic serum drug levels: 20 to 50 mcg/ml. Half-life is 18 to 50 hours.
Metabolism Oxidized and reduced to metabolites in the liver.
Excretion In urine.

Side Effects Common reactions include drowsiness (50%), ataxia (30%), and behavioral problems (25%). Respiratory effects include rales, shortness of breath, and depressed breathing. CNS disturbances include abnormal eye movements, diplopia, slurred speech, aphornia, dizziness, and coma.

Generic Name Diazepam
Trade Name Valium
Classification Anticonvulsant

Action CNS depressant with anticonvulsant properties similar to chlordiazepoxide (Librium), but has no peripheral autonomic blocking action and induces fewer extrapyramidal side effects. Large doses may cause ataxia. Has a depressant effect on the cardiovascular system and may cause apnea and/or cardiac arrest, particularly in the elderly and debilitated clients.

Indications for Drug Short-term control of status epilepticus, severe recurrent seizures.

Contraindications Hypersensitivity to benzodiazepines, acute narrow-angle glaucoma, untreated open-angle glaucoma. Tonic status epilepticus has been precipitated in clients treated with diazepam IV for petit mal seizure disorders. Causes local vein irritation and may cause thrombosis.

Forms of Drug Scored tablets containing 2, 5, or 10 mg; 2-ml ampules containing 5 mg/ml; 10-ml multi-dose vials containing 5 mg/ml.

Administration of Drug Adults: 5 to 10 mg slow IV bolus, repeat every 10 to 15 minutes times 2 doses, if necessary; Maximum dosage: 30 mg every 2 to 4 hours. Elderly, debilitated clients with hepatic impairment: 2 to 5 mg slow IV bolus, repeat every 10 to 15 minutes, or twice more, if necessary; Maximum dosage: 15 mg every 2 to 4 hours. Children: 0.1 to 0.3 mg/kg slow IV bolus, repeat every 10 to 15 minutes times 2 doses, if necessary; Maximum dosage: Under 5 years: 5 mg; Over 5 years: 10 mg.

Absorption Has a biphasic half-life: 7 to 10 hours; 2 to 8 days. Crosses placenta and enters breast milk.
Metabolism In the liver. One active metabolite, oxazepam, is produced. Oxazepam has sedative and muscle relaxant properties.
Excretion By the kidneys.

Interactive Effects There are numerous drug interactions reported for diazepam, primarily because of the drug's method of metabolism and slow excretion. Client should be monitored carefully for drug toxicity. Diazepam increases the effects of phenytoin and other anticonvulsants. Concurrent therapy has an additive CNS depressant effect. An increase in CNS depression occurs with concurrent use of alcohol, narcotics, other sedatives, antihistamines, phenothiazines, MAO inhibitors, and tricyclic antidepressants. Respiratory depression may occur when used concurrently with gallamine triethiodide and other neuromuscular blocking agents.

Nursing Considerations

1. Monitor blood pressure, pulse, and respiration continuously. Observe for toxicity (hypotension, apnea, arrhythmias, coma).
2. Complete blood cell count and SMA-12 should be done periodically. Dialysis is of no value for the treatment of toxicity.
3. If IV route is used:
   a. Administer slowly (5 mg per minute at most).
   b. Do not mix with other drugs or solutions because of possible incompatibilities.

OTHER ANTICONVULSANT AGENTS

Generic Name   Carbamazepine
Trade Name   Tegretol
Classification   Anticonvulsant

Action   Exact mechanism is unknown but this iminostilbene derivative is thought to have actions similar to phenytoin. It is not considered a drug of choice because of serious untoward reactions.

Indications for Drug   Psychomotor, grand mal, and mixed seizure disorders; trigeminal neuralgia.

Contraindications   History of bone marrow depression, hypersensitivity to carbamazepine or any tricyclic compound, concurrent therapy with MAO inhibitors. Safe use during pregnancy has not been established.

Forms of Drug   Scored tablets containing 200 mg. Chewable tablets containing 100 mg.

Administration of Drug   Adults and children over 12 years: Initial dosage: 200 mg po bid; then increase by 200 mg daily and give in divided doses q8h; Maximum dosage: Ages 12 to 15 years: 1000 mg/day; Over 15 years: 1200 mg/day; Adults: 1600 mg/day. Children 6 to 12 years: Initial dosage: 100 mg po bid; then increase by 100 mg daily and give in divided doses q8h, then q6h; Maximum dosage: 1000 mg/day.

Absorption   Half-life: Initially 25 to 65 hours, then 12 to 17 hours. Therapeutic serum drug levels: 4 to 12 mcg/ml.
Metabolism   In the liver.
Excretion   Primarily by the kidneys, some in feces.

Side Effects   Toxicity manifested by dizziness, ataxia, drowsiness, stupor, restlessness, agitation, disorientation, tremor, and coma. Additionally, nausea, vomiting, mydriasis, nystagmus, urinary retention, blood pressure changes, and cyanosis may occur. Serious blood dyscrasias, including aplastic anemia, agranulocytosis, leukopenia, and thrombocytopenia may develop.

Nursing Considerations

1. Periodic hepatic function tests are recommended, since hepatic impairment and tumors may occur.
2. Periodic eye examinations are recommended, since changes in the eye have occurred.
3. Complete blood cell count should be obtained every week, then monthly.
4. Drug should be discontinued if any of the following occur: red blood cell count less than 4,000,000/mm^3; hematocrit less than 32%; hemoglobin less than 11 g/dl; platelets less than 100,000/mm^3; reticulocytes less than 20,000/mm^3; serum iron greater than 150 mcg/dl.

Generic Name   Magnesium sulfate
Classification   Anticonvulsant

Action   Elevated serum magnesium levels cause CNS depression by blocking the release of acetylcholine and may desensitize muscles to neurologic impulses.

Indications for Drug   Eclampsia, control of preeclampsia, hypomagnesemic seizures.

Contraindications   Severe renal failure, congestive heart failure, heart block. Use with caution just prior to delivery because it will cause CNS depression in the newborn; be prepared to resuscitate the newborn. Complete heart block may occur in digitalized clients.

Forms of Drug   10% solution containing 1 g/10 ml; 50% solution containing 5 g/10 ml.

Administration of Drug   Loading dosage: 4 g of 10% solution slow IV bolus or in 100 to 250 ml of 5% D/W; then 4 g IM every 4 to 6 hours, as needed. Renal impairment: 1 to 2 g of 10% solution slow IV bolus or in 50 to 100 ml of 5% D/W; then 1 g every 4 to 6 hours, as needed.

695

When administering IV:
1. Use 10% solution only.
2. May be diluted in 50 to 250 ml of 5% D/W.
3. Administer slowly; do not exceed 150 mg/min. (1.5 ml 10% solution). Infusion pump is recommended.

When administering IM:
1. Use 50% solution only.
2. Inject deep into large muscle mass.
3. Rotate injection sites.

Absorption Onset of action occurs in: minutes (IV); about 1 hour (IM). Duration of action is: 30 to 60 minutes (IV); 3 to 4 hours (IM). Therapeutic serum drug levels: up to 12 mEq/l. Normal serum levels: 1.5 to 3 mEq/l. Crosses placenta.
Excretion By the kidneys.

Interactive Effects Heart block may occur in clients receiving digitalis glycosides. Profound CNS depression can occur if given concurrently with other anticonvulsants, anesthetics, barbiturates, narcotics, and other CNS depressants. Calcium gluconate can be used to counteract hypermagnesemia (antidote).

Nursing Considerations
1. Monitor serum magnesium levels frequently and have calcium gluconate available for testing magnesium toxicity.
2. Monitor blood pressure, respiration, and cardiac rhythm continuously; hypotension, heart block, and apnea may occur.
3. Monitor intake and output hourly. Output should be 30 ml/hour or more.
4. Check for toxicity frequently (every 30 to 60 minutes); absence of knee jerk reflex precedes toxicity.

Generic Name Paraldehyde
Trade Name Paral
Classification Anticonvulsant

Action Relatively nontoxic but potent CNS depressant with sedative and hypnotic properties similar to barbiturates. It has a strong odor and taste.

Indications for Drug Status epilepticus, seizures due to drug poisoning, refractory grand mal seizures.

Contraindications Asthma or other pulmonary disorders, severe hepatic impairment.

Forms of Drug Parenteral solution containing 1 g/ml; oral solution containing 1 g/ml. Deteriorates rapidly to acetic acid; refrigerate in airtight jars. Do not use if solution turns brown.

Administration of Drug Adults: 5 to 10 g IM; 200 to 400 mg slow IV in normal saline. Children: 15 mg/kg IM every 4 to 6 hours, as needed; 30 mg/kg as retention enema q1h prn (do not exceed 5g); continuous drip 5 g/hour or less, as needed.

1. Dilute rectal retention enema in 50 to 100 ml of cottonseed or olive oil or with 200 ml of normal saline.
2. When administering IM, inject deep into large muscle mass, since drug can be irritating to tissues and may cause abscesses. Do not deliver more than 5 ml to a site and rotate sites.
3. As drug reacts with plastic, use glass syringes and containers.
4. Add parenteral drug solution to 50 to 250 ml of normal saline (0.9% IV solution) and administer slowly.
5. Keep room well ventilated to remove drug in exhaled air.

Absorption Half-life is 8 hours. Crosses placenta.
Metabolism Primarily in the liver.
Excretion In urine and exhaled air.

Side Effects Toxicity may cause pulmonary edema, hypotension, and circulatory and respiratory collapse.

Nursing Considerations Observe client frequently for signs of toxicity.

Generic Name Phenacemide
Trade Name Phenurone
Classification Anticonvulsant

Action Elevates the seizure threshold and abolishes the tonic phase of maximal electroshock seizures. Particularly effective in controlling focal psychomotor seizures, but the drug is very toxic and causes serious, even fatal, untoward reactions.

Indications for Drug Refractory psychomotor seizures; grand mal, petit mal, and mixed seizure disorders.

Contraindications Safe use during pregnancy has not been established; may cause birth defects.

Forms of Drug Grooved tablets containing 500 mg.

Administration of Drug Adults: Initial dosage: 500 mg po tid at mealtime; then, if seizures are poorly controlled after 7 days, 500 mg po upon awakening (early A.M.) or at bedtime; dosage range: 2 to 3 g po daily. Children: Ages 5 to 10 years: ½ of adult dosage, same schedule.

Absorption Well absorbed from GI tract. Duration of action about 5 hours.
Excretion By the kidneys.

Side Effects GI disturbances (anorexia, weight loss), nephritis, headache, drowsiness, dizziness, ataxia, insomnia, paresthesia, psychotic behavior, and rashes have been reported. Fatal reactions: hepatitis, aplastic anemia, agranulocytosis, leukopenia.

Nursing Considerations Complete blood count and renal function test should be done regularly, at least once a month.

Generic Names Valproic acid, valproate sodium
Trade Name Depakene
Classification Anticonvulsant

Action Precise mechanism of action of this carboxylic acid derivative is unknown, but is thought to increase brain levels of gamma aminobutyric acid.

Indications for Drug Simple and complex petit mal seizures, as an adjunct in mixed seizures.

Contraindications Hepatic disease or impairment, hypersensitivity to valproic acid or its sodium salt. Safe use during pregnancy has not been established; may cause birth defects. Abrupt withdrawal may precipitate status epilepticus in clients being treated for grand mal disorders.

Forms of Drug Capsules containing 250 mg; syrup containing 250 mg per 5 ml.

Administration of Drug Adults: Initial dosage: 15 mg/kg/day; then increase 5 to 10 mg at 1-week intervals until desired effect; if total daily dose exceeds 250 mg, give in divided doses; Maximum dosage: 60 mg/kg/day.

Absorption Rapidly absorbed from GI tract. If taken with meals there is a slight delay in rate of absorption, but the total amount is absorbed. Peak levels occur in 1 to 4 hours. Therapeutic serum drug levels: 50 to 100 mcg/ml. Half-life is 8 to 12 hours and pKa is 4.8. About 90% bound to plasma proteins.
Metabolism In the liver; glucuronide conjugate and other metabolites are formed.
Excretion Primarily in urine, some in feces and exhaled air.

Side Effects Fatal hepatotoxicity has occurred within 6 months of initiating drug therapy and is usually preceded by loss of seizure control, malaise, weakness, lethargy, anorexia, and vomiting. Asymptomatic hyperammonemia may occur. Elevated serum transaminase levels are dose related.

Interactive Effects Marked CNS depression can occur when taken with barbiturates and alcohol.

Nursing Considerations Liver function tests should be done regularly, at monthly intervals. May give false positive results for urinary ketones.

697

ANTIPARKINSONIAN MEDICATIONS

Drugs that decrease the cholinergic activity in the basal ganglia or restore the inhibitory effects of dopamine receptor stimulation are effective in controlling the symptoms of parkinsonism. Until the late 1960s, only drugs with anticholinergic activity were available; as the client's symptoms progressed, the characteristic tremors could only be controlled by brain surgery. Levodopa, the precursor of dopamine, was released for use in 1970. Both levodopa and anticholinergic drugs are used today.

Anticholinergic agents, such as trihexyphenidyl, are effective in controlling the rigidity and tremors of parkinsonism. Drugs that block the brain's muscarinic receptor sites are particularly effective; unfortunately, these atropinelike drugs cause numerous untoward reactions, including dry mouth, constipation, blurred vision, and urinary retention. When necessary, the long-acting drug benztropine can be injected and is used for clients who are unable to take oral medication. The newer synthetic anticholinergic agents are effective in controlling akinesia, as well as rigidity and tremors.

Antihistamines, such as diphenhydramine, and the phenothiazine derivative ethopropazine have anticholinergic properties and are therefore useful in controlling symptoms of parkinsonism. The effectiveness of antihistamines and ethopropazine seems to be related to their anticholinergic properties. These drugs tend to cause drowsiness and other central nervous system disturbances.

Levodopa increases the amount of dopamine in the basal ganglia. Dopamine is unable to cross the blood-brain barrier, but levodopa can and is converted to dopamine by the nigrostriatal nerve endings. Although parkinsonism symptoms do not improve immediately, continued use of the drug will first result in improvement of akinesia and then rigidity and tremors. Levodopa does not cure the disease, it only replaces a necessary body substance. If the drug is not taken regularly, symptoms will reappear. Due to the high incidence of untoward reactions, levodopa treatment is initiated at relatively low dosages and the dosage is then gradually increased every 5 to 7 days until the maximum benefit is obtained with the minimum of untoward reactions, particularly nausea and orthostatic hypotension. As the effectiveness of levodopa varies from individual to individual, dosages are highly individualized.

Carbidopa prevents the degradation of levodopa by body tissues so that larger quantities of intact levodopa molecules are available to cross the blood-brain barrier. Since carbidopa is unable to cross the blood-brain barrier, its action is limited to tissues outside the brain. When carbidopa is administered concurrently with levodopa, lower dosages of levodopa are required to sustain therapeutic drug levels in the blood and therefore the brain.

Amantadine is actually an antiviral agent, but has been found to be effective in treating parkinsonism. Although the exact mechanism of action is unknown, amantadine is thought to stimulate the release of dopamine from nigrostriatal neurons, thus causing increased dopamine levels in the basal ganglia. Amantadine is effective within 2 to 4 weeks and causes few untoward reactions.

Bromocriptine has been found to be a potent stimulator of dopamine receptor sites in the corpus striatum and is therefore useful in the treatment of parkinsonism. Unfortunately, the drug is less effective than levodopa and can induce marked behavioral changes. However, combined therapy with levodopa permits smaller dosages of each drug to be used.

Since the advent of tranquilizers for the treatment of mental disorders, drug-induced extrapyramidal symptoms similar to parkinsonism have become a major concern. Phenothiazines and other tranquilizers block stimulation and dopamine receptor sites by dopamine. The drug effects cause extrapyramidal symptoms similar to parkinsonism.

ANTICHOLINERGIC AGENTS

Generic Name   Trihexyphenidyl hydrochloride
Trade Names   Artane, Hexyphen, Pipanol, Tremin, Trihexidyl
Classification   Anticholinergic agent

Action   Trihexyphenidyl, a synthetic tertiary amine, causes relaxation of smooth musculature through a direct action on the muscle tissue and indirectly by inhibiting the parasympathetic nervous system. Its antispasmodic activity is about one-half as effective as atropine; but trihexyphenidyl causes milder secondary effects, such as mydriasis, drying of secretions, and cardioacceleration. The drug is particularly effective in reducing the rigidity associated with all forms of parkinsonism and is effective in treating extrapyramidal disorders caused by CNS drugs, such as dibenoxazepines, phenothiazines, thioxanthenes, and butyrophenones. It is said to partially relieve some of the depression associated with parkinsonism.

Indications for Drug   Drug-induced extrapyramidal disorders, as an adjunct in the treatment of postencephalitic, arteriosclerotic, and idiopathic parkinsonism.

Contraindications   Although it is not contraindicated in hypertensive clients, these clients should be assessed frequently for untoward reactions. Use with caution in clients with glaucoma, obstructive disorders of the GI tract, and elderly clients with prostatic hypertrophy. Elderly clients (over 60 years) and clients with arteriosclerosis or a history of drug hypersensitivity may be hypersensitive to the drug's action and may require reduced dosages during long-term therapy. Incipient glaucoma may be precipitated.

Forms of Drug   Scored tablets containing 2 or 5 mg; elixir containing 2 mg/5 ml; sustained-release capsules containing 5 mg (used after desired dosage has been established).

Administration of Drug   Highly individualized. Reduced dosages are required in clients over 60 years.

- *Drug-induced extrapyramidal disorders:* If the dosage of the causative agent is reduced, less trihexyphenidyl is required to eliminate the extrapyramidal symptoms. Initial dosage: 1 mg po daily after a meal; 1 mg po bid after meals; then 1 mg po tid after meals; then increase by 1 to 2 mg po daily; Dosage range: 5 to 15 mg daily. Dosage may be reduced when the symptoms are controlled for several days.

■ *Idiopathic and postencephalitic parkinsonism:* Initial dosage: 1 mg po daily after meals; then increase by 2 mg daily every 3 to 5 days; give in 2 to 3 divided doses after meals; Dosage range for idiopathic: 6 to 10 mg daily; Dosage range for postencephalitic: 12 to 15 mg daily. Clients receiving other antiparkinsonian agents, particularly levodopa, may only require 3 to 6 mg daily.

1. Give after meals with a full glass of water.
2. Provide client with a full pitcher of ice water or other measures to control dry mouth.
3. Drug can be given 3 minutes before meals; but may cause nausea.

Absorption Rapidly absorbed from GI tract; may be irritating to GI tract. Onset of action is about 1 hour. Peak action occurs in 2 to 3 hours and duration of action is 6 to 12 hours.
Metabolism Unknown.
Excretion By the kidneys.

Side Effects Mild secondary reactions such as dry mouth, blurred vision, dizziness, nausea, and nervousness are experienced by 30% to 50% of clients. These symptoms tend to disappear during long-term therapy. Untoward reactions characteristic of atropine, including suppurative parotitis, skin rashes, colon dilation, paralytic ileus, delusions, and hallucinations, rarely occur. Dilation of the pupil and increased intraocular tension may progress to angle-closure glaucoma during long-term therapy. GI disturbances, including nausea, vomiting, and constipation, may occur. Urinary hesitancy and retention may occur, particularly in elderly males. Drowsiness, tachycardia, weakness, and headaches may occur. Elderly clients and clients with arteriosclerosis or a history of drug hypersensitivity may develop CNS disturbances, including confusion, amnesia, agitation, paranoid behavior, nausea, and vomiting.

Interactive Effects Concurrent therapy with antihistamines has additive anticholinergic effects and may cause excessive dryness of the mouth, loss of teeth, and suppurative parotitis. Concomitant therapy with amantadine may cause CNS disturbances, such as confusion, agitation, delusions, and hallucinations. The dosage of trihexyphenidyl should be reduced before instituting amantadine therapy.

Nursing Considerations
1. Assessment and planning
   a. Assess the amount of muscular rigidity, drooling, and other symptoms before instituting therapy.
   b. Gonioscopic evaluation and intraocular pressure should be determined before initiating therapy.
   c. Obtain history of drug hypersensitivities and the presence of urinary disturbances, particularly in elderly males.
2. Assessment and implementation
   a. Client may require cool drinks, ice chips, or sugarless gum to control dry mouth.
   b. Assess the type and severity of symptoms daily when drug is first instituted or dosage adjusted.
   c. Assess the presence daily of CNS disturbances in elderly clients when drug is first instituted or dosage is adjusted.
   d. Record intake and output. Notify physician if urinary retention occurs. Advise client to void before taking drug.
   e. Caution client against driving or engaging in other activities that require constant attention until dosage adjustment is complete.
3. Assessment and evaluation
   a. Tolerance to the drug may develop with long-term therapy. Assess the symptoms of parkinsonism regularly.
   b. Instruct client on long-term therapy to report the return of symptoms (muscular rigidity) to the health care provider.

Generic Name Benztropine mesylate
Trade Name Cogentin
Classification Anticholinergic agent

See trihexyphenidyl hydrochloride for contraindications, side effects, and drug interactions.

Action Benztropine exhibits anticholinergic and antihistaminic effects. This drug has the advantage of being injectable and can therefore be used in emergency situations for dystonia. (See trihexyphenidyl hydrochloride.)

Indications for Drug Parkinsonism, drug-induced extrapyramidal disorders, acute dystonia (except tardive dyskinesia).

Contraindications Children under 3 years, angle-closure glaucoma. May aggravate tardive dyskinesia and may cause paralytic ileus.

699

Forms of Drug   Tablets containing 0.5, 1, or 2 mg; 2-ml ampules containing 2 mg/ml.

Administration of Drug

- *Parkinsonism:* Initial dosage: 0.5 to 1 mg po at bedtime; then increase gradually; Usual dosage: 1 to 2 mg daily.
- *Drug-induced extrapyramidal disorders:* 1 to 2 mg IM; then 1 to 2 mg po bid to prevent recurrence.
- *Acute dystonia:* 1 to 2 mg IM or IV; then 1 to 2 mg po bid; may be gradually increased by 0.5 mg/day; Maximum dosage: 6 mg/day.

Absorption   Onset of action is: about 1 hour (po); within minutes (IM, IV). Duration of action is about 8 to 12 hours.

Nursing Considerations   Protect drug ampules from light. (See trihexyphenidyl hydrochloride.)

Generic Name   Biperiden hydrochloride
Trade Name   Akineton Hydrochloride
Classification   Anticholinergic agent

See trihexyphenidyl hydrochloride for drug interactions and nursing considerations.

Action   More effective than atropine in reducing akinesia, rigidity, and tremors. Weak action on intestinal mucosa and blood vessels and little mydriatic activity. Particularly effective in treating drug-induced akathisia, akinesia, dyskinetic tremors, rigidity, oculogyric crisis, and profuse sweating caused by reserpine and phenothiazines. May not be effective for arteriosclerotic parkinsonism.

Indications for Drug   Drug-induced extrapyramidal disorders, parkinsonism, spastic disorders (multiple sclerosis, cerebral palsy, spinal cord injuries).

Contraindications   Hypersensitivity to biperiden preparations. Safe use in children and during pregnancy and lactation has not been established.

Forms of Drug   Scored tablets containing 2 mg.

Administration of Drug   2 mg po tid or qid after meals or with food.

Absorption   Nearly 90% of drug is thought to be absorbed from GI tract.

Side Effects   Dry mouth and blurred vision are common. GI disturbances may occur, particularly when given on an empty stomach. Hypotension and dizziness may occur.

Generic Name   Biperiden lactate
Trade Name   Akineton Lactate
Classification   Anticholinergic agent

See trihexyphenidyl hydrochloride for contraindications and drug interactions. See biperiden hydrochloride for action.

Indications for Drug   Acute episodes of drug-induced extrapyramidal disorders.

Contraindications   Use with caution in clients with arrhythmias or prostatic hypertrophy.

Forms of Drug   Ampules of 1 ml containing 5 mg/ml.

Administration of Drug   5 mg slow IV bolus; may be repeated in 24 hours, or 2 mg IM or IV may be repeated every 30 minutes until resolution of symptoms; Maximum dosage: 8 mg/day.

Side Effects   Transient hypotension, confusion, euphoria, and disturbances of coordination may occur.

Nursing Considerations   (See trihexyphenidyl hydrochloride.)

1. Do not use if solution is discolored or if a precipitate has formed.
2. Monitor vital signs frequently, particularly in elderly and debilitated clients.
3. Have client void before administering drug, when possible.

700

Generic Name   Chlorphenoxamine hydrochloride
Trade Name   Phenoxene
Classification   Anticholinergic agent

See trihexyphenidyl hydrochloride for contraindications, drug interactions, and nursing considerations.

Action   Mild anticholinergic activity. Particularly effective in controlling rigidity. Tremors may be augmented.

Indications for Drug   All forms of parkinsonism.

Contraindications   Use with caution in clients with narrow-angle glaucoma, arrhythmias, or prostatic hypertrophy.

Administration of Drug   50 to 100 mg po tid or qid after meals.

Side Effects   Blurred vision, constipation, dry mouth, nausea, and vomiting. May cause drowsiness, particularly in the elderly.

Generic Name   Cycrimine hydrochloride
Trade Name   Pagitane Hydrochloride
Classification   Anticholinergic agent

See trihexyphenidyl hydrochloride for nursing considerations.

Action   Less than half as potent as atropine in reducing neuromuscular symptoms and is slightly more toxic. May not be well tolerated or effective in arteriosclerotic parkinsonism or the elderly. Ineffective for drug-induced extrapyramidal disorders.

Indications for Drug   Parkinsonism.

Contraindications   Safe use during pregnancy has not been established. Use with caution in the elderly and in clients with glaucoma, tachycardia, or urinary retention.

Forms of Drug   Sugar-coated tablets containing 0.25 or 2.5 mg.

Administration of Drug
- *Postencephalitic parkinsonism:* 5 mg po tid; then increase slowly.
- *Idiopathic and arteriosclerotic parkinsonism:* 1.25 mg po tid; then increase slowly; Maximum dosage: 20 mg/day.

Side Effects   Blurred vision, GI disturbances, and dry mouth are common. CNS disturbances may occur.

Generic Name   Procyclidine hydrochloride
Trade Name   Kemadrin
Classification   Anticholinergic agent

See trihexyphenidyl hydrochloride for drug interactions and nursing considerations.

Action   Relieves spasticity of voluntary muscles. Particularly effective in reducing rigidity, but may not reduce tremors.

Indications for Drug   Parkinsonism, drug-induced extrapyramidal disorders, sialorrhea.

Contraindications   Angle-closure glaucoma. Use with caution in clients with mental disorders, since psychotic reactions may be precipitated. Use with caution in the elderly and in clients with tachycardia, prostatic hypertrophy, or hypotension.
   Safe use in children and during pregnancy and lactation has not been established.

Forms of Drug   Scored tablets containing 2 or 5 mg.

Administration of Drug
- *Parkinsonism:* Initial dosage: 2 to 2.5 mg po tid after meals; then increase slowly; usual dosage: 15 to 30 mg daily.
- *Extrapyramidal disorders:* Initial dosage: 2 to 2.5 mg po tid after meals; then increase by 2 to 2.5 mg daily until desired effect; Usual dosage: 10 to 20 mg daily.

Absorption   Onset of action is about 30 minutes and duration of action is about 4 hours.

Side Effects   Low toxicity, but secondary reactions frequently occur with high dosages. Dry mouth, mydriasis, blurred vision, and nausea are common. Suppurative parotitis may occur. Constipation, epigastric distress, and vomiting are relatively common. Allergic skin rashes have occurred. Weakness, confusion, disorientation, agitation, and hallucinations have occurred.

701

Antihistamines

Generic Name   Diphenhydramine hydrochloride
Trade Names   Benadryl, Phenamine
Classification   Antiparkinsonian agent

Action   Has significant anticholinergic activity.

Indications for Drug   Parkinsonism in the elderly who are unable to tolerate other antiparkinsonian agents. Mild parkinsonism in all age groups except newborns. Sometimes used in conjunction with anticholinergic agents for parkinsonism.

Contraindications   Neonates, premature infants, breast-feeding mothers, clients with acute bronchial and other lower respiratory tract disorders, clients taking MAO inhibitors. Use with caution in young children and clients with hyperthyroidism, hypertension, or a history of bronchial asthma. Use with extreme caution in clients with narrow-angle glaucoma, peptic ulcer, pyloric obstruction, or urinary retention. Safe use during pregnancy has not been established.

Forms of Drug   Capsules containing 25 or 50 mg; Elixir containing 12.5 mg/ml and 14% alcohol; Multi-dose vials containing 10 mg/ml.

Administration of Drug   Adults: 25 ro 50 mg po tid or qid; Children under 12 years: 5 mg/kg po daily in 4 divided doses.

Absorption   Readily absorbed from GI tract. Peak action occurs in about 60 minutes. Duration of action is 4 to 6 hours. Crosses blood-brain barrier.
Metabolism   Mainly by liver; some by other tissues, including the kidneys and lungs.
Excretion   In urine, primarily as metabolites.

Side Effects   Photosensitivity, diplopia, nausea, dry mouth, constipation, dysuria, and nasal stuffiness are relatively common. Tends to cause drowsiness, particularly in the elderly.

Interactive Effects   Anticholinergic agents and MAO inhibitors may prolong and intensify the anticholinergic effects of antihistamines. Excessive sedation and other CNS disturbances may occur when alcohol, barbiturates, and CNS depressants are used concomitantly.

Nursing Considerations   Warn client against concurrent ingestion of alcohol. (See trihexyphenidyl hydrochloride.)

Generic Name   Orphenadrine hydrochloride
Trade Name   Disipal
Classification   Antiparkinsonian agent

See trihexyphenidyl hydrochloride for nursing considerations. See diphenhydramine hydrochloride for indications for drug, contraindications, and drug interactions.

Action   Low antihistaminic, but high anticholinergic action.

Forms of Drug   Tablets containing 50 mg.

Administration of Drug   50 mg po qid or 100 mg po bid.

Side Effects   Dry mouth, constipation, arrhythmias, urinary hesitancy, and paralytic ileus may occur. May cause some drowsiness, but this soon disappears with continued therapy.

Nursing Considerations   (See trihexyphenidyl hydrochloride.)

Phenothiazine Derivatives

Generic Name   Ethopropazine hydrochloride
Trade Name   Parsidol
Classification   Antiparkinsonian agent

See trihexyphenidyl hydrochloride for nursing considerations.

Action   Although the exact mechanism of action is unknown, ethopropazine is effective in controlling the neuromuscular symptoms of all forms of parkinsonism and extrapyramidal disorders induced by reserpine and phenothiazines. The drug exerts a significant anticholinergic and antihistaminic effect. Unlike many of the drugs used in the treatment of parkinsonism, ethopropazine is effective in controlling tremors in most clients. It is also effective in relieving rigidity, spasms, sialorrhea, oculogyric crises, and festination associated with parkinsonism. Unlike phenothiazines, ethopropazine does not potentiate CNS depressants or have an antiemetic effect.

Indications for Drug All forms of parkinsonism, drug-induced extrapyramidal disorders (reserpine, phenothiazines).

Contraindications Glaucoma, prostatic hypertrophy. Use with caution in clients with a history of hypersensitivity to anticholinergic agents. May precipitate toxic psychosis in clients with mental disorders. Safe use during pregnancy and lactation has not been established.

Forms of Drug Tablets containing 10 or 50 mg.

Administration of Drug Highly individualized. Initial dosage: 50 mg po daily or bid; may be gradually increased to 100 to 400 mg po daily in divided doses. Postencephalitic parkinsonism may require as much as 500 to 600 mg daily.

Side Effects Common secondary reactions include drowsiness, inability to think, lassitude, forgetfulness, and confusion. Anticholinergic secondary reactions include dry mouth, nausea, vomiting, blurred vision, diplopia, constipation, and urinary retention. These symptoms tend to disappear with dosage reduction. Mild, transient hypotension may occur when large dosages are administered. Other effects include epigastric distress, muscle cramps, paresthesia, sensation of heavy limbs, and skin rashes. Phenothiazine-related secondary reactions include seizures, slowing of EEG, tachycardia, agranulocytosis, pancytopenia, purpura, jaundice, hallucinations, and pigmentation of the cornea, lens, retina, or skin.

Interactive Effects Unlike other phenothiazines, ethopropazine does not potentiate CNS depressants. Atropine has an additive effect with ethopropazine in the control of oculogyric crises. May mask phenothiazine-induced extrapyramidal disorders, which may become permanent with prolonged phenothiazine therapy.

ANTIPARKINSONIAN AGENTS

Generic Name Levodopa
Trade Names Dopar, L-Dopa, Larodopa
Classification Antiparkinsonian agent

Action Levodopa is a synthetic levorotatory isomer of dihydroxyphenylalanine (dopa). The symptoms of Parkinson's disease are related to depletion of striatal dopamine in the CNS. Dopamine cannot be given to overcome the deficit since it is unable to cross the blood-brain barrier. However, the precursor of dopamine levodopa is able to penetrate the blood-brain barrier. Levodopa is thought to be converted to dopamine in the basal ganglia, thus relieving the symptoms of parkinsonism by restoring dopamine levels in extrapyramidal centers. Cardiac stimulation may occur due to action on beta-adrenergic receptors and the drug may alter glucose metabolism.

Indications for Drug Idiopathic Parkinson's disease (paralysis agitans), postencephalitic parkinsonism associated with carbon monoxide and magnesium poisoning, parkinsonism associated with cerebral arteriosclerosis.

Contraindications Hypersensitivity to levodopa, narrow-angle glaucoma, within 2 weeks of therapy with MAO inhibitors. Levodopa may activate malignant melanoma and should therefore not be used in clients with suspicious or undiagnosed skin lesions. Use with caution in clients with severe cardiovascular or pulmonary disease, bronchial asthma, wide-angle glaucoma, renal, hepatic, or endocrine disorders, and those receiving antihypertensive drugs. Use with extreme caution in clients with arrhythmias or a history of myocardial infarction. GI hemorrhage may occur in clients with a history of peptic ulcer disease. Psychotic and depressed clients may develop severe depression or suicidal tendencies. Safe use in children under 12 years and during pregnancy has not been established; animal studies indicate abnormal fetal growth and viability.

Forms of Drug Scored tablets containing 250, 500, or 1000 mg; capsules containing 250, 500, or 1000 mg.

Administration of Drug Highly individualized; the goal is to induce maximum improvement with the minimum of untoward reactions. Six months of therapy may be required for maximum therapeutic response. Initial dosage: 500 to 1000 mg po daily in 2 or 3 divided doses with food; then increase by 500 to 750 mg daily every 3 to 7 days as tolerated; Maximum dosage: 8 g daily.

Absorption Rapidly and completely absorbed from GI tract; may cause GI disturbances. Peak plasma levels occur in 1 to 3 hours. Therapeutic response lasts about 5 hours.
Metabolism Some converted to dopamine in GI tract and liver; may cause tachycardia and other systemic dopamine effects. Crosses blood-brain barrier; amount entering is variable; then converted to dopa decarboxylase.

Excretion Primarily by the kidneys as metabolites dopamine and homovanillic acid; some excreted in feces.

1. If client is unable to swallow the tablet or capsule, it can be crushed and taken with apple sauce or other food.
2. Give drug with meals.

Side Effects Adventitious movements, such as choreiform and/or dystonia, are common. Involuntary grimacing or head movements, ataxia, tremors, muscular twitching, and body jerks may occur. Bradykinetic episodes in which the adventitious movements are sometimes present and sometimes absent may occur. Other CNS disturbances include loss of memory, delirium, hallucinations, anxiety, nervousness, insomnia, nightmares, fatigue, and euphoria. Cardiac irregularities (arrhythmias) and orthostatic hypotension are relatively common. Changes in mental status are relatively common and include depression, paranoid reactions, and psychotic disturbances. Urinary retention, incontinence, priapism, and excessive or inappropriate sexual behavior may occur. GI disturbances, including nausea, vomiting, and anorexia, are relatively common. Dry mouth, abdominal discomfort, and dysphagia may also occur. Bitter taste, burning sensation of the tongue, diarrhea, and constipation have been reported. Visual disturbances, including blepharospasm, blurring, diplopia, dilated pupils, oculogyric crisis, and activation of latent Horner's syndrome, have occurred. A harmless dark discoloration of urine and sweat may occur. Hepatotoxicity may occur. Leukopenia has occurred and a reduction in hemoglobin and hematocrit has been reported.

Interactive Effects Pyridoxine (vitamin B_6) in dosages of 10 to 25 mg will reduce the therapeutic effects of levodopa rapidly. Drugs that decrease the therapeutic effectiveness of levodopa include anticholinergic agents, tricyclic antidepressants, phenothiazines, phenytoin, papaverine, and reserpine. Concomitant administration of antacids or propranolol may increase the therapeutic effects of levodopa. Concurrent therapy with MAO inhibitors is contraindicated within 14 days of levodopa therapy; hypertension may occur. Levodopa may alter the effects of antihypertensive agents and postural hypotension can occur.

Nursing Considerations
1. Assessment and planning
    a. Obtain history of GI, genitourinary, hepatic, ophthalmic, endocrine, and cardiovascular disorders.
    b. Diabetics should be well controlled before instituting drug.
    c. Intraocular pressure should be determined before initiating drug. If elevated, notify physician.
    d. Determine the potential for drug interactions (include multivitamin preparations).
    e. Record symptoms of parkinsonism and their severity.

2. Assessment and implementation
    a. Monitor vital signs periodically (q8h) during dosage adjustments.
    b. Muscular twitching and blepharospasm are early warnings of drug toxicity. If symptoms occur, notify physician.
    c. Monitor the occurrence of depression. Suicide precautions may be required. Notify physician, as indicated.
    d. Clients with glaucoma should have their intraocular pressure checked periodically.
    e. Check serum glucose of diabetic clients frequently during dosage adjustments. Urinary testing for sugar content may be unreliable.
    f. Dosage should be reduced if drug-induced involuntary muscle movements occur. More than 75% of clients may develop involuntary movements after 1 to 2 years of drug therapy.
    g. Clients receiving antihypertensive drugs may require dosage adjustments. Monitor blood pressure and notify physician, as indicated.
    h. If surgery is required during levodopa therapy, the drug should be stopped and reinstituted as soon as possible. Lower dosages may be required if client has been off drug for more than a few days.
    i. Warn client to change position slowly to avoid orthostatic hypotension.
    j. Instruct client and family members to administer drug regularly with meals, as prescribed.
    k. Warn client that interruptions in drug therapy can cause untoward reactions.
    l. Instruct client to consult physician before taking OTC drugs, since many contain drugs that interact with levodopa.
    m. Instruct client to consult physician before taking a multivitamin preparation.
    n. Inform client that physiotherapy and physical activity will assist in increasing abilities; but warn client to resume activities slowly.
3. Assessment and evaluation
    a. Periodic evaluations of hepatic, renal, hematopoietic, and cardiovascular function are recommended. Complete blood cell count, blood urea nitrogen, and other hepatic function tests should be taken every 1 to 6 months. If hepatotoxicity occurs, the drug should be discontinued.
    b. Stress the importance of periodic laboratory and medical checkups.
    c. Blood urea nitrogen, serum glutamic-oxaloacetic transaminase, serum glutamic-pyruvic transaminase, lactate dehydrogenase, bilirubin, alkaline phosphatase, uric acid, and protein-bound iodine may be elevated. A positive Coombs' test result may occur.

704

Generic Name   Levodopa/carbidopa
Trade Name   Sinemet
Classification   Antiparkinsonian agent

See levodopa for indications for drug, contraindications, and nursing considerations.

Action   Large dosages of levodopa are required to produce adequate drug levels in the CNS because large quantities are metabolized in the GI tract and liver. Carbidopa is a dicarboxylase inhibitor that is unable to cross the blood-brain barrier. When given in combination, carbidopa inhibits the metabolism of levodopa; thus leaving more intact levodopa available to cross the blood-brain barrier. Carbidopa increases the plasma half-life of both levodopa and homovanillic acid. Consequently, about 75% less levodopa is required to produce a therapeutic effect and fewer untoward reactions (GI disturbances, arrhythmias) occur. An added benefit of the combination drug is that pyridoxine intake does not alter the therapeutic effect of levodopa significantly. Pyridoxine increases the rate of decarboxylation and since carbidopa inhibits this process, pyridoxine supplements do not increase the metabolism of levodopa. Although the combination drug decreases the incidence of GI disturbances and dopamine-related reactions, it does not decrease CNS disturbances. More rapid titration of the drug is also possible. Levodopa must be discontinued at least 8 hours before instituting the combination drug. (See levodopa.)

Forms of Drug   10/100 tablets containing 10 mg carbidopa and 100 mg levodopa; 25/100 tablets containing 25 mg carbidopa and 100 mg levodopa; 25/250 tablets containing 25 mg carbidopa and 250 mg levodopa.

Administration of Drug   Highly individualized. Initial dosage: 1 to 2 25/250-mg tablets with meals; Maintenance dosage: 3 to 6 25/250-mg tablets daily in divided doses with meals; Maximum dosage: 8 tablets of 25/250 or 25/100 mg daily. If greater quantities of levodopa are needed, plain levodopa is added to the regimen. Maximum dosage of carbidopa: 200 mg daily.

Side Effects   Choreiform, dystonia, and other involuntary movements are common. Changes in mental status, including depression and psychosis, can occur. Convulsions have been reported, but rarely. Some nausea may occur. (See levodopa.)

Interactive Effects   Fewer drug interactions occur with the combination drug than with levodopa. Papaverine, diazepam, clonidine, and phenothiazines may antagonize the therapeutic effects of levodopa. (See levodopa.)

Generic Name   Amantadine hydrochloride
Trade Name   Symmetrel
Classification   Antiparkinsonian and antiviral agent

Action   Although amantadine was originally released as an antiviral agent, the drug was found to have an antiparkinsonian effect. The exact mechanism of action is unknown, but amantadine is thought to stimulate the release of dopamine from nigrostriatal neurons, since animal studies have demonstrated increased dopamine levels in the brain. Although the drug is less effective than levodopa and lacks anticholinergic activity, amantadine causes relatively fewer serious untoward reactions and therapeutic results occur relatively quickly, usually within 2 to 4 weeks. Amantadine is effective against influenza A virus. The drug apparently prevents the release of infectious viral nucleic acid into the host cell. The drug does not seem to interfere with the vaccine against influenza A virus and can therefore be used prophylactically in conjunction with the vaccine for high-risk clients exposed to the viral infection until adequate antibody formation has occurred.

Indications for Drug   Idiopathic Parkinson's disease (paralysis agitans), postencephalitic parkinsonism, drug-induced extrapyramidal reactions, parkinsonism associated with head injuries and cerebral arteriosclerosis. Respiratory infections caused by influenza A viral infections in susceptible clients, such as the elderly and debilitated clients.

Contraindications   Hypersensitivity to amantadine. Use with caution in epileptics and clients with seizure disorders, since seizure activity may increase; in clients with a history of congestive heart failure or peripheral edema, since congestive heart failure may be precipitated; in clients with hepatic disorders or with a history of eczematoid rashes. If used concurrently with anticholinergic drugs, the dosage of the latter drug should be reduced if untoward reactions characteristic of atropine occur. Use with caution during pregnancy; embryotoxic and teratogenic effects have occurred in animal studies. Safe use in infants under 1 year has not been established.

Forms of Drug   Capsules containing 100 mg; syrup containing 50 mg/5 ml.

705

Administration of Drug Highly individualized; drug's effectiveness may subside after a few months, necessitating an increase in dosage.

- *Parkinsonism:* Only drug used: 100 mg po bid; Maximum dosage: 400 mg daily in divided doses. Multiple drug therapy: 100 mg po daily for 1 week; then 100 mg po bid, as needed. Lower dosages may be required for debilitated clients.
- *Drug-induced extrapyramidal reactions:* 100 mg po bid; 300 mg daily may be required by some clients.
- *Prevention and treatment of influenza A virus infections:* Adults: 200 mg po daily or 100 mg po bid. Continuous drug therapy for 10 days after exposure to virus is required. When administered concurrently with vaccine it is given for 2 to 3 weeks. Children: Ages 1 to 9 years: 4.4 to 8.8 mg/kg/day; Ages 9 to 12 years: 100 mg po bid; Maximum dosage: 150 mg/day.

Absorption Fairly well absorbed from GI tract. Peak serum levels occur in 4 hours. Mean half-life is about 15 hours. Onset of therapeutic effect occurs in about 48 hours. Crosses placenta and enters breast milk; lactating mothers should bottle-feed their babies.
Metabolism None.
Excretion By the kidneys as unchanged drug at the rate of 5 mg/hour.

Side Effects CNS disturbances include depression, psychosis, hallucinations, confusion, anxiety, irritability, ataxia, dizziness, insomnia, headache, slurred speech, and visual disturbances. Cardiovascular disturbances include the development of peripheral edema, which may progress to congestive heart failure. Orthostatic hypotension occurs relatively frequently, as does urinary retention. GI disturbances include anorexia, nausea, vomiting, constipation, and dry mouth. Livedo reticularis frequently occurs, but eczematoid dermatitis is rare. Rare reactions include convulsions, leukopenia, neutropenia, and oculogyric reactions.

Interactive Effects No significant interactions known.

Nursing Considerations (See levodopa.)
1. Warn elderly and debilitated clients to change position slowly to avoid orthostatic hypotension.
2. Administer drug early in the day to avoid insomnia.
3. Give with a full glass of water.
4. Warn client about CNS disturbances and to avoid situations that require constant attention until CNS disturbances subside. If CNS disturbances persist with a one-day dosage schedule, a split dosage schedule may eliminate them.
5. Instruct client to inform physician of untoward reactions and worsening of parkinsonism (usually around 2 to 6 months after beginning drug).
6. Warn client against abrupt withdrawal of drug, as this may precipitate a parkinsonian crisis (rapid and marked deterioration).
7. Optimal therapeutic effect may not be apparent for 2 weeks.

Generic Name Bromocriptine mesylate
Trade Name Parlodel
Classification Antiparkinsonian and hyperprolactinemia agent

Action Bromocriptine, an ergot derivative, is a potent stimulant of dopamine receptor sites, including those in the corpus striatal region of the brain and in the tubero-infundibular process. Stimulation of the latter receptor sites inhibits the secretion of prolactin from the anterior pituitary gland, so the drug has been found effective in the short-term treatment of amenorrhea, galactorrhea, and infertility associated with hyperprolactinemia. The stimulation of dopamine receptor sites in the corpus striatal region causes an inhibitory response on cholinergic neurons in the area and is therefore effective in minimizing the symptoms of parkinsonism. Although the drug-induced untoward reactions tend to be mild and transient, there is a significantly higher incidence of untoward reactions during long-term therapy of parkinsonism than with levodopa/carbidopa drug therapy.

Indications for Drug Short-term treatment of hyperprolactinemia that results in amenorrhea, galactorrhea, and female infertility; prevention of lactation after an abortion, stillbirth, or childbirth when lactation is undesired or contraindicated; Idiopathic or postencephalitic parkinsonism, particularly in clients who experience end-of-dose-failure or on-off phenomenon with levodopa therapy.

Contraindications Hypersensitivity to ergot alkaloids. The presence of a pituitary tumor (Forbes-Albright syndrome) should be ruled out before instituting drug therapy. Although plasma prolactin levels are decreased by the drug, accepted therapies for destruction of the pituitary tumor must be instituted. Discontinue drug immediately if pregnancy occurs. Client should be assessed frequently for tiny prolactin-secreting adenomas that are not detectable by standard diagnostic measures, but which may grow and cause compression of the optic nerve during pregnancy. Vital signs must be stabilized after abortion or childbirth before the drug can be instituted, since hypotension may occur. Use with caution in clients receiving drugs that lower blood pressure and those with arrhythmias or a history of myocardial infarction. Safe use in children under 15 years and clients with hepatic or renal disorders has not been established. Safe use of drug beyond 2 years for parkinsonism has not been established. Contraceptive measures, other than oral contraceptives, should be used during drug therapy.

Forms of Drug Tablets containing 2.5 mg.

Administration of Drug
- *Amenorrhea, galactorrhea, infertility:* Initial dosage: 2.5 mg po daily with meals; dosage may be increased within 1 week; then 2.5 mg po bid or tid with meals for 14 days to 6 months. Do not exceed 6 months of therapy.
- *Prevention of lactation:* 2.5 mg po bid with meals for 14 to 21 days.
- *Parkinsonism:* Initial dosage: 1.75 mg po bid with meals; then increase by 2.5 mg every 14 to 28 days until desired effect.

Absorption Less than one-third of the oral dose is absorbed from the GI tract; GI disturbances are common. Some bound to serum albumin, but not significantly in vivo. Almost 96% bound to serum albumin in vitro.
Metabolism Completely metabolized in the liver and other tissues.
Excretion Primarily in bile and ultimately excreted in feces. Only 2% to 5.5% in urine. Completely excreted after 5 days.

1. Give drug with meals or a snack.
2. Tablet can be crushed and mixed with apple sauce for clients who have difficulty in swallowing.

Side Effects The incidence of untoward reactions varies according to the purpose of drug administration. Nausea and other GI disturbances occur more frequently in clients being treated for amenorrhea, galactorrhea, and female infertility. Hypotension, headache, and dizziness are common in clients receiving the drug for prevention of lactation. CNS disturbances are more common in parkinsonian clients.

Hypotension is a secondary reaction to the drug and may be symptomatic in some clients. Faintness, dizziness, fatigue, lightheadedness, vertigo, and syncope are common within the first few days of therapy; but the symptoms subside when the dosage is reduced. GI disturbances, including nausea, vomiting, abdominal cramps, diarrhea, and constipation, are common. CNS disturbances, including headache, hallucinations, and confusion, are common. Drowsiness, weakness, insomnia, depression, nervousness, lethargy, nightmares, and paresthesia have been reported. Abnormal involuntary movements and "on-off" phenomenon have emerged in clients being tapered off levodopa/carbidopa. Other reactions, including nasal stuffiness (common), urinary frequency, incontinence or retention, skin rashes, seizures, and ergotism, have occurred, but rarely.

Interactive Effects Symptomatic hypotension may occur if administered concurrently with antihypertensive agents. Pregnancy may occur if client relies on oral contraceptives.

Nursing Considerations
1. Assessment and planning
   a. Obtain history of symptoms for which the drug is to be administered.
   b. Baseline hepatic function tests (blood urea nitrogen, transaminases) should be obtained.
   c. Pregnancy test should be performed, when applicable.
   d. Obtain baseline blood pressure.
2. Assessment and implementation
   a. Warn client that lightheadedness and fainting may occur when drug is started and when dosage is increased. Client should change position slowly and report symptoms immediately.
   b. Instruct client to take medication with meals to avoid nausea.
   c. When appropriate, caution female clients to use contraceptive measures other than oral contraceptives to avoid pregnancy.
   d. Caution client against driving a car or engaging in activities that require constant attention until hypotension is well controlled.
3. Assessment and evaluation
   a. Obtain blood pressure before administering dose when drug is first initiated or dosage is adjusted.

b. In amenorrhea, menses may resume within 6 to 8 weeks of therapy.

c. In galactorrhea, breast secretions and inflammation are usually reduced by 75% after 8 to 12 weeks of therapy.

d. A pregnancy test is recommended every 4 weeks when drug is administered for hyperprolactinemia.

e. Pregnancy test should be done if menses do not commence within 3 days of expected date.

f. When long-term therapy is required, hepatic, hematopoietic, cardiovascular, and renal function tests should be done periodically.

g. Laboratory alterations include transient elevations in blood urea nitrogen, serum glutamic-oxaloacetic transaminase, serum glutamic-pyruvic transaminase, creatine phosphokinase, alkaline phosphatase, and uric acid.

ANTIPSYCHOTIC MEDICATIONS

The five major types of antipsychotic agents are (1) phenothiazines, (2) butyrophenones, (3) thioxanthenes, (4) dihydroindolones, and (5) dibenzoxazepines. Formerly called major tranquilizers, antipsychotic agents are also known as neuroleptics and ataractics.

Antipsychotic agents are sometimes termed chemical restraints, as they have made such physical restraints as straitjackets and hydrotherapy obsolete. The resulting reduction in the incidence and duration of violent behavior among the mentally ill receiving these drugs provided the means for their deinstitutionalization and return to community care.

Antipsychotic agents effectively decrease the severity of hallucinations, delusions, and the accompanying behavior. Clients who take these medications consistently as treatment measures are more amenable to participating in other modalities.

The usefulness of chlorpromazine in treating mental illness was discovered when antihistamine research was in progress. It has been widely used as an effective antipsychotic agent since 1951. A number of derivatives that provide the same therapeutic effects as chlorpromazine while minimizing side effects have also been developed. The phenothiazines act as sedative antipsychotic agents by depressing the subcortical centers of the brain, which are believed to be the seat of the emotions. Although vital centers of the brain are not depressed, the calmness produced is often sufficient to improve sleep problems. The exact mechanism of action is unknown, but the drugs apparently work by inhibiting dopamine receptors.

PHENOTHIAZINES

Generic Name Chlorpromazine hydrochloride
Trade Names Chlor-PZ, Promachel, Promapar, Sonazine, Thorazine
Classification Antipsychotic

Action Antipsychotic, antiemetic, hypothermic, sedative, antidopaminergic, and anticholinergic actions. Inhibits release of ACTH, growth hormone, and prolactin-inhibiting factor. Not effective in depression or retarded withdrawal states.

Indications for Drug Psychoses, hiccups, acromegaly, as an antiemetic. Also, during surgery, labor, and delivery, to enhance action of narcotics and hypnotics. In combination with analgesics for severe pain.

Contraindications Pregnancy, coma, glaucoma, prostatic hypertrophy, cardiovascular disease, convulsive disorders, infants under 6 months. Use with caution in women of childbearing age, elderly clients, and children (since they are more susceptible to acute dystonia than adults). Clients with cirrhosis are more susceptible to sedative effects. Clients with the following conditions should be evaluated frequently: renal, hepatic, cardiovascular, or respiratory disease, blood dyscrasias, cardiovascular accidents, hypoparathyroidism.

Forms of Drug Tablets containing 10, 25, 50, 100, or 200 mg; sustained-release capsules containing 30, 75, 150, or 200 mg; ampules of 1 or 2 ml containing 25 mg/ml; 10-ml vials containing 25 mg/ml; syrup containing 10 mg/5 ml; suppositories containing 25 or 100 mg.

Administration of Drug Adults: 30 mg to 1 g po, IM, or IV daily in divided doses; Rectal suppository: 100 mg every 6 to 8 hours. Children: 2 mg/kg po daily in divided doses.

1. Protect skin, eyes, and clothing from contact with drug.
2. When administering IM, drug should be slowly and deeply injected. The pain from injection can be alleviated by massaging the injection site.
3. Do not mix with other drugs.

Absorption Readily absorbed from parenteral sites; erratic absorption following oral administration. Peak action occurs in 1 to 3 hours and duration of action is 3 to 6 hours. Half-life is about 6 hours. Crosses placenta and blood-brain barrier.
Distribution Distributed to all body tissues with some distribution to brain. Concentrated in lungs and keratin structures.
Metabolism In the liver.
Excretion In urine and feces.

Side Effects Drowsiness is common; tolerance usually develops in 1 to 2 weeks. Hypotension, evidenced by dizziness and weakness on standing, is common. Extrapyramidal symptoms: uncoordinated spasmodic movements, involuntary motor restlessness, parkinsonism. Tardive dyskinesia, which is characterized by hyperkinetic activity in the oral region and for which there is no effective treatment, may appear after long-term use; has also been reported after low doses given for short periods. Autonomic nervous system effects: dry mouth, blurred vision, constipation, urinary disturbances, weight gain, delayed ovulation, amenorrhea, abnormal lactation, increased libido in women, decreased libido in men. Dermatologic effects: skin rash, skin discoloration on exposure to sunlight, phototoxicity (painful sunburn after brief exposure to sun). Visual changes: corneal and lens opacities. Toxic effects: obstructive jaundice, agranulocytosis, hepatitis, leukopenia.

Interactive Effects Potentiates hypotensive effects of methyldopa, reserpine, and beta blockers; potentiates the anticholinergic effects of tricyclic antidepressants and antiparkinsonian drugs. Enhances respiratory depression produced by meperidine. Blocks the hypotensive effects of guanethidine. Lithium, trihexyphenidyl, and antacids decrease plasma levels of chlorpromazine. Alcohol and sedatives potentiate sedative effects of chlorpromazine.

Nursing Considerations
1. Assessment and planning
   a. Caution client against activities requiring mental alertness and muscular coordination.
   b. Advise client to avoid alcohol, sedatives, and hypnotics.
   c. Advise client to change position gradually and to dangle legs for 1 minute before getting out of bed.
   d. Because of photosensitivity, client should be instructed to protect him- or herself from exposure to sun.
   e. Encourage high fluid intake and frequent rinsing of mouth.
2. Assessment and implementation
   a. Because orthostatic hypotension is common, the client's blood pressure should be monitored daily.
   b. Observe for dizziness and weakness.
   c. In severe cases of hypotension, put client in Trendelenburg's position and request administration of plasma expanders.
   d. Monitor intake and output; check frequency of bowel movements.
   e. Drug should be discontinued at least 48 hours prior to surgery.
   f. Protect elderly clients with bedrails; these clients are more prone to develop hypotension.
   g. Institute measures to prevent hyperthermia or hypothermia.
   h. If client develops extrapyramidal symptoms, reduce sensory stimuli.
3. Assessment and evaluation
   a. Report any visual changes and schedule regular eye examinations.
   b. Report sore throat or elevated temperature.
   c. Observe client for jaundice.
   d. Advise client not to discontinue drug without medical supervision.
   e. False-positive results may occur for urobilinogen, urine bilirubin, and pregnancy tests. May also affect results for urine catecholamines, ketones, and radioactive iodine uptake tests.

Generic Name Acetophenazine maleate
Trade Name Tindal
Classification Antipsychotic

See chlorpromazine for contraindications, drug interactions, and nursing considerations.

Action Acetophenazine has a stronger sedative effect than chlorpromazine. (See chlorpromazine.)

Indications for Drug Management of psychoses in the elderly, such as organic brain syndrome. Large dosages are needed to treat other psychoses.

Forms of Drug Tablets containing 20 mg.

Administration of Drug Adults: 40 to 80 mg po daily; Children: 0.8 to 1.6 mg/kg po daily in 3 divided doses.

Side Effects Produces fewer extrapyramidal symptoms than chlorpromazine. (See chlorpromazine.)

Generic Name Butaperazine maleate
Trade Name Repoise
Classification Antipsychotic

See chlorpromazine for contraindications, drug interactions, and nursing considerations.

Action Similar to chlorpromazine. (See chlorpromazine.)

Indications for Drug Treatment of paranoia and chronic brain syndrome.

Forms of Drug Tablets containing, 5, 10, or 25 mg.

709

Administration of Drug   Adults: 15 to 30 mg po daily in divided doses; can be increased to a maximum dosage of 100 mg/day. Geriatrics: ¼ to ½ of adult dosage.

Side Effects   Extrapyramidal symptoms occur frequently.

Generic Name   Carphenazine maleate
Trade Name   Proketazine
Classification   Antipsychotic

See chlorpromazine for indications for drug, contraindications, drug interactions, and side effects.

Action   Similar to other phenothiazines in the piperazine group. (See chlorpromazine.)

Administration of Drug   Adults: 75 to 150 mg po daily in divided doses; can be increased every 1 to 2 weeks by 25 to 50 mg; Maximum dosage: 400 mg/day. Geriatrics: ½ of adult dosage.

Forms of Drug   Tablets containing 12.5, 25, or 50 mg; concentrate containing 50 mg/ml.

Nursing Considerations   Full therapeutic effect may not be apparent for several months. (See chlorpromazine.)

Generic Names   Fluphenazine enanthate, fluphenazine decanoate
Trade Name   Prolixin
Classification   Antipsychotic

See chlorpromazine for contraindications and drug interactions.

Action   Similar to chlorpromazine. (See chlorpromazine.)

Indications for Drug   Treatment of outpatients whose compliance with a medication regimen is doubtful.

Forms of Drug   Vials of 10 ml containing 2.5 mg/ml; protect from light; if solution is darker than light amber, do not use. Tablets containing 1, 2.5, 5, or 10 mg; protect from light. Elixir containing 0.5 mg/ml; avoid freezing.

Administration of Drug   Adults: 2.5 to 10 mg po daily in divided doses; under close hospital supervision, clients can receive up to 20 mg daily; 25 mg IM every 1 to 3 weeks. Children: 0.25 to 3 mg po daily in divided doses.

Side Effects   This drug is very potent and has a high incidence of extrapyramidal symptoms. (See chlorpromazine.)

Nursing Considerations   (See chlorpromazine.)
1. Antiparkinsonian drugs may be needed to prevent extrapyramidal symptoms.
2. Geriatric clients are at a greater risk of developing extrapyramidal symptoms, especially women who have been medicated with phenothiazines for a long time.

Generic Name   Mesoridazine besylate
Trade Name   Serentil
Classification   Antipsychotic

See chlorpromazine for indications for drug, contraindications, side effects, drug interactions, and nursing considerations.

Action   Similar to chlorpromazine. Not effective in treatment of delirium tremens. (See chlorpromazine.)

Forms of Drug   Tablets containing 10, 25, 50, or 100 mg; 10-ml vials containing 25 mg/ml.

Administration of Drug   Adults: 100 to 400 mg po daily in divided doses; 25 to 200 mg IM daily in divided doses. Geriatrics: ¼ to ½ of drug dosage.

Generic Name   Perphenazine
Trade Name   Trilafon
Classification   Antipsychotic, antiemetic

See chlorpromazine for indications for drug, contraindications, drug interactions, and side effects.

Action   Similar to chlorpromazine, but six times more potent. (See chlorpromazine.)

Forms of Drug   Tablets containing 2, 4, or 8 mg; syrup containing 2 mg/5 ml; concentrate containing 16 mg/ml (diluted in 60 ml of fluid).

Administration of Drug   Adults: 16 to 64 mg po or IM daily in divided doses.

Nursing Considerations   (See chlorpromazine.)
1. May be used IV during surgery for hiccups or vomiting. Should not be given IV as an antipsychotic.
2. Dilute concentrate with water, milk, or orange juice. Do not mix with tea, coffee, cola, apple, or grape juice.

Generic Name   Piperacetazine
Trade Name   Quide
Classification   Antipsychotic

See chlorpromazine for contraindications, drug interactions, and nursing considerations.

Action   Similar to chlorpromazine. (See chlorpromazine.)

Indications for Drug   Schizophrenia characterized by agitation; most effective in treating acute rather than chronic schizophrenia.

Forms of Drug   Tablets containing 10 or 25 mg.

Administration of Drug   Adults: 20 to 40 mg po daily in divided doses; can be increased to 160 mg daily in divided doses. Geriatrics: ¼ to ½ of adult dosage.

Side Effects   Piperacetazine causes a higher incidence of extrapyramidal symptoms than most phenothiazines. (See chlorpromazine.)

Generic Name   Prochlorperazine maleate
Trade Names   Combid, Compazine
Classification   Antipsychotic, antiemetic

See chlorpromazine for indications for drug, contraindications, drug interactions, and nursing considerations.

Action   Prochlorperazine has greater antiemetic activity than most phenothiazines. It is also effective as an antipsychotic agent. (See chlorpromazine.)

Forms of Drug   Tablets containing 5, 10, or 25 mg; sustained-release capsules containing 10, 15, 30, or 75 mg; 10-ml vials containing 5 mg/ml; 2-ml ampules containing 5 mg/ml; suppositories containing 2.5, 5, or 25 mg; syrup containing 5 mg/ml; concentrate containing 10 mg/ml.

Administration of Drug
- *Antipsychotic:* Adults: 5 to 10 mg po or IM bid, tid, or qid; the dosage can be gradually increased to 75 to 150 mg daily in divided doses. Rectal suppository: 25 mg bid. Children: Ages 2 years and older: 0.4 mg/kg daily in divided doses.
- *Antiemetic:* Adults: Preoperative: 5 to 10 mg IM 1 to 2 hours before surgery; 5 to 10 mg IV 30 minutes before anesthesia. Postoperative: 5 to 10 mg IM.

Side Effects   The risk of developing extrapyramidal symptoms is greater for prochlorperazine than for other phenothiazines. (See chlorpromazine.)

711

Generic Name   Trifluoperazine hydrochloride
Trade Name   Stelazine
Classification   Antipsychotic

See chlorpromazine for contraindications and drug interactions.

Action   Trifluoperazine is fast acting and 10 times more potent than chlorpromazine. (See chlorpromazine.)

Indications for Drug   Treatment of psychoses where the client demonstrates withdrawal and apathy.

Forms of Drug   Tablets containing 1, 2, 5, or 10 mg; 10-ml vials containing 2 mg/ml; concentrate containing 10 mg/ml (dilute in 60 ml of fluid).

Administration of Drug   Adults: Oral: 2 to 5 mg bid or tid initially; then increase to 15 to 20 mg daily in 2 to 3 divided doses. Intramuscular: 1 to 2 mg every 4 to 6 hours; can be increased to 6 to 10 mg daily. Children: Ages 6 to 12 years: 1 to 2 mg po daily; Maximum dosage: 15 mg/day.

Side Effects   Extrapyramidal symptoms occur frequently. (See chlorpromazine.)

Nursing Considerations   The maximum therapeutic effect is reached in 3 weeks and is more prolonged than with chlorpromazine. (See chlorpromazine.)

Generic Name Triflupromazine hydrochloride
Trade Name Vesprin
Classification Antipsychotic

See chlorpromazine for indications for drug, contraindications, drug interactions, and nursing considerations.

Action Similar to chlorpromazine; fast acting. (See chlorpromazine.)

Forms of Drug Tablets containing 10, 25, or 50 mg; 10-ml vials containing 10 or 20 mg/ml; suspension containing 50 mg/5 ml.

Administration of Drug Adults: Determined individually; up to 150 mg daily. Children: Ages 6 to 12 years: 2 mg/kg po, or 0.25 mg/kg IM daily. Maximum dosage: 150 mg/day po, or 10 mg/day IM.

Side Effects Extrapyramidal symptoms are the most serious. (See chlorpromazine.)

Generic Name Thiopropazate hydrochloride
Trade Name Dartal
Classification Antipsychotic

See chlorpromazine for contraindications, side effects, drug interactions, and nursing considerations.

Action Similar to chlorpromazine. (See chlorpromazine.)

Indications for Drug Psychoses marked by hostility and aggression.

Forms of Drug Tablets containing 5 or 10 mg.

Administration of Drug Adults: 10 mg po tid; Maximum dosage: 100 mg/day.

Generic Name Thioridazine hydrochloride
Trade Name Mellaril
Classification Antipsychotic

See chlorpromazine for indications for drug, contraindications, drug interactions, and nursing considerations.

Action Thioridazine is one of the less potent tranquilizers. It has very little antiemetic activity and does not affect the temperature-regulating mechanism. It is considered to be a useful antipsychotic drug and a good basic tranquilizer. (See chlorpromazine.)

Forms of Drug Tablets containing 10, 25, 50, 100, 150, or 200 mg; concentrate containing 30 mg/ml.

Administration of Drug Adults: 20 to 800 mg po daily; Children: Over 2 years: 1 mg/kg po daily in 3 to 4 divided doses.

Side Effects Produces fewer extrapyramidal symptoms than chlorpromazine. Large dosages have reportedly produced pigmentary retinopathy. Sudden death has been reported following long-term use. (See chlorpromazine.)

BUTYROPHENONES

Generic Name Haloperidol
Trade Name Haldol
Classification Antipsychotic, antiemetic

See chlorpromazine for contraindications and drug interactions.

Action Similar to phenothiazines. (See chlorpromazine.)

Indications for Drug Control of hyperactivity that occurs in the manic phase of manic-depressive illness; acute psychiatric problems.

Contraindications Parkinsonism. (See chlorpromazine.)

Forms of Drug Tablets containing 0.5, 1, or 2 mg; concentrate containing 2 mg/ml; ampules containing 5 mg/ml.

Administration of Drug Adults: 2 to 8 mg po or IM daily; can be gradually increased 0.5 to 1 mg every 3 days; Maximum dosage: 15 mg/day.

Absorption Peak action occurs in 30 to 45 minutes.
Excretion Slowly in urine.

Side Effects Generally similar to phenothiazines, but there is a high incidence of extrapyramidal symptoms and less sedation, hypotension, hypothermia, and photosensitivity. Severe depression leading to suicidal tendencies may develop. (See chlorpromazine.)

Nursing Considerations There is a narrow margin between therapeutic and toxic dosages. (See chlorpromazine.)

THIOXANTHENES

Generic Name Chlorprothixene
Trade Name Taractan
Classification Antipsychotic, antiemetic

See chlorpromazine for contraindications, drug interactions, and nursing considerations.

Action Similar to phenothiazines, but a more powerful inhibitor of motor coordination and produces fewer antihistaminic effects. (See chlorpromazine.)

Indications for Drug Schizophrenia, acute depression, neurosis, withdrawal from alcohol, agitation.

Forms of Drug Tablets containing 10, 25, 50, or 100 mg; vials containing 12.5 mg/ml.

Administration of Drug Adults: 30 to 200 mg po or IM daily in divided doses; Children: 30 to 100 mg po daily.

Absorption Peak action occurs in 30 minutes.

Side Effects Drowsiness, orthostatic hypotension, and dry mouth occur frequently. Extrapyramidal symptoms, agranulocytosis, and cholestatic hepatitis are less likely to occur. (See chlorpromazine.)

Generic Name Thiothixene
Trade Name Navane
Classification Antipsychotic

See chlorpromazine for contraindications and drug interactions.

Action Similar to phenothiazines, but a more powerful inhibitor of motor coordination and produces fewer antihistaminic effects. (See chlorpromazine.)

Indications for Drug Acute and chronic schizophrenia.

Forms of Drug Capsules containing 1, 2, 5, or 10 mg; concentrate containing 5 mg/ml; vials containing 2 mg/ml.

Administration of Drug Adults: 6 to 15 mg po or IM daily in divided doses; can be gradually increased to a maximum oral dosage of 60 mg/day or a maximum intramuscular dosage or 30 mg/day.

Side Effects Insomnia and extrapyramidal symptoms occur frequently. (See chlorpromazine.)

Nursing Considerations There is a very narrow margin between therapeutic and toxic dosages. (See chlorpromazine.)

DIHYDROINDOLONES

Generic Name Molindone
Trade Names Lidone, Moban
Classification Antipsychotic

See chlorpromazine for contraindications and nursing considerations.

Action Similar to phenothiazines. (See chlorpromazine.)

Indications for Drug Acute schizophrenia.

Forms of Drug Tablets and capsules containing 5, 10, or 25 mg.

713

Administration of Drug
- *Mild schizophrenia:* Adults: 5 to 15 mg po daily in divided doses.
- *Moderate schizophrenia:* Adults: 10 to 25 mg po daily in divided doses.
- *Severe schizophrenia:* Adults: Up to 225 mg po daily in divided doses.

Side Effects Clients have experienced profound CNS depression while taking other drugs. (See chlorpromazine.) Excessive weight gain is less of a problem. (See chlorpromazine.)

DIBENZOXAZEPINES

Generic Name Loxapine
Trade Names Daxolin, Loxitane
Classification Antipsychotic

714

See chlorpromazine for contraindications, drug interactions, and nursing considerations.

Action Newly available tricyclic drug with actions similar to phenothiazines. (See chlorpromazine.)

Indications for Drug Schizophrenia.

Forms of Drug Capsules containing 5, 10, 25, or 50 mg; concentrate containing 25 mg/ml.

Administration of Drug Adults: 60 to 100 mg po daily in divided doses; can be gradually increased to a maximum dosage of 250 mg/day.

Side Effects Similar to phenothiazines, but less likely to produce the serious side effects, such as extrapyramidal symptoms. (See chlorpromazine.)

BARBITURATE MEDICATIONS

The major action of barbiturates is central nervous system depression. When used within prescribed dosage ranges, the effects can range from mild sedation to coma, depending on the particular barbiturate used, its duration of action, route of administration, and the client's clinical status. When used in high concentrations, barbiturates have a generalized depressant effect on most other body systems. With prompt treatment, these effects are reversible, but the danger of car-

diovascular collapse in acute barbiturate intoxication poses a serious threat while the drug is in the body.

Barbiturates also have subtle, long-lasting effects. There is evidence of impairment of fine motor functions and of judgment for as long as 20 hours after ingestion of a sleep-inducing dosage. Many individuals become irritable and/or emotionally labile during this period.

Although all barbiturates have anticonvulsant properties, phenobarbital has a specific effect on the motor cortex when given in small, nonsedative doses. It is most effective for the control of grand mal seizures, alone or in combination with other anticonvulsant drugs.

Barbiturates can produce physical and psychological dependence and tolerance. Physical tolerance develops for two reasons: (1) the production of enzymes in the liver is increased and results in more rapid metabolism of the drug, and (2) the central nervous system adapts to the drug. As tolerance develops, higher doses are required to maintain effective concentrations of the drug. Tolerance to a lethal dose does not increase proportionately, so that as physical tolerance escalates, the gap between the effective intoxicating dose and the fatal dose is narrowed. Another danger is that barbiturates, alcohol, and many other sedative drugs are cross-tolerant.

Barbiturate overdose produces symptoms that can range from slurred speech to cardiovascular collapse, respiratory depression, and coma and death. The greatest dangers of barbiturate poisoning are circulatory collapse, respiratory insufficiency, and renal failure. Emergency treatment is directed at preventing these complications. Long-term users who are physically dependent on barbiturates will suffer serious symptoms if their drug withdrawal is sudden. Psychoses, convulsions, and even death may result unless withdrawal takes place in a protected, medically safe environment. Despite their potential for misuse, barbiturates have legitimate therapeutic value if carefully administered and supervised.

ULTRA-SHORT-ACTING BARBITURATES

Generic Name Methohexital sodium
Trade Name Brevital Sodium
Classification Barbiturate anesthetic

Action CNS depressant. Induction dose with 1% solution will provide anesthesia for 5 to 7 minutes.

Indications for Drug Induction of anesthesia, anesthetic for short procedures, as a supplement to other anesthetic agents.

Contraindications Known hypersensitivity, severe cardiac disease, hepatic or renal impairment, Addison's disease, myxedema, anemia, asthma, increased intracranial pressure, history of porphyria. May be habit forming. Use with caution in clients with impaired or circulatory, respiratory, endocrine, hepatic, or renal function. Use with caution in pregnancy. Use with extreme caution in status asthmaticus.

Forms of Drug Vials and ampules containing 250 or 500 mg of dry powder.

Administration of Drug 5 to 12 ml (50 to 120 mg) of a 1% solution IV at a rate of 1 ml/5 seconds for induction; then 20 to 40 mg every 4 to 7 minutes for maintenance. Administration must be performed only by qualified anesthetists. Close observation of patient is necessary, since reactions to drug are highly individualistic. Oxygen and rescusitative equipment should be at hand.

Absorption Onset of action is 30 to 40 seconds after IV administration. Crosses placenta.
Distribution Stored in fatty tissues.
Metabolism In the liver.
Excretion By the kidneys.

Side Effects Circulatory depression, arrhythmias, respiratory depression, bronchospasm, nausea, vomiting, twitching, headache, hiccups, hypotension, rash, sneezing, coughing, hypersensitivity reactions.

Interactive Effects An increase in CNS depression occurs with concurrent use of alcohol, other sedatives, narcotics, antihistamines, phenothiazines, disulfiam, MAO inhibitors, procarbazine, and methotrimeprazine. By interfering with absorption and increasing liver enzyme activity barbiturates can decrease the effects of oral anticoagulants, corticosteroids, digitalis glycosides, estrogens, oral contraceptives, griseofulvin, lidocaine, phenytoin, carbamazepine, and methyldopa. Sulfonamides increase the effect of barbiturates by inhibiting protein binding.

Nursing Considerations
1. Contact with nonvascular tissues can cause necrosis. Intraarterial injection can cause gangrene. Incompatible in solution with lactated Ringer's solution and acid solutions, such as succinylcholine chloride, atropine, and metocurine iodide.
2. Dilute only in sterile water, 5% dextrose, or 0.9% sodium chloride IV solutions.
3. When reconstituted, solution should be clear. If dissolved in sterile water, solution is stable at room temperature for 6 weeks. If dissolved in dextrose or saline, solution is stable at room temperature for 24 hours only.

Generic Name Thiamylal sodium
Trade Names Surital, Thioseconal
Classification Barbiturate anesthetic

See methohexital sodium for indications for drug, contraindications, side effects, and drug interactions.

Action CNS depressant.

Forms of Drug Ampules and vials containing 1, 5, or 10g.

Administration of Drug 3 to 6 ml of a 2.5% solution IV at a rate of 1 ml/5 seconds for induction; then 1 drop/second for maintenance.

Nursing Considerations Solutions may be stored in refrigerator for 6 days or at room temperature for 24 hours. (See methohexital sodium.)

715

Generic Name Thiopental sodium
Trade Names Intraval, Pentothal
Classification Barbiturate anesthetic

See methohexital sodium for contraindications, side effects, and drug interactions.

Action CNS depressant.

Indications for Drug Control of convulsions following other anesthetics, reducing intracranial pressure during neurosurgical procedures, narcoanalysis and narcosynthesis in psychiatric disorders.

Forms of Drug Ampules and vials in a variety of dosages.

Administration of Drug 2 to 3 ml (50 to 75 mg) of a 2.5% solution IV for induction; then use a continuous drip of a 0.2% to 0.4% solution for maintenance or additional IV injections of 25 to 50 mg as necessary.

Nursing Considerations (See methohexital sodium.)
1. Reconstituted solutions should be used within 24 hours.
2. After induction of anesthesia, shivering sometimes occurs because of client's increased sensitivity to cold.

SHORT-ACTING BARBITURATES

Generic Name Pentobarbital sodium
Trade Names Nebralin, Nembutal, Pental
Classification Barbiturate sedative and hypnotic

See methohexital sodium for contraindications, side effects, and drug interactions.

Action CNS depressant. Onset of action is 15 to 30 minutes after oral administration. Duration of action is up to 4 hours.

Indications for Drug Sedation, hypnosis, preanesthesia, acute convulsive states.

Forms of Drug Elixir (5 ml unit dose) in pint and gallon bottles (20 mg/5 ml); capsules containing 30, 50, or 100 mg in bottles and unit-dose packages; tablets containing 100 mg; 2-ml ampules; vials of 20 or 50 ml; suppositories containing 30, 60, 120, or 200 mg.

Administration of Drug
- *Sedation:* Adults: 30 mg po tid or qid.
- *Hypnosis:* Adults: 100 to 500 mg IV; 150 to 200 mg IM; 120 to 200 mg rectally.

Dosage is individually adjusted according to age, weight, general condition, and purpose of administration.

Nursing Considerations
1. Assessment and planning
   a. Client should be warned that mental and/or physical abilities may be impaired for a 24-hour period following dosage.
   b. Oxygen and resuscitative equipment should be readily available when drug is administered IV.
2. Assessment and implementation
   a. Parenteral solutions should be clear.
   b. Extravasation and intraarterial administration must be avoided, since tissue necrosis can result.
   c. When administering IM, inject into large muscle mass with no more than 5 ml delivered to a site.

3. Assessment and evaluation
   a. Since reactions to drug are highly individualistic, clients should be assessed carefully for adverse effects.
   b. Vital signs should be monitored every 3 to 5 minutes when drug is administered IV.
   c. Some clients, particularly the elderly, may become restless and irritable after administration; appropriate precautions, including bedrails, should be instituted.
   d. Client should be advised that prolonged use can lead to physical and psychological dependence.
   e. Clients on prolonged therapy must be cautioned against discontinuing the drug abruptly, since withdrawal symptoms can be life threatening.

Generic Name Secobarbital sodium
Trade Name Seconal
Classification Barbiturate sedative and hypnotic

See methohexital sodium for contraindications, side effects, and drug interactions.

Action CNS depressant. Duration of action is up to 4 hours.

Indications for Drug Sedation, hypnosis, preanesthesia, acute convulsive states.

Forms of Drug Elixir in 16-oz bottles (22 mg/5 ml); capsules containing 30, 50, or 100 mg in bottles and unit-dose packages; tablets containing 100 mg; 20-ml ampules (50 mg/ml); suppositories containing 30, 60, 120, or 200 mg.

Administration of Drug
- *Sedation:* Adults: 30 to 50 mg po tid.
- *Hypnosis:* Adults: 100 to 200 mg IV (up to 250 mg); 50 to 150 mg IM; 150 to 250 mg rectally.

Dosages are adjusted for children according to age and body weight.

Nursing Considerations (See pentobarbital sodium.)
1. Ampules and suppositories must be refrigerated.
2. Aqueous solution must be used within 30 minutes after container is opened. Solution is mixed by rotating vial; do not shake. Solution should be clear.

INTERMEDIATE-ACTING BARBITURATES

Generic Name   Amobarbital sodium
Trade Names   Amytal, Tuinal
Classification   Barbiturate sedative and hypnotic

See methohexital sodium for contraindications, side effects, and drug interactions.

Action   CNS depressant. Duration of action is up to 8 hours.

Indications for Drug   Sedation, relief of anxiety, hypnosis, acute convulsive states, narcoanalysis and narcotherapy in psychiatric disorders.

Forms of Drug   Elixir in 16-oz bottles; capsules containing 65 or 200 in bottles and unit-dose packages; tablets containing 15, 30, 50, or 100 mg. Ampules containing 125, 250, or 500 mg of dry powder; dissolve in sterile water; may dissolve slowly.

Administration of Drug   Oral: 30 to 50 mg tid or 65 to 200 mg in one dose; Maximum dosage: 1 g in adults. Intramuscular: 65 to 500 mg (10% to 20% solution); Maximum dosage: 0.5 g in adults. Intravenous: 1 ml/min. of a 10% solution; must not exceed 1 ml/min.

Nursing Considerations   Aqueous solution must be used within 30 minutes after container is opened. Solution is mixed by rotating vial; do not shake. Solution should be clear. (See pentobarbital sodium.)

Generic Name   Aprobarbital
Trade Name   Alurate
Classification   Barbiturate sedative and hypnotic

See methohexital sodium for contraindications, side effects, and drug interactions. See pentobarbital sodium for nursing considerations.

Action   CNS depressant. Duration of action is up to 8 hours.

Indications for Drug   Sedation, insomnia.

Forms of Drug   Elixir in 16-oz and gallon bottles (40 mg/5 ml).

Administration of Drug   Adults: 5 ml (40 mg) po tid, 5 to 20 ml hs for sedation or insomnia.

Generic Name   Butabarbital sodium
Trade Names   Butisol, Butal, Buticaps, Sarisol
Classification   Barbiturate sedative and hypnotic

See methohexital sodium for contraindications, side effects, and drug interactions. See pentobarbital sodium for nursing considerations.

Action   CNS depressant. Duration of action is 5 to 8 hours.

Indications for Drug   Sedation, hypnosis.

Forms of Drug   Elixir in pint and gallon bottles (30 mg/5 ml); capsules and tablets containing 15, 30, 50, or 100 mg.

Administration of Drug
- *Sedation:* Adults: 15 to 30 mg po tid or qid; 50 to 100 mg preoperatively.
- *Hypnosis:* Adults: 50 to 100 mg hs.

LONG-ACTING BARBITURATES

Generic Name   Mephobarbital
Trade Name   Mebaral
Classification   Barbiturate sedative

See methohexital sodium for contraindications, side effects, and drug interactions.

Action   Duration of action is 10 hours or more.

Indications for Drug   Sedation, acute convulsive states (epilepsy).

Forms of Drug   Tablets containing 32, 50, 100, or 200 mg.

Administration of Drug   *Sedation:* Adults: 50 mg po tid or qid; Children: 16 to 32 mg po tid or qid.

Nursing Considerations   (See pentobarbital sodium.)

1. Does not generally cause clouding of mental faculties.
2. Possibility of cumulative drug action increases with the long-acting barbiturates. Client should be instructed to be alert for adverse reactions.
3. Drug should not be withdrawn abruptly, but tapered over a period of 1 to 2 weeks.

Generic Names   Phenobarbital; phenobarbital sodium
Trade Names   Eskabarb, Luminal, Solfoton; Sodium Luminal
Classification   Barbiturate sedative and hypnotic

See methohexital sodium for contraindications, side effects, and drug interactions.

Action   CNS depressant. Onset of action is 10 to 60 minutes and duration of action is 10 to 16 hours. Lowers bilirubin by stimulating production of glucuronyl transferase.

Indications for Drug   Sedation, hypnosis, acute convulsive states, neonatal hyperbilirubinemia.

Forms of Drug   Elixir containing 20 mg/5 ml; capsules (prolonged action) containing 65 or 100 mg; tablets containing 8, 16, 32, 65, or 100 mg. Vials containing dry powder must be reconstituted with sterile water. Solution should be clear; stable for 2 days.

Administration of Drug
- *Sedation:* Adults: 15 to 120 mg po bid or tid; Children: 15 to 50 mg po.
- *Hypnosis:* Adults: 100 to 320 mg po daily; 100 to 300 mg IM or IV daily. Children: 2 to 5 mg/kg IM or IV; 2 to 3 mg/kg rectally bid or tid.

1. Drowsiness may occur during early weeks of treatment.
2. Elderly patients may exhibit restlessness or excitability.
3. When administering IV, dose should not exceed 60 mg/min.
4. When administering IM, inject into large muscle mass with no more than 5 ml delivered to a site.

Nursing Considerations   (See pentobarbital sodium and mephobarbital.)

1. Long-term treatment may cause blood dyscrasias. Be alert for signs of infection or bleeding.
2. Hepatic function tests and blood counts should be done routinely for clients on prolonged therapy.

BARBITURATE COMBINATION PREPARATIONS

Trade Name   Antrocol
Classification   Anticholinergic

Indications for Drug   Peptic ulcer, GI disturbances.

Contraindications   May be habit forming. Do not use in glaucoma. Use with caution in clients who have a history of prostatic hypertrophy.

Forms of Drug   Generic contents in each tablet or capsule: atropine sulfate: 0.195 mg; phenobarbital: 16 mg.

Administration of Drug   2 to 8 tablets or capsules po daily.

Side Effects   May induce flushing, dry mouth, tachycardia, or urinary retention.

Trade Name   Arco-Lase Plus
Classification   Anticholinergic

Indications for Drug   Peptic ulcer, GI disturbances.

Forms of Drug   Generic contents in each tablet: amylolytic enzyme: 30 mg; proteolytic enzyme: 6 mg; cellulolytic enzyme: 2 mg; lipase: 25 mg; hyoscyamine sulfate: 0.1 mg; atropine sulfate: 0.02 mg; phenobarbital: 7.5 mg.

Administration of Drug   1 tablet po pc.

Side Effects   May induce dry mouth, tachycardia, or blurred vision.

Nursing Considerations   May be habit forming. Do not use in clients who have a history of glaucoma or prostate hypertrophy.

Trade Names   Bellermine-O.D., Bellergal-S
Classification   Anticholinergic

Indications for Drug   Management of disorders characterized by nervous tension and exaggerated autonomic response.

Contraindications History of peripheral vascular disease, coronary heart disease, impaired renal or hepatic function, or glaucoma; porphyria; pregnancy and lactation.

Forms of Drug Generic contents in each capsule or tablet: phenobarbital: 40 mg; ergotamine tartrate: 0.6 mg; belladonna alkaloids: 0.2 mg; Bellergal-S also contains FD&C No. 5 yellow.

Side Effects May induce tingling in the extremities, dry mouth, tachycardia, blurred vision, urinary retention, decreased sweating, or flushing.

Nursing Considerations Do not give concurrently with dopamine, since hypertension will occur. Additive effects occur if taken with other CNS depressants, alcohol, or sedatives. Phenobarbital content may lower plasma levels of dicumarol. Concomitant administration of tricyclic antidepressants may result in additive anticholinergic effects. May be habit forming.

Trade Name Bentyl with Phenobarbital
Classification Anticholinergic

Indications for Drug Possibly effective in the treatment of irritable bowel syndrome and acute enterocolitis.

Contraindications History of obstructive uropathy, paralytic ileus, severe ulcerative colitis, or myasthenia gravis. Use with caution in clients who have a history of glaucoma, prostatic hypertrophy, autonomic neuropathy, hyperthyroidism, or cardiac disease.

Forms of Drug Generic contents in each capsule: dicyclomine hydrochloride: 10, 20 mg; phenobarbital: 15 mg.

Administration of Drug 1 capsule po tid or qid.

Side Effects May induce urinary hesitancy, tachycardia, blurred vision, drowsiness, headache, nausea, or urticaria.

Interactive Effects Additive effects occur if taken with other CNS depressants, alcohol, or tranquilizers.

Nursing Considerations Caution client that heat prostration can occur in warm climates. May be habit forming.

Trade Name Cantil with Phenobarbital
Classification Anticholinergic

Indications for Drug Peptic ulcer.

Contraindications History of obstructive uropathy, paralytic ileus, severe ulcerative colitis, or myasthenia gravis; lactation. Use with caution in clients who have a history of renal or hepatic disease, autonomic neuropathy, mild ulcerative colitis, glaucoma, hyperthyroidism, or cardiac disease.

Forms of Drug Generic contents in each yellow tablet: mepenzolate bromide: 25 mg; phenobarbital: 16 mg. Also contains FD&C No. 5 yellow.

Administration of Drug 1 to 2 tablets po qid with meals and hs.

Side Effects May induce tachycardia, blurred vision, decreased sweating, urinary retention, drowsiness, headache, nausea, or urticaria.

Interactive Effects Additive effects occur if taken with other anticholinergic drugs.

Nursing Considerations Caution client that heat prostration can occur in warm climates.

Trade Name Chardonna-2
Classification Anticholinergic

Indications for Drug Possibly effective in the treatment of irritable bowel syndrome.

Contraindications History of glaucoma, prostatic hypertrophy, or porphyria.

Forms of Drug Generic contents in each tablet: belladonna extract: 15 mg; phenobarbital: 15 mg.

Administration of Drug 1 to 2 tablets po qid, given 30 minutes before meals and hs.

719

Side Effects May induce tachycardia, dry mouth, blurred vision, vertigo, flushing, drowsiness, headache, nausea, vomiting, or skin eruptions.

Interactive Effects Additive effects occur if taken with other CNS depressants, alcohol, or sedatives.

Nursing Considerations May be habit forming. Use with caution in clients who have a history of hepatic or renal disease.

Trade Name Isordil with Phenobarbital
Classification Antianginal

Indications for Drug Possibly effective in the treatment of angina pectoris.

Forms of Drug Generic contents in each orange scored tablet: isosorbide dinitrate: 10 mg; phenobarbital: 15 mg.

Administration of Drug 1 tablet po qid before meals and hs.

Side Effects May induce flushing, headache, dizziness, nausea, vomiting, or drug rash.

Interactive Effects Alcohol may enhance the hypotensive effects of this drug. Can act as a physiologic antagonist to norepinephrine, acetylcholine, and histamine.

Nursing Considerations May be habit forming. Tolerance to this and other nitrates and nitrites may occur.

720

Trade Name Phazyme-PB
Classification Antiflatulent

Indications for Drug Relief of gas pain associated with anxiety, as seen in aerophagia, postoperative distention, dyspepsia, and food intolerance.

Forms of Drug Generic contents in each yellow-coated, two-phase tablet: Outer-layer (releases in the stomach): simethicone: 20 mg; phenobarbital: 15 mg. Enteric-coated core (releases in the small intestine): simethicone: 40 mg; protease: 3000 U.S.P. units; lipase: 240 U.S.P. units; amylase: 2000 U.S.P. units.

Administration 1 to 2 tablets po qid with meals and hs.

Side Effects May induce drowsiness.

Nursing Considerations May be habit forming.

Trade Name Pro-Banthine with Phenobarbital
Classification Anticholinergic

Indications for Drug Possibly effective as adjunctive therapy in the treatment of peptic ulcer and irritable bowel syndrome.

Contraindications History of glaucoma, obstructive uropathy, paralytic ileus, severe ulcerative colitis, or myasthenia gravis. Use with caution in clients who have a history of autonomic neuropathy, hepatic, cardiac, or renal disease, hyperthyroidism, or hypertension.

Forms of Drug Generic contents in each tablet: propantheline bromide: 15 mg; phenobarbital: 15 mg.

Administration of Drug 1 tablet po 30 minutes before each meal and 2 tablets po hs.

Side Effects May induce tachycardia, dry mouth, blurred vision, drowsiness, headache, urticaria, or GI disturbances.

Interactive Effects Concurrent use of Pro-Banthine with slow-dissolving tablets of digoxin may cause increased serum digoxin levels. Additive effects occur if taken with other anticholinergic drugs or belladonna alkaloids.

Nursing Considerations Caution client that heat prostration can occur in warm climates. May be habit forming.

Trade Name Pyridium Plus
Classification Antispasmodic

Indications for Drug Relief of pain associated with irritation of the lower urinary tract mucosa.

Contraindications Do not give to clients who have a history of glaucoma, renal or hepatic insufficiency, or porphyria.

Forms of Drug Generic contents in each dark maroon tablet: phenazopyridine hydrochloride: 150 mg; hyoscyamine hydrobromide: 0.3 mg; butabarbital: 15 mg.

Side Effects May induce methemoglobinemia, hemolytic anemia, and renal and hepatic toxicity; may also induce dry mouth, blurred vision, drowsiness, or GI disturbances.

Nursing Considerations
1. Inform client that urine will turn a reddish orange.
2. Discontinue use if a yellowish tinge appears in the skin or sclera.
3. May be habit forming.

Trade Name Valpin 50-PB
Classification Anticholinergic

Indications for Drug Possibly effective as adjunctive therapy in the treatment of peptic ulcer and irritable or neurologic bowel disorders.

Contraindications History of glaucoma, obstructive uropathy, paralytic ileus, severe ulcerative colitis, myasthenia gravis, or porphyria. Use with caution in clients who have a history of autonomic neuropathy, hepatic, cardiac, or renal disease, hyperthyroidism, or hypertension.

Forms of Drug Generic contents in each white scored tablet: anisotropine methylbromide: 50 mg; phenobarbital: 15 mg.

Administration of Drug 1 tablet po tid.

Side Effects May induce tachycardia, blurred vision, urinary retention, drowsiness, headache, excitement, GI disturbances, or drug rash.

Interactive Effects Phenobarbital may decrease the prothrombin time response to oral anticoagulants. Additive effects occur if taken with other anticholinergic drugs.

Nursing Considerations Caution client that heat prostration can occur in warm climates. May be habit forming.

Trade Name WANS #1, #2
Classification Antiemetic

Indications for Drug Relief of nausea and vomiting.

Contraindications Pregnancy and lactation; infants under 6 months; clients with a history of drug dependence or suicidal tendencies; history of porphyria or CNS injury.

Forms of Drug Generic contents in each blue suppository for children: pyrilamine maleate: 25 mg; pentobarbital sodium: 30 mg. Generic contents in each pink No. 1 suppository: pyrilamine maleate: 50 mg; pentobarbital sodium: 50 mg. Generic contents in each yellow No. 2 suppository: pyrilamine maleate: 50 mg; pentobarbital sodium: 100 mg.

Administration of Drug Adults: No. 1 and No. 2: 1 suppository rectally every 4 to 6 hours, as needed; Maximum dosage: 4 doses. Children: Ages 6 months to 2 years: ½ suppository rectally every 6 to 8 hours, as needed; Ages 2 to 12 years: 1 suppository rectally every 6 to 8 hours, as needed; Maximum dosage: 3 doses.

Side Effects May induce tachycardia, dry mouth, blurred vision, drowsiness, urinary retention, GI disturbances, vertigo, tinnitus, or drug rash.

Interactive Effects Do not give with MAO inhibitors. Additive effects occur if taken with other CNS depressants, alcohol, or tranquilizers.

Nursing Considerations May be habit forming. There is some suspicion that central-acting antiemetics in combination with viral illnesses may contribute to the development of Reye's syndrome. Use with caution in clients who have a history of hepatic disease, fever, diabetes, hyperthyroidism, severe anemia, or congestive heart failure.

721

CEREBRAL STIMULANT MEDICATIONS

Drugs that stimulate the cerebral cortex are called *central* or *cerebral stimulants*, and include amphetamines, xanthines, and some sympathomimetics. All these drugs cross the blood-brain barrier, which is a prerequisite for any central nervous system stimulant. Cocaine and the hallucinogens are also classified as cerebral stimulants, although they have little or no therapeutic value.

Amphetamines, which are sympathomimetic amines, are potent cerebral stimulants. The dextro isomers of amphetamine are more potent than the levo isomers. Although they are chemically similar to ephedrine, tolerance to amphetamines can develop within a few weeks while tolerance to ephedrine preparations can take months.

Although xanthines induce central nervous system stimulation, these drugs are used more often for their diuretic effect. Caffeine is the most commonly used of the xanthine group.

Some sympathomimetics cross the blood-brain barrier and are effective in treating narcolepsy, minimal brain dysfunctions, and obesity. Hallucinogenic drugs are CNS stimulants of little proven therapeutic value and are often subject to abuse.

AMPHETAMINES

Generic Name Amphetamine sulfate
Trade Name Benzedrine
Classification Cerebral stimulant

Action Amphetamine is a synthetic sympathomimetic amine (noncatecholamine) similar to ephedrine that has a marked stimulatory effect on the CNS and has alpha- and beta-adrenergic activity. Although the exact mechanism of CNS stimulation is unknown, amphetamine is thought to stimulate alpha receptors in the CNS and to induce the release of norepinephrine and dopamine in the cerebral cortex and the reticular activating system. The drug-induced CNS stimulation results in wakefulness, diminished feelings of fatigue, mood elevation, self-confidence, and an enhanced ability to concentrate. Although work output may increase, the number of work errors seldom decreases. Amphetamine depresses the sense of smell and taste and is an effective appetite suppressant (central anorectic agent), but has limited therapeutic value because drug tolerance develops after a few weeks.

Indications for Drug Narcolepsy, hyperkinesis, minimal brain dysfunctions, as a short-term adjunct in exogenous obesity. Has been used to treat nocturnal enuresis and as an adjunct in the treatment of apathy, certain fatigue states, and psychomotor dysfunctions.

Contraindications Advanced arteriosclerosis, moderate or severe hypertension, hyperthyroidism, angina pectoris, symptomatic cardiovascular disorders, glaucoma, hypersensitivity to sympathomimetic amines, history of drug abuse, severe agitated state, concurrently or within 14 days of therapy with MAO inhibitors. Long-term effects in children have not been established; not recommended for children under 3 years. May inhibit physical growth in children. May exacerbate behavioral disturbances in psychotic children. Amphetamines are not appropriate for all children with minimal brain dysfunctions; careful assessment and evaluation are required. Tolerance, extreme psychologic dependence, and severe social disability have occurred; the lowest feasible dose should be prescribed or dispensed. Safe use during pregnancy has not been established. Insulin requirements in diabetic clients may be altered by drug therapy.

Forms of Drug Tablets containing 5 or 10 mg; sustained-release capsules containing 15 mg.

Administration of Drug

- *Narcolepsy:* Adults: 5 to 60 mg po daily in divided doses; Children: over 12 years: 10 mg po daily in divided doses; Ages 6 to 12 years: 5 mg po daily in divided doses.
- *Brain disorders:* Children: Over 5 years: 5 mg po daily; Ages 3 to 5 years: 2.5 mg po daily; dosage may be increased weekly until desired effect.
- *Obesity:* Adults and children over 12 years: 5 mg po tid 30 to 60 minutes before meals.

1. Give tablets with a full glass of water. Sustained-release capsules should be given in early A.M.
2. Schedule amphetamine administration in early A.M. (narcolepsy or minimal brain dysfunction) or before meals (appetite suppression). Last dose of day should be given in late afternoon to avoid insomnia.

Absorption Rapidly absorbed. Onset of appetite suppression is 30 to 60 minutes. Duration of action varies between 4 and 24 hours.
Distribution Widely distributed. High concentrations are found in the brain and cerebrospinal fluid. Crosses blood-brain barrier.
Metabolism Some in the liver.
Excretion Primarily by the kidneys. Urinary acidifiers increase drug excretion; but urinary alkalizers promote reabsorption of drug.

722

Side Effects Common reactions include tachycardia, palpitations, insomnia, talkativeness, and restlessness. Fatigue and mental depression may occur when drug is discontinued. CNS disturbances include dizziness, euphoria, dysphoria, tremor, and irritability. Psychotic episodes may occur, but rarely at recommended doses. Psychotic disturbances may occur with prolonged doses higher than those recommended. Confusion, schizophreniclike psychosis, combative behavior, delirium, paranoid delusions, vivid hallucinations, and panic states have been reported. Dermatitis and marked weight loss are associated with chronic intoxication. Fatalities from toxicity are a result of convulsions and coma due to cerebral hemorrhages. Cardiovascular disturbances include pallor or flushing, hypertension or hypotension, chills, arrhythmias, dry mouth, and metallic taste. Other reactions include impotence, excessive sweating, and alterations in libido. Hypersensitivity reactions, including urticaria, have been reported. Many individuals with narcolepsy will maintain clinical effectiveness from small doses (5 to 10 mg) for years; but tolerance to anorectic effect often develops within 3 to 6 weeks. If euphoria occurs, notify primary care provider since potential for abuse and/or tolerance is great.

Interactive Effects Hypertensive crisis may occur if amphetamines are administered concurrently or within 14 days of therapy with MAO inhibitors. Urinary alkalizers, including sodium bicarbonate and acetazolamide, will increase the renal reabsorption of amphetamines. Urinary acidifiers, including ascorbic acid and ammonium chloride, will promote excretion of amphetamines; ammonium chloride is often used to promote drug excretion during toxicity. Amphetamines will decrease the antihypertensive effects of guanethidine. Phenothiazines, reserpine, and haloperidol will decrease the effects of amphetamines. Caffeine and sympathomimetic amines may potentiate the CNS and/or peripheral effects of amphetamines.

Nursing Considerations
1. Assessment and planning
   a. Obtain history of neurological, cardiovascular, and renal disorders.
   b. Obtain baseline vital signs.
   c. Explore history of drug use and abuse.
   d. Determine all OTC or Rx drugs currently being used by client.

2. Assessment and implementation
   a. Emphasize the importance of schedule for drug administration to elicit best response without untoward reactions.
   b. Warn client to notify physician if drug tolerance occurs.
   c. Caution client against driving a car or engaging in hazardous activity.
   d. Emphasize the need for regular medical evaluation of drug's effectiveness. Encourage client to maintain appointments.
   e. Instruct client to obtain medical advice before taking OTC preparations.
   f. Instruct client to avoid caffeine drinks, since potentiation of drug action may occur.

3. Assessment and evaluation
   a. Obtain vital signs periodically, particularly when drug is first initiated or dosage is adjusted.
   b. Evaluate effectiveness of drug for narcolepsy. Flowcharts indicating the client's patterns of sleep, feelings of tiredness, and wakefulness are helpful.
   c. Evaluate effectiveness of drug as appetite suppressant. A flowchart showing caloric intake, activity level, and daily weight is helpful.
   d. Abrupt withdrawal of drug after prolonged use may result in severe psychotic disturbances. Gradual withdrawal is recommended.
   e. Monitor physical growth of children receiving long-term therapy.

Generic Name Amphetamine phosphate
Classification Cerebral stimulant

See amphetamine sulfate for contraindications, side effects, drug interactions, and nursing considerations.

Action The phosphate salt of amphetamine is more soluble than the sulfate salt and can therefore be given parenterally. It can also be given orally in the same dosages as the sulfate salt. (See amphetamine sulfate.)

Indications for Drug Narcolepsy, hyperkinesis, minimal brain dysfunctions, as a short-term adjunct in exogenous obesity.

Forms of Drug Vials of dry powder for reconstitution.

Administration of Drug 10 to 15 mg po or IM, as needed.

Generic Name   Dextroamphetamine phosphate
Classification   Cerebral stimulant

See amphetamine sulfate for contraindications, side effects, drug interactions, and nursing considerations.

Action   Dextro isomer of amphetamine with greater stimulatory effect than amphetamine sulfate. (See amphetamine sulfate.)

Indications for Drug   Narcolepsy, hyperkinesis, minimal brain dysfunctions, as a short-term adjunct in exogenous obesity.

Forms of Drug   Tablets containing 5 mg.

Administration of Drug   5 mg po every 4 to 6 hours, as needed.

Generic Name   Dextroamphetamine sulfate
Trade Name   Dexedrine
Classification   Cerebral stimulant

See amphetamine sulfate for contraindications, side effects, drug interactions, and nursing considerations.

Action   Dextro isomer of amphetamine with greater stimulatory effect than amphetamine sulfate. (See amphetamine sulfate.)

Indications for Drug   Narcolepsy, hyperkinesis, minimal brain dysfunctions, as a short-term adjunct in exogenous obesity.

Forms of Drug   Tablets containing 5 mg; sustained-release tablets containing 5, 10, or 15 mg; elixir containing 5 mg/ml with 10% alcohol.

Administration of Drug   2.5 mg po tid.

Generic Name   Benzphetamine hydrochloride
Trade Name   Didrex
Classification   Cerebral stimulant

See amphetamine sulfate for contraindications, side effects, drug interactions, and nursing considerations.

Action   Less potent than amphetamine sulfate. (See amphetamine sulfate.)

Indications for Drug   As a short-term adjunct in exogenous obesity.

Forms of Drug   Tablets containing 25 or 50 mg.

Administration of Drug   25 to 50 mg po daily, bid, or tid.

Generic Name   Levamfetamine succinate
Trade Name   Cydril
Classification   Cerebral stimulant

See amphetamine sulfate for contraindications, side effects, drug interactions, and nursing considerations.

Action   Levo isomer of amphetamine. Levamfetamine induces less CNS stimulation than the dextroamphetamines, but has a more potent vasopressor effect. It may delay the emptying of the stomach. (See amphetamine sulfate.)

Indications for Drug   As a short-term adjunct in exogenous obesity.

Forms of Drug   Tablets containing 7 mg.

Administration of Drug   7 mg po tid.

Generic Name   Methamphetamine hydrochloride
Trade Names   Desoxyn, Drinalfa, Methedrine, Obedrin
Classification   Cerebral stimulant

See amphetamine sulfate for contraindications, side effects, drug interactions, and nursing considerations.

Action   Methamphetamine is an analog of amphetamine with slightly greater stimulatory effect, but fewer cardiovascular effects. (See amphetamine sulfate.)

Indications for Drug Narcolepsy, hyperkinesis, minimal brain dysfunctions, as a short-term adjunct in exogenous obesity.

Forms of Drug Tablets containing 2.5 or 5 mg; sustained-release tablets containing 5, 10, or 15 mg; elixir containing 1 mg/ml.

Administration of Drug 2.5 to 5 mg po daily, bid, or tid.

COMBINATION AMPHETAMINE PREPARATIONS

Trade Name Biphetamine
Classification Cerebral stimulant

See amphetamine sulfate for contraindications, side effects, drug interactions, and nursing considerations.

Action Resin complexes of amphetamine and dextro-amphetamine. (See amphetamine sulfate.)

Indications for Drug Narcolepsy, minimal brain dysfunctions, as a short-term adjunct in exogenous obesity.

Forms of Drug Capsules containing 7.5, 12.5, or 20 mg. Generic contents in each 7.5-mg capsule: dextro-amphetamine: 3.75 mg; amphetamine: 3.75 mg. Generic contents in each 12.5-mg capsule: dextroampheta-mine: 6.25 mg; amphetamine: 6.25 mg. Generic contents in each 20-mg capsule: dextroamphetamine: 10 mg; amphetamine: 10 mg.

Administration of Drug 1 capsule po daily in early A.M.

Trade Name Obetrol
Classification Cerebral stimulant

See amphetamine sulfate for contraindications, side effects, drug interactions, and nursing considerations.

Action Combination of neutral salts of amphetamine and dextroamphetamine. (See amphetamine sulfate.)

Indications for Drug Narcolepsy, hyperkinesis, minimal brain dysfunctions, as a short-term adjunct in exogenous obesity.

Forms of Drug Tablets containing 10 or 20 mg. Generic contents in each 10-mg tablet: dextroampheta-mine saccharate: 2.5 mg; amphetamine aspartate: 2.5 mg; dextroamphetamine sulfate: 2.5 mg; amphetamine sulfate: 2.5 mg. Generic contents in each 20-mg tablet: dextroamphetamine saccharate: 5 mg; amphetamine aspartate: 5 mg; dextroamphetamine sulfate: 5 mg; amphetamine sulfate: 5 mg.

Administration of Drug
- *Narcolepsy:* 5 to 60 mg po daily in divided doses.
- *Hyperkinesis:* Children: Ages 3 to 5 years: 2.5 mg po daily; Ages 6 years and older: 5 mg po daily or bid.
- *Obesity:* Adults: 5 to 30 mg po daily in divided doses.

XANTHINES

Generic Names Caffeine, citrated caffeine, caffeine sodium benzoate
Classification Cerebral stimulant

Source Caffeine is found in coffee, tea, cocoa, and the kola nut, which is used in soft drinks. The content of caffeine in some dietary substances is: brewed coffee: 100 to 150 mg/cup; instant coffee: 60 to 150 mg/cup; tea: 40 to 100 mg/cup; cola drinks: 17 to 55 mg/80 ml.

Action Caffeine has a poor solubility in water; caffeine sodium benzoate has increased solubility. Caffeine is the most potent xanthine CNS and respiratory stimulant. Like other xanthines, caffeine produces diuresis, dilation of the coronary arteries, and stimulation of the myocardium, but to a lesser extent than theophylline or theobromide. Stimulation of skeletal and smooth muscles also occurs. Caffeine crosses the blood-brain barrier and stimulates the cerebral cortex and medullary respiratory, vasomotor, and vagal centers. Mental alertness and attention span increase while fatigue and drowsiness decrease. The rate and depth of respirations are increased. Vascular resistance decreases peripherally but increases in the cerebral vasculature. Cardiac output and metabolic rate increase. In excessive doses, caffeine will cause arrhythmias, irritability, and possibly convulsions resulting from stimulation of the spinal cord. Even small doses of caffeine stimulate the secretion of gastric juices and may produce epigastric discomfort or aggravate a peptic ulcer. The drug is often included in analgesic preparations to counteract analgesic-induced depression of the cerebral cortex.

Indications for Drug Mild to moderate respiratory depression induced by CNS depressants, such as barbiturates and narcotics; as an adjunct in restoring mental alertness and combating lethargy; headache caused by vascular congestion or spinal puncture. Has been used as a mild diuretic.

725

Contraindications   Hypersensitivity to caffeine or caffeine-containing substances, gastric or duodenal ulcer, acute myocardial infarction. Tolerance to the diuretic and vasodilator effects of caffeine will develop with prolonged use, but cerebral stimulation will still occur. Cross-tolerance between the xanthines may occur. Psychological dependence may occur with prolonged use. Ineffective for alcohol-induced and other types of severe respiratory depression.

Forms of Drug   *Caffeine:* Bitter powder. *Citrated caffeine* (caffeine and citric acid): Tablets containing 60 mg. *Caffeine and sodium benzoate:* Ampules containing NoDoz, Stimm 250, and Vivarin. Ingredient in several analgesics, including APC, Buff-A Comp, Cafamine, Cafergot, Rogesic, Soma Compound, and Vanquish.

Administration of Drug   Adults: Oral: 60 to 200 mg, as needed; Intramuscular, intravenous: 500 mg, as needed; Intravenous: 250 to 100 mg q4h, as needed; Maximum dosage: 1 g.

1. Medication may be injected deep into large muscle mass. Rotate sites when multiple injections are required.
2. May be given via IV bolus over 1 to 5 minutes. Do not mix with other medications.
3. Check expiration date of caffeine and sodium benzoate before administering.

Absorption   Rapidly absorbed from GI tract and parenteral sites. About 15% bound to proteins. Crosses placenta and enters breast milk; caffeine should be avoided by pregnant and lactating women. Crosses blood-brain barrier.
Metabolism   Unknown but probably oxidized and demethylated.
Excretion   In urine; 10% excreted as unchanged drug.

Side Effects   Tachycardia, diuresis, and insomnia are common. Acute toxicity causes insomnia, restlessness, excitability, delirium, sensory disturbances (ringing in ears, flashes of light), fine muscular tremors, twitching, tachycardia, arrhythmias, and diuresis; convulsions may follow. Death is unlikely but may be caused by respiratory failure. Short-acting barbiturates are effective in treating toxicity. Gastric irritation is common after oral administration. May aggravate existing gastritis or peptic ulcer. Abrupt withdrawal after chronic ingestion of large doses may cause irritability, nervousness, and headache.

Interactive Effects   Insignificant.

Nursing Considerations
1. Assessment and planning
   a. Determine what medication or chemical substance caused the respiratory depression. If alcohol was ingested, notify physician before administering drug.
   b. Gastric lavage is performed simultaneously, when indicated.
   c. Obtain baseline vital signs.
   d. Obtain history of cardiovascular disorders. Drug is usually avoided if acute myocardial infarction is suspected.
2. Assessment and implementation
   a. Indwelling urinary catheter insertion may be necessary.
   b. Equipment for mechanical ventilation should be readily available.
   c. Cardiac monitoring is recommended.
   d. Monitor vital signs.
   e. Monitor neurological signs.
   f. Monitor intake and output.
3. Assessment and evaluation
   a. Recognize that caffeine reduces client's response to superficial pain.
   b. Clients should be warned that excessive intake of caffeine can cause gastric irritation and cardiovascular dysfunction.
   c. Reassure clients that irritability, nervousness, and headache are common after abrupt withdrawal, but that these symptoms disappear within a few days.

SYMPATHOMIMETICS

Generic Name   Chlorphentermine hydrochloride
Trade Names   Chlorophen, Pre-Sate
Classification   CNS stimulant

Action   Appetite suppressant similar to amphetamine; but significantly less stimulation of CNS occurs. (See amphetamine sulfate.)

Indications for Drug   As a short-term adjunct in exogenous obesity.

Contraindications   Glaucoma, clients on MAO inhibitors, severe cardiovascular disorders. Tolerance to anorectic effect may develop within 4 to 8 weeks. Use with caution in clients with hypertension. Not recommended for children under 12 years. Safe use during pregnancy and lactation has not been established.

Forms of Drug   Sustained-release capsules containing 65 mg.

726

Administration of Drug   65 mg po daily before breakfast.

Side Effects   Insomnia, tachycardia, palpitations, and a slight increase in blood pressure are common. GI disturbances include nausea, an unpleasant taste, and either diarrhea or constipation. CNS disturbances include dizziness, nervousness, headache, and paradoxic sedation.

Nursing Considerations   (See amphetamine sulfate.) Monitor blood pressure and pulse periodically.

Generic Name   Clotermine hydrochloride
Trade Name   Voranil
Classification   CNS stimulant

Action   A sympathomimetic amine similar to amphetamine. It suppresses the appetite by inducing CNS stimulation and elevates blood pressure. (See amphetamine sulfate.)

Indications for Drug   As a short-term adjunct in exogenous obesity.

Contraindications   Hyperthyroidism, hypersensitivity to sympathomimetic amines, glaucoma, severe hypertension, concurrent use of MAO inhibitors. Tolerance to anorectic effect may develop within a few weeks. Use with caution in diabetic clients since insulin requirements may change. Safe use during pregnancy and lactation has not been established.

Forms of Drug   Tablets containing 50 mg.

Administration of Drug   Adults: 50 mg po daily in midmorning.

Side Effects   Insomnia, tachycardia, palpitations, restlessness, and a slight elevation in blood pressure are common. Hepatitis may develop if the drug is taken for longer than 8 weeks. Hypersensitivity reactions to FD&C No. 5 yellow have occurred. (See amphetamine sulfate.)

Nursing Considerations   Monitoring blood pressure and pulse periodically. (See amphetamine sulfate.)

Generic Name   Deanol acetamidobenzoate
Trade Names   Deaner, Deaner-250
Classification   CNS stimulant

Action   Psychomotor stimulant which is a nonquaternized precursor to choline. It is thought to cross the blood-brain barrier and serve as the choline precursor of acetylcholine in the brain. It has a low toxicity and induces mild untoward reactions. Unlike amphetamines, this drug does not suppress the appetite or induce nervousness.

Indications for Drug   Minimal brain dysfunctions, dyskinesia. Has been used for mild depressive states.

Contraindications   Grand mal epilepsy. Use with caution in clients with hypertension or diabetes mellitus.

Forms of Drug   Tablets containing 50 or 250 mg.

Administration of Drug   Children: Over 6 years: initial dosage: 500 mg po daily after breakfast; then 250 to 500 mg po daily. Depression: 25 to 150 mg po daily.

Side Effects   Headache, constipation, muscular tightness, twitching, and insomnia are relatively common. Dyspnea, irritability, rashes, and postural hypotension have been reported. Most untoward reactions disappear after several weeks of therapy.

Nursing Considerations   Beneficial response will not occur until after several weeks of therapy. (See amphetamine sulfate.)

Generic Name   Diethylpropion hydrochloride
Trade Names   Diethylpropion-TR, Tenuate, Tenuate Dospan, Tepanil, Tepanil Ten-Tab
Classification   CNS stimulant

See amphetamine sulfate for nursing considerations.

Action   A sympathomimetic amine similar to amphetamine, but less effective as an anorexiant. It causes CNS stimulation and elevates blood pressure.

Indications for Drug   As a short-term adjunct in exogenous obesity.

727

Contraindications   Advanced arteriosclerosis, hypersensitivity to sympathomimetic amines, agitated states, history of drug abuse, within 14 days of therapy with MAO inhibitors, epilepsy. Tolerance to anorectic effect may develop after 4 to 8 weeks. Use with caution in diabetic clients since insulin requirements may change.

Forms of Drug   Tablets containing 25 mg; sustained-release tablets and capsules containing 75 mg.

Administration of Drug   Adults: 25 mg po tid 60 minutes before meals; 75 mg sustained-release tablet po daily in midmorning.

Side Effects   Tachycardia, palpitations, elevation in blood pressure, and nervousness are common. CNS disturbances include dizziness, headache, and precipitation of a preexisting psychosis. Menstrual irregularities may occur. Bone marrow depression has been reported with prolonged use.

728

Generic Name   Fenfluramine hydrochloride
Trade Name   Pondimin
Classification   CNS stimulant

Action   A sympathomimetic amine that differs from amphetamine in that more CNS depression than stimulation occurs.

Indications for Drug   As a short-term adjunct in exogenous obesity.

Contraindications   Glaucoma, severe cardiovascular disorders, history of drug abuse or alcoholism, hypersensitivity to sympathomimetic amines, mental depression, concurrent use of MAO inhibitors. Tolerance to anorectic effect may develop within a few weeks. Use with caution in clients with hypertension or diabetes mellitus.

Forms of Drug   Tablets containing 20 mg.

Administration of Drug   Initial dosage: 20 mg po tid before meals; Maximum dosage: 40 mg.

Side Effects   Insomnia, palpitations, and alterations in blood pressure are common. GI disturbances include dry mouth, nausea, vomiting, diarrhea, and constipation. Genitourinary disturbances, including dysuria, urinary frequency, and impotence, may occur. Urticaria, sweating, fever, and eye irritation have been reported.

Nursing Considerations   Monitor vital signs and blood sugar periodically. (See amphetamine sulfate.)

Generic Name   Mazindol
Trade Names   Mazanor, Sanorex
Classification   CNS stimulant

See amphetamine sulfate for nursing considerations.

Action   An isoindole anorexiant with action similar to amphetamine. Stimulates the CNS, particularly the limbic system.

Indications for Drug   As a short-term adjunct in exogenous obesity.

Contraindications   Glaucoma, hypersensitivity to mazindol, agitated states, history of drug abuse, within 14 days of therapy with MAO inhibitors. Tolerance to anorectic effect may develop within a few weeks. Not recommended for children under 12 years. Safe use during pregnancy and lactation has not been established.

Forms of Drug   Tablets containing 1 or 2 mg.

Administration of Drug   1 mg po tid 60 minutes before meals or 2 mg po daily 60 minutes before lunch.

Side Effects   Nervousness, dry mouth, tachycardia, constipation, and insomnia are common. GI disturbances may occur. Overstimulation or drowsiness may occur. Corneal opacities have occurred with prolonged use in dogs.

Generic Name   Methylphenidate hydrochloride
Trade Names   Methidate, Ritalin
Classification   CNS stimulant

See amphetamine sulfate for nursing considerations.

Action   Piperidine derivative with actions similar to amphetamine. Stimulates the cerebral cortex and exerts mild stimulation of respirations.

Indications for Drug   Narcolepsy, attention deficit disorder, minimal brain dysfunctions, mild depression, withdrawn senile behavior.

Contraindications Glaucoma, marked anxiety or tension, agitation, within 14 days of therapy with MAO inhibitors, hypersensitivity to piperidine derivatives. Not effective for children with primary psychosis or secondary environmental behavioral disturbances. Not recommended for children under 6 years. Suppression of growth may occur but no cause and effect relationship has been found. Safe use during pregnancy and lactation has not been established.

Forms of Drug Tablets containing 5, 10, or 20 mg.

Administration of Drug Highly individualized. Adults (narcolepsy, depression): 10 mg po bid or tid 30 minutes before meals; Dosage range: 5 to 50 mg daily. Children: Ages 6 years and older: Initial dosage: 5 to 10 mg po daily before breakfast or lunch; then increase weekly, as needed; Maximum dosage: 60 mg/day.

Side Effects Insomnia, nervousness, tachycardia, palpitations, alterations in blood pressure, and transient headaches are common. GI disturbances, including dry mouth, nausea, anorexia, and weight loss, can occur. Exfoliative dermatitis, urticaria, and other rashes have occurred. Dyskinesia and blurred vision have been reported. Toxicity may cause convulsions.

Generic Name Pemoline
Trade Name Cylert
Classification CNS stimulant

Action Pemoline is an oxazolidinone compound that stimulates the CNS and has minimal sympathomimetic effects. Mechanism of action is unknown, but it is thought to stimulate dopaminergic neurons in the brain.

Indications for Drug Minimal brain dysfunctions, attention deficit disorder, hyperkinetic syndrome.

Contraindications History of drug abuse, children under the age of 6. Use with caution in clients with impaired renal or hepatic function. Safe use during pregnancy and lactation has not been established.

Forms of Drug Tablets containing 18.75, 37.5, or 75 mg; chewable tablets containing 37.5 mg.

Administration of Drug Children: Ages 6 years and over: Initial dosage: 37.5 mg po daily; then increase by 18.75 mg weekly; Dosage range: 56.25 to 75 mg; Maximum dosage: 112.5 mg/day.

Absorption Half-life is 12 hours. Steady-state levels reached in 2 to 3 days.
Excretion By the kidneys as unchanged drug (43%) and metabolites.

Side Effects May exaggerate a preexisting psychotic disturbance. Anorexia, transient weight loss, and insomnia may occur in the first few weeks of therapy. Nausea, stomach pain, irritability, dizziness, headache, depression, and hallucinations have been reported. Elevations in serum glutamic-oxaloacetic transaminase, serum glutamic-pyruvic transaminase, and lactate dehydrogenase have occurred after several months of therapy. Jaundice has also been reported. Dyskinetic movements have been reported and may be due to the drug. Toxicity causes agitation, restlessness, hallucinations, dyskinetic movements, and tachycardia.

Nursing Considerations (See amphetamine sulfate.)
1. Growth should be monitored during therapy.
2. Monitor hepatic function tests periodically.
3. Beneficial effects may not occur for 3 to 4 weeks.

Generic Name Phendimetrazine tartrate
Trade Names Bacarate, Bontril PDM, Melfiat, Plegine, Prelu-2, SPRX-105, Trimstat, Trimtabs, Wehless-35
Classification CNS stimulant

See amphetamine sulfate for nursing considerations. See phenmetrazine hydrochloride for contraindications and side effects.

Action Phendimetrazine tartrate is an analog of phenmetrazine. (See phenmetrazine hydrochloride.)

Indications for Drug As a short-term adjunct in exogenous obesity.

Forms of Drug Tablets containing 35 mg; sustained-release capsules containing 105 mg.

Administration of Drug Adults: 35 mg po bid or tid 60 minutes before meals; 105 mg sustained-release capsule po daily in midmorning.

Nursing Considerations Peak blood levels occur in about 1 hour for the regular tablet and the duration of action is 4 hours. Duration of action is about 12 hours for sustained-release capsules.

Generic Name Phenmetrazine hydrochloride
Trade Name Preludin
Classification CNS stimulant

See amphetamine sulfate for drug interactions.

Action Phenmetrazine is a sympathomimetic amine that belongs to the oxazine group of compounds. This drug has anorectic effects, similar to amphetamine. It stimulates the CNS and elevates blood pressure.

Indications for Drug As a short-term adjunct in exogenous obesity.

Contraindications Advanced arteriosclerosis, severe cardiovascular disorders, hypertension, hyperthyroidism, hypersensitivity to sympathomimetic amines, glaucoma, agitated states, history of drug abuse, within 14 days of therapy with MAO inhibitors. Tolerance to anorectic effect may develop after a few weeks. Safe use during pregnancy and lactation has not been established.

Forms of Drug Tablets containing 25 mg; sustained-release tablets containing 50 or 75 mg.

Administration of Drug Adults and children over 12 years: 25 mg po bid or tid 60 minutes before meals; 50 to 75 mg sustained-release tablets po daily.

Side Effects Insomnia, tachycardia, and elevation in blood pressure are common. CNS disturbances include overstimulation, restlessness, dizziness, euphoria, dysphoria, tremors, and headache; psychosis rarely occurs. GI disturbances include dry mouth, unpleasant taste, diarrhea, and constipation. Urticaria has been reported. Impotence and alterations in libido may occur.

Nursing Considerations Monitor vital signs periodically. (See amphetamine sulfate.)

Generic Name Phentermine hydrochloride
Trade Names Adipex-P, Anoxine, Fastin, Ionamine, Parmine, T-Diet, Teramine, Wilpo
Classification CNS stimulant

Action Similar to amphetamine.

Indications for Drug As a short-term adjunct in exogenous obesity.

Contraindications Hypertension, angina or severe cardiovascular disorders, glaucoma. Tolerance to anorectic effect may develop. Use with caution in clients with a history of drug addiction or hyperexcitability.

Forms of Drug Tablets containing 8 mg; sustained-release capsules containing 30 mg; sustained-release tablets containing 37.5 mg (free base bound to an ion exchange resin for delayed release).

Administration of Drug 8 mg po tid 30 to 60 minutes before meals; 30 or 37.5 mg of sustained-release form 15 to 30 minutes before breakfast.

Side Effects Tachycardia, palpitations, nervousness, and insomnia are common. Fatigue may develop as the effects of the drug subside. Dry mouth, nausea, and constipation may occur. Hypertension and dizziness have been reported. Impotence may occur.

Interactive Effects Urinary acidifiers enhance excretion of the drug. Urinary alkalizers enhance reabsorption and may result in prolonged drug effects. (See amphetamine sulfate.)

Nursing Considerations Monitor vital signs periodically. (See amphetamine sulfate.)

COMBINATION PREPARATIONS

Trade Name Efed II
Classification CNS stimulant

Action Produces CNS stimulation, bronchial dilation, and decongestion.

Indications for Drug Relieves fatigue, drowsiness, and stiffness; used to increase mental alertness. Has been used for bronchial asthma.

Contraindications Use with caution in elderly clients with prostatic hypertrophy, since urinary retention may occur, and clients with hypertension, cardiac disease, hyperthyroidism, or diabetes. Not recommended for children.

Forms of Drug Generic contents in each capsule: ephedrine sulfate: 25 mg; phenylpropanolamine hydrochloride: 50 mg; caffeine: 125 mg.

Administration of Drug Adults: 1 capsule po q4h; Maximum dosage: 4 capsules daily.

Side Effects May interfere with sleep if taken within 4 hours of bedtime.

Nursing Considerations Reduce dosage if nervousness, restlessness, or insomnia occur.

CEREBRAL STIMULANTS WITH LITTLE OR NO KNOWN THERAPEUTIC VALUE

Generic Name Bufotenine
Classification Cerebral stimulant

Source Occurs naturally in the skin secretions of toads and in the seeds of *Piptadenia peregrina*.

Action Bufotenine is an indole derivative of serotonin and has been used as a snuff by some South American Indians. It induces vivid hallucinations.

Generic Name Cocaine
Trade Name Cocaine Topical Solution
Classification Cerebral stimulant

Source Alkaloid obtained from the leaves of *Erythroxylon cocoa* or synthetically produced from ergonine.

Action Exists as levorotatory colorless crystals or a white crystalline powder, hence the street name "snow." Cocaine is an effective topical anesthetic with a duration of action of 60 minutes. It has limited use as an anesthetic for nasal, oral, and ophthalmic examinations or procedures. Little or no absorption occurs through the skin, but it is well absorbed through mucous membranes. Addicts sniff cocaine or inject it intravenously for its systemic effects, which include euphoria, feelings of physical superiority, and self-confidence. Paranoid delusions and hallucinations also occur.

Forms of Drug Topical solution 1%.

Nursing Considerations High abuse potential.

Generic Name Cocaine hydrochloride
Trade Name Cocaine Hydrochloride Topical Solution
Classification Cerebral stimulant

Source Salt of cocaine that is more soluble in water than plain alcohol.

Action Unstable at elevated temperatures; loses potency when sterilized by autoclaving. Bacteriological filtration is used to remove pathogens. It has limited use as an anesthetic for nasal, oral, and ophthalmic examinations or procedures.

Forms of Drug Topical solutions 2% to 10%.

Nursing Considerations High abuse potential.

Generic Name Dimethyltryptamine
Trade Names DET, DMT
Classification Cerebral stimulant

Action Induces vivid hallucinations for approximately 1 hour.

Side Effects Alterations in blood pressure, pulse, and respirations.

Generic Name Lysergic acid diethylamide
Trade Name LSD
Classification Cerebral stimulant

Action Potent hallucinogenic compound. Contains indole ethylamine and phenylethylamine. Has been taken orally as: a solution containing 100 to 400 mcg; a sugar cube in 100 to 400 mcg; with lactose in capsules or tablets; or in a solution dropped on a sugar cube.

Side Effects Initial reactions (within 30 to 40 minutes): anxiety, sweating, clouding of consciousness; then psychomimetic effects with disturbances of perception, vivid hallucinations, and euphoria, which last about 8 hours. May induce prolonged psychotic disturbances with flashes of light. Acute episodes can be terminated by phenothiazine tranquilizers.

731

Generic Name Mescaline
Trade Names DOM, Peace, Peyote, Serenity, STP, Tranquility
Classification Cerebral stimulant

Source Occurs naturally in the flowering heads (mescal buttons) of the Mexican cactus *Lophophora williamsii*.

Action Mescaline is an amine that is chemically related to lysergic acid diethylamide. It has been used in religious ceremonies by certain Mexican Indian tribes and Indians in the American Southwest.

Generic Name Psilocybin
Classification Cerebral stimulant

Source Active hallucinogenic principle found in certain Mexican mushrooms of the Psilocybe group.

Action Similar to mescaline and lysergic acid diethylamide. It has been used in religious ceremonies by Mexican Indians. Peak effects occur in 2 minutes, but they are of short duration.

A

abreaction
The process of bringing repressed material to conscious awareness, including the emotional response elicited by the recalled material.

abuse
Actions that mistreat, injure, or threaten oneself or others. Drug abuse inflicts injury on oneself; child abuse inflicts injury on children; spouse abuse inflicts injury on a husband or wife.

accommodation
The process of reorganizing information already known in order to include new information; adjusting to reality and unfamiliar experiences.

achieved role
A role conferred because of special skills or attributes of an individual; sometimes referred to as *assumed role*.

acrophobia
Extreme fear of heights.

acting out
Discharging tension by responding to the present situation as if it were a previous situation in which the response was initiated.

acute alterations
Changes in physiological structure or function characterized by severe symptoms and a relatively short course.

adaptation
Response to change within the organism or outside its boundaries. Adaptation requires mobilization of the organism in addition to processes of assimilation.

addiction
A behavioral pattern of drug use characterized by an overwhelming preoccupation with compulsive use of the drug and securing a supply and by a tendency to withdrawal symptoms upon abstinence.

adjustment
Modification of various aspects of the self in order to cope with the demands of daily life.

advocacy
See client advocacy.

affect
An emotional or feeling state.

affective disorders
Alterations in mood that may take the form of severe depression or elation.

aggression
Actions performed in order to gratify the need to excel, achieve, or compete within or separate from the group; aggressive actions may be positive or negative in nature.

agitation
Extreme restlessness and excitability.

agoraphobia
Extreme fear of open spaces.

akathisia
Sensations of restlessness and unease often caused by reactions to psychotropic medication.

alienation
Loss or lack of relationships with others.

alterations of degenerative origin
Changes due to deterioration of physiological structure or function, usually from a higher to a lower level or form.

altered patterns of relatedness
A term used in this textbook to describe behavioral alterations caused by anxiety and personality disorders that adversely affect interpersonal relationships.

altruism
Concern for the well-being of others without regard for personal gain.

Alzheimer's disease
A degenerative neurological disorder characterized by loss of mental powers, disorientation, and motor impairment; thought to be inherited.

ambivalence
Conflict resulting from simultaneous feelings of being attracted to and repelled by the same object, action, or goal; often expressed in approach-avoidance behavior.

amnesia
Loss of memory for events within a certain period of time; may be temporary or permanent.

amniocentesis
Drawing of amniotic fluid from the amniotic sac of a pregnant woman in order to examine fetal cells for chromosomal abnormalities. Down's syndrome, among other disorders, may be diagnosed in utero through this diagnostic technique.

anaclitic separation
Loss of the mother or mother figure by the infant during the first year of life, often resulting in developmental deficits or indications of depression.

anhedonia
Inability to experience pleasure or joy.

anomie
Absence or loss of meaningful relationships with other individuals or groups; absence or loss of social norms and values.

anorexia nervosa
Refusal to eat because of psychological factors such as distorted body image or control issues. May result in extreme emaciation and even death.

anxiety
A vague sense of apprehension or dread originating within the individual; it may not necessarily be generated by identifiable external stimuli.

anxiety disorders
A group of disorders manifested in various behavioral patterns that tend to be rigid and fixed; excessive anxiety is present and is handled by the appearance of maladaptive behavioral syndromes.

apathy
Lack of feeling, interest, or initiative.

ascribed role
A role conferred because of status, age, gender, or position and not because of attributes or qualities within the control of the individual.

assertiveness
The ability to express one's needs, goals, or preferences appropriately and effectively in interpersonal transactions.

assimilation
The process of integrating new information or experience into what is already known and understood.

ataxia
Deficient muscular coordination causing difficulty in walking.

attention deficit disorder
A behavioral problem characterized by chronic inattention, overactivity, and difficulty in dealing with multiple stimuli.

authenticity
Acting in accord with one's own attitudes, beliefs, and values.

autism
A disorder of childhood characterized by language deficits and inability to relate to others.

autistic thinking
Preoccupation with private, self-determined thoughts or actions without concern for reality or objective standards shared with others.

autonomic nervous system
The part of the peripheral nervous system that innervates internal organs; is subdivided into the sympathetic and parasympathetic nervous systems.

autonomy
Self-determination and self-reliance; the sense of being individual and independent.

aversion therapy
A form of behavior modification in which a painful stimulus is linked with a pleasurable stimulus, thereby causing dislike (aversion) for the stimulus previously associated with pleasure.

B

behavior modification
A therapeutic modality that uses stimulus and response conditioning in order to alter dysfunctional patterns of behavior.

bestiality
Sexual intercourse with animals; sometimes referred to as zoophilia.

biofeedback
Use of electrical devices to monitor autonomic physiological processes in order to produce relaxation and reduce tension.

biogenic amines
Organic substances that serve as transmitters or monitors of neural impulses.

bipolar disorder
A disturbance of mood and affect in which at least one manic episode can be identified; it may or may not be characterized by depressive episodes.

bisexuality
Sexual attraction toward both males and females.

blocking
Difficulty in communicating because channels of thought are obstructed or interrupted for emotional reasons.

body image
Internalized impressions and attitudes regarding one's physical self.

bonding
Attachment of a parent to an infant; any process in which individuals make a mutual commitment.

brief psychotherapy
Short-term therapy that usually focuses on restoring functioning and providing emotional support.

bulimia
Alternating episodes of overeating (binge eating) and deliberate, self-induced vomiting.

burnout
A reaction to stressful occupational conditions in which workers feel exhausted and depleted; often expressed behaviorally through anger, apathy, depression, or detachment.

C

caring
The act of attending to or being concerned with another person or persons; in a professional sense, the act of providing and being responsible for holistic health care.

case management
A nursing model in which one nurse is responsible for the comprehensive care of several clients, often with the assistance of other nurses accountable to the nurse charged with case management.

castration anxiety
In psychoanalysis, a threat to the masculinity or femininity of individuals.

catatonia
A state of muscular rigidity and inflexibility, often accompanied by symptoms such as tremor, excitability, or stupor.

catecholamines
A group of biogenic amines, including dopamine, epinephrine, and norepinephrine, that affect the neuronal systems.

cathexis
Psychoanalytic term used to describe a bond or attachment.

central nervous system
Neural structures of brain and spinal cord.

cerebral palsy
Partial paralysis and poor muscle coordination due to a defect, injury, or disease of nerve tissue in one or more areas of the brain, often caused at the time of birth because of anoxia, premature or difficult delivery, or blood type incompatibility.

chronobiology
study of the effect of time intervals on living systems or organisms.

circadian rhythms
Cyclical changes occurring within a period of 24 hours.

circumstantiality
A communication pattern in which tangential, trivial details are given. The purpose is usually to lower the anxiety of the speaker.

clanging
Rhyming speech patterns; often used by persons with schizophrenia.

classical conditioning
A behavioral procedure in which two stimuli are offered simultaneously or close together in sequence. One stimulus evokes a spontaneous reponse from the subject; the other does not. If the pairing is repeated, the stimulus that previously evoked no response will eventually elicit the spontaneous reponse from the subject. This conditioned response will appear even without the stimulus that was previously needed to arouse the response.

claustrophobia
Extreme fear of being confined in a small space.

client advocacy
Process in which professionals, paraprofessionals, and clients themselves attempt to improve the quality of care and protect the rights of persons receiving care.

client-centered therapy
Originated by Carl Rogers, a form of therapy that offers empathy and nonjudgmental acceptance to enable the client to embark on a journey of self-actualization or self-discovery.

cognition
The act, process, or result of knowing, learning, or understanding.

cohesion
Conditions of attraction among group members and between individual members and the group as a whole.

coitus
Sexual intercourse between persons of the opposite sex.

collaboration
The process of sharing information and working together, usually toward common or mutually acceptable goals.

coma
Deep stupor or loss of consciousness.

commitment
Hospitalization that was not sought by the client but was arranged by family members or by legal or medical officers when the client was considered a clear danger to himself or others.

community
Any group of people living in proximity, sharing certain interests regardless of spatial separation, working toward a common goal, or upholding certain values.

compulsion
An irrational, repetitive act that must be performed in order to control rising anxiety.

concrete operational stage
According to Piaget, the stage at which the child can begin to use and manipulate numbers; thinking tends to be concrete, and the abilities for abstract reasoning are absent or limited.

concrete thinking
Use of literal statements instead of abstract or symbolic forms of communication.

confabulation
Filling in lost memory gaps with manufactured details.

confidentiality
The responsibility of professionals to disclose no information about clients except to participating colleagues, and then only with the knowledge and consent of the client.

conflict
Discomfort (anxiety) experienced by persons torn between a wish for something and fear of the consequences if the wish is gratified; a clash between opposing intrapersonal or interpersonal forces.

confrontation
Communication designed to help others engage in reflection and self-examination of their motives and behaviors.

congruence
Agreement between verbal and nonverbal levels of communication.

consensual validation
Reinforcement of meanings and interpretations by evidence and corroboration from others.

consultation
A process in which a nurse or group of nurses seek remedial advice from a person, usually another nurse, who is a specialist in a particular area. The consultant works through the consultees and rarely gives direct, hands-on service.

context
The setting and circumstances in which an event or transaction occurs.

contract
Agreement between client and professional concerning therapeutic goals and regimen; usually developed collaboratively.

conversion disorder
Transformation of anxiety-producing thoughts and feelings into sensory or motor impairment; previously termed a hysterical reaction.

coping

Efforts directed toward managing various problems, events, and stressors.

correlation

Establishing of relationships between variables; a correlation shows connections but not cause and effect relationships between variables.

counter-transference

A phenomenon in which the person on whom transference thoughts and feelings are projected returns and reinforces the transference.

covert

Concealed; masked; not openly manifest.

crisis

Periods of vulnerability or disorganization that have the potential for growth and maturation.

crisis intervention

Therapeutic intervention designed to restore functioning at or above precrisis levels; usually time limited.

critical task

A developmental milestone that involves the acquisition and mastery of specific behaviors and competence.

culture

Sum of the customs, habits, and traditions of a particular ethnic or social group.

cunnilinguis

Oral contact with the vulva and clitoris.

cystic fibrosis

A congenital, general disorder of the exocrine glands resulting in accumulation of thick mucus and excessive secretion of sweat and saliva. The mucus secretion of persons with cystic fibrosis is tenacious and adhesive; the lungs are clogged and bacteria adhere to the tissues. Secretions also impede the flow of digestive enzymes from the pancreas to the small intestine. Infections, usually staphylococcal, recur repeatedly, leading to chronic lung damage. Poor transmission of digestive enzymes leads to malnutrition; fats are particularly hard for the person with cystic fibrosis to metabolize.

D

data base

The sum of information collected from which to make inferences, develop hypotheses, assess needs, and evaluate outcomes.

day hospital

Facility offering a therapeutic program for clients who attend during the day and return home at night; a form of partial hospitalization.

decompensation

Disorganization of the personality or ego during periods of overwhelming stress.

defense mechanisms

Unconscious intrapsychic processes used to reduce anxiety and emotional conflict.

deinstitutionalization

Return to community living of persons previously hospitalized for long periods; a movement emphasizing community aftercare rather than institutional care for clients.

deja vu

A sense of having experienced new events previously.

delinquency

Legally prohibited actions committed by a juvenile or minor.

delirium

Impairment of mental processes to the extent of confusion and disorientation, usually caused by a specific agent or stressor.

delirium tremens

State produced by withdrawal from alcohol, characterized by tremors, hallucinations, and occasionally convulsions.

delusion

A false belief maintained despite the absence of factual or corroborating evidence.

dementia

Absence, impairment, or reduction of cognitive and intellectual abilities.

dementia praecox

Outmoded term once applied to schizophrenia.

denial

Refusal to acknowledge the reality of certain events, thereby protecting the individual from the unwelcome recognition of such events.

dependency

The tendency to rely on others.

depersonalization

Feelings of unreality and disconnection from the self occurring as a result of personality disorganization.

depression

A psychological state characterized by dejection, lowered self-esteem, hopelessness, helplessness, indecision, and rumination.

desensitization

The reduction of intense reactions to various stimuli by repeated exposure to the stimuli in milder forms.

desocialization

Withdrawal from interaction with others, often attributable to autistic patterns of thinking and acting.

desymbolization

Loss of the ability to derive commonly understood meanings from well-known symbols; it often accompanies concrete thinking and the inability to think in abstract terms.

detoxification

Elimination of a toxic agent from the body via natural physiological processes or with the aid of medical and nursing measures.

deviance

Noncompliance with norms established and upheld by the group.

Diagnostic Related Group (DRG)

A group of disorders of similar severity that are deemed to require a stipulated number of hospital days for treatment and recuperation. Reimbursement to the treating agency would be made according to the number of days assumed to be necessary for the in-hospital stay of persons suffering disorders in the group. If the hospital stay proved more costly or exceeded the allowable time, the treating agency would suffer financial loss; if the hospital stay were less than the allowable time and less costly, the hospital would receive some financial benefit.

discrimination

Ability to differentiate between and respond differently to two or more stimuli.

disengagement
An interactional process characterized by withdrawal. The withdrawal is often reciprocal, as in the case of interactions between the elderly and society or in family situations where members maintain distance from each other.

disorientation
Confusion and impaired ability to identify time, place, and person.

displacement
A transfer of emotion or behaviors to an unrelated person or event; substituting one target of emotions or behavior for another target.

dissociative disorders
Reactions that protect the self from awareness of anxiety-producing stimuli. Amnesia, somnambulism, fugue states, and multiple personality are examples of dissociative reactions.

double bind
Communication in which a positive command is followed by a negative command; the recipient cannot obey both commands and therefore feels confused and trapped.

Down's syndrome
A form of mental retardation associated with chromosomal abnormalities.

drives
In psychoanalytic theory, instinctual urges and impulses arising from biological and psychological needs.

drug abuse
See abuse.

drug dependence
Physiological or psychological dependence on a chemical substance.

dyad
A two-person group.

dynamic formulation
Synthesis of a client's traits, values, behaviors, and conflicts for the purpose of explaining, understanding, and helping the client.

dynamics
Interactive forces within the individual, usually unconscious, that are manifested in thoughts, feelings, behavior, and symptomatology.

dyslexia
Impaired ability to read.

dyspareunia
Painful sexual intercourse. It occurs in both sexes but more often in women.

dystonia
Muscle spasms of the face, head, neck, and back; usually an acute side effect of antipsychotic medication.

E

echolalia
Automatic repetition of words and phrases recently heard.

echopraxia
Repetition of movements and actions recently observed in others.

ego
In psychoanalytic theory, the aspect of the personality that mediates between demands of the id and the superego; the aspect of the personality that deals with reality.

ego dystonic (ego alien)
Thoughts, feelings, impulses, and acts that are unacceptable to the ego and therefore produce anxiety.

ego ideal
The internalized image of the self as one would like to be.

ego syntonic
Thoughts, feelings, impulses, and acts that are acceptable to the superego and therefore do not produce anxiety.

electroconvulsive therapy (ECT)
Therapeutic seizures produced by means of electric current applied to the temporal areas under controlled conditions.

electroencephalogram (EEG)
A graphic record of the electrical activity of the brain obtained by means of electrodes applied to areas of the head.

empathy
The ability to understand the feelings of others and respond sensitively to their perceptions of experience.

encopresis
Soiling of the clothing by feces.

endocrine glands
Ductless glands that secrete hormones directly into the lymphatic or circulatory system.

endogenous
Originating in internal sources and causes.

endorphins
Opiumlike substances produced by the brain in response to stimulation of the pituitary gland and other areas.

eneuresis
Involuntary discharge of urine.

enmeshment
A maladaptive pattern of overinvolvement and intensity seen in families.

epidemiology
The study of the distribution of physical and mental disorders in a given population.

episodic
Tendency of events, conditions, symptoms, and disorders to abate and recur intermittently.

ethics
A system of professional standards, moral conduct, and accountability adhered to by an individual or group.

ethnocentrism
The belief that one's own group, race, or culture is superior to any other.

etiology
The systematic study of the cause of disorders.

eugenics
Utilization of selective breeding methods for the purpose of improving the species.

euphoria
An exaggerated sense of well-being and pleasure.

exhaustion
The final stage of the general adaptation syndrome; the organism no longer has the resources to react adaptively to stress. In extreme cases, exhaustion may result in death.

exhibitionism
Sexual gratification obtained through public exposure of the genitals.

exogenous
Originating in external sources or causes.

extended family
All persons related by birth, marriage, or adoption.

737

extinction

The gradual disappearance of a conditioned response; it occurs when the response is no longer reinforced.

extrapyramidal effects

Side effects of antipsychotic medication that resemble the symptoms of Parkinson's disease.

F

family therapy

A treatment modality that focuses on relationships within the family system.

fantasy

Unrealistic mental images based on conscious or unconscious wish fulfillment.

feedback

Process by which functioning is monitored, corrected if necessary, and maintained if appropriate.

fellatio

Oral sexual contact with the penis.

fetal alcohol syndrome

Fetal irregularities such as low birth weight, cardiac problems, and other congenital abnormalities caused by maternal alcohol ingestion during pregnancy.

fetish

An object or a part of the body to which sexual significance or meaning is attached.

fixation

Attachment to immature levels of thinking and acting instead of progressing developmentally.

flashback

Recurrence of an experience, often drug-induced, without further use of the substance; memory traces of intense experiences that continue to intrude on the individual and cause emotional discomfort.

flight of ideas

Rapid movement from one topic to another in response to stimuli from outside and from within the individual.

folie à deux

Interpersonal relationship in which two participants show psychotic characteristics; the irrational behavior of one person reinforces the irrational behavior of the other.

forensic psychiatry

The branch of psychiatry that deals with legal issues surrounding mental disorders.

formal operational stage

Piaget's final stage of cognitive development, during which abstract thinking exists, mental problems are often solved by sequential steps, and hypotheses may be formulated and tested.

free association

Psychoanalytic technique in which the client communicates whatever thoughts come to mind without interference from the therapist.

frustration

Curtailment of gratification by conditions of external reality or by internal controls.

fugue state

A mental state characterized by physical flight from the immediate surroundings and by total or partial amnesia.

G

gender

A person's biological maleness or femaleness.

gender identity

Psychological awareness of being male or female.

gender roles

Culturally determined rules about tasks, expectations, and feelings considered appropriate for each gender.

geneogram

A technique used in family counseling to record accurately and in some detail the intergenerational data of the original families of the partners.

general adaptation syndrome (GAS)

Physiological and structural changes produced in response to stress; the stages are alarm, resistance, and exhaustion of the organism.

genetics

The science of heredity.

geriatrics

The study and treatment of disorders associated with aging.

gerontology

Study of the aging process.

Gestaltists

Persons concerned with existentialism or self-determination. They emphasize human potential and authentic or genuine emotional expression.

goals

The ends or purposes that nurse and client endeavor to reach; usually goals or aims are stated in client-centered terms to facilitate evaluation of the client's progress.

grief

Mourning as a response to loss, actual or imagined, of a meaningful person, object, or situation.

grief work

The process of reacting to loss in which anger, denial, and idealization of what was lost may play a part before detachment and restitution can occur.

group

Collection of two or more persons who are interdependent to some extent and who share meaningful interaction.

group therapy

A treatment modality that involves several persons in the same session and that utilizes interpersonal group behaviors to produce corrective or supportive interactions.

guilt

A sense of culpability and self-blame due to transgressions against one's internalized values and principles.

H

habeus corpus

The right of persons who are detained involuntarily to a legal hearing to determine whether the detainment should continue.

hallucination

A false perception in the absence of any external sensory stimuli.

hallucinogen

A substance that produces a temporary psychotic state in which contact with and perceptions of reality are impaired.

helplessness

Belief on the part of individuals that they cannot help themselves.

hemiplegia
Paralysis of one lateral half of the body.

hemophilia
Impaired ability of the blood to coagulate; in its classic form the condition is hereditary, transmitted by females but limited to males.

hermaphrodite
An individual with genitals of both sexes.

holism
The study of the whole or total configuration of an organism; the view of human beings as unified biopsychosocial organisms interacting with their internal and external environments.

homeostasis
The tendency of organisms to maintain balance by preserving a constant internal environment.

homosexuality
Sexual attraction or preference for persons of the same sex.

hopelessness
Belief on the part of individuals that no one can help them.

hostility
Impulses or urges directed toward the destruction of a person or object.

Huntington's chorea
A hereditary disease characterized by rapid involuntary movements, speech disturbance, and mental deterioration due to degeneration of the cerebral cortex and basal ganglia. The condition appears in mature adulthood, with incapacitation and death occurring over a period of about fifteen years.

hyperactivity
Behavior characterized by high energy expenditure and excessive activity. Accelerated motor activity, emotional lability, and flight of ideas may be present.

hyperventilation
Rapid respiration due to high levels of anxiety.

hypochondriasis
A state of exaggerated concern for one's physical well-being in the absence of actual physiological problems.

hysteric
An individual who deals with anxiety by means of self-dramatization, excitability, and attention-seeking behavior.

I

id
In psychoanalytic theory, the component of the personality that is present at birth and is the repository of drives and instincts.

ideas of reference
The belief that certain events or objects have a special meaning or significance for oneself.

identification
A process in which the attributes and traits of another are adopted and made part of oneself.

identity
The sense of selfhood that makes possible and sustains an integrated, consistent personality structure.

ideology
A belief system.

illusion
Misinterpretation of a sensory stimulus.

implosive therapy
A desensitization process in which a technique called "flooding" is used; the subject confronts an anxiety-producing object or situation at full intensity for prolonged periods of time. Anxiety is thought to diminish with repeated exposure to the flooding process.

incest
Sexual relationships between persons related biologically.

incorporation
A process in which persons introject or make part of themselves the qualities and attributes of another.

individuation
A developmental process in which the person separates from others and develops a unique, distinct identity.

indoleamines
A group of biogenic amines, including serotonin.

inferiority complex
Intense, generalized feelings of inadequacy that influence the way an individual behaves and relates to others.

inhibition
Control or restraint imposed on an unacceptable impulse, thought, or action; usually but not always self-imposed.

insanity
A synonym for mental disorder or psychosis; rarely applied by professionals except in legal matters.

insight
The ability to recognize and understand the connection between behavior and underlying motives and feelings.

integrity
Commitment to honesty, ethics, and values in various aspects of life.

intellectualization
Use of rationalization to avoid uncomfortable insights or awareness.

intelligence quotient (IQ)
Originally, the mental age of an individual multiplied by 100 and divided by chronological age; an arbitrary measure obtained by standardized intelligence tests.

interdisciplinary
A team arrangement composed of members of different disciplines who engage in joint services and responsibilities.

interpersonal
Arising or generated between two or more persons.

intrapsychic
Arising, generated, or residing within the self.

introjection
A maladaptive variant of identification in which the qualities of another person are totally incorporated by the individual.

introspection
Self-examination of one's own mental processes and emotional reactions.

involutional melancholia
A form of affective disturbance that occurs in middle age; it may appear as agitated or retarded depression and is more common in women than men. Although self-limiting, the condition is severe; suicide potential is high, and various delusions may be present.

739

isolation
Separation of thoughts, ideas, or actions from their emotional aspects.

J

judgment
The ability to predict the consequences of an action and modify one's behavior accordingly; the ability to make rational decisions based on cognition and reality.

K

kinesics
Body movements that may be seen as a component of nonverbal communication.

Klinefelter's syndrome
A condition in which the testes are abnormally small, Leydig's cells are dysfunctional, and urinary gonadotropins are increased; the condition is associated with abnormality of the sex chromosomes.

Korsakoff's syndrome
An organic brain syndrome attributed to polyneuritis and thiamine deficits occurring as a result of alcoholism; amnesia, confusion, and confabulation are among the manifestations.

L

la belle indifference
A total lack of concern for the disabling effects of a conversion reaction.

labeling
Consigning an individual to a category or classification based on behavior patterns, personality configuration, or psychiatric diagnosis.

lability
Changeable and poorly controlled emotional states.

latent
Inactive or dormant, with the potential for becoming active or manifest.

learned helplessness
Attitudes and behaviors that indicate unreadiness or inability to participate or take responsibility for solving one's problems; causes vary from repeated failures, secondary gains, and depression to knowledge that someone else is available to help.

learning disability
An impairment in one or more cognitive processes such as attention, memory, visual perception, or written or spoken language. Examples are dyslexia and dysgraphia.

lesbian
Female homosexual.

liaison nursing
The linking of two or more nursing groups for the promotion of effective collaboration between the groups, resulting in improved client care.

libido
A psychoanalytic term applied to instinctual energy; it usually denotes sexual drive or energy.

limit setting
Actions that encourage others to respect rules and norms; consequences attached to failure to adhere to rules and norms.

lithium carbonate
A drug effective for the treatment of acute mania and a prophylactic for the prevention of depressive and manic recurrences.

local adaptation syndrome (LAS)
A stress reaction limited to a particular part of the body.

loose associations
Unrelated ideas or events that activate connections with other ideas and events; a frequent manifestation during schizophrenic episodes.

M

magical thinking
The belief that thinking about a possible occurrence can make it happen; a primitive, immature form of thinking.

malingering
Conscious, deliberate feigning or exaggeration of disability or incapacity.

malpractice
Actions that have been performed incorrectly, have not been performed in the best interests of the client, have violated agency policy, or have failed to adhere to current standards of the ANA or to conform to state or national legislation.

mania
A state of accelerated activity, mental and physical; generally thought to be a maladaptive defense against depression.

manipulation
Exertion of indirect control or influence over the actions of others in order to obtain one's own purpose.

marital schism
A dysfunctional form of family structure characterized by discordance and factionalism.

masochism
Gratification obtained by experiencing pain, abuse, or humiliation from others; usually applied to deviant sexual actions.

masturbation
Sexual gratification obtained by self-stimulation of the genitals.

maturation
Development resulting from heredity rather than learning.

maturational crisis
A developmental episode in which life transitions occur and the individual is vulnerable to disequilibrium.

mental retardation
Significantly subaverage general intellectual functioning existing concurrently with deficits in adaptive behavior and manifested during the developmental period.

mental status exam
A formal, structured format for assessing a client's intelligence, mood and affect, appearance, thought processes, and capacity for insight.

metacommunication
Communication about the messages being transmitted; includes connotative as well as denotative components of communication.

migraine

A severe form of headache, usually limited to one side of the head, often accompanied by nausea and vomiting; it is believed to be associated with the constriction or dilation of cerebral arteries. The condition is believed to have emotional components.

milieu

The immediate environment, physical and social, in which individuals function.

milieu therapy

A treatment modality that uses all aspects of the environment, physical and social, in order to promote adaptive change.

Minnesota Multiphasic Personality Inventory (MMPI)

A widely used, empirically validated measure of personality.

monamine oxidase (MAO) inhibitors

A group of antidepressants that act by blocking the metabolism of certain neurotransmitters, thereby increasing the amounts available. Although useful, these drugs require extensive dietary restrictions.

morbid

Unhealthy; pathological; unwholesome.

mourning

Psychological and physiological response of individuals to loss; a necessary process involving gradual renunciation of what was lost followed by the ability to form new attachments.

multidisciplinary

A team arrangement composed of members of different disciplines who provide discipline-specific services.

multiple personality

A reaction in which two or more different personality configurations are present in the same body.

mutations

Changes in a gene that can cause new characteristics to appear in offspring.

N

narcissism

Self-love or egocentricity.

narcolepsy

Periods of sleep or trancelike episodes that occur suddenly without intent or control by the affected individual.

necrophilia

Sexual gratification related to sexual acts performed on a corpse; fantasies of such acts may be sufficient to produce sexual arousal and orgasm.

negative reinforcers

The removal of undesirable consequences in order to increase the behaviors they follow.

negativism

Refusal to cooperate or follow directions; exhibiting behaviors contrary to what is desired or expected.

negligence

Failure to perform any of a wide range of actions in accord with the best interests of the client, agency policy, ANA standards, or with state or national legislation.

neologism

Coining of new words or phrases; the attribution of new, private meanings to familiar words and phrases.

neurasthenia

A condition characterized by mental and physical fatigue and vague complaints without organic basis; a disorder related to anxiety.

neurology

Study of the brain and nervous system; the branch of medicine concerned with disorders and dysfunctions of the nervous system.

neuron

An individual nerve cell.

neurosis

An emotional disturbance accompanied by various avoidance behaviors and actions aimed at the reduction of anxiety; manifestations vary, but contact with reality is not lost.

neurotransmitters

Chemical substances that transmit impulses from one neuron to another.

norm

A standard of behavior upheld by a family, group, or community.

normal distribution

The tendency for most persons in a population to cluster round a central point with the remaining persons scattered near opposing extremes.

nosology

Study of the classification of diseases.

nuclear family

A two-generational family consisting of parents and their offspring, natural or adopted; the family of procreation established by the parental dyad.

nursing care plan

A comprehensive guide for the therapeutic utilization of the nursing process. It is based on the nursing process and delineates the means by which the nurse hopes to preserve, promote, or improve the adaptive behaviors of the client. It is also a means of facilitating communication between care providers, evaluating and revising aspects of nursing process.

nursing diagnosis

The basic meaning of the term diagnosis is "through knowledge"; thus, nursing diagnosis is a problem-orientated statement of a client's needs based on accumulated data and the nurse's identification of significant factors affecting the client in the past, present, and future.

nursing intervention

The initiation of action by the nurse on behalf of the client. Intervention is a specific aspect of the implementation phase of the nursing process; it is a consequence of assessment, diagnosis, and planning and a precipitant of evaluation.

nursing process

A cooperative process enabling the nurse to involve clients in a systematic process of problem solving designed to maintain, restore, or enhance the health of the client, whether individual, family, or community. Nursing process includes the ongoing activities of assessment, nursing diagnoses, planning, implementation, and evaluation.

nursing research
A process involving scientific principles of research studies and data analysis in laboratory and clinical settings to solve problems, test hypotheses, and contribute to the growing body of nursing theory, with the ultimate goal of improving health care.

O

obesity
Excess weight that exceeds accepted standards by more than 20 percent.

obsession
A recurring thought or idea that cannot be removed from conscious awareness.

obsessive-compulsive disorder
A behavioral style characterized by perfectionism, rigidity, and excessive need for control of the self and the environment.

occupational therapy
A therapeutic method involving planned, purposeful activity in which tangible products or discernible goals are accomplished.

oculogyric reaction
Uncontrollable upward movement of the eyes due to the side effects of antipsychotic medication.

Oedipus complex
In psychoanalytic theory, the child's attachment to the parent of the opposite sex and hostility toward the parent of the same sex.

operant conditioning
Behavior modification that changes behavior by manipulating stimuli and the consequences of reactions to stimuli.

organic brain syndrome
Any mental disorder caused by or associated with impairment of brain tissue structure; it may be acute or chronic, reversible or irreversible; etiology may be endogenous or exogenous.

orientation
Awareness of time, place, and person.

orthostatic hypotension
A decrease in blood pressure due to postural changes; a frequent side effect of psychotropic medication.

overload
Sensory input or performance demands that are beyond the tolerance or capacity of the individual.

overt
Open; direct; unconcealed.

P

paleological thinking
Thought patterns in which connections are made not between topics or subjects of sentences but between predicates. This leads to incoherent thinking and incomprehensible communication.

panic attack
Severe disorganization caused by intense anxiety; characterized by cognitive, emotional, and behavioral distortion.

paranoia
Extreme suspiciousness of others; usually related to use of the defense mechanism projection, whereby anxiety-producing thoughts and feelings are disowned by the individual and attributed to other people.

paraphilia
Sexual deviance in which unusual objects, rituals, or events are employed to obtain full sexual gratification.

paraphrase
Restating of what has been communicated in order to validate the accuracy of one's understanding and comprehension.

paraprofessional
An individual who has experience or training in a field but is not a professional.

parataxic
A mode of experience that is individualistic and idiosyncratic and in which consensual language and capacity for symbolism are limited.

parasympathetic nervous system
A division of the autonomic nervous system that controls most of the metabolic processes needed for the maintenance of life.

Parkinson's disease
A progressive disease of later life characterized by a masklike facial expression, tremor of muscles at rest, slow voluntary movements, ataxia, and muscle weakness. Mental capacity is not usually affected. When the symptoms occur in response to medication or are secondary to another disorder, the resultant syndrome is called Parkinsonism.

passive-aggressive
Behavior employed to express hostility and aggression indirectly.

pedophilia
Sexual attraction of an adult toward children.

peer review
A system for evaluating professional practice within any health care discipline by a panel of peer reviewers concerned with admission criteria and continued stay review. In the review process, norms, criteria, and standards available in written form are used to screen large numbers of cases so as to identify appropriate and adequate care and to discover exceptions, if any.

perception
The individualistic process of viewing, comprehending, and interpreting the world and one's own experiences.

perseveration
Inappropriate repetition of a word or action once it is initiated.

personality
The accumulated configuration of traits, attributes, behaviors, qualities, and attitudes that characterize an individual.

personality disorders
A group of disorders, manifested in various behavioral patterns, in which the prevailing feature is relatively little anxiety and a tendency to project blame on others.

perversion
Deviation from what is considered normal and acceptable by the majority.

phallic
Pertaining to the penis.

phenylketonuria (PKU)
A congenital disease resulting from a defect in the metabolism of the amino acid phenylalanine; this hereditary condition is transmitted by recessive genes of parents apparently healthy but if tested shown to be carriers. If untreated, the disease causes mental retardation and other abnormalities.

phobia
An extreme, irrational fear of certain objects or circumstances.

pleasure principle
A psychoanalytic concept describing the tendency of the id to find gratification and avoid discomfort; it is gradually modified by the reality principle, which imposes delayed gratification on the individual.

positive reinforcers
Desirable consequences given as the result of a desirable behavior.

posttraumatic stress syndrome
A delayed reaction to overwhelming stress, such as war or rape. Emotional instability, psychic numbing, and flashbacks are aspects of the clinical picture.

premorbid
That which existed prior to the onset of a disorder.

preoperational stage
The second Piagetian developmental stage, during which the thinking of the child is egocentric and inflexible. The child at this stage achieves *object permanence*, or the realization that people and objects exist apart from the child. This stage also introduces symbolization into the child's thinking and language.

primal therapy
A form of therapy that reduces the defenses of the client, fostering regression so that the client may retrospectively experience painful events of the past, thus reducing residual tension, and putting the client in touch with the authentic, newly liberated self. The purpose of this therapy is to evoke pain and to elicit outcries known as "primal screaming." Some clients have reported reliving the traumatic experience of their own birth.

primary gain
A decrease in anxiety as a result of measures taken by individuals to deal with stress or conflict. The measures used include thoughts, actions, or reactions that may be conscious or unconscious but have the effect of lowering anxiety.

primary group
The social group, usually the family, that has the most profound influence on an individual.

primary nursing
A nursing model in which one nurse is responsible for the health care of a client 24 hours a day.

primary prevention
Measures used to promote health and reduce the incidence of disorder or dysfunction by opposing causative agents.

primary process thinking
Primitive, infantile thought processes that seek instant outlets; in psychoanalytic theory, those thought processes controlled by id forces.

progressive relaxation
A systematic technique to induce relaxation in various muscle groups of the body, progressing until total relaxation is achieved.

projection
Attribution of blame or responsibility for one's own acts and feelings to other people.

projective tests
Test forms in which ambiguous items are used to elicit information regarding psychological tendencies and personality traits of the subjects. The ambiguity of the items causes subjects to project aspects of themselves onto the answers, thus disclosing data that must be expertly interpreted and analyzed.

prototaxic
A mode of experience characteristic of the first months of life that is perceived by the infant as continuous, boundless, undifferentiated, and wordless.

proxemics
Spatial relationships in social interactions.

pseudohostility
Family dissension that avoids genuine sources of conflict.

pseudomutuality
Family harmony that is superficial and maintained at the expense of one or more family members.

psychic determinism
The psychoanalytic axiom that human behavior is neither random nor accidental but is determined by preceding experiences and events.

psychoanalysis
A theoretical and therapeutic approach that explores anxiety-producing events of early life. Through the defense mechanism of repression, the memory of such events becomes unconscious; the purpose of psychoanalysis is to bring repressed material into conscious awareness so that it may be dealt with adaptively.

psychodrama
The use of dramatization under professional direction in order to help clients act out life experiences before an audience of peers who offer constructive alternative suggestions for coping.

psychodynamic
Pertaining to the causes and consequences of behavior and experience, with attention to underlying motivation, conscious and unconscious.

psychogenic
Psychological in origin.

psychomotor retardation
Slowed motor activity, often seen in depressed persons.

psychopathology
Study of the causes and nature of abnormal behavior; in general, the study of psychiatric disorders.

psychosexual theory
A theoretical framework proposed by Freud and others pertaining to the interrelated psychological and sexual development of individuals.

psychosis
Any dysfunction in which the ability to recognize reality, communicate, and relate to others is seriously impaired, resulting in reliance on maladaptive defenses and inability to cope with life.

psychosocial theory

A theoretical framework proposed by Erikson and others pertaining to the interrelated psychological and social development of individuals. Implicit in Erikson's formulation is the physiological developmental influence.

psychosurgery

Surgical intervention for psychiatric disorders, usually involving neural pathways or areas of the brain.

psychotherapy

Measures and interventions employed to offer support or to modify maladaptive behavior. It may include identification of emotional problems troubling the client, goal setting, and negotiation of a therapeutic regimen.

psychotropic

Having an effect on the mind.

Q

quality assurance

A system of monitoring the level of health care by applying principles of internal accountability and self-regulation. Quality assurance uses peer review methods and utilization review to ensure that available services are being used properly and are of high quality as well as cost effective.

R

rape

Sexual intercourse with a minor (statutory rape); sexual intercourse without the consent of the partner (forcible rape).

rapport

Shared understanding and harmony between two people based on mutual trust.

rational emotive therapy

A treatment approach that emphasizes taking responsibility for one's own behavior, utilizing concepts based on existentialism.

rationalization

Fabrication of socially acceptable reasons to justify actions, thoughts, or feelings that might be unacceptable to the self or others.

reaction formation

Control or eradication of unacceptable ideas or impulses by engaging in opposite forms of behavior or attitudes.

reality

The world as it actually is; the external world as opposed to the internal world of daydreams and fantasy.

reality principle

A psychoanalytic concept applied to the gradual development of the ability to delay gratification and modify one's desires in accordance with the demands of society and external reality.

reality testing

An essential ego function that enables the individual to distinguish internal stimuli from external stimuli; differentiating subjective from objective experience.

reality therapy

A treatment approach that employs the existential concepts of responsibility, self-determination, and progress toward goals.

recidivism

Recurrence of delinquency or criminality despite punishment, incarceration, or treatment.

reciprocal inhibition

A behavior modification procedure in which an anxiety-producing stimulus is paired with an anxiety-reducing stimulus until anxiety is lowered to a comfortable level.

reference group

Any group with which one identifies and whose beliefs and values are influential.

reflection

A communication technique in which ideas or feelings expressed by one person are verbalized by the other in order to clarify meaning and encourage amplification.

regression

A retreat to less mature levels of thought and action in an attempt to deal with stressful or anxiety-producing situations.

reinforcement

The strengthening of behavior, particularly desirable behavior, by positive methods (rewards) or negative methods (removing punishments).

relationship therapy

A form of therapy often used by nurses to help clients establish trust and maintain contact with reality, thus fostering more adaptive patterns of thinking, feeling, and behaving.

relaxation therapy

Utilization of consciously induced states of relaxation in order to reduce tension and various maladaptive responses to stress.

reliability

Data, results, or scores that are dependable and consistent.

remotivation therapy

A therapeutic approach designed to stimulate the interest and promote the socialization of chronic clients.

repression

Removal of unpleasant, anxiety-producing thoughts, desires, or memories from conscious awareness.

resistance

The tendency to maintain maladaptive patterns of thinking and behaving despite therapeutic intervention.

reversal

Behavior in which instinctual feelings are expressed by opposing actions.

risk factors

Those factors—social, psychological, environmental, or physiological—that render certain individuals, families, or communities vulnerable to particular dysfunctions, disorders, or agents.

role

A set of behavioral expectations associated with an individual's status and functions in the family, group, or community.

role enactment

The performance of the functions, responsibilities, privileges, and obligations attached to the position or role one assumes in a family or group.

Rorschach test

A projective psychological test designed to reveal basic attitudes and conflicts by having the individual interpret a series of inkblots.

744

S

sadism

Gratification obtained by inflicting pain, abuse, or humiliation on others; usually applied to sexually deviant acts.

scapegoat

An individual who is the target of aggression from others but who may not be the actual cause of hostility or frustration in others.

schism

A term applied to families characterized by severe conflict and dissension.

schizophrenia

A psychotic disorder of thought and perception characterized by withdrawal, impaired social relationships, loose associations, flat affect, autism, ambivalence, and regression. Manifestations may vary from person to person depending on the defense mechanisms and coping ability of the client.

school phobia

Aversion to school often generated by fears of separation from parents; also known as school avoidance behavior.

seclusion

Placing an individual in a room away from others so as to reduce stimuli and foster self-control; seclusion rooms may or may not be locked.

secondary gain

An additional gain or reward, such as attention, derived from any illness or disability.

secondary prevention

Measures designed to reduce the prevalence of dysfunction and disorders through early detection and adequate care.

secondary process thinking

Rational, mature thought processes considered to be under the control of the ego.

security operations

Any behavior employed to increase psychological comfort and reduce anxiety; may be conscious or unconscious.

self-actualization

The process of reaching one's full potential.

self-awareness

Recognition of what one is experiencing and how one is reacting.

self-concept

The sum of an individual's knowledge and beliefs about the self and its relation to the physical and social environment.

self-differentiation

The extent to which the individual preserves a sense of identity and separateness from the group.

self-esteem

Feelings held by individuals regarding their own worth and value.

self-fulfilling prophecy

A phenomenon in which expectations shape and maintain behavior, events, and interpersonal transactions.

self-system

Term coined by H. S. Sullivan to describe the integration of the "good me," "bad me," and "nonme" aspects of self.

sensate focus

A therapeutic sexual technique in which the partners evoke erotic responses by fondling and touching without necessarily engaging in coitus.

sensorimotor stage

The initial stage in the cognitive development of the child as the child explores the environment through the senses and through motor activity, as described by Piaget.

sensory deprivation

Reduction of sensory input or stimuli below levels necessary to maintain self-awareness and support normal central nervous system function.

separation anxiety

Apprehension generated by loss or fear of loss of the mothering person; subsequent loss of significant persons or objects may reactivate separation anxiety.

sexual deviance

Sexual behaviors that do not conform to standards of the population majority.

sexual dysfunction

Impaired ability to give or receive sexual gratification.

shaping

A form of behavior modification in which any behaviors resembling the desired goal are rewarded (reinforced); eventually only the closest approximate behaviors are rewarded; finally only the desired behavior is rewarded.

sibling rivalry

Competition between brothers and sisters for recognition and affection.

sick role

Set of behaviors, privileges, and obligations expected from persons designated as being ill.

sickle cell anemia

A genetic defect commonly affecting blacks, characterized by abnormal hemoglobin, anemia, reticulocytosis, jaundice, recurrent fever, and pain. The name is derived from the crescent- or sickle-shaped erythrocytes caused by varying proportions of hemoglobin.

significant others

Essential persons, often but not always related to the individual, who are sources of support for the individual.

situational crisis

Disturbed equilibrium that develops as a result of the impact of a specific event.

skew

Term applied to families in which relationships are distorted.

socialization

The process of acquiring the values, attitudes, and behaviors considered appropriate in a particular culture.

sociogram

A technique used in family counseling to observe and note the routes and lines of communication between family members.

sodomy

Sexual intercourse involving the anus; anal penetration in sexual intercourse.

somnambulism

Sleepwalking.

spasm

Intense, involuntary contraction of muscles, usually accompanied by severe pain.

745

spasticity

Continued muscle contraction causing hypertonicity, rigidity, and coordination problems.

spina bifida

A defect of the spinal column resulting from imperfect union of paired vertebral arches, sometimes extensive enough to cause herniation of the meninges and spinal cord.

standardization

Utilization of methods designed to establish the expected range of scores on a test.

standards of practice

Authoritative statements or approved concepts that provide guidance to the nursing profession and its members in the actual delivery of care.

Stanford-Binet test

A standardized intelligence test for children.

stereotype

A generalization of how members of a particular group or category are likely to look or act.

stress

Any situation or condition requiring adjustment on the part of the individual, family, or group.

stressor

A stimulus, event, or experience that demands changed or new behavior. Stressors usually require expenditure of considerable energy, thus arousing alarm and mobilization responses.

sublimation

Conscious transformation of unacceptable drives and impulses into socially acceptable behavior in order to satisfy the drive or impulse.

successive approximation

See shaping.

superego

In psychoanalytic theory, the aspect of the personality that monitors thoughts and actions; comparable to the conscience or internal censor.

suppression

Conscious inhibition or control of certain desires, thoughts, or emotions.

symbol

The representation of an idea or concept by means of an object, sign, or signal that conveys connotative and denotative meanings.

sympathetic nervous system

That part of the autonomic nervous system that is activated by stressful conditions, actual or perceived.

syndrome

A grouping or cluster of symptoms that represent the usual clinical manifestations of a disorder.

syntaxic

A mode of experience that is characterized by shared, consensually validated language and meanings and by the capacity for abstract thinking.

system

A set of interrelated components defined by boundaries, interdependent and interacting in such a manner that any stimulus affecting one component affects every other component, as well as acting on the system as a whole.

systematic desensitization

The reduction of anxiety-laden responses by gradually exposing the subject to approximations of feared objects or situations until the subject can tolerate the actual object or experience.

systems theory

The interdependent behavior of various entities or components functioning in reciprocal interactions, usually for a common purpose.

T

tardive dyskinesia

An irreversible side effect of major tranquilizers that causes involuntary grimacing and disfiguring movements of the tongue, mouth, and lower jaw.

Tay-Sachs disease

An inherited recessive condition resulting in retardation and blindness of infants. Tests for the presence of the disease may be performed on the fetus at 14 weeks, when absence of the enzyme hexoaminidase shows conclusively the presence of Tay-Sachs disease. Carriers show lower levels of the enzyme; thus populations at risk may be screened. The disease is prevalent among Jewish infants; genetic counseling offers a form of primary prevention if screening indicates a risk.

team nursing

A hierarchical nursing model with the most experienced nurse usually acting as team leader and other team members performing tasks according to their ability and the clients' needs.

theoretical framework

A systematic formulation of concepts and principles related to phenomena that have been observed and verified to some extent.

theory

A systematic statement of related concepts and principles.

therapeutic community

A form of environmental interpersonal therapy that is much like milieu therapy but usually less hierarchical. Administration and planning are delegated to an interdisciplinary team rather than to an acknowledged leader.

time out

A behavioral technique used when an impasse develops in which reinforcers are not being used effectively to modify disruptive behavior. Taking "time out" from the interaction introduces an element of rationality. It allows disruptive behavior and dysfunctional exchanges to be terminated for a time.

token economy

A behavioral modification system in which desired objects, in the form of tokens or various privileges, are bestowed in return for desirable behavior. The granting of tokens is a form of positive reinforcement.

tolerance
A condition in which increasingly large doses of a drug or other substance must be taken to obtain the same effect previously produced with smaller doses or amounts.

transcultural nursing
A subspecialty within nursing concerned with identifying and meeting the special needs of cultural groups within this pluralistic society and acting when necessary as advocates on behalf of such diverse groups.

transference
A psychological distortion in which the client acts or feels as if another individual is a significant person from early life; the distortion is usually unconscious.

transsexual
Sex identity confusion in which the individual has a strong wish to belong to the opposite sex; also, a person who has undergone surgical and hormonal intervention to achieve this purpose.

transvestite
An individual who derives sexual pleasure from dressing in garments usually worn by the opposite sex.

tricyclic antidepressants
Antidepressants that prevent reuptake of neurotransmitters into the presynaptic cleft, thus increasing the amounts available.

Turner's syndrome
A condition characterized by retarded growth and sexual development; it is associated with absence or abnormality of the second X chromosome in females.

type A
A personality type characterized by traits of competitiveness, time urgency, and high tension levels; type A's are believed by some investigators to be prone to stress-related disorders.

U

undoing
Performance of activities designed to atone for errors or misdeeds, thus cancelling them.

unidisciplinary
A team arrangement composed of members of the same discipline.

unipolar disorder
A disorder of mood and affect in which only episodes of depression occur.

V

vaginismus
Involuntary muscle spasms of the vaginal orifice and wall preventing sexual penetration.

validity
Data, results, or scores that are sound, relevant, and convincing.

violence
Expression of aggressive impulses by acting destructively toward others.

visualization therapy
A form of self-hypnosis or conditioning used to promote relaxation or to mobilize the defenses of the individual against physical and psychological distress. The person using visualization therapy may depict in imagination a place of security and comfort or a state of active participation and assertiveness.

voluntary admission
Process in which individuals are admitted to a psychiatric hospital with their consent.

voyeurism
A sexual deviation in which gratification is obtained by witnessing sexual activities or by viewing sexually attractive persons, usually without their knowledge.

W

waxy flexibility
A condition seen in persons with catatonic schizophrenia; the individual retains a position or stance for long periods of time before gradually changing the position; also known as cerea flexibilitas.

Wechsler Intelligence Scale for Children
A standardized intelligence test for children.

Wernicke's syndrome
A complication of chronic alcoholism due to thiamine deficiency characterized by paralysis of the eye muscles and mental deterioration; it occasionally appears as a manifestation of other disorders.

withdrawal
Behaviors adopted to avoid interacting with others.

word salad
Incoherent use of words by disoriented or psychotic persons.

Z

zoophilia
See bestiality.

zygote
A fertilized cell formed by the union of male and female gametes.

747

A

abuse. *See* alcohol abuse; drug abuse
Abused Women's Aid in Crisis, 422
acalculia, 284
acceptance, 109, 112, 150
accountability, professional, 623–625
accreditation of hospitals, 638
acetylcholine, 283, 286
acknowledgment of client, 150
acquired immune deficiency syndrome (AIDS), 345
ACTH, 53, 306
acting out, 518
Action for Mental Health, 12
active listening, 113–114
adaptation, 55–58
    altered patterns of, 7
    characteristics of, 55
    disorders of, 309–331
    health as, 6–7
    modes of (Roy), 60
addiction, 219–220
addictive clients, care of, 220, 228–231, 239–242
Adler, Alfred, 571
adolescents, 385
    antisocial behavior in, 386–387
    body image distortion in, 387–388
    depression in, 163
    identity confusion in, 372, 385–386
    suicide and, 410
    working with, 388
adrenal glands, 306–307
adrenogenital syndrome, 348
adulthood, altered maturational patterns in, 390–395

advice, offering, 583
advocacy, client, 626–630
    for battered wives, 418
affect, 63, 140, 164
    See also mood and affect, altered patterns of
    blunted, 141
    flat, 141
    inappropriate, 141
    in schizophrenia, 140–141
affective disorders, 164–165
    See also mood and affect, altered patterns of
agent factors, 551–552
aggression, 412
    See also violence
    arthritis and, 321
    passive, 210
aggressive client, relationship therapy for, 585–586
aging, 396
    See also elderly
    degenerative disorders and, 281–282
    health and, 396–397
    maturational crises of, 395–398
agitated depression, 410
agnosia, 284
agranulocytosis, 146
Aguilera, Donna, 77
AIDS, 345
akathisia, 147, 149
akinesia, 147, 149, 285
alarm reaction, 306, 307, 308
Albrecht, G. L., 227
alcohol, 220–221
alcohol abuse
    See also alcoholism
    attitudes toward, 221
    culture and, 225
    personality and, 224–225
    physiological consequences of, 225–227

    prevalence of, 221
    violence and, 412–413, 424–425, 430
Alcoholics Anonymous (AA), 221, 231
alcoholism
    See also alcohol abuse
    aversion therapy for, 469
    causes of, 223–225
    classifications of, 222–223
    depression and, 163–164
    as disease, 221, 222
    nursing process and, 228–231
    phases of, 228
    physiological consequences of, 225–227
    prevalence of, 221
    progression of, 227–228
    role of spouse in, 231
    suicide and, 409
alcohol metabolism, 226
Alexander, Franz, 304, 305
allergy, asthma and, 313–316
Almond, R., 579
alpha-fetoprotein, 264
altruistic suicide, 406
aluminum levels, in brain, 283
Alzheimer, Alois, 282
Alzheimer's disease, 279, 281, 282–285, 287
Alzheimer's Disease and Related Disorders Association, 291
ambivalence, in schizophrenia, 140
American Association on Mental Deficiency, 253
American Group Therapy Association, 515
American Hospital Association, 619
American Nurses' Association, 618, 623, 638
American Nurses' Association Commission on Nursing Research, 643

American Psychiatric Association (APA), 15, 303
A Mind That Found Itself (Beers), 11
amines, 166
amnesia, 207
amniocentesis, 264
amoxapine, 178
amphetamines, 233
    See also stimulants
anaclitic depression, 167
anaclitic separation anxiety, 29
anal stage, 198
Anatomy of Melancholy, The (Burton), 10
androgyny, 356
anger, 413–414
    See also aggression; violence
    in depressed client, 168–169, 171
angry client, care of, 89–91
anhedonia, 169
anomia, 289
anomic suicide, 407
anorexia nervosa, 323–325, 387–388
anoxia, 252, 261
Antabuse, 230, 469
antianxiety drugs, 213–214
    abuse of, 235
anticholinergic agents, 148
anticipatory grief, 184
anticipatory guidance, 383, 449
antidepressant drugs, 176–179
    for phobias, 206
antipsychotic drugs, 145–149
antisocial behavior, adolescent, 386–387
antisocial personality disorder, 209–210, 350
anxiety, 84, 197, 202
    behavior therapy for, 467–468
    in Freud's theory, 29, 197–198
    hierarchy of, 468
    imagery for, 575
    implosion therapy for, 575
    separation, 29
    in Sullivan's theory, 198–199
    types of, 447
anxiety disorders, 202–203
    Janov's explanation of, 576–577
anxiety-provoking brief therapy, 448
anxiety-suppressive brief therapy, 448, 449
anxious client, care of, 84–86, 202–203, 447
apathy, 141
applied science, 474
Arieti, S., 137
Arnold, H. M., 150
Arnold Chiari malformation, 263
arthritis, 320–321, 322
assaultive behavior. See violence
assaultive client, 289
assertion training, 470
    for nurses, 605–606

assessment, 61, 78–79, 118–119
    of abused children, 423–424
    of alcoholic client, 228, 229
    of battered wife, 425, 426
    of child with congenital disorder, 269–270
    of client with chronic degenerative disorder, 292–293
    communication strategies in, 117
    in community mental health, 558
    in consultation process, 604
    of depressed client, 168–170
    for drug abuse, 239
    of elated client, 172–174
    of family, 379, 497–499, 502–503
    of family functioning, 489, 491–494
    guidelines for (Roy), 61
    of intelligence, 61–62
    of mental status, 62–64
    of personality, 64–67
    of potentially violent client, 413
    in primary nursing, 599
    in relationship therapy, 583–584
    in sexual counseling, 358
    of sexual health status, 360
    of suicidal client, 409–410
    in team nursing, 598
associations, loose, 140
asthma, 313–316
Atchley, R., 396
attachment, 379
attention deficit disorder, 257–258
auditory hallucinations, 141–142
audits, 638, 639, 640
authenticity, 109, 150, 583
authoritarian leadership, 526–528
autistic thinking, 144
autocratic leadership, 526–528
autoimmune disease, 320
    Alzheimer's disease as, 284
autonomic nervous system, 307
autorhythmometry, 42
aversion therapy, 468–469, 471–472
    for alcohol abuse, 230
avoidance model, 466

B

Bachrach, L. L., 557
bacterial endocarditis, 239
Baker, B., 606
Baldwin, B. A., 449–450
Bales Interaction Process Analysis, 535
barbiturates, 234–235, 238
Bateson, Gregory, 495
battered children. See child abuse
battered wives. See spouse abuse
Battered Wives (Martin), 417
Beall, L., 408
Beck, A. T., 169–170

bedwetting, 382
Beers, Clifford, 11
behavioral therapy, 461, 467–472
    limitations of, 472, 474
    for phobias, 206
behaviorism, 463
behavior modification, 461
    for childhood fears, 383
    for enuresis, 382
    guidelines for use of, 471–472
    for mentally retarded, 254
    for obesity, 323
    techniques for, 467–471
    underlying principles of, 462–467
    for weight loss, 323
beliefs, irrational, 572–574
Bell, A., 344–347
Benfer, B. A., 597, 598
bereavement. See grief
Berlo, D. K., 107
Bernard, Claude, 305
bestiality, 351
Bibring, E., 165, 182
binge eating, 323–324
bioamines, schizophrenia and, 133
biofeedback, 318
biogenic theories, 39–44
biological rhythms, 40–43
bipolar disorders, 164
    biochemical factors in, 40, 166
    existential factors in, 167
    genetic factors in, 167
    lithium therapy for, 179–181
    nursing care for, 172–175
    sexuality and, 350
birth defects. See congenital disorders
bisexuality, 347
blackouts, 226
Bleuler, Eugene, 131, 140
blood dyscrasias, 146, 148
blood pressure, high, 316–319
blunted affect, 141
body image, 143
    change in, 184
    distortion of, 387–388
    sexuality and, 349
body language, 108
body types, 39
bondage, 353
borderline conditions, 213
boundaries, 483–484, 489
    elastic, 487
Bourne, P., 552
Bowen, Murray, 489–494
Bowlby, J., 165, 167, 183
bradykinesia, 285
brain
    alterations in, in Alzheimer's disease, 282–283
    alterations in, in Huntington's chorea, 286
brainwashing, 420
Braun, P., 556, 557
Brigham, Amariah, 8
Brower, H., 628
bulimia, 323–324, 387–388
burnout, 606
    staff, 442, 452–453

Burrow, Trignant, 515
Burton, Robert, 10
Butler, R., 400

C

caffeine, 233
cancer, stress and, 326–327, 330–331
Cannon, Walter, 305
Caplan, Gerald, 13, 439, 601, 602–603, 604
cardiomyopathy, alcoholic, 227
cardiovascular disorders, stress and, 316–320
career crises, 390–391
caring behavior, 76, 105–106
Carroll, M. A., 621
case management, 598, 599
case method, 598
case mix, 635, 636
castration anxiety, 29
catatonic schizophrenia, 139
catchment areas, 12, 545
catecholamines, 40
    depression and, 166
    heart disease and, 319
    schizophrenia and, 133
celibacy, 347
cerebral palsy, 261–262
certification of psychiatric mental health nurses, 15
Challela, M., 597
Chapman, Jane Roberts, 421
child abuse, 422–424, 426, 427, 430
children
    See also family; parents
    asthma in, 313–315
    cognitive development in, 375–376
    depression in, 163
    developmental tasks of, 371–372
    divorce and, 391, 394
    eating disturbances in, 381–382
    fears and phobias in, 383
    moral development in, 372–375
    nursing care for, 383–385
    play therapy for, 515
    sleep disturbances in, 379–380
    urinary and excretory disturbances in, 382–383
Chinese immigrants, 546
chlorpromazine, 145–146
choreiform movements, 286
chromosomal abnormalities, 255, 264
chronic degenerative disorders, 280, 292
chronic illness, 251, 321
chronobiology, 40–43
CIC (clean intermittent catheterization), 263
circadian rhythms, 40–43
circumstantiality, 288
cirrhosis, alcoholic, 226–227

Ciske, K. L., 599
civil rights, 618–620
clang associations, 141
clarification, 115
clarifying expectations, 106
classical conditioning, 463–465
clean intermittent catheterization, 263
client advocacy, 554, 626–630
client-centered care, 78, 79, 81, 108
    advocacy and, 627–629
client-centered therapy, 461, 581–582
client education, 311, 599, 600, 629
    of adolescents, 388
    regarding sexuality, 360–361
client government, 579
client-nurse relationships. *See* nurse-client relationships
client's record, 118–124
client's rights, 618–623
    advocacy and, 626–628
clinical research in nursing, 641
clinical specialists, 15
clitoris, 337
cocaine, 233
Code for Nurses (ANA), 618
cognitive development, 375–376, 378
cognitive functions, assessment of, 64
cognitive impairment, in congenital disorders, 288–289
cognitive theory, 47, 472–473
cognitive triad of depression, 170, 171
cohesion, 520
cohesiveness, 374
coleadership, 529–530
colitis, ulcerative, 312–313
collaboration, 610
    in milieu therapy, 153
    nurse-client, 109–111, 117, 583–586
Comfort, Alex, 279
commitment, involuntary, 621–622
communication, 105
    cognitive approach to, 496
    in consultation process, 603, 604
    documentation of, 120–124
    dysfunctional, 498
    emotion and, 497
    in family, 494–499
    in groups, 534
    impaired, 289, 290
    in marriage, 358
    nonverbal, 107–108
    power and, 496–497
    in sexual relationships, 357
    suicide and, 408
    therapeutic, 106–109, 111–118
    in a therapeutic relationship, 582–583
communication patterns, 496, 498–499
communication techniques, 113–116, 582
    with clients who have degenerative disorders, 290

community, 545
    as culture, 548–550
    family and, 480, 481
    as group, 545–547
    as place, 547–548
    as social system, 554
    therapeutic, 579–581
community health care, 554–555
community mental health, 545
    epidemiological concepts applied to, 550–554
Community Mental Health Act, 12
community mental health centers, 555
community mental health movement, 12–13
community mental health nurses, 15, 557–558
community network, 516
community programs, evaluation of, 558–559
Community Support Systems Program (Denver), 580
compartmentalization, 201
complementary relationships, 496
compulsion, 203
compulsive behavior, 95
Compulsive Drug Abuse Control and Prevention Act, 233
compulsive drug use, 219
compulsive personality disorder, 209
concepts, 25
concrete operational stage, 376
concrete thinking, 144
concretization, 137–138
conditioning
    classical, 463–465
    operant, 465–467
confabulation, 288
confidentiality, 109
conflict, specific physical disorders and, 304
confrontation, 115–116
congenital disorders
    adaptation to, 267–268
    etiology of, 251–253
    impact of, on family, 264–267
    nursing process and, 269–274
    types of, 253–264
congenital origin, alterations of, 251–274
conjoint family therapy, 480
consciousness, expansion of, 76
consensual validation, 35, 136, 137
consent, written, 620
consistency, of nurse, 106, 584
constancies, perceptual, 143, 144
constipation, 382
constructs, 25
consultation, 601, 602
    comprehensive, 604
    goals of, 603
    implementation of, 603–605
    implications of, 605–607
    outcomes of, 605
    requests for, 607–610
    types of, 602–603
content analysis, 526

contract
    for crisis counseling, 446
    group, 520
    therapeutic, 110–111
control group, 644, 646
conversion disorders, 202, 206–207
coordination of client care, 599,
    600, 610, 612
coping behaviors, 56
    of family with disabled child,
        266–268
coping mechanisms, 440–441, 445
coronary artery disease, stress and,
    319–320
corticoids, 306
costs of health care, 635
counseling
    for battered wives, 427
    crisis, 445–448
    genetic, 268–269
    marital, 357–358
    premarital, 355–357
    for rape victims, 417
    sexual, 358–360
counter-conditioning, 467–468
countertransference, 30, 517–518
crisis, 439, 442
    anxiety in, 447
    assessment of, 444–445
    characteristics of, 439–440
    duration of, 442–443
    emergency and, 441–442
    opportunities in, 440–441
    perception of, 444–445
    reaction to, 443–444
    staff burnout as, 452–453
    stress and, 439, 442
    typology of, 449–452
crisis intervention, 427, 430,
    444–448
    theory of, 77
crisis work, 444–448
    types of, 448–449
critical tasks, 371, 376–377,
    482–483
cross-addiction, 220
cross-dressing, 348
Cry for Help, The (Farberow and
    Shneidman), 408
culture, 548
    alcohol abuse and, 225
    community and, 546, 548–549
    drug abuse and, 238
    family and, 378
    health care and, 76
    nursing and, 548–549
curative factors, in groups, 533–534
Curtin, L., 627
cyclazocine, 241
cyclothymic disorders, 164
cystic fibrosis, 259–260

D

data analysis, 647
data collection, 117, 646–647
Davis, D. S., 602

death and dying, 182, 397–398
decentralization of nursing depart-
    ments, 637
defense mechanisms, 29–30,
    201–202, 577
    in alcoholism, 225
    levels of, 56–57
    in obsessive-compulsive reac-
        tions, 203
    in phobias, 205
degenerative disorders, 279–281
    aging and, 281–282
    behavioral alterations in, 288
    cognitive alterations in, 288
    impact of, on nurse, 292
    impaired communication in,
        289
    impaired judgment in, 289
    impaired reality testing in,
        288–289
    memory impairment in,
        287–288
    nursing process and, 292–293
    self-care deficits in, 289–290
    social alterations in, 290–292
    types of, 282–287
degenerative origin, altered patterns
    of, 279–294
deinstitutionalization, 12, 555–557
delinquency, 386–387
delirium, 280
delirium tremens (DTs), 226
delusional client, care of, 86–87
delusional thinking, nursing care
    plan for, 82
delusions, 64, 86, 144, 168
    types of, 145
demanding client, 108
    care of, 87–89
dementia, 279, 280–281, 288
    Alzheimer's, 279, 282
    in Huntington's chorea, 286
    in Parkinson's disease, 285
dementia praecox, 131
democratic leadership, 526–528
denial, 30
dependency
    in clients with peptic ulcers,
        309–311
    in groups, 522–523
depersonalization, 143–144
depressant drugs, abuse of, 232,
    234–235
depressed client
    care of, 170–172
    referral of, 609
depression, 163
    See also mood and affect,
        altered patterns of
    agitated, 410
    alcoholism and, 225
    anaclitic, 167
    in anorexia nervosa, 325
    antihypertensive medication
        and, 317
    biochemical factors in, 40,
        166–167
    categories of, 164
    cognitive triad of, 170, 171

drug therapy for, 176–179
electroconvulsive therapy for,
    175–176
existential factors in, 167
genetic factors in, 167
manifestations of, 168–170
neurotic patterns and, 202
prevalence of, 163
psychodynamic factors in,
    165–166
suicide and, 406, 410
descriptive studies, 646
desensitization, 206, 467–468, 473,
    575, 585–586
desocialization, 138
desymbolization, 138
detoxification, of alcoholic, 228–229
development
    cognitive, 375–376
    family, 376–378
    moral, 372–375
    psychosexual, 28–29
    psychosocial, 31–34, 134,
        371–372
    theories of, 371–379
developmental crises, 371, 439, 451
developmental disabilities, 251
developmental tasks, 482–483
Diagnostic and Statistical Manual of
    Mental Disorders. See DSM-III
Diagnostic Related Groups (DRGs),
    635–637
diarrhea, 326
diet, PKU and, 259
differentiation of self, 491–492
disabled children, abuse of, 423
disaster, survival of, 444
discharge plan, 120, 609
discharge planning, 612, 637
discharge summary, 120, 121
discipline, parental, 385, 422
discrimination, 465, 466
disease, 76–77
    See also health; illness
Disease of Alcoholism, The (Jellinek),
    221
disequilibrium, 439, 440–441
disorganized schizophrenia, 139
displacement, 30, 205
dispositional crises, 450
disruptive client, care of, 174
dissociative disorders, 202, 207
disulfiram, 230, 469
divorce, 391
Dix, Dorothea, 11
Dobash, R. E., 422
Dobash, R. P., 422
documentation of care, 118–124,
    599
    auditing of, 639
Dollard, John, 467
dopamine, 40
    in Huntington's chorea, 286
    mood alteration and, 166
    in Parkinson's disease, 285–286
    schizophrenia and, 133, 145
double binds, 495–496
Down's syndrome, 255–256
    Alzheimer's disease and, 283

DRGs, 635–637
drug abuse, 219–220, 231–233, 237
  causes of, 236–238
  nursing process for, 239–242
  physiological consequences of, 238
  prevalence of, 232
  suicide and, 409
drug combinations, unsafe, 181
drug dependence, 219
drug-free communities, 241–242
drug interaction, 234–235
drug laws, 232–233
drugs
  antianxiety, 213–214
  antidepressant, 176–179
  antiparkinsonian, 148
  antipsychotic, 145–149
  for degenerative disorders, 288
  effects on fetus, 252
  lithium therapy, 179–181
  refusal to take, 620–621, 622
DSM-III, 15–17
  affective disorders in, 165
  alcohol abuse in, 223
  degenerative disorders in, 283
  drug abuse in, 237
  homosexuality in, 347
  learning disabilities in, 258
  mental retardation in, 258
  neurotic disorders in, 200
  psychophysiological disorders in, 303–304
  schizophrenia in, 139
  sexual deviance in, 351, 352
  sexual dysfunction in, 352
  suicide in, 409
  violence in, 414
Duke University, 602
Dunbar, F., 304, 305
Durel, S., 630
Durkheim, Emile, 406–407
Duvall, Evelyn, 376–378, 379, 482–483
dynamisms, 199
dyscrasia, 9
dysgraphia, 257
dyslexia, 257
dysthymic disorders, 164
dystonias, 147, 149

E

eating disorders, 322–325
  in adolescence, 387–388
  in childhood, 381–382
echolalia, 141, 284
eclectic approach, 585
ecology, 536
ECT. See electroconvulsive therapy
ectomorphy, 39
education, in consultant process, 605, 606
  See also client education
ego, 197
  according to Erikson, 32

according to Freud, 27–28, 32
ego boundaries, loss of, 143–144
egocentric roles, 530, 531
egocentrism, 375
ego dystonic (ego alien), 28
ego ideal, 27
egoistic suicide, 406
ego strength, 32
ego syntonic, 28
ejaculation, 339, 340
  rapid, 351
ejaculatory inhibition, 351
elated client, care of, 172–175
Elavil, 177
elderly
  See also aging
  depression in, 163
  maturational crises in, 395–400
  nursing care for, 398–400
  suicide and, 409
Electra conflict, 498
electroconvulsive therapy (ECT), 175–176
Ellis, Albert, 571–575
emergency, psychiatric, 452
emergency situations, 441–442, 443
emotional cutoff, 493
emotions, 140
  asthma and, 313–314
  cancer and, 326–327
  physical disorders and, 304, 309
  ulcers and, 309
empathy, 35, 112–113, 581–582, 583
empty nest syndrome, 395
encephalitis, 252
encopresis, 382–383
encounter groups, 516–517
endocarditis, 239
endocrine system
  alcohol and, 227
  response to stress, 306–307
endomorphy, 39
Engel, G. L., 5
enuresis, 382–383
environment
  community and, 547–548
  disease and, 551
eosinophilia, 146
ephredine, 177
Epictetus, 471
epidemiology, 550–554
epinephrine, 53
equifinality, 496
erectile inhibition, 350
Erikson, Erik, 31–34, 134, 166, 198, 371–372, 379, 388, 391, 482, 525
escape model, 466
ethics, 617
  nursing and, 617–623
ethnic groups, 545–549
eustressors, 308
evaluation, 80–81
  of community programs, 558–559
  of group progress, 521–522
  of nursing care plan, 117–118
  of nursing services, 637–641
  in relationship therapy, 586

exchange theory, 426–427
excretory disturbances in children, 382–383
exhibitionism, 352–353
existential theory, 44, 47
  of anxiety, 202
exorcism, 9–10
experimental design, 646
experimentation, 462–463
explosive disorder, 414
extended family, 481
externalization, 201
extinction, 465
extinction paradigm, 467, 468
extinction techniques, 467
extrapyramidal effects, 147

F

family
  alcohol abuse and, 230–231
  assessment of, 379, 481
  asthmatic child and, 314, 315
  blended, 394
  of client with degenerative disorder, 291–292
  communication in, 495–499
  community and, 480, 481
  conflict in, 378, 487
  cultural influences on, 378
  effect of disabled child on, 264–268
  false harmony in, 486–487
  Freud's view of, 486
  of heart attack victim, 320
  incest in, 354–355
  juvenile delinquency and, 386–387
  nature of, 480–481
  as primary group, 480, 514
  rape victim and, 416
  roles in, 500
  schizophrenia and, 135–136
  social class of, 549–550
  stress in, 377–378, 379
  subsystems in, 488–489
  suicidal client and, 411, 412
  as system, 483–486, 489
  variations in, 480, 481
family chronology, 497
family constellation, 493–494
family counseling, 387
family-focused nursing care, 481
family history, 269, 492
family life cycle, 376–378, 482–483
family patterns, dysfunctional, 135–137
family projection, 492
family structure, 488–489
family theory, 478, 479–481, 481
  approaches to, 501–502
  communication concepts in, 495–499
  developmental concepts in, 482–483
  functional concepts in, 489–495

family theory (*continued*)
  learning theory concepts in, 499–500
  psychodynamic concepts in, 486–488
  structural concepts in, 488–489
  systems theory concepts in, 483–486
family therapy, 427, 430, 478, 479, 502–507
  forms of, 480
family violence, 417
  child abuse, 422–424, 426, 427, 430
  nursing process and, 326–330
  spouse abuse, 417–422
fat cells, 322
fear, 197
  in childhood, 380, 383
Federal Narcotics Control Act, 232
feedback, 470
  in systems, 484–486
feminism
  psychoanalytic theory and, 31, 486
  spouse abuse and, 421
Fenichel, Otto, 224
fetal alcohol syndrome, 227, 252
fetal development, alterations in, 251–252
fetishism, 351
fight-or-flight response, 53, 307–308
fixation, 28
flashbacks, 204, 235
flat affect, 141
flooding, 575
focusing technique, 115
Fontaine, Karen, 356
formal operational stage, 376
Franklin, Benjamin, 10
free association, 30
Freud, Anna, 29
Freud, Sigmund, 11, 25–31, 182, 197–198, 224, 407, 412, 418, 486, 525
Friedman, Meyer, 305
friendships, associative, 395
friendships of reciprocity, 395
frigidity, 350
Fromm-Reichmann, F., 325
frustration, aggression and, 412
functional disorders, 195, 279
functional nursing, 598

G

gangrene, drug abuse and, 239
GAS (general adaptation syndrome), 306–308
gastrointestinal disorders, stress and, 309–313
gays. *See* homosexuality
Gelles, Richard, 417, 421, 425
gender, 348
gender identity, 348

gender roles, 348
  in marriage, 355–356, 358
  spouse abuse and, 422
geneogram, 492
general adaptation syndrome (GAS), 306–308
generalist nurses, 15
generalization, 465
general leads, 114
genetic counseling, 268–269
genetic factors, 553
  in affective disorders, 167
  in alcoholism, 223–224
  in Alzheimer's disease, 283
  in congenital disorders, 251–252, 255, 258, 259, 260–261, 262, 264
  in drug dependence, 238
  in Huntington's chorea, 286
  in mental disorder, 39
  in personality disorders, 208
  in schizophrenia, 132
genetic predisposition, 39
genital malformation, 348
genitals, 337–339
Giacquinta, B., 182
Gilligan, Carol, 375
Glasser, William, 569–571
glucocorticoids, 306–307
goal-directedness, 108–109
goals
  of community programs, 558
  of consultation, 603
  formulation of, 110–111, 584
  nursing, 79–80
Goffman, Erving, 12
government involvement in health care, 11–12, 554
Greeks, 8–9
grief, 181–182
  adaptive and maladaptive, 182–183, 186
  anticipatory, 184
  as crisis, 443–444, 449
  dealing with, 184–186
  in nurses, 606
  phases of, 183–184
  in termination phase of therapeutic relationship, 586, 589
grief work, 182, 183, 186
Griffin, J. Q., 183
group, community as, 545–547
Group Atmosphere Scale, 536
group cohesion, 520, 533
group contract, 520
group dynamics, 516
group membership, 519–520, 530–533
group norms, 523–524, 532
group pressure, 516
group process, 526
group research, 534–536
group rules, 523–524
groups
  categories of, 513–514
  curative factors in, 533–534
  development of, 521, 522–525
  environment and, 536

  heterogeneous versus homogeneous, 519
  leaderless, 525
  leadership in, 525–530
  membership roles in, 530–533
  organizing, 518–522
  psychodynamic issues in, 517–518
  size of, 520
  therapeutic, 513, 514–517
group therapy, 513, 515
  for alcoholics, 230
G-spot, 337
guilt, 27, 33
gustatory hallucinations, 142
Guthrie blood test, 259

H

Haley, Jay, 496
halfway houses, 153, 321
hallucinating client, care of, 89, 90
hallucinations, 64, 89, 138
  of alcoholic, 226
  types of, 141–143
hallucinogens, 235–236
hallucinosis, acute alcohol, 226
haloperidol, 288
Harrison Narcotics Act, 232
Hayter, J., 291
headache, 325–326
health
  as adaptation, 6–7, 77
  definition of, 5–6, 76
health care delivery, 554–555, 635–637
health care teams, 44, 597–598
health history, 118–119
health status profile, 118–119
hearing, impaired, 256, 289
heart
  alcohol and, 227
  drug abuse and, 239
heart disease
  personality and, 305
  stress and, 319–320
Helfer, R. E., 423
helplessness, learned, 420
hemodialysis, schizophrenia and, 133
hemophilia, 260–261
Henderson, V., 59
hepatitis, 239
  alcohol, 226
heredity, mental disorders and, 39
  See also genetic factors
heroin addiction, 232, 234, 239
heroin maintenance, 241
Hilberman, E., 419
Hippocrates, 8–9
Hirschfeld, M. H., 291
histrionic personality disorder, 209
holism, 5
holistic approach to mind-body interaction, 303–304
holistic interaction, 53–55
  modes of (Roy), 60–61

holistic nursing, 59
homeostasis, 41, 305, 308
    in families, 484, 496
homophobia, 343–344
homosexuality, 343–347
    AIDS and, 345
    aversion therapy for, 469
    psychiatry and, 347
homosexual relationships, 346
honesty, of nurse, 106
hormones, in response to stress, 306–307
Horney, Karen, 53, 197, 201
hospital costs, 635–636
host factors, 551
hostility, 413
    See also violence
    migraines and, 325
humanitarian movement, 581–582
Human Outreach and Achievement Institute (Boston), 348
human rights, 617–618
humors, bodily, 9
Huntington's chorea, 286–287, 295–296
Huxley, Thomas, 303
hydrocephalus, 263, 269
hyperactive client, nursing care plan for, 83
hypertension, 316–319, 321
hypervigilance, 83
hypnotic drugs, 234–235
hypochondriacal client, care of, 91–92, 207–208
hypochondriacal reactions, 207–208
hypothalamus, 306–307
hypotheses, 644, 645–646
    in group research, 534–535
hysterical personality disorder, 408
hysterical reactions, 207

I

id, 26–28, 197
ideas of reference, 145
identification, 30
identity confusion, 385–386
"I" language, 357
illness, 5
    chronic, 251
    as crisis, 439
    epidemiological approach to, 551
illusions, 64
imagery, 575–576
    See also visualization therapy
immigration, 546, 547
immune system, 320, 326–327
immunology, 551
implementation, 80
    of client care, 599
    of nursing care plan, 109, 117
implosive therapy, 468, 575–576, 585–586
impotence, 350
incest, 354–355

incidence, 551, 552
incompetency, legal, 621–622
incontinence
    in childhood, 382
    degenerative disorders and, 290
    disability and, 263, 267–268
indolamines, 133, 166
inductive reasoning, 462
infants. *See* children
inhalants, 236
inkblot test, 66
insight, 518
insomnia, 170–171
Institute for Living (Hartford, Conn.), 42
institutionalization
    See also deinstitutionalization
    of client with degenerative disorder, 292, 293
    of juvenile offenders, 387
    of suicidal client, 410–411
insurance, liability, 625–626
intake interview, 118
intellectualization, 30, 201
intelligence testing, 61–62
interaction
    dysfunctional, 53
    functional, 53, 61
    holistic, 53–55
    reciprocal, 54
interdisciplinary conferences, 600
interdisciplinary team, 13, 597–598
Interpersonal Relations in Nursing (Peplau), 14
interpersonal theory, 34–36, 75–76, 198–199
interpretation, 115, 152
intimacy crisis, 391
intoxication, pathologic, 226
introjection, 30
introspection, 112, 463
involuntary commitment, 621–622
involutional melancholia, 168
involvement with clients, 583
IQ, 61–62
    mental retardation and, 253, 254
Irish Americans, 546–547
isolation (defense mechanism), 30

J

Jackson, D. D., 496
Jakob-Creutzfeldt disease, 283–284
Janov, Arthur, 576–579
Jansen, E., 579
Jansson, D. P., 606
jaundice, 146, 149
Jellinek, E. M., 221, 222, 227
job stress, 390–391
Johnson, B. S., 602
Johnson, Dorothy, 77
Johnson, Virginia, 339
Joint Commission on Accreditation of Hospitals, 638

Jones, Maxwell, 579
judgment, impaired, 289
judgmental attitudes, 583
juvenile delinquency, 386–387

K

Kanfer, F. H., 472
Kaposi's sarcoma, 345
Karon, B., 408
Kaufman, I., 423
Kempe, Henry, 422, 423
Kennedy, John F., 12
King, Imogene, 6, 77
Kinlein, Lucille, 76
Kinsey, Alfred, 344, 347
Klinefelter's syndrome, 264
Kohlberg, Lawrence, 372
Kohnke, M., 628
Korsakoff's syndrome, 226
Kraepelin, Emil, 39, 131
Krauss, J. B., 557
Kübler-Ross, E., 183

L

la belle indifference, 206
laissez-faire leadership, 526–528
Lamb, H. R., 555
Langman-Dorwart, N., 605–606
language, alterations in, 141
Larsen, E., 641
law, nursing ethics and, 617, 618
law of effect, 465
Lazarus, Arnold, 467, 474
leader, of health care team, 597
leaders
    attitudes toward, 528–529
    in group work, 519, 521, 522–523
    types of, 525, 526–527
leadership, 525–530
leadership functions, 525
leadership interventions, 525
lead poisoning, 253
learned helplessness, 420
learning, in mentally retarded, 254
learning disabilities, 256–258
learning theory, 463–467
    of alcohol abuse, 225
    of family interaction, 499–500
    neurotic patterns in, 202
    of obsessive-compulsive behaviors, 203
    phobias in, 205–206
Leininger, Madeleine, 76, 548–549
levodopa, 286
Levy, J. S., 603
Lewin, Kurt, 516
Lewis, A., 603
liability, professional, 625–626
liability insurance, 625–626
liaison, 601
liaison team, 601

liaison work, 601–602
  implementation of, 603–605
  implications of, 605–607
Lidz, T., 487–488
life changes, 57–58
  physical disorders and, 304, 308
life cycle
  Erikson's stages of, 32–34
  family, 376–378
life review, 399–400
limit setting, 110, 116, 153, 584
Lindemann, E., 183, 443, 449
Lipowski, Z. J., 601
listening, active, 113–114
literature, review of, 645
lithium therapy, 179–181
Litman, R. E., 408
liver
  alcohol and, 226–227
  drug abuse and, 239
local adaptation syndrome, 306
Lofenalac, 259
logoclonia, 284
logo therapy, 47
loneliness, suicide and, 405
Loomis, M. E., 439
Loomis, M. K., 528, 534
loose associations, 140
loss, depression and, 164
loxapine, 288
LSD, 236
Lynn, M., 606

M

Madison, Wisconsin, 555–556
magical thinking, 140, 203, 571
mainstreaming, 255
maintenance roles, 530, 531
malingering, 206
malnutrition, alcohol abuse and, 227
malpractice, 625
mania. *See* bipolar disorder
manipulative client, care of, 92–93, 174
maprotiline, 178
Marcia, J., 386
marijuana, abuse of, 232, 235
marital counseling, 357–358
marital schism, 487
marital skew, 487–488
Marmor, J., 347
Marram, G. W., 525
marriage
  See also family
  crises in, 391–392
  dual-career, 391
  expectations for, 355–356
  homosexual-heterosexual, 346
  violence in, 417–422
Marsh, L. Cody, 514–515
Martin, Del, 417, 421
Marvin, L. K., 520
Maslow, Abraham, 5–6, 7, 53, 395, 516

masochism, 210, 353, 418
Masson, J. M., 486
Masters, William, 339
masturbatory ideologies, 572–574
Mattson, A., 314
maturational crises, 371
Mauksch, I., 627, 630
McLean Asylum, 10
mean rate, 552
medical model, 6, 44
medications. *See* drugs
Mellow, June, 14, 75
memory
  ECT and, 175–176
  impaired, in Alzheimer's disease, 284
  impaired, in degenerative disorders, 287–288
meningitis, 252
meningomyelocele, 262–264, 271–272
Menninger, Karl, 224, 407
Menninger Clinic, 578–579
mental disturbance
  as affliction, 10–11
  as psychodynamic, 11
  as supernatural, 8–10
mental health, definitions of, 7–8
mental health clients, rights of, 618–623
mental hospitals, 10–11, 555
Mental Hygiene Movement, 11
mental retardation, 253–255
  cerebral palsy and, 262
  classifications of, 253–254
  Down's syndrome and, 256
  nursing care for, 254–255
  PKU and, 259
mental status assessment, 62–64
Mereness, D., 557, 597
Merton, R., 225
mesomorphy, 39
metabolic encephalopathy, 280
methadone maintenance, 240–241
Middle Ages, 9–10
Midtown Manhattan study, 38
migraine headache, 325–326
milieu therapy, 12, 516, 578–581, 585
  for schizophrenic clients, 151–153
Miller, Neil, 467
Mills, T. M., 535
mind-body interaction, 303, 575–576
mineralocorticoids, 306
Minnesota Multiphasic Personality Inventory (MMPI), 64–65
Minuchin, S., 489
mirror gazing, 400
MMPI (Minnesota Multiphasic Personality Inventory), 64–65
mobility, physical, 267
modeling, 500
  in sex therapy, 358
molindone, 288
monoamine oxidase (MAO) inhibitors, 166, 176–177
mood, 63, 164

mood and affect, altered patterns of
  See also bipolar disorders; depression
  classification of, 164–165
  etiology of, 40, 165–167
  somatic treatment for, 175–181
moral development, Kohlberg's theory of, 372–375
moral therapy, 578
Moreno, Jacob, 515
Morgagni, Giovanni, 303
mosaicism, 255
mourning, 181–182, 183, 184, 398
mucoviscidosis, 259
multiaxial psychiatric diagnosis, 16
  See also DSM-III
multidisciplinary team, 13, 597
multigenerational transmission, 493
multiple personality, 207
muscles, alcohol and, 227
myoglobinuria, 227
myopathy, alcoholic, 227

N

nalorphine, 241
naloxone, 241
naltrexone, 241, 242
narcotics. *See* opiates
National Council on Alcoholism, 221
National Institute for Mental Health, 12
National Training Laboratory for Applied Behavioral Science, 516
necrophilia, 353
needs, Maslow's hierarchy of, 6, 7
negative reinforcement, 465, 466
negativism, as expression of ambivalence, 140
negligence, 625
neologisms, 141
neoplasm, stress and, 326–327
network family therapy, 480
neural tube defects, 262
neuritic plaque, 282
neurofibrillary tangles, 281, 282
neurons, alterations in, 281, 282
neurotic disorders, 195, 200
  characteristics of, 201–202
  compared with personality disorders, 199, 200
  compared with psychotic disorders, 199, 200
  drug therapy for, 213–214
  in DSM-III, 200
  nursing diagnoses for, 201
  psychoanalytic theory of, 197–198
  psychosocial theory of, 198
  Sullivan's explanation of, 198–199
  types of, 202–208
neurotransmitters, 40, 166
Newman, Margaret, 76–77
New York City, 556

Nightingale, Florence, 13, 303, 479, 642
nonverbal communication, 107–108
norepinephrine, 53, 133, 166
normalization, 254
norms, group, 523–524
North American Nursing Diagnosis Association, 18
nuclear family, 481
nuclear family emotional system, 489, 490, 492
nurse
    as advocate, 626–630
    as change agent, 630–631
    community mental health, 15, 557–558
    as interdisciplinary team member, 597–598
    political influence of, 630–631
nurse-client relationship, 14–15, 75–76, 582–586
    advocacy and, 627–630
    communication in, 105–109, 111–118
nurses
    accountability of, 623–625
    attitudes toward alcohol and drug abusers, 220
    attitudes toward clients with degenerative disorders, 292
    attitudes toward rape, 416
    attitudes toward sexuality, 360
    attitudes toward suicide, 409, 412
    attitudes toward violent clients, 413
    burnout in, 442, 452–453, 606
    changing role of, 579–580
    collaboration among, 610
    in community mental health movement, 13
    group therapy and, 519
    group work by, 513
    morale of, 330–331
    professional liability of, 625–626
    role in community, 554
    in therapeutic community, 579–580
    writing by, 647, 650
nurse-nurse consultation, 606–607
nursing
    consultation and liaison in, 601–607
    DRGs and, 636–637
    ethics and, 617–623
    primary, 598, 599–600, 601
    quality assurance and, 637–641
    role expansion in, 13–14
    team, 598–600, 601
    transcultural, 76, 548–549
nursing care
    client-centered, 78, 79, 81, 627–629
    costs of, 636–637
    documentation of, 118–124
    standards of, 624
nursing care delivery, models of, 598–600

nursing care plans, 80, 117, 118, 154
    evaluation of, 81–82
    format of, 82
    generic, 82–84
    purpose of, 81
    in therapeutic relationship, 584
nursing diagnoses
    applicable to neurotic patterns, 201
    official, 17, 18
    related to degenerative disorders, 283
    related to mental retardation and learning disabilities, 258
    related to suicide, 409
    related to violent client, 414
    for sexual problems, 360, 361
    validation of, 117
nursing diagnosis, 17, 79
nursing education, 609, 642
nursing functions, 13–14
nursing goals, 79–80
nursing homes, 293
nursing interventions, 14, 80
    in family, 502–507
nursing models, 59
nursing practice
    standards of, 623–624
    theoretical bases of, 75–77
nursing problems, 17, 18
nursing process, 77–78
    alcoholism and, 228–231
    child abuse and, 423–424
    for client with chronic degenerative disorder, 292–294
    components of, 78–81
    congenital disorders and, 269–274
    drug abuse and, 239–242
    rape and, 416–417
    in relationship therapy, 582–586
    in sexual health care, 360–361
    therapeutic communication and, 117–118
nursing research, 609, 641–642
    history of, 642–643
    methodology of, 643–647
    priorities for, 643
    quality assurance and, 641
    theory and, 25
Nursing Research, 642
nursing schools, 642
nursing theories, 75–77, 78
nursing therapy, 75
nutrition, aging and, 397

O

obesity, 322–323
objectives, of nursing care, 81
object permanence, 375
observation, 462–463
obsession, 203
obsessive-compulsive disorders, 199, 202, 203
occupational stress, 390–391

Oedipal conflict, 29, 418
olfactory hallucinations, 142
one genus postulate, 34, 136
O'Connor v. Donaldson, 621
operant conditioning, 465–467
operant techniques, 470–471
opiates, 234, 238
oral stage, 198
Orem, Dorothy, 76
organic brain disorders, 131
organic brain syndrome, 280
    violence and, 413
organic disorders, 195
organic mental disorder, 280
orgasm, 340, 342
orgasm difficulties, 350–351
orientation
    assessment of, 64
    in degenerative disorders, 288–289
Orlando, Ida, 14
Osler, Sir William, 320

P

Pagelow, M., 422
pain
    in headache, 325–326
    primal, 577–578
paleological thinking, 138
panic, 447
panic attacks, 202
paralysis, 263
paranoia
    alcoholic, 226
    violence and, 413
paranoid personality disorder, 210
paranoid schizophrenia, 139
paraphilias, 351–353
paraplegia, 263
parataxic mode, 35, 136
parents
    See also family; marriage
    abusing, 422–430
    children's eating disturbances and, 381–382
    children's sleep disturbances and, 380–381
    dysfunction in children and, 385
    effect of disabled child on, 264–268
    expectations of, 378, 423
    schizophrenogenic, 135
    strains on, 394
Parents United, 355
Parkinson, James, 285
Parkinson's disease, 285–286, 287
parkinsonism, drug-induced, 147, 148
Parsons, Talcott, 38, 206
passive-aggressive/passive-dependent personality disorder, 210
Patient's Bill of Rights, 619
patriarchal society, 420, 421, 422
Pavlov, Ivan, 463–465

peak experiences, 516
pedophilia, 352
peer review, 624–625
penis, 337, 339
Pennsylvania Hospital, 10
Peplau, Hildegarde, 14, 36, 37, 75–76, 625
Pepper, B., 555
peptic ulcer, 309–311, 312
perception
    alterations in, 141–143
    assessment of, 63–64
perceptual constancies, 143, 144
performance anxiety, 350, 358
perseveration, 284
personality
    alcoholic, 224–225
    of drug abusers, 237
    heart disease and, 319
    hypertension and, 317
    peptic ulcer and, 309–311
    physical disorders and, 304–305
    rheumatoid arthritis and, 320
    ulcerative colitis and, 312
personality assessment, 64–67
personality development
    according to Erikson, 31–34
    according to Freud, 28–29
    according to Sullivan, 35–36
personality disorders, 195, 208–213
    compared with neurotic disorders, 199, 200
    violence and, 413
personality structure, Freud's theory of, 26–28
personal space, 108
phallic stage, 198
phenylalanine, 258, 259
phenylketonuria (PKU), 258–259
Phillips, J. S., 472
phobias, 202, 204–206
    childhood, 383
phobic client, care of, 206
physical environment, of care facility, 152
physiology, as a science, 462
Piaget, Jean, 47, 375–376, 378
Pinel, Philippe, 10
pituitary gland, 306–307
Pizzey, Erin, 418
PKU. *See* phenylketonuria
planning client care, 79–80
    communication and, 117
    in primary nursing, 599
    in relationship therapy, 584
    in team nursing, 599
play therapy, 515
Pol, G. C., 608
political influence, of nurses, 630–631
population groups, 547
positive reinforcement, 116
posttraumatic stress syndrome, 203–204
poverty
    congenital disorders and, 253
    race and, 553

power struggle, in groups, 522–523
power tactics, 496
Pratt, Joseph, 514
preconscious, 28
predicate thinking, 138
prediction of client behavior, 599, 600
premarital counseling, 355–357, 427
premature infants, 252
prenatal development, alterations in, 252
prenatal diagnosis, 268–269
preoperational stage, 375
prevalence, 551, 552
prevention, levels of, 13
    group work and, 513, 514
priapism, 147
primal scream, 577–578
primal therapy, 576–579
primary group, 514
primary nursing, 598, 599–600, 601
primary prevention, 13
primary process thinking, 26
private duty nursing, 598
problem drinking, 222, 223, 227
problem list, 119
process analysis, 526, 535
process recording, 120–124
Professional Standards Review Organizations (PSROs), 638
progressive relaxation, 318
progressive teleological regression, 137
progress notes, 119–120
Prohibition, 221
projection, 30, 205, 492
projective tests, 65–67
prospective payment system, 635–637
prototaxic mode, 35, 136
pseudohostility, 487
pseudomutuality, 486–487
PSROs, 638
psychedelic drugs, 235–236
psychiatric care, trends in, 11–12
psychiatric diagnoses, 15–17
    See also DSM-III
psychiatric emergency, 452
psychiatric liaison nursing, 602–607
psychiatric mental health nurses, 15
psychiatric nursing, 14–15
    See also nurses; nursing
    advocacy and, 630
    clients' rights and, 618–623
    expanded role of, 75
    research in, 643
    theoretical bases of, 75–77
psychiatrists, referral to, 607, 609
psychic determinism, 30
psychic energy, 26
psychic numbing, 204
psychoanalysis, 11, 30–31, 461
psychoanalytic theory, 25–31
    of aggression, 412
    of alcoholism, 224
    of conversion reactions, 206
    of depression, 165–166

    of family dynamics, 486–488
    homosexuality in, 343
    learning theory and, 467
    of neurosis, 197–198
    of obsessive-compulsive behavior, 203
    of phobias, 205
    of schizophrenia, 137–138
    of spouse abuse, 418–419
    of suicide, 407
    applied to therapeutic groups, 517–518
psychodrama, 515
psychodynamic theory. *See* psychoanalytic theory; psychosocial theory
psychology, 462–463
psychopathological crises, 451
psychophysiological disorders, 303–304
psychosexual disorders, 352
psychosexual stages, 28–29
psychosexual theory, 25–31, 198
psychosocial stages, 371–372
psychosocial theory, 31–34, 134, 198, 371–372
psychosomatic disorders, 303–304
psychotherapy. *See* therapy
psychotic alterations, 199, 200
pulmonary embolism, 239
punishment, 466–467, 471–472
    of children, 422
Putt, A., 311

Q

quality assurance, 637–641
quasi-experimental design, 646
questioning, of clients, 114

R

race, poverty and, 553
racial discrimination, 546
racial groups, 547
random sampling, 644
rape
    attitudes toward, 416
    motivation for, 415
    nursing process and, 416–417
    reactions of victims, 415
rational emotive therapy (RET), 47, 571–575, 585
rationalization, 30, 201–202
reaction formation, 30
reaction time, 396
reality testing, 138
    impaired, 288–289
reality therapy, 47, 569–571, 585
reasoning, inductive, 462
reassurance, 582–583
reciprocal inhibition, 206, 467

reciprocal interaction, 54
reconstituted family, 481
reference groups, 38, 374, 514
referral process, 607–610
referral protocol, 608
referrals, 430
reflection technique, 114–115
refusal of treatment, 620–621, 622
regressed client, care of, 93–95
regression, 28, 30, 93, 382
    in schizophrenia, 137, 140, 152
    societal, 494
rehabilitation
    of alcoholic client, 229–231
    of drug-abusing client,
        239–242
reinforcement, 465–466, 470–471,
    500
    negative, 465–466
    positive, 116
Reisman, J., 395
relabeling, 496
relatedness, altered patterns of,
    195–214
relationship therapy, 582–586
    for schizophrenia, 148,
        150–151
relative intensity measures (RIMs),
    636
relaxation techniques, 318–319,
    467–468
reliability, 644
    of group data, 534
    of IQ tests, 62
    of mental status assessment, 64
remarriage, 391, 394
repression, 28, 29–30, 197–198,
    206
reproductive organs, 337–339
research. See nursing research
residual schizophrenia, 139
resistance, 518
respect for client, 106, 112
respiratory disorders, stress and,
    313–316
response discrimination, 466
responsibility, 569–571
restatement, 114–115
restraint measures, 414, 415, 621
restrictive treatment, 621, 622
RET (rational emotive therapy), 47,
    571–575, 585
retirement, 395–396
reward model, 466, 471
rheumatoid arthritis, 320–321, 322
Richards, Linda, 10
rights
    human, 617–618
    of mental health clients,
        618–623
right to refuse treatment, 620–621
RIMs, 636
risk factors, 552–553
ritualistic client, care of, 95–96, 203
rituals, 95
Rogers, Carl, 461, 581–582
Rogers, Martha, 5, 59
role assessment questionnaire, 356

role differentiation, 530
role enactment, 530
role function, 60
role playing, 470, 515
roles, 500
    gender, 348
    in groups, 530–533
    social, 38
role specialization, 530–531
Romans, 9
Rorschach test, 66
Rosenman, Ray, 305
Rotter, Julian, 474
Roy, Callista, 59–61
Roy, Maria, 422, 424
rubber fences, 487
Rubin, S., 183
Rush, Benjamin, 8, 10, 221
Ryglewicz, H., 555

S

sadism, 353
sadomasochism, 353–354
Satir, Virginia, 497–498
scapegoating, 265, 488–489,
    531–532
schismatic families, 487–488
schizoid personality disorder,
    208–209
schizophrenia
    behavioral manifestations of,
        150, 151
    biochemical basis of, 40, 133
    drug therapy for, 145–148, 149
    etiologic theories of, 132–138
    family and, 135–137, 479, 487,
        495
    family therapy for, 153
    genetic factors in, 39, 132
    milieu therapy for, 151–153
    nursing care plan for client
        with, 154
    prevalence of, 131
    primary manifestations of,
        140–141
    problems identifying, 131
    prognosis for client with,
        153–155
    relationship therapy for,
        148–151
    risk factors for, 133
    secondary manifestations of,
        141–144
    types of, 139
schizophrenic process, steps of, 139
schizophrenogenic parents, 135
Schoenberg, B., 182
Schutz, W. C., 525
scientific method, 462–463
seclusion, 621
secondary groups, 514
secondary prevention, 13
secondary process thinking, 26
secondary reinforcers, 465, 471
sedatives, 234–235

segregated neighborhoods, 547
self, sense of, healthy versus altered,
    196, 197
self-actualization, 6, 516
self-awareness
    encouraging, 112, 115–116, 448
    of nurse's own feelings, 150,
        292, 360, 583
self-care, 76
self-care deficits, 289–290
self-destructive clients, care of, 84,
    409–412
self-differentiation, 491–492
self-disclosure, 109, 529
self-esteem, 497–498
    of client with degenerative dis-
        order, 291
    disability and, 268
    in elderly, 398–399
self-help groups, for obesity, 323
self-image
    alterations in, 143–144
    idealized, 196
self system, 34
Seligman, Martin, 420
Selye, Hans, 305–308
senile dementia, 282
senile plaques, 281
sensate focusing, 358–359
sensitivity training, 516
sensitization, 469
sensorimotor stage, 375
sentence completion tests, 67
separation anxiety, 29, 379, 383
serotonin
    mood alteration and, 166
    schizophrenia and, 133
sex-change surgery, 349
sex chromosomes, 264
sex roles. See gender roles
sex roles, alternative. See homosex-
    uality; transsexualism
sex-role stereotypes, 356
sexual abuse, 353, 415–416
    of children, 352, 354–355
sexual activity, as coping mecha-
    nism, 342–343
sexual anatomy, 337–339
sexual behavior, inappropriate, in
    degenerative disorders, 289
sexual counseling, 358–360
    of cardiac clients, 320
sexual deviance, 351–353
sexual dysfunctions, 349–351, 352
    alcohol and, 227
    therapy for, 358–360
sexual expectations, 341–342
sexual harassment, 355
sexual interest
    decreased, 349–350
    increased, 350
sexuality, 337, 341–343
    nursing process and, 360–361
sexual response phases, 339–340
Shainness, N., 418
shame, 27, 33
shaping of behavior, 466, 469
Sheehy, G., 557

Sheldon, William, 39
sibling position, 493–494
sickle cell anemia, 261
sick role, 38, 206, 265
Sifneos, P. E., 448
silence, 107, 114, 582
  in groups, 532–533
Simon, Herman, 578
Simonton, O., 327, 330
Sinequan, 177
skewed families, 487–488
Skinner, B. F., 465–466, 499
Skinner box, 465, 466
Slavson, Samuel, 515
sleep disturbance
  in Alzheimer's victims, 284
  in children, 379
  depression and, 170–171, 172
sleep talking, 380
sleepwalking, 380
Smith, D. W., 444
Smith, S., 555
smoking, hypertension and, 318
social class, 549–550
  child abuse and, 422–423
  child-rearing practices and, 550
  congenital disorders and, 252
  deviant behavior and, 38
  family violence and, 421
  learning disability and, 257
  mental disorder and, 38
  mental health care and, 12
  obesity and, 322
  personality development and,
    38
  spouse abuse and, 417
social institutions, 37
socialization, 37
social learning, 499–500
social learning theory
  of aggression, 412
  of spouse abuse, 422
social mobility, 550
social-psychological theory of
  suicide, 408
Social Readjustment Rating Scale,
  57–58
social roles, 38
Social Security Act, 11–12
societal regression, 494
society
  patriarchal, 420, 421, 422
  suicide and, 406–407
  violence in, 420
Society for the Prevention of
  Cruelty to Children, 422
socioemotional leader, 525,
  529–530
sociogram, 498–499
sociological theories
  of family violence, 420–422
  of suicide, 406–407
solvents, 232, 236
somatic treatments, 11, 43
  See also drugs
  for affective disorders, 175–181
Sontag, Susan, 5
speech therapy, 289
spina bifida, 262–264, 271–272

Spitz, R., 167
spontaneous recovery, 465
spouse abuse, 417–422, 424–425
  nursing process and, 426–427,
    430
S-R relationships, 54–55, 464–465
St. Christopher's Hospice, 185
staff burnout, 442, 452–453, 606
standards of care, 624
standards of practice, 617, 623
Standards of Psychiatric and Mental
  Health Nursing Practice, 623
statistical analysis, 647
statistics, 644
Steinmetz, S., 419–420, 425
step-family, 394
stimulant drugs, 178, 258
  abuse of, 233–234
stimulus discrimination, 465
stimulus generalization, 465
Straus, M. A., 420, 421–422, 425
stress
  anorexia nervosa and, 323–325
  arthritis and, 320–321, 322
  asthma and, 313–316
  cancer and, 326–327, 330–331
  crisis and, 439, 442
  disabled child and, 266–267
  in family, 377–378, 379
  headache and, 325–326
  heart disease and, 319–320
  hypertension and, 316–319
  management of, 308–309
  obesity and, 322–323
  occupational, 390–391
  physical disorders and, 309
  schizophrenia and, 132–133
  spouse abuse and, 419
  suicide and, 410
  theories of, 306–309
  tolerance of, 307, 308
  ulcerative colitis and, 312–313
  ulcers and, 309–311, 312
stress management, 308–309,
  318–319, 320
stressors, 306, 308
sublimation, 30
subrogating the claim, 625
substance abuse. See alcohol abuse;
  drug abuse
suicidal client, care of, 409–412,
  447
suicide
  depression and, 170
  diagnoses related to, 409
  by drug overdose, 178
  grief and, 185
  historical attitudes toward, 405
  myths concerning, 407
  nursing attitudes toward, 409
  nursing process and, 409–412
  sex differences in, 405
  statistics on, 405–406
  theories of, 406–409
Sullivan, Harry Stack, 34–36,
  134–137, 198–199, 447, 479
summarizing, 116
sunlight sensitivity, 146, 148
superego, 27–28, 197

support groups, 394–395
  for battered wives, 427
  for nurses, 453
support systems, for family with disabled child, 267, 269
surveillance theory, 326–327
survey research, 646
survivors, 443–444
suspicious client
  care of, 96–97
  nursing care plan for, 83
Sydenham, Thomas, 10
symbolic interactionism, 37–38
symbols, 138
  learning of, 375
symmetrical relationships, 496
Symonds, A., 419
Symonds, M., 419
sympathetic nervous system, 53
sympathy, 583
Synanon, 241
synaptic transmission, 166
syntaxic mode, 35, 136
systematic desensitization, 467–468,
  473, 575, 585–586
systems theory, 58–61, 77
  as applied to family, 483–486
  basic terminology of, 58
  of family violence, 421–422
  principles of, 59
Szasz, Thomas, 8

T

tactile hallucinations, 142
taraxine, 133
tardive dyskinesia, 147–148, 149
task analysis, 254, 536
task leadership, 525, 529–530
task roles, in groups, 530, 531
TAT (Thematic Apperception Test),
  66–67
Tay-Sachs disease, 259
team approaches, 13, 44, 597–598
team nursing, 598–599, 601
tension headache, 325
terminal illness, 182, 183, 293
termination phase of relationship
  therapy, 586
tertiary prevention, 13, 153
testicles, 339
testicular feminization syndrome,
  348
tetracyclates, 176
tetrahydrocannabinol (THC), 235
T-groups, 516
Thematic Apperception Test (TAT),
  66–67
theme interference, 604
themes, in nurse-client interactions,
  75–76
theoretical frameworks, 25
theory, 25
therapeutic community, 515,
  579–581, 585
therapeutic contract, 110–111

therapeutic relationship, 582–586
    collaboration in, 109–111
    communication in, 106–109,
        111–118, 582–583
    establishment of, 105–106
therapy
    behavioral, 467–474
    brief, 448–449
    choice of, 569
    client-centered, 461, 581–582
    eclectic approach to, 569
    effectiveness of, 569
    implosive, 468, 575–576,
        585–586
    milieu, 12, 516, 578–581, 585
    primal, 576–578
    rational emotive, 47, 571–575,
        585
    reality, 47, 569–571, 585
    relationship, 148, 150–151,
        582–586
thinking, alterations in. *See* thought
    disturbance
thinking, magical, 140, 203, 571
thioridazine, 288
third-party payment, 635
Thollaugh, S., 628
Thorndike, Edward R., 465
thought disturbance
    See also schizophrenia
    etiologic theories of, 132–138
    nursing care plan for client
        with, 154
    primary manifestations of,
        140–141
    process of, 138–144
    secondary manifestations of,
        141–144
    therapeutic approaches to,
        144–155
    types of, 139
thought processes, assessment of, 63
thrombophlebitis, 239
time out, 470
Tofranil, 177
token economies, 470–471
tolerance, drug, 219
Toman, W., 493–494
Torrey, E., 569, 580, 581
toxic psychosis, 280
tranquilizers. *See* antianxiety drugs
transcultural nursing, 76, 548–549
transference, 30, 517
transitional crises, 450
translocation, chromosomal, 255
transmethylation, 40
transsexualism, 348–349
transvestism, 348
traumatic crises, 450–451
triangling, 492, 493
tricyclic antidepressants, 166,
    177–179
trisomy, 21, 255

trust
    between nurse and client, 105,
        584
    in infant, 371
tryamine, 177
tryptamine, 133
Tuckman, B. W., 525
Turner's syndrome, 264
twins
    alcoholism in, 224
    schizophrenia in, 132
type A personality, 305, 317,
    319–320
tyranny of the "shoulds," 201
tyrosine, 258

U

ulcerative colitis, 312–313
ulcers, 309–311, 312
unconditional positive regard, 461,
    581
unconscious, 28
undifferentiated ego mass, 489, 491
undifferentiated schizophrenia, 139
undoing, 30
unemployment, 553
unidisciplinary team, 13, 597
Uniform Narcotics Law, 232
urinary disturbances in children,
    382–383

V

vagina, 337
vaginal lubrication, inhibition of,
    350
vaginismus, 350
validation, 115
validity, 644
    of group data, 534
    of IQ tests, 62
values, 617
variables, 644, 645
victims
    of child abuse, 422–424
    of rape, 415–417
    of spouse abuse, 418–422
Viet Nam veterans, 203–204
violence, 412
    alcohol and, 412–413, 424–425
    family, 417–430
    nursing process for, 413–415
violent client
    care of, 448
    handling of, 413–415
vision, impaired, 289
visual hallucinations, 142–143

visualization therapy, 327, 330
voluntary organizations, 554
Von Bertalanffy, L., 483
voyeurism, 353

W

Wahl, C. W., 408
Walker, Lenore, 417, 420
Wang, H. S., 281
Ward Atmosphere Scale, 536
Watson, John, 463
weight loss, 323
Wellesley College, 516
wellness, high-level, 5
Wernicke's syndrome, 226
White, William A., 8
widowhood, 398
wife battering. *See* spouse abuse
witchcraft, 9–10
withdrawal symptoms, 219, 234, 235
withdrawn client, care of, 97–98
Wolff, I., 557
Wolff, P., 608–609
Wolpe, Joseph, 467–468
women
    anorexia nervosa in, 388
    eating disorders and, 324
    empty nest syndrome in, 395
    as rape victims, 415–417
    suicide and, 405
    as victims of spouse abuse,
        417–422
Women's Advocates, 418
Wood, D. J., 439
word association tests, 67
word salad, 141
working phase, of relationship ther-
    apy, 585–586
Working Women United Institute,
    355
World Health Organization, 5
writing, by nurses, 647, 650
Wundt, Wilhelm, 463
Wynne, L., 486–487

Y

Yale University, 635
Yalom, I. D., 521, 526, 533
"you" language, 357

Z

Zilboorg, G., 407
zoophilia, 351